FIFTH EDITION

TRANSCULTURAL NURSING

Assessment and Intervention

FIFTH EDITION

TRANSCULTURAL NURSING

Assessment and Intervention

Joyce Newman Giger, EdD, APRN, BC, FAAN

Professor and Lulu Wolff Hassenplug Endowed Chair in Nursing
University of California at Los Angeles
School of Nursing
Los Angeles, California

Ruth Elaine Davidhizar, DNS, RN, APRN, BC, FAAN

Dean and Professor
Division of Nursing
Bethel College
Mishawaka, Indiana

MOSBY

ELSEVIER

MOSBY
ELSEVIER

11830 Westline Industrial Drive
St. Louis, Missouri 63146

TRANSCULTURAL NURSING: ASSESSMENT AND INTERVENTION,   ISBN: 978-0-323-04811-8
FIFTH EDITION

Notice

Knowledge and best practice in this field are constantly changing. As new research and experience broaden our knowledge, changes in practice, treatment and drug therapy may become necessary or appropriate. Readers are advised to check the most current information provided (i) on procedures featured or (ii) by the manufacturer of each product to be administered, to verify the recommended dose or formula, the method and duration of administration, and contraindications. It is the responsibility of the practitioner, relying on their own experience and knowledge of the patient, to make diagnoses, to determine dosages and the best treatment for each individual patient, and to take all appropriate safety precautions. To the fullest extent of the law, neither the Publisher nor the Editors assumes any liability for any injury and/or damage to persons or property arising out or related to any use of the material contained in this book.

The Publisher

Photographs for Chapters 8, 9, 11, 13, 15–22, 24–26, and 28–30: Copyright © Dottie Kauffman

Library of Congress Control Number: 2007931686

Acquisitions Editor: Robin Carter
Developmental Editor: Deanna Davis
Publishing Services Manager: Melissa Lastarria
Senior Project Manager: Joy Moore
Cover Design Direction: Paula Catalano
Text Designer: Paula Catalano

Printed in the United States of America

Last digit is the print number: 9 8 7 6 5 4 3 2

**Working together to grow
libraries in developing countries**

www.elsevier.com | www.bookaid.org | www.sabre.org

ELSEVIER   BOOK AID International   Sabre Foundation

To Our Parents
The late Ionia Holmes Newman
Lucille & Ralph Holderman
and the late Naomi Holderman

To Our Husbands
Argusta Giger, Jr. and Ronald Davidhizar

To Our Mentors
Richmond Calvin, EdD; the late Frances P Dixon, BS;
and Angela Barron McBride, PhD, RN, FAAN

To the students of Bethel College, past, present, and future, and all
the nurses and students who seek a better way to render culturally
appropriate care

Contributors

Doris Bartlett, RN, MS
Adjunct Professor
Bethel College
Mishawaka, Indiana

Karen Chang, PhD, RN
Assistant Professor
Purdue University
West Lafayette, Indiana

Brenda Cherry, MSN, FNP-C
Associate Professor of Nursing
Georgia Perimeter
Clarkston, Georgia

Yoshiko Colclough, PhD, RN
Assistant Professor
College of Nursing
Montana State University–Bozeman
Bozeman, Montana

Nancy L. Conrad, BSN, MSN
Faculty Emerita
Southwestern College
Chula Vista, California

Robert E. Cosgray, BSN, MA
Surgical Nurse
St. Vincent's Hospital
Indianapolis, Indiana

Tina D. DeLapp, EdD, MSN, BSN
Emeritus Professor of Nursing
University of Alaska–Anchorage
Anchorage, Alaska

Dawn Liam Doutrich, PhD, RN, CNS
Interim Regional Director and Assistant Dean
Associate Professor
Intercollegiate College of Nursing
Washington State University
Vancouver, Washington

Jaibun Kim Earp, PhD, ARNP, FNP
Professor and Director
FAMU Wellness Center
Florida A&M University
Tallahassee, Florida

M. Christina R. Esperat, PhD, RN
Professor
School of Nursing
Texas Tech University Health Sciences Center
Lubbock, Texas

Ken Farr, MS, PMHCNS-BC
Instructor
School of Nursing
University of Alabama at Birmingham
Birmingham, Alabama

Miguel A. Franco, PhD, HSPP
Counseling Psychologist
University of Notre Dame
Notre Dame, Indiana

Elizabeth W. Gonzalez, PhD, APRN, BC
Associate Professor
College of Nursing and Health Professions
Drexel University
Philadelphia, Pennsylvania

Linda G. Haddad, RN, MSN, PhD
Associate Professor
Virginia Commonwealth University
Richmond, Virginia

Catherine E. Hanley, RN, BSN, MPH, FAAN, FACHE
Hospital and Health Care Consultant
Flagstaff, Arizona

Mervin R. Helmuth, RN, BSN, MN
Associate Professor of Nursing
Goshen College
Goshen, Indiana

Razia A. Iqbul, PsyD, MA, BA
Doctor of Psychology (Clinical Psychologist)
Kaiser Permanente
San Jose, California

Lisa Skemp Kelley, PhD, RN, BSN, MA
Assistant Professor
University of Iowa College of Nursing
Iowa City, Iowa

Kira Ann Lass, RN, BSN, MSN(c)
Critical Care Transport Nurse
American Medical Response
Contra Costa Country
Concord, California

Juliene G. Lipson, PhD, RN, FAAN
Professor Emerita
Mill Valley, California

**Cheryl M. Martin, BSN, MSN, PhD, WHNP,
CNE, RNC**
Educational Consultant
Educational Resources, Inc
Lenexa, Kansas

Scott Wilson Miller, BSN, MSN, FIHPS, RNC
Lead Clinical Instructor
American Medical Response
Northern California Critical Care Transport
San Jose, California

**Cordelia Chinwe Nnedu, PhD, RNC, ARNP,
WHCNP**
Associate Professor and Assistant Director
Tuskegee University School of Nursing
Tuskegee Institute
Tuskegee, Alabama

Patricia A. Omidian, PhD
Country Representative, Afghanistan
American Friends Service Committee
Kabul, Afghanistan

Donna C. Owen, PhD, RN
Professor
School of Nursing
Texas Tech University Health Sciences Center
Lubbock, Texas

Mary Reidy, RN, BN, MSc(app), PhD
Full Professor (Retired)
University of Montreal;
Professional Researcher
University of Quebec at Montreal
Montreal, Quebec

Enid A. Schwartz, RN, MS, MC, PhD
Registered Nurse
University of Phoenix
Sierra Vista, Arizona

Karon Schwartz, RN, BSN, MS, PhD
Graduate Nursing Program Director
Bethel College
Mishawaka, Indiana

Ruth A. Shearer, RN, MS, MSN
Associate Professor of Nursing
Bethel College
Mishawaka, Indiana

Cynthia C. Small, MSN, RN, APRN-BC, FNP
Lake Michigan College
Lakeland Regional Health Systems
Benton Harbor, Michigan

Linda S. Smith, BSN, MS, DSN, RN, CLNC
Director and Associate Professor
Idaho State University
Pocatello, Idaho

Ruth Yoder Stauffer, RN, BSN, MA
Virginia Mennonite Retirement Community
Harrisonburg, Virginia

Sara Torres, PhD
Professor
University of Medicine and Dentistry of New Jersey
Newark, New Jersey

Toni Tripp-Reimer, PhD, RN, FAAN
Professor and Associate Dean for Research
College of Nursing
University of Iowa
Iowa City, Iowa

Mary Grace Umlauf, RN, PhD
Professor
University of Alabama School of Nursing
Birmingham, Alabama

Anna R. Vance, PhD, RN, FNP
Denver Health and Hospital Authority
Denver, Colorado

Thad Wilson, RN, APRN, BC, PhD
Associate Dean
University of Missouri–Kansas City
Kansas City, Missouri

Yu Xu, PhD, MSN, MEd, BA
Associate Professor
School of Nursing
University of Nevada–Las Vegas
Las Vegas, Nevada

Foreword

Because racial/ethnic minorities tend to receive a lower quality of health care even when their access to services is similar to non-minorities and because the diversity of the U.S. population is growing, the Institute of Medicine (2003) has advocated cross-cultural education in the health professions as a key strategy in ending such disparities. Nursing has long focused on both personal and population-based caregiving issues (American Nurses' Association, 1980) and has a proud tradition of cross-cultural assessment and intervention dating back to the pioneering work of Leininger (1977). One of the first issues of the *Annual Review of Nursing Research* contained a chapter on cross-cultural nursing research (Tripp-Reimer & Dougherty, 1985).

Building on this proud tradition and mindful that there is an urgency all providers must demonstrate in addressing these disparities (Brach & Fraserirector, 2000). Giger and Davidhizer have published the fifth edition of their popular book on transcultural nursing. Their Transcultural Assessment Model, which has been used to develop effective educational interventions in the past (Smith, 2001), provides a framework for assessment that focuses on the six cultural phenomena believed to shape care—communication, space, social organization, time, environmental control, and biological variations. Many of the chapters specify how a particular racial/ethnic group (for example, African-Americans, Appalachians, Navajos, Eskimos, and Mexican-Americans) may vary in these six areas, after which they provide rich information as to how these variations may be taken into account in planning care. These examples also provide a model for looking at the experience of other populations not included in this book.

While it has become commonplace for nurses to urge culturally appropriate care, what that really means is not always clear, other than some general admonition to be aware that not all patients with the same medical diagnosis are likely to have the same experience. The notion that patients and their families make choices based on the unique meaning they assign to their experience is often discounted on a day-to-day basis when the prevailing emphasis seems to be more on the importance of procedures and coverage than on providing tailored interventions. That is why this volume can be so useful to students and seasoned clinicians alike, because it provides so many examples of how individual experience is likely to vary in ways that go well beyond the patterning of medical symptoms: Is this man one who responds well to frequent touching? Does this woman need considerable personal space? Will an effective intervention necessarily have to involve the patient's extended family? Is this person likely to make eye contact with a provider? What are this couple's beliefs about the nature of illness? What does well-oxygenated skin color look like when the infant being rated on the Apgar scale is dark skinned? Will the observation of certain rituals ease the anguish these parents feel at their child's death?

This edition, which draws on the clinical experience of many individuals, speaks to the needs of our pluralistic society by providing a wealth of insights about how cultural assessment is integral to understanding the meaning of behaviors that, if not understood within the context of ethnic values, might be regarded as puzzling or even negative. The editors are seasoned professionals who have constantly striven to update their insights to keep up with the times (Giger & Davidhizar, 2002). As a result they are able to provide details that make us sensitive to the concerns of a multitude of population groups, all the while providing us with a framework with broad generic applicability. This volume is part of the health care revolution that is critical of the professional who paternalistically sets out to do what is best for patients; instead, it wisely emphasizes the importance of the caregiver building on patients' concepts of what is good for them.

Angela Barron McBride, PhD, RN, FAAN
Distinguished Professor–University Dean Emerita
Indiana University School of Nursing
Indianapolis, Indiana

References

American Nurses' Association. (1980). *Nursing: a social policy statement.* Kansas City, MO: ANA.

Brach, C., & Fraserirector, I. (2000). Can cultural competency reduce racial and ethnic health disparities: a review and conceptual model. *Medical Care Research,* 57(Suppl 1), 181–217.

Giger, J. N., & Davidhizar, R. (2002). Culturally competent care: emphasis on understanding the people of Afghanistan, Afghanistan Americans, and Islamic culture and religion. *International Nursing Review,* 49, 79–86.

Institute of Medicine. (2003). In Smedley, B. D., Stith, A. Y., & Nelson, A. R. (Eds.), *Unequal treatment. Confronting racial and ethnic disparities in health care.* Washington, DC: The National Academies Press.

Leininger, M. (1977). In Leininger, M. (Ed.), *Transcultural care of infants and children: proceedings from the first transcultural conference.* Salt Lake City: University of Utah.

Smith, L. S. (2001). Evaluation of an educational intervention to increase cultural competence among registered nurses. *Journal of Cultural Diversity,* 8(2), 50–63.

Tripp-Reimer, T., & Dougherty, M. C. (1985). Cross-cultural nursing research. *Annual Review of Nursing Research,* 3, 77–104.

Preface

The concept of transcultural nursing is relatively new to the nursing literature. In fact, it has been only in the last three decades that nurses have begun to develop an appreciation for the need to incorporate culturally appropriate clinical approaches into the daily routine of client care. Although nurses have begun to recognize the need for culturally appropriate clinical approaches, the literature on the subject is either scanty or does not provide a systematic method for comprehensive assessment and intervention. However, a good foundation in transcultural nursing is essential for the nurse because it can provide a conceptual framework for holistic client care in a variety of clinical settings and assist the nurse throughout a nursing career.

When we were challenged almost 20 years ago by the nursing students at Bethel College to develop a systematic approach to client assessment for use with individuals from diverse cultural backgrounds, we had no idea how profoundly important this topic would become for all health care providers. The United States is rapidly becoming a multicultural, heterogeneous, pluralistic society. With changing demographics, it is imperative that nurses develop not only sensitivity, but also cultural competence to render safe, effective care to all clients.

When we were first challenged by the students at Bethel College, we discovered that the students had difficulty finding adequate literature to assist in planning for clients from diverse cultural backgrounds. We, like our students, had identified a similar need by virtue of our own diverse cultural backgrounds: one of us is African-American and was raised in the South, and the other is White and was raised in an Eskimo setting in Alaska. Thus, in response to both a personal interest and the need identified by our students, we set about to synthesize a body of literature that would assist students in developing the theoretical knowledge necessary to provide culturally appropriate care. Although the literature has vastly improved since the initial release of this text, there is still much work to be done in this area.

This text, like the four previous editions, is divided into two parts. The first part, which focuses on theory, includes an introduction and six chapters describing the six cultural phenomena that make up our transcultural conceptual theory of assessment. The six cultural phenomena that we have identified as being evidenced in all cultural groups are (1) communication, (2) space, (3) social organization, (4) time, (5) environmental control, and (6) biological variations. The chapters in Part One describe how these phenomena vary with application and utilization across cultures.

Part Two contains chapters by contributing authors in which the six cultural phenomena are systematically applied to the assessment and care of individuals in specific cultures. The cultures selected for inclusion represent those most likely to be encountered by a nurse practicing in the United States.

Now, as in the fourth edition, six chapters are available on the Evolve site via the Internet. In addition, a new NCLEX-RN Review test on Cultural Competency is available on the Internet.

In the fifth edition, we have once again selected contributing authors with expertise and clinical backgrounds in the care of selected cultural groups. As in our first four editions, many of our chapters were written by contributing authors who actually represent, by ethnic heritage, the cultural group described. Not only are unique and diverse cultures represented, but also the contributing authors span the North American continent with representation truly from coast to coast and from California to Alaska and Hawaii. Thus the assessment model is applied to persons in diverse cultural settings by nurses who have expertise and sensitivity in the cultural group and in the unique care strategies that a nurse should use in providing culturally appropriate and competent care.

Because our first edition was translated into French, we perceived a need to incorporate some of the cultural uniqueness of our neighbors to the north (the people of Québec in Canada). This perceived need led to a new book, *Canadian Transcultural Nursing*, published in 1998, which we urge our readers to review. Once again, in this fifth edition we have tried to select cultural groups who by virtual numbers reflect the greater percentage of our current population. We recognize and value the diversity of all the cultural groups found in the United States, but because of space and fiscal considerations, we have selected the most populous groups.

Since publication of the first edition, we have developed a quick reference, user-friendly assessment tool for use with clients in diverse clinical settings. In addition, in 2006, we developed the Giger and Davidhizar NCLEX-RN Review for Cultural Competency. The Answer Key to the Cultural Competency Skills Test will be provided for faculty only and can be found online at http://evolve.elsevier.com/Giger/. Our model has been cited, excerpted, or modified for inclusion in 490 new nursing textbooks. Our model has shown great applicability across clinical disciplines. As such, the text was included in the library of the Education Testing Service (ETS) for many years as the only text of its kind to validate test items developed for the former RN-NCLEX and the current RN-CAT. In the fifth edition, led by Ken Farr and Doris Bartlett, text questions designed for the current NCLEX-RN test

question format are added to allow the student and faculty to relate cultural context to a testing format. In addition, in this new edition, we have added clear and more concise definitions of health disparities and offer for the first time disabilities as a culture. In fact, Dr. Joan Earle Hahn developed a precise and understandable disability cultural schematic model based on Giger & Davidhizar that most health care professionals will find useful in their practice.

This book was written primarily for all nurses and nursing students who are interested in developing knowledge of transcultural concepts to apply to client-centered care. However, we believe our new edition will also be applicable across other disciplines, such as psychology, sociology, medicine, and anthropology, because it provides not only a nursing perspective, but also a historical and biotechnological approach to transcultural health care.

In our commitment to transcultural nursing, we have once again made every effort, through extensive research, to be as culturally sensitive as possible and not offend our readers or specific racial, cultural, ethnic, or religious groups. Despite our careful attention to detail to prevent this from happening, we realize that the presentation of literature and research findings is often interpreted differently by individuals. We apologize for any content that our readers may find insensitive and assure our readers that as nurse researchers, clinicians, and academicians, we have as our only intent the presentation of factual information.

Acknowledgments

We would like to acknowledge and thank our former editors: Linda Duncan, whose vision of the future allowed this project to come to fruition; Darlene Como, who took up the challenge to continue this project; Loren Wilson, who continued to challenge us to provide the best-referenced text on this subject; Michael Ledbetter, who worked diligently on past editions of this text, and finally to our new editor Robin Carter for working diligently to bring this project to completion. We would also like to thank Mary Parker for all of her assistance as we sought to develop this new edition. In addition, a special thanks to Deanna Davis, who diligently and painstakingly brought this edition to fruition.

We would like to thank Dr. Clyde Root, Director of Library Services, Bethel College, for the multitude of computer searches conducted on our behalf. A special recognition goes to the people who, by their religious affiliation, proved to be invaluable content experts in providing advice, counsel, and information on special religious groups. These individuals include Judy Mason, a member of the staff, University of Alabama at Birmingham, School of Nursing, whose expert advice on Jehovah's Witnesses proved to be invaluable. Similarly, we would like to thank Tamra Walters, a former baccalaureate nursing student at the University of Tulsa, Tulsa, Oklahoma, who read our first edition and graciously provided in-depth insight on the Church of Jesus Christ of Latter Day Saints (Mormons); Dr. Mary Grace Umlauf, who through her extensive travels to Jordan not only contributed to that chapter, but also helped us through her extensive ties to the Muslim world understand Islam as a world religion; Dr. Joan Earle Hahn, who developed for us a new disability cultural schematic model based on Giger & Davidhizar; Kenneth Farr and Doris Bartlett for all the attention to our new NCLEX-RN Cultural Competency Test Bank; and Karen Danz for working tirelessly with manuscript edits.

We wish to thank the many persons who took the photos and provided them for use in this textbook and all the individuals who posed for these pictures. A special thanks goes to Dottie Kauffman, our photographer, who has labored on this project for some 17 years. We also offer special thanks to Ruth Shearer, who has provided consistency to each of the care plans throughout the book. We thank our chapter contributors who believed in this project. Each of you has made invaluable contributions. Finally, we would like to acknowledge the friendship and respect that has grown over these 25 years. We believe that given the diversity of our heritages (one African-American and one White American), our ability to complement each other is a testimonial to the achievement of racial, ethnic, and cultural harmony across the United States, Canada, and countries throughout the world in this century. As we venture into the second half of the new millennium, we are hopeful that all health care providers will continue to strive to achieve cultural competence.

Joyce Newman Giger
Ruth Elaine Davidhizar

Special Acknowledgments

Since the last edition, I have been challenged to think about how precious life is. In 2006, I lost my mentor and best friend, Dr. Mary Starke Harper, one of the founders of the National Black Nurses Association. Although she was 86 years young, I thought, as did many others in the country, that she had many other contributions to make to the world. Like so many other African-Americans before her, I thought my friend and mentor had gone too soon, despite her advanced age, and that she had gone with so many things yet to do to teach the next generation about care and caring. Valuing diversity is essential, but understanding the challenges of cultural competence care is paramount to ending unequal treatment and the unequal burden of such diseases as cancer, diabetes, and heart disease.

It has been my pleasure to have traveled the road to discovery leading to more culturally competent care with such a wonderful friend as Ruth Davidhizar. We began this odyssey of discovery more than 25 years ago. Unlike most writing partners, I think we began as friends, and this relationship has grown stronger throughout the decades. Thanks for sharing this odyssey with me, Ruth. I lovingly dedicate this book to the memory of my mentor and friend, Dr. Mary Starke Harper, and all vulnerable populations who might suffer from culturally incompetent and unequal health care treatment throughout the world.

Love, Joyce

A special acknowledgment is made to Dr. Joyce Newman Giger, my friend and colleague, who some time ago was diagnosed with breast cancer.

Joyce, you are an amazing breast cancer survivor. It has seemed through almost every edition but this one, you have dealt with the effects of breast cancer. As an African-American woman, you defy the present statistics on survivability from this devastating condition. Nonetheless, through all of this, you maintained your steadfast faith in the goodness of God and your trust that His will would be done. Your hope in life and your knowledge that your life has a special plan not only saw us through this book, but also will see us through as we plan the next one. I know that you have recently lost one your mentors and best friend and a great African-American pioneer in nursing, Dr. Mary Starke Harper. I hope for a new and challenging treatment for breast cancer in our lifetime. On your behalf and on behalf of Dr. Karon Schwartz, author of the Amish chapter, and my secretary, Karen Danz, who worked tirelessly with manuscript edits, I dedicate this book to all the women of the world who are breast cancer survivors. May each and every woman with breast cancer continue to rise to enjoy all the precious moments of life.

With Love, Ruth

Contents

PART ONE **Framework for Cultural Assessment and Intervention Techniques**

1	Introduction to Transcultural Nursing	2
2	Communication	20
3	Space	47
4	Social Organization	68
5	Time	106
6	Environmental Control	129
7	Biological Variations	145

PART TWO **Application of Assessment and Intervention Techniques to Specific Cultural Groups**

8	African-Americans	190
9	Mexican Americans	239
10	Navajos	276
11	Appalachians	300
12	American Eskimos: The Yup'ik and Inupiat	323
13	Japanese Americans	357
14	Afghans and Afghan Americans	394
15	Russian Americans	410
16	Chinese Americans	442
17	Filipino Americans	467
18	Vietnamese Americans	494
19	East Indian Hindu Americans	537
20	Haitian Americans	563
21	Jewish Americans	592
22	Korean Americans	619
23	French Canadians of Québec Origin	642
24	Puerto Rican Americans	670

Appendix A:	Answer Key for NCLEX-RN Review Questions	A–1
Index		I–1

The following chapters can be found online at http://evolve.elsevier.com/Giger/

25	Nigerian Americans	
26	Ugandan Americans	
27	Jordanian Americans	
28	Cuban Americans	
29	Amish Americans	
30	Irish Americans	

PART ONE

Framework for Cultural Assessment and Intervention Techniques

CHAPTER 1 Introduction to Transcultural Nursing

Theories of transcultural nursing with established clinical approaches to clients from varying cultures are relatively new. According to Madeleine Leininger (1977), who founded the field of transcultural nursing in the mid-1960s, the education of nursing students in this field is only now beginning to yield significant results. Today, nurses with a deeper appreciation of human life and values are developing cultural sensitivity for appropriate, individualized clinical approaches. Transcultural nursing concepts are being incorporated into the curricula for student nurses in the United States and Canada.

The Transcultural Nursing Society, founded in 1974, is promoting interest in transcultural concepts and the education of transcultural nurses at the graduate level (Giger & Davidhizar, 1990; Wenger, 1989). Since its inception, the society has promoted such efforts at annual transcultural nursing conferences in different worldwide locations. The society also implemented the first certification plan in transcultural nursing. Through the efforts of the society, a number of U.S. and Canadian nurses have received certification. Other international conferences, such as that supported by the Rockefeller Foundation in October 1988 in Bellagio, Italy, have sought to promote international health care management. The society also publishes the *Transcultural Nursing Society Newsletter* and *The Journal of Transcultural Nursing*. Additionally, other transcultural publications include the *International Journal of Nursing Studies* and the *International Nursing Review*. Although the literature on patient approaches in culturally diverse situations is mushrooming and nurses are beginning to do transcultural research studies, up to now relatively few theories on transcultural nursing have provided a systematic method for comprehensive nursing assessment (Brink, 2001a, 2001b; Leininger, 1985a, 1985b, 1991; Spector, 1996; Tripp-Reimer, 1984a,

1984b; Tripp-Reimer & Dougherty, 1985; Tripp-Reimer & Friedl, 1977).

CULTURE DEFINED

Culture is a patterned behavioral response that develops over time as a result of imprinting the mind through social and religious structures and intellectual and artistic manifestations. Culture is also the result of acquired mechanisms that may have innate influences but are primarily affected by internal and external environmental stimuli. Culture is shaped by values, beliefs, norms, and practices that are shared by members of the same cultural group. Culture guides our thinking, doing, and being and becomes patterned expressions of who we are. These patterned expressions are passed down from one generation to the next. Other definitions of culture have been offered by Leininger (1985a, 1985b, 1991), Leininger and McFarland (2002), Spector (2001, 2004), and Andrews and Boyle (2003). According to Leininger (1985a, 1985b, 1991) and Leininger and McFarland (2002), culture is the values, beliefs, norms, and practices of a particular group that are learned and shared and that guide thinking, decisions, and actions in a patterned way. Spector (2001, 2004) contends that culture is a metacommunication system based on nonphysical traits, such as values, beliefs, attitudes, customs, language, and behaviors, that are shared by a group of people and are passed down from one generation to the next. According to Andrews and Boyle (2003), culture represents a unique way of perceiving, behaving, and evaluating the external environment and as such provides a blueprint for determining values, beliefs, and practices. Regardless of the definition chosen, the term culture implies a dynamic, ever-changing, active, or passive process.

Cultural values are unique expressions of a particular culture that have been accepted as appropriate over time. They guide actions and decision making that facilitate self-worth and self-esteem. Leininger (1985a) postulates that cultural values develop as a direct result of an individual's desirable or preferred way of acting or knowing something that is often sustained by a culture over time and that governs actions or decisions.

THE NEED FOR TRANSCULTURAL NURSING KNOWLEDGE

It is believed that demography is destiny, demographic change is reality, and demographic sensitivity is imperative. The United States is rapidly becoming a multicultural, pluralistic society. In 2002, 70.18% of the population in the United States was White of European descent; 12.3%, African-American; 12.52%, Hispanic American; 4.1%, Asian American; and 0.9%, American Indian (*Time Almanac with Information Please*, 2006; U.S. Department of Commerce, Bureau of the Census, Summary File 3, 2002a). It is projected that by the year 2020, only 53% of the U.S. population will be White of European descent. It is further projected that by the year 2021, the number of Asian Americans and Hispanic Americans will triple, while the number of African-Americans will double (U.S. Department of Commerce, Bureau of the Census, 2002b).

If the 2000 census data on fertility, birth, and mortality are correct, it is conceivable that it will be almost impossible to isolate and identify a "pure" race of Whites of European descent by the year 2070 (U.S. Department of Commerce, Bureau of the Census, 2002b). In light of these statistical data, it is imperative that the nursing workforce rapidly adapt itself to a changing, heterogeneous society.

Providing culturally appropriate and thus competent care in the 21st century will be a complex and difficult task for many nurses. In many professional health career programs, such as nursing, medicine, and respiratory therapy, students are rarely taught culturally appropriate and competent care techniques. Thus, when these individuals encounter clients from culturally diverse backgrounds in the clinical setting, they are often unable to accurately assess and provide the kind of interventions that are culturally appropriate.

The burden of teaching nurses culturally competent care techniques will rest not only with the individual programs of practice development but also with the health care agency itself. Regardless of who is responsible for this task, nurses must develop an understanding about culture and its relevance to competent care.

A nurse who does not recognize the value and importance of culturally appropriate care cannot possibly be an effective care agent in this changing demographic society. If nurses do not recognize that the intervention strategies planned for an African-American client with diabetes are uniquely different from those planned for a Vietnamese American, an Italian American, and so forth, they cannot possibly hope to change health-seeking behaviors or actively encourage the wellness behaviors of this client or any client. When nurses consider race, ethnicity, culture, and cultural heritage, they become more sensitive to clients. This is not to suggest that there is a cookbook approach to delivering care to clients by virtue of race, ethnicity, or culture. There is as much variation within certain races, cultures, or ethnic groups as there is across cultural groups. When the informed nurse considers the significance of culture, clients are approached with a more informed perspective.

The time to learn differing perspectives about culture is at hand. As professional health care providers, nurses will be asked to step forward to provide the leadership to ensure that all people have equal access to high-quality, culturally appropriate, and culturally competent health care. This task can be accomplished only through culturally diverse nursing care.

CULTURAL ASSESSMENT
Using Non-Nursing Models

In a pluralistic society, nurse practitioners need to be prepared to provide culturally appropriate nursing care for each client, regardless of that client's cultural background. To provide culturally appropriate nursing care, nurses must understand specific factors that influence individual health and illness behaviors (Tripp-Reimer, Brink, &

Saunders, 1984). According to Affonso (1979), cultural assessment can give meaning to behaviors that might otherwise be judged negatively. If cultural behaviors are not appropriately identified, their significance will be confusing to the nurse.

Although transcultural nursing theories have appeared in the literature (Affonso, 1979; Leininger, 1985a, 1985b), adequate nursing assessment methods to accompany these theories have not been consistently provided. One of the most comprehensive tools used for nursing cultural assessment is the *Outline of Cultural Materials* by Murdock et al. (1971); however, this tool was developed primarily for anthropologists who were concerned with ethnographic descriptions of cultural groups. Although the tool is well developed and contains 88 major categories, it was not designed for nurse practitioners and thus does not provide for systematic use of the nursing process. Another assessment tool is in Brownlee's (1978) *Community, Culture, and Care: A Cross-Cultural Guide for Health Workers.* Brownlee's work is devoted to the process of practical assessment of a community, with specific attention given to health areas. The work deals with three aspects of assessment: what to find out, why it is important, and how to do it. Brownlee's assessment tool has been criticized as being too comprehensive, too difficult, and too detailed for use with individual clients. Although this tool was developed for use by health care practitioners, it is not exclusively a nursing assessment tool.

Using Nursing-Specific Models

Transcultural nursing as defined by Leininger (1991) is a "humanistic and scientific area of formal study and practice which is focused upon differences and similarities among cultures with respect to human care, health (or well-being), and illness based upon the people's cultural values, beliefs, and practices." According to Leininger (1991), the ultimate goal of transcultural nursing is use of relevant knowledge to provide culturally specific and culturally congruent nursing care to people. From this theoretical perspective, Leininger (1985a, 1985b; Leininger & McFarland, 2002) provides a comprehensive transcultural theory and assessment model. For more than 30 years, this model has helped nurses discover and understand what health care means to various cultures. Leininger's sunrise model symbolizes the rising of the sun (care). The model depicts a full sun with four levels of foci. Within the circle in the upper portion of the model are components of the social structure and worldview factors that influence care and health through language and environment. These factors influence the folk, professional, and nursing systems or subsystems located in the lower half of the model. Also included in the model are levels of abstraction and analysis from which care can be studied at each level. Various cultural phenomena are studied from the micro, middle, and macro perspectives (Leininger, 1985a, 1985b). Leininger's model has served as the prototype for the development of other culturally specific nursing models and tools (Bloch, 1983; Branch & Paxton, 1976; Orque, 1983; Rund & Krause, 1978).

An Analysis of Culturally Specific Models and Tools

Tripp-Reimer, Brink, and Saunders (1984) analyzed selected culturally appropriate models and tools to determine whether the models significantly differed. They concluded that most cultural assessment guides are similar because they all seek to identify major cultural domains that are important variables if culturally appropriate care is to be rendered. Nine culturally appropriate models or guides were analyzed: Aamodt (1978), Bloch (1983), Branch and Paxton (1976), Brownlee (1978), Kay (1978), Leininger (1977), Orque (1983), Rund and Krause (1978), and Tripp-Reimer (1984b). In analyzing the models, Tripp-Reimer, Brink, and Saunders (1984) concluded that the same two limitations existed in each guide. The first limitation was the tendency to include too much cultural content, ultimately negating the "heart of the matter," which is the process itself. The second limitation was that it is often impossible to separate client-specific data from normative data.

Using Nursing Diagnoses

The relative significance of culturally appropriate health care cannot be understood if the nurse does not understand the value of culturally relevant nursing diagnoses. Geissler (1991) reported a study to determine the applicability of the North American Nursing Diagnosis Association (NANDA) taxonomy as a culturally appropriate assessment tool for use with diverse populations. In the study, three nursing diagnoses were analyzed to validate their cultural appropriateness: (1) impaired verbal communication, (2) social isolation, and (3) noncompliance in culturally diverse situations. Participants in the study ($n = 245$ nurses) were experts in the field of transcultural nursing and were members of either the Transcultural Nursing Society or the American Nurses Association Council on Cultural Diversity (Geissler, 1991). Findings from this study also indicate that nursing diagnoses tend to (1) focus on the client rather than the provider and therefore do not acknowledge the existence of other culturally relevant viewpoints (such as those expressed by the provider); (2) be generalized and, as a result, increase the likelihood, when applied in diverse cultural settings, for stereotyping and victimization because so-called non-Western medical models are believed to be "abnormal" and thus require necessary interventions; and (3) involve mislabeling phenomena, which in actuality arise as expressions of cultural dissonance rather than expressions of political, social, psychological, or economic factors.

In the study reported by Geissler (1991), the NANDA nursing diagnosis "impaired communication, verbal, related to cultural differences" is an excellent example of a client-oriented diagnosis that does not recognize linguistic cultural differences. The study concludes that the NANDA diagnosis of "impaired verbal communication" connotes that the client's verbal communication and ability to understand and use language are impaired in some way. This diagnosis does not consider the causative factors creating the impairment (Giger, Davidhizar, Evers, & Ingram, 1994). It is apparent that individuals who speak a language different from that used by health care providers or nurses may be very capable of both use and comprehension of a specific language when interacting with persons fluent in that language (Giger, Davidhizar, Evers, & Ingram, 1994). According to Geissler (1991), if the client

in this situation is "verbally impaired," the nurse is equally impaired. Geissler also concludes that the NANDA diagnosis of "impaired verbal communication" does not adequately address the issue of nonverbal communication, which was identified in the earlier nursing literature as an essential assessment factor (Giger & Davidhizar, 1990, 1994).

According to Geissler (1991), nursing diagnoses related to social isolation and noncompliance need further defining characteristics for use with culturally diverse populations. Rather than use the term *noncompliance*, Geissler (1991) suggests that the term *nonadherence* may be more appropriate because this term may more accurately reflect behavior resulting from cultural dissonance. At the same time, the use of *nonadherence* may remove the stigma of guilt experienced by the health care recipient who is inappropriately labeled noncompliant.

GIGER AND DAVIDHIZAR'S TRANSCULTURAL ASSESSMENT MODEL

In response to the need for a practical assessment tool for evaluating cultural variables and their effects on health and illness behaviors, a transcultural assessment model is offered that greatly minimizes the time needed to conduct a comprehensive assessment in an effort to provide culturally competent care. The metaparadigm for the Giger and Davidhizar Transcultural Assessment Model includes (1) transcultural nursing and culturally diverse nursing, (2) culturally competent care, (3) culturally unique individuals, (4) culturally sensitive environments, and (5) health and health status based on culturally specific illness and wellness behaviors.

Transcultural Nursing Defined

In the context of Giger and Davidhizar's Transcultural Assessment Model (1990), transcultural nursing is viewed as a culturally competent practice field that is client centered and research focused. Although transcultural nursing is viewed as client centered, it is important for nurses to remember that culture can and does influence how clients are viewed and the care that is rendered.

Every individual is culturally unique, and nurses are no exception to this premise. Nonetheless, nurses must use caution to avoid projecting on the client their own cultural uniqueness and worldviews if culturally appropriate care is to be provided. Nurses must carefully discern personal cultural beliefs and values to separate them from the client's beliefs and values. To deliver culturally sensitive care, the nurse must remember that each individual is unique and a product of experiences, beliefs, and values that have been learned and passed down from one generation to the next.

According to Stokes (1991), nursing as a profession is not "culturally free" but rather is "culturally determined." Nurses must recognize and understand this fact to avoid becoming grossly ethnocentric (Stokes, 1991). Because there is a contingent relationship between cultural determination and the delivery of culturally sensitive care, the transcultural nurse must be guided by acquired knowledge in the assessment, diagnosis, planning, implementation, and evaluation of the client's needs based on culturally relevant information. This ideology does not presuppose that all individuals within a specific cultural group will think and behave in a similar manner with relative predictability. The astute nurse must remember that there is as much diversity within a cultural group as there is across cultural groups. Nonetheless, the goal of transcultural nursing is the discovery of culturally relevant facts about the client to provide culturally appropriate and competent care.

Although transcultural nursing is becoming a highly specialized field of specially educated individuals, every nurse, regardless of academic or experiential background, must use transcultural knowledge to facilitate culturally appropriate care. Regardless of preparation in the field of transcultural nursing, every nurse who is entrusted with care of clients must make every effort to deliver culturally sensitive care that is free of inherent biases based on gender, race, or religion.

Culturally Diverse Nursing Care

Culturally diverse nursing care refers to the variability in nursing approaches needed to provide culturally appropriate and competent care. Nurses need to utilize transcultural knowledge in a skillful and artful manner to render culturally appropriate and competent care to a rapidly changing, heterogeneous client population. Culturally diverse nursing care must take into account six cultural phenomena that vary with application and use yet are evident in all cultural groups: (1) communication, (2) space, (3) social organization, (4) time, (5) environmental control, and (6) biological variations (Figs. 1-1 and 1-2).

Culturally Competent Care Defined

As a heightened awareness of transcultural health care has been espoused, so too has been the widened use of the term *cultural competence*. There are as many varying definitions for this term as there are for the term *culture*. Purnell and Paulanka (2003) note that *cultural competence* is the act whereby a health care professional develops an awareness of one's existence, sensations, thoughts, and environment without letting these factors have an undue effect on those for whom care is provided. Further, they conclude that cultural competence is the adaptation of care in a manner that is congruent with the client's culture. In this sense, cultural competence is a conscious process and as such cannot be necessarily viewed as linear (Purnell & Paulanka, 2003).

According to Smith (1998b), cultural competence is a continuous process of awareness, knowledge, skill, interaction, and sensitivity that is demonstrated among those who render care and the services they provide. Smith concludes that cultural competence requires continuous seeking of skills, practices, and attitudes that enable nurses to transform interventions into positive health outcomes, such as improved client morbidity and mortality, as well as augmenting client and professional levels of satisfaction.

Cultural competence is a dynamic, fluid, continuous process whereby an individual, system, or health care agency finds meaningful and useful care-delivery strategies based on knowledge of the cultural heritage, beliefs, attitudes, and behaviors of those to whom they render care. To develop

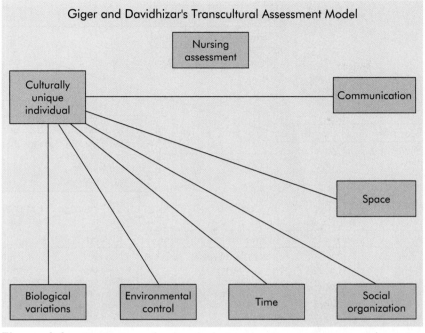

Figure 1-1   Application of cultural phenomena to nursing care and nursing practice.

cultural competence, it is essential for the health care professional to utilize knowledge gained from conceptual and theoretical models of culturally appropriate care. In addition, cultural competence connotes a higher, more sophisticated level of refinement of cognitive and psychomotor skills, attitudes, and personal beliefs. Attainment of cultural competence can assist the astute nurse in devising meaningful interventions to promote optimal health among individuals, regardless of race, ethnicity, gender identity, sexual identity, or cultural heritage. It is interesting to note that in searching for an adequate definition for *cultural competence*, Cohall and Bannister (2001), writing in a seminal text done by Braithwaite and Taylor (2001), used the *cultural competency* definition proposed by Giger and Davidhizar.

Culturally Unique Individuals

To provide culturally appropriate and competent care, it is important to remember that each individual is culturally unique and as such is a product of experiences, cultural beliefs, and cultural norms. Cultural expressions become patterned responses and give each individual a unique identity (see Fig. 1-2). Although there is as much diversity within cultural and racial groups as there is across and among cultural and racial groups, knowledge of general baseline data relative to the specific cultural group is an excellent starting point to provide culturally appropriate care.

Culturally Sensitive Environments

Culturally diverse health care can and should be rendered in a variety of clinical settings. Regardless of the level of care—primary, secondary, or tertiary—knowledge of culturally relevant information will assist the nurse in planning and implementing a treatment regimen that is unique for each client.

In response to the apparent lack of practical assessment tools available in nursing for evaluating

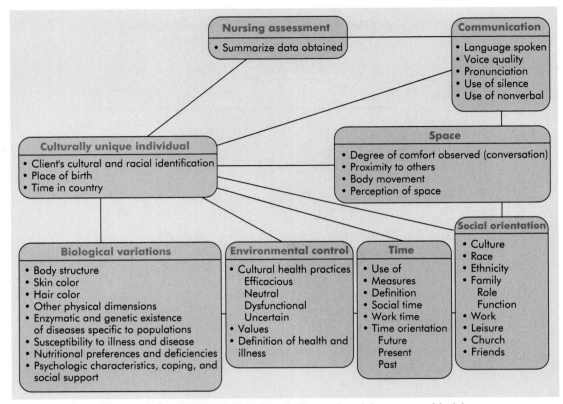

Nursing assessment
• Summarize data obtained

Communication
• Language spoken
• Voice quality
• Pronunciation
• Use of silence
• Use of nonverbal

Culturally unique individual
• Client's cultural and racial identification
• Place of birth
• Time in country

Space
• Degree of comfort observed (conversation)
• Proximity to others
• Body movement
• Perception of space

Social orientation
• Culture
• Race
• Ethnicity
• Family
  Role
  Function
• Work
• Leisure
• Church
• Friends

Biological variations
• Body structure
• Skin color
• Hair color
• Other physical dimensions
• Enzymatic and genetic existence of diseases specific to populations
• Susceptibility to illness and disease
• Nutritional preferences and deficiencies
• Psychologic characteristics, coping, and social support

Environmental control
• Cultural health practices
  Efficacious
  Neutral
  Dysfunctional
  Uncertain
• Values
• Definition of health and illness

Time
• Use of
• Measures
• Definition
• Social time
• Work time
• Time orientation
  Future
  Present
  Past

Figure 1-2   Giger and Davidhizar's Transcultural Assessment Model.

cultural variables and their effects on health and illness behaviors, this text provides a systematic approach to evaluating the six essential cultural phenomena to assist the nurse in providing culturally appropriate nursing care. Although the six cultural phenomena are evident in all cultural groups, they vary in application across cultures. Thus, an individualized assessment of these areas is necessary when working with clients from diverse cultural groups (Fig. 1-3).

DEVELOPMENT AND REFINEMENT OF GIGER AND DAVIDHIZAR'S TRANSCULTURAL ASSESSMENT MODEL

Clinical Application

Since its introduction in 1991, Giger and Davidhizar's Transcultural Assessment Model has been applied to the care of clients in a variety of clinical specialties, including the maternity client (Giger, Davidhizar, & Wieczorek, 1993), the operating room client (Bowen & Davidhizar, 1991), and the psychiatric client (Giger, Davidhizar, Evers, & Ingram, 1994).

In 1993, Spector illustrated the model's utility by combining it with the Cultural Heritage Model. The combination of these two models (Fig. 1-4), which appears in Potter and Perry's *Fundamentals of Nursing* textbook, is unique because it provides a holistic method of providing culturally competent care. In addition, using Giger and Davidhizar's six cultural phenomena, though in a different hierarchical arrangement, Spector (1996) created a unique quick reference guide for cultural assessment of people from a variety of racial and cultural groups (Table 1-1).

Table 1-1   Cross-Cultural Examples of Cultural Phenomena Impacting Nursing Care

Nations of Origin	Communication	Space	Time Orientation	Social Organization	Environmental Control	Biological Variations
Asia China Hawaii Phillippines Korea Japan Southeast Asia (Laos, Cambodia, Vietnam)	National language preference Dialects, written characters Use of silence Nonverbal and contextual cuing	Noncontact people	Present	Family: hierarchical structure, loyalty Devotion to tradition Many religions, including Taoism, Buddhism, Islam, and Christianity Community social organizations	Traditional health and illness beliefs Use of traditional medicines Traditional practitioners: Chinese doctors and herbalists	Liver cancer Stomach cancer Coccidioidomycosis Hypertension Lactose intolerance
Africa West coast (as slaves) Many African countries West Indian Islands Dominican Republic Haiti Jamaica	National languages Dialect: pidgin, creole, Spanish, and French	Close personal space	Present over future	Family: many female, single-parent Large, extended family networks Strong church affiliation within community Community social organizations	Traditional health and illness beliefs Folk medicine tradition Traditional healer: root-worker	Sickle cell anemia Hypertension Cancer of the esophagus Stomach cancer Coccidioidomycosis Lactose intolerance

(Continued)

Table 1-1   Cross-Cultural Examples of Cultural Phenomena Impacting Nursing Care—Cont'd

Nations of Origin	Communication	Space	Time Orientation	Social Organization	Environmental Control	Biological Variations
Europe Germany England Italy Ireland Other European countries	National languages Many learn English immediately	Noncontact people Aloof Distant Southern countries: closer contact and touch	Future over present	Nuclear families Extended families Judeo-Christian religions Community social organizations	Primary reliance on modern health care system Traditional health and illness beliefs Some remaining folk medicine traditions	Breast cancer Heart disease Diabetes mellitus Thalassemia
American Indian 500 American Indian tribes Aleuts Eskimos	Tribal languages Use of silence and body language	Space very important and has no boundaries	Present	Extremely family oriented Biological and extended families Children taught to respect traditions Community social organizations	Traditional health and illness beliefs Folk medicine tradition Traditional healer: medicine man	Accidents Heart disease Cirrhosis of the liver Diabetes mellitus
Hispanic countries Spain Cuba Mexico Central and South America	Spanish or Portuguese primary language	Tactile relationships Touch Handshakes Embracing Value physical presence	Present	Nuclear family Extended families *Compadrazgo;* godparents Community social organizations	Traditional health and illness beliefs Folk medicine tradition Traditional healers: *curandero, espiritista, partera, señora*	Diabetes mellitus Parasites Coccidioidomycosis Lactose intolerance

Compiled by Rachel Spector, RN, PhD. In Potter, P.A., & Perry, A. G. (1997). *Fundamentals of nursing: concepts, process, and practice* (ed. 4). St. Louis: Mosby.

Table 1-2	Cultural Behaviors Relevant to Health Assessment	
Cultural Group	**Cultural Variations (Common Belief/ Practice)**	**Nursing Implications**
African-Americans	Dialect and slang terms require careful communication to prevent error (e.g., "bad" may mean "good").	Question the client's meaning or intent.
Mexican Americans	Eye behavior is important. An individual who looks at and admires a child without touching the child has given the child the "evil eye."	Always touch the child you are examining or admiring.
American Indians	Eye contact is considered a sign of disrespect and is thus avoided.	Recognize that the client may be attentive and interested even though eye contact is avoided.
Appalachians	Eye contact is considered impolite or a sign of hostility. Verbal patter may be confusing.	Avoid excessive eye contact. Clarify statements.
American Eskimos	Body language is very important. The individual seldom disagrees publicly with others. Client may nod yes to be polite, even if not in agreement.	Monitor own body language closely as well as client's to detect meaning.
Jewish Americans	Orthodox Jews consider excess touching, particularly from members of the opposite sex, offensive.	Establish whether client is an Orthodox Jew and, if so, avoid excessive touch.
Chinese Americans	Individual may nod head to indicate yes or shake head to indicate no. Excessive eye contact indicates rudeness. Excessive touch is offensive.	Ask questions carefully and clarify responses. Avoid excessive eye contact and touch.
Filipino Americans	Offending people is to be avoided at all cost. Nonverbal behavior is very important.	Monitor nonverbal behaviors of self and client, being sensitive to physical and emotional discomfort or concerns of the client.
Haitian Americans	Touch is used in conversation. Direct eye contact is used to gain attention and respect during communication.	Use direct eye contact when communicating.
East Indian Hindu Americans	Be aware that men may view eye contact by women as offensive. Avoid eye contact.	Women avoid eye contact as a sign of respect.
Vietnamese Americans	Avoidance of eye contact is a sign of respect. The head is considered sacred; it is not polite to pat the head. An upturned palm is offensive in communication.	Limit eye contact. Touch the head only when mandated and explain clearly before proceeding to do so. Avoid hand gesturing.

From Giger, J., & Davidhizar, R. (1995). *Transcultural nursing* (ed. 2). St. Louis: Mosby; also appears in Kozier, B., Erb, G., Blaise, K., Johnson, J. Y., & Smith-Temple, J. (1993). *Techniques in clinical nursing* (ed. 2). Reading, Mass., Addison-Wesley.

Application to Other Disciplines

The model is broad enough in scope to be recognized for applicability by many other health care professions (for example, medical imaging, dentistry, education and training departments, and hospital administration) (Dowd, Giger, & Davidhizar, 1998). This model has had numerous applications in medical imaging: a description of its use in dealing with diversity in radiology departments (Davidhizar, Dowd, & Giger, 1997a); a proposal for its use in the theory base of the profession of radiography (Davidhizar, Dowd, & Giger, 1997b);

and a method for how to deal with cultural differences affecting pain response (Davidhizar, Dowd, & Giger, 1997c). Dental hygienists are also involved with clients from diverse cultures. "Transcultural Patient Assessment, a Method of Advancing Dental Care," published in *Dental Assistant* (Davidhizar & Giger, 1998a, 1998b) illuminates how awareness of the behavior of clients in the dental office is often culturally motivated. The model is also described in journals that cross health care professions, such as *Hospital Topics* (Davidhizar & Giger, 1996), *Community Health: Education and Promotion Manual*

(Giger, Davidhizar, Johnson, & Poole, 1996), and *Health Care Traveler* (Giger, Davidhizar, Johnson, & Poole, 1997). Application of Giger and Davidhizar's model to diverse clinical settings is quickly producing a way for staff across disciplines to understand cultural diversity and learn techniques of culturally competent care. In addition, Giger and Davidhizar's Transcultural Assessment Model has also been shown to be applicable to the analysis of current trends in multiculturalism in health care (Smith, 1998a).

Refinement Through Research

Refinement of Giger and Davidhizar's Transcultural Assessment Model is also being enhanced through the research efforts of various individuals. For example, in 1992, a graduate student from the University of Kansas completed a master's thesis titled "Utilizing Giger and Davidhizar's Transcultural Assessment Model for the Cultural Assessment of Farm Families" (Daugherty, 1992). In 1993, a graduate student at Georgia Southern University at Statesboro conducted a research study on the health beliefs and self-care practices of hypertensive African-American women by using Giger and Davidhizar's Transcultural Assessment Model as a theoretical framework to guide and evaluate research findings (Walthour, 1993). In addition to these master's theses, several doctoral dissertations have been completed using the model. In 1995, a group of interdisciplinary researchers (nursing, behavioral medicine, lipoprotein research, human genetics, preventive medicine, nutrition, biostatistics) at the University of Alabama at Birmingham and at Emory University received $750,000 from the Uniformed Health Sciences, University of the Health Sciences, Tri-Services Nursing Military Research Group, Department of Defense, to identify behavioral risk-reduction strategies and chronic indicators for premenopausal African-American women with coronary heart disease or associated risk factors. The model served as the overarching theoretical framework to test its usefulness as an educational tool to enhance and promote compliance. The study is titled "Behavioral Risk Reduction Strategies for Chronic Indicators and High Risk Factors for Premenopausal African-American Women (25–45) with Coronary Heart Disease" (Giger & Strickland, 1995).

In 1998, Linda Smith, a doctoral student at the University of Alabama at Birmingham, completed a pilot study guided by Giger and Davidhizar's Transcultural Assessment Model as the overarching theoretical framework. The primary purpose of this descriptive correlational study was to describe the relationship among scores and subscores on scales measuring concepts of cultural competence. A secondary purpose of this study was to develop reliability and validity data on each of three cultural scales for a population ($n = 51$) of hospital-based registered nurses. These three scales were (1) the Cultural Attitude Scale (CAS), originally developed by Bonaparte (1977, 1979) and modified by Rooda (1990, 1992); (2) the Cultural Self-Efficacy Scale (CSES), developed by Bernal and Froman (1987); and (3) knowledge base questions (Rooda, 1990). Each of the scales had previously reported reliability and validity data but was administered to populations potentially different from hospital-employed registered nurses. Giger and Davidhizar's Transcultural Assessment Model served as the theoretical foundation, and the CSES, the CAS, and the knowledge base questions were the chosen instruments. Analysis of the data indicates that, for this study population, the reliability analysis scale (alpha) was 0.9778 for the 58-item CSES, 0.6412 for the 40-item CAS, and 0.6038 for the 22 knowledge base questions. Canonical correlation analysis was performed between a set of attitude variables and a set of self-efficacy variables. Both sets of variables demonstrated statistically significant relationships (at an *a priori* alpha of 0.05) to each other (with an approximate eta-squared value for practical significance of 0.365), providing sufficient evidence to reject the nonrelationship null hypothesis. For this sample and for these data, cultural self-efficacy toward Asian, African-American, and Hispanic clients and self-efficacy regarding nursing skills when caring for diverse clients related to cultural attitudes and cultural self-efficacy. Nursing care, cultural health beliefs, and cultural health attitudes are related to attitudes toward care of diverse clients.

Both sets of variables relate to each other as qualities of culturally competent nursing care (Smith, 1998b).

In 1998, Sharon S. Mullen and Carla G. Phillips at Ohio University School of Nursing also utilized Giger and Davidhizar's Transcultural Assessment Model as the overarching theoretical framework to explore the cultural beliefs of Appalachians from southeastern Ohio (Mullen & Phillips, 1998). The primary purpose of the qualitative ethnographic study was to identify cultural beliefs as a means of providing culturally competent nursing care. Giger and Davidhizar's Transcultural Assessment Model was used to identify cultural beliefs from six phenomena of interest: (1) communication, (2) space, (3) social organization, (4) time, (5) environmental control, and (6) biological variations. The participants were 14 adults who were native to southeastern Ohio and who had resided in the area their entire lives. Giger and Davidhizar's Transcultural Assessment Model, which also included interview questions and observational guidelines, was used for structured interviews. Findings from this study suggest that these individuals were more socially inclined, communicated more openly, had more of an internal locus of control, had fewer personal space needs, were more future oriented, used no significant home remedies, were more conscientious about getting to appointments on time, and were more likely to follow medical protocols than Appalachians in general. However, findings also suggest that these individuals still resembled the mainstream Appalachian population in that they tended to have a strong character, tended to be stoic and nonassertive, and also tended to have a strong belief in a Supreme Being.

ORGANIZATION OF THE TEXT

In this book, the six cultural phenomena (communication, space, social organization, time, environmental control, and biological variations) are presented in individual chapters with areas that must be assessed when working with clients from multicultural populations. In addition, these six phenomena are applied to the care and management of clients in 16 subcultural groups found in the United States and throughout the world. The Web site used in the fourth edition has been further refined to assist in the clinical application of Giger and Davidhizar's Transcultural Assessment Model, which has been applied to six additional ethnic and cultural groups. At the end of each chapter, test questions based on the NCLEX-RN review format are found. In addition, *http://evolve.elsevier.com/Giger/* provides a user-friendly cultural competency test based on the NCLEX-RN test format with supporting key for faculty use. This tool is based on Giger and Davidhizar's Transcultural Assessment Model. The newly created test was developed by Kenneth Farr, Doris Bartlett, Joyce Newman Giger, and Ruth Davidhizar. Concept analyses of individual items were done by the developers, and the concepts were found to be valid. Ambiguous or difficult concepts were discarded or reworded after concept analyses. To date, 108 nursing faculty have taken the test as a pre- and post-test to establish reliability. Reliability of this instrument ranged from .82 to .91 on the pre-test and .91 to .94 on the post-test. In the future, reliability and validity of the test will be further assessed. It is important to remember that a comprehensive nursing assessment is necessary for both the nurse practitioner and the researcher to provide culturally appropriate nursing care.

References

Aamodt, A. M. (1978). The care component in a health and healing system. In Bauwens, E. (Ed.), *The anthropology of health*. St. Louis: Mosby.

Affonso, D. (1979). Framework for cultural assessment. In Clark, A. L. (Ed.), *Childbearing: a nursing perspective* (ed. 2) (pp. 107–119). Philadelphia: F.A. Davis.

Andrews, M., & Boyle, J. (2003). *Transcultural concepts in nursing care* (ed. 4). Philadelphia: Lippincott, Williams & Wilkins.

Bernal, H., & Froman, R. (1987). The confidence of community health nurses in caring for ethnically diverse populations. *Image: Journal of Nursing Scholarship*, 19(4), 201–203.

Bloch, B. (1983). Bloch's assessment guide for ethnic/cultural variations. In Orque, M. S., Bloch, B., & Monrroy, L. S. A. (Eds.), *Ethnic nursing care: a multicultural approach* (pp. 49–75). St. Louis: Mosby.

Bonaparte, B. H. G. (1977). *An investigation of the relation between ego defensiveness and open-closed mindedness of female registered professional nurses and their attitude toward culturally different patients.* Unpublished doctoral dissertation. New York: New York University.

Bonaparte, B. H. G. (1979). Ego defensiveness, open-closed mindedness, and nurses' attitude toward culturally different patients. *Nursing Research,* 28(3), 166–172.

Bowen, M., & Davidhizar, R. (1991). Communication with the client in the OR. *Today's OR Nurse,* 1, 11–14.

Braithwaite, R., & Taylor, S. (2001). *Health issues in the Black community* (ed. 2). San Francisco: Jossey Bass.

Branch, M. F., & Paxton, P. P. (Eds.) (1976). *Providing safe nursing care for ethnic people of color.* Englewood Cliffs, N.J.: Prentice-Hall.

Brink, P. J. (2001a). *Transcultural nursing: a book of readings.* Prospect Heights, Ill.: Waveland Press.

Brink, P. J. (2001b). Cultural diversity in nursing: how much can we tolerate? In McCloskey, J. & Grace, H. (Eds.), *Current issues in nursing* (ed. 6). St. Louis: Mosby.

Brownlee, A. T. (1978). *Community, culture, and care: a cross-cultural guide for health workers.* St. Louis: Mosby.

Burk, M., Wieser, P., & Keegan, L. (1995, June). Cultural beliefs and health behaviors of pregnant Mexican-American women: implications for primary care, *Advances in Nursing Science,* 17(4), 37–52.

Cohall, A., & Bannister, H. (2001). The health status of children and adolescents. In Braithwaite, R., & Taylor, S. (Eds)., *Health issues in the Black community.* San Francisco: Jossey-Bass Publishers, 13–43.

Daugherty, B. (1992). *Utilizing Giger and Davidhizar's transcultural assessment model for the cultural assessment of farm families.* Unpublished master's thesis Lawrence, Kans.: University of Kansas.

Davidhizar, R., Dowd, S., & Giger, J. (1997a, January–February). Managing a multicultural radiology staff. *Radiology Management,* 19(1), 50–55.

Davidhizar, R., Dowd, S., & Giger, J. (1997b, January–February). Model for cultural diversity in the radiology department. *Radiologic Technology,* 68(3), 233–238.

Davidhizar, R., Dowd, S., & Giger, J. (1997c, March–April). Cultural differences in pain management. *Radiologic Technology,* 68(4), 345–348.

Davidhizar, R., & Giger, J. (1996, Summer). Reflections on the minority elderly in health care. *Hospital Topics,* 74(3), 20–24.

Davidhizar, R., & Giger, J. (1998a). Caring for the patient from another culture. *Journal of the Canadian Dental Association,* 39(1), 24–27.

Davidhizar, R., & Giger, J. (1998b, November–December). Transcultural patient assessment: a method of advancing dental care. *The Dental Assistant* 39(1), 40–43.

Dowd, S., Giger, J., & Davidhizar, R. (1998, July–August). Use of the Giger and Davidhizar Model by other health professions: contributions of nursing science. *International Nursing Review,* 45(4), 119–203.

Geissler, E. M. (1991). Transcultural nursing and nursing diagnosis. *Nursing and Health Care,* 12(4), 190–203.

Giger, J., & Davidhizar, R. (1990). Transcultural nursing assessment: a method for advancing practice. *International Nursing Review,* 37(1), 199–203.

Giger, J., & Davidhizar, R. (1994). Transcultural nursing: have we gone too far or not far enough? In Strickland, O., & Fishman, D. (Eds.), *Nursing issues in the 1990s* (pp. 491–504). New York: Delmar.

Giger, J., & Davidhizar, R. (1998). *Canadian transcultural nursing, assessment, and intervention.* St. Louis: Mosby.

Giger, J., Davidhizar, R., Evers, S., & Ingram, C. (1994). Cultural factors influencing mental health and mental illness. In Taylor, C. M. (Ed.), *Merness' essentials of psychiatric nursing* (ed. 14) (pp. 217–236). St. Louis: Mosby.

Giger, J., Davidhizar, R., Johnson, J., & Poole, V. (1996). Health promotion in minority populations. In Schust, C. S. (Ed.), *Community health: education and promotion manual.* Gaithersburg, Md.: Aspen.

Giger, J., Davidhizar, R., Johnson, J., & Poole, V. (1997, January). The changing faces of America: using cultural phenomena to improve care. *The Health Care Traveler,* 4(4), 10–40.

Giger, J., Davidhizar, R., & Wieczorek, S. (1993). Culture and ethnicity. In Bobak, I., & Jensen, M. (Eds.), *Maternity and gynecological care* (ed. 5) (pp. 43–67). St. Louis: Mosby.

Giger, J., & Strickland, O. (1995). *Behavioral risk reduction strategies for chronic indicators and high risk factors for premenopausal African-American women (25–45) with coronary heart disease.* Grant Number N95–019. Bethesda, Md.: Department of Defense, Uniformed Health Services, University of the Health Sciences, Tri-Service Nursing Research.

Kay, M. (1978). Clinical anthropology. In Bauwens, E. E. (Ed.), *The anthropology of health* (pp. 3–11). St. Louis: Mosby.

Kozier, B., Erb, G., Blaise, K., Johnson, J., & Smith-Temple, J. (1993). *Techniques in clinical nursing* (ed. 2). Reading, Mass.: Addison-Wesley.

Kozier, B., Erb, G., Blaise, K., & Wilkinson, J. (2004). *Fundamentals of nursing* (ed. 7). Upper Saddle River, N. J.: Prentice Hall Health.

Leininger, M. (1977). Transcultural nursing and a proposed conceptual framework. In Leininger, M. (Ed.), *Transcultural nursing care of infants and children: proceedings from the first transcultural conference.* Salt Lake City: University of Utah.

Leininger, M. (1985a). *Qualitative research methods in nursing.* Orlando, Fla.: Grune & Stratton.

Leininger, M. (1985b). Transcultural care, diversity and universality: a theory of nursing. *Nursing and Health Care,* 6(4), 209–212.

Leininger, M. (1991). Transcultural nursing: the study and practice field. *Imprint,* 38(2), 55–66.

Leininger, M., & McFarland, M. (2002). *Transcultural nursing: concepts, theory, research, and practice* (ed. 3). New York: McGraw-Hill Professional.

Mosby's medical, nursing, and allied health dictionary (2002) (ed. 6.) St Louis: Mosby.

Mullen, S., & Phillips, C. (1998). *Cultural beliefs of southeastern Ohio Appalachians. Proceedings of the Fourth International and Interdisciplinary Health Research Symposium 1998 Health Care and Culture.* Morgantown, Va.: School of Nursing, West Virginia University.

Murdock, G. P, et al. (1971). *Outline of cultural materials.* (ed. 4). New Haven, Conn.: Human Relations Area Files.

Orque, M.S. (1983). Orque's ethnic/cultural system: a framework for ethnic nursing care. In Orque, M. S., Bloch, B., & Monrroy, L. S. A. (Eds.), *Ethnic nursing care: a multi-cultural approach* (pp. 5–48). St. Louis: Mosby.

Purnell, L.D., & Paulanka, B.J. (Eds.), (2003). Transcultural health care (ed. 2). Philadelphia: F.A. Davis.

Rooda, L. (1990). *Knowledge and attitudes of nurses toward culturally diverse patients.* Unpublished doctoral dissertation. West Lafayette, Ind.: Purdue University.

Rooda, L. (1992). Attitudes of nurses toward culturally diverse patients: an examination of the social contact theory. *Journal of the National Black Nurses Association,* 6(1), 48–56.

Rund, N., & Krause, L. (1978). Health attitudes and your health programs. In Bauwens, E. E. (Ed.), *The anthropology of health* (pp. 73–78). St. Louis: Mosby.

Sheridan, D., & Zimbler, E. (1993). *Nursing management skills: a modular self-assessment series, module IV, transcultural nursing.* New York: National League for Nursing.

Smith, L. (1998a). Trends in multiculturalism in health care. *Hospital Material Management Quarterly,* 20(1), 61–69.

Smith, L. (1998b). Concept analysis: culture competence. *Journal of Cultural Diversity,* 5(1), 4–10.

Spector, R. (2001). Culture, ethnicity, and nursing. In Potter, P., & Perry, A. (Eds.), *Fundamentals of nursing: concepts, process, and practice* (ed. 5). St. Louis: Mosby.

Spector, R. (2004). *Cultural diversity in health and illness.* (ed. 6). Upper Saddle River, N.J.: Pearson Prentice Hall.

Stokes, G. (1991). A transcultural nurse is about. *Senior Nurse,* 11(1), 40–42.

Time almanac with information please. (2006). Boston: Information Please.

Tripp-Reimer, T. (1984a). Research in cultural diversity. *Western Journal of Nursing Research,* 6(3), 353–355.

Tripp-Reimer, T. (1984b). Cultural assessment. In Bellack, J. P., & Bamford, P. A. (Eds.), *Nursing assessment: a multidimensional approach* (pp. 226–246). Monterey, Calif.: Wadsworth.

Tripp-Reimer, T., Brink, P., & Saunders, J. (1984). Cultural assessment: content and process. *Nursing Outlook,* 32 (2), 78–82.

Tripp-Reimer, T., & Dougherty, M. C. (1985). Cross-cultural nursing research. *Annual Review of Nursing Research,* 3, 77–104.

Tripp-Reimer, T., & Friedl, M. (1977). Appalachians: a neglected minority. *Nursing Clinics of North America,* 12(1), 41–54.

U.S. Department of Commerce, Bureau of Census. (2002a). *Population profiles by age, sex, race, and Hispanic origin, Summary File 3.* Washington, D.C.: U.S. Government Printing Office.

U.S. Department of Commerce, Bureau of Census. (2002b). *Population projection of the United States by age, sex, race, and Hispanic origin: 2000 to 2050.* Washington, D.C.: U.S. Government Printing Office Internet update.

Walthour, E. (1993). *Health beliefs and self-care practices of hypertensive African-Americans.* Unpublished master's thesis Statesboro, Ga.: Georgia Southern University.

Wenger, F. (1989). President's address. *Transcultural Nursing Society Newsletter,* 9(1), 3.

CHAPTER 2 Communication

Behavioral Objectives

After reading this chapter, the nurse will be able to:

1. Describe the importance of communication as it relates to transcultural nursing assessment.
2. Delineate barriers to communication that hinder the development of a nurse–client relationship in transcultural settings.
3. Understand the importance of dialect, style, volume, use of touch, context of speech, and kinesics and their relationship to transcultural nursing assessment and care.
4. Describe appropriate nursing intervention techniques to develop positive communication in the nurse–client relationship.
5. Understand the significance of nonverbal communication and the use of silence and their relationship to transcultural nursing assessment and care.
6. Explain the significance of the structure and format of names in various cultural groups.
7. Explain the significance of variations in word meanings across and within various cultural and ethnic groups.

The word *communication* comes from the Latin verb *communicāre*, "to make common, share, participate, or impart" (Guralnik, 1989). Communication, however, goes further than this definition implies and embraces the entire realm of human interaction and behavior. All behavior, whether verbal or nonverbal, in the presence of another individual is communication (Potter & Perry, 2005; Watzlawich, Beavin, & Jackson, 1967).

As the matrix of all thought and relationships among people, communication provides the means by which people connect. It establishes a sense of commonality with others and permits the sharing of information, signals, or messages in the form of ideas and feelings. Communication is a continuous process by which one person may affect another through written or oral language, gestures, facial expressions, body language, space, or other symbols.

Nurses have long recognized the importance of communication to health. Effective communication of health care information motivates individuals to work with their health care providers to manage their health. Giorgianni (2000) notes that individuals who have had effective health care communication are better informed and more confident in pursuing health care. Communication received increased visibility nationally with the inclusion of an entire chapter on health communication in *Healthy People 2010* (U.S. Department of Health and Human Services, 2000). Among the six national objectives were increased access to the Internet from home, increased satisfaction by individuals in the communication skills of their health care providers, and increased research on health communication. Effective communication of health care information is critical if individuals are to take action on behalf of their own health, the strategic goal of *Healthy People 2010.*

Communication is the core of most nursing curricula. However, if effective communication is to occur in today's multicultural setting, nursing curricula not only need to provide skills in communication but also must teach diversity as a value (Cook & Cullen, 2000). To accomplish this, nursing curricula are increasingly reflecting integration of culture as a central concept (Davidhizar & Eshleman, 2006; Davidhizar & Giger, 2001; Wood, 2001). Furthermore, to promote effective communication, health care settings are modifying the climate of units and organizations to accommodate multiculturalism (Buerhaus & Auerbach, 1999; Byrne, 2002; Davidhizar, Dowd, & Giger, 1998; Davidhizar, Shearer, & Giger, 2002; Davidhizar & Shearer, 2005).

Nevertheless, communication frequently presents barriers between nurses and clients, especially when the nurses and the clients are from different cultural backgrounds. If the nurse and the client do not speak the same language or if communication styles and patterns differ, both the nurse and the client can feel alienated and helpless. When communication is impaired, the physical healing process may be impaired. Nurses may also feel angry and helpless if their communication is not understood or if they cannot understand the client. With ineffective communication, certain physiological problems such as pain may not be controlled (Davidhizar & Hart, 2005). Nurses need to have not only a working knowledge of communication with clients of the same culture but also a thorough awareness of racial, cultural, and social factors that may affect communication with persons from other cultures. Communication with family members is also crucial to client and family satisfaction. When Shields and King (2001) interviewed family members in four countries, all the respondents identified the importance of communication with family members in the provision of care.

Nurses must have an awareness of how an individual, though speaking the same language as the nurse, may differ in communication patterns and understandings as a result of cultural orientation. Nurses must also have communication skills in relating to individuals who do not speak a familiar language (Davidhizar & Brownson, 2000; Ericksen, 2002; Sieh & Brentin, 1997). Nurses generally assume that their perceptions and assessment of the client's health status are accurate and congruent with those of the client. However, there is evidence that discrepancies in perceptions persist and may interfere with the provision of care to special populations with higher than average risk of developing health problems (Crump, Bartman, Walker, & Mitchell, 2000). Many factors obstruct high-quality client care, including cost, fear, poor communication, noncompliance with the treatment regimen, inadequate or unnecessary treatment, and ethical problems. All these factors combine to create discrepancies in perceptions between nurse and client (Andrews & Boyle, 2003; Crump, Bartman, Walker, & Mitchell, 2000; Giger, Davidhizar, Johnson, & Poole, 1997; Lester, 1998).

COMMUNICATION AND CULTURE

Communication and culture are closely intertwined. Communication is the means by which culture is transmitted and preserved (Delgado, 1983). Culture influences how feelings are expressed and what verbal and nonverbal expressions are appropriate. Americans may be more likely to conceal feelings, and the United States is generally considered a low-touch culture, whereas a member of an Eastern culture may be open and loud with expressions of grief, anger, or joy and may use touch more (Davidhizar & Giger, 2002; Hall, 1966; Thayer, 1988). Other cultural variables, such as the perception of time, bodily contact, and territorial rights, also influence communication. The cultural differences in contact can be quite dramatic. In a classic study, Sidney Jourard (1972) reported that when touch between pairs of people in coffee shops around the world was studied, there was more touch in certain cities. For example, it was reported that touch occurred as frequently as 180 times an hour between couples in San Juan, Puerto Rico, and 110 times an hour in Paris, France. In other cities there was less touch; specifically, touch occurred twice an hour between couples in Gainesville, Florida, and zero times an hour in London, England.

Cultural patterns of communication are embedded early, typically by age 5, and are found in childrearing practices (Anderson, 2003; Capirci, Iverson, Pizzuto, & Volterra, 1996). Gibson (1984) studied the playgrounds and beaches of Greece, the Soviet Union, and the United States and compared the frequency and nature of touch between caregivers and children ranging from 2 to 5 years of age. The analysis of data indicates that although rates of touching for retrieving or punishing the children were similar, rates of touching for soothing, holding, and playing were dissimilar. American children were less likely to be touched than children from other cultures. The communication practices of persons in different cultural groups affect the expression of ideas and feelings, decision making, and communication strategies. The communication of an individual reflects, determines, and consequently molds the culture (Hedlund, 1993; Krech, Crutchfield, & Ballachey, 1962). In other words, a culture may be limited and molded by its communication practices. Sapir (1929) proposed that individuals are at the mercy of the particular language that has become the medium of expression of their society. Experiences are determined by language habits that predispose the individual to certain conceptions of the world and choices of interpretation. Kayser (1996) noted that educational programming that is provided to children of different cultural and linguistic backgrounds is critical for the successful implementation of language interventions. Focusing on English-language development while minimizing learning opportunities limits children who do not speak English as their first language from development of higher-level cognitive skills.

Variations in communication may be limited to specific meanings for a few individuals in a small group, for example, a family. On the other hand, unique communication patterns are frequently found among persons from the same ethnic and cultural group, such as the Gypsies or the Amish (Banks & Banks, 1995; Beachy, Hershberger, Davidhizar, & Giger, 1997). Some persons consider the deaf a cultural group. In any case, persons who are deaf have a unique language and communication patterns that require nurses to use special communication approaches (McLeod & Bently, 1996). However, the nurse must be cautious about assuming that a certain communication pattern can be generalized to all persons in a designated cultural group because communication patterns are often unique. In assessing the client, the nurse should keep in mind common cultural patterns and approach the client as an individual who should not be categorized because of cultural heritage.

LINGUISTICS

Because communication is a broad concept and encompasses all human behavior, it has been conceptualized in many ways. One way is to consider the structure of communication, as in linguistics. The major focus on the structure of communication has been developed within the fields of ethnomethodology in sociology and of linguistics in anthropology. Structure may be perceived as a form of language and the use of words and behaviors to construct messages. The role of ethnomethodologists is to consider the structure and effects of communication and to look at rules of communication and the consequences of breaking these rules. Ethnomethodologists not only have emphasized the study of the structure and rules of language but also have studied the structure and rules of nonverbal communication (Sudnow, 1967). Linguistics is the area within anthropology concerned with the study of the structure of language. Linguistic patterns represent more than the use of grammatically nonequivalent words; these patterns can create real disparity in social treatment.

FUNCTIONS OF COMMUNICATION

Another way to think about communication is to consider what it achieves or accomplishes in human interaction. Consideration of the functions of communication refers to examining what the communication accomplishes rather than how the communication is structured. A relationship exists between communication structure and communication function in the sense that structure does affect function.

As a part of human interaction, communication discloses information or provides a specific message. Messages can be sent with no expectation of a response. Included in the disclosure of information may be an element of self-disclosure. Communication may or may not be intended as a method of self-disclosure or a means to provide information about the self or the individual's perception of self (Hedlund, 1993; Luft & Ingham, 1984). Perceptions of self include acts that describe the self and estimations of self-worth. In some situations self-awareness may be achieved through communication. This function of communication involves interaction with people (Davidhizar & Dowd, 2005). Through communication with others, an individual may become more aware of personal feelings. Communication can also serve the important interpersonal functions of conveying respect and giving or taking away power (Beutter & Davidhizar, 1999; Davidhizar & Dowd, 2004; Miller & Davidhizar, 2001).

PROCESS OF COMMUNICATION

Communication may be conceptualized as a process that includes a sender, a transmitting device, signals, a receiver, and feedback (Varcarolis, 2006). A sender attempts to relay a message, an idea, or information to another person or group through the use of signals or symbols. Many factors influence how the message is given and how it is received. For example, physical health, emotional well-being, the situation being discussed and the meaning it has, other distractions, knowledge of the matter being discussed, skill at communicating, and attitudes toward the other person and the subject being discussed may all affect the communication that takes place (Box 2-1). In addition, personal needs and interests; background, including cultural, social, and philosophical values; the senses and their functional ability; a personal tendency to make judgments and be judgmental of others; the environment in which the communication takes place; and experiences that relate or are related to the present situation may all affect the message that is received. The receiver then interprets the message. Feedback is given to the sender about the message, and more communication may occur. If no feedback is given, there may be no reciprocal interaction. Cultures such as the mainstream U.S. culture may be low-context whereas the Asian cultures are high context, that is, very little of the message is the coded, explicit, transmitted part of the message. Members of individualistic cultures have a tendency to communicate in a more direct

---

> **Box 2-1**
>
> ## FACTORS INFLUENCING COMMUNICATION
>
> 1. Physical health and emotional well-being
> 2. The situation being discussed and its meaning
> 3. Distractions to the communication process
> 4. Knowledge of the matter being discussed
> 5. Skill at communicating
> 6. Attitudes toward the other person and toward the subject being discussed
> 7. Personal needs and interests
> 8. Background, including cultural, social, and philosophical values
> 9. The senses involved and their functional ability
> 10. Personal tendency to make judgments and be judgmental of others
> 11. The environment in which the communication occurs
> 12. Experiences that relate to the current situation

---

manner that has relatively low dependence on context, while members of collectivistic cultures use high-context message in a more indirect fashion (Xu & Davidhizar, 2005).

Although the process of communication is universal, nurses should be aware that styles and types of feedback may be unique to certain cultural groups. For example, before the assimilation of the Alaskan Eskimo into the American culture, the Alaskan Eskimo would indicate that a message was received by blinking rather than by making a verbal response (Davidhizar & Giger, 2000). Nonverbal responses are also found in the Vietnamese. Vietnamese persons may smile, but the smile may not indicate understanding. A Vietnamese person may say yes simply to avoid confrontation or out of a desire to please. A smile may cover up disturbed feelings. Nodding, which nurses commonly interpret as understanding and compliance, may, for a Vietnamese individual, simply indicate respect for the person talking (Hoang & Erickson, 1982; Lindsay, Narayan, & Rea, 1998). The nurse may be surprised later when the Vietnamese client who smiled and nodded does not follow through with the instructions given.

In today's health care system, optimal communication includes use of technology. E-mail, cell phones, voice mail, and PDAs have greatly improved timeliness in communication (Davidhizar & Dowd, 2006). E-mail messages can be printed to provide hard copy for documentation purposes. Notebook computers with cell phone modem connections to access clinical information can be used in a client's home in a rural setting to give clients more efficient service. Past health records can be accessed via the computer to be viewed by health professionals. Nurses can use the Internet and search Web sites to keep up to date on health care information and to print health education material for clients. Clients can be assisted to find age—and language—appropriate TV programs as well as Web sites for health information (Jones, 2000). Health promotion strategies can include CD-ROMs, health consumer e-journals, toll-free telephone numbers, and DVDs.

Linguistic Isolation in the United States

In the United States, some 43 million adults are linguistically isolated, do not speak English well, or speak a language other than English at home (U.S. Department of Commerce, Bureau of Census, Summary File 3, 2002). Table 2-1 shows some of the languages spoken in the United States.

VERBAL AND NONVERBAL COMMUNICATION

Another way to conceptualize communication is in terms of verbal and nonverbal behavior (Box 2-2). Communication first of all involves language or verbal communication, including vocabulary or a repertoire of words and grammatical structure (Barkauskas, 1994).

Although foreign-born persons need to demonstrate English proficiency to obtain U.S. citizenship, the nurse may encounter many persons in the United States who are not fluent in English. In 2000, 31.1 million (10.4%) of the U.S. population were foreign-born, representing 11.1% of the total U.S. population. It is interesting to note that between 1990 and 2000, the foreign-born population increased by 11.3 million people. This figure represents a 57.4% increase. Among the foreign

Table 2-1	Languages Other than English Spoken by Persons Residing in the United States
Language Spoken at Home for Persons Over 18 Years of Age	**Number**
Spanish or Spanish Creole	21,270,952
Chinese	1,705,037
French (including patois, Cajun)	1,411,142
German	1,218,418
Tagalog	1,096,451
Vietnamese	804,562
Korean	737,983
Japanese	422,442
African languages	350,232
Navajo	135,458
Mon-Khmer, Cambodian	123,950
Laotian	111,001
Miao, Hmong	85,410

Adapted from the U.S. Department of Commerce, Bureau of Census, Summary File 3, 2002.

Box 2-2

VERBAL AND NONVERBAL COMMUNICATION

LANGUAGE OR VERBAL COMMUNICATION

Vocabulary	Rhythm
Grammatical structure	Speed
Voice qualities	Pronunciation
Intonation	Silence

NONVERBAL COMMUNICATION
Touch
Facial expression
Eye movement
Body posture

COMMUNICATIONS THAT COMBINE VERBAL AND NONVERBAL ELEMENTS
Warmth
Humor

---

born in 2000, 51.0% were born in Latin America, 25.5% were born in Asia, 15.3% were born in Europe, and approximately 8.1% were born in other regions of the world. In fact, among the foreign-born, the top three countries representing the greatest number of the foreign-born were Mexico, China, and the Philippines. Of the total number of foreign-born, 40.3% are U.S. citizens and 17.9% live in poverty (*Time Almanac with Information Please*, 2006; U.S. Department of Commerce, Bureau of Census, 2000).

Among the foreign-born, four of every five speak a language other than English at home. This translates roughly to 83% of the foreign-born older than 5 years of age who speak a language other than English at home. This figure includes 52.3% who speak Spanish, 21.9% who speak other Indo-European languages, and 21.6% who speak Asian or Pacific Island languages. In 2000, of the number of foreign-born who spoke a language other than English at home, only 38.5% spoke English "very well," while 12.2% of the foreign-born did not speak English at all. Among the foreign-born who speak Spanish at home, only 52% speak English very well (*Time Almanac with Information Please*, 2006; U.S. Department of Commerce, Bureau of Census, 2000).

According to the 2000 census, 184,859,425 persons older than 5 years of age spoke English at home; 26,424,495 spoke Spanish, 1,702,000 French, 1,547,000 Italian, 1,249,000 Chinese, 843,000 Tagalog, and 723,000 Polish. Vietnamese was spoken by 507,000, Portuguese by 430,000, Japanese by 428,000, Greek by 388,000, Arabic by 355,000, and Hindi by 331,000. Russian, Yiddish, Thai, Persian, French Creole, Armenian, Navajo, Hungarian, Hebrew, Dutch, Khmer (Cambodian), and Gujarati were all spoken by at least 100,000 people. In addition to these persons registered as living in households, many other non–English-speaking persons are in the United States as visitors, on temporary visas, or illegally. Approximately one sixth (31,845,000) of the population reported that they spoke another language besides English in the home, yet only a small minority of caregivers speak a language other than English (U.S. Department of Commerce, Bureau of Census, Summary File 3, 2002).

It is important to appreciate that along with language, significant communication cues are received from voice quality, intonation, rhythm, and speed, as well as from the pronunciation used. Dialect may differ significantly among persons both across and within cultures. Silence during communication may itself be a significant part of the message.

Communication involves nonverbal messages, which include touch, facial expressions, eye behavior, body posture, and the use of space (Giger & Davidhizar, 1990a). Spatial behavior also affects communication and encompasses a variety of behaviors, including movement and proximity to others and to objects in the environment (see Chapter 3). Although nonverbal communication is powerful and honest, its importance and meaning vary among and within cultures; therefore, it is essential that the nurse has an awareness and appreciation of the role that body language may have in the communication process. In addition, some communications combine nonverbal and verbal components in the message that is sent. Two examples of combination messages are warmth and humor.

Language, or Verbal Communication

Language is basic to communication. Without language, the higher-order cognitive processes of thinking, reasoning, and generalizing cannot be attained. Words are tools or symbols used to express ideas and feelings or to identify or describe objects. Words shape experiences and influence cultural perceptions. Words convey interpretations and influence relationships (Pirandello 1970; Talbot, 1996; Varcarolis, 2006). Although words provide a special way of looking at the world, the same words often have different meanings for different individuals within cultural groups. In addition, word meanings change over time and in different situations. It is important to ascertain that the message is received and understood as the sender intended. As early as 1954, Sullivan emphasized the importance of ongoing validation in a therapeutic relationship to verify interpretations made on the behavior and words of another. Even today, this validation remains relevant in a nurse–client relationship in which many experiential, educational, and cultural differences are present. Smith and Cantrell (1988) reported a study comparing the effect of personal questions and physical distance on anxiety rates. Pulse rates were higher when the investigator asked personal questions, regardless of the physical distance from subjects. Although the data from this study indicate that the most important part of a message may be verbal, the opposite has also been found to be true. Thus, both verbal and nonverbal communication must be considered before a conclusion about the true meaning of a message can be determined.

To provide culturally appropriate nursing care, nurses must separate values based on their own cultural background from the values of the clients to whom care is given. Transcultural communication and understanding break down when caregivers project their own culturally specific values and behaviors onto the client. Thiederman (1986) has suggested that projection of values as well as hindering care may actually contribute to noncompliance.

Vocabulary. Even though people may speak the same language, establishing communication is often difficult because word meanings for both the sender and the receiver vary according to past experiences and learning. Words have both denotative and connotative meanings. A denotative meaning is one that is in general use by most persons who share a common language. A connotative meaning usually arises from a person's personal experience. For example, although all Americans are likely to share the same general denotative meaning for the word *pig,* depending on the occupation and cultural perception of the person, the connotation may be entirely different and precipitate completely different reactions. The word *pig* will invoke either negative or positive reactions from certain people on the basis of occupation and culture. For example, an Orthodox Jew's reactions will differ from those of a pig farmer. For an Orthodox Jew, the word *pig* is synonymous with the word *unclean* or *unholy* and thus should be avoided. On the other hand, for a pig farmer the word *pig* implies a clean, wholesome means of making a living. Numerous conflicts resulting from differences in word meaning among various ethnic and racial groups are reported in the literature. Among her many famous cultural studies, Margaret Mead (1947) reported on

the different meanings that the word *compromise* carries for an Englishman and an American:

In Britain, the word *compromise* is a good word, and one may speak approvingly of any arrangement which has been a compromise, including, very often one in which the other side has gained more than fifty percent of the points at issue. Where, in Britain, to compromise means to work out a good solution, in America it usually means to work out a bad one, a solution in which all the points of importance are lost.

Often people who have learned a language have learned the meaning for the word in only one context. For example, Díaz-Duque (1982) reported that a Hispanic person who was told he was going "to be discharged tomorrow" somehow interpreted this to mean that he was going to develop "a discharge from below." Díaz-Duque also indicated that for Hispanics problems arise with cognates such as *constipation* because for Hispanics this term generally refers to nasal congestion rather than intestinal constipation. Lunsford (2006) recounts the story of Xial Ming Li, now a college teacher, who came to the United States from China where she had been a good writer. However, in college in the United States she struggled to understand what faculty expected of her writing. Although she used appropriate words and sentence grammar, she needed tutors to assist her to write in the "U.S.A. style" that was expected.

Although barriers exist when people speak the same language, more profound barriers are present when different languages are spoken. Each language has a whole set of unconscious assumptions about the world and life. Understanding differences in the meaning of words can provide insight into people of different cultures. For example, many English-speaking Americans are puzzled by what seems to be a different time orientation among Hispanic peoples. An understanding of the meaning of the word *time* helps provide insight into this different orientation. In Spanish, time is defined as "passing"—a clock "passes time" or "moves," whereas in English a clock "runs." If time is moving rapidly, as English usage declares, we must hurry. On the other hand, the Spanish definition allows for a more leisurely attitude (Randall-David, 1989). Such cultural understandings can provide insight into the reasons why Spanish individuals are often late for health care appointments.

Language reflects the dominant concerns and interests of a people, which can be noted in the number of words for certain things. Some classic studies have reported that certain cultures use many words to describe a particular object of importance. Boas (1938) pointed out that Eskimos have 20 or so words for snow depending on consistency and texture. The language of a people is a key that unlocks their culture. A nurse who is familiar with the language of clients will have the best chance of gaining insight into their culture.

Names. Names have a special psychological and cultural significance. All people have names, and in every culture naming a newborn is considered important. The considerations that go into the naming process vary greatly from culture to culture. For example, in Roman tradition there is a given name for boys; a family name, which is second; and a third name that specifies an extended family unit. The name Caius Julius Caesar illustrates the importance of tribal connections as well as male chauvinism (Clemmens, 1988). In Roman times girls had only one name, the female version of the family name; for example, Caesar's sister was Julia, as were his father's sister and other relatives. During the early Roman times, women lacked individuality and thus in Roman society were not worth being named.

The Hebrew tradition has a patrilineal way of looking at names, that is, a given name plus "son of." Mothers' names are not included. A spiritual and traditional continuity is evidenced in this system of naming. The Hebrew tradition can be seen today in Iceland, where all males have their given names, followed by their father's given name, ending in "son." In contemporary Western society as well, there are systems of naming. The most common one in the dominant culture in the United States is a patrilineal succession plus one or more given names. In the United States, the middle name is often one that relates to the family, such as the mother's maiden name.

The Russian system of naming provides a clue to the significance placed on relating son and father, as well as daughter and father. The mother is left out, with Russians habitually addressing each other by the individual's given name together with the patronymic. The family name is omitted. Spaniards and Latin Americans include women more than other cultures, with children carrying their father's name first and their mother's name second. The mother's name usually appears only on documents and for formal occasions because the addition of the mother's name makes the name quite long. Another variation is seen in the Dutch, who have the option of using both the husband's and the wife's family names jointly. Among the various cultures the most common theme of naming is pride in lineage (Clemmens, 1985, 1988).

Grammatical Structure. Cultural differences are reflected in grammatical structure and the use and meaning of phrases. "That's all right" is a phrase frequently used by African-Americans when they actually mean "I have some plans, but I am not telling you what they are" (Mitchell, 1978). In another example, for some Hispanic American women, having a stillborn baby or a miscarriage does not equate with a pregnancy—rather, pregnancy is equated only with a successful live birth (Haffner, 1992). It is important for nurses to keep in mind that there is little validity in generalizations about the meaning of phrases by persons in varying cultures.

Length of sentence and speech forms may vary not only with culture but also with social class. For example, Argyle (1992) noted that persons from the lower class commonly use short, simple sentences and are more direct than are persons with more education. Word choice, grammatical structure, speech fluency, and articulation provide cues to social status and class. Jargon is also a speech variation that may prove to be a barrier to communication. Nurses frequently have difficulty expressing things in simple, jargon-free language (without medical terms) that clients can understand. On the other hand, a nurse who does not know the jargon used by the clients served may have a difficult time relating to them.

For some cultures, patterns of social amenities can create communication problems. Small talk, social chitchat, and discussion of mundane topics that may appear to "kill time" are sometimes necessary as preliminaries for more purposeful discussion. Yet the busy nurse seeking short, succinct answers to questions may be annoyed by the amount of anecdotal information that a Hispanic American client gives. Many clients tend to add irrelevant material because it lessens embarrassment. They may be more comfortable if attention is not focused on their medical problems, and so they may intersperse actual symptoms with other biographical data. Cultural factors may also play a role in what seems to be verbal rambling. Patients who are used to folk healers believe that information on the weather, the environment, and eating habits are really important pieces of information for the health professional.

Voice Qualities. Paralinguistics, or paralanguage, refers to something beyond the words themselves. Voice quality, which includes pitch and range, can add an important element to communication. The commonly used phrase "Don't speak to me in that tone of voice" indicates the significance of this aspect of the communication message.

The softer volume of Asian American or American Indian speech may be interpreted by the nurse as shyness. On the other hand, the nurse's behavior may be viewed as loud and boisterous if the volume is loud and if there is a deliberate attempt to accent particular words. Sometimes people who speak softly, slowly, and without emphasis on particular words are viewed as wishy-washy. When the nurse cannot hear what the client is saying, there is a tendency for the nurse to speak louder. It is important to remember that amplifying the volume does not necessarily equate with being understood or understanding. Nurses must remember when they are assessing the client that paralinguistic behavior is an important cultural consideration. The nurse can recognize this behavior by listening to tone of voice, quality of voice, and nonword vocalizations, such as sobbing, laughing, and grunting.

Intonation. Intonation is an important aspect of the communication message. When people say they feel "fine," they may mean they genuinely do or they may mean they do not feel fine but do not wish to discuss it. If said sarcastically, it may also mean they feel just the opposite of fine. There is often a latent or hidden meaning in what a person is saying, and intonation frequently provides the clue that is needed to interpret the true message.

Techniques of intonation vary among cultures. For example, Americans put commands in the form of suggestions and often as questions, whereas Arabic speech contains much emphasis and exaggeration (Argyle, 1992). Some cultures value indirectness and subtlety in speech and may be alienated by the frankness of Western health care professionals. Asian clients, for example, may interpret this method of communication as rude, immature, and lacking finesse. On the other hand, health care professionals may label Asian clients as evasive, fearful, and unable to confront problems (Sue & Sue, 1999).

Rhythm. Rhythm also varies from culture to culture; some people have a melodic rhythm to their verbal communication, whereas others appear to lack rhythm. Rhythm may also vary among persons within a culture. For example, some African-American ministers use a singsong rhythm to deliver fiery sermons.

Speed. Rate and volume of speech frequently provide a clue to an individual's mood. A depressed person will tend to talk slowly and quietly, whereas an aggressive, dominating person is more apt to talk rapidly and loudly.

Pronunciation. Persons from some cultural groups may be identified by their dialect, such as Black dialect or Black English, Irish brogue, or a Brooklyn accent. Black English includes words and expressions not commonly found in Standard English and is sometimes spoken by African-Americans. It ranges on a continuum from being more to less Africanized, with the mild end of the continuum being much like Standard English (Taylor, 1976). However, even persons with dialects at the mild end of the continuum may have a "Black sound" that identifies them as African-American. A person may hear a boil called a "raisin" or difficult breathing called "the smothers" (Snow, 1976); dentures may be called "racks" (Dillard, 1973). Some African-Americans speak in dialect when they do not want others to understand what is being said. One function of the Black dialect may be to enhance the in-group solidarity of African-Americans (Taylor, 1976).

"Ahs," "ers," and grunts also provide important dimensions to communication. Although hesitations may indicate a person who is unsure and slow to make a commitment, for some cultures this can have the opposite meaning.

Silence. The meaning of silence varies among cultural groups. Silences may be thoughtful, or they may be blank and empty when the individual has nothing to say. A silence in a conversation may also indicate stubbornness and resistance, apprehension, or discomfort. Silence may be viewed by some cultural groups as extremely uncomfortable; therefore, attempts may be made to fill every gap with conversation. Persons in other cultural groups value silence and see it as essential to understanding a person's needs. Many American Indians have this latter view of silence, just as some traditional Chinese and Japanese persons have. Therefore, when one of these persons is speaking and suddenly stops, what may be implied is that the person wants the nurse to consider the content of what has been said before continuing. Other cultures may use silence in yet other ways. For example, English and Arabic persons use silence for privacy, whereas Russian, French, and Spanish persons may use silence to indicate agreement between parties. Some persons in Asian cultures may view silence as a sign of respect, particularly toward an elder. Mexicans may use silence when instructions are given by a person in authority rather than showing the disrespect of disagreement (Quarnero, 2005).

Nurses need to be aware of possible meanings of silence so that personal anxiety does not promote the silence to be interrupted prematurely or to be nontherapeutic. A nurse who understands the therapeutic value of silence can use this understanding to enhance care of clients from other cultures.

Nonverbal Communication

Hall (1969) suggested that 65% of the message received in communication is nonverbal. Through body language or motions (kinetic behavior), the person conveys what cannot or may not be said in words. For a message to be accurately interpreted, not only must words be translated but also the meaning held by nuances, intonation patterns, and facial expressions. Just as verbal behavior may undo nonverbal behavior, nonverbal behavior may repeat, clarify, contradict, modify, emphasize, or regulate the flow of communication. Nonverbal behavior is less significant as an isolated behavior, but it does add to the whole communication message. To understand the client, the nurse may wish to validate impressions with other health team members, since different people often interpret nonverbal behavior differently. It is important for the nurse to be aware not only of the client's nonverbal behavior but also of personal nonverbal behavior that may add to, undo, or contradict verbal communication (Reusch, 1961).

Touch. Touch, or tactile sensation, is a powerful form of communication that can be used to bridge distances between nurse and client (Bronstein, 1996; Davidhizar & Giger, 1988; Giger, Davidhizar, & Wieczorek, 1993). Touch has many meanings (Box 2-3). It can connect people, provide affirmation, be reassuring, decrease loneliness, share warmth, provide stimulation, and increase self-concept. Being touched can be highly valued and sought after. On the other hand, touch can also communicate frustration, anger, aggression, and punishment; invade personal space and privacy; and convey a negative (such as a subservient) type of relationship. In certain situations touch can be disconcerting because it signals power. In a study reported by Thayer (1988), higher-status individuals were found to enjoy more liberties concerning touch than their lower-status associates. It is generally considered improper for individuals to put their hands on superiors.

Touching or lack of touch has cultural significance and symbolism and is a learned behavior. Cultural uses of touch vary. Each culture trains its children to develop different kinds of thresholds to tactile contacts and stimulation so that their organic, constitutional, and temperamental characteristics are accentuated or reduced. Some cultures

---

Box 2-3

MEANINGS OF TOUCH

Touch may:

1. Connect one individual with another, both literally and figuratively, by indicating availability
2. Provide affirmation and approval
3. Be reassuring by providing empathy, interest, encouragement, nurturance, caring, trust, concern, gentleness, and protection
4. Decrease loneliness by indicating a relationship with another
5. Share warmth, rapport, love, intimacy, excitement, and happiness
6. Provide stimulation by being a mode of sensation, perception, and experience
7. Increase self-concept
8. Communicate frustration, anger, aggression, or punishment
9. Invade personal space and privacy by physical and psychological assault or intrusion
10. Convey a negative type of relationship with another
11. Cause sexual arousal
12. Allow a person to perform a functional or professional role, such as a physician, barber, or tailor, and be devoid of personal message
13. Reflect cordiality, such as a handshake by business associates and among strangers and acquaintances

---

are characterized by a "do not touch me" way of life. These persons may view fondling and kissing as embarrassing. Some cultures include every possible variation on the theme of tactility. In the United States, the dominant culture generally tolerates hugs and embraces among intimates and a pat on the shoulder as a gesture of camaraderie. The firm, hearty handshake is symbolic of good character and a sign of strength. In some American Indian groups, however, the hand is offered in some interpersonal interactions, but the expectation is different. Rather than a firm handshake, there is a light touch or grasp or even just a passing of hands. Some American Indians interpret vigorous handshaking as an aggressive action and are offended by a firm, lengthy handshake (Montagu, 1986).

Americans often give a lingering touch a sexual connotation. For some Americans, even casual

touching is considered taboo and may be a result of residual Victorian sexual prudence (DeThomaso, 1971). Other cultures also consider touching taboo; the English and Germans carry untouchability further than Americans do. On the other hand, highly tactile cultures do exist, such as the Spanish, Italians, French, Jews, and South Americans (Montagu, 1986). However, generalizations about diverse national or ethnic groups in the area of touch can be problematic. For example, Shuter (1976) reported on studies of touch in Costa Rica, Colombia, and Panama. Findings from this study indicate that Latin Americans are commonly oriented toward high contact. Thayer (1988) also compared couples in Costa Rica, Colombia, and Panama and found that partners in Costa Rica were touched and held more often than partners in the other two countries.

Most cultures give touch different rules and meanings depending on the sex of the persons involved. Whitcher and Fisher (1979) reported that women in a hospital study had a strikingly positive reaction to being touched, with subsequent lowered blood pressure and anxiety before surgery, whereas men found the same experience upsetting, with a subsequent increase in blood pressure and anxiety. Thayer (1988) reported on a study at the Kansas City International Airport that found women greeted women and men more physically, with lip kisses, embraces, and more kinds of touch and holding and for longer periods than did men. For men a more common greeting was to shake hands. Regardless of sex, some research has shown that people who are most uncomfortable with touch are also uncomfortable with communicating through other means and have lower self-esteem (Thayer, 1988). Other studies have shown that people who touch more are less afraid and suspicious of other people's motives and intentions and have less anxiety and tension in their everyday lives. In some cultures, leaning back, showing the palm of the hand, and fussing with the other person's collar may be perceived as possible courting behaviors because they may convey an invitation for closeness or affiliation. Touching behaviors such as reaching out during conversation to poke the other person in the chest may be viewed as domineering behavior. However, laughing while being poked may be a way to submit to and at the same time trivialize or eliminate the other person's aggressive intent (Scheflen & Scheflen, 1972).

In some cultures touch is considered magical and healing (Mackey, 1995). For example, some Mexican Americans and American Indians view touch as symbolic of "undoing" an evil spell, as a means for prevention of harm, or as a means for healing (Montagu, 1986). On the other hand, Vietnamese Americans may find touching shoulders with another to be anxiety producing, since they believe that the soul can leave the body on physical contact and that health problems may result (Rocereto, 1981). The Vietnamese regard the human head as the seat of life and therefore highly personal. Procedures that invade the surface or any orifice of the head can frighten the Vietnamese, who fear that these procedures could provide an escape for the essence of life (Stauffer, 2005).

Nurses must be alert to the rules of touch for individuals encountered in the work role. Lane (1989) found that nurses perceive male clients as being less receptive to touch and closeness than their female counterparts, which could be attributed to the fact that males generally have a larger personal space than females have. Thus it is believed that people generally maintain a greater distance from males (Insel & Lindgren, 1978; Sommer, 1959). Lane concluded that there may be a double standard concerning touch because of societal norms and expectations: male clients may be more receptive to touch than are female nurses, but female nurses are perhaps more comfortable with the closeness and touch of female clients.

Although the rules of touch may be unspoken and unwritten, they are usually visible to the observer. A nurse should stay within the rules of touch that are culturally prescribed. It is essential that the nurse uses touch judiciously and avoids forcing touch on anyone. Nurses must keep in mind that the message conveyed through touch depends on the attitude of the other person involved and on the meaning of touch both to the person touching and to the person being touched. Generally,

the need for intimacy and touch is so strong that the satisfaction of that need is a greater influence on behavior than fears about its inappropriateness (Johnson, 1965). A momentary and seemingly incidental touch can establish a positive, temporary bond between strangers, making them more compliant, helpful, positive, and giving. In all cases, touch needs to be applied deliberately, with empathy, and with close attention to the person's particular needs. All cultural groups have rules, often unspoken, about who touches whom, when, and where. To avoid being perceived as intrusive, the astute nurse must be mindful of the client's reaction to touch.

Facial Expression. Facial expression is commonly used as a guide to a person's feelings. Research shows that generally, in Americans, facial expression is used as a part of the communication message. A constant stare with immobile facial muscles indicates coldness. During fear, the eyes open wide, the eyebrows rise, and the mouth becomes tense with the lips drawn back. When a person is angry, the eyes become fixed in a hard stare with the upper lids lowered and the eyebrows drawn down. An angry person's lips are often tightly compressed. Eyes rolled upward may be related to tiredness or may show disapproval. Narrowed eyes, a curled upper lip, and a moving nose commonly signal disgust. A person who is embarrassed or self-conscious may turn the eyes away or down; have a flushed face; pretend to smile; rub the eyes, nose, or face; or twitch the hair, beard, or mustache. A direct gaze with raised eyebrows shows surprise (Ekman & Friesen, 1975; Polhemus, 1978).

Facial expression also varies with culture. Italian, Jewish, African-American, and Hispanic persons smile readily and use many facial expressions, along with gestures and words, to communicate feelings of happiness, pain, or displeasure. Irish, English, and northern European persons tend to have less facial expression and are generally less responsive, especially to strangers. Facial expression can also be used to convey an opposite meaning of the one that is felt; for example, in Asia negative emotions may be concealed with a smile (Sue & Sue, 2003).

Eye Movement. Research on eye movement has vastly increased as a result of the development of computer-based data collection and analysis routines. Recording techniques for eye movements provide a vast array of data to the researcher (Grainger, 1992; Rayner, 1992; Shapiro, 1991).

Eye movement is an important aspect of interpersonal communication. Generally, during social interaction, most people look each other in the eye for short periods (Argyle & Dean, 1965; Davidhizar, 1988a). People use more eye contact while they are listening and may use glances of about 3 to 10 seconds. When glances are longer than this, anxiety is aroused.

Eye contact is an important tool in transcultural nursing assessment and is used both for observation and to initiate interaction. In the United States, those of the dominant culture (predominately Whites) value eye contact as symbolic of a positive self-concept, openness, interest in others, attentiveness, and honesty. Eye contact can communicate warmth and bridge interpersonal gaps between people. A nurse who wears glasses and wants to make a point may increase the intensity of eye contact by taking off the glasses. The removal of glasses has also been cited as a technique that can humanize an individual's face, since barriers to eye contact are removed (Giger & Davidhizar, 1990b).

Lack of eye contact may be interpreted as a sign of shyness, lack of interest, subordination, humility, guilt, embarrassment, low self-esteem, rudeness, thoughtfulness, or dishonesty. In social interaction the speaker glances away from the listener to indicate collecting of thoughts or planning of what is to be said. If contact is not resumed, lack of interest may be interpreted. Pupil dilation and constriction can also be a clue to anxiety level and positive response (Hess, 1965, 1975).

Most Mexican American and African-American clients are comfortable with eye contact (Guruge & Donner, 1996; Murray & Huelskoetter, 1991). In contrast to this view, others have suggested that through a process of socialization in a "minority status" of relative powerlessness, some African-Americans have learned to deliberately avoid eye contact with others (Giger, Davidhizar, Evers, & Ingram, 1994). In fact, in the United States avoidance of eye contact is sometimes considered rude, an indication of lack of attention, or a sign of mental illness (Bigham, 1964; Paynich, 1964). On the other hand, McKenzie and Chrisman (1977) reported that, for some Filipinos, eye contact that turns away is associated with the possibility of being a witch. Other groups who find eye contact difficult include some Asian people and some American Indians, who relate eye contact to impoliteness and an invasion of privacy. Many American Indians regard eye contact as disrespectful because it is believed that "looking in an individual's eyes" is "looking into an individual's soul" (Galanti, 2003; Giger & Davidhizar, 2001; Henderson & Primeaux, 1981; Poole, Davidhizar, & Giger, 2003).

Persons in certain Indian cultures avoid eye contact with persons of a higher or lower socioeconomic class. The Vietnamese generally practice less eye contact (Rocereto, 1981), and prolonged eye contact is also avoided by some African-Americans (Giger & Davidhizar, 1990b). In some Indian cultures eye contact is given a special sexual significance. Some Orthodox Jews also attribute a sexual significance to eye contact by an elderly man with a woman other than his wife (Sue & Sue, 1999). Some Appalachian people tend to avert their eyes because for them eye contact is related to hostility and aggressiveness (Tripp-Reimer & Friedl, 1977). Certain cultures place more focus on the eyes than others; for example, in India and Greece the use of the eyes is all-important (Eibl-Eibesfelt, 1972).

Body Posture. Communication is also affected by body posture. A nurse can bridge distance in an interaction by placing the forearms on the table, palms up. In Western culture, palms up can send a message of acquiescence even while disagreeing. However, the nurse should also recognize that palms up in other cultures may have a sexual implication. Therefore, the decision to use this gesture should be weighed carefully.

Body posture can provide important messages about receptivity. In some Western cultures, such as among Whites in the United States, the closer a listener's overall posturing matches the posture of the speaker, the higher the likelihood of receptivity.

If the individuals' unconscious gestures differ, probably their perspective on the matter at hand is also different. Matching body movements to those of another person can communicate a sense of solidarity, even if solidarity is not present. Body posture can also communicate attitude toward a person. For example, within the dominant culture of Whites in the United States, an attentive posture is indicated by leaning toward a person. Attentive posture is used toward people of higher stature and toward people who are liked (Mehrabian, 1968, 1981). An American man may indicate sexual attraction by placing his arms in front of his body with his legs closed. An American woman, on the other hand, indicates attraction by a more open posture, that is, arms down at the side (Hall, 1966). Physical pain is communicated by rigid muscles, flexed body, and cautious movements. Argyle et al. (1970) reported that in England dominance is communicated when the dominant person stands or sits more erectly than the compliant or submissive person. Knowledge of sociocultural heritage is essential in interpreting body language, since various body parts are used differently in different cultures.

Communications that Combine Verbal and Nonverbal Elements

Many interpersonal communications combine both verbal and nonverbal elements. The communications of warmth and humor are two of these.

Warmth. Warmth is a quality or state that promotes feelings of friendship, well-being, or pleasure. Warmth can be communicated verbally ("You really lay still during the procedure, and that surely helped us to do it as quickly as possible") and may also be communicated nonverbally, as by a pat on the shoulder or a gentle smile.

Although warmth is also a matter of perception, communication that focuses on human needs is more likely to be related to warmth in the speaker. Statements that show respect, address the human need to be needed, and promote self-acceptance will usually be interpreted positively and can increase motivation, morale, and cooperation. Personal recognition and concern also communicate warmth. Verbal recognition (for example, a hello on meeting) or a statement of genuine concern (for example, "How are you feeling?") can convey interest and may facilitate a positive relationship between client and family and the nurse (Davidhizar, 1989).

The nurse's communication of warmth is an important and dynamic aspect of a therapeutic nurse–client relationship. If the client is from another culture and is having difficulty with understanding communication, the nurse's warmth may be vital to promoting a positive relationship. Graham-Dickerson (1996) suggests that the healing process is promoted by the interrelation between the nurse and the client, and without this relationship the client from another culture may not be engaged in the healing process.

Humor. Humor is a powerful component of verbal and nonverbal communication. Humor can create a bond of shared pleasure between people, decrease anxiety and tension, build relationships, promote problem solving and learning, provide motivation, and enable personal survival. As a healthy and constructive coping mechanism, humor can provide a discharge for aggressive feelings in a more or less acceptable way and can enable management of stressful situations (Davidhizar, 1988b). Humor that is therapeutic does not ridicule and rarely uses cynicism (Huckaby, 1987). Personality, culture, background, and levels of stress and pain may influence reactions to humor. When people are from a different culture, humor must be used in a limited and deliberate manner since humor can be an obstacle to a relationship if it is misunderstood. The nurse must carefully assess the individual client and the situation to decide if humor is appropriate. Humor not only can improve communication when used appropriately but may also affect the immune system by promoting the body's ability to combat such problems as cancer and diseases of the connective tissue, such as arthritis and lupus (Simonton, Simonton, & Creighton, 1978).

When the individual spoken with does not have a full grasp of the language and the nuances and puns that are often involved in humor, jokes, and statements meant humorously may not be understood or may be misinterpreted. It is also important for an individual who tries to speak in another language to be prepared to precipitate laughter. A statement meant to be serious may be perceived as comical. The ability to laugh at oneself and with others can ease the anxiety that may be present in an intercultural situation.

IMPLICATIONS FOR NURSING CARE

Guidelines for Relating to Patients from Different Cultures

Nurses commonly relate to clients in an interview setting. The nurse may also relate during the process of client care or at a more informal level on the hospital unit or in the clinic. Although cultural issues may cause the client to interpret the nurse's behavior from a unique perspective, adherence to the following guidelines will increase the likelihood that the nurse–client relationship will be positive (Box 2-4).

1. Assess Personal Beliefs of Persons from Different Cultures. Awareness of the nurse's personal beliefs is vital in relating to clients from diverse cultural backgrounds (Boone, 2005). A nurse working with a client from another background should carefully review personal beliefs and experiences to determine conscious and unconscious attitudes. It is important for the nurse to set aside personal values, biases, ideas, and attitudes that are judgmental and may negatively affect care. The nurse can learn to control personal reactions by a broadened understanding of others' beliefs and behaviors (Winans-Orr & McIntosh, 1996). Leininger & McFarland (2006) contend that there is a major crisis in nursing in that most nurses are unprepared to function effectively with migrants and cultural strangers. Understanding of other cultures can be enhanced through immersion in another culture. Additionally, use of cultural assessment tools provides a method to assess personal attitude (Anthony, 1997).

2. Assess Communication Variables from a Cultural Perspective. To communicate with a client from another culture, it is essential to assess each client from a cultural perspective. Oxendine (2000) reports a health education project in which Zuni, Pueblo, Hopi, and Navajo women showed no interest in breast cancer brochures with pictures of breasts on the cover. The women said they found the pictures of breasts unsuitable and wanted the term *breast health* rather than *breast cancer* used. When a contest was held to pick new cover art for the brochure, 120 American Indian artists entered. Carneiro (2000) describes a health education program for a Hispanic Latino community in which a video featured a slim, blond, blue-eyed model who did not look at all Latino. The educators did not appreciate that in the Latino communities, being chubby is viewed by some as being healthier and that some Latino parents still associate a skinny baby with not having enough money to feed the child. The nurse must also assess whether the individual is from a culture in which priority is given to context versus content since this will influence communication style (Goldman & Schmalz, 2005; Xu & Davidhizar, 2005). The cultural phenomena of communication cannot be minimized when providing culturally appropriate nursing care. The nurse who understands differences in communication variables can attempt to transcend communication barriers to provide high-quality client care.

It is important to realize that cultural assessment does not require information on every aspect of a specific culture. However, data should elicit ethnic identity, including generation in the United States (that is, first or second generation); the beliefs of a first-generation immigrant, regardless of ethnic heritage, may differ from those of a second-generation person. Whenever possible, the client should be used as the primary informant, since others, even though close to the client, may have different ideas and beliefs.

After a careful assessment of cultural factors that may enter into a relationship, the nurse must respond appropriately. For example, for African-Americans and Mexican Americans who tend to value eye contact, it is important for the nurse to use eye contact (Kendall, 1996). On the other hand, when relating to Filipino Americans who are afraid of eye contact, the nurse should avoid eye contact. When relating to Southeast Asians, it is important to remember that persons from this cultural background usually are very formal in their language.

Box 2-4

GUIDELINES FOR RELATING TO PATIENTS FROM DIFFERENT CULTURES

1. Assess your personal beliefs surrounding persons from different cultures.
   - Review your personal beliefs and experiences.
   - Set aside any values, biases, ideas, and attitudes that are judgmental and may negatively affect care.
2. Assess communication variables from a cultural perspective.
   - Determine the ethnic identity of the patient, including generations in the United States.
   - Use the patient as a source of information when possible.
   - Assess cultural factors that may affect your relationship with the patient and respond appropriately.
3. Plan care according to the communicated needs and cultural background.
   - Learn as much as possible about the patient's cultural customs and beliefs.
   - Encourage the patient to reveal cultural interpretation of health, illness, and health care.
   - Be sensitive to the uniqueness of the patient.
   - Identify sources of discrepancy between the patient's and your own concepts of health and illness.
   - Communicate at the patient's personal level of functioning.
   - Evaluate effectiveness of nursing actions and modify nursing care plan when necessary.
4. Modify communication approaches to meet cultural needs.
   - Be attentive to signs of fear, anxiety, and confusion in the patient.
   - Respond in a reassuring manner in keeping with the patient's cultural orientation.
   - Be aware that in some cultural groups discussion with others concerning the patient may be offensive and impede the nursing process.
5. Understand that respect for the patient and communicated needs is central to the therapeutic relationship.
   - Communicate respect by using a kind and attentive approach.
   - Learn how listening is communicated in the patient's culture.
   - Use appropriate active listening techniques.
   - Adopt an attitude of flexibility, respect, and interest to help bridge barriers imposed by culture.
6. Communicate in a nonthreatening manner.
   - Conduct the interview in an unhurried manner.
   - Follow acceptable social and cultural amenities.
   - Ask general questions during the information-gathering stage.
   - Be patient with a respondent who gives information that may seem unrelated to the patient's health problem.
   - Develop a trusting relationship by listening carefully, allowing time, and giving the patient your full attention.
7. Use validating techniques in communication.
   - Be alert for feedback that the patient is not understanding.
   - Do not assume meaning is interpreted without distortion.
8. Be considerate of reluctance to talk when the subject involves sexual matters.
   - Be aware that in some cultures sexual matters are not discussed freely with members of the opposite sex.
9. Adopt special approaches when the patient speaks a different language.
   - Use a caring tone of voice and facial expression to help alleviate the patient's fears.
   - Speak slowly and distinctly, but not loudly.
   - Use gestures, pictures, and play acting to help the patient understand.
   - Repeat the message in different ways if necessary.
   - Be alert to words the patient seems to understand and use them frequently.
   - Keep messages simple and repeat them frequently.
   - Avoid using medical terms and abbreviations that the patient may not understand.
   - Use an appropriate language dictionary.
10. Use interpreters to improve communication.
    - Ask the interpreter to translate the message, not just the individual words.
    - Obtain feedback to confirm understanding.
    - Use an interpreter who is culturally sensitive.

It is essential that courtesy be shown by use of the family name or a title until one is given permission to address the client by a given name. Asians also use an indirect approach to obtaining information, and so direct questions are not received well; such questions are considered rude, and the interviewer is not likely to receive the information sought (Hagen, 1988; Mattson, 1995). If communication is to be effective in today's multicultural society, relating in a culturally sensitive manner is essential (Campinha-Bacote, 1995).

3. Plan Care Based on the Communicated Needs and Cultural Background. Care for persons from other cultures must be consistent with the client's lifestyle and unique needs that have been communicated by the client to the nurse and mutually agreed on (Geissler, 1991; Grossman, 1996). To establish an appropriate plan, it is essential to improve personal knowledge about the customs and beliefs of the culture of the clients receiving care. The nurse should encourage the client to communicate interpretations of health, illness, and health care since culture influences what are considered appropriate approaches to health, wellness, illness, and death (Sieh & Brentin, 1997). A client's perception of illness will affect not only communication but also the care that is planned. Sensitivity to the uniqueness of each client is required if the nurse is to work effectively, particularly with clients from different cultures. This sensitivity can be gained only through appropriate communication techniques. Additionally, nurses who cannot communicate and correctly interpret cultural behavior will feel inadequate and helpless and quickly experience stress and burnout (Scholz, 1990). It is important to remember that the best teacher in learning about culture is people themselves. Individuals must be communicated with at their personal level of functioning. Values and beliefs of persons from different cultures may affect the way care is delivered. Many cultures have similar idiosyncrasies that must be considered. Finally, it is important to evaluate the effectiveness of nursing actions with clients from diverse culture groups. It may be necessary to modify the plan of care to provide an effective intervention based on communicated needs.

4. Modify Communication Approaches to Meet Cultural Needs. A factor that commonly interferes with care delivery to a person from another culture is confusion and fear about the treatment process. The nurse must be attentive to signs of anxiety and respond in a reassuring manner in keeping with the client's cultural orientation. When English is the client's second language, the nurse should be alert to the fact that meanings of words and how facts are presented may vary according to the family and culture of origin (Davidhizar & Brownson, 2000).

Some cultures are primarily oral and do not rely on a written form of communication. In such a society, the spoken word holds greater meaning and power. For example, Hmong are considered an oral cultural group. For these individuals, the formation of and acceptance in a social group is primarily dependent on the spoken word (Shadick, 1993). When interacting with individuals from an oral culture, the nurse must remember that if the teaching–learning process is to be effective, instruction must be oral.

Some Muslim sects do not believe in prevention and thus are unwilling to perform the most basic health intervention and promotion activities. Taking active measures to prevent disease is thought to go against the wishes of Allah (Carneiro, 2000; Davidhizar & Giger, 2002). The nurse must appreciate the impact of this cultural belief on health behavior in order to think of communication strategies to respond to health needs.

5. Understand that Respect for the Client and Communicated Needs Is Central to the Therapeutic Relationship. The need to communicate respect for the client is a nursing concept that crosses all cultural boundaries and conserves use of resources (Purnell, 2001). Regardless of the language spoken or the cultural orientation, the nurse whose approach focuses on individuals and their emotional and physical needs increases communication and reduces interpersonal distance. Communication of respect is central to a focus on emotional needs. Respect for clients is communicated by a kind and attentive approach in which the client is heard. Active listening techniques are used, such as encouraging clients to share thoughts and feelings by reflecting back what has been heard. The nurse should be attentive to how listening is communicated in the client's culture. For example, for some persons, listening may be indicated by eye contact, whereas for others listening may mean having the listener turn a listening "ear." Predictions about what the client is trying to express may be made to encourage elaboration. At the heart of the task of hearing is the art of listening (Martin, 1995). Listening communicates genuine interest and caring. The feeling of being heard is powerful, reducing distance and drawing people together into positive interpersonal interactions. An attitude of flexibility, respect, and interest can bridge the artificial barriers of distance imposed by culture and role.

6. Communicate in a Nonthreatening Manner. The interview should be started in an unhurried manner, with adherence to acceptable social and cultural amenities. It is usually wise to start with general social topics and to make some connection with the individual before asking questions (Wissing, 2000). Being aware of and using cultural information provides a valuable base from which to proceed (Sieh & Brentin, 1997). During the information-gathering stage, general rather than specific questions should be asked. The interviewer should allow time for the respondent to give what appears to be unrelated information. For many persons a direct approach appears rude and uncaring. For example, persons of European background and Hispanic individuals often value "small talk" and will not relate optimally to the nurse who talks only about illness-related matters. Many persons, specifically Asian and Spanish-speaking persons, respond better to a nondirective approach with open-ended questions than to direct questions (Giger & Davidhizar, 1990b). Storytelling (Evans & Severtsen, 2001), photography (Killion, 2001), and literature (Barton & Richardson, 1998; Studer, 2002) can provide important information to assist in understanding individuals and their cultural orientation.

7. Utilize Strategies to Develop Trust. When personal matters are discussed, it is important to allow time for the development of a relationship. In a significant book on cultural perspective, *The Spirit Catches You and You Fall Down*, Fadiman (1997) provides an example of a health care worker visiting a pregnant Hmong woman with tuberculosis who was refusing her medication. The interpreter stopped the caregiver from starting on this topic but rather started the conversation by wishing the patient's family well and initiating conversation with the husband. Once friendly contact had been established, the social worker inquired as to why the wife was not taking medications and was told that they feared that the baby would be born without arms and legs. When this misunderstanding was corrected, she took her medication. It is essential to first communicate a positive attitude in order to promote trust and confidence if collaboration about health care needs is to occur (Jenkins & Fallowfield, 2000). The appearances of being too busy, of not having time to listen, of not giving sufficient time for an answer, and of not really wanting to hear are equally effective in cutting off the client. Research has demonstrated that racial and ethnic minorities have lower levels of trust in health care providers than do White Americans (Satcher & Pamies, 2006). For example, LaVeist, Nickerson, & Bowie (2000) reported that African-Americans were more likely to perceive racism in the health care system and report distrust.

When working with persons from diverse cultural backgrounds, the astute nurse must recognize that the communication process may be impeded by hesitancy to speak to Westerners about health concerns. Some American Indians are becoming more confident and willing to speak out about their personal needs. However, Hagey and Buller (1983) noted that the Ojibway people traditionally avoided direct oral questioning by health care workers and viewed it as a violation of dignity and thus inappropriate. Such questions could be met with complete silence and meaningless answers. For some Ojibway, in response to a question, it would be entirely acceptable for an answer to be given in a few days or weeks. It is critical that the nurse serve as a client advocate to provide culturally sensitive care. It is also essential that the nurse learn to appreciate a value held by some Ojibway that espouses deep-rooted ideals of noninterference, which may be found among some Native and ethnic groups (Grypma, 1993; Reimer & Redskye, 1998). Regardless of cultural background, listening is one of the most effective therapeutic techniques (Potter & Perry, 2005).

8. Use Validating Techniques in Communication. Although validating techniques are always important, they are especially important when the client is from a different culture. The nurse should be alert for feedback that the client is not understanding and should use restating and validating techniques, such as "Did I hear and understand you correctly?" When the nurse has difficulty understanding, it may help to find out precisely what the topic is, such as "Are you telling me where you're having pain?" By determining the topic, the number of words can be decreased. If the message is not understood, it may be helpful to have the client try to convey the message in another way—for example, through pointing or imitation. The nurse should never pretend to understand a message. People usually know when they are understood. By pretending, the nurse conveys that the message is not really important (Pore, 1995).

9. Be Considerate of Reluctance to Talk When the Subject Involves Sexual Matters. Hispanic and Indian clients, who tend to be hesitant to talk about sexually related matters, may talk more freely to a nurse of the same sex. When talking about sexual matters with a male child from certain cultures (such as Spanish, Pakistani, or Arabic), it is important to have the father rather than the mother present.

10. Adopt Special Approaches When the Client Speaks a Different Language. A client who enters the health care system without being able to speak the dominant language of the caregivers enters a frightening and frustrating world. This may also be true for clients whose first language differs from that of the nurse (Davidhizar, Shearer, & Giger, 2002). The nurse should keep in mind that for clients who cannot speak the language of the professionals encountered, basic procedures such as registering at the emergency desk or for a diagnostic procedure may be very anxiety producing. Clients who do not understand are more likely to be hostile and belligerent, to be uncooperative, or to withdraw (Spector, 2004).

The nurse should be alert for the client who pretends to understand to please the caregiver and gain acceptance. This patient will usually say yes to all questions. Without the availability of words, the nurse must relate to a client at an affective level. A tone and facial expression of caring can be vital in alleviating a client's fear.

If an interpreter is not available and the client seems to have some understanding of the language, speaking slowly and distinctly, using a lot of gestures, acting out, using pictures, and repeating the message several times in different ways may enable the client to understand what is being said. The nurse should be alert for words that the client seems to understand so that these words can be used more frequently. Messages should be kept simple and stated sentence by sentence, not paragraph by paragraph. Clients who appear to be having difficulty understanding should be asked to provide feedback on what they have heard to provide opportunity for further clarification.

It is especially necessary to avoid using medical terms and jargon when speaking to a client with only a partial understanding of the language. Abbreviations such as TPR and BP should be avoided. An individual usually first understands standard words and picks up slang expressions and professional terms at a much later stage of language acquisition.

The nurse should select a dictionary that has both the language the nurse speaks and the language the client speaks, such as a Spanish–English, English–Spanish dictionary. In addition, standard nursing references, such as *Taber's Cyclopedic Medical Dictionary* (Venes, 2005) and *Mosby's Medical, Nursing, and Allied Health Dictionary* (Anderson, Keith, Novak, & Elliot, 2005), have sections that give common medical statements and questions in several languages. Nursing textbooks are increasingly adding sections related to speaking to non–English-speaking clients. For example, Ignatavicius and Workman's *Medical-Surgical Nursing* (2006) contains a communication reference for Spanish-speaking clients.

In addition to assessing how much English a client knows, it is important to assess whether the client can read English or is literate in the language spoken so that appropriate printed information on the agency, consent forms, and health information can be obtained. With on-line technology, multilingual and even age-specific communication can automatically happen, making health care and prescription drug information available in whatever language is selected (Giorgianni, 2000). However, as Mika, Kelly, Price, Franquiz, and Villarreal (2005) note, a significant portion of the U.S. population has serious problems with both literacy and understanding how to effectively use health-related information. An adult literacy survey found that 45% of the adult population in the United States had limited literacy skills (Kirsch, Jungeblut, Jenkins, & Kolstad, 1993).

The cultural orientation of the client also affects such factors as assignment of caregivers. For example, for conservative Arab, Afghan, or other Muslim clients, females giving instructions to males may not be effective (Davidhizar & Giger, 2002). If a male nurse is providing services to a female Arab client, strict rules would require that a family member always be present. Older Arab clients may not comply with direct instructions given by a young staff member; with these clients, indirect requests and suggestions are the desired methods (Nellum-Davis, 2002; Wilson, 1996).

11. Use Interpreters to Improve Communication

When the client and nurse do not speak the same language, an interpreter must be obtained. When a medical interpreter is not available, a family member may be utilized. However, use of a child should be avoided since a child may not adequately understand or explain technical information (Davidhizar & Brownson, 2000). The nurse should evaluate whether having a family member interpret is satisfactory to the client because some clients may not be willing to confide certain information to a family member (Clark, 1995). Hallenbeck (2004) notes that if a family member serves as translator, family values such as not talking openly about

cancer or death may affect the translation. The interpreter should be able to translate not only the literal meaning of the words but also the nonverbal messages that accompany the communication. Interpreters who act out their message through intonation, facial expression, or gestures are more likely to be effective in getting the message across. Even when every effort is made to ensure effective interpretation, neither the nurse nor the interpreter can be completely sure that accurate communication has been accomplished; therefore, obtaining feedback remains essential. Communication through a third party compounds the problem of sending a message clearly. Interpreters often face the difficulty of interpreting versus translating. Although a message may be translated into another language, helping another understand is much more complex and involves interpreting the message into understandable terms. An interpreter must have transcultural sensitivity, understand how to impart knowledge, and understand how to be a client advocate to represent the client's needs to the nurse. Interpreting with cultural sensitivity is much more complex than simply putting the words into another language (Díaz-Duque, 1982; Wolfson, 1996). Monolingualism in multicultural practices frequently presents ethical dilemmas. If the nurse, the interpreter, and the client's views on the ethical principles regarding care differ, problems can be compounded (Kaufert & Putsch, 1997). Boston (1993) conducted a study of Italian immigrant families in Montreal to determine whether they felt frustration with their caregivers because of language barriers. Findings from this study indicated that respondents expressed fear and helplessness about their treatment because of the language barriers. Even when an interpreter was provided, family members believed that their own deeper concerns and fears were not adequately communicated. Communication extends beyond conveying information and must include methods of conveying emotional and social support (Papadopoulos & Lees, 2004). England, Doughty, Genc, and Putkeli (2003) also reported that even when interpreters are provided, staff should be concerned that communication problems related to other social issues may remain unaddressed.

When the health professional can speak the language of the client, cultural barriers will be lowered. Even if the nurse knows only key words or phrases, this can significantly affect communication and satisfaction with care (Burnard & Naiyapatana, 2004; Powell, 2005).

Case Study

A 35- to 37-year-old Black woman who has been recently diagnosed as having hypertension is admitted for a medical work-up examination. Her history reveals that she has recently moved from New Orleans to New York. The nurse is having difficulty communicating with the client because she not only speaks in Black English but also has a heavy Southern drawl and tends to speak in pidgin English. Another factor complicating the development of the nurse–client relationship is that not only does the client not understand the hospital jargon and medical terms but also word meanings for the nurse and the client vary. For example, when the nurse asks if the client likes her physician, she responds, "He's bad." Only later does the nurse discover that the client was speaking in an argot that is a special linguistic code for some Blacks. The client appears very fearful and anxious about being in the hospital. When questioning the client, the nurse finds that the fear and anxiety are related to the connotative and denotative meanings of the word "hospital." In this case, the client believes that hospitals are associated with death and that she may not leave the hospital alive. When the nurse communicates with the client, she speaks very loudly and repeats the same words again and again.

✳ STUDY QUESTIONS

1. Describe at least two problems encountered by the nurse when giving nursing care to persons who do not speak English as their primary language.
2. Describe four communication approaches that the nurse can use to give culturally appropriate care.
3. Describe approaches the nurse can use when relating to a client whose primary language is not English.
4. Describe at least two nonverbal indicators of anxiety the nurse may encounter when dealing with a client who does not speak English.
5. List at least two problems encountered by the nurse who assumes that speaking louder will improve communication.

NCLEX-RN REVIEW QUESTIONS

1. While assessing a client who does not speak English, the nurse is aware of nonverbal indications of anxiety that include:
   A. Being uncooperative and withdrawn.
   B. Looking directly at the nurse and nodding yes.
   C. Looking at the blood and nodding no.
   D. Being cooperative and outgoing.

2. When analyzing the assessment data on the admissions of a client with limited English skills, the nurse realizes the client has answered yes or nodded the head indicating yes to all questions. The nurse interprets this as indicating:
   A. The client "intended to" answer all questions yes.
   B. The client nodded the head and responded yes to indicate cooperation.

C. The nurse should repeat the questions more loudly so the client will hear.

D. The nurse should get an interpreter to assist with the assessment.

3. The nurse plans to use an interpreter when teaching a Spanish-speaking client about diabetes mellitus. The best interpreter for the nurse to select is:

A. A family member who lives with the client.

B. One who translates not only the words but the nonverbal messages too.

C. One who can translate the words into Spanish.

D. One who can translate the words into oral and written format.

References

Anderson, D., Keith, J., Novak, P., & Elliot, M (2006). *Mosby's dictionary of medical, nursing, and health professions* (ed. 6 revised). St. Louis: Mosby.

Anderson, M. (2003). Transcultural perspectives in the nursing care of children. In Andrews, M., & Boyle, J. (Eds.), *Transcultural concepts in nursing care*. Philadelphia: Lippincott Williams & Wilkins.

Andrews, M. M., & Boyle, J. S. (2003). *Transcultural concepts in nursing care* (ed. 4). Philadelphia: Lippincott Williams & Wilkins.

Anthony, M. (1997). A cultural values assessment tool. *Journal of Cultural Diversity*, 4(2), 49–52.

Argyle, M. (1992). *The social psychology of everyday life*. New York: Routledge.

Argyle, M., & Dean, J. (1965). Eye-contact, distance, and affiliation. *Sociometry*, 28, 289–304.

Argyle, M., Salter, H., & Nicholson, N., et al. (1970). The communication of inferior and superior attitudes by verbal and nonverbal signals. *British Journal of Social and Clinical Psychology*, 9, 221–231.

Banks, A., & Banks, S. (1995, November). Cultural identity, resistance, and "good theory": implications for intercultural communication theory from Gypsy culture. *Howard Journal of Communication*, 6(3), 146–163.

Barkauskas, P. (1994). *Quick reference to cultural assessment*. St. Louis: Mosby.

Barton, G., & Richardson, L. (1998, First Quarter). Using literature to create cultural competence. *Image: Journal of Nursing Scholarship*, 30(1), 75–79.

Beachy, A., Hershberger, E., Davidhizar, R., & Giger, J. (1997). Cultural implications for nursing care of the Amish. *Journal of Cultural Diversity*, 4(4), 118–128.

Beutter, B., & Davidhizar, R. (1999, September). A home care provider's challenge: caring for the Hispanic client in the home. *Journal of Practical Nursing*, 49(3), 26–36.

Bigham, C. (1964). To communicate with Negro patients. *American Journal of Nursing*, 64(9), 113–115.

Boas, F. (Ed.) (1938). *General anthropology*. Boston: D.C. Heath.

Boone, S. (2005). Talk directly to patients about beliefs, practices. *Hospital Care Management*, 13(6), 95–96.

Boston, P. (1993). Culture and cancer: the relevance of cultural orientation within cancer education programmes. *European Journal of Cancer Care*, 2, 72–76.

Bronstein, M. (1996). Healing hands. *The Canadian Nurse*, 92(1), 32–34.

Buerhaus, P., & Auerbach, D. (1999). Slow growth in the United States of the number of minorities in the RN workforce. *Image: Journal of Nursing Scholarship*, 31(2), 179–183.

Burnard, P., & Naiyapatana, W. (2004). Culture and communication in Thai nursing: a report of an ethnographic study. *The International Journal of Nursing Studies*, 41(7), 755–765.

Byrne, M. (2002, April). Diversity and the subculture of healthcare. *Healthcare Traveler*, 9(6), 14–16, 59, 60.

Campinha-Bacote, J. (1995, October–December). The quest for cultural competence in nursing care. *Nursing Forum*, 30(4), 19–24.

Capirci, O., Iverson, J., Pizzuto, E., & Volterra, V. (1996). Gestures and words during the transition in two-word speech. *Journal of Child Language*, 23, 645–673.

Carneiro, J. (2000). Know the audience. *The Pfizer Journal: Innovations in Communication*, 4(3), 19–27.

Clark, C. (1995, September–October). Enhancing communication with families. *Health Traveler*, 3(2), 34.

Clemmens, E. (1985). An analyst looks at languages, cultures, and translations. *American Journal of Psychoanalysis*, 45(4), 310–321.

Clemmens, E. (1988). Some psychological functions of language. *American Journal of Psychoanalysis*, 43(4), 294–304.

Cook, P., & Cullen, J. (2000, July–August). Diversity as a value in undergraduate education. *Nursing and Health Care Education*, 21(4), 178–183.

Crump, R., Bartman, B., Walker, D., & Mitchell, J. (2000). Special populations: who are they and what makes them so special? *Community Health Forum*, 2(2), 35–37.

Davidhizar, R. (1988a). Distance in managerial encounters. *Today's OR Nurse*, 10(10), 23–29.

Davidhizar, R. (1988b). Humor—no nurse should be without it. *Today's OR Nurse*, 10(1), 18–20.

Davidhizar, R. (1989). Developing managerial warmth. *Dimensions of Critical Care*, 8(1), 28–34.

Davidhizar, R., & Brownson, K. (2000). Literacy, cultural diversity, and client education. *Home Health Care Management Practice*, 12(2), 38–44.

Davidhizar, R., & Dowd, S. (2004). When your boss is evil. *RT*, 17(40), 4–7.

Davidhizar, R., & Dowd, S. (2005). The trick about leadership is to make it look easy. *Healthcare Traveler*, 13(2), 2631.

Davidhizar, R., & Dowd, S. (2006). Taking criticism. *Journal of Practical Nursing*, 56(2), 21–24.

Davidhizar, R., Dowd, S., & Giger, J. (1998). Prepare now to work with diverse staff. *Case Management Advisor*, 9(9), 149–151.

Davidhizar, R., & Eshleman, J. (2006). Strategies for developing cultural competency in an RN-BSN program. *Journal of Transcultural Nursing*, 17(2), 179–183.

Davidhizar, R., & Giger, J. (1988). Managerial touch. *Today's OR Nurse*, 10(7), 18–23.

Davidhizar, R., & Giger, J. (2000, January–February). Culture and care: profiling Alaskan Eskimos. *Healthcare Traveler* 7(4), 12, 43–47.

Davidhizar, R., & Giger, J. (2001, September). Teaching culture within the nursing curriculum using the Giger-Davidhizar model of transcultural nursing assessment. *Journal of Nursing Education*, 40(6), 282–284.

Davidhizar, R., & Giger, J. (2002, January 21). Cultural issues: using a transcultural assessment model to understand Afghanis and Islamic culture and religion. *Advances for Nurses*, 37–38.

Davidhizar, R., & Hart, A. (2005). Pain management. *Healthcare Traveler*, 13(6), 3–41.

Davidhizar, R. & Shearer, R. (2005). When your nursing student is culturally diverse. *Health Care Manager*, 24(4), 356–363.

Davidhizar, R., Shearer, R., & Giger, J. (2002). The challenges of cross-cultural communication. *RT Image*, 15(11), 18–23.

Delgado, M. (1983). Hispanics and psychotherapeutic groups. *International Journal of Psychotherapy*, 33(4), 507–520.

DeThomaso, M. (1971). Touch power and the screen of loneliness. *Perspectives in Psychiatric Care*, 9(3), 112–117.

Díaz-Duque, O. F. (1982). Overcoming the language barrier: advice from an interpreter. *American Journal of Nursing*, 82(9), 1380–1382.

Dillard, J. (1973). *Black English: its history and usage in the United States.* New York: Vintage Books.

Eibl-Eibesfelt, I. (1972). Similarities and differences between cultures in expressive movements. In Hinde, R. A. (Ed.), *Nonverbal communication* (pp. 297–312). Cambridge, England: Cambridge University Press.

Ekman, P., & Friesen, W. (1975). *Unmasking the face: a guide recognizing emotions from facial clues.* Englewood Cliffs, N.J.: Prentice Hall.

England, R., Doughty, K., Genc, S., & Putkeli, Z. (2003). Working with refugees: Health education and communiation issues in a child health clinic. *Health Education Journal*, 62(4), 359–368.

Ericksen, A. (2002, March). Culturally speaking. *Healthcare Traveler*, 9(6), 8–12, 59–60.

Evans, B., & Severtsen, B. (2001, July/August). Storytelling as cultural assessment. *Nursing and Health Perspectives*, 22(4), 180–183.

Fadiman, A. (1997). *The spirit catches you and you fall down: Hmong child, her American doctors, and the collision of two cultures.* New York: Noonday Press.

Galanti, G. (2003). *Caring for patients from different cultures: case studies from American hospitals* (ed. 3). (pp. 26–27). Philadelphia: University of Pennsylvania Press.

Geissler, E. (1991). Transcultural nursing and nursing diagnosis. *Nursing and Health Care*, 12(4), 190–192.

Gibson, J. (1984, January). As they grow: 1 year olds. *Parents*, 128.

Giger, J., & Davidhizar, R. (1990a). Culture and space. *Advancing Clinical Care*, 6(6), 8–10.

Giger, J., & Davidhizar, R. (1990b). Transcultural nursing assessment: a method for advancing nursing practice. *International Nursing Review*, 37(1), 199–202.

Giger, J., & Davidhizar, R. (2001). Diversity in caring. In Potter, P., & Perry, A. (Eds.), *Fundamentals of nursing* (ed. 5). St. Louis: Mosby.

Giger, J., Davidhizar, R., Evers, S., & Ingram, C. (1994). Cultural factors influencing mental health and mental illness. In Taylor, C. (Ed.), *Mereness' essentials of psychiatric nursing* (pp. 214–238). St. Louis: Mosby.

Giger, J., Davidhizar, R., Johnson, J., & Poole, V. (1997). Health promotion among ethnic minorities: the importance of cultural phenomena. *Rehabilitation nursing*, 22(6), 303–307, 310, 336.

Giger, J., Davidhizar, R., & Wieczorek, S. (1993). Culture and ethnicity. In Bobak, I. M., & Jensen, M. (Eds.), *Maternity and gynecological care* (ed. 5) (pp. 43–67). St. Louis: Mosby.

Giorgianni, S. (2000). Activating the health consumer. *The Pfizer Journal: Innovations in Communication*, 4(3), 4–36.

Goldman, K., & Schmalz, K. (2005). E=MC2: Effective multiple competence. *Health Promotion Practice*, 6(3), 237–239.

Graham-Dickerson, P. (1996, Summer). Healing through discourse for culturally diverse people within the health care system. *The Journal of Multicultural Nursing and Health*, 2(3), 33–37.

Grainger, R. (1992). Eye movements: a new psychotherapeutic tool. *American Journal of Nursing*, 92(5), 18.

Grossman, D. (1996, July). Cultural dimensions in home health care nursing. *American Journal of Nursing*, 96(7), 33–36.

Grypma, S. (1993, September). Culture shock. *The Canadian Nurse*, 33–36.

Guralnik, D. (Ed.) (1989). *Webster's new world dictionary: student edition* (ed. 3). New York: Prentice Hall.

Guruge, S., & Donner, G. (1996, September). Transcultural nursing in Canada. *The Canadian Nurse*, 34–39.

Haffner, L. (1992). Translation is not enough: interpreting in a medical setting. *Western Journal of Medicine*, 157(3), 248–254.

Hagen, E. (1988, July 8). *Southeast Asians in the United States: an overview of belief systems, and the refugee experience*. Paper presented at the seminar Working with the Southeast Asian Health Consumer, St. Mary Medical Center, Long Beach, Calif.

Hagey, R., & Buller, E. (1983). Drumming and dancing: a new rhythm in nursing care. *The Canadian Nurse*, 79(4), 28–31.

Hall, E. T. (1966). *The silent language*. New York: Anchor Books.

Hallenbeck, J. (2004). Communication across cultures. *Journal of Palliative Medicine*, 7(3), 477–480.

Hedlund, N. (1993). Communication. In Rawlins, R. P., Williams, S., Beck, C. K. (Eds.), *Mental health–psychiatric nursing: a holistic life approach* (ed. 3). St. Louis: Mosby.

Henderson, G., & Primeaux, M. (1981). *Transcultural health care*. Menlo Park, Calif.: Addison-Wesley.

Hess, E. H. (1965). Attitude and pupil size. *Scientific American*, 212, 46–54.

Hess, E. H. (1975). The role of pupil size in communication. *Scientific American*, 233(5), 110–119.

Hoang, G., & Erickson, R. (1982). Guidelines for providing medical care to Southeast Asian refugees. *Journal of the American Medical Association*, 248(6), 710–714.

Huckaby, D. (1987). Take time to laugh. *Nursing*, 87, 17, 81.

Ignatavicius, D., & Workman, M. (2006). *Medical-surgical nursing* (ed. 5). Philadelphia: W.B. Saunders.

Insel, P. M., & Lindgren, H. C. (1978). *Too close for comfort: the psychology of crowding*. Englewood Cliffs, N.J.: Prentice Hall.

Jenkins, V., & Fallowfield, L. (2000). Reasons for accepting or declining to participate in randomized clinical trials for cancer therapy. *British Journal of Cancer*, 82, 1782–1788.

Johnson, B. (1965). The meaning of touch in nursing. *Nursing Outlook*, 13(2), 59–60.

Jones, R. (2000, May). Developments in consumer health informatics in the next decade. *Health Libraries Review*, 17(1), 26–31.

Jourard, S. (1972). *The transparent self: self disclosure and well-being* (revised ed.). New York: Van Nostrand-Reinhold.

Kaufert, J., & Putsch, R. (1997, Spring). Communication through interpreters in healthcare: ethical dilemmas arising from differences in class, culture, language, and power. *The Journal of Clinical Ethics*, 8(1), 71–87.

Kayser, H. (1996, October). Cultural/linguistic variations in the United States and its implications for assessment and intervention in speech-language pathology: an epilogue. *Language, Speech and Hearing Services in Schools*, 27(4), 385–387.

Kendall, J. (1996, June). Creating a culturally responsive psychotherapeutic environment for African-American youths: a critical analysis. *Advances in Nursing Science*, 18(4), 11–28.

Killion, C. (2001). Understanding cultural aspects of health through photography. *Nursing Outlook*, 49(1), 50–54.

Kirsch, I., Jengeblut, A., Jenkins, L, & Kolstad, A. (1993). *Adult literacy in America: a first look at the results of the National Adult Literacy Survey*. Washington, D.C.: National Center for Education Statistics, U.S. Dept. of Education.

Krech, D., Crutchfield, R., & Ballachey, E. (1962). *Individual in society: a textbook of social psychology*. New York: McGraw-Hill.

Lane, P. (1989). Nurse-client perceptions: the double standard of touch. *Issues in Mental Health Nursing*, 10, 1–13.

LaVeist, T, Nickerson, K., & Bowie, J. (2000). Attitudes about racism, medical mistrust, and satisfaction with care among African American and white cardiac patients. *Medical Care Research Review*, 57(Suppl 1), 146–161.

Leininger, M., & McFarland, M. (2006). *Culture care diversity and universality* (ed. 2). Sudbury, MA: Jones and Bartlett.

Lester, N. (1998, August). Cultural competence: a nursing dialogue. *American Journal of Nursing*, 98(8), 26–33.

Lindsay, J., Narayan, M., & Rea, K. (1998, October). Nursing across cultures: the Vietnamese client. *Home Healthcare Nurse*, 16(10), 693–700.

Luft, J., & Ingham, H. (1984). The Johari window: a graphic model of awareness in interpersonal relations. In Luft, J. (Ed.), *Group processes: an introduction to group dynamics* (ed. 3). Palo Alto, Calif.: Mayfield Pub. Co.

Lunsford, A. (2006). *Easy writer: a pocket reference* (ed. 3). Boston: Bedford/St. Martin's.

Mackey, R. (1995, April). Discover the health power of therapeutic touch. *American Journal of Nursing*, 95, 27–32.

Martin, B. (1995, December 12). The difficult art of listening. *Gospel Herald*, 88(48), 1–2.

Mattson, S. (1995, May). Culturally sensitive perinatal care for Southeast Asians. *Journal of Obstetric and Gynecological Neonatal Nursing*, 24(4), 335–341.

McKenzie, J., & Chrisman, N. (1977). Healing herbs, gods, and magic folk health beliefs among Filipino-Americans. *Nursing Outlook*, 25(5), 326.

McLeod, R., & Bently, C. (1996, Fall). Understanding deafness as a culture with a unique language. *Advanced Practice Nursing Quarterly*, 2(2), 50–58.

Mead, M. (1947). The application of anthropological technique to cross-national communication. *Transcultural New York Academy of Science, Series II*, 9, 4.

Mehrabian, A. (1968). The influence of attitudes from the posture, orientation, and distance of a communicator. *Journal of Consulting Clinical Psychology*, 32, 296–308.

Mehrabian, A. (1981). *Silent messages: implicit communication of emotions and attitudes*. Belmont, Calif.: Wadsworth.

Mika, V., Kelly, P., Price, M., Franquiz, M., & Virrarreal, R. (2005). The ABCs of health literacy. *Family Community Health*, 28(4), 351–357.

Miller, S., & Davidhizar, R. (2001, June). Sociocultural aspects of adherence to medical regimens for Mexican Americans. *Journal of Care Management*, 7(3), 44–48.

Mitchell, A. (1978). Barriers to therapeutic communication with Black clients. *Nursing Outlook*, 26, 109–112.

Montagu, A. (1986). *Touching: the human significance of the skin* (ed. 3). New York: Columbia University Press.

Murray, R., & Huelskoetter, N. (1991). *Psychiatric/mental health nursing: giving emotional care* (ed. 3). Norwalk, Conn.: Appleton & Lange.

Nellum-Davis, P. (2002). Clinical practice issues. In Battle, D. E. (Ed.), *Communicationdisorders in multicultural populations* (ed. 3). Boston: Andover Medical Publishers.

Oxendine, J. (2000, January). Creating culturally-sensitive health materials for American Indians. *Closing the Gap*, 12.

Papadopoulos, I., & Lees, S. (2004). Cancer and communications: Similarities and differences of men with cancer from six different ethnic groups. *European Journal of Cancer Care*, 16, 154–162.

Paynich, M. (1964). Cultural barriers to nurse communication. *American Journal of Nursing*, 64(2), 87–90.

Pirandello, L. (1970). Language and thought. *Perspectives in Psychiatric Care*, 8(5), 230.

Polhemus, T. (Ed.) (1978). *The body reader: social aspects of the human body*. New York: Pantheon Books.

Poole, V., Davidhizar, R., & Giger, J. (2003). Cultural aspects of psychiatric nursing. In Keltner, N., Schwecke, L., & Bostrom, C. (Eds.), *Psychiatric nursing* (ed. 4). St. Louis: Mosby.

Pore, S. (1995, July). I can't understand what my patient is saying. *Advance for Nurse Practitioners*, 3, 47–48.

Potter, R., & Perry, A. (2005). *Fundamentals of nursing* (ed. 6). St. Louis: Mosby.

Powell, K. (2005). Personal conversation. Goshen, Ind.

Purnell, L. (2001, January). Guatemalans' practices for health promotion and the meaning of respect afforded them by health care providers. *Journal of Transcultural Nursing*, 12(1), 40–47.

Quarnero, P. (2005). Mexicans. In Lipson, J., & Dibble, S. (Eds.), *Culture and clinical care.* School of Nursing, University of California, San Francisco: UCSF Nursing Press.

Randall-David, E. (1989). *Strategies for working with culturally diverse communities and clients [Brochure].* Washington, D.C.: Association for the Care of Children's Health.

Rayner, K. (1992). *Eye movements and visual cognition: scene perception and reading.* New York: Springer-Verlag.

Reimer, J., & Redskye, C. (1998). The Canadian Ojibwa. In Davidhizar, R., & Giger, J. (Eds.), *Canadian transcultural nursing: assessment and intervention.* St. Louis: Mosby.

Reusch, J. (1961). *Therapeutic communication.* New York: W.W. Norton.

Rocereto, L. (1981). Selected health beliefs of Vietnamese refugees. *Journal of School Health,* 51(1), 63–64.

Sapir, E. (1929). The status of linguistics as a science. *Language,* 5, 207–214.

Satcher, D., & Pamies, R. (2006). *Multicultural medicine and health disparities.* New York: McGraw-Hill.

Scheflen, A., & Scheflen, A. (1972). *Body language and social order.* Englewood Cliffs, N.J.: Prentice Hall.

Scholz, J. (1990). Cultural expressions affecting patient care. *Dimensions in Oncology Nursing,* 4(1), 16–20.

Shadick, K. (1993). Development of a transcultural health education program for the Hmong. *Clinical Nurse Specialist,* 7(2), 48–53.

Shapiro, F. (1991, May). Eye movement desensitization and reprocessing procedure: from EMD to EMD/R—a new treatment model for anxiety and related traumata. *The Behavioral Therapist,* 133–135.

Shields, L., & King, S. (2001, June). International pediatric nursing: qualitative analysis of the care of children in hospital in four countries. *Journal of Pediatric Nursing: Nursing Care of Children and Families,* 16 (3), 206–213.

Shuter, R. (1976). Proxemics and tactility in Latin America. *Journal of Communication,* 26(3), 46–52.

Sieh, A., & Brentin, L. (1997). *The nurse communicates.* Philadelphia: Saunders.

Simonton, O. C., Simonton, S., & Creighton, J. (1978). *Getting well again: a step-by-step, self-help guide to overcoming cancer for patients and their families.* New York: Bantam Books.

Smith, B., & Cantrell, P. (1988). Distance in nurse-patient encounters. *Journal of Psychosocial Nursing,* 26(2), 22–26.

Snow, L. (1976, June). "High blood" is not "high blood pressure." *Urban Health,* 5(3), 54–55.

Sommer, R. (1959). Studies in personal space. *Sociometry,* 22, 247–260.

Spector, R. (2004). *Cultural diversity in health and illness* (ed. 6). Upper Saddle River, N.J.: Pearson Prentice Hall.

Stauffer, R. (2005). *Personal communication.* Harrisburg, VA.

Studer, C. (2002). Reflections: body language—melting pain into song. *American Journal of Nursing,* 102(1), 45.

Sudnow, D. (1967). *Passing on: the social organization of dying.* Englewood Cliffs, N.J.: Prentice Hall.

Sue, D. W., & Sue, D. (2003). *Counseling the culturally diverse: theory and practice* (ed. 4). New York: John Wiley.

Sullivan, H. (1954). *The interpersonal theory of psychiatry.* New York: W.W. Norton.

Talbot, L. R. (1996). The power of words. *Canadian Journal of Nursing Research,* 28(1), 9–15.

Taylor, C. (1976). Soul talk: a key to Black cultural attitudes. In Luckroft, D. (Ed.), *Black awareness: implications for Black patient care.* New York: American Journal of Nursing Company.

Thayer, S. (1988, March). Close encounters. *Psychology Today,* 31–36.

Thiederman, S. (1986). Ethnocentrism: a barrier to effective health care. *Nurse Practitioner,* 11(8), 52–59.

Time almanac with information please (2006). Boston: Information Please, Inc.

Tripp-Reimer, T., & Friedl, M. (1977). Appalachians: a neglected minority. *Nursing Outlook,* 32(2), 41–45.

U.S. Department of Commerce: Bureau of Census. (2000, March). *The foreign-born population in the United States: Current Populations Reports* (pp. 20–534). Washington, D.C.: U.S. Census Bureau.

U.S. Department of Commerce: Bureau of Census. (2002). *Population profiles by age, sex, race, and Hispanic origin.* Summary File 3, Washington, D.C.: U.S. Government Printing Office.

U.S. Department of Health and Human Services (2000). *Healthy people 2010.* Washington, D.C.: U.S. Government Printing Office.

Varcarolis, E. (2006). The clinical interview and communication skills. In *Foundations of psychiatric mental health nursing* (ed. 5). Philadelphia: W.B. Saunders.

Venes, D., (2005). *Taber's cyclopedic medical dictionary* (ed. 20). Philadelphia: F.A. Davis.

Watzlawich, P., Beavin, J., & Jackson, D. (1967). *Pragmatics of human communication: a study of interactional patterns, pathologies, & paradoxes.* New York: W.W. Norton.

Whitcher, S. J., & Fisher, J. D. (1979). Multidimensional reaction to therapeutic touch in hospital setting.

Journal of Personality, Sociology, and Psychology, 37(1), 87–96.

Wilson, M. (1996, August). Arabic speakers: language and culture, here and abroad. *Topics in Language Disorders,* 18(4), 65–80.

Winans-Orr, P., & McIntosh, M. (1996, April). Putting control theory to work. *The Canadian Nurse,* 51.

Wissing, D. (2000, January). Respect is key to great people pictures. *Journey,* 12.

Wolfson, L. (1996, January). Breaking the language barrier. *Hemispheres,* 37–38.

Wood, D. (2001, Spring). Learning about difference. *Minority nurse,* 45–50.

Xu, Y., & Davidhizar, R. (2005). Intercultural communication in nursing education: when Asian students and American Faculty converage. *Journal of Nursing Education,* 44(5), 209–215.

CHAPTER 3

Space

Behavioral Objectives

After reading this chapter, the nurse will be able to:

1. Discuss factors related to distance and immediate receptors that influence spatial behavior.
2. Define the term *personal space* and relate its significance to care plan development for clients from varying cultures.
3. Explain how actions of the nurse may contribute to feelings of anxiety and loss of control for clients from transcultural backgrounds.
4. List actions the nurse can take to promote feelings of autonomy and self-worth when caring for clients from transcultural backgrounds.
5. Delineate the difference between tactile space and visual space and show their relationship to transcultural nursing care.

Personal space is the area that surrounds a person's body; it includes the space and the objects within the space. Personal space can also describe inner space that filters the incoming stimuli that a person receives (Scott & Dumas, 1995). Scott (1988) defines *inner personal space* as dynamic, invisible lines of demarcation that can be divided into four concentric areas of space: (1) the inner spirit core, (2) an area of thoughts and feelings perceived as unacceptable, (3) an area of thoughts and feelings perceived as acceptable, and (4) an area of superficial public image. An individual's comfort level is related to both inner and outer personal space; discomfort is experienced when personal space is invaded. Although personal space is an individual matter and varies with the situation, dimensions of the personal space comfort zone also vary from culture to culture (Davidhizar, Shearer, & Giger, 2002).

Traditionally, nursing research paid little attention to geographical approaches and the dynamics of nursing and space. However change is occurring and research is beginning on the relationship between nursing, space, and place as an emerging geography of nursing and a health geography sub-discipline (Andrews, 2003; Halford & Leonard,

2003). Andrews postulates that from a disciplinary perspective, studying the geography of nursing can explain the relationship between health geography and mainstream health service and medical concerns in a place-sensitive, patient-sensitive, and qualitative form (Andrews, 2002; Andrews & Andrews, 2003; Andrews and Phillips, 2002). Nevertheless, nurses have long drawn from the social science disciplines and appreciated that spatial behavior is an important consideration in measuring distance in relationships. Since spatial behavior is usually judged to be spontaneous and unintentional, individuals are typically more likely to trust the accuracy of actions rather than words as a reflection of true feelings. Although a large percentage of spatial behaviors are spontaneous and unintentional, communication in this domain can be managed to promote favorable and desired impressions. For example, a nurse may choose to stand when greeting a client to show respect.

To understand human behavior, one must understand something of the nature of our receptor systems and how the information received by these systems is modified by culture. Because spatial behavior is a response to sensory stimulation in the internal and the external environment, the phenomenon of space can be understood only as an integral part of the sensory systems, that is, sight, sound, touch, and smell. Spatial behavior encompasses a variety of behaviors, including proximity to others, objects in the environment, and movement.

PERCEPTION OF SPACE

Sensory apparatuses fall into two categories:

1. *Distance receptors* are concerned with the examination of distant objects. The sensory receptors for distance include the eyes, ears, and nose.
2. *Immediate receptors* are used to examine the world up close. Sensory receptors used to examine the world up close include touch, which is the sensation received from the skin membranes (Hall, 1969, 1977).

These two classifications can be broken down even further to facilitate the nurse's understanding of the phenomenon of space. For example, the skin is the chief organ of touch and is sensitive to heat gain and heat loss; both radiant and conducted heat are detected by the skin. Therefore, the skin must be perceived as both an immediate receptor and a distance receptor. (In general, there is a relationship between the evolutionary age of the receptor system and the amount and quality of information it can convey to the central nervous system.) Many psychologists estimate that the touch system is as old as life itself (Hall, 1966). Because the ability to respond to stimuli is based on touch, the response to touch is one of the basic criteria for the maintenance of life. In comparison, sight is believed to be the last and most specialized sense to develop in humans. From an anthropological view, vision became more important than olfactory response when our ancestors left the ground and took to trees in search of food and safety. Stereoscopic vision became essential for primitive humans because without it jumping from branch to branch was difficult and dangerous.

Distance Receptors

Distance receptors include sensory apparatuses for visual, auditory, and olfactory perception. It is essential that the nurse understand the relationship between sight, touch, and smell and how the reaction to these stimuli can be modified by culture.

Visual and Auditory Perception. As indicated earlier, vision was the last of the senses to evolve. However, it is by far the most complex. Seemingly, more data are fed to the nervous system through the eyes at a much greater rate than through the senses of touch or hearing. For example, the information a blind person can gather outdoors is limited to a circle of 20 to 100 feet because a blind person can perceive by way of auditory or olfactory stimuli only what is immediately surrounding him or her. However, with sight a person can see the stars if they are out. Even very talented blind persons are limited to an average speed of perception of 2 to 3 miles an hour over familiar territory. In contrast, with sight a person has to fly faster than sound before additional visual aids are needed to avoid bumping into things. The amount of information that can be gathered by the eyes as contrasted to the ears cannot be precisely calculated. Such a calculation would require not only a translation process but also the knowledge of precisely what to count. A general notion held by most scientists is that the relative complexities of the two systems, visual and auditory, can be obtained by comparison of the size of the nerves connecting the eyes and the ears to the centers of the brain (Brown, Leavitt, & Graham, 1977).

The optic nerve contains roughly 18 times as many neurons as the cochlear nerve; therefore, one might assume that it transmits at least that much more information. The eyes may act as a defense mechanism because they normally alert us to danger; the eyes may be as much as a thousand times more effective than the ears in gathering information to protect us from harmful stimuli. The area that the unaided ear can effectively cover in the course of daily living is quite limited. The ear is very efficient, but only up to a distance of 20 feet. At about 100 feet, one-way vocal communication is possible but at a somewhat slower rate than at a conversational distance. Although two-way conversation is also possible at this distance, it is considerably altered. Beyond this distance the auditory cues begin to break down rapidly. The unaided eye, on the other hand, can gather an extraordinary amount of information within a 100-yard radius and is efficient for human interaction at up to a mile (Hall, 1969).

The impulses that activate the eyes and the ears differ in speed and quality. For example, at a temperature of $0°$ C $(32°$ F$)$ at sea level, sound waves can travel 1100 feet per second and be heard in frequencies of 50 to 1500 cycles per second (Hertz). On the other hand, light rays can travel 186,000 miles (300,000 km) per second and thus are visible at a maximal frequency of 500 trillion at yellow-green (Hall, 1969).

Many complex and remarkable instruments have been invented to extend the eyes and ears. Radio, television, and the Internet have revolutionized the perception of space and shortened distances between people worldwide. During World War II, radio was relied on quite extensively to bring news from the occupied countries to parts of the free world. Perhaps one of the most famous broadcasts of this period was done by Tokyo Rose, whose broadcasts, which were reported to be untrue, influenced many people in the listening audience about the nature and direction of World War II. However, radio lacked the visual stimuli offered later by television, which filled in perception gaps left by radio. Television came of age in the 1960s, when for the first time, brighter, clearer, and bolder pictures were offered to viewers. The addition of color filled another perception gap and enhanced our receptor fields. For the first time in history, from their living rooms, the people of the United States could view their president doing the ordinary, the extraordinary, and the unusual. For example, the people of the United States were informed about the Cuban missile crisis by U.S. President Kennedy on television. They were also able to see this president playing with his children in the Oval Office. In 1963, when President Kennedy was assassinated, little was left to the imagination of the people of the United States, who were mesmerized by complete television coverage from assassination to burial. Because of television, the nation and the world at large experienced grief still present today and mourned collectively. The development of cyberspace technology has added another visual

dimension to space. On September 11, 2001, the nation and the world collectively experienced shock as terrorists crashed airplanes into the World Trade Center and the Pentagon. Not only did many view the disasters as they happened on television and on the Internet, but also horrific images and reports of the September 11th terrorist attacks were broadcast for weeks. Technology also allowed the world to visually see the emotional reactions of others to the disaster and in turn precipitated responses of condolence. Immediately, e-mail messages offering sympathy to grieving Americans poured in from friends around the world. Cyberspace technology united the world in grief as memorials on each continent were displayed on the Internet. The visual impressions provided by technology enabled persons who did not directly experience the disaster to be profoundly disturbed by it (Davidhizar & Shearer, 2002). In 2005, the nation experienced a similar phenomenon with the devastation of Hurricane Katrina that became a part of the lived experience of persons who had access to television or the Internet (Thomas, 2006). The Internet and multimedia technologies provide a range of quasi-public spaces that encouraged debate and active citizenship to assess the reaction of the government and the nation to this event (Thomas, 2006).

In summary, visual space has an entirely different character from that of auditory space. The overriding quality that differentiates visual space from auditory space is that visual information tends to be less ambiguous and more focused than auditory information. Therefore, visual information is less subject to external manipulation than is auditory information. One major exception to this rule is the blind person who has learned to understand selectively the higher audio frequencies, which can assist him or her in locating objects within a familiar or unfamiliar room. For example, a blind person may know where the door is in a room by the relationship of the sound that comes from that direction.

Even today it is not known what effects the incongruities between auditory and visual space have on individuals. Some data indicate that auditory space is a factor in performance. J.W. Black, a phonetician, demonstrated that the size and reverberation (vibrations of external sounds) of a room can affect an individual's reading rate. In a classic study, Black (1950) found that people read more slowly in larger rooms, where the reverberation time, or circulation of sound, is slower than that in smaller rooms. Hall (1966, 1969) interviewed subjects in regard to the slowing of reverberation time in a larger room. Among the interviewees was a gifted English architect who improved the performance of a malfunctioning committee by simply blending the auditory and visual worlds of the conference chamber where the committee met. The complaint the architect had received was that the chairman was inadequate and was about to be replaced. However, the architect had reason to believe that the difficulties this committee encountered were caused by more in the environment than just the chairman. In this situation the meeting room was next to a busy street, and traffic noises were intensified by reverberations from the hard walls and rugless floors inside the building and particularly in the meeting room. The architect was able to adjust the room by adding an acoustic ceiling, carpet, and soundproof walls. Once interferences were reduced, the chairman was able to conduct the meeting without undue strain, and complaints about the chairman ceased.

People who are brought up in different cultures learn unknowingly to screen out various bits of information and to sort information into relevant or irrelevant categories, and once set, these perceptual patterns remain stable throughout life. For example, Japanese individuals tend to give meaning to spaces that a Westerner may classify as empty (Gregg, 1996). Japanese readers expect to be presented with the parts first and then the whole rather than getting the "big picture" and then a breakdown of material into its component parts (Davidhizar, Dowd, & Bowen, 1998; Simply Stated, 1985). Additionally, Japanese people screen visually in a variety of ways and are more perceptive to visual stimuli. Japanese people are therefore perfectly content with paper walls as acoustic screens. A Westerner who finds himself in a Japanese inn where a party is going on next door may be in for a new sensory experience since only paper-thin walls separate each room. In contrast, German and Dutch people depend on double doors and thick walls to screen out sound and may have difficulty if they must rely on their own powers of concentration to do so. If two rooms are the same size and one screens out sound and the other one does not, a sensitive German or Dutch person who is trying to concentrate will feel less intruded on in the former and thus less crowded (Hall, 1966, 1969). Cultural patterning of space can also be seen in the arrangements of urban space in different cultures. For example, U.S. cities are usually laid out along a grid with the axis generally north-south and east-west. In Paris, main streets are laid out radiating from centers with no grid system (Gregg, 1996). The layout of French cities is only one aspect of the theme of centralization that characterizes French culture. In French offices, the most important person has the desk in the middle of the office.

Yet another aspect of cultural patterning of space is function of space. For example, space in India is sometimes related to concepts of superiority and inferiority. In Indian cities, villages, and even homes, spaces may be designated as inferior or polluted. Spaces in India are divided so that high and low castes, secular and sacred activities, and male and female can be kept segregated (Gregg, 1996).

Olfactory Perception. Some cultures place more importance on olfactory perceptions than do others. For example, Hall (1966, 1969) found Americans culturally underdeveloped in the use of their olfactory apparatuses. Hall (1966) contended that the deprivations of the olfactory stimulus are a result of the extensive use of deodorants and the suppression of odors in public places, which has resulted in a land of olfactory blandness and sameness that is difficult to duplicate anywhere else in the world.

People in the United States are continuously bombarded with commercials for room deodorizers, antiperspirants, mouthwashes, carpet deodorizers, and so on. All of these factors result in bland, undifferentiated spaces and deprive many people in the United States of the richness and variety of life. For example, if one is cooking with garlic, a room deodorizer may be used during the cooking process, causing the garlic smell to be eliminated. It is this type of behavior on the part of people of the United States that obscures memories. It is believed that smells evoke much deeper memories than either vision or sound; when the sound or the sight of what has happened has passed, the memory of the smell lingers on. Even today many U.S. citizens equate certain holidays, such as Christmas, with certain smells. For example, because Christmas is traditionally equated with the smell of baked goods, holly, pine, and fruit, today many people in the United States try to reproduce these smells at Christmas. An individual who has an artificial Christmas tree may buy a pine-scented spray to create the effects of a fresh tree. Another old-fashioned scent for many U.S. citizens is country potpourri, which has now been simulated in aerosol cans for easy dispensing. A new car odor can be simulated by a car spray that smells like new leather. Soap may be purchased to recreate a desired feeling; for example, the soap Mother used at home may create a feeling of hominess. Smells may also create a negative reaction; for example, an individual who washes with lye soap may be thought to have body odor because the smell is unusually strong and medicinal. A medicinal smell is perceived by most individuals in the United States to be appropriate for a hospital room but not elsewhere.

Odor is perhaps one of the most basic methods of communication. It is primarily chemical in nature and is therefore referred to in a chemical sense. The olfactory sense has diverse functions and not only differentiates individuals but also makes it possible to identify the emotional state of others. Even an infant can learn to identify his or her parents through the sense of smell. Although the young infant has not learned to see and discriminate patterns well, the infant can distinguish identity through the olfactory sense.

In a hospital setting an employee who has an unpleasant odor creates a real management dilemma. The supervisor may counsel and even reprimand the employee for poor hygiene. Employees who have the smell of alcohol may be sent home. It is important that the nurse appreciate that odors may be pathological, as in certain diabetic states,

or the result of certain mouthwashes or soaps. If a client has an unpleasant odor, the nurse should first assess whether some pathological condition is present, such as an inflammatory process. In a psychiatric hospital a client's odor could be associated with a condition such as schizophrenia, and although there is some thought that such an odor may be pathological, it is more likely to be related to a lack of motivation for self-care skills.

Immediate Receptors

Immediate receptors are those that examine the world up close, such as tactile stimuli received by way of the skin membranes. It is important that the nurse appreciate the effect culture may have on an individual's reaction to these stimuli and how these stimuli can be modified by cultural influences.

Skin Membranes. Human beings receive a tremendous amount of information from the distance receptors, which include the eyes, ears, and nose. Because of the vast amount of information that is received from the distance receptors, few people think of the skin as a major sense organ. However, if we humans lacked the ability to perceive heat and cold, we would soon perish. Without the ability to perceive heat and cold and to react appropriately to these stimuli, we would freeze in the winter and become overheated in the summer. The skin, as a major sense organ, is so grossly overlooked that even some of its subtle sensing and communicating qualities go unnoticed. Nerves called *proprioceptors* keep us informed as to exactly what is happening as we work our muscles. These nerves provide the feedback that enables us to move our bodies smoothly; thus they occupy a key position in kinesthetic space perception. The body also has another set of nerves called *exteroceptors,* which are located in the skin and convey the sensations of heat, cold, touch, and pain to the central nervous system. In light of the fact that two different systems of nerves are employed in the perception of space, kinesthetic space is considered qualitatively different from thermal space. However, nurses must remember that these two systems work together and are mutually reinforcing most of the time.

It has been only in modern scientific times that some remarkable thermal characteristics of the skin have been discovered. The capacity of the skin for emitting and detecting radiant or infrared heat is extraordinarily high. One might assume that is so because it was important to survival in the past and most certainly had a significant function in early human beings. Although the discovery of the thermal characteristics of the skin has been only within recent times, the nurse should not overlook the importance of the skin as an immediate receptor.

Humans are well equipped to send and receive messages concerning emotional states based on changes in skin temperature. Skin temperature can give very important clues to the emotional state of the individual. A common indicator of embarrassment or anger in fair-skinned individuals is blushing. However, dark-skinned people also blush. Therefore blushing cannot be perceived as simply a matter of change in skin coloration. The nurse must carefully observe dark-skinned persons when looking for changes in emotional state, such as embarrassment or anger, by noting a swelling of regions of the forehead. The additional blood to these areas will raise the temperature, and these areas will appear flushed. Therefore, even if there is no significant change in color to these areas in dark-skinned individuals, these areas will feel warm to the touch.

Many novel instruments have been developed to make it possible to study heat emission. These instruments should make it possible to study the thermal details of interpersonal communication, an area not previously accessible to direct observation. Thermographic devices (infrared-detection devices and cameras) that were originally developed for satellites and homing missiles have been used for recording subvisual phenomena. Photographs taken in the dark using radiant heat of the human body have shown that an inflamed area of the body actually emits more heat than the surrounding areas. Diagnosis of cancer is also possible with thermographic devices that measure blocked circulation of blood. Thermographic devices have been useful in health care delivery because skin color does not affect the amount of heat delivered; dark skin does

not emit more or less heat than light skin. Thus the observable phenomenon in all individuals regarding heat emission is the blood supply in a given area of the body.

Increased heat on the surface is detected in three ways:

1. Thermal detectors in the skin, particularly if two individuals are close enough to each other.
2. Intensified olfactory interactions, which are augmented when skin temperature rises. Perfumes and lotions may be smelled at a greater distance when the body temperature is increased.
3. Visual examination, which can give clues to an increase or decrease in body temperature. For example, an individual who is pale may have a decrease in body temperature, whereas a person who appears flushed may have an increase in body temperature.

Certain individuals or racial groups are more aware of subtle changes in skin temperature. In addition, some persons accentuate or take advantage of this medium of communication. For example, an individual knowledgeable about variations in skin temperature according to location may apply perfume to certain parts of the body. The phenomenon of crowding is a chain reaction set in motion when there is not enough space to dissipate the heat within a crowd and the heat intensifies. A hot crowd will require more room than a cool crowd if they are to maintain the same degree of comfort and lack of involvement. It is important for the nurse to remember that when thermal spaces overlap and people can smell each other, they become more involved and may even be under the chemical influences of each other's emotions. Some individuals by virtue of cultural heritage have trouble with the phenomenon of crowding. These individuals are more likely to be unable to sit in a chair soon after someone else has vacated it. An example of this phenomenon is often given by sailors on submarines who are forced to participate in "hot bunking," the practice of sharing a bunk as soon as someone gets out of it. It is not understood why one's own heat is not objectionable whereas a stranger's may be. It may be attributable in part to the fact that humans have a great sensitivity to small differences; therefore, individuals respond negatively to a heat pattern that is not familiar (Hall, 1966, 1969).

Body-heat regulation lies deep in the brain and is controlled by the hypothalamus. Culture affects attitudes in regard to the perception of skin temperature changes. Human beings exert little or no conscious control over the heat system of the body. Many cultural groups tend to stress phenomena that can be controlled and deny those that cannot. In other words, because some individuals by virtue of their cultural heritage have been taught to ignore certain uncontrollable stimuli, they experience body heat as a highly personal stimulus. Body heat is therefore linked to intimacy as well as to the experiences of childhood. An adult who as a child was used to close personal contact with parents and other loved ones may have a pleasant association when in a crowded environment where heat and warmth are radiated. On the other hand, an adult who was subjected to discomfort in close relationships or who was not exposed to closeness as a child may experience a great deal of difficulty and anxiety when in a close environment, for example, an overcrowded bus.

A person born in a heavily populated country where closeness was necessitated by overcrowding may experience conscious discomfort in moving to another locality where closeness is not the norm. On the other hand, persons born in thinly populated countries may have a conscious feeling of overcrowding in a country where closeness is the norm. For example, a tourist from the United States visiting a country such as Jamaica or China or a city such as Hong Kong, all of which are extremely overpopulated, may quickly react to the experience of closeness and associate the country or this particular city with unpleasantness. This experience is not limited to different cultures but may also be noted when a rural person visits an urban setting, such as a person from rural Mississippi visiting New York City.

The English language is full of expressions that relate to skin sensation and body temperature changes. For example, it is not uncommon in the United States to hear individuals say that another person made them hot under the collar, gave them a cold stare, involved them in a heated argument, or warmed them up. These expressions may be more than just a figure of speech; they may be a way of recognizing the changes in body temperature that occur both personally and in other people. Thus these common experiences have been incorporated into language in the United States.

Relationship Between Tactile Space and Visual Space

Touch and visual spatial experiences are so interwoven that they cannot be easily separated. Young children and infants learn to reach, grasp, fondle, and mouth everything in the environment. Teaching children the relationship between tactile and visual space is a difficult task that requires many years of training for children to subordinate the world of touch to the visual world. Visual and tactile space can be distinguished by the fact that tactile space separates the viewer from the object, whereas visual space separates objects from each other. As early as 1945, Michael Baliant described two different perceptual worlds: sight oriented and touch oriented. According to Baliant, the touch-oriented world is both immediate and friendlier than the sight-oriented world, in which space is friendly but filled with dangerous and unpredictable objects, namely, people. Using Baliant's definition of tactile space, it is difficult to conceive that designers and engineers have failed to grasp in all of their scientific research the deep significance of touch, particularly active touch (actually contacting others or objects). Individuals incorporate both tactile and visual stimuli in relating to the world. For example, although automakers tend to rely heavily on visual perception when designing a particular car, they are also concerned with tactile perception, as evidenced by their attention to such things as luxury upholstery, automatic windows, doors, gas-cap locks, ornate trimmings, and carpeting. In response to such stimuli, prospective buyers touch both the car's interior and exterior before making a purchase.

Some objects in the environment are appraised and appreciated almost entirely by touch, even when these objects are visually presented, such as objects made from wood, cloth, or ceramics. The Japanese are very conscious of the significance of texture. Emphasis is placed on the smoothness of the item being crafted. It may be perceived that it requires more time to make a smooth-textured item than a rough-textured item and that the time spent on the crafted item is related to the care and concern of the craftsman. The objects that are produced by Japanese people may be perceived as being made by caring craftsmen.

Touch is the most personal of all the sensations. Touch is sometimes described as the most important sense because it confirms the reality perceived through the other senses (Montagu, 1986). As discussed in Chapter 2, touch is central to the human communication process and is often used to communicate messages. Touch is a part of most intimate relationships, which are increasingly recognized as integral to health. While relationships can exist without touch, distance creates loneliness, which has been related to lack of health (Cacioppo, Ernst, Burleson, et al., 2000). James Lynch, author of *The Broken Heart: The Medical Consequences of Loneliness,* noted that there is a cardioprotective nature of community life and loving relationships (Lynch, 1998). In fact, studies have found that loneliness at the time of surgery is a contributor to death at both 30 days and 5 years following coronary artery bypass grafting and that the recurrent cardiac event rate at 6 months after initial myocardial infarction was significantly higher among those who lived alone (Herlitz, Wiklund, Caidahl, et al., 1998; Case, Moss, Case, McDermott, & Eberly, 1992). Positive intimate relationships increase longevity, lower morbidity, and increase personal happiness (Giorgianni, 2000).

In contrast to tactile space is the phenomenon of visual space. To understand visual space, the nurse must understand that people do not see exactly the same thing when actively using their eyes in a natural situation; people do not relate to the world around them in exactly the same way. For example, different persons will visually notice different objects because of perceptual differences (Davidhizar, Dowd, & Giger, 1997). It is important for the nurse to recognize these differences and at the same time be able to translate from one perceptual world to another. The distance between the perceptual worlds of two persons of the same culture may be considerably less than the distance between the perceptual worlds of two persons of different cultures. There is significant evidence that people brought up in different cultures live in different perceptual worlds. North Americans tend to have a more linear perceptual field. This difference is demonstrated in art and architectural design. American artists prefer designs that are linear, whereas Chinese and Japanese artists prefer depth and maintaining constancy in a design.

SPATIAL BEHAVIOR

Spatial behavior is often described in nursing literature in relation to the universal need for territoriality (Allekian, 1973; Brant, 1983; Davidhizar, 1988; Davidhizar & Giger, 1998; Oland, 1978). People by nature are territorial. Territoriality refers to a state characterized by possessiveness, control, and authority over an area of physical space. If the need for territoriality is to be met, the person must be in control of some space and must be able to establish rules for that space. The need for territoriality cannot be fully met unless individuals can defend their space against invasion or misuse by others (Roberts, 1978). Hayter (1981) has suggested three important aspects of territoriality to consider when planning nursing care: a physical space of one's own, a personal space, and the territory of expertise or role. One can also relate territoriality needs to spatial behaviors of or proximity to others, to objects in the environment, and to body movement or position. Territoriality serves to achieve diverse functions for individuals, including meeting needs for security, privacy, autonomy, and self-identity. Group rights must also be considered in relation to space. In cultures where priority is given to the group over the individual (Asian cultures, many Latino and Mediterranean cultures, most Arab cultures, and cultures of Africa and the Middle East), group rights and shared space are important considerations. In cultures where priority is given to the individual rather than the group (United States,

Canada, cultures of North and West Europe, Australia, and New Zealand), privacy is more likely to be valued (Goldman & Schmalz, 2005). In a culture where priority is given to the individual, a person may choose to be alone when feeling ill or in pain (Davidhizar & Hart, 2005). Palos, a multicultural researcher at the Department of Symptom Research at the University of Texas M.D. Anderson Cancer Center and School of Public Health in Houston, states that finding 20 relatives at the bedside arises out of the concept of collectivity rather than polarity and may be a strange concept to health care professionals oriented to the biomedical model based on autonomy (Kaegi, 2004). It is important for the nurse to understand the effect such variables may have on spatial behavior and the ethical implications (Piaschenko, 1997).

Proximity to Others

Proxemics is the term for the study of human use and perception of social and personal space (Hall, 1974). Individuals tend to divide surrounding space into regions of front, back, right, and left (Franklin, Henkel, & Zangas, 1995). The front region is considered the most important, is the largest, is recalled with the greatest precision, and is described with the greatest detail. Proxemics has been shown to allow one to predict self-esteem and self-evaluative moods, even after controlling for the contribution of the personality dimensions of neuroticism, extroversion, and agreeableness (Hart, Field, Garfinkle, & Singer, 1997). Physical distancing from others varies with setting and is culturally learned (Murray & Huelskoetter, 1991). Generally, in Western culture there are three primary dimensions of space: the intimate zone (0 to 18 inches), the personal zone (18 inches to 3 feet), and the social or public zone (3 to 6 feet) (Hall, 1966). The intimate zone may be used for comforting, protecting, and counseling and is reserved for people who feel close. The personal zone usually is maintained with friends or in some counseling interactions. Touch can occur in the intimate and personal zones. The social zone is usually used when impersonal business is conducted or with people who are working together. Sensory involvement and communication are often

less intense in the social zone. Wide variations to these general dimensions do occur and are often influenced by cultural background (Giger & Davidhizar, 1990). Montagu (1986) has suggested that childrearing practices affecting sleep behavior may have an effect on the use of space, especially as it determines acceptable interaction distance. He reported on varying cultural approaches apparently related to family group sleeping arrangements and the Western middle-class practice of separating the child from parents for sleep. According to Oland (1978), the Western practice of putting small children in a room of their own, which separates them from other family members, may enculturate children to desire isolation and separation and cause or facilitate a desire for more extensive territory.

Among the Eskimos and Northern Indians of Canada, the practice of separate bedrooms varies dramatically because living quarters are often small, with all persons sleeping in the same room (Burke, Maloney, Pothaar, & Baumgart, 1988; Giger & Davidhizar, 1998; Young, 1988). For these individuals, proximity to others in small living quarters is often a necessity for survival since staying inside and near the body heat of others may be necessary to avoid freezing in the frigid arctic temperatures. The need for space also varies for many Southeast Asian immigrants who have come to the United States as refugees. These individuals are also accustomed to living in crowded living situations. Therefore, for some Southeast Asian Americans, spacious living accommodations may cause discomfort (Van Esterik, 1980). Sinha and Mukherjee (1996) investigated college students at Dayalbagh, India, and noted that more roommates led to larger space requirements, decreased tolerance for crowding, and a more negative attitude toward room environment. However, high cooperation among roommates moderated the effects of crowding. Walkey and Gilmour (1984) noted that a preferred interpersonal distance score in inmates was effective in predicting prison fighting behavior with a 71% degree of success.

Spatial needs and the desire for a certain proximity to certain people continue through life and have been studied in the elderly. In nursing homes, elderly clients may have certain chairs identified as theirs and become upset when a stranger sits in that chair or in the seat nearby that is reserved for a special friend. Moving from household to household to stay with adult children on a rotating basis, rather than being viewed as a pleasant variation, is also likely to be upsetting to older people. Since the elderly are more likely to experience separation from others through the death of a spouse and the moving away of offspring, their spatial needs may appear to change; that is, they may withdraw or may reach out more for others (Ittelson, Proshansky, Rivlin, & Winkel, 1974).

Interpersonal messages are communicated not only by body proximity but also by the location and availability of the nurse during the day. A client who knows that the nurse will answer when the call bell is pressed feels differently from the client who does not understand how the call bell works or feels that it is an imposition to ask for help and waits for the nurse to ask what can be done (Schuster & Ashburn, 1992).

Individuals have different requirements for sensory stimulation. Either overstimulation, as by crowding, or understimulation, as by isolation, may cause an untoward reaction. For example, in times of disaster, overstimulation induced by crowding can be so extreme that it can result in insanity or death. In this example, a person is perceived as being in a little black box and unable to move about freely, which causes the person to jostle, push, and shove. How the individual responds to jostling and therefore to the enclosed space depends on how he or she feels about being touched by strangers. It is this constant touching and being touched that may result in widespread panic and "freezing" in disaster situations (Hall, 1966).

An enclosed space requirement can also be overstimulating. For example, a client who must remain in a hospital room in bed and in isolation for a lengthy period can be overstimulated because of the spatial limits presented by the boundaries, including bed rest and the four walls of the room. Nursing interventions for this client include opening curtains, frequently calling by intercom to check

on the client, and stopping by to see the client as often as possible. A client in isolation can suffer from understimulation in regard to tactile stimulation. The few people who do enter the room may hesitate to touch the client out of fear of contracting the illness. One of the greatest problems expressed by clients with acquired immunodeficiency syndrome (AIDS) is the isolation they experience because of physical distance from others. Family members afraid of catching AIDS may hesitate to touch, hug, or kiss the AIDS victim. Caregivers also may show their fear by standing a greater distance from the client, wearing gloves, and having less frequent encounters with the client (Zook & Davidhizar, 1989). How individuals perceive and interact with HIV risk varies by a myriad of social, contextual, and setting-related issues (Brown & Maycock, 2005). The strong link between curing, the major focus of health care, and caring by health care practitioners has been emphasized by Leininger and McFarland (2006), who cite touch as one of the special constructs of the caring process. As a therapeutic element of human interaction, touch can help the nurse to show caring. Marx, Wener, and Cohen-Mansfield (1989) noted a divergent response to touch among elderly in a nursing home. For some, touching was interpreted as a violation of personal space, while at other times touching was perceived as a comforting form of communication.

Today, the image of the nurse as someone standing close to the bedside and having physical proximity is changing. Within the wider discourse of fiscal restraint on health care spending, professional nurses need not be in physical proximity for meanings to be generated, to be acted upon, and to have effects in the present. Modern technology is redefining the need for physical proximity. The needs of modern health care are redefining where the nurse's presence needs to be to accomplish the needs of professional nursing (Purkis, 1996).

Cultural Implications

Watson (1980) noted that although there are variations in spatial requirements from person to person, individuals in the same cultural group tend to act similarly. For example, nomads do not seem to desire a permanent territory but are content with establishing a temporary territory and then moving on. Because individuals are usually not consciously aware of their personal space requirements, they frequently have difficulty understanding a different cultural pattern. What may be considered an act of friendliness by one person (such as standing close to another person) may be perceived by the other as a threatening invasion of personal space. A person who wishes to maintain distance will indicate this by body language. Clients who step back, do not face the nurse directly, or pull their chair back from the nurse are sending messages indicating additional space requirements. The nurse's responsiveness to the client's spatial requirements is an important factor in the client's emotional comfort. It is important that the nurse be cognizant of the effects of culture on the client's spatial needs and use sensitivity in responding to the client's need for personal territory. Subtle cultural variations in the use of nonverbal signals often lead to misunderstanding; thus, to meet the client needs, it is essential that the nurse have knowledge of cultural variations in spatial requirements.

Nurses and clients from the population groups of American Indians, Appalachians, Japanese Americans, and Mexican Americans often find a comfortable position between the personal and social distance (Tripp-Reimer & Lively, 1993). Watson (1980) studied cultural differences in the use of personal space. He compiled a range of space by nationality and found that persons in the United States, Canadians, and the British require the most personal space, whereas Latin Americans, Japanese, and Arabic persons need the least. These latter groups seemingly have a much higher tolerance for crowding in public spaces than some other cultural groups, such as North Americans and northern Europeans, but they also appear to be more concerned about their own requirements for the space they live in. In particular, the Japanese tend to devote more time and attention to the proper organization of their living space for perception by all the senses (Hall, 1966). Asians are generally more sensitive to personal space and are more likely

to feel comfortable conversing from a distance of 5 or 6 feet. Maintaining distance for some Asian Americans is an indication of respect. Therefore, it is important to remember to avoid invading the personal space of these individuals. Some West Indians maintain little space between friends when communicating, but for some West Indians, an outsider is expected to maintain some distance when interacting (Carson, 2000). Arab Americans value modesty and privacy, particularly with strangers. Comfort and personal disclosure are increased if the care provider is of the same sex (Davidhizar & Giger, 2002; Giger, Davidhizar, & Wieczorek, 1993; Meleis, 2006).

A White American female nurse from a nontactile culture may experience discomfort when a male client from a tactile culture, such as the Latin American, African-American, or Indonesian cultures, stands in the intimate zone while describing symptoms (Rawlins, Williams, & Beck, 1993; Tripp-Reimer & Friedl, 1977). Touching between persons of the same sex, including men, is more common among Arabs than it is among Americans. However, among some Asian cultures, touch between women is less common. For example, in some Asian cultures women do not shake hands with each other or with men (Randall-David, 1989). In the United States the kind of familiarity common among Arabs may be considered a homosexual pass (Hall, 1966). Hall and Whyte (1990) note that a handshake in Latin America, particularly between two men, is seen as cold and impersonal. For some Latins, the *doble abrazo,* in which two men embrace by placing their arms around each other's shoulders is the accepted form of greeting. On the other hand, touching the shoulders of a Japanese man is seen as a humiliation and an unpardonable breach of traditional etiquette. Argyle and Dean (1965) reported that members of some societies in Africa and Indonesia also came closer and maintained body contact during conversation.

Abuse and violence involve intrusion on the physical, personal, or cognitive space (verbal functioning or mental strategizing) of another. However, violence is interpreted in a cultural context and according to cultural norms (Burlae, 2004).

Wife beatings may not be considered abuse in some cultures. Violence can be more subtle. A contemptuous boss may give a female employee an office in the basement or a desk in a public area while male employees have private offices near the employer. This invasion of space carries with it an innuendo that can lead to violence (Burlae, 2004).

In the Thai and Vietnamese cultures, the head is sacred, and patting the head of a small child is considered offensive. For these individuals the head is considered to be the "seat of life." When the head is touched, it is believed that the spirit leaves through this channel. Therefore, when the head needs to be touched for medical reasons, it is important to explain the reason and to ask permission of the adults (Carson, 2000; Randall-David, 1989).

In the United States, a person who stands at a slight angle to another person indicates a body position of readiness to communicate. A desire to exclude a third person can be shown by two persons who face each other directly and have ongoing eye contact. Rejection is also communicated by a person who stands at a right angle to another (Scheflen & Scheflen, 1972). The position of the toes can create distance by communicating rank. A person who feels subordinate will usually stand with the toes inward, whereas a person who feels superior will stand with the toes facing out (*Personal Report*, 1987). A comparison of the movie shown in the United States, *Three Men and a Baby,* and the French comedy on which it was based, *Three Men and a Cradle,* illustrates the differences in responses in the two cultures. In the French version, when the natural father returns to the two bachelors who have been inconvenienced by the care of the baby, icy silence occurs. The two men sit stiffly in their chairs and refuse to answer their friend's questions or even acknowledge his presence. In the version seen in the United States, when the natural father returns, he is pummeled and a loud scene occurs (Grosvenor, 1989).

Territoriality influences relationships between people. Some German people tend to need a larger space and are less flexible in their spatial behavior than some American, French, and Arab people.

Differences in spatial patterns between persons in different cultures apply not only to their body proximity but also to such behavior as changing geographic location. For example, Germans often live in the same house their entire lives, whereas Americans tend to change houses approximately every 5 years, and nomads are content with temporary territories rather than permanent ones. According to Evans and Howard (1973), some Puerto Ricans and African-Americans may have different perspectives about space. Some African-Americans have more eye contact when they speak, have greater body activity, and have a closer personal space (Sue & Sue, 2003). However, as indicated in Chapter 2, some African-Americans have been socialized through a long history of hostile, punitive interactions with Whites to avoid direct eye contact. This behavior may also influence personal space zones (Giger, Davidhizar, Evers, & Ingram, 1994).

OBJECTS IN THE ENVIRONMENT

Objects in the environment offer additional dimensions to communication and can provide both positive and negative qualifiers to verbal communication. Easily movable chairs in a waiting room or office can be pulled together to provide physical closeness or separated to provide distance. Positioning chairs at a 90-degree angle can communicate a cooperative stance, whereas a side-by-side arrangement of chairs can decrease communication. Discomfort and, consequently, emotional distance can be created by uncomfortable furniture. The nurse's position during the conversation (such as sitting behind a desk or leaning against the corner of the desk while looking down on the client seated at a lower level) can also promote the perception of psychological distance. Health care icons, such as stethoscope, name tag, uniform, a nurse's cap, or a lab coat, are also objects that can convey a message to the client about the nurse's authority (Bechtel & Davidhizar, 1998). However, all icons can have positive and negative associations for different individuals—for example, a stethoscope can be associated with a person who cares for a patient, or it may be associated with a stranger who invades personal space (Andrews, 2003). The nurse must be aware of the effect culture may play on the client's reaction to objects in the environment and should respond in a way that increases client comfort. The nurse dealing with Eskimos should appreciate the value Eskimos place on objects they possess. These individuals tend to highly value generosity and a sense of sharing, as in "What is mine is here for all." For some of these people, only what is needed for the present is taken and used. This can be a problem for the Eskimo who is diabetic because if food is available, it will be shared with anyone, regardless of the special health needs (Davidhizar & Giger, 2000).

Cleanliness in the environment may also be a significant factor in creating a healthy and comfortable milieu. This is particularly true in surgical areas, where space is used in designing a physical layout that will allow for maintaining aseptic technique (Fox, 1997). Comfortable air conditioning in a client waiting room on a hot day can facilitate a client's ease and decrease anxiety. On the other hand, when the air conditioning is absent or malfunctioning on a hospital ward on a hot day, client and staff anxiety can escalate.

Structural Boundaries

The term *personal boundaries* is sometimes used to describe the use of structural boundaries in the environment. A boundary separates a person from others and also helps define a person's space. Fences, doors, curtains, walls, desks, chairs, and other objects may create boundaries between persons (Scott, 1988). The purpose of a boundary is to facilitate individuation or separation from the environment. Developmentally, this concept begins at approximately 6 months of age. Mahler, Pine, and Bergman (1975) described an infant's first attempts at separation or individuation as behaviors such as pulling at the parent's hair, ears, or nose and pushing the body away from the parent to get a better look at him or her. At 7 to 8 months of age the infant begins to differentiate self from the parent. The child may examine the parent's jewelry or glasses and is anxious around others. These crucial developmental steps are indicative of the child's beginning formation of boundary, which

continues through the toddler stage. By 3 years of age the toddler has a fairly stable sense of identity and self-boundaries.

Doors, walls, glass panels, and waist-high partitions serve as structural boundaries for nurses' territories in health care settings. Doors, curtains, and furniture arrangements may define client territories. Structural boundaries can help the individual adapt to both internal and external stresses. On the other hand, when structural boundaries are violated, anxiety may increase. The nurse needs to assess whether the client has rigid or flexible boundaries. If a client has open boundaries, less anxiety will be encountered in interactions with health professionals that may violate personal boundaries. If the client has rigid boundaries, the nurse should guard against approaches that may be perceived as threatening.

The use of restraints with agitated clients involves physical invasion of both intimate space and body boundaries. Patients who resist restraints and become aggressive and combative may be viewed as resisting this personal invasion.

Just as individuals can be described by personal boundaries that determine comfort levels in relation to others, territoriality also describes an interpersonal phenomenon in the environment. As indicated earlier, territoriality is a state characterized by possessiveness, control, and authority over an area of physical space (Hayter, 1981). For the need for territoriality to be met fully, the person must be in control of some space, be able to establish rules for that space, and be able to defend it against invasion or misuse by others. In addition, the person's right to do things in the space must be acknowledged by others (Roberts, 1978). For example, a hospitalized client needs not only a personal sleeping area but also a place to put and arrange personal belongings without fear that they will be disturbed by others. The nurse should respect patient privacy and knock before entering the room (Stuart, 2005).

Nurses also have professional territorial imperatives. Nurses' stations and lounges may be designated as staff territory. When a psychiatric unit is renovated and the staff are asked by administration to change from a locked-nursing station to an open-nursing station so that clients may come to an open half wall to interact openly with staff who may be inside, the staff may find this very intrusive of "their" territory and object to this invasion of their space. Nursing staff may also fear personal assault (Croker & Cummings, 1995; Roberts, 1989, 1991). McMahon (1994) noted that, for psychiatric staff, space in the ward office serves several significant functions, including the opportunity for informal contact between nurses and a place to have a liaison with visiting professionals, to store possessions, to provide a "patient-free" zone, and to serve as a communication center. Staff needs for territory must be considered when unit staff and clients' areas are designed. Restricting certain staff from certain hospital areas (such as the mailroom or the copy machine room) may be seen as punitive and dehumanizing. Thus it is essential that explanations given for this restriction be clearly understood to avoid paranoid interpretations of this action.

Cultural Implications

Color is a phenomenon with cultural implications. In many North American cultures, warm colors such as yellow, red, and orange tend to stimulate creative and happy responses. In some Asian countries, white is associated with a funeral. In many African countries, red symbolizes witchcraft and death (Carson, 2000). In the dominant culture in the United States, good mental health is often associated with the ability to coordinate the color of one's wardrobe (Ramírez, 1991). In contrast, in some countries, including those in Africa, the Caribbean, and the South Pacific, bright, multiple colors are the accepted norm of dress (Carson, 2000). Leff and Isaacs (1996) noted that a scarf tied around the forehead may not indicate "royalty" or schizophrenia but the cultural response by a West Indian to a headache. In Western culture, cool colors such as blue, green, and gray tend to encourage meditation and deliberation and thus may have a dampening effect on communication. The nurse should plan color in the environment to be therapeutic in an effort to enhance communication (Bartholet, 1968; Mufford, 1992).

For clients who have a chronic disability with difficulty in moving, it is important that space in the living environment be arranged to maximize power and use of resources (Moss, 1997). Access and ability to negotiate space in the living environment can be critical to quality of life and maximum independence (Useh, Moyo, & Munyonga, 2001). Space can also be used to promote health. Andersen, Franckowiak, Snyder, Bartlett, and Fontaine (1998) reported that signs promoting the health and weight-control benefits of stair use as a community intervention significantly increased the physical activity of 17,901 persons in a shopping mall. However, more lean persons as compared with overweight persons, and more Whites than Blacks, changed their behavior as a result of the sign intervention.

BODY MOVEMENT OR POSITION

Body movement or position can also communicate a message to others. This concept has been well documented by the pioneering work of Efron (1941), Birdwhitstell (1970), Scheflen and Scheflen (1972), Ekman and Friesen (1975), and Ekman (2001) and by recent reviews of the state of the art in this field (Bull, 1983; Davis, 1975; Davis & Skupien, 1982; Hickson & Stacks, 2002; Leathers, 1997; Wolfgang, 1984). This information has also been applied to counseling and psychotherapeutic techniques through the work of Moreno (1946), Gendlin (1969), Steere (1982), Marcus (1985), and Perls, Hefferline, and Goodman (1983), all of whom made body movement and awareness central aspects of their therapeutic approach. Thus, a broad body of knowledge supports the premise that through body movement a person may convey what is not verbalized.

It is well known that body movements may be of particular importance during periods of stress. Expressions of self through movement are learned before speech; therefore, when stress is experienced, a person may revert to a form of expression used at an earlier level. Attention to body movement can facilitate understanding of a person experiencing stress. There are endless expressions of body movement, such as finger pointing, head nodding, smiles, slaps on the back, head and general body movements, and even body sounds, including belching, knuckle cracking, and laughing. A seemingly insignificant act, such as how a doorbell is rung, may bear the stamp of an individual's personality, as well as an emotional state. For example, the doorbell may be rung loudly, impatiently, repetitively, tentatively, feebly, or aggressively (Bendich, 1988).

The nurse must also consider the effect of slow versus fast movements (Newman, 1976). In an emergency, rapid movements are essential. On the other hand, a young child in the hospital for the first time may be frightened by a health professional who enters the room quickly, approaches the child rapidly, and immediately picks up the child. In another situation, an agitated psychiatric client who is approached slowly and with a quiet voice may be calmed by the slow movements of the nurse, which are seen as reassuring.

Nurses are also exploring movement as a therapeutic medium, such as movement therapy for the aged (Goldberg & Fitzpatrick, 1980; Stevenson, 1989), movement therapy after inactivity or infection (Folta, 1989; Kasper, 1989), dance and movement therapy, and exercise to music. It has been thought that movement therapy can provide a way to communicate when the ability to communicate feelings is limited. Movement therapy has also been used for relaxation and to provide relief of blocked emotion.

Body motions, or kinetic behaviors, can be categorized as follows (Knapp & Hall, 1992):

1. *Emblems.* Nonverbal actions that have a verbal translation into a word, phrase, or symbol. They include sign language used in the operating room or the gesture of thumb and forefinger to form a circle to say "A-OK" in the United States or to indicate an obscenity in Brazil.
2. *Affect displays.* Facial expressions, such as a frown, a smile, or lips pulled down at the corners.
3. *Illustrations.* Nonverbal acts accompanying speech. Examples include an upturned thumb to indicate that a ride is desired or pointing a finger to indicate a direction.
4. *Adapters.* Nonverbal behavior that modifies or adds to what is being said. For example, folded arms may indicate disgust or that a person is feeling closed to others; a wave may be used as a friendly greeting; leg swinging and finger tapping may indicate anxiety.
5. *Regulators.* Movements that maintain interaction and provide feedback. Head nods or changing gaze can indicate that it is the other person's turn to talk. A head nod can also indicate listening.

Cultural Implications

Body movement is also related to culture. For example, in the United States head nodding is common, whereas in Africa the torso is frequently moved (Eibl-Eibesfeldt, 1972). Gestures are used by Americans and the British to denote activity and by Italian or Jewish persons to emphasize words (Bigham, 1964). In some cultures, certain actions are not considered proper with strangers, such as touching, standing close to, or looking directly at the individual. Some cultures give certain body movements a sexual interpretation. In the Western culture, stroking the hair, adjusting the clothes, or changing position to accent maleness or femaleness may have or be given a sexual connotation (Scheflen & Scheflen, 1972). Although a kiss is often given a sexual connotation in the United States, the Japanese kiss to show deference to superiors (Sue & Sue, 1999). When Brazilian clients were compared with American clients for space and motion discomfort in relation to anxiety disorders, a country bias was noted. Brazilian clients were more likely than American clients to endorse symptoms, thus showing a transcultural bias (Romas, Jacob, & Lilienfeld, 1997).

IMPLICATIONS FOR NURSING CARE

Nurses can create a healing environment by influencing a client's inner personal space as well as by creating a therapeutic outer space for the client to occupy (Birx, 2002). It is important for the nurse to remember that the need for space serves four functions: security, privacy, autonomy, and self-identity (Oland, 1978). The nurse needs an understanding of cultural diversity and culturally appropriate behaviors in relation to these functions. Security includes actual safety from harm and giving the person a feeling of being safe. The nurse must also remember that if a client is in a place where a feeling of control is experienced, the client will feel safer, less threatened, and less anxious (Sheeshka, Potter, Norrie, et al., 2001). People generally tend to feel safer in their own territory because it is arranged and equipped in a familiar manner. In addition, most people believe there is a degree of predictability associated with being in one's own personal space and that this degree of predictability is hard to achieve elsewhere. Nurses must also remember that the anxiety level of a client is increased when the client is hospitalized. However, the same client may experience a decrease in anxiety if the client is allowed to return home, even if still sick. Some terminally ill clients request to go home because of the feeling of security experienced in one's own personal space.

In addition to security, personal space provides privacy and at the same time protected communication. Most people believe it is not necessary to be on guard or to keep up pretenses—not be themselves—in the security of one's personal space. The fulfillment of the desire to be oneself contributes to feelings of decreased anxiety and promotes relaxation. Many people may complain of feeling tense and tired after a long day at work but may experience relaxation and ease of tension as soon as they get home. Contributing to these feelings are the fact that activities at home are different from those at work and that people experience more relaxation in their personal space (Hayter, 1981). In some instances, hospital staff members tend to treat elevators as private space and make inappropriate comments while riding back and forth on them. Hospital employees need to be very careful to consider certain hospital locations, such as elevators, as public spaces and to guard against violation of client privacy (Ubel, Zell, Miller, et al., 1995). If it becomes necessary to transfer a client from one room to another or from one floor to another, the nurse should remember that the client may

experience increased anxiety because of the loss of security and privacy of the room to which the client has become accustomed (Smith, 1976). This feeling of loss of security and privacy can also be related to nursing practice. For example, a nurse manager who returns from vacation to find office furniture rearranged may feel unsettled until the furniture is returned to a familiar arrangement. The nurse should remember that clients may already be experiencing feelings of anxiety that are related to the reasons for seeking health care. Additional anxiety invoked by issues involving territoriality can be minimized by the nurse who develops an understanding of culture and its implications for territoriality or interpersonal space.

Another important aspect of territoriality for nurses is the function of autonomy. Autonomy is the means by which a person controls what happens. In personal territory a person may feel free to ask questions, resist suggested actions, hold out for those things that are most important personally, and share personal feelings. A client, on the other hand, is out of personal territory and lacks control. Therefore, it is important for the nurse to determine if the client has an adequate understanding of the treatment regimen and is not submitting to treatment merely because of a lack of control of territory. Statements to the client that maximize feelings of control, such as "How do you want to arrange the room?" or "Are you concerned about your treatment? We can walk down the hall to the visiting room, where it is private, to discuss your feelings" should promote feelings of security and autonomy for the client. Feelings of autonomy are also evidenced in nursing practice. For example, when a nurse manager needs to counsel an employee, the manager's control will be maximized if the counseling occurs in the manager's office. On the other hand, a manager who is viewed as too controlling may intentionally select a more neutral territory for the counseling, such as a conference room.

It is essential to remember that having personal space promotes self-identity by affording opportunities for self-expression and that personal well-being is often related to the critical distance a person keeps from others (Giger & Davidhizar, 2001; Giger, Davidhizar, Johnson, & Poole, 1997; Wilson & Kneisl, 1995). Another way to define self-identity in relation to personal space is to view self-identity as a mode of individuality. The personal space over which a person has jurisdiction often becomes a personal extension of self and a reflection of characteristics, personality, and interest. A nurse may communicate warmth and reduce feelings of anxiety by moving close to a client. On the other hand, rapidly moving toward an anxious client may dramatically increase the client's anxiety. People have a need to organize and arrange personal space so that it maximizes functioning and at the same time meets needs. For example, when a person purchases a new home, it becomes essential for that home to take on the person's identity. This is evidenced by the desire of the new occupants to change such items as the wallpaper, colors of the walls, carpet, lighting fixtures, and draperies. Regardless of whether these items are new, each person has a need for self-expression or individuality. When clients set out personal pictures of their family and other personal items from home and wear their own sleepwear, self-identity is enhanced. Therefore, changing items to reflect this individuality becomes an essential aspect of personal security and autonomy. Self-identity is also created by the nurse when he or she is negotiating symbolic space.

Case Study

Mr. Bernhard Wolfgang, a 56-year-old German immigrant who works as an engineer, is admitted with chest pain and shortness of breath. Mr. Wolfgang is admitted to the coronary care unit to rule out myocardial infarction. Immediately after admission, Mr. Wolfgang's wife comes to the coronary care unit with personal items such as family portraits, some roses from the client's garden, and some personal clothing. However, since the coronary care unit is restricted in space, personal items are not allowed, and the wife is instructed to take the items home. On admission, Mr. Wolfgang's vital signs are stable and his color is good. He reports that the chest pain is not debilitating and is more or less an occasional dull ache. After 2 days the diagnosis of myocardial infarction is confirmed, and Mr. Wolfgang remains restricted to bed but is transferred to a semiprivate room in the coronary care step-down unit. After admission to the coronary care step-down unit, the nurse observes that Mr. Wolfgang is anxious, somewhat withdrawn, and unable to express his needs and feelings.

STUDY QUESTIONS

1. When assessing Mr. Wolfgang, the nurse should realize that some German people have specific needs that are related to territoriality and space. Name at least two factors that affect some Germans and their spatial behavior.
2. List ways the nurse could enable Mr. Wolfgang to meet his needs for privacy and autonomy while in a semiprivate room.
3. Identify markers that would indicate Mr. Wolfgang's need for the establishment of a temporary territorial space.
4. Identify ways in which illness and hospitalization could threaten Mr. Wolfgang's personal sense of territoriality.
5. Identify factors present in a coronary care unit that could negatively affect spatial behavior.
6. List two factors related to perceptual and visual stimuli that adversely affect some German clients.
7. List ways the nurse could control perceptual and verbal stimuli that may affect Mr. Wolfgang.

NCLEX-RN REVIEW QUESTIONS

1. Encouraging clients to set out personal items and wear their own sleep wear is a means of promoting:
   A. Personal space
   B. Self-identity
   C. Visual space
   D. Autonomy

2. In the Vietnamese culture, because touching the head has specific meaning, before measuring the head circumference of a child, the nurse should:

A. Explain the procedure and ask permission of the parent.
B. Play a game with the child.
C. Provide privacy by pulling the curtains.
D. Sit the child on the parent's lap.

3. When assessing an Asian client the best way to obtain information is to:
   A. Use an interest approach to get information.
   B. Ask question through an interpreter.
   C. Ask family members to answer question.
   D. Ask short-answer questions.

References

Allekian, C. E. (1973). Intrusions of territory and personal space. *Nursing Research*, 22, 236–241.

Andersen, R., Franckowiak, S., Snyder, J., Bartlett, S., & Fontaine, K. (1998). Can inexpensive signs encourage the use of stairs? Results from a community intervention. *Annals of Internal Medicine*, 129, 363–369.

Andrews, G. (2002). Towards a more place-sensitive nursing research: An invitation to medical and health geography. *Nursing Inquiry*, 9(4), 221–238.

Andrews, G. (2003). Locating a geography of nursing: Space, place and the progress of geographical thought. *Nursing Philosophy*, (4), 231–248.

Andrews, G. J. P., & Andrews, G. J. (2003). Life in a secure unit: The rehabilitation of young people through the use of sport. *Social Science and Medicine*, 56, 531–550.

Andrews, G. J., & Phillips, D. (2002). Changing local geographies of private residential care for older people 1983–1999: lessons for social policy in England and Wales. *Social Science and Medicine*, 55, 63–78.

Argyle, M., & Dean, J. (1965). Eye-contact, distance, and affiliation. *Sociometry*, 28, 289–304.

Baliant, M. (1945). Friendly expanses—hard empty spaces. *International Journal of Psychoanalysis*, 4, 38–46.

Bartholet, M. (1968). Effects of color on dynamics of patient care. *Nursing Outlook*, 6(10), 51–53.

Bechtel, G., & Davidhizar, R. (1998). Culture, personal space, and health. *Competence matters*, Birmingham, Ala.: University of Alabama at Birmingham.

Bendich, S. (1988). Appreciating bodily phenomena in verbally oriented psychotherapy sessions. *Issues in Mental Health Nursing*, 9, 1–7.

Bigham, C. (1964). To communicate with Negro patients. *American Journal of Nursing*, 64(9), 113–115.

Birdwhitstell, R. (1970). *Kinesics and context: essays on body motion communication*. Philadelphia: University of Pennsylvania Press.

Birx, E. (2002). *Healing Zen.*. Ontario, Canada: Viking Compass.

Black, J. W. (1950). The effect of room characteristics on vocalizations and rate. *Journal of Acoustical Society in America*, 22, 174–176.

Brant, C. (1983). *Native ethics and rules of behavior*. London, Ontario: University of Western Ontario.

Brown, G., & Maycock, B. (2005). Different spaces, same faces: Perth gay men's experiences of sexuality, risk and HIV. *Culture, Health, and Sexuality*, 7(1), 59–72.

Brown, J. W., Leavitt, L., & Graham, F. (1977). Response to auditory stimuli in six- and nine-week-old infants. *Developmental Psychobiology*, 10, 255–266.

Bull, P. (1983). *Body movement and interpersonal communication*. New York: John Wiley & Sons.

Burke, S., Maloney, R., Pothaar, D., & Baumgart, A. (1988). *Four views of childbearing and child health care: northern Indians, urban natives, urban Euro-Canadians and nurses*. A report for the National Health Research Development Program, Health and Welfare Canada.

Burlae, K. (2004). The theory of mindful space. *Identifying, understanding, and preventing violence*, 19(1), 85–98.

Cacioppo, J., Ernst, J., & Burleson, M., et al. (2000). Lonely traits and concomitant physiological process: The MacArthur social neuroscience studies. *International Journal of Psychophysiology*, 35, 143–154.

Carson, V. (2000). *Mental health nursing: the nurse-patient journey* (ed. 2). Philadelphia: W.B. Saunders.

Case, R., Moss, A., Case, N., McDermott, M., & Eberly, S. (1992). Living alone after myocardial infarction. *Journal of the American Medical Association*, 267, 515–519.

Croker, K., & Cummings, A. (1995). Nurses' reactions to physical assault by their patients. *Canadian Journal of Nursing Research*, 27(2), 81–93.

Davidhizar, R. (1988). Distance in managerial encounters. *Today's OR Nurse*, 10(10), 23–30.

Davidhizar, R., Dowd, S., & Bowen, M. (1998, July–August). The educational role of the surgical nurse with the multicultural patient and family. *Today's Surgical Nurse*, 20(4), 20–22.

Davidhizar, R., Dowd, S., & Giger, J. (1997). Model for cultural diversity in the radiology department. *Radiology Technology*, 68(3), 233–240.

Davidhizar, R., & Giger, J. (1998). *Canadian transcultural nursing: assessment and intervention*. St. Louis: Mosby.

Davidhizar, R., & Giger, J. (2000, January–February). Culture and care: profiling Alaskan Eskimos. *Health Traveler: The Magazine for Healthcare Travel Professionals*, 7(4), 12, 43–47.

Davidhizar, R., & Giger, J. (2002, January). Cultural issues. *Advances for Nurses*, 37–38.

Davidhizar, R., & Hart, A. (2005). Pain management. *Healthcare Traveler*, 13(6), 3–41.

Davidhizar, R., & Shearer, R. (2002, March). Helping children cope with public disasters. *AJN*, 102(3), 26–32.

Davidhizar, R., Shearer, R., & Giger, J. (2002, March 18). The challenges of cross-cultural communication. *RT Image*, 15(11), 18–20.

Davis, M. (1975). *Towards understanding the intrinsic in body movement*. New York: Ayer.

Davis, M., & Skupien, J. (1982). *Body movement and nonverbal communication: an annotated bibliography, 1971–1981*. Bloomington, Ind.: Indiana University Press.

Efron, D. (1941). *Gesture and environment: a tentative study of the spatio-temporal and "linguistic" aspects of the gestural behavior of Eastern Jews and Southern Italians in New York City living in similar as well as different environmental conditions*. New York: King's Crown Press.

Eibl-Eibesfeldt, I. (1972). Similarities and differences between cultures in expressive movements. In Hinde, R. A. (Ed.), *Nonverbal communication* (pp. 297–312). Cambridge, England: Cambridge University Press.

Ekman, P. (2001). *Telling lie: clues to deceit in the marketplace, politics, and marriage*. New York: W.W. Norton.

Ekman, P., & Friesen, W. (1975). *Unmasking the face: a guide to recognizing emotions from facial clues*. Englewood Cliffs, N.J.: Prentice Hall.

Evans, G. W., & Howard, R. B. (1973). Personal space. *Psychological Bulletin*, 80, 335–344.

Folta, A. (1989, April 3). *Exercise and functional capacity after myocardial infarction*, Paper presented at the 13th annual Midwest Nursing Research Society Conference, Cincinnati, Ohio.

Fox, N. J. (1997, September). Space, sterility, and surgery: circuits of hygiene in the operating theater. *Social Science & Medicine*, 45(5): 649–657.

Franklin, N., Henkel, L., & Zangas, T. (1995, July). Parsing surrounding space into regions. *Memory and Cognition*, 23(4), 397–407.

Gendlin, E. T. (1969). Focusing. *American Journal of Psychotherapy*, 1, 1–18.

Giger, J., & Davidhizar, R. (1990). Culture and space. *Advancing Critical Care*, 5(8), 8–11.

Giger, J., & Davidhizar, R. (1998). *Canadian transcultural nursing, assessment, and intervention*. St. Louis: Mosby.

Giger, J., & Davidhizar, R. (2001). Diversity in caring. In Potter, P., & Perry, A. (Eds.), *Fundamentals in Nursing* (ed. 5). St. Louis: Mosby.

Giger, J., Davidhizar, R., Evers, S., & Ingram, C. (1994). Cultural factors influencing mental health and mental illness. In Taylor, C. (Ed.), *Mereness' essentials of psychiatric nursing* (ed. 14) (pp. 215–238). St. Louis: Mosby.

Giger, J., Davidhizar, R., Johnson, J., & Poole, V. (1997). The changing face of America. *Health Care Traveler*, 4(4), 11–17.

Giger, J., Davidhizar, R., & Wieczorek, S. (1993). Culture and ethnicity. In Bobak, I., Jensen, M., & Lowdermilk, D. (Eds.), *Maternity and gynecologic care: the nurse and the family* (ed. 5). St. Louis: Mosby.

Giorgianni, S. (2000). *Intimate relationships: a vital component of health*. New York: Pfizer.

Goldberg, W., & Fitzpatrick, J. (1980). Movement therapy with the aged. *Nursing Research*, 29, 339–346.

Goldman, K., & Schmalz, K. (2005). E=MC2: Effective multicultural communication. *Health promotion practice*, 6(3), 237–239.

Gregg, J. (1996). *Communication and culture: a reading and writing text* (ed. 4). Boston: Heinle.

Grosvenor, G. M. (1989, July). Viva la différence [President's editorial]. *National Geographic*, 15.

Halford, S., & Leonard, P. (2003). Space and place in the construction and performance of gendered nursing identities. *Journal of Advanced Nursing*, 42(2), 20208.

Hall, E. T. (1966). *The silent language.* New York: Anchor Books.

Hall, E. T. (1969). *The hidden dimension.* New York: Anchor Books.

Hall, E. T. (1974). Proxemics. In Weitz, S. (Ed.), *Nonverbal communication* (ed. 2). New York: Oxford University Press.

Hall, E. T. (1977). *Beyond culture.* New York: Anchor Books.

Hall, E., & Whyte, W. (1990). Interpersonal communication: a guide to men of action. In Brink, P. J. (Ed.), *Transcultural nursing: a book of readings* Prospect Heights, Ill.: Waveland Press.

Hart, D., Field, N., Garfinkle, J., & Singer, J. (1997). Representations of self and others: a semantic space model. *Journal of Personality,* 65(1), 77–105.

Hayter, J. (1981). Territoriality as a universal need. *Journal of Advanced Nursing,* 6, 79–85.

Herlitz, J., Wiklund, I., & Caidahl, K., et al. (1998). The feeling of loneliness prior to coronary artery bypass grafting might be a predictor of short- and long-term postoperative morbidity. *European Journal of Vascular and Endovascular Surgery,* 16, 120–125.

Hickson, M. L., & Stacks, D. W. (2002). *Nonverbal communication: studies and applications* (ed. 4). Los Angeles: Roxbury.

Ittelson, W., Proshansky, H., Rivlin, I., & Winkel, H. (1974). *An introduction to environmental psychology.* New York: Holt, Rinehart, & Winston.

Kaegi, L. (2004, Summer). What color is your pain? *Minority Nurse,* 28–35.

Kasper, C. (1989, April 3). *Exercise-induced degeneration of skeletal muscle following inactivity.* Paper presented at the 13th annual Midwest Nursing Research Society Conference, Cincinnati, Ohio.

Knapp, M., & Hall, J. (1992). *Nonverbal communication in human interaction* (ed. 3). New York: Holt, Rinehart, & Winston.

Leathers, D. B. (1997). *Successful nonverbal communication: principles and applications* (ed. 3). Boston: Allyn & Bacon.

Leff, J., & Isaacs, A. (1996). *Psychiatric examination in clinical practice* (ed. 3). Boston: Blackwell Scientific.

Leininger, M., & McFarland, M. (2006). *Cultural care diversity and universality* (ed. 2). Sudbury, Mass: Jones and Bartlett.

Lynch, J. J. (1998). Decoding the language of the heart: developing a physiology of inclusion. *Integrative Physiological and Behavioral Science,* 33, 130–136.

Mahler, M., Pine, F., & Bergman, A. (1975). *The psychological birth of the human infant: symbiosis and individuation.* New York: Basic Books.

Marcus, N. (1985). Utilization of nonverbal expressive behavior in cognitive therapy. *American Journal of Psychotherapy,* 39(4), 467–478.

Marx, M., Wener, P., & Cohen-Mansfield, J. (1989, June). Agitation and touch in the nursing home. *Psychological Reports,* 64(3, Pt 2), 1019–1026.

McMahon, B. (1994). The functions of space. *Journal of Advanced Nursing,* 19, 362–366.

Meleis, A. (2006). Arabs. In Lipson, J., & Dibble, S. (Eds.), *Culture and clinical care.* San Francisco: UCSF Nursing Press.

Montagu, A. (1986). *Touching: the human significance of the skin.* New York: Harper & Row.

Moreno, J. L. (1946). *Psychodrama* (vol. 1). New York: Beacon House.

Moss, P. (1997, July). Negotiating spaces in home environments: older women living with arthritis. *Social Science Medicine,* 45(1), 23–33.

Mufford, C. (1992, October). A cure of many colors. *New Physician,* 14–19.

Murray, R., & Huelskoetter, M. (1991). *Psychiatric-mental health nursing: giving emotional care* (ed. 3). Norwalk, Conn.: Appleton & Lange.

Newman, M. (1976). Movement therapy and the experience of time. *Nursing Research,* 25, 273–279.

Oland, L. (1978). The need for territoriality. In Yura, H., & Walsh, M. B. (Eds.), *Human needs and the nursing process.* Norwalk, Conn.: Appleton-Century-Crofts.

Perls, F. S., Hefferline, R., & Goodman, P. (1983). *Gestalt therapy.* New York: Dell.

Personal Report for the Executive. (1987, July 15). New York: National Institute of Business Management.

Piaschenko, J. (1997). Ethics and the geography of the nurse-patient relationship: spatial vulnerable and gendered space. *Scholarly Inquiry of Nursing Practice,* 11(1), 45–59.

Purkis, M. E. (1996). Nursing in quality space. *Nursing Inquiry,* 3(2), 101–111.

Ramírez, M. (1991). *Psychotherapy and counseling with minorities.* New York: Pergamon Press.

Randall-David, E. (1989). *Strategies for working with culturally diverse communities and clients [Brochure].* Washington, D.C.: U.S. Department of Health and Human Services.

Rawlins, R., Williams, S., & Beck, C. (1993). *Mental health-psychiatric nursing: a holistic life cycle approach* (ed. 3). St. Louis: Mosby.

Roberts, S. (1989). *The effects of assault on nurses who have been physically assaulted by their clients.* Unpublished master's thesis. Toronto, Ontario: University of Toronto.

Roberts, S. (1991). Nurse abuse: a taboo topic. *The Canadian Nurse,* 87(3), 23–25.

Roberts, S. L. (1978). *Behavioral concepts and nursing throughout the life span.* Englewood Cliffs, N.J.: Prentice Hall.

Romas, R. T., Jacob, R. G., & Lilienfeld, S. O. (1997). Space and motion discomfort in Brazilian versus American patients with anxiety disorders. *Journal of Anxiety Disorders,* 11(2), 131–139.

Scheflen, A., & Scheflen, A. (1972). *Body language and social order: communication as behavioral control.* Englewood Cliffs, N.J.: Prentice Hall.

Schuster, C., & Ashburn, S. (1992). *The process of human development: a holistic lifespan approach* (ed. 3). New York: Lippincott.

Scott, A. (1988). Human interaction and personal boundaries. *Journal of Psychosocial Nursing,* 26(8), 23–28.

Scott, A., & Dumas, R. (1995). Personal space boundaries: clinical applications in psychiatric mental health nursing. *Perspectives in Psychiatric Care,* 31(3), 14–19.

Sheeshka, J., Potter, B., & Norrie, E., et al. (2001, February 17). Women's experiences breastfeeding in public places. *Journal of Human Lactation,* 17(1), 81–88.

Simply Stated. (1985, July). *Writing user manuals for Japanese readers.* No. 57.

Sinha, S., & Mukherjee, N. (1996, October). The effect of perceived cooperation on personal space. *Journal of Social Psychology,* 136(5), 655–657.

Smith, M. (1976). Patient responses to being transferred during hospitalization. *Nursing Research,* 25, 192–196.

Steere, D. A. (1982). *Bodily expressions in psychotherapy.* New York: Brunner/Mazel.

Stevenson, J. (1989, April 3). *Exercise in frail elders: findings and methodological issues,* Paper presented at the 13th annual Midwest Nursing Research Society Conference, Cincinnati, Ohio.

Stuart, G. (2005). Therapeutic nurse patient relationship. In Stuart, G., & Larai, M. (Eds.), *Principles and practice of psychiatric nursing* (ed. 8) St. Louis: Elsevier.

Sue, D. W., & Sue, D. (2003). *Counseling the culturally diverse: theory and a holistic life cycle approach* (ed. 4). New York: John Wiley.

Thomas, E. (2006, January 2). Taken by storm. *Newsweek,* 46–66.

Tripp-Reimer, T., & Friedl, M. (1977). Appalachians: a neglected minority. *Nursing Clinics of North America,* 12(41), 41–54.

Tripp-Reimer, T., & Lively, S. (1993). Cultural considerations in mental health-psychiatric nursing. In Rawlins, R., Williams, S., & Beck, C. (Eds.), *Mental health-psychiatric nursing* (ed. 3). St. Louis: Mosby.

Ubel, P., Zell, M., & Miller, D., et al. (1995, August 1). Elevator talk: observational study of inappropriate comments in a public space. *American Journal of Medicine,* 99(2), 190–194.

Useh, U., Moyo, A., & Munyonga, E. (2001, July 20). Wheelchair accessibility of public buildings in the central business district of Harare, Zimbabwe. *Disability and Rehabilitation,* 23(11), 490–496.

Van Esterik, P. (1980). Cultural factors affecting adjustment of Southeast Asian refugees. In Tepper, E. (Ed.), *Southeast Asian exodus: from tradition to resettlement* (pp. 151–172). Ottawa, Ontario: The Canadian Asian Studies Association.

Walkey, F., & Gilmour, R. (1984, September). The relationship between interpersonal distance and violence in imprisoned offenders. *Criminal Justice and Behavior,* 11(3), 331–340.

Watson, O. M. (1980). *Proxemic behavior: a cross-cultural study.* The Hague, the Netherlands: Mouton.

Wilson, H., & Kneisl, C. (1995). *Psychiatric nursing* (ed. 5). Reading, Mass: Addison-Wesley.

Wolfgang, A. (Ed.) (1984). *Nonverbal behavior: perspectives, applications, and intercultural insights.* Lewiston, N.Y.: C.J. Hogrete.

Young, T. (1988). *Health care and cultural change: the Indian experience in the central subarctic.* Toronto: University of Toronto Press.

Zook, R., & Davidhizar, R. (1989). Caring for the psychiatric inpatient with AIDS. *Perspectives in Psychiatric Nursing Care,* 25(2), 3–8.

CHAPTER 4

Social Organization

Behavioral Objectives

After reading this chapter, the nurse will be able to:

1. Describe how cultural behavior is acquired in a social setting.
2. Define selected terms unique to the concept of social organization, such as *culture-bound, ethnocentrism, homogeneity, bicultural, biracial, ethnicity, race, ethnic people of color, minority,* and *stereotyping.*
3. Describe significant social organization groups.
4. Define family groups, including nuclear, nuclear dyad, extended, alternative, blended, single parent, and special forms of family groups.
5. List at least two primary goals inherent in the American culture in regard to the family as a unit.
6. Describe the significant influence that religion may have on the way individuals relate to health care practitioners.

Cultural behavior, or how one acts in certain situations, is socially acquired, not genetically inherited. Patterns of cultural behavior are learned through a process called *enculturation* (also referred to as *socialization*), which involves acquiring knowledge and internalizing values. Most people achieve competence in their own culture through enculturation. Children learn to behave culturally by watching adults and making inferences about the rules for behavior (Nolt, 1992). Patterns of cultural behavior are important to the nurse because they provide explanations for behavior related to life events. Life events that are significant transculturally include birth, death, puberty, childbearing, childrearing, illness, and disease. Children learn certain beliefs, values, and attitudes about these life events, and the learned behavior that results persists throughout the entire life span unless necessity or forced adaptation compels them to learn different ways. Patterns of cultural behavior are also apparent in rituals. Some commonly observed rituals include weddings, funerals, and special holiday meals (Bonder, Martin, & Miracle, 2002). It is important for the nurse to recognize the value of social organizations and their relationship to physiological and psychological growth and maturation.

CULTURE AS A TOTALITY

Most anthropologists believe that to understand culture and the meaning assigned to culture-specific behavior, one must view culture in the total social context. The concept of holism requires that human behavior not be isolated from the context in which it occurs. Therefore, culture must be viewed and analyzed as a totality—a functional, integrated whole whose parts are interrelated and yet interdependent. The components of culture, such as politics, economics, religion, kinship, and health systems, perform separate functions but nevertheless mesh to form an operating whole. Culture is more than the sum of its parts (Goldsby, 1977; Henderson & Primeaux, 1981).

Culture-Bound

As children grow and learn a specific culture, they are to some extent imprisoned without knowing it. Some anthropologists have referred to this existence as "culture-bound." In this context the term *culture-bound* describes a person living within a certain reality that is considered "the reality." Most people have learned ways to interpret their world based on enculturation. Thus, although certain interpretations are understandable and persuasive to persons brought up to share the same frame of reference, other people may not share these interpretations and therefore may make little sense out of the context. Shipler (1997), who has traveled extensively around the United States, notes that connecting across racial lines is among the most difficult things on earth. In a perceptive work, *A Country of Strangers*, he notes, "Even as we look upon each other like strangers from afar, we are trapped in each other's imaginations." In *Liberal Racism*, Sleeper (1997) suggests that rather than trying to overcome racism and create a color-blind world, individuals should fight for equality on non-racial terms. In fact, in polls most Americans agree that people should be judged for themselves, not for their race (Sniderman & Carmines, 1997).

Nurses are also culturally bound within the profession because they are likely to bring a unique scientific approach—the nursing process—to determining and resolving health problems. Many nurses are likely to consider the nursing process the best and only means of meeting the needs of all clients, regardless of their cultural heritage. However, clients may view this modern scientific approach differently, believing that the nursing process meets their needs in some ways but not in others. The nursing process may not consider alternative health services, such as folk remedies, holistic health care, and spiritual interventions. In these cultures, medicine is often practiced in unscientific ways, according to the Western viewpoint. Therefore, desirable outcomes for treatment may occur independently of medical and health care interventions.

Traditionally, American nurses have been socialized to believe that modern Western medicine is the answer to all humanity's health needs. Most illnesses have been attributed to a biological cause (Grypma, 1993). More recently, Americans have been moving toward a more harmonious relationship with nature in which there is a growing sensitivity to the environment. Traditional attitudes toward disease are being reassessed. Today, more attention is given to the concept of the individual as an organic whole. Nurses are beginning to study and assess options outside of Western medicine that have been used by other cultures, such as Zen meditation, a Buddhist practice (Birx, 2002), or tai chi, an exercise treatment used in China for hundreds of years to reduce chronic pain in older adults (Adler, Good, Roberts, & Snyder, 2000). Many nursing leaders in America are calling for a change in nursing paradigms from scientific to holistic (Davidhizar, King, Bechtel, & Giger, 1998; Guruge & Donner, 1996; Thomas, 2001).

Culture-Bound Syndromes

The nurse should appreciate that some illnesses are uniquely found in a given cultural group. *Culture-bound syndromes* is a term that refers to "diseases" that seem to be specific to a single culture or a group of related cultures. Culture-bound syndromes are generally limited to specific societies or culture areas and are localized, folk, diagnostic categories that frame coherent meanings for a pattern of sets of experiences (American Psychiatric Association, 2000). In some cases the "illness" may be linked to a category in the *Diagnostic and Statistical Manual of Mental Disorders* (APA, 2000) but have symptoms, a course, and social responses that are influenced by local cultural factors. Examples are *amok*, a mental or emotional affliction known in the Philippines that causes one to become a killer, and *susto*, an ailment widely associated with Spanish-speaking groups in which the soul is believed to leave the body as a result of a frightening event (Bonder, Martin, & Miracle, 2002).

Ethnocentrism

For the most part, people look at the world from their own particular cultural viewpoint. "Ethnocentrism" is the perception that one's own way is best. Even in the nursing profession, there is a tendency to lean toward ethnocentrism. Nurses must remain cognizant of the fact that their ways are not necessarily the best and that other people's ideas are not "ignorant" or "inferior." Nurses must remember that the ideas of laypersons may be valid for them and, more importantly, will influence their health care behavior and consequently their health status. In contrast to the term *ethnocentrism* is the word *ethnic*, which relates to large groups of people classed according to common traits or customs. In populations throughout the world, people are bound by common ties, elements, life patterns, and basic beliefs germane to their particular country of origin.

In general, the medical paradigm used in Western culture views health, illness, and dying as biophysical realities. However, the meaning a nurse places on life can affect relationships with clients. For example, a nurse's belief that there is no relationship between illness and evil may conflict with a client's belief that illness is a punishment from God or the work of spirits (Gregory, 1988; Grypma, 1993; Zola, 1972). On one hand, some Puerto Ricans believe that sickness and suffering are a result of one's evil deeds; on the other hand, many Ugandans believe that an infant's illness or death is the result of a neighbor's curse (Grypma, 1993).

It is also important for the nurse to be aware of treatment practices clients may present that do not appear in Western medicine and may seem shocking. For example, female genital cutting, which may range from a ceremonial pricking of the genitalia to the removal of the clitoris, occurs in 28 African countries with prevalence rates estimated at 50% (Natinsky, 2001). Yet another concept that the nurse should appreciate is that moral definitions of an illness may arise from particular historical, social, or medical circumstances that are different in each society. For example, in some societies leprosy is common and considered just another debilitating illness, which many families tolerate. In other societies leprosy has been stigmatized, and lepers are quickly divorced, are pushed out of their homes, and end up as beggars (Wexler, 1981).

Homogeneity

It is difficult to find a homogeneous culture in the United States. If a homogeneous culture did exist, all individuals would share the same attitudes, interests, and goals—a phenomenon referred to as

"ethnic collectivity." People who are reared in ethnic collectivity share a bond that includes common origins, a sense of identity, and a shared standard for behavior. These values are often acquired from experiences that are perceived to be cultural norms and determine the thoughts and behaviors of individual members (Harwood, 1981; Saunders, 1954). The ultimate consequences of enculturation are carried over to health care and become an important influence on activities relative to health and illness behaviors. In the American culture there is a tendency to speak of culture as if it included a set of values shared by everyone. However, even within an ethnic collectivity, intraethnic variations occur and are obvious in health behaviors. For example, intraethnic variations are seen in the concept of mental illness (Guttmacher & Elinson, 1972; Berry, 1988; Sands & Berry, 1993), in cultural definitions of health and illness, in skepticism about medical care and consequently the use or lack of use of health care services (Berkanovic & Reeder, 1973; Spector, 2004), and in the willingness of the individual to assume a dependent role when ill (Suchman, 1964). Since there may not be obvious clues (for example, language, physical appearance, clothing) to alert the nurse to intraethnic variations, it is essential to be alert to the presence of differences and to be sensitive in interactions with the client when nurse–client variations become evident (Bonder, Martin, & Miracle, 2002).

Bicultural

The term *bicultural* is used to describe a person who crosses two cultures, lifestyles, and sets of values. Some children of African-American, Hispanic, Asian, and American Indian heritage are socialized to be bicultural—that is, to acquire skills to function in both a minority and a majority culture (Andrews & Boyle, 2003; Zayas & Solari, 1994).

Ethnicity

Ethnicity is frequently and perhaps erroneously used to mean "race," but the term *ethnicity* includes more than the biological identification. Ethnicity in its broadest sense refers to groups whose members share a common social and cultural heritage passed on to each successive generation. The most important characteristic of ethnicity is that members of an ethnic group feel a sense of identity.

Race

In the last decade, efforts to precisely delineate the term *race* have been made by many scientists (American Association of Physical Anthropologists [AAPA], 1996). The AAPA suggests that race, in a pure sense of genetically homogeneous populations, does not exist in any human species today. Freeman (1998) also proposes that the biological concept previously held to be the "one drop rule" is dated and as such is no longer tenable in today's society. Nonetheless, many biological scientists suggest that while socioeconomic status may have a more profound effect on health status, *race* is a viable term that merits attention. Thus, in contrast to the term ethnicity is the term *race*, which is related to biology. Members of a particular race share distinguishing physical features, such as skin color, bone structure, or blood group. Ethnic and racial groups can and do overlap because in many cases the biological and cultural similarities reinforce one another (Bullough & Bullough, 1982). A more precise definition of race is a breeding population that primarily mates within itself (Giger, Davidhizar, & Wieczorek, 1994). There are very few races that still mate largely within the group, but some pure-blooded lineages are found in certain parts of the world, such as some of the descendants of West Africans who live along the Georgia and South Carolina seacoasts in the United States. These people have protected their lineage because they have refused to intermarry. These individuals are known as the Gullah people, who have not only their own lineage but also their own distinct dialect of English (Wolfram & Clark, 1971). It is important for the nurse to remember that regardless of race, all people have a cultural heritage that makes them ethnic. It is also important to appreciate that race has an interrelational effect with family structure and income that can influence health and academic and professional achievement (Blum, Buehring, & Rinehart, 2000).

Biracial

When an individual crosses two racial and cultural groups, the individual is considered "biracial." To be both biracial and bicultural often creates an almost insurmountable dilemma for an individual. Physical attributes such as color, shape of eyes, or hair may have a profound influence on others' acceptance of the "biracial" individual. One problem associated with biracialism is the inability of the individual to identify or find acceptance in any one of the biologically related racial groups (Giger, Davidhizar, Evers, & Ingram, 1994). It is the total exclusion and the sense of not belonging to either of the racial or cultural groups that often create the dilemma. For example, an African-American who is an "octoroon," a person with one-eighth African-American blood, may have difficulty being accepted as African-American because of the lightness of the skin. Conversely, this same individual might be ostracized by some Whites because of the "blackness of the blood lineage." While interracial marriages are on the rise, issues of discrimination still occur. Golf champion Tiger Woods revealed in 1997 that in spite of his national stature, his mixed-race origin of White, Black, Indian, and Asian was sometimes met with hostility (Cose, 2000). Cose suggests that even in the emerging U.S. mestizo future, if the Latin American experience is a guide, people who are whiter will still have the advantage. Even in Brazil, where racial mixing is sometimes celebrated, status and privilege are still related to lighter skin. For some people of color, there is a perception that White America believes that color is the difference that makes the differences (Giger, Johnson, Davidhizar, & Fishman, 1993).

Minority

A minority can consist of a particular racial, religious, or occupational group that constitutes less than a numerical majority of the population. With use of this definition for the term *minority*, it is obvious that all types of people can belong to various kinds of minorities (Bullough & Bullough, 1982). Often a group is designated *minority* because of its lack of power, assumed inferior traits, or supposedly undesirable characteristics. In any society, cultural groups can be arranged in a hierarchical power structure. Dominant groups are considered to be powerful, whereas those in minority groups are considered inferior and lacking in power.

The term *minority* is not synonymous with numbers. In the United States, people of color (African-Americans, Latin Americans, Asian Americans) are considered minorities. However, when the population of the world is considered in its aggregate, it is obvious that people of color are in the majority.

Gender is another example of how the term *minority* is used erroneously. Females in the United States are a larger numerical percentage (50.9%) than males (49.1%) but are considered to be in the minority because of their underrepresentation in high-level managerial positions in the workplace.

The significance of the term *minority* cannot be overemphasized. The central defining characteristic of any minority group, according to Adams (1995, p. 6), is its "experience with various disadvantages at the hands of another social group."

Ethnic Minority

The term *ethnic minority* is often used because it is less offensive to people of color than other terms. Supposedly it takes into account ethnicity, race, and the relative status of the groups of persons included in the category. Were it not for the use of the word minority, perhaps this terminology would be less culturally offensive to some groups of people (that is, ethnic people of color). According to Gary (1991), use of the term *people of color* might be the preferable option, particularly in situations where sensitivity to racial preferences needs to be heightened. It is estimated that by the year 2050 about half of the total American population will be nonwhite, thus eliminating the meaning of the term *ethnic minority* (Kunen, 1996; U.S. Department of Commerce, Bureau of the Census, Summary File 3, 2002).

Stereotyping

Stereotyping is the assumption that all people in a similar cultural, racial, or ethnic group are alike

and share the same values and beliefs. For example, stereotyping occurs when an African-American nurse is assigned to care for an African-American client simply because of ethnicity and race. It is stereotypical when the assumption is made that all African-Americans are alike and therefore the African-American nurse is more likely to be more sensitive to the needs of the African-American client. Race and ethnicity do not, in and of themselves, make persons "resident experts" on the belief and value systems of other persons. Whether stereotyping is engaged in as a result of scientifically proved, research-based data or because of past associations and experiences, stereotyping can ultimately lead to faulty data gathering and wrong interpretations.

Role of Gender and Cultural Significance

In traditional Chinese society, women have held subordinate roles to men, a belief that dates back to the first millennium B.C. (Mo, 1992). Traditional Chinese believe that the universe developed from two complementary opposites: *yin* (Cantonese, *yam*), the female, and *yang* (Cantonese, *yeung*), the male. For some traditional Chinese Americans, the *yin* represents the dark, cold, wet, passive, weak, feminine aspect of humankind. In stark contrast, the *yang* represents the bright, hot, dry, active, strong, masculine aspect of humankind (Mo, 1992). In traditional societies, there are written and unwritten roles that dictate behavior of girls and women (Strickland & Giger, 1994). Although some countries in North America are highly evolved technologically, traditional beliefs about the role of women in society still persist throughout many regions of America. Peitchinis (1989) noted that discrimination exists for women in the workplace because women are viewed as having a higher absentee rate than their male counterparts. For many women, discrimination creates a barrier to entrance into the workplace and even more importantly places a "glass ceiling" on advancement that their male counterparts need not overcome (Misener, Sowell, Phillips, & Harris, 1997). According to a General Accounting Office study in 2000 (Associated Press, 2000), salaries of women and men in managerial jobs were even farther apart in 2000 than in 1995 in 7 of the 10 industries that employ the most women in the United States. In 1995 female managers in entertainment earned 83 cents for every dollar earned by a male manager; by 2000 female managers in the industry earned only 62 cents. On the other hand, although women have tended to be an oppressed group in the workplace, numerous studies have indicated efforts by industries to implement policies and procedures to prevent discrimination on the basis of sex. For example, women may have access to benefits such as child care leave, alternative working arrangements, child care arrangements, special brief leaves to deal with family problems, and free prenatal classes (Danyliw, 1997). Because breast-feeding reduces the incidence and severity of diarrhea, ear infections, allergies, and sudden infant death syndrome and lessens the risk of ovarian and breast cancer in mothers, programs that allow mothers to do so can result in significant savings for companies in medical claims (Danyliw, 1997).

In some cultures nursing is a low-status occupation. For example, in Saudi Arabia and Kuwait, care for the sick is carried out by health care providers hired from abroad for the purpose of caring for the bodily needs of the sick (Andrews & Boyle, 2003). Clients or physicians from a culture where nurses are in the lower class may have difficulty accepting the nurse as being in a role of authority and as having expertise. In many parts of the world, female purity and modesty are major values, and disregard of these values can cause distress. For example, female purity is especially important in the Middle East and other Muslim countries. In some cultures it is preferable to assign nurses of the same gender as care providers (Habel, 2001). If the nurse is female and the client is male and is from a cultural group where touch is permitted only between members of the same sex and where direct eye contact is avoided, special modifications in care may be needed (Kulwicki, 2003; Meleis, 2006).

Role of Disability and Culture

Today almost exclusively more attention has been directed towards a definition of culture that included groups of people by such characteristics of race/ ethnicity, religion, and cultural heritage. In addition, the same is true for the term "health disparities." Statistical data now suggest that other population data, not just race and ethnicity, should now be used to define cultures of people, including those living with health disparities. Disabled people, for example, can now be considered a cultural group that lives with a number of health disparities. A person with a long-lasting condition or disability can be described as suffering from a health disparity. The 2000 census identified 49.7 million individuals with disabilities in the United States (2000 Census Briefs). Kinne, Patrick, and Doyle (2004) reported a two to three times greater likelihood that individuals with disabilities would suffer from each of 16 secondary conditions, including falls or other injuries, respiratory infections, asthma, sleep problems, chronic pain, and periods of depression. Individuals with disability are also at higher risk for preventable physical, mental, or social disorders that may result from the initial disabling condition. Individuals with disabilities are more likely to report that their health is poor or fair (44.8%) than are individuals without disabilities (9.4%) (U.S. Department of Health and Human Services, 2000). These individuals are less likely to be involved in physical activity and more likely to smoke and be overweight (U.S. Department of Health and Human Services, 2000). Negative social and economic circumstances are also more likely among individuals with disabilities, including decreased participation in social relationships, decreased employment, and decreased income for those employed (U.S. Department of Health and Human Services, 2000). Thus, it is important to assess the individual with a disability by using the six phenomena of the Giger and Davidhizar model to determine the specific difficulties that this culturally unique individual may experience (Hahn, 2006) (Figure 4-1).

SOCIAL ORGANIZATION GROUPS AS SYSTEMS

Social organizations are structured in a variety of groups, including family, religious, ethnic, racial, tribal, kinship, clan, and other special interest groups. Groups are dependent on particular persons and are more affected by changes in members

Figure 4-1 Hahn's Culture and Disability Assessment Model (Adapted from Giger, J.N., & Davidhizar, R. [2004]. *Transcultural Nursing Assessment and Intervention*, St Louis: Mosby.)

1. Americans with Disabilities Act. 42 U. S. C. § 12102(2).
2. Lipson, J. G., Rogers, J. G. (2000). Cultural aspects of disability. *Journal of Transcultural Nursing*, 11, 212-219.
3. Eddey, G. E., Robey, K. L. (2005). Considering the culture of disability in cultural competence education. *Academic Medicine*, 80, 706-712.
4. Giger, J. N., Davidhizar, R. (2002). The Giger and Davidhizar Transcultural Assessment Model. *Journal of Transcultural Nursing*, 13, 185-188.
5. Gill, C. J. (1995). A psychological view of disability culture. *Disability Study Quarterly*, 15, 16-19.
6. Smeltzer SC, et al. (2004). Accessible online health promotion information for persons with disabilities. *Online J Issues Nurs*. 2004 Jan 31;9(1):11.
7. Mele, N., Archer, J., Pusch, B.D. (2005). Access to breast cancer screening services for women with disabilities. *JOGNN*, 34, 453-464.
8. Pope, A. M. (1992). Preventing Secondary Conditions. *Mental Retardation*, 30, 347-354.
9. Nosek, M. A., Hughes, R. B., Howland, C. A., Young, M. E., Mullen, P. D., Shelton, M. L. (2004). The meaning of health for women with physical disabilities: a qualitative analysis. *Family Community Health*, 27, 6-21.
10. Treloar, L. L. (1999). People with disabilities—the same, but different: implications for health care practice. *Journal of Transcultural Nursing*, 10, 358-364.
11. MacIntyre, *A. Dependent Rational Animals: Why Human Beings Need the Virtues*. Chicago: Open Court.
12. Meleis, A. (1999). Theoretical considerations of health care for immigrant and minority women. In P. F. Hill, J. G. Lipson, & A. I. Meleis [eds.] *Caring for Women Cross-Culturally*. Philadelphia: F. A. Davis.
13. Soderberg, S. (1999). Sturgling for dignity: the meaning of women's experiences of living with fibromyalgia. *Qualitative Health Research*, 9, 575-587.
14. Jha, A., Patrick, D. L., Maclehose, R. F., Doctor, J. N., Chan, L. (2002). Dissatisfaction with medical services among Medicare beneficiaries with disabilities. *Archives of Physical Medicine and Rehabilitation*, 1335-1341.
15. Administration on Developmental Disabilities (ADA), Administration for Children and Families, U. S. Department of Health and Human Services (n.d.). The American Dream Belongs to Everyone: A Report to Congress, the President, and the National Council on Disability.

Reference for *Culture and Disability Assessment Model* developed by J. E. Hahn, 2006.

than are other systems. In most groups, except for racial and ethnic groups, members may come and go. Thus, the formation and the disintegration of groups are more likely to occur during the members' lifetimes than are the formation and the disintegration of other systems.

According to general systems theory, social organization groups are characterized by a steady state and a sense of balance or equilibrium that is maintained even as the group changes. Most groups form, grow, and reach a state of maturity. Social organization groups begin with a variety of elements that include individuals with unique personalities, needs, ideas, potentials, and limits. In the course of development of the group, a pattern of behavior and a set of norms, beliefs, and values evolve. As the group strives toward maturity, parts become differentiated, and each member assumes special functions.

Family Groups

One group of paramount concern for the nurse when working transculturally is the family. In fact, as the family goes, so goes the health care system. Nevertheless, a consensus about the definition of the word "family" does not exist. *Merriam-Webster's Dictionary* (2003 online edition) offers 21 definitions of family. In terms of the U.S. Census, the term *family households* is defined as "people who occupy a housing unit" (U.S. Department of Commerce, Bureau of the Census, Summary File 1, 2000). In 2000, there were 72,261,780 family households and 41,165,148 nonfamily households, representing 68.1% and 31.9% of all U.S. households, respectively. Married couples maintained 51.7% of all families, whereas women with no husband maintained 12.2% (U.S. Department of Commerce, Bureau of the Census, Summary File 3, 2002).

Regardless of cultural background or the nature of the family, the family is the basic unit of society in the United States. From a sociological perspective, *family* may be defined as a social unit that interacts with a larger society. The discipline of economics may define *family* in terms of how it works together to meet material needs. From a psychological perspective, *family* may be defined as a basic unit for personality development and the development of subgroup relationships, such as parent–child relationships. Still another definition is offered from a biological perspective, which conceptualizes the family as a unit with the biological function of perpetuating the species. However, even while families deliver most of health care and at one time being in a family was expected, today not being in a family is both common and accepted and has profound implications for health care delivery (Giorgianni, 2003).

Types of Family Structures

Traditional Nuclear Family. According to Virginia Satir (1983), the traditional nuclear family consists of one man and one woman of the same race, religion, and age who are of sound mind and body and who marry during their early or middle twenties, are faithful to the other for life, have and raise their own children, retire, and finally die. This definition appears narrow; however, it has maintained popularity over the years and is still seen by many persons as the most desirable family form. Today a more current definition of the nuclear family allows for more variation: a family of two generations formed by a married woman and man with their children by birth or adoption (Jones, 2003). Within this particular family form, as within all identified family forms, the assigned roles and functions performed by each member vary. One common family structure has the father working outside the home and the mother working at home taking care of the children and household tasks. However, today the traditional nuclear family often finds both mother and father working outside the home. Thus, childrearing and child care may be shared by both parents as well as by others outside the family, such as a day care center.

The most common type of household, married-couple families, changed from 55% to 53% of all households from 1990 to 2003. In the United States in 2003, 57 million or 53% of persons were part of a married couple family, with an additional 4% of households headed by males and 12% of households headed by females with no spouse present (*Time Almanac with Information Please*, 2006).

The number of married-couple households varies by state, with the highest number in Utah and Idaho and in the West Central section of the country (*World Almanac*, 2006). A total of 44% of married-couple families have children under age 18 in their home. The average size of the nation's households declined from 2.63 persons in 1990 to 2.57 persons in 2003. In 2004, first marriage occurred at age 25.8 years for women and 27.4 years for men. An increasing and less stigmatized trend today is for adult children to live at home. In 2004 2.72 millions males and 1.56 million females between the ages of 25 and 34 were still living at home. This is approximately double the number in 1970 (Jayson, 2006). Certain ethnic groups, including Asians, African-Americans, and Hispanics, are more likely to stay home longer and are less likely to move far away.

The median age of the U.S. population in 2000 was 35.3 years, the highest it has ever been, up from 32.9 years in 1990. As the median age rose, so did the age of first marriage. The average age at first marriage in 2000 was 26.9 for men and 25.1 for women, and has been creeping upward (U.S. Department of Commerce, Bureau of the Census, Summary File 3, 2002). As the population continues to age, relatively fewer families will have children—a projected 41% in 2010, down from 50% in 1994. Among families with children, a lower proportion is expected to include two married parents—a projected 72% in 2010, down from 74% in 1994. It is estimated that fewer than 14% of American children living today are growing up in two-parent nuclear families (Kadis & McClendon, 2003). While the number of children in a family is decreasing, increasing numbers of married and unmarried Americans are seeking children to adopt. In 1998 a survey of American women found just 200,000 considering adoption; in 2000, by contrast, 500,000 wanted to adopt a child. Because fewer children are available in the United States, there has been a concomitant sharp increase in foreign adoptions, with 18,441 in 2000 (Clark & Shute, 2001).

Interestingly, although the nuclear family is on the decline, immigration laws still lean toward "family preference." In the interest of keeping families together, U.S. policy allows an unlimited number of visas to certain relatives of U.S. citizens and of permanent resident aliens. Thus, an illiterate laborer with no skills but with a parent in the United States has a better chance of immigration than a graduate school–educated foreigner with no family or employer in the United States. In 1995, about 68% of immigrants came to the United States through the family preference, and about 10% of them came as adult siblings. People born in Mexico, which sends more legal immigrants—18%—to the United States than does any other country, have responded to family preference in particularly high numbers, and they are more likely to use ties to extended family members than any other group. The result is a family-based immigrant population that, for Mexicans and Central Americans at least, is skewed toward unskilled labor (Headden, 1998).

The second most common type of household, consisting of people living alone, rose from 25% to 28.15% of all households in 2000 for a total of 27.2 million (U.S. Department of Commerce, Bureau of the Census, Summary File 1, 2000).

Nuclear Dyad Family. The nuclear dyad family consists of one generation and is made up of a married couple without children. In the United States, 54 million people (19.4% of the population) report that they live in a household with only a spouse (U.S. Department of Commerce, Bureau of the Census, Summary File 1, 2000). There are numerous reasons why a family may remain childless: the family may have chosen not to have children, they may not be able to have children or to adopt them, or the children may have died. Unlike their parents, couples who married in the United States in 2002 are more likely to delay having children (Orecklin, 2002). In some cultures this family form is considered a beginning point for the formation of the family. However, in other cultures the nuclear dyad family is considered a part of the mainstream of the social organization of the family.

Extended Family. The extended family is multigenerational and includes all relatives by birth, marriage, or adoption. The family group includes grandparents, aunts, uncles, nieces, nephews, cousins, brothers, sisters, and in-laws. In today's society there is a tendency for children to leave the homes and communities of their parents, which has resulted in a separation of the nuclear family from the extended family. As longevity in America increases, increasing numbers of people are elderly. In 2002, 11.4% of Americans were over age 65. Concomitantly, the number of multigenerational or extended family households is increasing. In 2000, more than 24 million (23.4%) households included individuals 65 years of age and older. The elderly are increasingly living alone. More than 9 million (9.2%) persons 65 years of age and older were in nonfamily households (U.S. Department of Commerce, Bureau of the Census, Summary File 1, 2000).

Skip-Generation Family. Grandparents who are taking care of grandchildren are a growing family group. With increasing numbers of parents dying of AIDS and single parents who are not interested in child care, grandparents are finding themselves in the role of primary caregiver (McMahon, 1997). An estimated 5.5 million of America's children live with their grandparents (U.S. Bureau of the Census, 2002).

Alternative Family. The alternative family consists of adults of a single generation or a combination of adults and children who live together without the social sanction of marriage. The alternative family is often either a communal arrangement—composed of roommates who might be either homosexual or heterosexual—or a love relationship between a man and a woman. Unmarried partners form 5.5 million households in the United States, including 4.9 million of the opposite sex and 600,000 of the same sex. These unmarried-partner households made up 9.1% of all households in 2000, an increase from 4% in 1990 and 2% in 1980 (*World Almanac*, 2006).

Single-Parent Family. The single-parent family consists of two generations and is made up of a mother or a father and children by birth or adoption. The reasons for a single-parent family include electing to be a single parent, divorce, death, separation, or abandonment. The prevalence of the single-parent family is increasing because of such factors as divorce and the acceptability of being a single parent. In the 2000 census, families maintained by women with no husband present remained constant at 12.2%, for a total of 12.9 million. Among female-headed households, 7.5 million or 7.2% of all households had children under age 18 years (U.S. Department of Commerce, Bureau of the Census, Summary File 3, 2002). For more than the past decade, about a third of all babies have been born to unmarried women, compared with 3.8% in 1940 (Kantrowitz & Wingert, 2001). However, the median age of the unmarried mothers is in the late twenties, they may be divorced or never married, and 40% are living with a man who may be the father of one or more of the children (U.S. Department of Commerce, Bureau of the Census, Summary File 1, 2000). More than half of the youngsters born in the 1990s are predicted to spend at least part of their childhood in a single-parent home. Single fathers account for 4.4 million households, an increase from 3% to 4% in the last decade (U.S. Department of Commerce, Bureau of the Census, Summary File 1, 2000).

Reconstituted or Blended Family. The reconstituted or blended family is formed by "put-together parts" of previously existing families with the intention of forming a new nuclear family (Satir, 1983). The blended family, like the traditional nuclear family, is two-generational. However, the blended family differs in form and may consist of a single person who marries a person with children or of a man and a woman, both of whom have children, who marry. This family form may also yield biological children; thus, there may be children who are "yours," "mine," and "ours" in the family. The blended family can become very complicated because of the composition of family members, which may include stepbrothers, stepsisters, stepparents, and stepgrandparents. Unipolar blended and bipolar blended describe whether one or both parents bring stepchildren to a marriage. If one parent's children do not live with the family, the family is a secondary-step, bipolar family. If one parent brings children from two previous marriages, the term *double-step family* is used (Rosemond, 1994). Nearly 25% of all minor children live in a stepfamily (Jones, 2003).

Special Forms of Families: Communal Families and Gay Families. In some cultures, an even wider array of family forms occurs, particularly if ideas about marriage and the requirement that the nuclear family is essential to family definition are disregarded. These groups function as families and therefore must be recognized. These special forms of families may be either unigenerational or multigenerational. Two or more adults constitute these special family forms, and they may or may not be of the same sex.

A commune is a group of people that intertwines husband–wife, parent–child, and brother–sister types of relationships of individuals who have elected to live together in one household or in closely adjoining structures. Family members in a commune must express a feeling of commitment to others in the group. Assigned family roles as well as responsibilities are divided among the members of the group. Generally there are specific rules and expectations for each member of the group. A commune may be formed when people have a common goal, such as a religious, philosophical, or political goal, or a common need, such as an economic, social, or physical need. Examples of communes include Israeli kibbutzim, religious cults, retirement homes for the elderly, and households where couples share resources.

Some gay households consist of two persons and generally function as a nuclear dyad. Other gay households may consist of more members, such as a commune. Today, perhaps as a result of the gay rights movement, homosexual couples have openly taken up residence together. Nevertheless, many members of society continue not to accept this particular family form, as indicated in a survey by the *Washington Post*, Harvard University, and the Henry J. Kaiser Family Foundation (1999) in which 53% of respondents stated they believed sexual relationships between two adults of the same sex were always wrong. To combat discrimination against gays and lesbians, legislation regarding the workplace, marriage, and adoption is increasingly being enacted at the state and federal level. In 1996, Congress passed a bill dubbed the "Defense of Marriage Act," which prohibited federal benefits for spouses in same-sex marriages and guaranteed that no state shall be required to legally recognize same-sex unions. Thus, 32 states specifically prohibit same-sex marriages. However, in July 2000 Vermont became the first state in the nation to recognize civil unions between two people of the same sex. In 2003 the Massachusetts Supreme Judicial Court also passed a "right to marry" act for gay couples (*Time Almanac with Information Please*, 2006). In 1997, a New Jersey gay couple was allowed to jointly adopt a child, as New Jersey became the first state to explicitly allow lesbian and gay couples to adopt children jointly, just as married couples do. As gay and lesbian baby boomers enter their golden years, the estimated current number of 1 to 3 million gay and lesbian seniors is expected to skyrocket. Gay retirement communities are being developed from Boston to Palm Springs to offer retirees the opportunity to be part of a like-minded community that stands against discrimination (Rosenberg, 2001). Young gays are disclosing their sexual orientation earlier. Whereas in 1997 there were approximately 100 gay–straight alliances (clubs for gays and gay-friendly kids) on U.S. high school campuses, today there are nearly 3000 (Cloud, 2005). The nursing literature is increasingly addressing variations in sexual orientation and encouraging nurses to come to terms with their own feelings about homosexuality and to practice unconditional acceptance of the individual regardless of sexual orientation (Townsend, 2006).

Characteristics of a Family System

According to general systems theory, a system is a group of interrelated parts or units that form a whole. When general systems theory is applied to the family, the individual family members are those units that make up the identifiable family system. These parts or units act as one or more subsystems within the larger system. Within the family system, the subsystems refer to the ways in which the members align themselves with one another. For example, in the family system, the parents may be one subsystem and the children another subsystem. At the same time, males and females of the family system may be two other subsystems. A subsystem may consist of any number of members who are linked by some common factor. Within the family system, membership in a particular subsystem may be determined by generational considerations, sexual identity, areas of interest, or a specifically designated function. Individual family members may belong to several different subsystems. Family members also belong to external systems, such as the community system, the school system, and career systems. Subsystems may be constructed to ensure that important functions within the family system are carried out to maintain the overall family structure.

Fawcett (1975) studied the family as a living open system and thus viewed family nursing as an emerging conceptual framework for nursing care. Nurses have cared for families for years; however, it is only recently that nurses have begun to study the family as a whole (Finkleman, 2000; Kearney, York, & Deatrick, 2000).

Family as a Behavioral System. The family is conceptualized as a behavioral system with unique properties inherent to the system. A close interrelationship exists between the psychosocial functioning of the family as a group and the emotional adaptation of individual family members. A distinguishable link exists between disorders of family living and disorders of family members. This link can best be understood in the context of systems theory. Systems theory is an orientation whereby people are recognized and defined by who they are in the context of their relationship with family, friends, and the society in which they live. Family systems theories were developed in the 1950s on both the East and West coasts of the United States. On the West Coast, a group of people that included Jackson, Haley, and their associates in Palo Alto, California, explored the notions of communication theory and homeostasis applied to the family with a schizophrenic member (Bateson, Jackson, Haley, & Weakland, 1968; Satir, 1983). On the East Coast, in Washington, D.C., Bowen (1985) conceptualized a family systems theory based on a biological systems model. In Philadelphia, Minuchin (1974) used a systems model in his research with families with psychosomatic disorders.

Lewis, Beavers, Gossett, and Phillips (1976) and Caplan (1976) explored both disturbed families and healthy families from a systems perspective. A system is a whole that consists of more than the sum of its parts; a system can be divided into subsystems, but the subsystems are not representative pieces of the whole. To study the family from a cultural perspective, one must understand the basic characteristics of a family system and of a living system. Today in nursing, the family nursing process is the same whether the focus is on the family as the client or the family as the environment. Therefore, the nursing process used in family nursing is the same as that used with individuals, that is, assessment, nursing diagnosis, planning, intervention, and evaluation. According to Friedman (1986), the only distinguishable difference is that both the individual and the family receive care simultaneously. There are some inherent underlying assumptions germane to the family approach to the nursing process, including the beliefs that all individuals must be viewed within their family context, that families have an effect on individuals, and that individuals have an effect on families. As nursing becomes more involved in the delivery of care in the community, it is imperative to strengthen nursing expertise in the delivery of care to the entire family (Hitchcock, 2003).

Independent Units. All systems have basic units that make functioning possible. Within the structure of the family system, the basic interdependent units are the individual family members. As in any open system, change within one family member affects the entire family system. For example, when one family member becomes physically or emotionally ill, the entire family system is changed in some way. Additional alterations in the family system occur because of the changing composition of family membership as a result of events such as birth, divorce, death, hospitalization, leaving home for college, or marriage. All these variables, whether positive or negative, may bring about disruption and disequilibrium in the family system. All family systems have dynamic characteristics that must be used when disruption or disequilibrium occurs if the family system is to be permitted to return to equilibrium as matter, energy, and information are exchanged (Lewis, 1979).

The number of adults who are unmarried (never married, widowed, or divorced) is dramatically increasing in the United States. In 2003 there were 51.9 million (27.9% of males and 21.1% of females) who were never-married compared with 32.3 million in 1980 (*Time Almanac with Information Please*, 2006). Widowed persons represented 13.8 million (2.3% of males and 10.3% of females) of the population while divorced individuals represented 21.5 million (8.8% of males and 11.5% of females) of the population (*Time Almanac with Information Please*, 2006).

Environment. As with all open systems, an internal and external environment controls the direction of growth of the family system. The internal environment involves the social and physical factors within the family boundaries, the quality of which is reflected by such factors as (1) marital relationship, (2) location of power, (3) closeness of family members, (4) communication, (5) problem-solving abilities, (6) free expression of feelings, (7) ability to deal with loss, (8) family values, (9) degree of intimacy, and (10) autonomy of family members. Within the family system, the external environment is the social and physical world outside the family, such as church, neighbors, extended family, school, friends, work, health care system, political system, and recreation.

Boundaries. Within the family system, the "boundary" is the imaginary line or area of demarcation that keeps the family system separate and unique from its external environment. As with all open systems, energy, in the form of information, material goods, and feeling states, passes among family members and the external environment. Openness and closeness in a family system are governed by the degree of information or energy that is exchanged and the nature of the boundaries. Information coming into the family system provides the family with information about the environment and about family functioning. If the family accepts the information, it may be used to formulate and respond to the environment, assist the family in coping with disequilibrium, or rejuvenate the family. Energy coming into the family can also be stored until needed. Finally, energy or information coming into the family can be rejected or ignored (Satir, 1983).

As with all open systems, the amount of energy or information that enters and leaves the system must be balanced within certain limits to maintain a steady state of functioning or homeostasis if proper adaptation of the system is to occur. Any system can become dysfunctional if the system is allowed to become too open or too closed. No truly closed systems exist, except in a theoretical sense. On the other hand, if a family system were totally open, the family system would probably lose its identity as a system separate from other systems to which family members belong. Therefore, the family members might suffer from alienation, rootlessness, and a lack of belonging. The opposite extreme, a theoretically closed family system, would have very rigid boundaries, and family members would become enmeshed, fixed, and unable to move out, grow, or change.

Communication Within the Family System

The verbal and nonverbal interaction among family members is communication. Factors that contribute to the family members' patterns of communication include (1) the pattern of members in acknowledging each other's verbal and nonverbal messages; (2) the degree of responsibility each member takes for expressing individual feelings, thoughts, and reactions in a constructive way; (3) the extent to which the family encourages a clear exchange of words; (4) the extent to which family members are allowed to talk for themselves; and (5) the patterns of spontaneous talking. Bonding among family members results from the form of communication patterns that exist.

Roles in the Family

Family member roles are patterns of wants, goals, beliefs, feelings, attitudes, and actions that family members have for themselves and others in the family. Roles are both assigned and acquired, and they specify what individuals do in the family. Although they are usually dependent on social class and cultural norms, roles are dynamic and change in response to factors both within the family and without. Roles are reciprocal and complement roles taken by other family members. Family equilibrium is dependent on how well roles in the family are balanced and reciprocated (Duvall & Miller, 1985; Friedman, 1986).

The way in which a family member assumes a particular role is influenced by various factors, including temperament, height, weight, gender, birth order, age, and health status. Certain roles, however, depend solely on the sex of the family member. Females can be sister, daughter, wife, mother, or girlfriend, whereas males can be brother, son, father, husband, or boyfriend. Other roles, such as breadwinner, child rearer, homemaker, cook, handyman, and gardener, are performance roles and depend on the person's ability to perform a certain task. In contrast to performance roles are emotional roles, such as leader, nurturer, scapegoat, caretaker, jester, arbitrator, or martyr, which may be adopted at certain times as a means of adjusting to the demands of a family system, to an extended family crisis such as a long-term family illness, or to long-term family conflict. The functions of emotional roles are to reduce conflict among family members and to promote temporary adaptation among family members. However, consistent use of emotional roles may impair adaptation, thus hindering the growth of the family. An example is when one family member, perhaps the oldest child, assumes the role of family caretaker, supporting other members and arbitrating disputes. The role may take on negative characteristics in this instance because the family caretaker may appear outwardly strong and capable but inwardly have unrealistic feelings, such as "I can't fail" or "I can't be weak." In this emotional role, this person may function under pressure to be perfect but at the same time have feelings of self-doubt and fear. It is important for the nurse to remember that roles have a significant effect on individual adjustment. Role function is influenced by the values of social groups to which the individual belongs. For example, in an international study by Vehvilainen (1998), Finnish Lutheran women placed less value on bearing and rearing children than other groups studied (American Mormons and Canadian Orthodox Jews).

Family Organization

To understand family organization, the nurse must remember that structuring of both functions and goals must be addressed. It is also important for the nurse to remember that most families are dynamic, endlessly adaptable, and continuously evolving in both structure and function. The functional ability of a family depends in part on the individual needs and wants of the members. If the nurse is unable to assist family members in meeting needs within the family structure, pain may be felt and confusion may exist. The nurse must keep in mind that, in the American culture, families are expected to be self-perpetuating and at the same time be the primary system for the transfer of social values and norms.

In the American culture, two primary goals are inherent in the family: (1) the encouragement and nurturance of each individual and (2) the production of autonomous, healthy children (O'Brien, 1992). Marital partners are expected to be supportive and protective of each other. Both the husband and the wife are expected to share a sense of meaning and emotional closeness within the boundaries of their relationship, thus fostering the goal of personality development. In families in which supportive relationships do not exist, the achievement of the first goal (the encouragement and nurturance of each individual) is not attainable. The second goal of the family includes encouraging children to develop their own identity and individuality by allowing them to develop ideals, feelings, and life directions. At the same time, children are encouraged to sense both similarities to and differences from others and to be able to initiate activities based on this information (Lewis, 1979). Factors that must be addressed to determine the degree to which the family will accomplish these two primary goals include the patterns of relationship and adaptive mechanisms that are present. There are many reasons why some families fail to accomplish these two primary goals, including psychiatric disturbance of family members, incomplete maturation of children, and disintegration of the family system. When the family uses adaptive mechanisms, internal equilibrium may result. These adaptive mechanisms are dependent on (1) the level of communication skills within the family; (2) the individual contributions of each family member to the family welfare; (3) the mutual respect and love within the family; (4) the type, kind, and amount of stressors encountered; (5) the response pattern to stressors encountered in the internal and external environment; and (6) the support or resources available and the opportunity to participate in support systems (Ackerman, 1984; Black, 2001). For example, a family that has an alcoholic father may not be able to accomplish goals because this problem may result in psychiatric disturbances in the wife and children, and ultimately the family system may disintegrate. The reasons for the disintegration of this family include not only the individual psychiatric disturbances but also accompanying difficulties, such as incomplete maturation of children and adult members, financial instability, inability to adapt successfully to stressors, and, more importantly, the inability of each family member to perceive the family unit as caring and loving (Brown, 1986).

Levels of Functioning. Four levels of family functioning that have been identified form a continuum in increasingly abstract levels (Box 4-1): (I) family functions and activities, (II) intrafamilial interactions, (III) interpersonal relationships, and (IV) the family system (Averaswald, 1973).

To understand the family from a cultural perspective, it is essential that the nurse recognize that

---

Box 4-1

LEVELS OF FAMILY FUNCTIONING

LEAST ABSTRACT
Level I: Family functions and activities
Level II: Intrafamilial interactions
Level III: Interpersonal relationships

MOST ABSTRACT
Level IV: The family system

Level I deals with family affairs and functions. Included in this level are tangible, pragmatic activities that are observable or easily identified; more important, these are things that family members are most comfortable discussing. Four categories of family functioning have been identified in Level I:

1. **Activities of family living.** Families are expected to provide physical safety and economic resources. Included in this category is the ability of family members to obtain such necessities as food, clothing, shelter, and health care.
2. **Ability of the family members to assist one another.** Included in this category is the family's ability to assist other members in developing emotionally and intellectually and at the same time attaining a personal as well as a family identity.
3. **Reproduction, socialization, and release of children.** Included in this category are functioning goals that allow the family to become closely aligned, thereby allowing the transmission of subcultural roles and values.
4. **Integration between the family, its culture, and society.** Included in this category is the ability of the family to use external environmental resources for support and feedback.

Level II deals with communication and various interactions between family members, including what is said, how it is said, patterns of communication over time, the ability of each family member to communicate, and the quality of communication skills. Also included in this level is the transfer of information from family member to family member.

Level III deals with the way family members interact in relationships that occur within the family constellation. The dimensions of closeness and power and the degree of empathy, support, and commitment among family members are important. How the family functions in regard to decision making and problem solving is included in this level.

Level IV deals with the concepts of the family system, as well as how the family functions as a system. Level IV is the most abstract level of family functioning. It encompasses the concepts of wholeness, openness or closedness, homeostasis, and rules.

Data obtained from Schneider, R. (1980, June). Conceptual scheme of family organization and function. Paper presented at St. Louis University Medical Center conference, St. Louis, Missouri.

family relationships are stronger among some ethnic or cultural groups than among others. However, the importance of socioeconomic class cannot be overlooked. According to Casavantes (1976), a pattern of strong family relationships exists, particularly among poor people, who have few resources and must rely on the support of the family kinship network to meet physical and emotional needs. Middle- or upper-class people often have resources that extend beyond the extended family and are therefore able to avail themselves of physical and emotional support within the community. It is often believed that when people do not have money or other available resources for recreation and social activities in the community, they tend to spend more time together and depend on the family group for recreational and social outlets.

Regardless of socioeconomic class, families must organize and structure themselves. Structure refers to the organization of the family and includes the type of family, such as nuclear or extended. The value system of the family dictates the roles assigned in the family, communication patterns within the family, and power distribution within the family (Friedman, 1986; Schneflen, 1972). The basic beliefs about humankind, nature, the supernatural (fate), time, and family relationships constitute a family's value system. Value systems are often clustered by socioeconomic status or ethnic groups. For example, families from lower socioeconomic groups tend to have a present-time orientation and view themselves as being subjugated by the environment or the supernatural (fate). Often the family relationships are disrupted by desertion of a spouse or by the early emancipation of the children because of severe economic difficulties. These families have been able to survive and adapt by taking in children of other extended family members; for example, a grandmother may provide direct assistance by raising her son's or daughter's children. In these families, power is usually authoritarian or not exerted at all.

Middle- and upper-class families in the United States for the most part espouse the Protestant work ethic values, which dictate the importance of working and planning for the future. These values encompass the belief that although man is somewhat evil, his behavior is changeable by hard work. In the middle- and upper-class family structure, financial stability and success are viewed as rewards for hard work. Within these classes, family relationships center on the nuclear family, socialization occurs with work-related or neighborhood friends, and power may be more egalitarian than in the lower-class family. Power tends to become more male dominated as the economic level of a family rises. Middle- and upper-class families often see themselves as able to control or have mastery over their environment (O'Brien, 1992).

When typical White American families are compared with Asian American families, some differences can generally be noted. The typical White American family defines itself by the present generation, is fiscally independent, has the core relationship as husband–wife, emphasizes happiness of the individual, and is more feeling oriented. In contrast, the Asian family is defined by past, present, and future generations; feels economic obligations to kin; has parent–child as the core relationship; emphasizes the welfare of the family; and is more task oriented (Hsu, 1985). The Asian client's explanatory model of illness is greatly influenced by the family (Smart, 1991), and the discussion of illness is related to a sense of obligation to family (Nilchaikovit, Hill, & Holland, 1993).

The nurse must keep in mind that these statements on structure and organization of a family by class are broad generalizations of social class values and in themselves cannot account for cultural differences. For example, many ethnic groups, such as the Newfoundland Inuit family, regardless of socioeconomic status, place great importance on extended family relationships rather than on the individualism valued by White, Protestant, middle-class Americans. A family with a good income but with a time orientation in the present, such as that commonly found among persons in the lower socioeconomic class, may fail to recognize the importance of saving money and thus may always struggle financially. To understand whether a family system organizes itself around a family unit, such as the extended family, or tends to be a more individualistic system, such as the nuclear family, the nurse must assess the family as a group. The American family is composed of diverse multicultural populations and is defined by three criteria: kinship, function, and location.

Kinship

In the first criterion, kinship, there are three dyads that imply the existence of or location for the individual within the family structure: husband–father, wife–mother, or child–sibling. There are several conventional forms of family structures that are composed of these positions, including the nuclear family and the stem family. The nuclear family, which was discussed earlier, may consist of a husband, a wife, and their nonadult children and is based on all three dyads, with their marital, parental, and sibling elements. Whereas the nuclear family is restricted to a depth of two generations, the stem family encompasses three generations: grandparents, parents, and children.

Function

The second criterion, function, describes the purpose, goals, and philosophy of the family organization. *Family function* is defined as the expected action of an individual in a given role. In a description of family organization, the term *function* is used to depict family roles and the assigned tasks for those roles. Every family has unit functions that must be performed to maintain the integrity of the family unit and to meet the needs of the family. If individual family members' needs and societal expectations are to be met, the functioning role of the family must be clearly delineated. In family systems with two or more individuals, the family members have unit functional responsibilities related to their social positions. Depending on position within the family structure, an individual may function in a variety of roles, such as companion, decision maker, health motivator, or sexual partner. It is important for the nurse to remember that the maintenance of the family system is dependent on these various roles. Some cultural groups function in traditional ways in which the family is viewed as a holistic functioning unit. Other cultural groups

may function as a disaggregate unit, meaning that the family does not function as a unit but members function independently.

When the nurse is providing care, it is particularly important to assess who has the decision-making function in the family. For example, a decision about consent to treatment, receiving care or teaching, or whether to follow instructions may need to be made individually (Haddad, 2001). On the other hand, a client may not feel comfortable in making a health care decision without the spouse or family. In some situations the client may defer to the spouse for decision making (Dowd, Davidhizar, & Giger, 2007). In still other situations, another individual or group, such as a deacon or a church, may need to be involved. In a traditional Mexican family, the man is the decision maker. When a decision regarding health care is needed, a woman may defer any decision until her husband can arrive (Bechtel & Davidhizar, 1998). Consideration for families' decision-making style is included in the recent additions to the standards of the Joint Commission for the Accreditation of Healthcare Organizations, which acknowledge the autonomy of the client and/or of the family in the health care decision-making process (JCAHO, 2000). Decisions about who makes decisions regarding the end of life may also be culturally determined, although it can never be assumed that all members of the group will act the same or share the same beliefs. For example, among Asian and Pacific Island cultures, the interaction of Buddhism, Confucianism, and Christianity generally supports filial piety. While the family assumes the decision-making role, terminating treatment for a parent can influence the fate of the living and be equated with ancestor murder. Thus, many families will want to provide artificial feedings and hydration to the terminally ill and to demented patients not taking food and fluids orally since they feel that only God decides when it is time to die (Mitty, 2001).

Another family function that the nurse needs to examine is family functions in relation to the family's physical, affectional, and social properties (Murray, Meili, & Zentner, 1993). Physical functions include providing food, clothing, and shelter;

protecting against danger; and providing health care. Affectional functions include meeting emotional needs. Social functions include providing social togetherness, fostering self-esteem, and supporting creativity and initiative. Another approach to examining family functions views the family from a task-oriented perspective (Sussman, 1971). Tasks include socialization of children, strengthening competency of family members in relation to their adjustments within organizations, appropriate use of social organizations, providing an environment that fosters the development of identities and affectional behavior, and creating a satisfying, emotionally healthy environment essential to the family's well-being. Adaptation is essential to the family's ability to carry out functions and tasks and to meet the changing needs of society and other social systems, such as political and health–illness systems.

One of the most significant dimensions affecting childrearing practices in America today is managing children's time with computers, TV, and video games. It is estimated that the average American child in 2002 spent an average of 4.5 hours a day at home in front of a screen, an increase of 30 minutes from the previous year. The average American child grows up in a home with two TVs, two VCRs, three audiotape players, two CD players, one video-game player, and one computer, according to a Kaiser Family Foundation study; children have an increasingly sedentary lifestyle and increased exposure to violent and sexual images (Kaiser Family Foundation, 1999). Parents are challenged to protect their children online by software packages such as Cyber Patrol, Net Nanny, and Cybersitter, but nothing is promoted as perfect, and children remain vulnerable to pornography and sex predators on the Internet (Dunnewind, 2001; Nordland & Bartholet, 2001).

Location

Family location is also a significant criterion for understanding the family. Martin (1978) and Leininger (1995)discussed the variations that occurred among values of African-American families when families were evaluated in urban versus rural settings. Martin found that when families moved from rural to urban settings, there was an erosion of values emphasizing "mutual aid" and a contrasting increase in individualism, materialism, and secularism. When urban African-Americans are compared with their rural counterparts, it appears that urban African-Americans may view their counterparts as lacking the toughness and sophistication needed to make headway in a dominant urban culture. Despite the variations that occur with location changes, geographical separation does not mean a severing of kinship ties, according to Martin; rather, geographical separation may strengthen the emotional bonds between relatives. Today there is a tendency among African-Americans, whether urban or rural, toward a migration back home and getting back to their people. For some African-Americans there has been an increasing awareness that the urban centers have not met their hopes and aspirations. From the 1940s to the 1970s, there was a migration by some African-Americans away from the rural South. In the 1980s there was a trend toward migration of some African-Americans away from the urban North back to the urban South. For example, significant numbers of urban Northern African-Americans have migrated to such cities as Atlanta, Dallas, and Houston (Kunen, 1996).

Religious Groups

According to many sociologists, religion is a social phenomenon (Carroll, Johnson, & Marty, 1979). Religious practices, therefore, are usually rooted in culture, and each culture typically has a set of beliefs that define health and the behaviors that prevent or treat illness (Davidhizar, Bechtel, & Cosey, 2000). However, many persons, particularly those with religious convictions, tend to think of religion in an entirely different way. For some people religion is seen in the context of a person's communion with the supernatural, and religious experiences fall outside ordinary experiences, whereas other people view religion as an expression of an instinctual reaction to cosmic forces (Johnstone, 2007). Another worldview of religion depicts it as an explicit set of messages from a deity. For the most part, all these beliefs tend to de-emphasize, ignore, and perhaps even reject the sociological dimensions of religion. Nevertheless, whether it is being considered in general, in regard to a particular religious family such as Christianity or Buddhism, or in regard to a very specific religious group, such as Baptists, religion is believed to interact with other social institutions and forces in society and to follow and illustrate sociological principles and laws. In other words, regardless of what religion is or is not, it is a social phenomenon and as such is in a continual reciprocal, interactive relationship with other social phenomena.

Regardless of its definition, be it theological or sociological, many different kinds of groups are based on religion. Generally, religious structures fall into two basic types: the church type and the withdrawal-group type. The church type of structure is broadly based and represents the normative spiritual values of a society that most people adhere to by virtue of their membership in the society, such as Hinduism in India or Catholicism in Spain. For the most part, membership in certain societies dictates the faith that the person should belong to if that person has not made a conscious, deliberate choice to adhere to something else. The church type of structure is generally a comprehensive system that allows for individual variations and in practice does not make extremely rigorous demands on its members. In the United States, the church type of structure is encompassed within numerous major denominations. This denominational structure is in sharp contrast with the church type of structure in other countries, such as India or Spain, where most of the people belong to one faith and one church. In some countries, particularly the United States, individual churches are often closely identified with an ethnic group rather than with a social class, and churches thrive, more or less, as a means of asserting ethnic identity. For example, the Black church, regardless of denominational faith, has become synonymous with the Black life experience. The Amish people, on the other hand, subscribe to one denominational belief; however, the belief is synonymous with the Amish life experience.

The second type of religious structure is the withdrawal group, which expresses the beliefs of those for whom personal commitment and experience are more important than the family and the community functions of religion (Ellwood, 2005). Withdrawal groups meet the needs of those who believe that the majority's faith or lack of faith is not for them. Persons involved in withdrawal groups define themselves by making a separate choice. These groups include the Amish or Jehovah's Witnesses, which tend to represent a more intense or unbending commitment than that held by the average person adhering to a religion. These groups may be called *sects*. Groups that combine separation with syncretism and new ideas and that emphasize mystical experience are often referred to as *cults*. However, the word *cult* is often used in Western society with caution because it has acquired a negative connotation. In some religious groups, such as the Church of Jesus Christ of Latter-Day Saints (Mormons), Muslims, Jehovah's Witnesses, Seventh-Day Adventists, Buddhists, or Hindus, as well as that of the Gypsy culture, the extended social organization of the religion is considered more important than membership in the individual family. It is essential to remember that while this view is held by some theological scholars (Ellwood, 2005), many members of these religious groups do not necessarily share this belief. For example, in the Church of Jesus Christ of Latter-Day Saints (the Mormon Church), children are taught at a very young age that families are eternal. In this sense, the family is viewed as a stable, cohesive group bonded by love and as such is one of the most important units on earth today (Sheler, 2000).

As persons from different religions increasingly intermarry, it is becoming more common for parents not to share the same faith. The proportion of Jews who married Gentiles, around 10% for the first half of the century, according to the American Jewish Committee, doubled in 1960, doubled again by the early 1970s, and in the 1990s has leveled off at just over 50%. Approximately one of three American Jews lives in an interfaith household (Wingert, Springen, Stone, et al., 1997). Comparable figures are 21% for Catholics, 30% for Mormons, and 40% for Muslims. Thus, a new form of religious identification in America is developing that is analogous to a "mixed race." However, although diversity is increasingly acceptable among American religions, observances inevitably involve some sectarianism. Even though raising children in two faiths promotes diversity, it is sometimes confusing for the children, who may feel that they are not as good as their all-Jewish or all- Christian cousins. Although attitudes toward intermarriage are becoming more liberal, for some it creates confusion over which holidays to celebrate and which church children should attend. On the other hand, intermarriage is not completely accepted in the United States. There are conservative sects, such as Old Colony Mennonites and Missouri Synod Lutherans, who are less tolerant of intermarriage and insist on born-again spouses (Wingert, Springen, Stone, et al., 1997).

There are 215 distinct church traditions represented in the United States. Many of these groups represent the process of dividing and reuniting that has been a characteristic of religious life in America (Lindner, 2004). According to the *Yearbook of American and Canadian Churches* (Lindner, 2004), there were 163,128,935 persons in the United States in 2005 who considered themselves members of a church; this is up from 2000, when more than 152 million claimed membership (Lindner, 2004). The denomination with the largest membership is the Catholic Church, with 66.4 million members; the Southern Baptist Convention has 16.2 million (all Baptists, including Southern Baptists, total 32.2 million), the United Methodist Church has 8.25 million, and the Church of God in Christ has 6.4 million. The Church of Jesus Christ of Latter-Day Saints ranks fifth, with a membership of 5.4 million, but is noted to have had a very brisk increase in membership since its origin in 1830. The Church of God in Christ, which has historically been the largest Black Pentecostal church, is now among the five largest denominations, indicative of the growth of Pentecostal churches (Lindner, 2004) (Tables 4-1 and 4-2).

Table 4-1 Largest Denominational Families in the United States

Denomination	2001 Estimated Adult Population
Roman Catholic Church	66,407,000
Baptist	32,432,000
Methodist/Wesleyan	11,001,000
Lutheran	7,551,000
Church of God in Christ	6,448,000
Church of Jesus Christ of Latter-day Saints	5,411,000
Presbyterian	3,407,000
Assemblies of God	2,687,000
Episcopal	2,334,000
Churches of Christ	1,072,000
Congregational/United Church of Christ	1,378,000
Jehovah's Witnesses	1,022,000
Seventh-Day Adventist	919,000
Orthodox Church in America	900,000
Christian Churches (Disciples of Christ)	786,000

Data reported via self-identification in the American Religious Identification Survey.

Worldwide, the vitality of Christianity is fading in the West, especially in Europe, where Christians often do not go to church. The center of Christianity is shifting to the developing world, as persons in Nigeria and India embrace the faith (Woodward, 2001). Christianity's identification with the poor is drawing the impoverished and the downtrodden. Christianity in the United States is attracting many young believers with an entertainment explosion. Alternative rock is just one part of the entertainment-led revolution that spans from the popular "Left Behind" novels, which have sold 28.8 million copies, to live festivals with Grammy-winning singers (Ali, 2001). Some 79% of Americans describe themselves as "spiritual"; 64% say they are "religious" (Underwood, 2005). Sixty-seven percent believe that when they die their souls will go to heaven or hell; 24% do not believe that heaven or hell exists. Beliefnet.com, a religious Web site, sends out more than 8 million daily e-mails of spiritual wisdom in various flavors to more than 5 million subscribers. Generic "inspiration" is the most popular

Table 4-2	Largest Organized Religions in the United States	
Religion	**2001 Estimated Adult Population**	**% of U.S. Population, 2001**
Christianity	159,030,000	76.7
Judaism	2,831,000	1.4
Islam	1,104,000	0.5
Buddhism	1,082,000	0.5
Hinduism	766,000	0.4
Unitarian Universalist	629,000	0.3
Wiccan/Pagan/Druid	307,000	0.1
Spiritualist	116,000	*
American Indian Religion	103,000	*
Baha'i	84,000	*

*Less than 0.05%.
Data reported via self-identification in the American Religious Identification Survey. Nonreligious, Atheist, and Agnostic categories have been dropped from this list.

type of e-mail (2.4 million), followed by the Bible (1.6 million), but there are 460,000 subscribers to the Buddhist thought for the day, 313 Torah devotees, 268,000 subscribers to Daily Muslim Wisdom, and 236,000 who get the Spirtual Weight Loss message. Islam is the fastest-growing religion in the world, with more than 7 million American believers (Ali, 2005). Campo-Flores (2004) describes the increasing number of Christian nightclubs that are proliferating in Dallas, Nashville, and Tamarac, Florida, along with the "Get your praise on" Christian movement.

Over the past decades, there has been a trend within nursing theory to separate religion from spirituality and to make spirituality the legitimate focus of nursing care (Kirkham, Pesut, Meyerhoff, Sawatzky, 2004). A priority in spiritual care is end-of-life care. Interest in transcultural nursing toward dying, death, and bereavement has dramatically increased in recent years (Fordham, Giger, & Davidhizar, 2006). Of particular interest are the disadvantaged dying: those who are older and are dying with other long-term degenerative and ultimately fatal illnesses; these patients are unlikely to be given the label of "terminally ill" or to be aware of their prognosis (Exley, 2004).

JEHOVAH'S WITNESSES

Although each group has unique practices that should be considered by the nurse, two groups with particular significance for the nurse are Jehovah's Witnesses and Seventh-Day Adventists.

The founder of the Watchtower Bible and Tract Society, which is the legal corporation now used by Jehovah's Witnesses, was Charles Taze Russell. The name "Jehovah's Witnesses" was taken in Columbus, Ohio, in 1931 in an attempt to differentiate between the Watchtower Tract Society and the true followers of Russell, who were represented by the Dawn Bible Students and the Layman's Home Missionary Movement. From 1876 to 1879, Russell served as pastor of a Bible class he organized in Pittsburgh, Pennsylvania, and was also the assistant editor of a small monthly magazine in Rochester, New York. However, he resigned from the editorial position in 1879 when controversy arose over his counterarguments on the atonement of Christ. In 1879 he founded the magazine *Herald of the Morning*, which developed into the magazine that is distributed today as *The Watchtower Announcing Jehovah's Kingdom*. This magazine has grown from a circulation of 6000 to 20.9 million per month and is published in 125 languages. Today there is another Watchtower periodical titled *Awake*; it has a circulation of 18.3 million issues twice a month and is published in 81 languages (*Jehovah's Witnesses 1997 Yearbook*, 1997).

In 1884 Russell incorporated Zion's Watchtower Tract Society, in Pittsburgh, which published a series of seven books. Russell himself wrote six of these books. The seventh volume, *The Finished Mystery*, caused a split in the group that culminated in a clean division. The larger portion of the group followed Joseph Franklin Rutherford, whereas the smaller portion subsequently became known as the Dawn Bible Students Association. Under Rutherford's leadership, the Watchtower Bible Society began to attack the doctrines of organized religion. This group eventually became known as the present-day Jehovah's Witnesses and has branches in 233 countries with 5.9 million members. According to 2004 statistics, there are 1,022,000 Jehovah's Witnesses in the United States (Lindner, 2004). The U.S. headquarters is located in Brooklyn, New York (Lindner, 2004).

Modern-day Jehovah's Witnesses still await the millennium. They regard Christ as a creature who will come to destroy the forces of evil at Armageddon, and they teach that sinners who are not saved will perish, whereas the faithful will enter into the Kingdom of Joy and Happiness. Because they believe in the Second Coming of the Kingdom, they undertake no military service. They also hold the belief that the institutions of government are under the control of Satan. It is this belief that has been the basis for some of the persecution they have undergone over the years. One view of this group is that Jehovah's Witnesses are peaceful but somewhat fanatical and that they know their Bible backward and forward (Smart, 1991). Some theologians believe that this religion appeals to persons of very modest education (Smart, 1991). The Jehovah's Witness faith is based on the doctrines presented in Box 4-2.

Implications for Nursing Care

There are many implications for the nurse who provides culturally appropriate nursing care to a Jehovah's Witness. The paramount concern for the nurse is that Jehovah's Witnesses are opposed, on the basis of scripture and Christian history, to homologous (amologous) blood transfusions (blood obtained from a blood bank or through donations). Blood that is precollected from the client for future use and is stored as either whole blood or as packed cells is also not acceptable (Watchtower, 1989). Jehovah's Witnesses hold the view that "God's determination is that blood represents life and thus is sacred" (Watchtower, 1989). They believe that it is God's commandment that no human should sustain life by taking blood. Jehovah's Witnesses believe that if blood is taken from a creature and not used for sacrifice, it should be disposed of and covered with dust. People who subscribe to this belief are likely to refuse any surgical or medical interventions that will require homologous blood transfusion. Even in the face of ominous danger and with the impending threat of loss of life, a Jehovah's Witness will refuse treatment for self and family members if a homologous transfusion is the only plausible blood replacement option available. However, many but not all Jehovah's Witnesses will submit to certain types of autologous blood transfusions (autotransfusion). Whether autologous blood transfusions will be accepted by a Jehovah's Witness depends on the type of autologous transfusion—one type that might be acceptable is blood retrieved through induced hemodilution at the start of surgery (blood that is directed to storage bags outside the client's body while plasma expanders [perfluorocarbons] are given to maintain blood volume). The blood is then reinfused toward the end of surgery or during the postoperative period. Although this type of autologous transfusion might be acceptable, other types, such as use of blood collected from a wound by aspiration, pumped through a filter or a centrifuge to remove debris and clots, and then returned to the client would not be an acceptable alternative (Watchtower, 1989). Many Jehovah's Witnesses carry a card stating that they refuse blood in all circumstances and the type of blood expander that is acceptable. The caregivers should ask the client for this extremely important card or, if the client is unconscious, examine the client's personal belongings to find it. When autologous blood transfusions or blood volume expanders are not plausible alternatives, many physicians look to alternatives during major surgery that are acceptable to Jehovah Witnesses, including colloids or colloid replacement fluids, electrocautery, hypotensive anesthesia, or

---

Box 4-2

BELIEFS OF JEHOVAH'S WITNESSES

1. Jehovah's Witnesses believe that there is one solitary Being from all eternity and that that Being is Jehovah, God, the creator and preserver of the universe in all things that are visible and invisible.
2. Jehovah's Witnesses do not believe in the Holy Trinity of three Gods in one—God the Father, God the Son, and God the Holy Ghost—who are equal in power, substance, and eternity (Watchtower Bible & Tract Society, 1953). Rather, they believe that Satan is the originator of the Trinity doctrine and that this doctrine is just another of Satan's attempts to keep people from learning the truth about Jehovah and his Son, Christ Jesus, which is that there is no Trinity (Watchtower Bible & Tract Society, 1953).
3. Jehovah's Witnesses believe that there is only one God and that he is greater than his Son. They believe that the Son, the first-born and only begotten, was sent by God but is not God himself and is not equal with God.
4. On the subject of the virgin birth, Jehovah's Witnesses believe that Jehovah God took the perfect life of his only begotten Son and transferred it from heaven to the womb of the unmarried virgin, Mary. They believe that Jesus' birth was not an incarnation but that he was emptied of all things heavenly and spiritual. This was a miracle in the sense that Jesus was born a man (and was flesh) instead of a spirit–human hybrid (Martin, 2003).
5. Jehovah's Witnesses believe that the human life that Jesus Christ laid down in sacrifice must be viewed as exactly equal to the life that Adam forfeited for all of his offspring. Thus, Jesus' life must be viewed as a perfect human life, no more and no less (Watchtower Bible & Tract Society, 1955).
6. Jehovah's Witnesses believe that immortality is a reward for faithfulness and that it does not come automatically to a human at birth (Watchtower Bible & Tract Society, 1953).
7. On the subject of the resurrection of Christ, Jehovah's Witnesses believe that Christ was raised from the dead, not as a human creature, but as a spirit (Watchtower Bible & Tract Society, 1953).
8. Jehovah's Witnesses believe that Christ Jesus will return again, not as a human but as a glorious spirit. National flags or symbols of the sovereign power of a nation are forbidden by Exodus 20:2–6. Thus, those who believe and ascribe salvation only to God may not salute a national emblem without violating Jehovah's commandments against idolatry (Watchtower Bible & Tract Society, 1953).
9. Jehovah's Witnesses believe that the hell mentioned in the Bible is mankind's common grave and that even an honest child can understand it. Thus, the doctrine of a burning hell where the wicked are tortured after death cannot be true.
10. Jehovah's Witnesses believe that man is a combination of two things: dust of the ground and breath of life. The combining of these two things produces a living soul, or a creature called man.
11. Jehovah's Witnesses believe that the undefeatable purpose of Jehovah God is to establish a righteous kingdom in these last days and that this purpose has already been fulfilled.
12. Jehovah's Witnesses believe that the Levitical commandments given by God to Moses included the commandment that no one in the House of David should eat blood or he would be cut off from people.

---

hypothermia. Researchers continue to seek a red cell substitute that is practical and safe, but the products that have been tried have not been pronounced successful. Many legal battles have been waged in the courts with regard to parents' refusal to allow surgical or medical interventions in their minor children. The consensus of the court in some countries, such as the Supreme Court in the United States, has been that a person of adult majority age has the right to refuse treatment but cannot withhold treatment from a minor child.

A second concern for the nurse is the refusal of Jehovah's Witnesses to eat certain foods to which

blood has been added, such as some sausages and lunch meats. The nurse must take extra care to ensure that blood has not been added to foods that are served to Jehovah's Witnesses. Because Jehovah's Witnesses are pacifists and conscientious objectors, the nurse must also take extra care to avoid raising such issues during interaction. In general, topics related to politics, government rule, and the like should be avoided. Because Jehovah's Witnesses do not observe any national holidays or ceremonies, including Christmas, the nurse should avoid any attempts to involve the client in preparations for such celebrations.

SEVENTH-DAY ADVENTISTS

The Seventh-Day Adventist religion sprang from the "Great Second Advent Awakening" that shocked the religious world just before the middle of the 19th century. During this period, reemphasis on the second advent of Jesus Christ was rampant in England and in Europe. It was not long before many of the Old World views and prophetic interpretations crossed the Atlantic and began to penetrate American theological circles (Martin, 2003). The American Seventh-Day Adventist group began in upper New York (Ellwood, 2005).

The first leader of the Seventh-Day Adventists was William Miller, a Baptist minister from Lower Hampton, New York. The Seventh-Day Adventist religion is based largely on the apocalyptic books of Daniel and Revelation. Many of the early students of the Seventh-Day Adventist religion, following the chronology of Archbishop Ussher, interpreted the 2300 days of Daniel as 2300 years, and thus they concluded that Christ would come back in about the year 1843. In 1818 Miller taught many of his followers that in about 25 years (1843), Jesus Christ would come again. Miller and his associates pinpointed October 22, 1843, as the specific final date on which Jesus Christ would return for his saints, visit judgment on sin, and establish the Kingdom of God on earth. Many theologians disagreed with Miller's contentions because they believed that Miller was teaching in contradiction to the Word of God. According to biblical scripture, "the day and hour knoweth no man, no, not the angels of heaven but God alone" (Matthew 24:36). Because of Miller's early teaching, the first group of Seventh-Day Adventists were called Millerites. However, the mistake of setting an exact date for Christ's Second Coming led to failure for the first Seventh-Day Adventist movement in the United States.

The modern Seventh-Day Adventist movement is based on the prophecy of Ellen G. White. White made an early assertion about Miller's prophecy that supported it and gave a date that she considered to be correct: October 22, 1844. Despite this failure in prediction, the group has grown and been active in evangelism. Today Seventh-Day Adventists believe that Christ will return again very soon and that Christians have an obligation to keep some of the laws of Moses, including worship on Saturday, the old Sabbath. Thirteen issues on doctrine that give direction for living and that are upheld by the Seventh-Day Adventist Church are presented in Box 4-3.

There were 914,106 members of the Seventh-Day Adventist Church in North America in 1999. The Seventh-Day Adventist Church is one of the fastest-growing churches in the world today, passing the 10 million mark in 1998 (General Conference of the Seventh-Day Adventists, 2002). The worldwide Seventh-Day Adventist Church headquarters are located in Washington, D.C.

Implications for Nursing Care

The religious doctrines of Seventh-Day Adventists teach that the body is a temple of God and thus should be kept healthy. Persons who subscribe to this faith may avoid such items as seafood, meat, caffeine, alcohol, drugs, and tobacco in all forms. To provide culturally appropriate nursing care to a Seventh-Day Adventist, the nurse must know and understand the religious doctrines of the Seventh-Day Adventist Church. A Seventh-Day Adventist may refuse surgical intervention on a Friday evening or Saturday morning or afternoon because the client may interpret such an intervention as being in direct conflict with religious doctrines. This same client may also refuse other medical interventions that might normally take place at these times, such as respiratory or physical therapy.

The religious doctrine regarding unclean foods may cause some clients to refuse to eat certain foods with shells, such as lobster or crab; scavenger fish, such as catfish; or certain meats. This refusal to eat some foods high in iodine or protein may cause these clients to have iodine and protein deficiencies; thus, it is important for the nurse to teach these clients that iodine and protein substitutes are necessary in the diet. Some specialty shops that have a Seventh-Day Adventist clientele stock a variety of protein substitutes for meats. These substitutes are often made from vegetables such as soybeans and

---

Box 4-3

BELIEFS OF SEVENTH-DAY ADVENTISTS

1. **Inspiration and authority of the scriptures.** Seventh-Day Adventists believe that the scriptures of both the Old Testament and the New Testament were inspired by God and constitute the very Word of God. They hold the Protestant position that the Bible is the sole root of the faith and practice of Christians.
2. **The nature of Christ.** Christ, called the Second Adam, is pure and holy, connected with God, and beloved by God. Seventh-Day Adventists believe that Christ is God and that he has existed with God for all eternity (Martin, 2003).
3. **The Atonement.** Seventh-Day Adventists do not believe that Christ made partial or incomplete sacrificial atonement on the cross. The all-sufficient sacrifice of Jesus was completed on the cross at Calvary.
4. **The Resurrection.** Seventh-Day Adventists believe that Jesus rose from the grave, ascended literally and bodily into heaven, and serves before God. They believe that there will be a resurrection of both the just and the unjust. For the just, this resurrection will take place at the Second Coming of Christ, whereas the resurrection of the unjust will take place 1000 years later, at the close of the millennium (Revelation 20:5–10).
5. **The Second Coming.** Seventh-Day Adventists believe that Jesus Christ will assuredly come the second time and that his second advent will be visible, audible, and personal.
6. **The plan of salvation.** Seventh-Day Adventists believe that one must be born again and fully accepted by the Lord. They believe that there is nothing an individual can ever do that will merit the salvation of God. Salvation is by grace (Romans 3:20).
7. **The spiritual nature of man.** Seventh-Day Adventists believe that man rests in the tomb until the resurrection of the just, when the righteous will be called forth by Christ (Revelation 20:4–5). It is at this point that the just will enter into everlasting life in their eternal home in the Kingdom of Glory.
8. **Punishment of the wicked.** Seventh-Day Adventists reject the doctrine of eternal torment because everlasting life is a gift from God (Romans 6:23). The wicked do not possess this and therefore shall not have eternal life (John 3:36).
9. **Sanctuary and investigative judgment.** Seventh-Day Adventists believe that the acceptance of Christ at conversion does not seal a person's destiny; rather, it determines his life's work after conversion. Man's record is closed when he comes to the end of his days; he is responsible for his influences during life and is likewise responsible for his evil influences after he is dead.
10. **Scapegoat teaching.** Seventh-Day Adventists repudiate the idea that Satan is the sin bearer.
11. **The Sabbath and the Mark of the Beast.** This doctrine is based on the Bible as interpreted by Seventh-Day Adventists and not according to Ellen White's writings. Seventh-Day Adventists do not believe that keeping the Sabbath is a means of keeping salvation or willing merit before God. They believe that man is saved only by grace.
12. **The question of unclean food.** Seventh-Day Adventists refrain from eating certain foods, not because of the laws of Moses but because it is a Christian duty to preserve the body in the best of health for the service and glory of God (1 Corinthians 3:16).
13. **The "remnant church."** Seventh-Day Adventists believe God has a precious remnant, a multitude of earnest and sincere individuals, in every church. The majority of God's children are scattered throughout the world and may practice their religion on Sunday.

---

may take the place of meats such as ground beef. These substitutes should be encouraged, particularly when they appear to be free of preservatives.

The nurse and the nurse manager should also be aware that a colleague who is a Seventh-Day Adventist may refuse to accept assignments on Friday evenings or Saturday during the day, since the Sabbath begins on Friday at dusk and extends to Saturday at dusk. It is important for the nurse who is a Seventh-Day Adventist to ascertain at the time of employment whether working on Friday evenings or Saturday during the day is a requirement of the job. On the other hand, it is also important for the nurse manager to include staff in making nondiscriminatory policies in this regard. Inclusion of staff in policy making may minimize implementation difficulties.

ISLAM: THE RELIGION*

According to a recent study of mosques (Bagby, Perl, & Froehle, 2001), Islam is the fastest-growing religion in the United States. Between 1994 and 2000, the number of mosques increased from 962

*The section on Islam (Muslims) was written by Mary Grace Umlauf, Ph.D., RN.

to 1209, an increase of 25%. Much of the growth in these congregations has occurred in less than 20 years; about one third of mosques were established in the 1980s and another third in the 1990s. The ethnic distribution of members of the average mosque is 25% Arab, 33% South Asian, and 30% African-American. Most organizations are involved in some outreach activities, 70% provide some type of assistance for the needy, and 20% have full-time schools for children. Based on the 2 million persons associated with a mosque in this study, the total U.S. Muslim population is estimated at 6 to 7 million persons and growing. Part of this increase in numbers is attributed to conversion to Islam, which has been estimated at 17% to 30% of membership.

The three major monotheistic religions of the world, Judaism, Christianity, and Islam, share common cultural roots and history. All three originated in the Middle East, and each developed and dispersed globally in response to cultural influences and world politics. The Arabic word *Islam* means "peace, submission, and obedience." Islam is a monotheistic religion that recognizes Muhammad as the last of the great prophets, following in the footsteps of Noah, Abraham, Moses, and Jesus. The life and writings of Muhammad, the Qur'an, serve as a template for Muslims to worship, pray, raise their families, and conduct daily life. The tenets of Islamic life are described as the "Five Pillars of Islam." Although religious groups often become well known by the actions of their extremist members, Islam is not typically practiced as a fundamentalist religion. The practice of Islam is less well known because Muslims are a religious minority primarily represented by immigrant populations. This demographic is changing with the increase in membership by African-Americans.

The Five Pillars of Islam

1. The declaration of faith: The first article of faith in Islam is to recognize the existence of one Supreme Being. Muslims bear witness that there is none worthy of worship except Allah and that Muhammad is his messenger to all humanity until the day of judgment. The prophethood of Muhammad obliges Muslims to follow his exemplary life as a model.
2. Daily prayers: Muslims offer prayers five times a day as part of their religious duty to remain focused on spiritual connectedness. These prayers are scheduled throughout the day at designated times and are observed at work, in school, and at home. The result is a rhythm of daily life that is punctuated with communal religious devotion.
3. Fasting during Ramadan: Islam employs both solar and lunar calendars, and the observance of daytime fasting occurs during the ninth lunar month, Ramadan. During this 28-day period Muslim adults abstain from food and drink from dawn to sunset. The purpose of this communal fast, known as *sawm*, is to develop restraint, self-control, self-discipline, and self-obedience. Pregnant or lactating women, children, the sick, and the elderly are excused from fasting, but those who can afford it may be expected to provide a meal to a poor person for each day they cannot fast.
4. Giving alms to the poor: *Zakat* is an annual payment or tithe of a percentage of income given to the poor or needy. All Muslims are bound by this religious duty, although the amount is based on the individual's ability to pay.
5. Pilgrimage to Mecca: Each Muslim is obligated to perform hajj, a pilgrimage to the holy city of Mecca in Saudi Arabia. Hajj is required once during a lifetime, provided that the individual Muslim is physically and financially able.

Common Muslim Phrases

"God willing" or "If God wills it" (إِنْ شَاءَ اللّٰه pronounced *in sha'allah*) is a common phrase used regarding future events to acknowledge the limited control of humans and the supremacy of Allah in daily life. For example, one person asks, "When will you return?" The respondent will often say something like "God willing, I will come again tomorrow."

"Thanks be to God" (الحمد لله pronounced *hamdu'allah*) is a phrase commonly used to acknowledge the hand of God in all things good. For example, when common greetings are exchanged, such as "How are you today?" the response is often "I am doing well. Thanks be to God." (Also see Box 4-4 for common Islamic terms.)

Social Differences in Islamic Culture

Apart from religious adherence, Islamic culture manifests itself in many ways that are similar to other cultural groups in the United States. The importance of the extended family unit is a pervasive theme among Muslims and other persons who come from countries that are historically Islamic. Social customs, such as styles of women's clothing, are distinct, but the theme of modest clothing for women is common to many other faiths and communities, such as the Amish and Orthodox Jews. Likewise, the prohibition against eating pork is also held in common with Judaism.

Emphasis on Family

In the context of Islamic culture, the value of the family group supersedes the importance of the individual. Individuals draw their identity and strength from their families. Family can be counted upon to provide nurturing, social support, economic assistance, and caregiving. Children are highly valued and lavished with affection by all members of the family. Children are more often cared for by family

---

Box 4-4

COMMON ISLAMIC TERMS

Allah: The Supreme Being, the one and only God, the same God as that worshiped by Jews and Christians.

Azan: The call for daily prayers, broadcast five times a day in Arabic over a loudspeaker in the minaret, or tower, of the mosque.

'Eid: A religious festival. There are two main celebrations in Islam. The 'Eid Al Fitr marks the end of Ramadan, a month of fasting. The 'Eid Al-Adhha is the Feast of Sacrifice in memory of when the prophet Abraham was asked to sacrifice his son Ishmael.

Hadith: A collection of sayings and traditions of the prophet Muhammad that are used to guide daily life, dietary practices, and social interactions.

Halal: A term meaning "lawful," which refers to compliance with the Qur'an and the Hadith. In Muslim communities, grocery stores advertise halal meat for sale. Like the Jewish Kosher tradition, these vendors have followed the Islamic practices required in the preparation and killing of animals.

Haram: The converse of halal, unlawful according to the tenets of the Qur'an and the Hadith. Eating pork is considered haram for Muslims. Sex outside of marriage is also haram or forbidden.

Imam: A religious leader who leads congregational prayers at the mosque. This person is not viewed as infallible. The imam is not ordained or assigned to a particular mosque by any higher religious authority.

Jihad: An Arabic word derived from the word jahada, which means to strive for a better way of life or endeavor, strain, exertion, effort, diligence, or fighting to defend one's life, land, and religious freedom. Extremists may use this concept as justification for violence, whereas most Muslims understand this concept to mean the intrapersonal struggle to overcome evil and to live a just and good life.

Masjid: The Arabic word for "mosque." The three holiest mosques are located in the Middle East. Al-Masjid Al-Haram and Al-Masjid Al-Nabawi are located in Mecca and Madinah, Saudi Arabia, where Islam originated. The third is Al-Masjid Al-Aqsa in Jerusalem.

Muhammad: The last and final prophet who established the monotheistic religion of Islam in the midst of a climate of political polytheism. He was born in 570 and died in 632 A.D. He was a husband, father, religious leader, political leader, and reformer. The contents of the Qur'an were revealed to him at the age of 40 through the angel Gabriel.

Muslim (or Moslem): A believer in Islam. The term "Mohammadan" is viewed as incorrect and inappropriate to Muslims because it implies that they worship Muhammad in the way Christians worship Christ. Moslems assert, as a primary article of faith, that they believe in Allah and do not deify Muhammad.

Qur'an (or Koran): The holy scripture of Islam revealed by Allah to Muhammad over a period of 23 years. The Qur'an is maintained in Arabic and studied in its original form. Translation of the text is said to dilute or reinterpret the original meaning of the text.

Zakah: Giving alms, one of the five pillars of Islam. The money collected is to be used for the welfare of society in the following categories: the poor, the needy, the sympathizers, the captives, the debtors, the cause of Allah, the wayfarers, and those who collect it. The amount collected ranges from 2.5% to 10%, depending upon the resources of the individual.

members and are seldom cared for by unrelated persons. Adolescents and young people develop strong bonds with other members of the family of the same sex, who provide career guidance and mentoring. Primary allegiance is deferred to parents, who make important decisions such as advanced schooling or career selection on behalf of the child, even into adulthood. This is not to say that the child has no input in decision making or that personal skill or ability is not considered. Typically, the parent and child discuss the pros and cons of a given course of action. The parent ultimately confirms or negates a decision, and the child is usually persuaded to accept the outcome. After marriage, this pattern of decision making is more consultative in nature. Marriage partners confer with each other, while also taking input from the other family members into account.

Social Support

Because family members prefer to live in close proximity and typically spend a lot of time together, the extended family can provide a great deal of support if there are problems in the nuclear family. For example, if a married couple is experiencing problems, it is usually apparent or known to some degree. Individually, the husband or wife will often confer with a trusted family member about the problem. Regardless of the nature of the problem, the family mobilizes to problem-solve or to reconcile differences between the partners. Although divorce is permitted in Islam, divorce is not preferable when children are involved. In general, problems of an individual or an individual nuclear family are also the concerns of the family group.

The Crisis of Infertility

Among families that are newly emigrated from Islamic countries, fertility problems are viewed as particularly disastrous for married partners. Because of the high value placed on children in the family, infertility may be an acceptable justification for divorce in an immigrant's country of origin. Some Islamic countries recognize polygamy as a social tradition that can remedy this problem for the male partner who is fertile. In those countries

he can retain an infertile wife and marry another wife who is likely to be fertile. However, polygamy is not permitted in the United States. Thus, an infertile Muslim woman may be at risk for an unwanted divorce because she now lives in the United States. An infertile man is also at risk of being rejected by his wife, who is likely to have full support of her family for this action. Medical interventions for infertility that involve sperm or egg donation are unacceptable under Islamic law because they violate the primary recognition of family membership. Each child must carry the name of his father and family. Anonymous donation of genetic material violates this essential directive. Adoption outside the family unit is not an attractive option for infertile couples for the same reason. Conversely, adoption of orphaned family members is viewed as a family obligation and right.

Covered Women

One of the most noticeable differences about practicing Muslims is the way some of the women dress. As Muslim girls are growing up, they are taught the importance of *hijab*, or modesty. Modesty, particularly the covering of the hair and arms when in public, is meant to avoid pride or showiness in outward appearance, much like the practice of Amish women or religious orders of Catholic women. As a matter of religious preference, when a girl reaches puberty, she can choose to cover herself when in public by wearing a headscarf and long-sleeved clothing. Typically, Muslim women also wear longer skirts or long pants. At home and in the presence of family members or groups of women only, these same women do not cover. Even though a woman may be dressed in a scarf and a somber-colored full-length dress in public, underneath she may be wearing the latest fashion and the brightest colors. Although the practice of *hijab* is viewed as a form of modesty and religiosity, becoming covered also marks a rite of passage and evolving membership for young women in the family and social group. Thus, very young girls make a very demur debut as young women in the Muslim community when they begin to cover.

Women who practice *hijab* are also likely to avoid situations where they must touch or be in very close proximity to men. These women may avoid shaking hands with men and will avoid sitting next to a man on public transportation, such as a bus or plane. Male health care providers may not be able to perform physical assessments or provide personal care to these women because of their commitment to modesty. A female nurse may have to perform breast or pelvic exams in lieu of a male physician or male nurse.

Sex and Marriage

Along with the emphasis on family and on modesty among women, sex outside of marriage is highly discouraged. Young people are encouraged to maintain strong social ties with others of the same sex. Activities sponsored by mosques and related organizations will congregate men with men and women with women. Only infrequently will there be activities that include a mixed group. Even wedding celebrations will provide separate but adjoining halls or ballrooms for men and women to congregate separately, and the children often migrate between rooms at will. In the more traditional families, dating does not begin unless there is an interest in marriage and the woman's family has approved beginning a relationship. The selection of a marriage partner is a planned activity, and the extended family may be called upon to identify well-qualified marriage partners. Families try to identify potential marriage partners with a good family background, a good education, a good job, and a compatible temperament who are also Muslim. In general, Muslim families will accept a marriage with a non-Muslim, but Christian families from an Islamic background will not accept a marriage with a Muslim. Families do not arrange marriages per se, but there is an active interest in making sure that the wrong type of person is not considered. Because this is an acceptable practice in Islamic cultures, there is less pressure for dating and premarital sex among young people. Concurrently, there is greater communal support for having a good reputation, an education, and a good job, as well as a good family background.

Stereotypes About Muslims

1. All Arabs are Muslims, all Muslims are Arabs: Arabs may be of any faith, and many are Orthodox Christians. Muslims may be from any ethnic group. Many U.S. converts to Islam are African-Americans. However, converts must learn Arabic to study the Qur'an.
2. Most Muslims are from the Middle East: There are more Muslims in Indonesia than in all Arab countries combined. Many Muslims also come from Asia and sub-Saharan Africa, or they may be American residents who have recently converted to Islam.
3. Islam promotes violence, or Muslims are violent people: Most Muslim immigrants come from developing countries with unstable political and economic systems. Many come to the United States to avoid the strife of war and to live peaceful lives with their families.
4. Muslims do not recognize the rights of women to go to school or to have jobs: Social custom or political oppression should not be confused with religious and cultural practices. Although there have been recent examples of the oppression of women in a few Islamic countries, the Qur'an does not deny women the freedom to learn, to be productive, or to own property.
5. Family violence is common among Muslims: Family violence can occur in any household regardless of religious background or economic status. Although no data are available, marital conflicts may occur more often among new immigrant families because they lack the economic and social support offered by extended families in their home countries. In response to this need, many mosques have initiated programs to address this problem. For example, the Islamic community in Oakland, California, has developed an outreach program called "Muslims against Family Violence" that includes public education, a toll-free number for assistance, and a Web site that describes their prevention program. This Web site also provides additional links for information and support (http://www.mcadsv.org/mrcdsv).

ETHNIC GROUPS IN RELATION TO FAMILY IN THE UNITED STATES

In 2000, there were an estimated 300 million people living in the United States (U.S. Department of Commerce, Bureau of the Census, Summary File 3, 2002). Of these, 34,361,740 (12.3%) were Black, 2,447,989 (0.9%) were American Indian/Eskimo-Aleuts, 10,171,820 (3.6%) were Asian, and 378,782 (0.3%) were Pacific Islander. Additionally, 35,238,481 (12.52%) were Hispanic. About 195 million (70.38%) of the total population classified themselves as non-Hispanic White (U.S. Department of Commerce, Bureau of the Census, Summary File 3, 2002). It is estimated that by 2050, the United States will have 393.9 million people, 40% more than the population today. It is also estimated that the population will be more diverse. The non-Hispanic White share of the population is projected to fall from the current 70.38% to 53% by 2050. Meanwhile, persons of Hispanic origin will increase from 12.5% to 24% of the population. Asians and Pacific Islanders will see their population climb from 3.75% to 9%. Increases are expected to be smaller for American Indian, Eskimo, and Aleut populations, from slightly under 1% and for African-Americans from 12.3% to 16% (U.S. Department of Commerce, Bureau of the Census, Summary File 3, 2002). Two ethnic groups will be discussed in relation to family as follows.

American Indians

According to the 2000 census, there are 2,423,457 American Indians living in the United States (U.S. Department of Commerce, Bureau of the Census, Summary File 3, 2002.) Because there are more than 500 different federally recognized tribes of American Indians and an additional 200 who do not benefit from federal recognition, it is difficult to predict patterns of residency unless one is dealing with specific tribes (Palacios, Butterfly, & Strickland, 2006). The 2000 census reported that the 10 states with the largest American Indian populations, in order, were California, Oklahoma, Arizona, Texas, New Mexico, New York, Washington, North Carolina, Michigan, and Alaska. Florida was the only other state with more than 100,000 American Indians. These 11 states are home to 62% of the total U.S. American Indian population (U.S. Department of Commerce, Bureau of the Census, Summary File 1, 2000). In the United States, Indian reservations are places where very slow and very rapid changes are occurring simultaneously. It is estimated that 72% of Navajo homes still do not have a telephone and that many homes lack plumbing. On the other hand, among American Indians type 2 diabetes mellitus and obesity have suddenly appeared with the highest incidence in the world (Reid, 2000). Providing culturally appropriate nursing care is complicated because each nation or tribe of American Indians has its own language and religion, and belief system practices differ significantly among groups as well as among members of the same tribe (Palacios, Butterfly, & Strickland, 2006).

The American Indian family is frequently composed of extended family members who may encompass several households. Through various religious ceremonies, other individuals can become the same as a parent in the family network. In some American Indian tribes, grandparents are viewed as the family leaders, and respect for individuals increases with their age. In some tribes, the family is viewed as important, particularly in periods of crises, when family members are expected to serve as sources of support and security. It is important for the nurse to remember that because some American Indian tribes tend to place great emphasis on the extended family as a unit, the opinions and ideas of the family members should be solicited in order to give culturally appropriate nursing care. Even though physicians and hospitals may be available to American Indians, some families may still hold traditional healing ceremonies in high regard, and it may be important to incorporate old ways to treat illnesses for a treatment plan to be effective.

The Hmong

The Hmong are of Asian descent and are an ethnic–cultural group of people who originally lived in the rural highlands of Laos (Johnson & Hang, 2006;

Lester, 2006). Many of the Hmong living in the United States today were displaced from their homeland because of their alignment with the United States during the Vietnam War (Johnson & Hang, 2006). There are 169,428 Hmong residing in the United States (U.S. Department of Commerce, Bureau of the Census, Summary File 3, 2002). Although the data are not available from the 2000 census by individual Asian groups, the mean age for Asian Americans was 32.7 years. In contrast, in 1995, the median age of Hmong who made the United States their home was 12.5 years. Hmong, by median age, are reported to be the youngest ethnic cultural group in the United States (U.S. Department of Commerce, Bureau of the Census, 1993a and 1993b). Not only are Hmong one of the youngest cultural groups residing in this country but also they tend to have larger families (6.6 persons) than other Asian Americans (3.8 persons) and the general U.S. population (3.2 persons) (U.S. Department of Commerce, Bureau of the Census, 1993b). Of the Hmong residing in the United States who are 25 years of age or older, 44.1% of men and 19.0% of women hold a high school diploma. Similarly, in this same age group, 7.0% of men and 3.5% of women hold a bachelor's degree or higher. Of the Hmong in the United States, 96.9% speak an Asian or Pacific Island language at home, 65.0% do not speak English well, and 43.9% are reported to be linguistically isolated (U.S. Department of Commerce, Bureau of the Census, 1993b).

The Hmong are primarily an oral cultural group, a statement implying that some Hmong have never learned to read Hmong or any other language (Shadick, 1993). In the 1950s, French missionaries introduced to the Hmong a form of written Hmong, which is based on the Roman alphabet (Shadick, 1993). There are two major dialectal variations in the oral Hmong language, Hmoo Daw (White Hmong) and Hmoo Ntsua (Blue Hmong) (Dunnigan, 1986). According to Catlin (1982), Hmong is spoken by using one of eight tones. For some Hmong, the oral word holds greater meaning and power than does the written word (Shadick, 1993). Some Hmong consider the spoken word to be the primary tool and mechanism for passing on traditions, rituals, and information to future generations (Shadick, 1993). It is important for the nurse to remember this when interacting with Hmong clients. Because they tend to be primarily an oral cultural group, culturally appropriate care is hindered when treatment plans and protocols are given to the client in a written form (even when the client does speak English). Hmong shaman are influential individuals within their community and often serve as resources for health information (Hensel, Mochel, & Bauer, 2005).

Special Interest Groups

Special interest groups are a significant part of the social structure of the United States. Individuals may join a group for many reasons, including support and self-help. Support groups provide the opportunity to increase the participant's social network, share solutions to common problems, and reshape perceptions of self and the environment. Examples of support groups include quality-of-life groups, caregiver support groups, and bereavement support groups (McMahon & Presswalla, 1997). Self-help groups are attractive to members because they promote well-being. Self-help groups are usually focused on particular clinical states, such as chronic mental illness; a particular social state, such as divorce; or special psychosocial issues, such as chemical dependency. Examples include Alcoholics Anonymous (AA), Narcotics Anonymous (NA), and Overeaters Anonymous (OA). Support groups may replace or augment the family or formal health care system and generally aim to link health behaviors with everyday existence. Self-help groups foster self-reliance and are a form of healing (McMahon & Presswalla, 1997). A network of friends, relatives, and neighbors can be crucial to psychological well-being and can relieve social isolation, promote mental health, facilitate coping, alleviate problems by preventive problem solving, and assist persons in preparing for stressful events in life (Brown, 1990).

Implications for Nursing Care

When nurses provide care to clients from a sociocultural background other than their own, they must have an awareness of and a sensitivity to the client's sociocultural background, including knowledge of family structure and organization, religious values and beliefs, and how ethnicity and culture relate to role and role assignment within group settings. Friedman (1986) contends that nursing care must be directed to the family as a whole as well as to the individual family member. The nurse must therefore view the family as having two separate entities, the first being the family as an environment and the second being the family as the client. Both approaches to client care can be useful when the nurse attempts to provide culturally appropriate nursing care.

If the family is viewed as an environment, the primary focus of nursing care is the health and development of individual family members within a very specific environment. In this context it is important for the nurse to assess the extent to which the family provides the individual basic needs of each person. It is also essential that the nurse remember that individual needs vary, depending on developmental level and the current situation. The nurse should recognize that families provide more than just the physical necessities; the ability of the family to help the client meet psychosociological needs is paramount.

When families are viewed as an environment, it is extremely important for the nurse to recognize that other family members may also need intervention. For example, when a child is hospitalized, the parents may feel anxiety and stress; therefore, intervention with them is just as important as intervention with the hospitalized child (Davidhizar, Havens, & Bechtel, 1999; Sydnor-Greenberg & Dokken, 2000).

When families are viewed as clients, it is important to assess crucial factors that are germane to family structure and organization. For example, if a hypertensive client is admitted to a hospital unit, it is crucial that the nurse assess several factors related to the family, including the following:
1. The family's current dietary patterns
2. The family's desire, as well as resources, for changing the dietary patterns
3. The family's knowledge about hypertension and its effects on the body
4. The family's capabilities to support a hypertensive family member
5. The family's ability to cope with and manage stress and anxiety

Whether the family is viewed as an environment or as the client, it is essential to incorporate cultural concepts when the nursing plan of care is being developed. The nursing process is used regardless of whether the family is viewed as an environment or as the client. The delineations or differences that occur in the nursing process are the result of cultural variables and beliefs that are germane to a particular ethnic or cultural group. Therefore, it is essential that the nurse incorporate cultural beliefs and concerns shared by family members into the plan of care.

Case Study

Susie Chung, a 24-year-old Chinese American, is admitted with right lower-quadrant abdominal pain. Within a few hours Miss Chung is taken to surgery for an appendectomy. When she returns to the floor, her vital signs remain stable. The nurse notes that even though Miss Chung is rapidly recovering, her immediate and extended family appear to hover about her. The nurse also notes that it is very difficult to administer nursing care because of the number of family members who are keeping a constant vigil.

✳ STUDY QUESTIONS

1. List at least three social organization factors that influence the interactions between members of the same ethnic group or members of varying ethnic groups.
2. List at least two social organization factors that contribute to the development of cultural behavior.
3. Explain the role that religion may play for Susie Chung with regard to sociopsychological adaptation to her illness.
4. List at least three nursing interventions that minimize the confusion caused by the large number of family members who are keeping constant vigil in Susie Chung's room.
5. List at least two reasons why the family members of Susie Chung have congregated in the hospital room.
6. List at least three factors that would support Susie Chung's family being defined as a behavioral system.
7. List at least two imaginary and two real boundaries that would be found within Susie Chung's family structure.
8. List at least two roles that Susie Chung may take on in a social context within her family structure.

NCLEX-RN REVIEW QUESTIONS

1. When planning to teach an Islamic client, the nurse needs to be aware that:
   A. Decision making tends to be male dominated.
   B. Decision making tends to be female dominated.
   C. Decision making tends to be generally consultative between spouses.
   D. Decision making tends to be consultative with the entire family.

2. When planning care for the patient who is a Jehovah's Witness and may need blood in an upcoming surgery, the nurse should be aware that:
   A. The patient will not accept whole blood.
   B. The patient will not accept predeposited autologous blood.
   C. The patient may accept autologous blood through induced hemodilution.
   D. The patient will accept wound-aspirated blood that has been filtered.

3. In developing a culturally sensitive care plan for a Hmong (Asian-American) psychiatric patient, which of the following would be inappropriate:
   A. Including the family in the plan of care.
   B. Showing respect by avoiding eye contact.
   C. Avoiding touching the head.
   D. Communicating all instructions in a written form.

References

Ackerman, N. (1984). *The theory of family systems*. New York: Gardner Press.

Adams, D. (1995). Cultural diversity and institutional inequity. In Adams, D. L. (Ed.), *Health issues for women of color*. Thousand Oaks, Calif.: Sage.

Adler, P., Good, M., Roberts, B., & Snyder, S. (2000, Fourth Quarter). The effects of Tai Chi on older adults with chronic arthritis pain. *Journal of Nursing Scholarship*, 32(4), 377–378.

Ali, L. (2001, July 16). The glorious rise of Christian pop. *Newsweek*, 38–41.

Ali, L. (2005, September 5). New welcoming spirit of the Mosque. *Newsweek*, 52.

American Association of Physical Anthropologists. (1996). AAPA statement on biological aspects of race. *American Journal of Physical Anthropology*, 101, 569–570.

American Psychiatric Association. (2000). *Diagnostic and statistical manual of mental disorders, text revision*.

(ed. 4.). Washington, D.C., American Psychiatric Association.

Andrews, M., & Boyle, J. (2003). *Transcultural concepts in nursing care*. (ed. 4.). Philadelphia: Lippincott.

Associated Press. (2000, January 24). Study: earnings gap between genders growing. *USA Today*, 1.

Averaswald, E. (1973). Families, change and the ecological perspective. In Ferber, A. (Ed.), *The book of family therapy*. New York: J. Aronson.

Bagby, I., Perl, P. M., & Froehle, B. T. (2001). *The mosque in America: a national portrait*. Washington, D.C.: Council on American-Islamic Relations.

Bateson, G., Jackson, D., Haley, J., & Weakland, J. (1968). Toward a theory of schizophrenia. In Jackson, D. D. (Ed.), *Communication, family and marriage*. Palo Alto, Calif.: Science & Behavior Books.

Bechtel, G., & Davidhizar, R. (1998, November). Mexicans in the psychiatric care setting. *Psychosocial Nursing and Mental Health Services*, 36(11), 20–27.

Berkanovic, E., & Reeder, L. G. (1973). Ethnic, economic and social psychological factors in the source of medical care. *Social Problems*, 21, 246–259.

Berry, J. (1988). Acculturation and psychological adaptation: a conceptual overview. In Berry, J. W., & Annis, R. C. (Eds.), *Ethnic psychology: research and practice with immigrants, refugees, native peoples, ethnic groups and sojourners*. Amsterdam: Swets & Zeitlinger.

Birx, E. (2002). *Healing Zen*. Ontario, Canada: Viking Compass.

Black, C. (2001). *It will never happen to me* (ed. 2.). Center City, Minn.: Hazelden.

Blum, R., Buehring, T., & Rinehart, P. (2000). *Protecting teens: beyond race, income, and family structure*. Minneapolis: Center for Adolescent Health, University of Minnesota.

Bonder, B., Martin, L., & Miracle, A. (2002). *Culture in clinical care*. Thorofare, N.J.: Slack.

Bowen, M. (1985). *Family therapy in clinical practice*. Northvale, N.J.: Jason Aronson.

Brown, R. (1990). Self-help and therapy groups. *The Marshall Cavendish encyclopedia of personal relationships: human behavior*, New York: Marshall Cavendish.

Brown, S. (1986). Children with an alcoholic parent. In Estes, N., & Heinemann, M. (Eds.), *Alcoholism: development, consequences, and interventions* (ed. 3.) (pp. 207–220). St. Louis: Mosby.

Bullough, V. L., & Bullough, B. (1982). *Health care for the other Americans*. East Norwalk, Conn.: Appleton-Century-Crofts.

Campo-Flores, A. (2004, April 19). Get your praise on. *Newsweek*, 56.

Caplan, G. (1976). The family as a support system. In Caplan, G., & Killilea, M. (Eds.), *Support systems and mutual help: multidisciplinary exploration*. New York: Grune & Stratton.

Carroll, J., Johnson, D., & Marty, M. (1979). *Religion in America: 1950 to present*. New York: Harper & Row.

Casavantes, E. (1976). Pride and prejudice: a Mexican American dilemma. In Hernandez, C. A., Haug, M. J., & Wagner, N. N. (Eds.), *Chicanos: social and psychological perspectives* (ed. 2.) (pp. 9–14). St. Louis: Mosby.

Catlin, A. R. (1982). Speech surrogate systems of the Hmong: from singing voices to talking reeds. In Downing, B. T., & Olney, D. P. (Eds.), *The Hmong in the West* (pp. 170–197). Minneapolis: Center for Urban and Regional Affairs, University of Minnesota.

Clark, K., & Shute, N. (2001, March 12). The adoption maze. *U. S. News*, 130(10), 60–64.

Cloud, J. (2005, October 10). The battle over day teens. *Time*, 43–51.

Cose, E. (2000, January 1). Our new look: the colors of race. *Newsweek*, 28.

Danyliw, N. (1997, December 15). Got mother's milk? *U.S. News and World Report*, 123(23), 79.

Davidhizar, R., Bechtel, G. & Cosey, E. (2000, December 25). Hospital extra: the spiritual needs of hospitalized patients. *American Journal of Nursing*, 25, 282–289.

Davidhizar, R., Havens, R., & Bechtel, G. (1999, July–August). Assessing culturally diverse pediatric clients. *Pediatric Nursing*, 25(4), 371–376, 393–394.

Davidhizar, R., King, V., Bechtel, G., & Giger, J. (1998). Nursing clients of Greek ethnicity at home. *Home Healthcare Nurse*, 16(9), 618–623.

Disability Status 2000. (2005). Census 2000 Brief. Washington, DC: U.S. Department of Commerce: Economics and Statistic Administration, U.S. Census Bureau. Available at http://www.census.gov/hhes/www/disability/disabcps.html.

Dowd, S., Davidhizar, R., & Giger, J. N. (2007). The mystery of altruism and transcultural nursing. *Health Care Manag (Frederick)*, 26(1), 64–67.

Dunnewind, S. (2001, December 25). Saturated. *Pittsburgh Post-Gazette AP from the Seattle Times*, E-2.

Dunnigan, T. (1986). Process of identity maintenance in Hmong society. In Hendricks, G. L., Downing, B. T., & Deinard, A. S. (Eds.), *The Hmong in transition* (pp. 41–53). Staten Island, N.Y.: Center for Migration Studies.

Duvall, E., & Miller, B. (1985). *Marriage and family development* (ed. 6.). New York: Harper & Row.

Ellwood, R. (2005). *Many peoples, many faiths* (ed. 8.). Upper Saddle River, N.J.: Pearson Prentice Hall.

Exley, C. (2004). Review article: the sociology of dying, death, and bereavement. *Sociology of health and illness,* 26(1), 110–122.

Fawcett, J. (1975). The family as a living open system: an emerging conceptual framework for nursing. *International Nursing Review,* 22, 113.

Finkleman, A. (2000). Psychiatric patients and families: moving from catastrophic event to long-term coping. *Home Care Providers,* 5(4), 142–147.

Fordham, P., Giger, J., & Davidhizar, R. (2006). Multicultural and multi-ethnic considerations and advanced directives: developing cultural competency. *Journal of Cultural Diversity,* 13(1), 3–9.

Freeman, H. P. (1998). The meaning of race in science—considerations for cancer research: concerns of special populations in the National Cancer Program. *Cancer,* 82, 219–225.

Friedman, M. M. (1986). *Family nursing: theory and assessment* (ed. 2.). East Norwalk, Conn.: Appleton-Century-Crofts.

Gary, F. (1991). Sociocultural diversity and mental health nursing. In Gary, F., & Kavanaugh, C. (Eds.), *Psychiatric nursing* (pp. 138–163). Philadelphia: J.B. Lippincott.

General Conference of the Seventh Day Adventists. (2002). *Facts and figures,* Retrieved May 16, 2002, from http://www.adventist.org/worldchurch/factsandfigures.html.

Giger, J., Davidhizar, R., Evers, S., & Ingram, C. (1994). Cultural factors influencing mental health and mental illness. In Taylor, C. (Ed.), *Mereness' essentials of psychiatric nursing* (ed. 14.) (pp. 215–238). St. Louis: Mosby.

Giger, J., Davidhizar, R., & Wieczorek, S. (1994). Transcultural nursing: have we gone too far or not far enough? In Strickland, O., & Fishman, D. (Eds.), *Nursing in a diverse society.* Albany, N.Y.: Delmar Publications.

Giger, J., Johnson, J., Davidhizar, R., & Fishman, D. (1993, March). Strategies for building a supportive faculty. *Nursing and Health Care,* 14(3), 144–159.

Giorgianni, S. (2003). How families matter in health. *The Pfizer Journal,* 7(1), 1.

Goldsby, R. A. (1977). *Race and races* (ed. 2.). New York: Macmillan.

Gregory, D. (1988). Nursing practice in native communities. In Baumgart, A., & Larson, J. (Eds.), *Canadian nursing faces the future* (ed. 2.) St. Louis: Mosby.

Grypma, S. (1993, September). Culture shock. *The Canadian Nurse,* 89(8), 33–36.

Guruge, S., & Donner, G. (1996, September). Transcultural nursing in Canada. *The Canadian Nurse,* 92(8), 36–40.

Guttmacher, S., & Elinson, J. (1972). Ethno-religious variation in perception of illness: the use of illness as an explanation for deviant behavior. *Social Science Medicine,* 5(2), 117–125.

Habel, M. (2001, February 12). Caring for people of many cultures. *Nurse Week,* 20–22.

Haddad, A. (2001, March). Ethics in action . . . competent, elderly Chinese woman . . . can't give consent because she must wait for her family to arrive to give approval. *RN,* 64(3), 21–2224.

Hahn, J. (2006). Hahn's culture and disability assessment model. Adapted from Giger and Davidhizar (2004). Unpublished.

Harwood, A. (Ed.). (1981). *Ethnicity and medical care.* Cambridge, Mass.: Harvard University Press.

Headden, S. (1998, January 5). Favor aliens with job skills. *U.S. News and World Report,* 123(25), 83–85.

Henderson, G., & Primeaux, M. (1981). *Transcultural health care.* Reading, Mass.: Addison-Wesley.

Hensel, D., Mochel, M., & Bauer, R. (2005). Chronic illness and Hmong shaman. *Journal of Transcultural Nursing,* 16(2), 150–154.

Hitchcock, J. (2003). Framework for assessing families. In Hitchcock, J., Schubert, P., & Thomas, S. (Eds.), *Community health nursing caring in action* (ed. 2.) San Francisco: Delmar Publishers.

Hsu, J. (1985). Asian family interaction patterns and their therapeutic implications. In Pichot, P., Berner, P., Wolf, R., & Thau, K. (Eds.), *Psychiatry: the state of art* (vol. 8) (pp. 599–606). New York: Plenum Press.

Jayson, S. (2006, March). Is "failure to launch" really a failure? *USA Today,* D1.

Jehovah's Witnesses 1997 yearbook. (1997). New York: Watchtower Bible and Tract Society.

Johnson, S., & Hang, A. (2006). Hmong. In Lipson, J. & Dibble, S. (Eds.), *Culture and clinical care*. San Francisco: UCSF Nursing Press.

Johnstone, R. (2007). *Religion in Society* (ed. 7.). Upper Saddle River, N.J.: Pearson Prentice Hall.

Joint Commission of Accreditation of Healthcare Organizations. (2000). *Accreditation manual for hospitals*. Oakbrook Terrace, Ill.: Joint Commission of Accreditation of Healthcare Organizations.

Jones, A. (2003). Reconstructing the stepfamily: old myths, new stories. *Social work*, 48(2), 228–234.

Kadis, L., & McClendon, R. (2003). Marital and family therapy. In Hales, R., Yadofsky, S., & Talbot, J. A. (Eds.), *The American Psychiatric Press textbook of psychiatry* (ed. 4.) Washington, D.C.: The American Psychiatric Press.

Kaiser Family Foundation. (1999, November). *Kids and media at the new millennium: a comprehensive national analysis of children's media use*. Menlo Park, Calif.: The Henry J. Kaiser Family Foundation.

Kantrowitz, B., & Wingert, P. (2001, May 28). Unmarried, with children. *Newsweek*, 46–52.

Kearney, M., York, R., & Deatrick, J. (2000, Fourth Quarter). Effects of home visits to vulnerable young families. *Journal of Nursing Scholarship*, 32(4), 309–314.

Kinne, S., Patrick, D. L., & Doyle, D. L. (2004). Prevalence of secondary conditions among people with disabilities. *American Journal of Public Health*, 94(3), 443–445.

Kirkham, S., Pesut, B., Meyerhoff, H., & Sawatzky, R. (2004). Spiritual caregiving at the juncture of religion, culture, and state. *CJNR*, 36(4), 148–169.

Kulwicki, A. P. (2003). People of Arab heritage. In Purnell, L., & Paulanka, B. (Eds.), *Transcultural health care: a culturally competent approach* (ed. 2.) Philadelphia: F.A. Davis.

Kunen, J. (1996, April 29). The end of integration. *Time*, 39–44.

Lester, M. (2006, September 11). MCC workers help preserve Hmong culture. *Mennonite Weekly Review*, 6.

Lewis, H. (1979). *How's your family?*. New York: Brunner/Mazel.

Lewis, J. M., Beavers, W. R., Gossett, J. T., & Phillips, V. A. (1976). *No single thread: psychological health in family systems*. New York: Brunner/Mazel.

Lindner, E. (2004). *Yearbook of American and Canadian Churches*. Nashville: Abingdon Press.

Martin, E. P. (1978). *The Black extended family*. Chicago: University of Chicago Press.

Martin, W. (2003). *The kingdom of the cults* (revised ed.). Minneapolis: Bethany House.

McMahon, A. (1997). Working with families. In Haber, J., Krainovich-Miller, D., McMahon, A., & Price-Hoskins, P. (Eds.), *Comprehensive psychiatric nursing*. St. Louis: Mosby.

McMahon, A., & Presswalla, J. L. (1997). Working with groups. In Haber, J., Krainovich-Miller, B., McMahon, A., & Price-Hoskins, P. (Eds.), *Comprehensive psychiatric nursing* (ed. 4.) St. Louis: Mosby.

Meleis, A. I. (2006). Arabs. In Lipson, J., & Dibble, S. (Eds.), *Culture and health care*. San Francisco: UCSF Nursing Press.

Minuchin, S. (1974). *Families and family therapy*. Cambridge, Mass.: Harvard University Press.

Misener, T., Sowell, R., Phillips, K., & Harris, C. (1997, July–August). Sexual orientation: a cultural diversity issue in nursing. *Nursing Outlook*, 45(4), 178–182.

Mitty, E. (2001, First Quarter). Ethnicity and end of life decision making. *Reflections on Nursing Leadership*, 46, 28–31.

Mo, B. (1992, September). Modesty, sexuality, and breast health in Chinese American women. *The Western Journal of Medicine*, 157, 260–264.

Murray, R., Meili, P., & Zentner, J. (1993). The family—basic unit for the developing person. In Murray, R., & Zentner, J. (Eds.), *Nursing concepts for health promotion* (ed. 5.) Englewood Cliffs, N.J.: Prentice Hall.

Natinsky, P. (2001, September–October). Female genital cutting: why are women mutilated? *Community Health Forum*, 2(5), 41–43.

Nilchaikovit, T., Hill, J. M., & Holland, J. C. (1993). The effects of culture on illness behavior and medical care: Asian and American differences. *General Hospital Psychiatry*, 15(1), 41–50.

Nolt, S. (1992). *A history of the Amish*. Intercourse, Pa.: Good Books.

Nordland, R., & Bartholet, J. (2001, March 19). The web's dark secret. *Newsweek*, 44–50.

O'Brien, S. (1992, Fall). Gender bias in family benefit provision. *Canadian Journal of Community Mental Health*, 11(2), 163–186.

Orecklin, M. (2002, February). If at first you don't succeed. *Time*, 14.

Palacios, J., Butterfly, & Strickland, C. (2006). American Indians. In Lipson, J., Dibble, S., & Minarik, P. (Eds.),

Culture and clinical care. San Francisco: UCSF Nursing Press.

Peitchinis, S. (1989). *Employment standards handbook.* Toronto: McClelland Stewart.

Reid, R. (2000, September–October). American Indian health. *Medicine of the Americas,* 1(1), 53.

Rosemond, J. (1994, August). Stepfamilies: a family by any other name. *Hemispheres,* 93.

Rosenberg, D. (2001, January 15). A place of their own. *Newsweek,* 54–56.

Sands, E., & Berry, J. (1993). Acculturation and mental health among Greek-Canadians in Toronto. *Canadian Journal of Community Mental Health,* 12(2), 117–124.

Satir, V. (1983). *Conjoint family therapy* (ed. 3.). Palo Alto, Calif.: Science & Behavior Books.

Saunders, L. (1954). *Cultural differences and medical care.* New York: Russell Sage Foundation.

Schneflen, A. (1972). *Body language in social order.* Englewood Cliffs, N.J.: Prentice Hall.

Schneider, R. (1980, June). *Conceptual scheme of family organization and function,* Paper presented at St. Louis University Medical Center Conference, St. Louis, Missouri.

Shadick, K. (1993). Development of a transcultural health education program for the Hmong. *Clinical Nurse Specialist,* 7(2), 48–53.

Sheler, J. (2000, November 13). The Church of Latter-Day Saints grows by leaps and bounds. *U.S. News and World Report,* 129(19), 59–65.

Shipler, D. (1997). *A country of strangers.* New York: Alfred A. Knopf.

Sleeper, J. (1997). *Liberal racism.* New York: Viking Press.

Smart, N. (1991). *The religious experience of mankind* (ed. 4.). New York: Macmillan.

Sniderman, P. M., & Carmines, E. G. (1997). *Reaching beyond race.* Cambridge, Mass.: Harvard University Press.

Spector, R. (2004). *Cultural diversity in health and illness* (ed. 6.). Upper Saddle River, N.J.: Pearson Prentice Hall.

Strickland, O., & Giger, J. (1994). Women's health in the decade of the woman. In Strickland, O., & Fishman, D. (Eds.), *Nursing issues and ethics* (pp. 362–399). Albany, N.Y.: Delmar.

Suchman, E. A. (1964). Sociomedical variations among ethnic groups. *American Journal of Sociology,* 70, 319–331.

Sussman, M. B. (1971, July). Family systems in the 1970s: analysis, politics, and programs. *Annals of American Academy of Political Social Science,* 396, 40–56.

Sydnor-Greenberg, N., & Dokken, D. (2000). Family focus. Communicating information at diagnosis: helping families and children manage asthma. *Journal of Child and Family Nursing,* 3(4), 290–295.

Thomas, N. (2001, January). The importance of culture throughout all of life and beyond. *Holistic Nursing Practice,* 15(2), 40–46.

Time almanac with information please. (2006). Boston, Information Please, Inc.

Townsend, M. (2006). *Psychiatric mental health nursing concepts of care* (ed. 5.). Philadelphia: F.A. Davis.

Underwood, A. (2005, September 5). Spirituality in America. *Newsweek,* 45–64.

U.S. Department of Commerce, Bureau of the Census. (1993a). *Current population reports: population profile of the United States, 1993,* Special Studies P23–P185. Washington, D.C.: Government Printing Office.

U.S. Department of Commerce, Bureau of the Census. (1993b). *We the American Asians.* Washington, D.C.: U.S. Government Printing Office.

U.S. Department of Commerce, Bureau of the Census. (2000). *Population and housing data by race and Hispanic origin, Summary File 1.* Washington, D.C.: U.S. Government Printing Office.

U.S. Department of Commerce, Bureau of the Census. (2002). *Population profiles by age, sex, race, and Hispanic origin, Summary File 3.* Washington, D.C.: U.S. Government Printing Office.

U.S. Department of Health and Human Services. (2000). *Healthy People 2010: Understanding and improving health* (ed. 2.). Washington, D.C.: U.S. Government Printing Office.

Vehvilainen, K. (1998, Second Quarter). Wake up to Finnish nursing. *Reflections in Nursing Leadership,* 28–29.

Watchtower. (1989, March 1). Questions from readers. *Watchtower,* 30–31.

Watchtower Bible & Tract Society. (1953). *Let God be true.* (revised ed.) New York: Author.

Watchtower Bible & Tract Society. (1955). *You may survive Armageddon into God's new world.* New York: Author.

Wexler, N. E. (1981). Learning to be a leper. In Mishler, E. G., et al. (Eds.). *Social context of health, illness and patient care.* Cambridge, England: Cambridge University Press.

Wingert, P., Springen, K., & Stone, B., et al. (1997, December). A matter of faith. *Newsweek,* 49–53.

Wolfram, W. A., & Clark, H. (Eds.) (1971). *Black–White speech relationships.* Washington, D.C.: Center for Applied Linguistics.

Woodward, K. (2001, April 16). The changing face of the church. *Newsweek,* 45–50.

World almanac. (2006). New York: World Almanac Books.

Zayas, L., & Solari, F. (1994). Early childhood socialization in Hispanic families: context, culture, and practice implications. *Professional Psychology: Research and Practice,* 25(3), 2100–2206.

Zola, I. (1972). The concept of trouble and sources of medical assistance to whom one can turn with that. *Social Science and Medicine,* 6, 673–679.

CHAPTER 5 Time

Behavioral Objectives

After reading this chapter, the nurse will be able to:

1. Postulate an adequate definition for the term *time* in relation to transcultural nursing care.
2. Understand the significant role that culture plays in the understanding and perception of time.
3. Understand the significant role that the developmental process plays in the understanding and perception of time.
4. Understand the significance of the measurement of time and the relationship to transcultural nursing care.
5. Differentiate the terms *social time* and *clock time*.
6. Describe the worldview of clock time and social time.
7. Define the three broad areas of the structure of social time: temporal patterns, temporal orientation, and temporal perspectives.

Since the beginning of life on earth, time has been the greatest mystery of all. The mystery of time becomes evident as soon as thought is given to the concept. Our experience with time continuously leads us into puzzles and paradoxes. According to Wessman and Gorman (1977), it is through an awareness and conception of time that the products of the human mind, that is, time itself, seem to possess an existence apart from time's passage, which is perceived as personal and inexorable. We measure time, and time measures us. It is this intimate and personal yet aloof and detached character that constitutes the paradox of human time.

CONCEPT OF TIME

The concept of the passage of time is very familiar to most people regardless of cultural heritage. The days and nights come and go, and with each passing day and night humankind grows older. In today's highly mechanized world, there are numerous clocks and watches that ceaselessly tick away time and determine the schedules by which hundreds of millions of people live. Thus it would seem that the concept of the passage of time should be second nature to humankind and thoroughly understood by all people (Spector, 2004).

However, developing an awareness of the concept of time is not a simple phenomenon but a gradual process (Hymovich & Chamberlin, 1980). Most people, regardless of cultural heritage, remember a time when their perception of the passage of time was altered. Such occasions might have been during times of boredom or of highly emotional and stressful events. During these events time might have seemed to have passed very slowly, or it might have seemed to have passed all too quickly. It must be remembered that a sense of time is not innate but is developed early as a result of everyday experiences that are common to all people. Thus, a sense of time results from learning. It becomes a part of human nature before one is conscious of its presence. Even infants perceive the essence of time. Infants are fed on demand or according to a strict timetable and experience the succession of day by night. Infants are thereby exposed to regular rhythmic changes that are reflected in rhythmic changes in bodily conditions, including being sated, awake, or asleep. Thus, one phenomenon of time is its association with rhythm and change.

Infants grow, develop, and begin to move through crawling. The speed with which crawling occurs determines the time it takes to get from one place to another. Thus, even this simple task makes individuals aware that time is associated with speed and velocity, which is the second phenomenon of time. As individuals grow older, they learn speech as they listen to stories that begin with "once upon a time." It is through these story-telling sessions that children learn that things did happen before they were born; thus, time is associated with history and goes backward as well as forward with the succession of events. As the growth and development of the child continue, an awareness of punctuality is developed. Children may be punished for being slow or late, and regardless of their reaction to it, the punishment contributes to the formation of character and the development of the understanding of time. Therefore, the third phenomenon of time is its association with social behavior (Sideleau, 1992).

The child begins to become conscious of time and asks questions such as, "Where was I before I was born?" and "What did God do before he created the world?" and "What will happen to me after I die?" Such questions lead to an understanding that time is associated with philosophy and religion. Children are taught to read time on a clock, and as they grow to adulthood, they learn that the clock is ubiquitous and that life is governed by the clock. Thus, there is an erroneous identification of time with the clock. Through questioning, individuals begin to contemplate existence on earth and to develop an understanding that time is associated with something external over which there is no control and that appears absolute (Elton, 1975; Sideleau, 1992).

Developing an understanding of the definition of time by looking at the developmental process is clearly too simple. The development of the awareness of time is directly influenced by earlier ideas and prejudices that are mostly unconscious. However, because it is the nature of humankind to have a questioning frame of mind, ideas and prejudices may become conscious.

Other considerations concerning time include the question of whether time is concrete or abstract. Time is perceived as real in the sense of being concrete and having direct effects, or it is regarded as not real in the sense of being abstract. The mathematical and physical sciences adopt the view that time is an abstract dimension with only a locational or reference function (McGrath & Kelly, 1986). On the other hand, the biological sciences adopt the view that time is an essential ingredient in many life and behavioral processes, such as gestation, healing, and metamorphosis. This difference in conceptualization of time may be related to an obvious difference between the physical and biological sciences and how each treats the concept of entropy. For the physical sciences, entropy, or randomness, continuously increases over time, whereas the biological sciences see organization, structure, and information residing within the organism and in the organism's relation to its environment as increasing over time.

MEASUREMENT OF TIME

Time has two distinct, though related, meanings. The first meaning is that of duration, which is an interval of time. The second meaning is that of specified instances, or points in time. These two meanings are related because a point in time is identified as being the end of a time interval that starts at an arbitrary or fixed reference point, such as the founding of Rome or the birth of Christ. Thus, if one asks the question, "What is the time?" and the answer given is "It is 10:00 A.M.," this answer refers to a point in time. At the same time, the answer refers to a time interval, since it indicates the time from a certain reference point, which in this case is midnight the previous night (Elton, 1975; Sideleau, 1992). The two meanings are quite different and must not be confused with each other. Measuring devices are meant to determine intervals of time, and clocks and watches are designed to read direct points in time. Clocks and watches therefore have to be standardized against a standard clock. The purpose of a standard clock is to measure accurately the time interval up to the present time. This phenomenon goes back to one universal standard clock against which all standard clocks are calibrated.

The purpose of a universal standard clock is to define operational time in terms of both time interval and point in time (Landes, 2000). The purpose of measuring devices is to define time; however, people need to have intuitive ideas about time to specify the properties of the instrument. Measuring devices of a phenomenon such as time are more accurate than measuring devices of some other phenomena. For example, if a person wanted to measure the weight of another person, this weight could be defined operationally as a point or reading on a scale. Thus a good scale would give accurate weight, just as any good clock would give accurate time. On the other hand, if an individual wanted to define a person's intelligence quotient (IQ) as the score obtained on an intelligence test but there was no general agreement about what constituted intelligence and what constituted a good intelligence test, the scores would not be so relevant or so meaningful as the weight or time measures.

Throughout the history of humankind, there have been two obvious standards of time: the day and the year. The day is a remarkably easy period of time to recognize because of the experience of daylight and darkness, which result from the earth's spinning on its axis. The year is also easy to recognize because of the passage of the seasons, which are caused by the tilting of the earth's axis. Thus a day is the period of time for one complete revolution of the earth about its axis, whereas a year is the time taken for the earth to move one complete revolution around the sun, which takes just under 365.25 days. Therefore, it is completely natural that we choose to mark the passage of time by first marking the days and then marking the years. Time measurement during the day has been divided into hours, and the hours in turn have been divided by 60 to give minutes. The minutes have been divided by 60 to give seconds.

Very early in the history of civilization, the middle of each day was determined as the point when the sun was at its highest point during the day. This point was defined as noon, and clocks were made to read 12 when it occurred. Thus, if it is noon in one place, it is midnight at the opposite side of the earth and different times at other places on the earth. To understand how time varies, the earth must be viewed as a circle that passes through both the North Pole and the South Pole.

Traditionally in science, Greenwich, the observatory in London, has been taken to have 0 degrees of longitude; the longitudes of all other places on earth are given as so many degrees east or west of Greenwich. Therefore, one half of the earth's surface has a longitude of up to 180 degrees east of Greenwich, whereas the other half has a longitude of up to 180 degrees west of Greenwich. The times of all places east of Greenwich are ahead of that of Greenwich, and the times of all places west of Greenwich lag behind that of Greenwich. For example, if a person started from Greenwich and traveled eastward to a longitude of 45 degrees, the time would be 3 hours ahead of Greenwich time. The converse is that if a person started at Greenwich and traveled westward to a longitude of 180 degrees, the time would be 12 hours behind that of Greenwich. In simpler terms, if it is 2 A.M. on Sunday morning at Greenwich, it is 2 P.M. on Sunday at a longitude 180 degrees east of Greenwich and 2 P.M. on Saturday at a longitude 180 degrees west of Greenwich (Elton, 1975).

This phenomenon of time presents some interesting effects on persons who travel great distances. For example, it is possible for an international traveler to have two birthdays (birthday anniversaries); that is, if a person crosses the international date line traveling eastward at 2 A.M. Sunday morning, at which point it suddenly becomes 2 A.M. Saturday, that person has Saturday all over again and thus is able to celebrate the birthday again. If this same international traveler who is about to celebrate a birthday on Saturday leaves from the point of origin at 2 A.M. on Saturday but crosses the international date line westward, the traveler suddenly finds that it is 2 A.M. Sunday morning, and apparently almost the entire day of Saturday and the birthday have been missed (Elton, 1975).

Clocks

According to historians and philosophers, the earliest clocks were undoubtedly sundials of various kinds, which were probably followed by devices that used the regular flow of a substance such as water, oil, or sand, or the steady combustion of oil or candles. The earliest clocks have been dated back to 1600 B.C. in Egypt, and clocks were used throughout classical times and the Middle Ages.

The 13th century saw the invention of a rhythmic motion clock, which was a saw-toothed crown wheel. However, the most important development in clock construction occurred with the introduction of the pendulum, which was discovered by Galileo in 1581. Galileo found that a swinging pendulum would readily tick away a unit of time by a specific number of swings and that even if the swings gradually died, the unit of time would remain relatively unaffected. Thus, for the first time in history, time was measured more accurately.

Tropical Years

An important distinction that scientists have made is the difference between a calendar year and a tropical year. According to scientists, a calendar year consists of 365 days, whereas a tropical year consists of 365.242199 solar days. (The word *tropical* in this instance has nothing to do with a hot climate.) The difference between these two numbers (tropical year and calendar year) is the reason for the necessity of leap years. Time that is based on the length of a tropical year is called *ephemeris time*. One tropical year is defined in terms of having 31,556,925.9747 seconds. Today, atomic clocks have replaced the old, outdated pendulum and weight- and gravity-driven clocks. Atomic clocks are so accurate that in due course scientists speculate that the difference between atomic time and ephemeris time will become very apparent. In fact, atomic clocks are said to be 10 million times more accurate than any other clock on earth and are never more than 1 billionth of a second off. Atomic clocks are considered to be so accurate that the exact second of an event can be obtained at the time of the event.

Solar Time

Solar time is perhaps the earliest way that time was measured (Dossey, 1993). Solar time considers a focal point, 12:00 noon, which is precisely the point at which the sun passes directly overhead (vertically above the meridian). The time between successive crossings of the sun directly over the same meridian is called a *solar day*. However, this measurement of time is not without its problems. When days are measured in this way, they turn out to be not exactly constant. A solar day varies slightly in length throughout the year because of the orbiting of the earth around the sun.

The concept of solar time has many implications for nurses who work at extreme southern or northern points of the earth, for example, at the North or South Pole. A nurse working in the northernmost part of Canada may find Indians operating on "Indian time" because the sun remains up during most of the summer and down during much of the winter. Activities requiring daylight can therefore be done anytime during a 24-hour period. Staying up much of the night and sleeping in the daytime is consistent with an orientation to do what feels right at the present time. On the other hand, "White man's time" is more future oriented and adheres to clocks and schedules rather than to the sun (England, 1986; Wuest, 1992; Young & Hayne, 1988). Generally, Whites who have not grown up in the northernmost part of Canada but have relocated to this area tend to work during familiar working hours and to sleep during familiar sleeping hours. However, this pattern may not necessarily correlate with the same time orientation for others who are native to the northernmost part of Canada.

Calendar

Inventing a simple yet efficient calendar has presented difficulties since the invention of the first calendar. Scientists believe that these difficulties lie in the fact that the three obvious periods are due to the rotation of the earth about the sun. These three revolutional periods are not simply related one to the other. In fact, they have obvious differences. For example, 1 tropical year equals 365.224 solar days, and 1 month is considered to be the observed time between one full moon and the next, or 29.5306 solar days.

Throughout history we have measured time by counting the months and the calendar years and combining the two. However, this combination of months and years has proved to be most confusing. Even if we ignored the moon, there would still be the problem of the solar year not being a whole number of days, though this problem has conceivably been dealt with by the system of leap years. With so many different civilizations contributing to the development of the calendar, it is no wonder that we are left with a complicated system that children and even adults, regardless of ethnic or cultural heritage, find difficult to remember or understand. Many of the significant events linked with the calendar can be traced to specific persons in history, such as Julius Caesar, who decreed that months should alternately have 30 and 31 days with the exception of February (which at that time was the last month of the Roman calendar). Historians believe that all would have been well with the calendar if Julius Caesar had not decided to call the fifth month Julius in his honor. The problem began when Augustus followed Julius Caesar and also wanted a month. He promptly chose the month that followed Julius and named it "Augustus." However, he very soon realized that his month was shorter than Julius Caesar's month and promptly took a day from February, added it to his month, and readjusted the rest of the year. The result was that there were three long months in succession, that is, June, July, and August. Even today, because of the vanity of Emperor Augustus, children continue to chant, "Thirty days hath September."

According to the earlier decree by Julius Caesar, September would have been an alternate month with 31 days if August had been given 30 days as originally planned (Elton, 1975). Although there have been attempts over the last 50 years to standardize the calendar by international agreement through the League of Nations and the United Nations, these attempts have uniformly failed. For example, the day that is considered the beginning of the New Year in the United States is January 1, but the beginning of the New Year is different in many countries.

SOCIAL TIME VERSUS CLOCK TIME

The word *time* immediately presents an image of a clock or calendar. However, the term *social time* is not equivalent with clock time. Social time refers to patterns and orientations that relate to social processes and to the conceptualization and ordering of social life. For centuries, many of the great thinkers have argued that social time must be distinguished from clock time. As early as 1910, Henri Bergson insisted that the homogeneous time of Newtonian physics was not the time that revealed the essence of humankind. On the other hand, Phillip Bock (1964), an anthropologist, showed that an Indian wake could be meaningfully analyzed in terms of "gathering time," "prayer time," "singing time," "intermission time," and "meal time." None of these times has a particular relationship to clock time. They all simply imply the passage of the mourner from one time to another by consensual feelings rather than by the clock.

According to some sociologists, certain kinds of psychological disorders may be viewed in terms of the individual living wholly in the present, the implication being that the past and the future are completely severed from consciousness. The difference, therefore, between social time and clock time is that the former is a more inclusive concept whereas the latter may or may not be. Hoppe and Heller (1974) conducted a study on Mexican Americans and proposed that Mexican Americans have a present-time orientation that may account for the tendency to be late for appointments. It is believed that present-time orientation, particularly in high-risk settings such as mental health facilities, may result in a crisis approach rather than a preventive one. For example, a client who has an immediate need at home may be late for appointments at the clinic or hospital, or may miss them altogether. The nurse should also keep in mind that clients with a present-time orientation may be reluctant to leave an appointment simply because the time is up.

This same lack of correlation between social time and clock time can be seen in mystical beliefs. According to mystical thought, magic can be employed to negate the temporal order that infers causality. For example, an Indian warrior who is wounded by an arrow may attend to his pain by hanging the arrow up where it is cool or by applying ointment to the arrow. What the Indian warrior is attempting to do is to reverse the clock time, that is, wrench the present back into the past to alter the course of events. For people who have mystical beliefs, temporal intervals are not simple, homogeneous series; rather, they contain an inherent quality and meaning or an essence and efficacy of their own (Cassirer, 1992). Therefore, the objectivity represented by clock time is unknown to a person with mystical beliefs.

Many sociologists believe that people who lack or minimize clock time also lack regularity or temporal measurement. The natural and social phenomena may dictate regularity and measurement. Ariotti (1995) provides several examples of natural events that have been used to time human activities: (1) The arrival of the cranes in ancient Greece marked the time for planting; (2) the return of the swallow marked the time for the end of pruning; (3) the South African Bushmen note the rising of Sirius and Canopus and are able to depict the progress of winter by the movement of these celestial bodies across the night sky.

Archeologists have been able to piece together the history of humankind by measuring the passage of time, using the method of geologists. This measure of time is based on rates of deposits to and erosion of natural early elements. An example of this kind of measurement is tree-ring chronology (Weyer, 1961).

WORLDVIEW OF SOCIAL TIME VERSUS CLOCK TIME

People throughout the world view social time and clock time differently (Davidhizar, Dowd, & Giger, 1997). For example, Sorokin (1964) noted that the division of time by weeks reflects social conditions rather than mechanical Newtonian divisions. Most societies have some kind of week, but the weeks vary in length from 3 to 16 or more days. In most cases, weeks reflect the cycle of market activities. The Khasi people have an 8-day week because they hold market every eighth day, and they have named the days of the week after the places where the principal markets occur (Sorokin, 1964).

Some cultural groups exhibit a social time that not only is different from clock time but also is actually scornful of clock time. For example, there are peasants in Algeria who live with a total indifference to the passage of clock time and who despise haste in human affairs. They have no notion of exact appointment times, they lack exact times for eating meals, and they have labeled the clock as the "devil's mill" (Thompson, 1967). Some Amish keep "slow time." When those around them adjust their time to go from daylight savings time to standard time, the Amish set clocks a half-hour ahead (Gingerich, 1972; Nolt, 1992; Randall-David, 1989; Wenger, 2006). This has important implications for the nurse who is trying to emphasize the importance of keeping medical appointments.

Despite the way people in various cultures view clock time as opposed to social time, the nurse must remember that clock time should not be regarded as unimportant or irrelevant. Although for some people in some cultural groups there is no necessary correlation of clock time and social time, clock time does not take on paramount importance in a social context such as the modern Western world, where the watch or the clock can become something of a tyrant. In Jonathan Swift's *Gulliver's Travels,* Gulliver never did anything without looking at his watch, which he called his "oracle." He said that his watch pointed out the time for every action of his life. Because of Gulliver's obsession with his watch, the Lilliputians concluded that the watch was Gulliver's god.

Aside from literature, many actual examples of human obsessive behavior in regard to clock time can be found. Lebhar (1958) wrote that he was exactly 43 years old and had probably only 227,760 hours to live, and he proceeded to detail how he would maximize the use of those remaining hours of his life. He concluded that if he reduced his sleep time from 8 hours to 6 hours, the 2 hours a day saved from sleeping would amount to 18,980 hours over a period of 26 years. If this savings were converted into 18-hour days, which is the equivalent of about 2 years and 11 months, he could virtually lengthen his remaining time alive by 2 years and 11 months. This example illustrates how human life can be turned into a lengthy succession of minutes and hours, with the individual's existence reduced to a compulsive and frantic effort to avoid waste.

Gilles and Faulkner (1978) conducted a study of the role of time in television news work. They found that time is a major factor in the production of unscheduled "hard" news. The definition for "hard" news refers to events such as fires, homicides, and accidents, which have a certain urgency to them. They summarized the findings of their research in three propositions. In the first proposition they concluded that the news value of an event is directly proportional to the time invested in covering it. An event may turn out to be relatively minor in the sense of not involving the trauma or shock value that was anticipated, but this factor is not considered when a film crew has invested time in the event, and the story is likely to be used in the evening news program anyway. They found in the second proposition that what is considered news by the news crew depends on when it happens and how long it lasts. Although viewers tend to believe that what they see on the evening news is a compilation of the universal news events for that particular day, what is telecast each evening is actually a compilation of news events that the news crew was able to learn about, get a story line on, capture on film, and then process and edit on film. The researchers found in the third proposition that bias in the news reflects occupational assumptions and temporal constraints more than it does the political or social views of the news crew. More important than political and social biases are the assumptions that the news crew makes about what will make good news on television and the severe time constraints on those persons assigned to locate film and write about events in time for the evening news program. The researchers concluded that because of deadline pressures, it is inevitable that events are reduced to surface actions and that the visuals seen each evening are of only the most dramatic events.

In today's modern technological society, clock time is of paramount importance. However, we must remember that even in a modern society the clock may be a relatively peripheral part of social life. Not all people in a modern technological society function under the inevitable tyranny of the clock. In a survey of a representative sample of the French population, approximately 21% of the respondents indicated a belief that there was no urgency about being punctual and also stated that they had not experienced the feeling of wasting time (Stoetzel, 1953). It is the perception of some people in some cultural groups that there is little correlation between being punctual and wasting time (Hein, 1980). Hein further postulated that assumptions and definitions in regard to time are determined by culture and cultural variables and are reflected in interactions with others, personal views concerning punctuality, use or waste of time, and value and respect for time or a lack thereof. Waiting is a cultural counterpart to time because a particular behavior, person, or event is anticipated within a particular time frame. Waiting may have a meaning similar to that of time for some African-American clients. The nurse may schedule an appointment for an African-American client and wait for the client to arrive for the appointment. However, the client may not arrive for several hours, or perhaps even a few days, because of other important issues that in the client's mind took precedence over the appointment. Although the nurse viewed this time as waiting and therefore wasting time, the client for whom the appointment was made was not wasting time (Randall-David, 1989).

In some cultures, for example, among some persons of Asian origin, time is viewed as flexible, and so there is no need to hurry or be punctual except in extremely important cases. Asians may spend hours getting to know people and view predetermined abrupt endings as rude (Stauffer, 1995). Nonetheless, the nurse should emphasize the importance of keeping scheduled appointments. Hispanics or Latinos as well often have difficulty with scheduled appointments and are sometimes said to be on "Latin time." However, this is sometimes explained by Hispanics as the result of consideration for others who were not ready to leave for the appointment (Hoppe & Heller, 1974; Ruiz, 2003; Ruiz & Padella, 1977).

In the American nursing profession, many nurses have related professionalism and success in their careers to a sense of precision about clock time. For example, in many health care facilities, a medication error is considered to occur when a medication is not given within 30 minutes of the prescribed time, even when the medication is given daily and is not a time-released medication. Thus the nurse must complete a medication error form for not giving a routine daily medication such as a vitamin or laxative, which is neither time released nor urgent.

Most agencies relate medication errors to disciplinary action and dismissal. In some facilities the nurse is expected to complete all morning or evening care in a precise time frame, even though many clients may not operate in the same time sphere as the facility schedule for client care. For example, a client may become upset when the night nurse refuses to help the client to shower at 3 A.M. because showering is a stated day-shift activity. In this case the client may be used to starting the day at 3 A.M. and unwilling to wait until 7 A.M. to do so. Another example is early-morning vital signs, which may be taken by the night nurse to facilitate a timely assessment of the client's condition for the physician who makes early morning rounds. The client may be annoyed at being awakened for such a brief procedure and then instructed by the nurse to return to sleep.

According to Zerubavel's (1979) analysis of the temporal order of the hospital, any unit of clock time is equal to any other unit, whether one is talking about minutes, hours, days, or weeks. However, Zerubavel concluded that different days mean quite different things to different people. Because people perceive days differently, it is important to remember that some days are more or less desirable for some people. For example, some health care personnel may perceive the fact of working two weekends in succession as unfair. Similarly, evening or night duty is usually considered less desirable than day duty. Thus it is important for hospital administrators to understand the necessity for fairness in scheduling. Some hospitals have a policy that all personnel are expected to work their share of the less desirable times. In other hospitals the staff are paid differentials for working what are perceived as the less desirable times, that is, evenings, nights, weekends, and holidays.

STRUCTURE OF SOCIAL TIME

The structure of social time is a complex phenomenon. To understand it, three broad areas of social time must be analyzed: temporal pattern, temporal orientation, and temporal perspective.

Temporal Pattern

Hawley (1986) identified the temporal pattern of social time as one of the most important aspects of ecological organization. He concluded that there are five basic elements in the temporal pattern of any social phenomenon: periodicity, tempo, timing, duration, and sequence.

Periodicity. *Periodicity* refers to the various rhythms of social life and is characterized by activities related to both the needs and the activities of people. For example, every community has a functional routine that is supposedly peculiar to that community, such as the search for food, shelter, and mates, which occurs more or less with regular periodicity. People also have transcendental needs that are pursued with regular periodicity. For example, people may attend church weekly in pursuit of satisfying transcendental needs. Even physical functions of the body occur in a periodic manner. There are cyclical variations in physiological functions of the body, such as body temperature, blood pressure, and pulse.

Nelkin (1970) studied the behavior patterns of migrant workers and found several daily, weekly, and seasonal rhythms that were germane to their existence. Nelkin concluded that these migrant workers seemed to alternate between compact and diffuse time. Migrant time was seen to be very present-oriented, irrational, and highly personal. Nelkin concluded that migrant time was in sharp contrast to the typical time perception, which was future-oriented, rational, and impersonal. Findings from the study indicate that social time for the migrants differed because it was a series of disconnected periods rather than a continuous and predictable process, which in part accounted for maladaptive behaviors such as excessive drinking, gambling, volatile social relationships, and apathy.

Periodicity is also considered important at the managerial level. An important aspect of managerial life concerns the periodicity of meetings. For example, it is inappropriate for managers of a volunteer organization to plan frequent meetings for the membership. It is believed that a volunteer organization can engage in systematic self-destruction and ensure itself of a high turnover of membership if the group seeks to gather its members too often. These organizations must justify their demands on the members' time and at the same time create the novelty necessary to maintain the interest of the membership. In contrast to this are nonvoluntary groups, such as those that are part of a job assignment. For example, in nursing administration, regular meetings are necessary as part of the required management structure and are not usually planned with the intent of being novel and interesting. Because the management structure requires regular meetings, the meetings are planned regardless of specific agenda items.

Periodicities are also noted at the individual level. It is believed that when people are able to control their own work patterns (periodicity), satisfaction and productivity are maximized (Strauss, 1963). Some individuals spontaneously choose to alternate bouts of intense work with periods of idleness.

It is important for the manager to realize that productivity is cyclic and that equal periods of productivity cannot always be maintained. For example, after a period in which a nursing care unit experiences high client acuity, necessitating an extremely heavy work load for staff, employees will need to recover with a period of less intense pressure. It is unwise to follow a period of high acuity with another assignment that requires major time on the task. However, some work environments by their very nature cannot provide for individual periodicity. For example, industrial workers often must work at a continuous rhythmic pace, such as that seen on an automobile assembly line.

To understand periodicity, the nurse must remember that it is an important aspect of human life and the first aspect of the temporal pattern. Periodicity therefore refers to the recurrence of a social phenomenon with some kind of regularity that can be measured by clock time or by comparison of the social phenomenon with other social phenomena.

Tempo. Tempo is the second aspect of the temporal pattern and refers to rate (Morgenstern, 1960). Tempo may refer to the frequency of activities in some unit of social time or to the rate of change of some phenomenon. An example is the industrialization of the United States, which differs from that of Russia and China because of different rates (Gioscia, 1971). In a study done by the Southern Illinois University Foundation (Veterans World Project, 1972), it was suggested that one major problem among Vietnam veterans resulted from the rapidity with which they were brought home. The study concluded that the sudden transition from combat back to the United States by way of jet flights required a psychological adjustment that was often quite traumatic for these veterans.

Tempo also includes perceived rapidity of time and experience and the rapidity of various modes of social life, such as urban versus rural and work versus leisure. For example, the tempo of life in a large city such as Chicago or New York is much different from the tempo of life in a small, rural Midwestern town. Thus a person who relocates may have difficulty adjusting to the different tempo.

Tempo has several important consequences at the individual level because control of the tempo of one's work seems to be important for a healthful self-concept (Kohn, 1977). The tempo of change in social order appears to be related to emotional health; thus, the more rapid the change, the greater the stress of the individual. This thought became the theme of Alvin Toffler (1970), who coined the term "future shock"—the psychological disruptions that result from experiencing too much change in too short a time. An example of this is noted with Japanese people, who traditionally have had to change their culture and society at a very rapid pace. The very rapid tempo of the deliberate transformation of the Meiji era in Japan produced considerable stress for the Japanese people. Some historians have concluded that the 1878 revolution in Japan did save Japan from Western domination, but the generations that followed experienced the brunt of the hectic rate of change and suffered extraordinary mental agonies as a result of these forced changes (Pyle, 1969).

Timing. Timing is the third element in the temporal pattern and is referred to as *synchronization*. Timing involves the adjustment of various social units and processes with each other. The necessity for synchronization has led to the emphasis on clock time in modern society. Timing can be a crucial factor in the initiation of planned social changes and is of obvious importance in numerous social contexts, such as industrial processes, military campaigns, and political campaigns. A presidential candidate who supports a particular view that is not popular or timely may lose an election but win at a later time when the view becomes popular or another view emerges. For example, Richard Nixon ran for president of the United States in 1960 and lost. Eight years later he ran for president again at the height of the Vietnam War, and because the issue of the war was a timely one, he campaigned on this issue and won. Success is related to being at the right place at the right time with popular ideas.

Another example of the importance of timing is provided by research data on institutionalized disturbed children. These children, because of their psychological limitations, can be permitted to engage in activities such as competitive sports for only limited amounts of time. The restrictions on time are necessary because the process of the game and the psychological processes can mesh for only limited periods of time before the two processes begin to conflict and lead to destructive behavior (Doob, 1971).

Some researchers have concluded that one of the most serious problems of the modern American family is the difficulty of synchronizing family life because of the diverse activities in which each member is engaged. Another difficulty that has emerged over the years lies in the efforts of rural immigrants to adjust to the stringent demands of industrial life. Some researchers have suggested that habitual functioning of these rural immigrants must be synchronized with the industrial process and that such synchronization disallows the individual's self-actualization.

Duration. Duration is the fourth element of the temporal pattern. It has been the concern of psychologists more than it has been the concern of sociologists. The psychological concern about duration is related to the duration of which the individual is conscious, or to what has been referred to as the "spacious present." According to the classic early work of James (1990), one of the early writers in the field of social psychology, longer or shorter periods are conceived symbolically by adding to or dividing the vaguely bound unit that is the spacious present.

Duration has significance beyond the psychological level, however. Some noted sociologists have set forth a number of laws that relate to duration and behavior in organizations (Parkinson, 1970). Parkinson developed the laws of triviality and delay. The law of triviality states that the amount of time spent on any item in the agenda of an organizational meeting is inversely proportional to the money involved with that item. People may quibble far more about an item costing $50 than about an item costing $10,000. For example, in professional staff meetings at a state psychiatric hospital, an inordinate amount of time was spent discussing the purchase of a 75-cent plastic receptacle for holding clients' personal items such as toothbrushes and soap. A year later, when some plastic lids were missing, several meetings were devoted to developing a strategic nursing procedure for safeguarding these "valuable plastic receptacles." The policy developed to safeguard these receptacles mandated that the staff send a written requisition to the director of nursing, who in turn was required to write a written justification for replacement of the receptacle or the lid. The law of delay asserts that delay is the deadliest form of denial. In addition, duration is perceived as a useful variable.

Researchers continue to investigate the effects of various phenomena such as perceived importance of time, anxiety, and boredom on the perception of time. For example, researchers have concluded that workers' morale may be improved if time is subjectively made to pass more quickly and if there are several methods whereby the apparent length of a period of time can be manipulated (Meade, 1960).

Sequence. Sequence is the fifth element of the temporal pattern and is derived from the fact that there are activities requiring order. An obvious evidence of the utility of sequence is the measuring of values. For example, work before play is an ordering of activities that reflects a valuing hierarchy. In a classic 1972 study, Friedman measured values relating to physical activities, theoretical–scientific interests, and aesthetic interests and found that study participants made similar choices on both time and money scales. Friedman concluded that when cost and time are equalized, similar preferential orderings are made for various activities.

In modern American society, time is indeed money. It is conceivable, however, that the sequential ordering of activities may reflect necessity rather than values as an industrial process. Conflict may also arise over whether the sequence actually does represent necessity rather than values. Generally, this kind of conflict is more common in organizational settings in which disputes arise over the necessity of sequential orderings that are demanded by bureaucratic rules.

Finally, sequential ordering may reflect habit. Rituals of primitive societies are ordered in accordance with custom. Modern rituals also fall in this category, even though some are more appropriately viewed as reflections of values. For example, the ritual of a man removing his hat before entering a room or elevator is a habitual sequence. However, the ritual of the same man removing his hat before the national anthem is played is a sequence demanded by values.

Temporal Orientation

Temporal orientation refers to the ordering of past, present, and future and to the fact that individuals and groups may be differentiated according to whether behavior is primarily related to the past, present, or future. Psychologists and sociologists, however, have raised objections to this particular ordering. One objection is that past, present, and future are perceived to make up an organic whole that cannot be separated (Cassirer, 1992; Sideleau,

1992). A second objection involves variations in the ordering of past, present, and future among various groups. For example, the argument is made that an actor's orientation to a situation always contains an "expectancy aspect," which implies that all orientations are to a future state of a situation as well as to the present. However, this may be true only in a limited sense because actors generally do not anticipate their demise in the situation. It is also untrue that orientation to the future is a universal and inherent aspect of all social action.

Future orientation refers to the fact that the future is a dominant factor in present behavior, and as such this kind of orientation is by no means universal. For example, the Navajo Indians' view of time does not include the expectancy aspect. In years past, efforts to get the Navajo Indians to engage in range control and soil conservation programs were extremely frustrating for government employees because the Navajos simply do not have a view of temporality that would lead them to act on the basis of an expected future (Hall & William, 1960). For the Navajo people the only real time, like the only real space, is that which is here and now (Iverson, 1992). For some Navajo Indians there is little reality of the future; thus the promise of future benefits is not worth thinking about (Hall & William, 1960). It is important for the nurse to remember that the way in which a society, group, or individual orders past, present, or future will be consequential for behavior.

Kluckhohn and Strodtbeck (1973) have argued that the knowledge of rank ordering of these three modes can tell much about a social unit and the direction of change for that unit. Some Americans have typically placed a dominant emphasis on the future, which does not imply that they ignore either the past or the present. Although there are some undesirable connotations for the label "old-fashioned," few Americans express total contentment with the present state of affairs. According to Kluckhohn and Strodtbeck, American values change easily as long as the change does not contradict what is perceived as the American way of life. There is a direct relationship between the extended future orientation and the amount of change. However, the change perceived is not expected to be the kind that threatens the existing order.

Generally speaking, resistance to change should be expected where there is a past orientation. Thus it should be expected that serious problems would arise in efforts to industrialize a society that lacks a future orientation. For example, in a classic 1953 study, Ritzenhaler found that among the Chippewa Indians, who traditionally lack any concern for the future, there were serious problems when attempts were made to industrialize their work. Ritzenhaler also noted that the Chippewa Indians quit work as soon as they had sufficient money for immediate needs.

Temporal orientations are not immutable; they can change, and along with change come various behavioral changes. Therefore, a shift of orientation to the present may have significant consequences in several contexts (Ketchum, 1951). For example, in a crowd situation the orientation may be drawn to the present, wherein some of the typical behaviors of crowds may manifest themselves as overreacting behaviors, such as struggling at a department store sale, racing to the exit doors in a fire, or panicking in an airplane during turbulence. Similarly, in a marriage or relationship where the partners perceive the relationship to be of uncertain duration, they may begin to act in accordance with feelings rather than stable values. For example, one of the partners may transfer joint banking accounts and charge card accounts to individual status. In other words, when situations are structured so that people function in a present orientation that lacks future and past orientations, a variety of self-destructive and self-limiting behaviors may result.

Whenever a change is anticipated, individuals or groups may resist orientation to the change, and serious consequences generally follow. The intermingling of traditional orientation, which is somewhat past-oriented, with the pressures manifested by modernization, which may be somewhat present- or future-oriented, may cause societal agony. For example, many problems arose in a factory in Cantal, Guatemala, because the management refused to be sensitive to market variations or to the problem of obsolete equipment (Nash, 1967). Worse

situations occurred in Iran, which is a past-oriented society. In past-oriented societies, the past is of primary importance and the future of minimal significance. In Iran, businessmen invested considerable sums of money in factories without any real plan for how to use these factories (Hall & William, 1960).

Temporal orientation is an important variable in societal behavior and is also significant at the societal level. Some psychological studies indicate that temporal orientation may be directly related to various kinds of emotional disorders, such as alcoholism, and to certain kinds of deviant behaviors, such as juvenile delinquency.

Temporal Perspective

Temporal perspective refers to the image of past, present, and future that prevails in a society, a social group, or individuals. The rank ordering of past, present, and future is of significance, yet it is insignificant in gaining an adequate understanding of social time. For example, if a particular group is future-oriented—that is, it ranks the future highest in its hierarchy of values—its behavior will depend largely on the way it perceives the future. If people in a society perceive that they may be extinct in the future, efforts may be made to ensure survival. The converse of this is that if people in a society perceive that they do not have a future (for example, they will be eradicated in a nuclear holocaust), they may adopt a present orientation, desiring to live life now to its fullest. An excellent example of this is found with the dying client's perception of time. For the dying client, living in the present is very important; however, the nurse should recognize other realms of time perception. The nurse should ascertain precisely how the client views the past, present, and future because these views may assist the nurse in helping the client cope with death and the challenges faced in the process (Maguire, 1984). An image of the future functions to direct present behavior in accordance with specific values, and some sociologists view a society as being magnetically pulled toward a future fulfillment of their own image of the future as well as being pushed from behind by their past (Polick, 1973).

A future orientation to illness, disease, and health care is essential to preventive medicine. Actions are taken in the present to safeguard the future, particularly regarding certain disease conditions, such as using condoms to prevent AIDS, practicing safe sex, adhering to a diet to prevent elevated cholesterol or blood glucose levels, not driving while under the influence of alcohol, and using seat belts.

TIME AND HUMAN INTERACTION

Up to this point, an effort has been made to create an awareness that social time arises out of interaction. Regardless of the cultural heritage of an individual or group, there is no kind of time that is natural to humans. Instead, time is a result of the structuring and functioning of social order. When a particular temporality emerges, it tends to persist and to influence subsequent interaction. Various cultural groups construct systems of time that have diverse meanings and therefore diverse consequences on social interactions. The most fundamental differences in the meaning of time occur when cultural groups measure time predominantly by either social events or the clock.

Cultural groups that measure time predominantly by social events construct time according to the activities of the group. Conversely, cultural groups that measure time by the clock schedule activities according to the clock. In this regard, time is perceived basically as qualitative for those who measure time by social life and activities and as quantitative for those who measure time by the clock. When measured by social activities, time has significance only in terms of the activities that are occurring. When time is measured by the clock, it has significance only in terms of money, which is perceived to be a scarce commodity, and all activities that take place do so in the shadow of the clock.

Few cultural groups or societies could be characterized as bound exclusively by the clock or as wholly independent of any constraints of temporality. How a group perceives time, nevertheless, has implications for interactions. For example, the Balinese people have a detemporalizing concept of time (Geertz, 1975). For these people social time includes a calendar with a complex system of periodicities. According to Geertz, this is called a "premutational calendar" because it contains 10 different cycles of days ranging in length from 1 to 10 days. Although this is a complex system, it nevertheless serves various religious and practical purposes; it identifies nearly all the holidays and temple celebrations and at the same time guides the individual in daily activities. According to Geertz, the structure of this complex system allows and disallows certain activities on certain days. For example, certain days are good or bad for building a house, starting a business enterprise, moving from one location to another, going on a trip, and harvesting and planting crops.

In contrast to the belief of the Balinese people is the belief held by some Americans that time is money and therefore a scarce commodity. Thus human interactions are controlled in accordance with some notion of the appropriate amount of time for a particular situation. For example, some Americans distinguish the amount of time that can rightfully be consumed by strangers from that which can be given to friends and relatives. Weigert (1981) concluded that interaction time is a measure of the meaning of the relationship between two persons. In the event that two casual acquaintances meet somewhere, it is unlikely that they will take more than a few minutes to express recognition or perhaps exchange a pleasantry or two; therefore, the interaction time for such a meeting is limited. The converse of this is that if two good friends meet and one of the friends attempts to limit the interaction, the other friend may feel rejected. Therefore, the violator is expected to account for the behavior, and if this accounting is not forthcoming, the friendship may be severely strained. A single logical conclusion is that interaction can be evaluated in terms of time consumption.

In the United States, methods to save time or to use time more effectively are in high demand. Numerous books, articles, workshops, tapes, and seminars imply that most Americans value time but at the same time do not think they use it wisely. Many busy professionals feel torn between wise use of time and taking time for interpersonal relationships with fellow workers or friends. For example, a dilemma may arise when a person is busy and a coworker drops in and asks, "Do you have a minute?" If time is considered money, a minute is costly. Because this worker values time, a reply of "yes" may be viewed as costly and thus unjustifiable. On the other hand, "no" may be perceived by the other person as a lack of sensitivity, coldness, and a lack of interest. Therefore, much of the advice given by time-efficiency experts can do much to depersonalize human interactions. A person who follows the advice of these experts to the letter may have far more hours in which to accomplish tasks but at the same time may have fewer friends and fewer intimate relationships.

Drucker (1993) called the executive a captive because everyone can move in on an executive's time, and, generally speaking, everybody does. An executive's time is often preempted by matters that are important to other people; therefore, the executive has little or no time for self. A nurse manager who is responsive to others may find there is little time to do paperwork in the office and thus may take a lot of work home. A nurse manager's personal priorities are often modified when employees present "more urgent" problems.

CULTURAL PERCEPTIONS OF TIME

Appreciating cultural differences regarding time is important for the nurse in relating to both peers and clients. When people of different cultures interact, as is frequently the case in health care settings, there is a great potential for misunderstanding. If nurses are to avoid misreading issues that involve time perceptions, they must understand how other persons in different cultures view time (Tripp-Reimer & Lively, 1993).

Campinha-Bacote (1997) compared time orientation among certain groups in relation to future-time and present-time orientation:

- Dominant American: future over present
- African Black: present over future
- Puerto Rican American: present over future
- Mexican American: present
- Chinese American: past over present
- American Indian: present

Individuals with Future-Oriented Perceptions

Most middle-class Americans, regardless of ethnic or cultural heritage, tend to be future oriented (Tripp-Reimer & Lively, 1993). For example, some middle-class Americans tend to defer gratification of personal pleasure until some future objective has been met, such as advanced education. Thus they delay starting families, purchasing homes, buying an expensive car, or investing money until they have prepared for a profession through advanced education. Another noted difference among members of the dominant American culture is that these individuals tend to structure time rigidly. For these people, adhering to a time-structured schedule is a way of life, regardless of whether the schedule involves work or leisure. For the nurse who works with future-oriented individuals, it is important to talk about events in relation to the future and to adhere to the schedule for planned events in a timely and precise manner.

Individuals with Present-Oriented Perceptions

Present-oriented individuals do not necessarily adhere strictly to a time-structured schedule. The present takes precedence over the future and the past for these individuals. More specifically, whatever is occurring at a precise moment may be more important than a future appointment. It is important for the nurse to avoid labeling such individuals as lazy, disrespectful, or lacking interest. Hoppe and Heller (1974) concluded that present-time orientation may be a reason why some Hispanic clients are late for appointments. Carter (1979) noted that it is important to gain an awareness of differences in values for African-Americans from low socioeconomic groups and proposed that instead of labeling tardiness as a blatant disregard for time, problems related to health, economics, and transportation should be considered with these individuals. Another explanation of individuals with present-time orientation is that they tend to react to time in a linear fashion. Because they perceive time as being on a straight plane, they believe that a present moment spent on a particular task or with a particular individual cannot be regained: "We will never have this moment again" or "We must do it now because we'll pass this way only once." This idea is in contrast to the thoughts held by persons with circular-time orientation, who say, "I'll get back with you" or "We can do it later." The implication of these latter statements is that both persons will be around and the essence of the moment can be relived. In relation to health care, present-oriented individuals are not likely to be involved in preventive care; however, they will seek out emergency care in acute care facilities (Grypma, 1993; Guruge & Donner, 1996). Grypma (1993) notes that after setting up a prenatal class for some American Indian women residing on a reservation, although these individuals had preregistered for the class and confirmed their appointments, they did not keep the appointment. The reason given by these women for not attending the class was a sudden weather shift and the low tide, which provided optimal conditions for picking abalone at islands nearby. For these women, the present-oriented need for food took precedence over planning for the future event of having a baby (Thompson & McDonald, 1989).

A common belief shared by some African-Americans and Mexican Americans is that time is flexible and events will begin when they arrive. For African-Americans this belief has been translated through the years as a perception of time wherein lateness of 30 minutes to an hour is acceptable. Mbiti (1990) traced this perception of time back to West Africa, where the concept of time was elastic and encompassed events that had already taken place, as well as those that would occur immediately.

Many American Indians and Inuits believe that only what is needed for the day should be used and that nature will continue to provide for future needs (McRae, 1994). Atcheson (1987) noted that health, and therefore life, is a spiritual experience for Indians, and the gifts of the Great Spirit should never be abused. Some American Indians and Inuits believe that the person who gives the most to others should be respected. This is also in keeping with the notion of being present-oriented. Many American Indians and Inuits have been taught to live in the present and not be concerned with the future. Therefore they share what they have today (Hagey & Buller, 1983; McRae, 1994; Young, Ingram, & Swartz, 1990).

It is important for the nurse to remember that time perception may also be related to socioeconomic status. For example, although some African-Americans and Mexican Americans can be characterized as present-oriented individuals, others have been assimilated into the dominant culture, are very time-conscious, and take pride in punctuality. These African-Americans and Mexican Americans are more likely to be future-oriented and therefore are more likely to save and plan for important events. They are also likely to be well educated and to hold professional positions. This may not always be the case, since some individuals may not be well educated or hold professional positions yet may value time and have future hopes for themselves and their children. According to Pouissant and Atkinson (1970), these individuals are more likely to encourage their children to seek higher education and to begin saving for the future.

Time perception may also be related to religious orientation. Some American Indians, Mexican Americans, and African-Americans hold strong religious beliefs, and their concept of time is therefore very future-oriented. These individuals, who may come from all socioeconomic and educational levels, have in common the belief that life on earth, with all of its pain and suffering, is bearable only because of the chance for future happiness after death. Such individuals, according to Smith (1976), may plan future activities related to their deaths; for example, they may plan their funeral, including their eulogy; purchase a grave plot; make a will; and otherwise prepare to die. Such individuals may also threaten heirs with disinheritance and talk about what the heirs will do with their hard-earned money.

Levine and Wolff (1985), with the assistance of colleagues Laurie West and Harry Reis, compared the time sense of male and female students in Niterói, Brazil, with similar students at California State University at Fresno. A total of 91 Brazilian students and 107 students from California were surveyed. The universities selected in Brazil and

California were similar in academic quality and size, and the cities in which they were located were secondary metropolitan centers with populations of approximately 350,000. The researchers asked students about their perception of time in several situations, including what they considered late or early for a hypothetical lunch appointment with a friend. According to the data, the average Brazilian student defined lateness for the hypothetical lunch as 33 minutes after the scheduled lunchtime, whereas the Fresno students defined lateness for the hypothetical lunch as 19 minutes after the scheduled lunchtime. The Brazilian students allowed an average of 54 minutes before they considered someone early for an appointment, whereas the Fresno students drew the line for earliness at 24 minutes. When the Brazilian students were asked to give typical reasons for lateness, they were less likely to attribute it to a lack of caring than their North American counterparts were. Instead, the Brazilian students pointed to unforeseen circumstances that an individual could not control without prior knowledge. In addition, the Brazilian students appeared less inclined to feel personally responsible for their own lateness. The question that comes to mind for the nurse is "Are Brazilians more flexible in their concepts of time and punctuality?" Another question for the nurse to consider is "If Brazilians are more flexible in their concepts of time and punctuality, how does this relate to the stereotypical picture of the fatalistic and irresponsible temperament associated with Latins?" This example illustrates the need for nurses to guard against formulating stereotyped images of persons from other cultures. Instead, the nurse must have an understanding of cultural variables that differ among cultures, such as the variation in viewing time.

Levine and Wolff (1985) found similar differences in how students from North America and Brazil characterize people who are late for appointments. In the survey, the Brazilian students indicated that a person who is consistently late is probably a person who is more successful than one who is consistently on time. These students seemed to accept the premise that someone of great stature is expected to arrive late; therefore, a lack of punctuality is a badge of success. In contrast, according to the North American students, persons who arrive late for scheduled appointments, rush in late to meetings, turn in assignments late, or fail to notify others when they find that they are going to be late are generally unorganized, have trouble with priorities, are inconsiderate, and thus will fail to advance professionally and will be less successful. Popular literature in the United States on creating a successful business and professional image espouses the need for continued punctuality.

PHYSIOCHEMICAL INFLUENCES IN RELATION TO TIME

Research on biological rhythms has found that internal body rhythms fluctuate within a 24-hour period. Biological capacities for some individuals are at a low ebb in the daytime, whereas for others, they are at a high level during the day (*Biological Rhythms*, 1970; Yogman, Lester, & Hoffman, 1983; Ziac, 1984). Research has shown that the time of day in which medication is given influences its effectiveness and its side effects; drugs may be more potent when biological capacities are at a low ebb. However, it is important for the nurse to remember that although drugs might be more potent with low biological capacities, the treatment may be less therapeutic. Health care professionals often fail to take into account the client's biological rhythms when scheduling surgical procedures and diagnostic tests. For example, surgical interventions should be avoided when a client's biological capacities are low. Persons who are at a low ebb of biological functioning may be at greater risk for an exaggerated response to anesthesia or may be less able to respond to blood loss (Bremner, Vitiello, & Prinz, 1983; Sideleau, 1992). Evidence also exists that diagnostic tests and treatments may be tolerated better by certain clients when they are timed according to biological rhythms. Hormones and other homeostatic physiological mechanisms fluctuate in the body in a rhythmic way. The timing of the collection of blood and urine samples is important and influences the interpretation of the information obtained.

Physiochemical levels also are related to age. Children have a higher metabolic rate, which tends to make time appear to move more slowly for children. On the other hand, older individuals have a slower metabolic rate, which results in time appearing to move more quickly.

Body rhythms may influence waking at a preselected time. Waking, however, is also a conditioned response. Body systems, including the nervous and endocrine systems, are the result not only of internal biological rhythms but also of psychological phenomena, such as the time or date of previous traumatic events.

Psychological phenomena can greatly affect the client's time perception. For example, according to Sideleau (1992), persons with psychiatric problems can manifest several types of time impairments, including the following:

1. Perception as related to rate and flow of time; that is, a sense that time passes too quickly or too slowly.
2. Failure to recognize finite division of time, which is manifested by confusion related to the inability to distinguish night from day.
3. Attention or inattention to time; that is, adhering too rigidly to schedules or the complete disregard for the value of time constraints or schedules.

It is important for the nurse to carefully discern whether the client's time perception is attributable to cultural phenomena or to some biochemical or psychological manifestation. For example, drug abusers tend to have an altered sense of time. If a hallucinogenic or excitatory drug is being used, the individual may experience temporal contraction and spatial expansion. For these persons, the distortion in time is so profound that they often arrive early for appointments (Sideleau, 1992). In stark contrast, individuals who are influenced by the effects of tranquilizers experience time expansion and space contraction. These individuals are more likely to arrive late for an appointment. Although all these phenomena can be experienced by clients who have a biochemical imbalance or a psychological disorder, the nurse must carefully determine if the faulty perception is caused by the disorder or

by a cultural phenomenon (Giger, Davidhizar, Evers, & Ingram, 1994; Giger, Davidhizar, Johnson, & Poole, 1997).

IMPLICATIONS FOR NURSING CARE

The nurse who gains an understanding of time as a cultural variable with a significant effect on clients and ultimately on client care must also gain an understanding of how time is managed to give high-quality client care. A general attitude shared by health care professionals is that time is irreplaceable and irreversible and that to waste time is to waste life. Moreover, there is no such thing as a lack of time; regardless of the way individuals spend time, it goes at the same pace (Salmond, 1986). That is, each individual has 168 hours to live per week, no more and no less. As health care needs have changed over the years, so have the demands that are placed on nurses. Nurses are constantly being challenged to work in a more time-efficient manner, causing high levels of stress. Some nurses maintain that they are losing control and lack personal satisfaction and thus are becoming burned out. However, it is important for the nurse to remember that one way to remain in control and to have personal satisfaction as opposed to burnout is to adopt an efficient system of time management. Getting organized and precisely articulating priorities are related to job satisfaction (Feldman, Monicken, & Crowley, 1983; MacStavic, 1978; McNiff, 1984). Nurses have long known the importance of working smarter rather than longer or harder (Barros, 1983).

Conflicts between nurses and physicians are sometimes complicated by differences in time perception. Nurses tend to operate on an hourly time sense with adherence to rigid schedules to complete client care assignments. Physicians tend to measure time with the client not in actual time spent with the client, which often is quite brief, but in the duration of the illness or its treatment. Physicians are less likely to schedule time strictly and often appear not to appreciate the nurse's sense of time (Sheard, 1980; Young & Hayne, 1988).

For the nurse, time-management issues involve how to manage both personal time and time at work to meet professional goals. In addition, as cost-containment issues are gaining increased attention in nursing, time-management concerns also necessitate precise assessment of client care needs to plan the hours of nursing time required to meet these needs and to manage the time of staff who are supervised in the delivery of care (Vestal, 1987). In the 1970s the concern with cost-effectiveness of client care and the realization that census may not be an adequate determinant of the demand for care prompted the development of client classification systems. These classification systems were used initially in general hospitals to determine needs for nursing resources by grouping clients into categories that reflected the magnitude of nursing care time. By 1979, over 1000 hospitals reported using some method of classifying levels of care and the time required (Schroder, Washington, Deering, & Coyne, 1986). In 1983 the development of client classification systems received a significant impetus when the Joint Commission on Accreditation for Hospitals and American Hospital Association Standards recommended client classification systems in all hospitals. As psychiatric hospitals began to seek accreditation under the American Hospital Association Standards, increasing attention was given to client classification systems in psychiatric hospital settings.

Appropriate grouping of clients in a hospital (such as having a unit for colostomy clients) can contribute to effective use of staff time. In addition, grouping client activities into a logical sequence (such as changing the client's bed after the colostomy irrigation is finished) can save the nurse time.

Organization of supplies and tasks is important when activities are grouped together. Organizing items prevents multiple interruptions during a procedure to collect things that were forgotten. A nurse who must leave a procedure to get items that are needed but were forgotten not only wastes time but also appears incompetent.

Nursing efforts to reduce hospitalization time are a serious concern today as health care costs spiral (Midgley & Osterhage, 1973). Yet another dimension of time management for nurses today involves appropriately timed data collection to determine client needs and to collect data about the nursing process (Felton, 1970; Polit & Hungler, 2004). If assessment of client and nursing needs is inadequately timed, inaccurate solutions may be planned. The nurse who is aware of the importance of time must also consider the time constraints of data collection. Although a 24-page nursing assessment may provide optimal client data, if the time taken to collect these data would result in other client care being neglected, time constraints will by necessity influence the length of the assessment. Time constraints also influence data collection for research purposes in a health care setting. If financial restraints prohibit additional staff for research purposes, a decision must be made about the priority of the research versus the priority of other nursing staff duties (Monette, Sullivan, & Dejong, 2008).

As change agents, nurses are also concerned with time in relation to change. According to organizational change theory, if change merely involves knowledge, change can be achieved in a short time with little difficulty. If attitudes are involved, somewhat longer periods of time are needed. If the behavior of an individual is involved, a moderate amount of time is required, and moderate difficulty may be encountered. If the behavior of a group is involved, a large amount of time may be required and a high level of difficulty may be encountered (Hersey & Blanchard, 2001).

Lest the nurse stereotype all persons in the United States as valuing timeliness, it must be emphasized that time and punctuality vary considerably from place to place and region to region. Each region and even each city has its own rhythm and rules. Words such as *now* and *later* can convey vastly different meanings. *Now* and *later* may also be interpreted differently by persons from different ethnic or cultural groups. For some African-Americans, *now* may not really imply "immediately"; rather, *now* may mean "soon," so that it could be hours before an action is taken. For the same African-American, *later* may not really imply "within a few hours," but "when you get around to it" (Mbiti, 1990). In contrast, for some future-oriented Americans, *now* means "immediately," and thus action is expected at once. For these same persons, *later* means "within a few hours."

For Americans who travel abroad, major differences encountered, surpassed only by language problems, are the contrasting paces of life and the punctuality differences of people from other countries. These differences can also be noted in the United States when one travels from region to region. For example, in the South, regardless of whether the area is rural or urban, the general pace of life is slow and laid back, and punctuality is not of paramount importance; thus people from this region may be stereotyped as "country." In contrast, in a large metropolitan area such as New York City, the pace of life is associated with more rapid activity, such as walking fast, talking fast, and making decisions quickly. Time differences are also seen in various agencies and among various health professionals. For example, the nurse may find that a more rapid pace is required in a particular hospital setting. The pace may also vary in different clinical disciplines. Duties may differ, and the pace may be more accelerated in high-risk areas such as the intensive care unit, coronary care unit, emergency department, operating room, and psychiatric unit. On the other hand, these areas also experience "slow time" or "down time" when the census is low.

When caring for clients who may have present-oriented time perceptions, such as some African-Americans, some Americans from Puerto Rico, some American Indians, some Mexican Americans, and some Chinese Americans, the nurse must remember that it is necessary to avoid adhering to time as a fixed resource. (An example would be rigid schedules for nursing care procedures such as baths, medications, and meals.) In this case the nurse may find that the standards of the institution regarding time and the time orientation of the client may be in conflict. Again, it is important for the nurse to remember that such persons may perceive time as flexible and that what is happening now is more important than what is going to happen in the future. Therefore, the nurse must be able to adapt client care within a range in time rather than according to fixed hours. It is important for the nurse to recognize that time is perceived differently by some individuals from diverse ethnic, cultural, age, and socioeconomic groups (Gaglione, 1988). Accepting that there are different ways of perceiving time is the first step to increasing tolerance for time-related cultural behaviors. The nurse should appreciate the breadth of factors that affect perception of time. For example, Carter, Green, Green, and Dufour (1994) noted that homeless individuals are very present-oriented. This can significantly affect follow-up care and adherence to treatment recommendations. On the other hand, certain illnesses may affect time perception. Individuals with schizophrenia tend to be present-oriented and have a limited ability to focus on the future. This can significantly affect adjustment to the hospital and community living situations (Suto & Frank, 1994). Chronic illness may affect perception of time for the future. For some persons, hope is important for an orientation to the future (Alberto, 1990).

Case Study

Miss Susie Jones is a 37-year-old Black American client who has been coming to the hospital's outpatient clinic because she has brittle diabetes. Miss Jones's diabetes was diagnosed 6 months previously; however, the diabetes remains uncontrolled by insulin. The client was put on a regimen of 40 units of lente insulin with 5 units of regular insulin at 7 A.M. and at 4 P.M. When Miss Jones comes to the clinic today, she relates to the nurse that she had an episode of "blacking out," or an "insulin reaction," because she forgot to eat after taking her morning insulin. This morning, as frequently in the past, Miss Jones is at least 1 hour late for her scheduled appointment. The following questions relate to variable time and its significance in relation to Susie Jones.

✳ STUDY QUESTIONS

1. List at least two things in relation to the perception of time and culture that may be contributing factors in Susie Jones's tardiness for appointments.
2. List at least two things that the nurse could suggest to Susie Jones that would assist her in being on time for future clinic appointments.
3. List at least two factors about time that contribute to Susie Jones's nonadherence to the medical regimen.
4. Identify ways that the nurse could assist Susie Jones in developing an understanding about time and its relationship to important medications such as insulin.
5. Identify a contributing factor to the insulin reaction that was described to the nurse by Susie Jones.

NCLEX-RN REVIEW QUESTIONS

1. In teaching a patient with present time orientation, the nurse should understand that it may:
   A. Result in taking medication in a timely manner.
   B. Result in adherence to a preventive health regimen.
   C. Result in the patient's attending to other events that are happening rather than focusing on times medication is to be taken.
   D. Influence actions related to a future benefit.

2. A nurse doing discharge teaching with a Navajo diabetic patient should recognize that the patient:
   A. May have trouble with keeping appointments.
   B. Will adhere to taking medication by associating it with meal times.
   C. Is future oriented and therefore motivated to be adherent.
   D. Is likely to perform illness prevention activities to be in harmony with nature.

3. When a nurse is discussing a medication home regimen with an Alaskan Eskimo patient, the nurse might expect the patient to be:
   A. Focused on present events.
   B. Focused on the benefit of present events as they affect the future
   C. Primarily concerned with past historic events
   D. Unaffected by time orientation.

References

Alberto, J. (1990). A test of a model of the relationships between time orientation, perception of threat, hope, and self-care behaviors of persons with chronic obstructive pulmonary disease. Doctoral dissertation, Indiana University School of Nursing, Bloomington, Indiana.

Ariotti, P. E. (1995). The concept of time in Western antiquity. In Fraser, J. T., & Lawrence, N. (Eds.), *The study of time* (Vol. 3) (pp. 69–80). New York: Springer-Verlag.

Atcheson, J. (1987). Traditional health beliefs and compliance in Native American tuberculosis patients. Unpublished master's thesis, Hamilton, Ontario: McMaster University.

Barros, A. (1983, August). Time management: learn to work smarter, not longer. *Medical Laboratory Observer*, 107–111.

Biological rhythms in psychiatry and medicine. (1970). Chevy Chase, Md.: U.S. Department of Health, Education, and Welfare, National Institute of Mental Health.

Bock, P. (1964). Social structure and language structure. *Southwestern Journal of Anthropology*, 20, 393–403.

Bremner, W. J., Vitiello, M. V., & Prinz, P. N. (1983). Loss of circadian rhythmicity in blood testosterone levels with aging in normal man. *Journal of Clinical Endocrinology and Metabolism*, 56(6), 1278–1281.

Campinha-Bacote, J. (1997). Understanding the influence of culture. In Haber, J., Krainovich-Miller, B., McMahon, A., & Hoskins, P. (Eds.), *Comprehensive psychiatric nursing* (ed. 5) (pp. 76–90). St. Louis: Mosby.

Carter, J. (1979). Frequent mistakes made with Black clients in psychotherapy. *Journal of the National Medical Association*, 71(10), 56–64.

Carter, K., Green, R., Green, L., & Dufour, L. (1994). Health needs of homeless clients accessing nursing care at a free clinic. *Journal of Community Health Nursing,* 11(3), 139–147.

Cassirer, E. (1992). *An essay on man.* New Haven, Conn: Yale University Press.

Davidhizar, R., Dowd, S., & Giger, J. (1997). Model for cultural diversity in the radiology department. *Radiology Technology,* 68(3), 233–240.

Doob, L. (1971). *Patterning of time.* New Haven, Conn.: Yale University Press.

Dossey, L. (1993). *Healing words.* San Francisco: Harper.

Drucker, P. (1993). *The effective executive.* New York: Harper Business.

Elton, L. (1975). *Time and man.* New York: Pergamon Press.

England, J. (1986). Cross-cultural health care. *Canada's Mental Health,* 34(4), 13–15.

Feldman, E., Monicken, L., & Crowley, M. (1983). The systems approach to prioritizing. *Nursing Administration Quarterly,* 7(2), 57–62.

Felton, J. S. (1970). Communicating in writing I and II. *Occupational Health Nursing,* 18(5), 13–19; 18(6), 13–25.

Friedman, B. (1972). *Foundations of the measurement of values.* New York: AMS Press.

Gaglione, B. (1988). *Cognitive orientations of three healthy retired American men.* Doctoral dissertation, New Brunswick, N.J.: Rutgers–The State University of New Jersey.

Geertz, C. (1975). *The interpretation of cultures.* London: Hutchinson.

Giger, J., Davidhizar, R., Evers, S., & Ingram, C. (1994). Cultural factors influencing mental health. In Taylor, C. (Ed.), *Essentials of psychiatric nursing* (ed. 14) (pp. 215–238). St. Louis: Mosby.

Giger, J., Davidhizar, R., Johnson, J., & Poole, V. (1997). The changing face of America. *Health Traveler,* 4(4), 11–17.

Gilles, R., & Faulkner, R. (1978). Time and television news work: task temporalization in the assembly of unscheduled events. *Sociological Quarterly,* 19, 89–102.

Gingerich, O. (1972). *The Amish of Canada.* Waterloo, Ontario: Conrad Press.

Gioscia, V. (1971). On social time. In Yaker, H., Osmond, H., & Cheek, F. (Eds.), *The future of time* (pp. 73–141). Garden City, N.Y.: Doubleday.

Grypma, S. (1993). *Culture shock.* The Canadian Nurse, 89(9), 33–37.

Guruge, S., & Donner, G. (1996). Transcultural nursing in Canada. *The Canadian Nurse,* 92(9), 34–39.

Hagey, R., & Buller, E. (1983). Drumming and dancing: a new rhythm in nursing care. *The Canadian Nurse,* 79(4), 28–31.

Hall, E., & William, F. (1960). Intercultural communication: a guide to men of action. *Human Organization,* 19, 7–9.

Hawley, A. (1986). *Human ecology.* Chicago: Chicago University Press.

Hein, E. C. (1980). *Communication in nursing practice* (ed. 2). Boston: Little, Brown & Co.

Hersey, P., & Blanchard, K. (2001). *Management of organizational behaviors* (ed. 8). Upper Saddle River, N.J.: Prentice Hall.

Hoppe, S., & Heller, P. (1974). Alienation, familism, and the utilization of health services by Mexican Americans. *Journal of Health and Social Behavior,* 15, 304.

Hymovich, D. P., & Chamberlin, R. W. (1980). *Child and family development.* New York: McGraw-Hill.

Iverson, P. (1992). *The Navajos.* New York: Chelsea House Publishers.

James, W. (1990). *Principles of psychology* (Vol. 1) (ed. 2). Chicago: Encyclopedia Britannica.

Ketchum, J. D. (1951). Time, values, and social organization. *Canadian Journal of Psychology,* 5, 97–109.

Kluckhohn, F., & Strodtbeck, F. (1973). *Variations in value orientation.* Westport, Conn.: Greenwood Press.

Kohn, M. (1977). *Class and conformity* (ed. 2). Chicago: University of Chicago Press.

Landes, D. (2000). *Revolution in time (revised ed.).* Cambridge, Mass.: Harvard University Press.

Lebhar, G. (1958). *The use of time* (ed. 3). New York: Chain Store.

Levine, R., & Wolff, E. (1985, March). Social time: the heartbeat of culture. *Psychology Today,* 29–35.

MacStavic, R. E. (1978). Setting priorities in health planning: what does it mean? *Inquiry,* 45(1), 20–24.

Maguire, D. C. (1984). *Death by choice.* Garden City, N.Y.: Image Books.

Mbiti, J. S. (1990). African religions and philosophies (ed. 2). Portsmouth, N.H.: Heineman.

McGrath, J., & Kelly, J. (1986). *Time and human interaction.* New York: Guilford Press.

McNiff, M. (1984). Getting organized—at last. *RN,* 47, 23–24.

McRae, L. (1994). Cultural sensitivity in rehabilitation related to native clients. *Canadian Journal of Rehabilitation,* 7(4), 251–256.

Meade, R. (1960). Time on their hands. *Personnel Journal,* 39, 130–132.

Midgley, J. W., & Osterhage, R. A. (1973). Effect of nursing instruction and length of hospitalization on postoperative complications in cholecystectomy patients. *Nursing Resident,* 22(1), 69–72.

Monette, F. C., Sullivan, T., & Dejong, C. (2008). *Applied social research* (ed. 7). Belmont, Calif: Thomson Higher Education.

Morgenstern, I. (1960). *The dimensional structure of time.* New York: Philosophical Library.

Nash, M. (1967). *Machine age Maya.* Chicago: University of Chicago Press.

Nelkin, D. (1970). Unpredictability and life style in a migrant camp. *Social Problems,* 17, 472–487.

Nolt, S. (1992). *A history of the Amish.* Intercourse, Pa.: Herald Press.

Parkinson, C. (1970). *The law of delay.* London: John Murray.

Polick, F. (1973).*The image of the future,* (vols. 1–2). San Francisco, Jossey-Bass.

Polit, D., & Hungler, B. P. (2004). *Nursing research: principles and methods* (ed. 7). Philadelphia: Lippincott Williams & Wilkins.

Pouissant, A., & Atkinson, C. (1970). Black youth and motivation. *Black Scholar,* 1, 43–51.

Pyle, K. (1969). *The new generation of Meiji Japan.* Stanford, Calif: Stanford University Press.

Randall-David, E. (1989). *Strategies for working with culturally diverse communities and clients [Brochure].* Washington, D.C.: U.S: Department of Health and Human Services.

Ritzenhaler, R. (1953). The impact of small industry on an Indian community. *American Anthropologist,* 55, 143–148.

Ruiz, R. (2003). Cultural and historical perspectives in counseling Hispanics. In Sue, D. (Ed.), *Counseling the culturally diverse: theory and practice* (ed. 4). New York: Wiley.

Ruiz, R. A., & Padella, A. M. (1977). Counseling Latinos. *The Personnel and Guidance Journal,* 55, 401–408.

Salmond, S. (1986). Time management: the time is now. *Orthopedic Nursing,* 5(3), 25–32.

Schroder, P. J., Washington, W. P., Deering, C. D., & Coyne, L. (1986). Testing validity and reliability in a psychiatric patient classification system. *Nursing Management,* 17(1), 49–54.

Sheard, T. (1980). The structure of conflict in nurse–physician relations. *Supervisor Nurse,* 11(8), 14–16.

Sideleau, B. (1992). Space and time. In Haber, J., Leach-McMahon, A., Price-Hoskins, P., & Sideleau, B. (Eds.), *Comprehensive psychiatric nursing* (ed. 4) St. Louis: Mosby.

Smith, J. A. (1976). The role of the Black clergy as allied health care professionals in working with Black patients. In Luckraft, J. D. (Ed.), *Black awareness:* *implications for Black care* (pp. 12–15). New York: American Journal of Nursing Company.

Sorokin, P. (1964). *Sociocultural causality, space, time.* New York: Russell & Russell.

Spector, R. (2004). *Cultural diversity in health and illness.* (ed. 6). Upper Saddle River, N.J.: Pearson Prentice Hall.

Stauffer, R. (1995). Personal communication. Harrisburg, Virginia.

Stoetzel, J. (1953). The contribution of public opinion research techniques to social anthropology. *International Social Science Bulletin,* 5, 494–503.

Strauss, G. (1963). Group dynamics and intergroup relations. In Lewis Jr., A. O. (Ed.), *Of men and machines* (pp. 321–327). New York: E.P. Dutton.

Suto, M., & Frank, G. (1994). Future time perspective and daily occupations of persons with chronic schizophrenia in a board and care home. *American Journal of Occupational Therapy,* 48(1), 7–18.

Thompson, E. (1967). Time, work-discipline, and industrial capitalism. *Past and Present,* 38, 58–59.

Thompson, P., & McDonald, J. (1989). Multicultural health education: responding to the challenge. *Health Promoting,* 28(2), 8–11.

Toffler, A. (1970). *Future shock.* New York: Random House.

Tripp-Reimer, T., & Lively, S. H. (1993). Cultural considerations in mental health–psychiatric nursing. In Rawlins, R. P., Williams, R. S., & Beck, C. K., (Eds.), *Mental health–psychiatric nursing* (ed. 3.) (pp. 166–177). St. Louis: Mosby.

Vestal, K. (1987). *Management concepts for the new nurse.* Philadelphia: J.B. Lippincott.

Veterans World Project. (1972). *Wasted men: the reality of the Vietnam veteran.* Edwardsville, Ill.: Southern Illinois University Foundation.

Weigert, A. (1981). *Sociology of everyday life.* New York: Longman.

Wenger, A. (2006). The culture care theory and the older order Amish. In Leininger, M. (Ed.), *Cultural care diversity and universality: a theory of nursing* (ed. 2) Sudbury, Mass.: Jones and Bartlett.

Wessman, A., & Gorman, B. (1977). The emergence of human awareness and concepts of time. In Gorman, B. S., & Wessman, A. E. (Eds.), *Personal experience of time*(p. 3). New York: Plenum Press.

Weyer, E. (1961). *Primitive peoples today.* Garden City, N.Y.: Doubleday.

Wuest, J. (1992). Joining together: students and faculty learn about transcultural nursing. *Journal of Nursing Education,* 31(2), 90–92.

Yogman, M. W., Lester, B. M., & Hoffman, J. (1983). Behavioral rhythmicity and circadian rhythmicity during mother, father, stranger, infant social interaction. *Pediatric Research*, 17(11), 872–876.

Young, D. E., Ingram, C., & Swartz, L. (1990). *Cry of the eagle: encounters with a Cree healer.* Toronto: University of Toronto Press.

Young, L., & Hayne, A. (1988). *Nursing administration: from concepts to practice.* Philadelphia: W.B. Saunders.

Zerubavel, E. (1979). *Patterns of time in hospital life.* Chicago: University of Chicago Press.

Ziac, D. C. (1984). Menstrual synchrony in university women. *American Journal of Physical Anthropology*, 63(2), 237.

CHAPTER 6 Environmental Control

Behavioral Objectives

After reading this chapter, the nurse will be able to:

1. Recognize relevant cultural factors that affect health-seeking behaviors related to environmental control.
2. Recognize relevant cultural factors that affect illness behaviors related to environmental control.
3. Identify various types of cultural folk health practices and the effect on health-seeking behaviors.
4. Recognize the relationship between external locus of control and fatalistic or health-seeking behaviors.
5. Recognize factors affecting external locus of control for persons in selected cultural groups.

Environmental control refers to the ability of an individual or persons from a particular cultural group to plan activities that control nature. Environmental control also refers to the individual's perception of ability to direct factors in the environment. This definition in itself implies that the concept of environment is broader than just the place where an individual resides or where treatment occurs. In the most practical sense, the term *environment* encompasses relevant systems and processes that affect individuals (Sideleau, 1997).

Systems are organized structures that may influence and be influenced by individuals. Processes may be viewed as organized, purposeful patterns of operations. Processes generally include the dynamics and interactions between families, groups, and the community at large. On the basis of these definitions, it is evident that the environment and humans have a reciprocal relationship in the sense that humans and the environment are constantly exchanging matter and energy. When this exchange has purpose and is goal directed, the interaction and exchange processes are considered functional and useful. However, when the exchange has no purpose and lacks goal direction,

a dyssynchronous relationship occurs (Haber & Giuffra, 1997).

In the broadest sense, health may be viewed as a balance between the individual and the environment. Health practices such as eating nutritiously, subscribing to preventive health services available in the community, and installing hazard- and pollution-control devices are all believed to have a positive effect on the individual, who in turn can positively affect the environment (Spector, 2004).

Complex systems of health beliefs and practices exist across and within cultural groups. In addition, variations, whether extreme or modest, to cultural beliefs and practices are found across ethnic and social class boundaries and even within family groups. Today the most widely accepted approach to health care is the biomedical model. This model emphasizes biological concerns, which are considered by those who support this model as more "real" and significant than psychological and sociological issues (Kleinman, Eisenberg, & Good, 1978).

Today in modern Western society, health care practitioners remain primarily interested in abnormalities in the structure and function of body systems and in the treatment of disease. According to

Kleinman, Eisenberg, and Good (1978), the biomedical approach is culture-specific, culture-bound, and value-laden. The biomedical model represents only one end of a continuum. At the opposite end of the continuum is the traditional model, which espouses popular beliefs and practices that diverge from medical science (Chrisman, 1977). Persons who subscribe to beliefs encompassed in the traditional model have varying health beliefs and practices, including folk beliefs and traditional beliefs that are also shaped by culture (Spector, 2004).

DISTINCTION BETWEEN ILLNESS AND DISEASE

During the last decade, scientists and anthropologists began to make a distinction between the terms *illness* and *disease*. The individual experiences that relate to illnesses do not necessarily correlate with the biomedical interpretation of disease. Illness can be defined as an individual's perception of being sick. On the other hand, disease is diagnosed when the condition is a deviation from clearly established norms based on Western biomedical science (Fabrega, 1971). Illness can and does occur in the absence of disease; approximately 50% of visits to physicians are for complaints without a definite basis. According to Kleinman, Eisenberg, and Good (1978), illness is culturally shaped in the sense that it is individually perceived. In other words, how one experiences and copes with disease is based on the individual's explanation of sickness. Disease is described in detail in medical–surgical nursing textbooks. However, nurses need to remember to incorporate both personal and cultural reactions of the client to illness, disease, and discomfort to give culturally appropriate nursing care.

Just as culture influences health-related behavior, it also has a profound effect on the expectations and perceptions of sickness that shape the labeling of sickness and on how, when, and to whom communication of health problems occurs (Campinha-Bacote, 1997). The astute nurse must keep in mind the fact that perceptions of health and illness are shaped by cultural factors. As a direct result of cultural shaping, individuals vary in health care behaviors, health status, and health-seeking attitudes (Grypma, 1993; Guruge & Donner, 1996; McRae, 1994; Thompson, 1993).

The term *health care behavior* is defined as the social and biological activities of an individual that are based on maintaining an acceptable health status or manipulating and altering an unacceptable condition (Bauwens & Anderson, 1992). The term *health status*, on the other hand, is defined as the success with which an individual adapts to the internal and external environment (Bauwens & Anderson, 1992). Thus health care behavior influences health status, which in turn influences health care behavior. Because health care behavior and health status are reciprocal in nature, they both can be affected by sociocultural forces, such as economics, politics, environmental influences, and the health care delivery system itself (Elling, 1977).

CULTURAL HEALTH PRACTICES VERSUS MEDICAL HEALTH PRACTICES

Cultural health practices are categorized as efficacious, neutral, dysfunctional (Pillsbury, 1982), or uncertain.

Efficacious Cultural Health Practices

According to Western medical standards, efficacious cultural health practices are beneficial to health status, though they can differ vastly from modern scientific practices. Because efficacious health practices can facilitate effective nursing care, nurses need to actively encourage these practices among and across cultural groups. Nurses must keep in mind that a treatment strategy that is consistent with the client's beliefs may have a better chance of being successful. For example, persons from cultural groups who subscribe to the theory of hot and cold, such as some Mexican Americans, may actually benefit from this particular belief. Individuals who subscribe to this theory may avoid hot foods in the presence of stomach ailments such as ulcers, a practice that is consistent with the bland diet used in a medical regimen for the treatment of ulcers. Thus scientific health care practices may be blended with efficacious cultural health practices.

Neutral Cultural Health Practices

Neutral cultural health practices have no effect on the health status of an individual. Although some health care practitioners may consider neutral health practices irrelevant, the nurse must remember that such practices may be extremely important because they might be linked to beliefs that are closely integrated with an individual's behavior (Pillsbury, 1982). Greene (1981) cited several examples of neutral practices, including "the ritual disposal of the placenta and cord," interpretation of signs in the cord, avoidance of sexual activity during various stages of pregnancy, certain hygiene practices, and avoidance of exposure to luminous rays of the moon during a lunar eclipse. Many Southeast Asian women believe that sitting in a door frame or on a step while they are pregnant will complicate labor and delivery. In waiting and examination rooms, these women avoid areas near doors. These women may also think that overeating or inactivity during pregnancy will cause a difficult delivery and that sleeping late or during the day will have the same effect. Hill tribeswomen (Hmong and Mien) avoid contact with scissors and knives because they fear sharp instruments may cause cleft lip or abortion. There is a general belief among these women that reaching overhead for something or working too hard may cause miscarriage or birth defects (Lew, 1989; Mattson, 1995). Although these practices require no planned nursing interventions, the astute nurse must recognize their significance and respect the client's right to subscribe to and practice such beliefs.

Dysfunctional Cultural Health Practices

Dysfunctional cultural health practices are harmful. An example of a dysfunctional health care practice found in the United States is the excessive use of such items as overrefined flour and sugar. The nurse must be aware of practices that are dysfunctional and should work to establish educational training programs that help individuals identify dysfunctional health practices and develop beneficial practices. A dysfunctional health care practice was noted among women of various racial, ethnic,

and cultural groups in British Columbia in Canada (Hislop, Deschamps, Band, et al., 1992). Findings from this study noted that implementation of a population-based cervical cytology screening program in British Columbia that began in 1955 decreased the mortality from invasive squamous cervical cancer by more than 70%. However, the mortality from cervical cancer, despite the implementation of this innovative program, remained high among the Canadian Native population (Inuits, Indians, Métis). In fact, the mortality was four times higher among Canadian Native women than among their non-Native counterparts (Threlfall, 1986). Although approximately 85% of the women in the general population complied with screening recommendations, the compliance by Native women was approximately 30% less. Whether this underparticipation by Native woman resulted from beliefs and attitudes or from lack of availability of resources was not determined.

Uncertain Cultural Health Practices

In 1994, Williams and Jelliffe developed a cultural assessment system that included a category of cultural health practices with unknown effects. Classified as uncertain, these practices included such things as swaddling a newborn infant to maintain body temperature and using an abdominal binder for mother and infant to prevent umbilical hernias.

The nurse must remember that in most instances health practices do not fit perfectly into one category or another. According to Greene (1981), health practices are subjectively evaluated as more or less beneficial or harmful when they are compared with the alternative practices available to the user.

VALUES AND THEIR RELATIONSHIP TO HEALTH CARE PRACTICES

Values may be viewed as individualized sets of rules by which people live and are governed. They serve as the cornerstone for beliefs, attitudes, and behaviors. Cultural values are often acquired unconsciously as an individual assimilates the culture throughout the process of growth and maturation. It is important for the nurse to recognize that because cultural values are believed to exist almost solely on an unconscious level, they are the most difficult to alter. Cultural values therefore have a pervasive and profound influence on the individual (Giger, Davidhizar, Johnson, & Poole, 1997).

Value Orientations

Kluckhohn and Strodtbeck (1973) defined *value orientations* as "complex but definitely patterned principles which give order and direction to the ever-flowing stream of human acts and thoughts as they relate to the solution of common human problems." Kluckhohn and Strodtbeck also proposed that it is entirely possible for an individual to hold a value orientation different from the rest of the same cultural group. However, they concluded that despite differences in value orientation within a cultural group, dominant value orientations can be identified for most persons of a particular cultural group.

Kluckhohn and Strodtbeck (1973) compared the way people in different cultural groups organize their thinking about such things as time, personal activity, interpersonal relationships, and their relationship to nature and the supernatural. They developed an orientation framework that includes temporal, activity, relational, people-to-nature, and innate human nature orientations.

Temporal Orientation

Temporal orientation refers to the method by which persons from particular cultural groups divide time. Time is generally divided into three frames of reference: past, present, and future. According to Kluckhohn and Strodtbeck (1973) and Haber and Giuffra (1997), most cultures combine all three orientations, but one is more likely to dominate than another.

Activity Orientation

Activity orientation refers to whether a cultural group is perceived as a "doing"-oriented culture, which is oriented toward achievement, or as a "being"-oriented culture, which values "being" and views people as an important link between generations. In other words, the "doing"-oriented culture values accomplishments, whereas the "being"-oriented culture values inherent existence.

Relational Orientation

Relational orientation from a cultural perspective distinguishes interpersonal patterns. More specifically, relational orientation refers to the way in which persons in a culture set goals for individual members. Relational orientations are found in three modes: lineal, individualistic, and collateral.

Lineal Mode. When the lineal mode is dominant within a particular cultural group, the goals and welfare of the group are viewed as major concerns. Other major concerns are the continuity of the group and the orderly succession of the group over time. Cultures that are perceived as subscribing to the lineal mode view kinship bonds as the basis for maintaining lineage.

Individualistic Mode. Cultures in which the dominant mode is individualistic value individual goals over group goals. Thus each individual is responsible for personal behaviors and ultimately is held accountable for personal accomplishments.

Collateral Mode. When the collateral mode is dominant in a cultural group, the goals and welfare of lateral groups such as siblings or peers are of paramount importance. Examples are found in Russia and in Israel, where the goals of individuals are subordinate to those that affect the entire lateral group.

People-to-Nature Orientation

People-to-nature orientation implies that people dominate nature, live in harmony with nature, or are subjugated to nature. The conceptual framework of people dominating nature is based on the view that humans dominate nature and further indicates that humankind can master or control natural events. When people live in harmony with nature, there is an integration among them, nature, and the universe. When the view that humans are subjugated to nature is held, a philosophy of fatalism is adopted; that is, fate is considered inevitable, and individuals perceive themselves as having no control over nature or their future—they consider themselves powerless to guide personal destiny.

An example is the belief held by some Appalachian people that "If I'm going to get cancer, I'm going to get it," so that taking preventive measures to avoid cancer would be of no benefit. This fatalistic attitude, however, is not completely consistent because most Appalachian people will go to a physician or hospital if they believe they are extremely ill.

Innate Human Nature Orientation

The innate human nature orientation distinguishes an individual's human nature as being good, evil, or neutral. Some cultural groups view human beings as having a basic nature that is either changeable or unchangeable. For example, an individual may be viewed as evil and unchangeable, evil but changeable, or neutral (subject to both good and negative influences).

LOCUS-OF-CONTROL CONSTRUCT AS A HEALTH CARE VALUE

The locus-of-control construct, which originated in social learning theory, is defined as follows:

When a reinforcement is perceived as following some action but not being entirely contingent upon (personal) action then in our culture it is typically perceived as a result of luck, chance, and fate, as under the control of powerful others, or unpredictable because of the great complexity of the forces surrounding [the individual]. When the event is interpreted in this way by an individual, this is labeled as a belief in external control. If a person perceives that the event is contingent upon his own behavior or his own permanent characteristics, we have termed this a belief in internal control. (Rotter, 1966)

This definition presupposes that individuals who believe that a contingent relationship exists between actions and outcomes have internal feelings of control and thus act to influence future behaviors and situations. Individuals who believe that efforts and rewards are uncorrelated, and who thus have external feelings of control, view the future as the result of luck, chance, or fate and are less likely to take action to change the future. The locus-of-control construct can be applied to a variety of phenomena, including the weather, preventive health, curative health actions, and feelings of well-being. For example, individuals who believe

that a contingent relationship exists between compliance to preventive and treatment regimens and health have an internal locus-of-control and are likely to respond positively to affect the future and thus promote good health. On the other hand, individuals who believe that compliance behaviors and health are unrelated have an external locus of control and have little motivation to develop behaviors that could affect the future and enhance good health. Rotter (1975) concluded that the locus of control does not in itself represent a behavior trait and can be modified by interaction with others.

While the locus-of-control construct originates in social learning theory (Rotter, 1966, 1975, 1992), it is essential to note that Siegleman (1992) believed that locus of control is often too general and tends to collapse good and bad events. However, in contrast, Peterson & Stunkard (1992) noted that thousands of researchers have scientifically examined the locus-of-control construct. In fact, Phares (1978), in summarizing the multitude of investigations on the locus-of-control construct, noted that compared with the external, the internal is often resistant to such factors as social pressure and is frequently dedicated to the pursuit of excellence. While Phares (1978) has been quick to add a disclaimer that internality is not necessarily good, the remainder of the research indicates that in a responsive environment, individuals who have an internal locus of control have been able to benefit from such beliefs (Peterson & Strunkard, 1992). Rotter (1992) noted that his 1966 monograph had been cited more than 4700 times in literature, thereby giving credence for its validity as an applicable construct. Some cultural experts in nursing, such as Giger, Davidhizar, and Turner (1992), continue to espouse the usefulness of the locus-of-control construct to understand individuals from diverse cultural backgrounds.

The astute nurse should recognize that persons who subscribe to an external locus of control tend to be more fatalistic about nature, health, illness, death, and disease. For example, some Hispanics, Appalachians, and Puerto Ricans are reported to have an external locus of control. Some American Indians, Chinese Americans, and Japanese

Americans or Japanese Canadians are said to be more or less in harmony with nature; therefore, their cultural beliefs fall outside the locus-of-control construct. However, northern European Americans and African-Americans are reported to fall within both the internal and the external locus-of-control construct (Kluckhohn & Strodtbeck, 1973). The nurse can help the client modify behaviors that fall within the realm of the external locus-of-control construct by showing the effects of certain behaviors on illnesses, health, and disease and thus promote the development of an internal locus of control.

FOLK MEDICINE

Folk medicine, or what is commonly referred to as "Third World beliefs and practices," is often called strange or weird by nurses and other health professionals who are unfamiliar with folk medicine beliefs (Giger, Davidhizar, & Turner, 1992; Snow, 1981). In reality, whether or not something seems "strange or weird" depends on familiarity with the beliefs. In most instances folk medicine practices do not seem strange or weird once health care providers become familiar with them.

The astute nurse must distinguish between practices that are familiar and practices that are desirable, since becoming familiar with something does not imply acceptance. In this situation, tolerance becomes a two-way process: people who subscribe to folk medicine practices need not feel compelled to abandon these beliefs and practices when they become familiar with modern medicine, and health care practitioners should not feel compelled to abandon modern medical practices when they become familiar with folk medicine practices.

An individual's worldview largely determines beliefs about disease and the appropriate treatment interventions. For example, a belief in magic may lead to the assumption that a disease is a result of human behavior and that a cure can be achieved by magical techniques. A religious belief may lead to the assumption that the disease is a result of supernatural forces and that a cure can be achieved by appealing to supernatural forces. The scientific view may lead to the assumption that the disease

is a result of the cause-and-effect relationship of natural phenomena and that a cure is achieved by scientific medicine (Henderson & Primeaux, 1981).

Folk Medicine Beliefs as a System

The folk medicine system classifies illnesses or diseases as natural or unnatural. This division of illnesses or diseases into natural and unnatural phenomena is common among Haitians, persons from Trinidad, Mexicans and Mexican Canadians, African Canadians, and some Southern White Americans (Snow, 1981).

Distinction Between Natural and Unnatural Events

The simplest way to distinguish between natural and unnatural illnesses is that, according to this belief system, natural events have to do with the world as God made it and as God intended it to be. Thus natural laws allow a measure of predictability for daily life. Unnatural events, on the other hand, imply the exact opposite because they upset the harmony of nature. Unnatural events can therefore be viewed as events that interrupt the plan intended by God and at their very worst represent the forces of evil and the machinations of the devil. Unnatural events are frightening because they have no predictability. They are outside the world of nature, and so when they do occur, they are beyond the control of ordinary mortals.

Germane to the tendency to view phenomena in terms of opposition, such as good versus evil and natural versus unnatural, is the belief held by some folk medicine systems that everything has an exact opposite. For example, some African Canadians who subscribe to a folk medicine system believe that for every birth there must be a death, for every marriage there must be a divorce, and for every person with good health there must be someone with bad health. This belief is so encompassing that such individuals believe that every illness has a cure, every poison has an antidote, every herb has a healing purpose, and so forth (Snow, 1981). Because of this belief, some cultural groups do not accept the chronicity of such diseases as AIDS, herpes, or syphilis.

Today, herbal medicine is enjoying a "rebirth" (French, 1996). Eisenberg, Kessler, Foster, et al. (1993) noted that 34% of all U.S. citizens use herbal products in some way. In 1990 they spent $13.7 billion on "unconventional" therapy, with 75% of this cost being out-of-pocket. Canadians are also participating in this resurgence with an increased use of herbal medicines (Abarts, 1995).

Distinction Between Natural and Unnatural Illnesses

Illnesses are generally classified as natural or unnatural, which affects the type of cure or practitioner sought. All illnesses can be viewed as representing disharmony and conflict in some particular area of life and thus tend to fall into two general categories: natural illnesses as environmental hazards and unnatural illnesses as divine punishment.

Natural Illnesses as Environmental Hazards. Natural illnesses in the folk medicine belief system occur because of dangerous agents, such as cold air or impurities in the air, food, and water. Natural illnesses are based on the belief that everything in nature is connected and that events can be both interpreted and directed by an understanding of these relationships. Sympathetic magic, the basis for popular folk medicine beliefs and practices, can be divided into two categories: contagious and imitative magic. At the root of contagious magic is the premise that the parts do represent the whole. Many witchcraft practices are based on contagious magic, including such practices as an evildoer obtaining a lock of the victim's hair or shavings from the victim's skin to do harm. Imitative magic, on the other hand, is based on the premise that like will follow like. For example, a knife under the bed will cut labor pains. To assist the client in preventing natural illnesses, the nurse must comprehend the direct connections between the body and natural phenomena, such as the phases of the moon, the position of the planets, and the changing of the seasons. Because in this belief system good health is contingent on these phenomena, it is imperative that one be able to read these signs if the body is to remain in harmony with nature.

Unnatural Illnesses as Divine Punishment. Unnatural illnesses are believed to occur because a person has become so grave a sinner that the Lord withdraws his favor. In fact, illnesses may be attributed to punishment for failure to abide by the proper behavior rules given to man by God (Gregory, 1992). The cause of unnatural illnesses, for those who subscribe to these beliefs, is based on the continual battle between the forces of good and evil as personified in God and the devil. Evil influences may be blamed for any unnatural illness, which may range from nightmares to tuberculosis to cancer (Boston, 1993). An example of a person subscribing to this belief would be a diabetic African-American woman who consistently refuses to inject herself with insulin because she believes her illness is the direct result of punishment by the devil for her sinful youth. However, unnatural illnesses are also believed to result from witchcraft. Witchcraft is based on the belief that there are individuals who have the ability to mobilize unusual powers for good and evil.

Comparison of the Folk Medicine System and Other Medical Systems

To develop an understanding of folk medicine as a system, the system itself must be examined, along with the ecological model, the Western medical system, alternative therapies, and religious systems. Every medical system is based on the philosophy of survival of the human organism. According to the classic work of Thomas Weaver (1970), both folk practices and Western medical practices are social systems with interdependent parts or variables that include beliefs, attitudes, practices, and roles associated with the concepts of health and disease and with the patterns of diagnoses and treatment.

All medical systems have an adaptive nature. As such, the term *medical system* can be defined as the pattern of cultural tradition and social institutions that evolves from deliberate behavior to improve health status, regardless of the outcome of a particular behavior (Dunn, 1998).

To achieve good health, an individual must develop an idea of what constitutes disease, with its counterpart conditions of pain and suffering. Once an individual adopts a philosophy of health, various health roles are delineated. These health roles require specific health care practitioners who are duly initiated into the rites of practice. Practitioner status may be granted by medical societies or, in the case of folk medicine practices, by supernatural forces. The body is an integral part of each individual; therefore, all medical systems use body parts or excreta for diagnostic purposes. In addition, folk medicine practices, in most cases, prescribe medicine to rub into the skin, to irrigate the body, or to anoint the sick.

Ecological Model. The ecological model is closely related to the folk medicine system. Kay (1979) defined *ecology* as having three foci: (1) biological, or the branch of biology that deals with the relationship between organisms and the environment; (2) social, or the relationship between people and institutions and the interdependence between the two; and (3) cultural, or the relationship between culture and the environment, which also includes culture and societies in the environment. Ecological dimensions of health care can assist the nurse in providing plausible explanations as to why certain individuals contract specific diseases and why other individuals do not. Over the past decade, health care practitioners have become increasingly concerned with the ecological dimensions of race and ethnic minority group health problems such as AIDS and sickle cell anemia.

Western Medical System. In contrast to the folk medicine system, which attempts to explain illness in terms of balances between an individual and the physical, social, and spiritual worlds, is the Western medical system of diagnoses and scientific explanations for illness. Western medical practices focus on preventive and curative medicine, whereas folk medicine practices focus on personal rather than scientific behavior. In the folk medicine system, it may make all the sense in the world to burn incense and to avoid certain individuals, cold air, and the "evil eye." According to Kay (1979), one person's religion is another person's magic, witchcraft, or superstition. However, it is very difficult for health care professionals to see these entities as directly relevant to medical practice or to recognize that for some cultural groups religion is the equivalent of a science.

Although many differences in focus can be seen when Western and folk medicine health practices are compared, some of these differences may not be that significant. For example, Western medical relationships are generally dyads, such as physician–client, physician–nurse, and nurse–client relationships, whereas folk medicine networks are generally multiperson health care networks that may consist of parents, other relatives, and nonrelatives as health care givers. However, today multiperson health care networks are no longer dismissed by Western health care practitioners as irrelevant and thus dysfunctional. In fact, multiperson networks are slowly being incorporated into the Western medical system of health care.

Ethnic diets are an important aspect of human ecology, and health care providers are beginning to incorporate the use of ethnic diets into practice and to understand their significance. A person, regardless of ethnic group, must consume enough food to meet nutritional requirements for energy, fat, protein, vitamins, and minerals to keep the body functioning. Rittenbaugh (1992) noted that very little is known regarding the range of human variability both among and within human populations, particularly regarding common parameters such as nutritional requirements, physiological response to malnutrition, and digestive capabilities. It is perhaps this lack of knowledge that has in the past resulted in Western-oriented health care providers prescribing diets unacceptable to persons from diverse and multicultural backgrounds. In fact, some individuals from diverse cultural backgrounds may have physical incompatibility with certain Western foods. Therefore, the nurse must consider factors regarding ethnic diets and other such folk practices when developing care plans for culturally specific nursing care.

Alternative Therapies. In 1990, 34% of Americans, approximately 61 million people, used one or more nonmedical forms of therapy to treat illness. Most of these individuals used these alternative therapies without informing their health practitioner

(Eisenberg, Kessler, Foster, et al., 1993). In contrast, William LaValley, founder of the Nova Scotia Medical Society's Complementary Medicine Section, estimates that 25% of the Canadian population seeks health care from alternative practitioners (University of Calgary–Complementary Medicine Seminar, 1995). Other presenters at the University of Calgary–Complementary Medicine Seminar (1995) reported that 18% of patients seen at the Calgary HIV/AIDS clinic and 27% of those seen at the University of Calgary gastroenterology clinic had tried alternative therapies. Some 44% of physicians from Alberta indicated that they made referrals to practitioners of alternative therapies, even though only 10% considered themselves informed on the subject (Peterson, 1996). Although Western medicine tends to focus on illness care, alternative therapy addresses the whole patient (Peterson, 1996). In alternative therapy, symptoms are seen as the tip of the iceberg and the body's means for communicating to the mind that something needs to be changed, removed, or added to one's life (Peterson, 1996). In alternative therapy, the mind and the body are seen as a whole. Acupuncture, holistic healing, therapeutic touch, aromatic therapy, meditation, guided imagery, and a variety of other techniques prevail as feasible alternative therapies (Barnum, 1994). Practitioners of alternative therapies include homeopaths, naturopaths, massage therapists, and reflexologists (Cronsberry, 1996). According to Dossey (1993), scientists working in the new field of psychoneuroimmunology have demonstrated the existence of intimate links between parts of the brain concerned with thought and emotion and the neurological and immune systems. Based on these discoveries, Dossey (1993) concluded that thought can become biology. Although the scientific value of alternative, or complementary, therapies is yet to be proved, there is a psychological component that allows the client to have a sense of control. For this reason, nurses should be well informed about nontraditional methods (Cronsberry, 1996).

Religious Systems. Some religious groups have elaborate rules concerning health care behaviors, including such things as the giving and receiving of health care. Religious experiences are based on cultural beliefs and may include such things as blessings from spiritual leaders, apparitions of dead relatives, and even miracle cures. Healing power based on religion may also be found in animate as well as inanimate objects. Religion can and does dictate social, moral, and dietary practices that are designed to assist an individual in maintaining a healthy balance and in addition plays a vital role in illness prevention. Examples of religious health care practices include illness prevention through such acts as the burning of candles, rituals of redemption, and prayer. Religious practices such as the blessing of the throats on St. Blaise's feast day are performed to prevent illnesses such as sore throats and choking. Baptism may be seen as a ritual of cleansing and dedication, as well as a prevention against evil. In addition to its meaning as dedication to God's will and a preparation for death, anointing the sick is related by some religious and cultural groups to recovery and may be performed in the hope of a miracle. Circumcision is also a religious practice in that it may be viewed as having redemptive values that may prevent illness and harm (Morgenstern, 1966; Spector, 2004).

It is important for the nurse to learn to distinguish between a shaman and a priest. A shaman derives power from the supernatural, whereas a priest learns a codified body of rituals from other priests and from biblical laws. In traditional folk medicine systems, some of the most significant religious rituals are those that mediate between events in the here and now and events in the hereafter or "out there" in the netherworld (Morley & Wallis, 1978).

Another example of a religious system is the Amish. For the Amish, religion and custom are inseparable and blend into a way of life (Randall-David, 1989). Religious considerations determine hours of work, occupation, means, destination of travel, and choice of friends and mates. The Amish value the importance of working with the elements of nature rather than mastery over these elements. Closeness to soil, animals, plants, and weather is valued. Salvation is viewed as obedience to the community (Wenger, 2006). The Amish have the belief that the human body was created by God and should not be tampered with. Some Amish believe that although medication may help, it is God who heals (Randall-David, 1989).

Many Amish have been increasingly influenced by special health food interests, vitamins, and food supplement industries (Wenger, 1988). Folk medical practices and opposition to health care seems to be dominant in some family systems (Hostetler, 1980). Egeland (1967) hypothesized that there is a relationship between the concept of family culture and health behavior. Clusters of family cultures serve as basic socializers of health (Egeland, 1967). *Friendshaft*, a concept that crosses distinct church lines, produces distinct patterns of behavior and personality in the Amish community related to choice of type of physician. It also influences choice of curative diet therapy, folk remedies, and family coding of preference of treatment in reference to the presumed cause of symptoms (Brewer & Bonalumi, 1995; Wenger, 1995).

Death and Dying and End-of-Life Decision Making Across Cultures

Some researchers have noted that grieving and death rituals vary across cultures and for the most part are often heavily influenced by religion (Chachkes & Jennings, 1994; Younoszai, 1993). It is essential to remember that how and to what extent rituals regarding death and dying are practiced will certainly vary and will depending on the country of origin and level of acculturation into the mainstream of U.S. society. Clements and colleagues (2003) also noted that the duration, frequency, and intensity of the grief process by various cultural groups is often also based on the manner in which death is experienced and the family cultural beliefs (Clements et al., 2003).

Cultural Beliefs and Advanced Directives. The United States health care system is based on three values:

1. Life is sacred and should be preserved at all costs.
2. Autonomous decision making should be maintained an all times.
3. Above all, it is important that no individuals suffer needlessly (Kagawa-Singer, 1998).

It is interesting to note that findings from some studies suggest that there are cultural variations in attitude towards concepts such as truth-telling, life-prolonging techniques, and decision-making styles at the end of life that are obvious between and across cultures (Giger, Davidhizar, & Fordham, 2006). Advanced directives are suggested for those who want to maintain some autonomy and decision making about their health care, yet some cultural groups have been slow to embrace this concept. For example, some African-Americans continue to distrust the health care system. This distrust is perhaps the result of such things as the Tuskegee Syphilis Study. While decision making for many African-Americans certainly varies by virtue of individual history, religiosity, and socioeconomic status, a great number of African-Americans may regard an advanced directive as a way to legalize neglect, perhaps deny treatment, and commit genocide of the race (DeSpelder & Strickland, 2005).

Autonomy in Decision Making and Truth-Telling About Death and Dying. In the United States, the value of autonomous decision making is valued by many persons from diverse cultures (Giger, Davidhizar, & Fordham, 2006). Blackhall, Murphy, Frank, Michel, and Azen (1995) found that when it comes to decision making in the case of the terminally ill, some Korean Americans and Mexican Americans subscribe to a family-centered model of decision making as opposed to a patient-centered model. For example, they noted that some Korean Americans may seek to avoid the unnecessary suffering of a loved one, particularly if they believe that more negative results would occur if a loved one were told of an unfavorable prognosis. In this case, the family serves as a group decision maker. Examples of other cultural groups that may subscribe to such beliefs include some Japanese Americans and Hispanic individuals (Giger, Davidhizar, & Fordham, 2006; Kagawa-Singer, 1996, 1998).

Findings from one study suggested that Mexican Americans and Korean Americans are significantly less likely than Whites and African-Americans to believe that a family member should be told of a diagnosis, particularly a diagnosis such as metastatic cancer (Blackhall, Murphy, Frank, Michel, & Azen, 1995). In fact, Koreans (47%) and Mexican Americans (65%) were significantly less likely than Whites (87%), and African-Americans (88%) to believe that a loved one should be told of a diagnosis such as metastatic cancer. A surprising finding from this study (Blackhall, Murphy, Frank, Michel, & Azen, 1995) was that Korean Americans (28%) and Mexican Americans (41%) tended to hold an overriding belief that loves one should not be allowed to make decisions about life-supporting measures as compared with 56% of Whites and 60% of Whites. In fact, some researchers suggest that among Mexican Americans there is a belief that the dying should be protected from knowing the prognosis. Yet when it comes to the decision of quality over quantity of life, some cultural groups also vary in this regard. For example, Blackhall, Murphy, Frank, Michel, and Azen (1995) noted that some African-Americans are about only half as likely as their White counterparts to opt for pain medications that might improve the quality of their lives at the expense of the length of life, even if it means that the physiological pain might be constantly present. On the other hand, Whites are more likely to refuse such life-sustaining measures as intubation than their Hispanic or African-American counterparts (Giger, Davidhizar, & Fordham, 2006).

The astute nurse who works with persons from diverse cultural backgrounds must be cognizant of the variations not only in the beliefs about death and dying but also about such keys issues as advanced directives, truth-telling, and autonomy in decision making.

IMPLICATIONS FOR NURSING CARE

The nurse must keep in mind that regardless of whether a client believes in internal or external locus of control or whether the client uses a folk medicine system, religious system, or ecological system, there is still safety in harmony and balance, and there may be danger in anything that is done to the extreme. In other words, it is bad for the body to eat too much, drink too much, stay out too late, and so on. In a classic 1972 study in Harlem, it was reported that 90% of African-American adolescents surveyed believed that good health was largely a matter of looking after oneself. These adolescents concluded that the results of excess may not be immediately visible but sooner or later will affect the individual because the body has become weakened (Brunswick & Josephson, 1972).

There seemingly is a gender and age differential that is associated with strengths and weaknesses among individuals. Generally speaking, strength is correlated with a person's ability to withstand illness, whereas weakness is correlated with a person's heightened susceptibility. For example, strength has been related to the male of our species. In Canada, females are generally regarded as weaker than their male counterparts, and as a result women are generally perceived as being more prone to illness, primarily because of functional blood loss and anatomical differences. Certain age groups have also been related to individual strength and weakness. Infants and unborn fetuses are considered the weakest of all and are perceived to be at the mercy of the mother's behavior, including prenatal behavior. During pregnancy, harmony and moderation are the keys to a healthy baby; thus the pregnancy period carries the greatest taboos among most cultural groups. For example, some Mexican Americans, Amish, Hutterites, and both Whites and African-Americans subscribe to the doctrine of maternal moderation in pregnancy (Bauer, 1969). It is even believed that the mother's emotional state during pregnancy may affect the baby, particularly in the case of pity, fear, mockery, or hate. For example, some southern African-Americans believe that feelings of hate for a particular individual may cause the baby to resemble that person or that a child could be subject to seizures if the mother saw someone having a seizure and felt pity. Some African-Americans, persons from the southern United States, and Mexican Americans also believe that when a pregnant woman makes fun of someone with a physical affliction, the baby may be born with the same affliction, thus punishing the mother for lack of charity (Snow, 1981).

Because some cultural groups believe in a direct connection between the body and the forces of nature, it is important for the nurse to recognize the relevance of natural phenomena such as phases of the moon, positions of the planets, and seasons of the year.

In the rural South in the United States, there is a dependence on natural signs to regulate behavior. Some of these people rely on the *Old Farmer's Almanac* to guide such events as planting crops, setting hens' eggs, destroying weeds, weaning babies, and fishing. The *Almanac* is consulted for many health needs, such as the best time to extract teeth or to have teeth filled. (According to the *Almanac*, the best time to have teeth extracted is during the moon's increase, and the best time to have teeth filled is during the moon's decrease.) The *Almanac* may also be used to determine the optimal time to undergo surgical procedures. The nurse must remember that the *Almanac* is used not only by rural Southern people but also in Northern urban areas, where many African-American pharmacists give copies of the *Almanac* as gifts to their customers for the New Year. Interestingly, the first *Old Farmer's Almanac* is reported to have been written by a physician in 1897.

It is also important for the nurse to remember that many people from diverse cultural groups use the zodiacal signs to manipulate health regimens but do not mention this practice to health professionals for fear of being ridiculed. Use of zodiacal signs illustrates how external forces are brought to bear on the individual; these signs are the basis for a lively practice of self-medication, dietary regulation, and behavior modifications. The nurse should remember that some of these practices are harmful, some are neutral, and some are beneficial. For example, it would be extremely detrimental for a client in need of a life-saving surgical procedure to wait for a full moon to have the procedure done. It is important for the nurse to devise training programs that will teach clients to manipulate behaviors and interpret zodiacal signs in a way that will maintain health and prevent illness and disease.

The nurse should also appreciate that dreams may have a role in health. Many Haitians believe that dreams are important events that allow the individual to communicate with inhabitants of the supernatural world. When dead relatives appear in a dream, they bring messages from the other world, which the Haitian individual is likely to see as reliable (Holcomb, Parsons, Giger, & Davidhizar, 1996; Randall-David, 1989).

In a study of the folk medicine system, it may become obvious that this system reflects a view of the world as a dangerous place, where the individual must be constantly on guard against nature, other persons, and possible punishment from God. This worldview teaches the individual that it is best to look out for oneself and that mistrust is wiser than trust. For example, Hispanics or Latinos may believe that illness has its roots in physical imbalances or supernatural forces that include God's will, magical powers, evil spirits, powerful human forces, or emotional upsets. For some Hispanics or Latinos, treatment comes primarily through a variety of healers that include the *curandero* (healer who uses prayer and artifacts), *yerbero* (herbalist), *espiritista* (practitioner of *espiritismo*, a religious cult concerned with communication with spirits and the purification of the soul through moral behavior), and *santero* (practitioner of *Santería*, a religious cult concerned with teaching people how to control or placate the supernatural) (Randall-David, 1989; Richardson, 1982; Ruiz, 1985; Wanderer & Rivera, 1986; Weclew, 1975). It may be necessary to involve spiritual healers and priests in crisis intervention therapy to treat the client.

The presence of an alternative medical (folk medicine) system that is different from and possibly in direct conflict with the Western medical system can complicate matters. Not only is it a matter of offering health care in the place of no health care, or offering superior health care in lieu of inferior health care, but also the nurse must remember that persons from diverse cultural backgrounds have deeply ingrained beliefs about how to attain and maintain health. These beliefs, which may be linked to the natural and supernatural worlds, may adversely affect the physician–client and nurse–client relationships and thus influence the individual's decision to follow or not follow prescribed treatment regimens. For example, in certain cultures, the occurrence of cancer may be attributed to insufficient use of herbal medicine, an insult to an ancestor, or a perceived punishment. Thus, standard Western medical approaches may not always appear relevant to certain clients in multicultural populations (Boston, 1993).

The nurse might correctly assume that when a low-income African-American, southern White American, Puerto Rican, or Mexican American arrives for professional care, every home remedy known to the client has already been tried. It is important for the nurse to determine what the client has been doing to combat the illness. If the home remedy is harmless, it is best left in the treatment plan with the nurse's own suggestions added. However, harmful practices must be eliminated. One of the best ways for the nurse to eliminate harmful practices is to inquire whether the practice has worked. If the client assumes that it has not worked, the nurse can simply suggest that something else be tried. If the client perceives that a harmful practice is beneficial, the nurse must provide education that will illuminate the dangers of this harmful practice.

Nurses have recently begun to explore the relationship of person and environment in nursing research. An exploratory study by Pyles (1989) related Etzioni's compliance theory to satisfaction by nursing employees in a school of nursing. Data from the study indicated that a normative power structure in the school and the resultant moral involvement profile in the faculty were compatible for an organization such as a university, which displays cultural goals. In a more clinical study, Gould (1989) studied 112 elderly residents in three metropolitan nursing homes. The data indicated that life satisfaction is an indicator of well-being, which is useful as a measure of quality of care because of its linkage to health. The data additionally indicated that bonding develops between institutionalized elderly persons and their caregivers, which precludes the drive for self-determination. Thus, the data explained why lower-income elderly persons demonstrated high levels of life satisfaction despite low levels of perceived influence over the institutional environment.

Case Study

Martha Brown is a 27-year-old woman who lives in the hills of northern Kentucky in a small cabin that has no indoor plumbing. She lives with her husband and six small children. The public health nurse makes a home visit after three of the children have been diagnosed by the school nurse as having lice. While the nurse is explaining the use of Rid (lice treatment) to the mother, she notes that Mrs. Brown has a persistent cough that she states she has had for 2 years. The nurse notes that the cough is productive, that Mrs. Brown looks emaciated, and that her color is extremely ashen. She tires easily. Although health insurance is a benefit of her husband's job in a nearby mine, Mrs. Brown's children were born at home, and she has never had a complete physical. When asked why she has not gone to a nearby free health clinic, Mrs. Brown replies, "Sickness is God's will, and he will cure me if he wants to. Anyway, my family comes first, and I don't have the time. Besides, doctors can't be trusted. My Aunt Jane went to one once, and she died the next week."

✳ STUDY QUESTIONS

1. Based on the fact that Mrs. Brown is Appalachian and taking into consideration the fact that every individual is unique, decide whether Mrs. Brown is more likely to be "being" oriented or "doing" oriented in regard to activity orientation.

2. Decide what the relational orientation is for Mrs. Brown, based on her reply to the public health nurse about why she has not sought treatment.

3. Based on Mrs. Brown's reply to the public health nurse and the fact that she is Hispanic, what

people-to-nature orientation is she likely to have?

4. Decide, on the basis of Mrs. Brown's comment and the fact that she is Hispanic, what view of human nature she is likely to hold.

NCLEX-RN REVIEW QUESTIONS

1. A nurse is teaching an Appalachian patient who says, "Whatever will be, will be." The nurse understands:
   A. External feelings of control are related to compliance.
   B. Internal feelings of control are related to compliance.
   C. A fatalistic point of view is related to taking preventative health care actions.
   D. Feelings of internal control are not necessary for compliance.

2. When caring for the patient who believes there is a relationship between outcomes and internal feelings of control, the patient can be expected to:
   A. Follow directions given for health care

5. List at least three reasons why Mrs. Brown might be apprehensive about seeking medical help.

   B. View the future as a result of luck, chance, or fate.
   C. Believe compliance behaviors and health are unrelated
   D. Adhere to beliefs of external control.

3. The nurse who is caring for a patient with an external locus of control can anticipate that:
   A. The patient will be more likely to be fatalistic about nature and illness.
   B. The patient is more likely to feel in control of events that affect him or her.
   C. The patient will expect to be able to modify behaviors to reach health goals.
   D. The patient will desire help to control health and illness outcomes.

References

Abarts, L. (1995, February). University of Calgary hosts complementary medicine society. *Holistic and Complementary Medical Society of Alberta Newsletter*, 1(1), 1.

Barnum, B. S. (1994). *Nursing theory* (ed. 4). Philadelphia: J. B. Lippincott Co.

Bauer, W. W. (1969). *Potions, remedies, and old wives' tales*. Garden City, NY: Doubleday.

Bauwens, E., & Anderson, S. (1992). Social and cultural influences on health care. In Stanhope, M., & Lancaster, J. (Eds.), *Community health nursing: process and practice for promoting health* (ed. 3). (pp. 89–108). St. Louis: Mosby–Year Book.

Blackhall, L. J., Murphy, S. T., Frank, G., Michel, V., & Azen, S. (1995). Ethnicity and attitudes towards patient autonomy. *Journal of the American Medical Association*, 274, 820–825.

Boston, P. (1993). Culture and cancer: the relevance of cultural orientation within cancer education programmes. *European Journal of Cancer Care*, 2, 72–76.

Brewer, J. A., & Bonalumi, N. M. (1995). Cultural diversity in the emergency department. *The Journal of Emergency Nursing*, 2(6), 494–497.

Brunswick, A. F., & Josephson, E. (1972). Adolescent health in Harlem. *American Journal of Public Health*, 72(suppl.), 7–47.

Campinha-Bacote, J. (1997). Understanding the influence of culture. In Haber, J., Krainovich-Miller, B., McMahon, A., & Price-Hoskins, P. (Eds.), *Comprehensive psychiatric nursing* (ed. 5). St. Louis: Mosby.

Chachkes, E., & Jennings, R. (1994). Latino communities: coping with death. In Dane, B., & Levine, C. (Eds.), *AIDS and the new orphans: coping with death*. Westport, Conn: The Greenwood Press, pp. 77–100.

Chrisman, N. J. (1977, April). The health seeking process. *Culture and Medicine in Psychiatry*, 1, 351–377.

Clements, P. T., Vigil, G. J., Manno, M. S., Henry, G. C., Wilks, J., Das, S., et al. (2003). Cultural perspectives of death, grief, and bereavement. *Journal of Psychosocial Nursing*, 41(7), 18–26.

Cronsberry, T. (1996, April). Alternative cancer therapies. *The Canadian Nurse*, 92(4), 35–38.

DeSpelder, L., & Strickland, A. (2005). *The last dance: encountering death and dying.* (ed. 7). Boston: McGraw-Hill.

Dossey, L. (1993). *Healing words.* San Francisco: Harper.

Dunn, F. L. (1998). Transcultural Asian medicine and cosmopolitan medicine as adaptive systems. In Leslie, E. (Ed.), *Asian medical systems: a comparative study* (p. 135). Delhi: Motilal Banarsidass Publishers.

Egeland, J. (1967). *Belief and behavior as related to illness: a community case study of the old order Amish (Doctoral dissertation, Yale University).* Dissertation Abstracts International, X, Ann Arbor, Mich: University Microfilms International.

Eisenberg, D., Kessler, R., & Foster, C, et al. (1993). Unconventional medicine in the United States: prevalence, costs, and patterns of use. *New England Journal of Medicine*, 328(4), 246–252.

Elling, R. H. (1977). *Socio-cultural influences on health and health care.* New York: Springer Publishing.

Fabrega, H. (1971). Medical anthropology. In Siegel, B. J. (Ed.), *Biennial review of anthropology.* Stanford, Calif.: Stanford University Press.

French, M. (1996, July). The power of plants. *Advances for Nurse Practitioners*, 16–18.

Giger, J. N., Davidhizar, E., & Fordham, P. (2006). Multicultural and multi-ethnic considerations and advanced directives: developing cultural competency. *Journal of Cultural Diversity*, 13(1), 3–9.

Giger, J., Davidhizar, R., Johnson, J., & Poole, V. (1997). The changing face of America. *Health Traveler*, 4(4), 11–17.

Giger, J., Davidhizar, R., & Turner, G. (1992). Black American folk medicine. *The ABNF Journal*, 42–46.

Gould, M. (1989). *The relationship of perceived social-environmental factors and functional health status to life satisfaction in the elderly.* Presented paper. Indianapolis, Ind.: Sigma Theta Tau International Conference.

Greene, L. (1981). *Social and biological predictors of nutritional status, physical growth, and neurological development.* New York: Academic Press.

Gregory, D. (1992). Nursing practice in native communities. In Baumgart, A., & Larson, J. (Eds.), *Canadian nursing faces the future* (ed. 2). St. Louis: Mosby–Year Book.

Grypma, S. (1993, September). Culture shock. *The Canadian Nurse*, 89(8), 33–37.

Guruge, S., & Donner, G. (1996, September). Transcultural nursing in Canada. *The Canadian Nurse*, 92(8), 36–40.

Haber, J., & Giuffra, M. (1997). Sociocultural issues. In Haber, J., Hoskins, P., Leach, A., & Sideleau, B.

(Eds.), *Comprehensive psychiatric nursing* (ed. 5). St. Louis: Mosby.

Henderson, G., & Primeaux, M. (1981). *Transcultural health care.* Reading, Mass.: Addison-Wesley.

Hislop, T. G., Deschamps, M., & Band, P. R., et al. (1992). Participation in the British Columbia Cervical Cytology Screening Programme by Native Indian women. *Canadian Journal of Public Health*, 83(5), 344–345.

Holcomb, L. O., Parsons, L. C., Giger, J. N., & Davidhizar, R. (1996). Haitian American: implications for nursing care. *Journal of Community Health Nursing*, 13(4), 249–260.

Hostetler, J. (1980). *Amish society* (ed 3). Baltimore: The Johns Hopkins University Press.

Kagawa-Singer, M. (1996). Cultural systems related to cancer. In McCorkle, R., Grant, M., Grant-Strong, M., & Brains, S. B. (Eds.), *Cancer nursing* (ed. 2). (pp. 38–52). Philadelphia: Saunders.

Kagawa-Singer, M. (1998). The cultural context of death rituals and mourning practices. *Oncology Nursing Forum*, 25(10), 1725–1756.

Kay, M. (1979). Clinical anthropology. In Bauwens, E. E. (Ed.), *The anthropology of health* (pp. 3–11). St. Louis: Mosby.

Kleinman, A., Eisenberg, L., & Good, B. (1978). Culture, illness and care. *Annals of Internal Medicine*, 88, 251–258.

Kluckhohn, K., & Strodtbeck, F. (1973). *Variations in value orientations.* Westport, Conn.: Greenwood Press.

Lew, L. (1989). *Southeast Asian Health Project: application for mother, children and infants demonstration grant.* Unpublished manuscript (grant proposal), Ottawa.

Mattson, S. (1995). Culturally sensitive perinatal care for southeast Asians. *Journal of Obstetric and Gynecological Neonatal Nursing*, 24(4), 335–341.

McRae, L. (1994). Cultural sensitivity in rehabilitation related to native clients. *Canadian Journal of Rehabilitation*, 7(4), 251–256.

Morgenstern, J. (1966). *Rites of birth, marriage, death, and kindred occasions among the Semites.* Chicago: Quadrangle (1973, New York: Ktav Publishing House).

Morley, P., & Wallis, R. (1978). *Culture and caring.* London: Peter Owen.

Peterson, B. (1996). The mind-body connection. *The Canadian Nurse*, 92(1), 29–31.

Peterson, C., & Stunkard, A. (1992). Cognates of personal control: locus of control, self-efficacy, and explanatory style. *Applied & Preventive Psychology*, 1, 111–117.

Phares, E. (1978). Locus of control. In London, H., & Exner, J. (Eds.) *Dimensions of personality* (pp. 263–304). New York: Wiley.

Pillsbury, B. (1982). Doing the month: confinement and convalescence of Chinese women after childbirth. In Kay, M. (Ed.), *Anthropology of human birth.* Philadelphia: F.A. Davis.

Pyles, C. (1989). *Power compatibility profile in a school of nursing.* Presented paper. Indianapolis, Ind.: Sigma Theta Tau International Conference.

Randall-David, E. (1989). *Strategies for working with culturally diverse communities and clients* [Brochure]. Washington, D.C.: U.S. Department of Health and Human Services.

Richardson, L. (1982). Caring through understanding: part 2. Folk medicine in the Hispanic population. *Imprint,* 29(2), 21.

Rittenbaugh, C. (1992). Human foodways: a window on evolution. In Bauwens, E. E. (Ed.), *The anthropology of health* (ed. 3). St. Louis: Mosby–Year Book.

Rotter, J. B. (1966). Generalized expectancies for internal versus external control of reinforcement. *Psychological Monographs,* 80(1), 1–28.

Rotter, J. B. (1975). Some problems and misconceptions related to the construct of internal versus external control of reinforcement. *Journal of Consulting and Clinical Psychology,* 43, 56–67.

Rotter, J. B. (1992). Some comments on the "Cognates of personal control." *Applied & Preventive Psychology,* 1, 127–129.

Ruiz, P. (1985). Cultural barriers to effective medical care among Hispanic-American patients. *Annual Review of Medicine,* 36(63).

Sideleau, B. (1997). Space and time. In Haber, J., McMahon, A., Price-Hoskins, P., & Sideleau, B. (Eds.), *Comprehensive psychiatric nursing* (ed. 5). St. Louis: Mosby.

Siegleman, M. (1992). Power and powerlessness: comments on "Cognates of personal control," *Applied & Personal Psychology,* 1, 119–120.

Snow, L. F. (1981). Folk medical beliefs and their implications for the care of patients: a review based on studies among Black Americans. In Henderson, G., & Primeaux, M. (Eds.), *Transcultural health care.* Reading, Mass.: Addison-Wesley.

Spector, R. (2004). *Cultural diversity in health and illness.* (ed. 6). Upper Saddle River, N.J.: Pearson Prentice Hall.

Thompson, K. (1993). Self-governed health. *The Canadian Nurse,* 89(8), 29–32.

Threlfall, W. J. (1986). Cancer patterns in British Columbia Native Indians. *Medical Journal,* 28, 508–510.

University of Calgary–Complementary Medicine Seminar (1995). Calgary, Alberta: University of Calgary.

Wanderer, J., & Rivera, G. (1986). Black magic beliefs and white magic practice: the common structures of intimacy, tradition and power. *Social Science Journal,* 23 (4), 419.

Weaver, T. (1970). Use of hypothetical situations in a study of Spanish-American illness referral systems. *Human Organisms,* 29, 141.

Weclew, R. V. (1975). The nature, prevalence, and level of awareness of curanderismo and some of its implications for community mental health. *Community Mental Health Journal,* 11(2), 145–154.

Wenger, A. (1988). *The phenomenon of care in a high context culture: the old order Amish. Doctoral dissertation.* Detroit, Mich.: Wayne State University.

Wenger, A. (1995). Cultural context, health, and health care decision making. *The Journal of Transcultural Nursing,* 7(1), 3–14.

Wenger, A. (2006). The culture care theory and the older order Amish. In Leininger, M. (Ed.), *Cultural care diversity and universality: a theory of nursing* (ed. 2). Sudbury, Mass: Jones and Bartlett.

Williams, C., & Jelliffe, D. (1994). *Mother and child health: delivering the services.* (ed. 3). New York: Oxford University Press.

Younoszai, B. (1993). Mexican American perspectives related to death. In Irish, D. P., Lundquist, K. F., & Nelson, V. J. (Eds.), *Ethic variations in dying, death, and grief.* Washington, DC: Taylor & Francis.

CHAPTER 7 Biological Variations

Behavioral Objectives

After reading this chapter, the nurse will be able to:

1. Articulate biological differences among individuals in various racial groups.
2. Relate the importance of knowledge of biological differences that may exist among individuals in various racial groups to the provision of health care by the nurse.
3. Describe nursing implications that may arise when providing care for individuals in different cultural and racial groups.
4. Describe nutritional preferences and deficiencies that may exist among persons in different cultural groups.
5. Explain how psychological characteristics may vary from one culture to another.
6. Explain how susceptibility to disease may differ among individuals in different racial groups.

It is a well-known fact that people differ culturally. Cultural differences are evident in communication, spatial relationships and needs, social organizations (family, kinships, and tribes), time orientation, and ability or desire to control the environment. Less recognized and understood are the biological differences among people in various racial groups. It is becoming more evident to nurses that a body of scientific knowledge does exist about biological cultural differences. References to and information about biocultural differences are mushrooming in the literature and have resulted in a field of study known as *biocultural ecology* (Bennett, Osborne, & Miller, 1975), which focuses on human adaptation and homeostasis. The purpose of biocultural ecology is to transcend the fragmentation inherent in the separation of culture, human biology, and ecology and the environment. Biocultural ecology is an examination of diverse human populations by means of this three-way interaction system and focuses on specific, localized individuals and populations within a given environment. Data relative to all the variables significant to people within a racial group are essential for complete understanding of the people. Not only are no two persons alike but also no two cultural or racial groups are alike, and all phenomena relative to both individuals and cultural or racial groups must be understood.

Although the significance of biocultural ecology concepts has been studied in other disciplines, such as sociology and medical anthropology, the nursing literature has only recently documented the importance of this field for nurses. A focus on transcultural issues that began in the mid-1960s with the impetus of nurses such as Madeleine Leininger (1970) has helped nurses to develop cultural insights and a deeper appreciation for human life and values from a cultural perspective. However, despite the introduction of transcultural nursing concepts, the nursing literature remains scanty on biological variations among people in various racial groups. The strongest argument for including concepts on biological variations in nursing education and subsequently nursing practice is that scientific facts about biological variations can aid the nurse in giving culturally appropriate health care. Nurses who care for people transculturally need to be cognizant of certain basic biological differences to give nonharmful and competent care.

Most nurses in the United States have been educated in a system of nursing practice based on biological baselines of the dominant White race. Because studies on biological baseline data in growth and development, nutrition, and other biological phenomena have been conducted with White subjects, standardized norms available to the nurse do not reflect biological variations among different racial groups. That people in various racial groups differ tremendously is evidenced externally and is related to biogenetic variations that have occurred internally. Therefore, values uniracially normed are inappropriate when applied across racial groups. In the United States, White-standardized values for factors related to growth and development, nutrition, and susceptibility to disease are often applied to African-Americans, Asians, and American Indians. Therefore, significant deviations from the norm that may be labeled "nonnormal" might be more appropriately labeled "non-White" (Overfield, 1977, 1995). In fact, biological variations among racial groups are so diverse that multiple dimensions are encompassed.

DIFFERENTIATION BETWEEN HEALTH DISPARITIES, HEALTH CARE DISPARITIES, HEALTH INEQUALITIES, AND HEALTH INEQUITIES

To understand the significance of biological variations, it is essential to understand other key terms, such as *health disparities, health care disparities, health inequities,* and *health inequalities.* These terms have augmented significance when health care professionals attempt to render culturally competent care to diverse, multicultural groups of people.

Health Disparity

A health disparity can be defined from a sociological, population-specific, or biopsychosocial perspective.

For example, from a sociological perspective, health disparity can be viewed as a chain of events signified by a difference in: (1) environment; (2) access to, utilization of, and quality of care; (3) health status; and (4) health outcome.

On the other hand, in its broadest sense, a health disparity can be defined as a "population-specific difference in not only disease, but health outcomes, or access to health care" (HRSA, 2004). In fact, the first National Institutes of Health (NIH) Working Group on Health Disparities succinctly narrowed the definition somewhat by defining health disparities as "differences in the incidence, prevalence, mortality, and burden of disease and other adverse health conditions that exist among specific population groups in the US" (First National Institutes of Health Work Group on Healthy Disparities, 2002). It is essential to remember that because the impact of health care on health disparities is an important factor, a definition of racial and ethnic health care disparities was provided by the Institute of Medicine's Committee on Understanding and Eliminating Racial and Ethnic Disparities in Health Care (Smedley, Stith, & Nelson, 2003). The committee unequivocally noted that a health disparity "more likely than not is a racial and ethnic difference in the quality of health care usually arising as a result of access-related factors or clinical needs, preferences and appropriateness of the intervention" (Smedley, Stith, & Nelson, 2003). In fact, the committee unequivocally noted that disparities in healthcare for the most part are consistent regardless of the nature of the illness of the time of services rendered (Smedley, Stith, & Nelson, 2003).

It is interesting to note that neither the sociological nor population-specific definitions allow for the inclusion of biological variations that may occur in groups of people regardless of race, ethnicity, socioeconomic status, and access to care issues. With this thought in mind, another approach to health disparity from a biopsychosocial perspective is offered that works in tandem with the concept of biological variations. From a *biopsychosocial* perspective, genes and biology, environment, and behavior all come together in a cataclysmic way to create a health disparity. It is essential to note that socioeconomic status plays a major contributing factor in unequal treatment, particularly where ethnic minorities are concerned. While this new definition does take into account the issue of vulnerability or race and ethnicity, socioeconomic status, geographical location, and access to care issues (Appel, Giger & Davidhizar, 2005), Braithwaite and Taylor (2002) noted that even if income levels were standardized and all impediments regarding access to care were eliminated, disparities in health outcomes might still exist. They contend that this argument gives credence to the need to eliminate cultural incompetence among health care providers. The biopsychosocial perspective does not negate the fact that certain groups, including specific racial and ethnic groups, persons residing in certain geographic locations, the poor and underserved, and the disabled, are more likely to suffer disproportionately from health disparities (Atrash & Hunter, 2006). It is also interesting to note that the term *disparity* is almost exclusively used in the United States, while the terms *health inequality* or *inequity* are more commonly used outside of the United States.

Health Care Inequality

Inequality, particularly when referring to health care, is a term used to refer to differences in age, rank, condition, lack of excellence in treatment, or dissimilitude (vast differences) in services available. *Inequity* is similarly defined as a condition of "being unequal" or "lack of opportunity, treatment or status." Yet another view of the term *health disparity* is that in the context of public health and the social sciences, the term has begun to take on a meaning of injustice (Atrash & Hunter, 2006). In fact, Atrash and Hunter (2006) contend that in the United States that there is growing concern that even when there are equivalent levels of access to care, most racial and ethnic minorities continue to experience a lower quality of health services and are therefore likely to receive needed routine medical procedures than their White counterparts. For example, African-Americans are less likely to receive peritoneal dialysis and kidney transplants for end-stage renal disease than their White counterparts (Kasiske, 1998; Barker-Cummings, McCellen, Soucie, et al., 1995). Similarly, some data suggest that African-Americans and Hispanic clients with long-bone fractures who are seen in the emergency department are far less likely than their White counterparts to receive necessary analgesics to suppress the pain (Todd,

Deaton, D'admao, et al., 2000). Yet another example of health care disparities include studies suggesting that African-American Medicare patients with congestive heart failure or pneumonia, for example, are more likely to receive a poorer quality of care than their White counterparts (Ayanian, Weissman, Chasan-Taber, et al., 1999).

DIMENSIONS OF BIOLOGICAL VARIATIONS

A direct relationship exists between race and body structure, skin color, other visible physical characteristics, enzymatic and genetic variations, electrocardiographic patterns, susceptibility to disease, nutritional preferences and deficiencies, and psychological characteristics. Differences among people in various racial groups in each of these areas are discussed in the following sections.

Body Structure

One category of difference between racial groups is body structure, which includes both body size and body shape. Newborn body proportions differ among racial groups. Although research on this topic remains scanty, it has been postulated that newborn body proportions appear to be genetically programmed to conform to the pelvic shape of the mother (Overfield, 1977, 1995).

Body structure as well as bone density also differs among adults. For example, the prevalence of osteoporosis and the incidence of vertebral fractures are both reported to be substantially lower in African-American women than in White American women (Cummings, Kelsey, Nevitt, & O'Dowd, 1985; Gilsanz, Roe, Mora, et al., 1991; Melton & Riggs, 2000; Pollitzer & Anderson, 1990). This finding is generally attributed to racial differences in adult bone mass (Pollitzer & Anderson, 1990).

Among adults, bone density is greater in African-Americans than in White Americans of either sex (Reid, Cullen, Schooler, et al., 1990). However, differences in adult bone density are not necessarily confined to these two racial groups. In fact, the bone density of adult Polynesians is reported to be greater than that of age-matched Whites (Reid, Cullen, Schooler, et al., 1990). In contrast, Asian

Americans generally have lower values for bone density than other racial groups (Reid, Cullen, Schooler, et al., 1990).

Biological markers that account for the variations in adult bone mass among racial groups are unknown. In addition, the time of life at which these differences are manifested is uncertain. According to Li, Specker, Ho, and Tsang (1989), prepubertal African-American children tend to have higher values for bone density than do their White counterparts. Some researchers (Garn, Nagy, & Sandusky, 1972; Li, Specker, Ho, & Tsang, 1989) have speculated that such findings indicate that racial differences in skeletal mass develop early in childhood and persist throughout life.

In regard to body structure and size, the face is perhaps one of the most fascinating areas of the body because it has many parts that combine to make the whole. The face tends to be the one prominent area that can visibly categorize people by race. For example, eyelids vary from racial group to racial group. In some racial groups the eyelids droop over the cartilage plate above the eye, and in other racial groups the eyelids do not droop. The epicanthic fold, another variation of the eyelids, is found predominantly in persons with Oriental characteristics but may be present in other racial groups.

Ears are another fascinating part of the face because they have a variety of shapes. Earlobes can be free and floppy, or attached close to the face as if the intent were to make sure the lobe stayed in place. Earlobes that are free and floppy are very handy for attaching earrings. When earlobes are attached, they are the least defined, and the wearing of objects such as earrings may be difficult.

Noses come in all sizes and shapes; however, nose size and shape correlate directly with one's racial ancestry. It has been postulated that small noses were an evolutionary result of living in cold climates, such as the classic Oriental nose, and that noses with high bridges were a result of living in climates that were dry, such as the classic Iranian and American Indian noses. People who lived in moist, hot climates developed broad, flat noses, such as those found on Africans and African-Americans (Overfield, 1977, 1995).

Teeth offer another important variation in body size and shape. Tooth size, which is important because the teeth help shape the size of the lower face, varies among racial groups. For example, Australian aborigines have the largest teeth in the world, as well as four extra molars. Oriental Americans and African-Americans have very large teeth, whereas White Americans have very small teeth. People with very large teeth tend to have their jaws projecting beyond the upper part of the face. This projection tends to be a normal variation and not an orthodontic problem. There is also a tendency among some racial groups for fewer teeth. For example, some racial groups do not have a third molar or maxillary lateral incisors. Peg teeth are sometimes a step in the evolutionary process that facilitates the presence or absence of a particular type of tooth (Overfield, 1977, 1995).

As teeth vary among racial groups, so do tongues. The most common variances are scrotal tongues, which occur in 5% of the population in some racial groups; geographic tongues, which occur in 3% of the population in some racial groups; and fissured tongues, which occur in 5% to 40% of the population in some racial groups (Witcop et al., 1963).

The mandibular or palatine torus is also of concern to the nurse when inspecting the mouth. The torus is a bony protuberance, and the palatine torus occurs on the midline of the palate, whereas the mandibular torus occurs as a lump on the inner side of the mandible near the second molar. Tori are fairly common, with palatine tori occurring in up to 25% of the population in most racial groups studied. Mandibular tori occur in 7% of Whites, 2% of African-Americans, and 40% of Orientals (Jarvis, 1972).

Another variation in body size and structure is attributable to muscle size and mass. In certain racial groups, specific muscles are absent altogether. The peroneus tertius muscle, which is found in the foot, and the palmaris longus muscle, which is found in the wrist, are absent in individuals in some racial groups. However, muscle absence in general does not appear to be more prevalent in any particular racial group, nor does absence of a particular muscle correspond with absence of another muscle.

Numerous studies have investigated inheritability of stature (Overfield, 1995). In general, the studies conclude that people vary in height as a result of race and that in the United States, African-Americans and White Americans are the tallest, American Indians are either similar in height or a few inches shorter than Mexican Americans, and Asian Americans are the shortest. Individuals of higher socioeconomic status in all ethnic groups are taller (Overfield, 1995). In regard to physical growth and developmental rates, African-Americans are generally advanced, whereas Orientals are generally retarded when these groups are compared with White norms.

Body Weight

It is a well-known fact that weight differs in individuals both by race and by gender. African-Americans and Whites are less similar in weight than they are in height. This is believed to occur because African-Americans have heavier bone and muscle mass than Whites (Greaves, Puhl, Baranowski, et al., 1989; Kuh, Power, & Rodgers, 1991; Laor, Seidman, & Danon, 1991; Ortiz, Russell, Daley, et al., 1992). On the average, African-American men weigh less than their White counterparts (166.1 compared to 170.6 pounds) (Najjar, 1987). In stark contrast, African-American women are consistently heavier at every age group than their White American counterparts (149.6 compared to 137.0 pounds). In addition, African-American women average about 20 pounds heavier than their White American counterparts from 35 to 65 years of age (Greaves, Puhl, Baranowski, et al., 1989; Haffner, Stern, Hazuda, et al., 1986). Similarly, Mexican American Whites, on the average, weigh more than non-Hispanic Whites as result of truncal fat (Greaves, Puhl, Baranowski, et al., 1989; Haffner, Stern, Hazuda, et al., 1986). On average, obesity is more pronounced in the lower class, less pronounced in the middle class compared with their lower-class counterparts, and even less pronounced in the upper class compared

with their middle-class counterparts (Garn, Sullivan, & Hawthorne, 1989).

Childhood Obesity.* If the health care statistics in Healthy People 2010 are dismal for African-American, Hispanic, and American Indian women and men, they are even worse for their children (U.S. Department of Health and Human Services, 2000). If being overweight is a common problem in the general U.S. population, it is said to be at epidemic proportions for children in this country (Strauss & Pollack, 2001). Data from the Youth Risk, Behavioral Surveillance (YRBS) 2003 survey indicated that the prevalence of overweight among children was higher among non-Hispanic Black (16.2%) and Hispanic children (16.4%) than non-Hispanic White children (10.4%), and higher among non-Hispanic black female (14.2%) and Hispanic female (11.5%) than White female 6.5%) students (Ogden et al., 2006). In a comparison of obesity rates in male students, the highest rate was in Hispanic (21.3%) and non-Hispanic Blacks (18.2%) than in Whites (14.0%). Nonetheless, childhood obesity continues to increase steadily and rapidly among African-American children (Strauss & Pollack, 2001). Some researchers conclude that childhood obesity often serves as a primary marker for high-risk dietary and physical inactivity practices (Crawford, Story, Wang, Ritchie, & Sabry, 2001). Childhood obesity can also contribute to the development of metabolic syndrome (syndrome X), also referred to as insulin resistance.

The Development of the Metabolic Syndrome (Syndrome X) from Childhood to Adolescence.* The metabolic syndrome (syndrome X) is a clustering of abnormalities characterized by the primary defect of compensatory insulin resistance, glucose intolerance, dyslipidemia, and centrally distributed obesity (Matthews, Hosker, Rudenski,

---

*Portions of the section on Childhood Adiposity and Metabolic Syndrome (Syndrome X) are excerpted with permission from a prior publication by Giger, J., Richardson, J., & Jones, D. (2002, July), African-American children: a precious commodity at risk. *Journal of the National Black Nurses Association* (editorial), 13(1), vii–viii.

et al., 1985). Chen, Bao, Begum, et al. (2000) conducted a study to examine the age-related patterns of cardiovascular risk factor clusters relative to metabolic syndrome (syndrome X) among African-American and White children. The clusters in this study for metabolic syndrome (syndrome X) included (1) insulin resistance index, (2) body mass index (BMI), (3) triglycerides:HDL cholesterol ratio, and (4) mean arterial pressure. Regardless of age, four mediating factors contribute to the development of coronary heart disease: hyperinsulinemia (metabolic syndrome [syndrome X]), hypercholesterolemia, hypertension, and obesity. A sedentary life-style, the large amount of fat consumed per day by some children (such as African-Americans), and the prevalence of obesity may all contribute to the development of metabolic syndrome (syndrome X). In other words, African-American, Hispanic, or American Indian children are not exempt because of their tender years from developing metabolic syndrome (syndrome X) and starting the downward spiral toward diabetes and ultimately coronary heart disease.

It is interesting to note that findings from the study of Chen, Bao, Begum, et al. (2000) suggest that overall, White children had a higher total of adverse clusters among the four indices measured (9.8; $P < 0.01$) than their African-American counterparts (7.4; $P < 0.01$). These follow-up findings to the Bogalusa Heart Study are interesting. Previous and recent analyses of these data sets suggest that while predictability of childhood adiposity and insulin resistance syndrome is difficult to determine with certainty in children, the contributions of these adverse clusters can provide convincing evidence for the future development of metabolic syndrome (syndrome X), thereby leading to the development of coronary heart disease in adulthood (Srinivasan, Myers, & Berenson, 2002). As African-Americans age, the adverse clusters outrank those of their White counterparts, and this ultimately leads to the development of metabolic syndrome (syndrome X) and coronary heart disease in adulthood (Giger, Richardson, & Jones, 2002). Srinivasan, Myers, and Berenson (2002) examined the contributions of childhood adiposity and

insulin as weighted predictors to adulthood risk of developing metabolic syndrome (syndrome X) among African-American and White children with baseline ages of 8 to 17 years. Using a logistic regression model, these researchers noted that childhood BMI and insulin resistance served as significant predictors of adult clustering for metabolic syndrome (syndrome X). In this study, BMI was the strongest indicator, exhibiting a curvilinear relationship. Further findings from this study also suggest that childhood obesity often is a powerful predictor of the development of metabolic syndrome (syndrome X) later in life. These findings suggest that children, and particularly ethnic minorities such as African-American children, can benefit tremendously from programs that underscore the importance of weight control and increased physical activity (Srinivasan, Myers, & Berenson, 2002). Nurses must rise to the challenge of helping these vulnerable families reduce the epidemic of childhood obesity among children. Strategies to reduce childhood obesity appear obvious but often are ignored by parents and even health care practitioners. These strategies include increasing the physical activity of vulnerable children, reducing the amount of television watched each day, and restricting the amount of fat consumed, particularly in nonefficacious foods (Davis, Northington, & Kolar, 2000). Lindquist, Reynolds, and Goran (1999) found that there are obvious sociocultural determinants of physical activity among children. Findings from this study suggest that while there is greater television viewing among children from single-parent homes, there is more vigorous exercise among these same children. This finding seems contradictory in terms of the amount of television watched. However, it is plausible to assume that in single-parent homes children are often responsible for themselves while the parent works. Although these children tend to watch more television, they also tend to engage in more outdoor activities because they do not have to seek permission to do so. Further findings from this study also suggest that there is less habitual physical activity among girls and less mandatory physical exercise among African-American children, particularly from single-parent homes (Lindquist, Reynolds, & Goran, 1999). There appears to be no plausible explanation for why some ethnic minority children such as African-American children engage in less physical exercise as mandated in many school systems. Nurses must rise to the clarion call of assisting parents and their children in developing an understanding about the importance of physical activity, proper dietary intake, and methods to increase the amount of fiber and fruits consumed per day. In addition, it is essential for nurses to underscore to parents the importance of limiting harmful activities, such as extensive television viewing.

Skin Color

When working with people from diverse cultural backgrounds, the nurse should understand how different races evolved in relation to the environment. Biological differences noted in skin color may be attributable to the biological adjustments a person's ancestors made in the environment in which they lived. For example, it has been scientifically postulated that the original skin color of humans was black (Overfield, 1977, 1995) and that white skin was the result of mutation and environmental pressures exerted on persons living in cold, cloudy northern Europe. The mutation is believed to have occurred because light skin was better able to synthesize vitamin D, particularly on cloudy days. It is believed that black skin became a neutral trait in climates where protection from the sun and heat of the tropics was not a factor (Overfield, 1977, 1995).

Skin color is probably the most significant biological variation in terms of nursing care. Nursing care delivery is based on accurate client assessment, and the darker the client's skin, the more difficult it becomes to assess changes in color. When caring for clients with highly pigmented skin, the nurse must first establish the baseline skin color, and daylight is the best light source for doing so. If possible, dark-skinned clients should always be given a bed by a window to provide access to sunlight. When daylight is not available to assess skin color, a lamp with at least a 60-watt bulb should be used. To establish the baseline skin color, the nurse must observe skin surfaces that have the least amount of pigmentation, which include the volar surfaces of the forearms, the palms of the hands, the soles of the feet, the abdomen, and the buttocks. When observing these areas, the nurse should look for an underlying red tone, which is typical of all skin, regardless of how dark its color. Absence of this red tone in a client may indicate pallor. Additional areas that are important to assess in dark-skinned clients include the mouth, the conjunctivae, and the nail beds. Generally speaking, the darkness of the oral mucosa correlates with the client's skin color. The darker the skin, the darker the mucosa; nevertheless, the mucosa is lighter than the skin.

The nurse must be aware that oral hyperpigmentation can occur on the tongue and the mucosa and can alter the value of the oral mucosa as a site for observation. The occurrence of oral hyperpigmentation is directly related to the darkness of a person's skin. Oral hyperpigmentation appears in 50% to 90% of African-Americans, compared with 10% to 50% of Whites. Another important consideration for the nurse is the appearance of a hard palate because it takes on a yellow discoloration, particularly in the presence of jaundice. The hard palate is frequently affected by hyperpigmentation in a manner similar to that of the oral mucosa and the tongue. The nurse should also assess the lips because they may be helpful in assessing skin-color changes (such as jaundice or cyanosis). It is important for the nurse to remember, however, that the lips of some Black people have a natural bluish hue (Rouch, 1977). Thus it is important for the nurse to have established the baseline color of the lips if they are to be of value in detecting cyanosis (Branch & Paxton, 1976).

It is also important for the nurse to establish the normal color of the conjunctivae when working with persons from transcultural populations. The conjunctivae will reflect the color changes of cyanosis or pallor and is a good site for observing petechiae. Another excellent source for determining the presence of jaundice is the sclera. The nurse should first establish a baseline color for the sclerae because the sclerae of dark-skinned persons often have a yellow coloration caused by subconjunctival fatty deposits. A common finding in persons with highly pigmented skin is the presence of melanin deposits or "freckles" on the sclerae.

The final area of assessment should be the nail beds, which are useful for detecting cyanosis or pallor. In dark-skinned persons, it is difficult to assess the nail beds because they may be highly pigmented, thick, or lined or contain melanin deposits. Regardless of color, for baseline assessment, it is important for the nurse to notice how quickly the color returns to the nail bed after pressure has been released from the free edge of the nail (Rouch, 1977). A slower return of color to the nail bed may indicate cyanosis or pallor. It is also difficult to detect rashes, inflammations, and ecchymoses in dark-skinned persons. It may be necessary to palpate rashes in dark-skinned persons because rashes may not be readily visible to the eye. When palpating the skin for rashes, the nurse should notice induration and warmth of the area.

Other Visible Physical Characteristics

In addition to looking for pallor and cyanosis, the nurse should note other aberrations in the skin. For example, mongolian spots may be present on the skin of African-American, Asian American, American Indian, or Mexican American newborns. Mongolian spots are bluish discolorations that vary tremendously in size and color and are often mistaken for bruises. Another aberration that is more common in African-Americans than in other racial groups is keloids. These ropelike scars represent an exaggeration of the wound-healing process and may result from any type of trauma, such as surgical incisions, ear piercing, or insertion of an intravenous catheter.

Enzymatic and Genetic Variations

The basic genetic makeup of an individual is determined from the moment of conception. Then, among other things, the upper limits of achievement are set; the "map," so to speak, is drawn. In other words, a person can be only what he or she is genetically determined to be. More specifically, growth and development cannot go beyond what the genes make possible. An individual will not grow 1 inch taller than the genetic structure allows, regardless of the amount of exercise or vitamins consumed. By the same token, an individual will be no more intelligent than genetic structure allows, despite the amount of tutoring or special schooling the individual receives (Burt, 1966; Lorton & Lorton, 1984).

In medical terms, a person's race represents his or her genetic makeup. Although race may be irrelevant in some situations, knowing the racial predisposition to a certain disease is often helpful in evaluating clients and diagnosing their illness, as well as in assessing risks (Divan, 1989). The genetic and enzymatic predisposition to certain diseases is discussed in this chapter under the heading "Susceptibility to Disease"; lactose intolerance and glucose-6-phosphate dehydrogenase deficiency are discussed under "Nutritional Deficiencies."

Genes are the working subunits of chemical information that carry a complete set of instructions for making the needed protein for a cell (Lewis, 2007). It is essential to remember that genes contain a particular set of instructions by way of coding for a particular protein (Collins, 1997). These coded instructions are known as deoxyribonucleic acid (DNA). DNA is composed of two long, paired strands that are spiraled into what is known as a *double helix* (Collins, 1997). Although there are only four different chemical bases in DNA—adenine, thymine, cytosine, and guanine—the order in which these bases occur determines specifically what information is available in a manner similar to the way in which the specific letters in the alphabet combine to form particular words and connect to form sentences (Collins, 1997). DNA itself resides in a core, or what is known as the *nucleus* of each of the cells in the body. In fact, every human cell, with the one notable exception of mature red blood cells, which have no nucleus, has the same DNA. All somatic cells have 46 molecules of double-stranded DNA. Likewise, each molecule consists of 50 to 250 million bases, which are housed in a chromosome (Collins, 1997).

There are several levels of genetic investigation, including molecular genetics and cytogenetics. *Molecular genetics* is the study of genes at a biochemical or cellular level (Lewis, 1997). A gene and its effects are often separable, and, as such, geneticists are able to distinguish the gene responsible for a trait or illness from the actual expression of a particular trait or illness (Lewis, 1997). For example, the genes themselves compose what is termed the *genotypes*, whereas the actual expression of these genes is called the *phenotype*. In contrast to molecular genetics, *cytogenetics* is the study of genes that involves matching phenotypes to chromosomal variants. As the twentieth century progressed, cytogenetics rapidly matured as geneticists built upon the mapping of all four chromosomes of the fruit fly. By 1950, the arduous task of mapping genes on the 22 pairs of autosomes was begun (Lewis, 1997). Today this process of sequencing a genetic map is known as the Human Genome Project (Collins, 1997). The purpose of the Human Genome Project was to identify the 3 billion–code letters of a representative human genome by the year 2005 (Collins, 1997). At the same time, geneticists were to identify the exact location of all genes on the sequencing map. Work relative to the 15-year international Human Genome Project was officially inaugurated in the United States on October 1, 1990. The U.S. project is currently jointly funded by the National Institutes of Health (through the National Center for Human Genome Research) and the Department of Energy (Collins, 1997). On April 14, 2003, work relative to the sequencing of the Human Genome Project was finally completed a full 2 years ahead of schedule.

Another area of genetic study is termed *population genetics*. Population genetics is the study of allele frequencies in populations (Lewis, 1997). Population genetics is extremely important because human beings tend to marry or mate with people primarily like themselves, that is, the same racial, ethnic, and cultural groups. Because of this there is a tendency for a frequency of certain alleles in that given population. For example, although 1 of 800 women in the general United States population are affected by the *BRCA1* breast cancer gene, this figure climbs dramatically to 1 of every 100 women among Ashkenazi Jews (Lewis, 1997).

Today the relative role that genetics plays in understanding the etiology of disease is becoming evident. It is important to remember that all diseases, except for trauma, have a genetic linkage. The earliest introduction to the concept of genetic inheritance comes from the nineteenth-century work of Gregor Mendel. Mendel's work involved the identification and breeding of a variety of pea plants (Overfield, 1995). From his work, Mendel noted that these pea plants had two different expressions of an inherited trait. For example, Mendel noted that when short plants were bred with short plants they were "true breeding," that is, giving rise to the production of only short plants. However, when tall plants were bred with short plants or another tall plant, the next generation resulted in only tall offspring. This phenomenon indicates that a gene can and does exist in alternative forms. In genetics, these alternative forms are called *alleles* (Lewis, 1997).

Ordinarily a gene is a stable entity, but over the course of time a gene can suffer a change in sequence (Lewis, 1997). This change is termed a *mutation*. The new form of the gene is inherited in a stable manner, as in the case of the previous form (Lewis, 1997). When a mutation occurs, the organism carrying the altered gene is called a *mutant*, whereas the organism that carries the normal, or unaltered, gene is called the wild type. The term *wild type* is used to describe either the genotype or the phenotype.

To understand how copies of a gene are transmitted, it is necessary to understand that the life cycle of an organism passes through a diploid phase and essentially has two copies of each gene. At conception, one of two copies is passed from the parent to a gamete (a germ cell, egg or sperm). At this point, the gamete contains one copy of each gene of the organism, and this is called the *haploid set*. Consequently, the alternative types of gametes produced by the parents unite to form what is called the *zygote* (the fertilized egg) (Lewis, 1997).

With a mutation, new alleles arise. Generally, when a mutation occurs, the particular frequency is represented by only one copy among all the copies of that particular gene in the population (Thompson, McInnes, & Willard, 1991). The probability that a new mutation will survive from one generation to the next is largely dependent on both chance and natural selection. From one generation to the next, depending on chance, allele frequencies fluctuate (Thompson, McInnes, & Willard, 1991). This entire phenomenon is termed *genetic drift*.

When an individual has two identical alleles for a gene, this individual is said to be *homozygous* for that gene. Similarly, an individual with two different alleles is *heterozygous*. In other words, a person inherits essentially one allele from each parent. These alleles can be the same or different. Therefore, at any locus on a chromosome pair, there is a gene composed of two alleles. For example, the blood types A, B, and O are the alleles for the ABO blood type locus (Overfield, 1995). If there is only one allele at a particular locus, then the gene is said to be *monomorphic*. In contrast, when there are multiple alleles at a particular gene locus, the gene is said to be *polymorphic* (Overfield, 1995). An excellent example of this concept is found in the enzyme deficiency disorder glucose-6-phosphate dehydrogenase (G-6-PD) deficiency, which is said to be caused by the most polymorphic genes known, with more than 320 alleles (Luzzato, 1986).

In Mendel's classic work, he noted that each of the genes identified had two alleles, which is suggestive of two obvious expressions. A gene may have many alleles (variants) as a result of changes in any of the hundreds or thousands of DNA base pairs that make up a gene. However, because the concept of DNA and DNA sequencing had not yet been identified, Mendel was able to detect a gene variant only if the phenotype was altered. For example, if a green pea produced a yellow pea, this phenomenon would be a phenotypic alteration (Lewis, 1997). As Mendel continued his work, he noted that in some instances one gene could mask the expression of another. In this case, the gene that masks the expression of the other is considered to be completely *dominant*, whereas the mask allele is considered to be *recessive*. An excellent example of this concept was noted when Mendel crossed a "true-breeding" tall plant with a short plant. In this case, the tall plant (or the tall allele) was completely dominant to the short plant (short allele), and thus all the plants in the next generation were tall (Lewis, 1997; Overfield, 1995).

An inherited trait is said therefore to be either dominant or recessive. Whether this trait is dominant or recessive depends on the particular nature of the phenotype. Often the heterozygote, on a biochemical level, is actually intermediate, or a mixture of the homozygous dominant and homozygous recessive, though the heterozygote and the homozygous-dominant genotypes are indistinguishable (Lewis, 1997; Overfield, 1995). For example, in the case of Tay-Sachs, a genetically inherited disease commonly found among Jews, the heterozygote (with one dominant and one recessive allele) actually produces half the normal amount of the enzyme that the gene encodes, yet this amount appears to be sufficient for normal function, and so that person remains as healthy as a person with two dominant alleles. A phenotypic (disease itself) expression of the gene would occur only if a person inherited two recessive alleles.

How a person inherits a particular gene depends on two basic characteristics: (1) the dominant or recessive nature of the allele and (2) the type of chromosome that the gene in question is part of (Lewis, 1997). If a person has dominant alleles—that is, has only one copy of the gene—this dominant allele can affect the phenotype. In contrast, a person who has a recessive allele must have two copies of the gene if the phenotype is to be expressed. For example, the cancer-predisposing alleles *BRCA1* and *BRCA2* are dominant. Therefore, an individual would need to inherit one copy of the gene from one parent to have a 1 in 2 chance of developing the disease. The second mode of inheritance depends on the chromosome location that the particular gene is a part of. For example, human beings have 46 chromosomes, including two that determine sex—X and Y (sex chromosomes). The presence or absence of a single gene on the Y chromosome is responsible for determining sex. The remaining chromosomes are termed *non-sex chromosomes*, or *autosomes*. Specifically, a female has 44 autosomes and two X chromosomes. In contrast, a male has 44 autosomes and one X and one Y chromosome. In other words, there are actually 23 pairs of chromosomes consisting of 22 pairs of autosomes, and one pair of X and Y chromosomes (Harper, 1993, Lewis, 1997). Because there is a difference in sex chromosome constitution, it is believed that genes on the sex chromosomes follow different, sex-linked, patterns of inheritances in the two sexes. In the case of X-linked dominant inheritance, it is essential to remember that male-to-male transmission never occurs because men cannot pass their X chromosomes to their sons. In addition, all daughters of an affected male with an X-linked gene will actually receive the gene either in a recessive or a dominant form (Harper, 1993). For example, if the father passes an X-linked recessive gene to his daughter, the daughter will be a carrier. However, if the father passes an X-linked dominant gene to his daughter, the daughter will be affected (Harper, 1993). Thus, modes of inheritance of a particular trait can depend on the recessive and dominant characteristics of the allele or on whether the gene is located on the sex chromosome or on an autosomal chromosome (Saito, Okui, Tokino, et al., 1992).

To understand the significance of genetics, it is essential to develop an awareness of the relative role of single Mendelian traits in humans. Single Mendelian traits in humans are associated with disorders or traits linked to a single gene. For example, the most prevalent Mendelian disorders are believed to be cystic fibrosis, Tay-Sachs disease, and Duchenne muscular dystrophy (Lewis, 1997). Yet, although these Mendelian traits are considered prevalent, they are extremely rare, affecting 1 in 10,000 or fewer births (Lewis, 1997). Today, about 2500 Mendelian disorders are known, and some 2500 other identifiable conditions are suspected to be Mendelian related because of their recurrence patterns in large families (Lewis, 1997).

Some disease cannot be explained by the single-gene Mendelian-trait theory. Although every individual has two alleles for any autosomal gene (one allele for each chromosome), a gene can exist in a given population in more than two allelic forms (Lewis, 1997). This different allele combination often leads to variations in phenotype (Harper, 1993; Lewis, 1997). In addition, there is a difference in the dominance relationship of an allele. For example, as previously indicated, in the case of complete dominance, one allele is expressed, and the other is not. However, in some instances, some genes demonstrate what is termed *incomplete dominance*, which occurs when the heterozygous phenotype is intermediate between that of either homozygote (Harper, 1993; Lewis, 1997). For example, in the case of familial hypercholesterolemia, an individual with two disease-causing alleles actually lacks the liver receptors that take up cholesterol from the bloodstream (Lewis, 1997). In this case, the phenotype will actually parallel the number of receptors. Individuals with one mutant allele die in young adulthood, and those with two of the wild type (the most common expression of a particular gene in a given population) do not develop this inherited form of heart disease (Lewis, 1997).

Understanding genetics and its transcultural and racial implications is of paramount importance. Understanding race and the genetic implications is also important. There are scientists who recognize only Black, White, and Asians/American Indians as racial groups (Brues, 1977; Overfield, 1995; Polednak, 1971). Asians and American Indians are often placed by these scientists in one major group because of some genetic similarities (Brues, 1977; Overfield, 1995). *Race* is an important term because races of people are not static. What is implied by this is that all races have evolved over time as a direct response to environmental stimuli. Thus the characteristics that define a race will not necessarily define any specific individual from that particular race of people (Overfield, 1995). For example, the Yupik Eskimos are said to have a 75% gene frequency of M in the MN blood system and 61% in the O, 25% in the A, and 16% in the B within the ABO blood groups (Overfield, 1995). These same individuals are believed to have no prevalence for Rh-negative blood (Overfield, 1995). A health care professional working with this group of people might assume incorrectly that therefore the most common array of traits for the Yupiks would be blood types M and O and that these individuals would be invariably Rh positive. Although some Yupiks might actually display this array of traits, it must be remembered that because of genetic heterogeneity, some individual Yupiks might differ (Overfield, 1995).

It has been reported that the incidence of dizygotic twinning is highest in African-Americans, occurring in 4% of births. Dizygote twinning occurs in approximately 2% of births in Whites and in 0.5% of births in Asians (Bulmer, 1970; Giger, Davidhizar, & Wieczorek, 1993).

Some research interpretations (Jensen, 1969, 1974, 1977) have indicated that the small but persistent differences between the average intelligence quotients (IQs) of African-American children and those of White children reflect a genetic difference. Jensen (1969) claimed to have controlled for variables, including income and education. He reported that he found a difference in IQ that he believed to indicate a genetic difference. Others have refuted Jensen's claim (Kamlin, 1974). In 1977 Jensen conducted a study of children between 5 and 16 years of age in the rural South indicating that the IQs of African-American children, but not those of White children, drop substantially as they grow older. Jensen believed that this contrast between African-Americans and Whites possibly meant that the decrement in IQ was genetically determined. This has not been supported by others' research.

Drug Interactions and Metabolism

Reactions to drugs vary with race. Some evidence indicates that drugs are metabolized by different races in different ways and at different rates (Echizen, Horai, & Ishizaki, 1989; Weber, 1999). For example, Zhou, Koshakji, Silberstein, et al. (1989) demonstrated that Chinese subjects are more sensitive to the cardiovascular effects of propranolol than White subjects are. In the body there are three classes of reactions to foreign chemicals or drugs: hydrolysis, conjugation, and oxidation (Kalow, 1982, 1986, 1989; Weber, 1999). The following are examples of reactions to specific drugs.

Isoniazid is a drug commonly used to treat tuberculosis. People metabolize this drug in one of two ways: they inactivate it very slowly or very rapidly. Those who inactivate this drug very slowly are at risk for developing peripheral neuropathy during therapy (Vessell, 1972). Rapid inactivation of this drug occurs in 40% of Whites, 60% of African-Americans, 60% to 90% of American Indians and Eskimos, and 85% to 90% of Orientals (Vessell, 1972). Pyridoxine is given with isoniazid, and the doses are spaced at larger intervals for slower reaction during treatment for tuberculosis. Primaquine is metabolized by oxidation and is used to treat malaria. When this drug is given to individuals who lack the enzymes necessary for glucose metabolism of the red blood cells, hemolysis of the red blood cells occurs. Approximately 100 million people in the world are affected by this particular enzyme deficiency and thus are unable to ingest primaquine. Approximately 35% of African-Americans have this particular enzyme deficiency.

Succinylcholine is a muscle relaxant used during surgery. It is inactivated by hydrolysis by the enzyme pseudocholinesterase. In most individuals it is rapidly inactivated, but some individuals have the atypical form of the enzyme and suffer prolonged muscle paralysis and an inability to breathe after administration of the drug. African-Americans, Asians, and American Indians are at risk for having pseudocholinesterase deficiency; Whites have a slightly higher risk than these groups. Some Jews and Alaskan Eskimos have a considerably greater risk: 1 of 135 Alaskan Eskimos cannot metabolize the drug succinylcholine normally (Kalow, 1982, 1986, 1989; Vessell, 1972).

Alcohol is metabolized differently, depending on race. There are two enzymes involved in the metabolism of alcohol: alcohol dehydrogenase (ADH) and acetaldehyde dehydrogenase (ALDH). Alcohol metabolism is a two-step process: ADH converts alcohol to acetaldehyde, and acetaldehyde ALDH converts acetaldehyde (a toxic substance) to acetic acid (a nontoxic substance). Both of these enzymes have more than one variant. ADH has a high-activity type, which converts alcohol to acetaldehyde rapidly, and a low-activity variant, which converts it slowly (Kalow, 1972, 1986; Weber, 1999). ALDH has four variants (ALDH-1 through 4). ALDH-1 is considered "normal"; other types are less efficient in their ability to metabolize acetaldehyde (Goedde, 1983, 1986).

In Whites with "normal" levels of both ADH and ALDH-1, alcohol is metabolized fairly efficiently. In contrast, American Indians and Asians have an excessive level of high-activity ADH and a low level of ALDH-1. Consequently, persons in these groups metabolize alcohol to acetaldehyde rapidly. However, the metabolism to acetic acid is delayed. Because acetaldehyde is toxic and acetic acid is not, the net result is unpleasant effects, such as facial flushing and palpitations (Keltner, 1994; Kudzma, 1992). Data from some studies indicate that American Indians and Asians experience noticeable facial flushing and other vasomotor symptoms after ingesting alcohol; in contrast, Whites and African-Americans experience less severe reactions. Facial flushing after ingestion of alcohol occurs in 45% to 85% of Asians versus 3% to 29% of Whites (Chan, 1986).

In regard to alcohol use, recent data suggest that Hispanic Americans and Black Americans are also at an increased risk for death from liver cirrhosis. While the reasons for this remain largely unknown, one study compared racial and ethnic aspartate aminotransferase and gamma-glutamyltransferase level elevations among these individuals who drank (Stewart, 2002). Findings from this study suggest that among current drinkers, Black and Mexican Americans were more likely to have a twofold elevation of aspartate aminotransferase level than their White counterparts. These elevated levels were even more pronounced among those who drank more frequently (Mexican American: odds ratio, 9.1 [95% confidence interval, 3.9–21.0]; Black Americans: odds ratio, 3.1 [95% confidence interval, 1.4–6.8]) than among those who drank less frequently or were abstainers (Stewart, 2002).

Caffeine, a component of many drugs as well as coffee, tea, and colas, appears to be metabolized and excreted faster by Whites than by Asians (Grant, Tang, & Kalow, 1983). It is thought that the differences noted in caffeine metabolism are directly correlated with liver enzyme differences (Kudzma, 1992).

Antihypertensives are another category of drugs that is metabolized differently depending on race. Several studies suggest that there are notable differences between African-Americans and their White counterparts in the metabolism of antihypertensive drugs (Freis, 1986; Moser & Lunn, 1982; Zhou, Koshakji, Silberstein, et al., 1989). Freis (1986) noted that African-Americans tend to need higher doses of beta-adrenergic receptor–blocking agents such as propranolol (Inderal). In contrast, Moser and Lunn (1982) found that angiotensin-converting enzyme inhibitors (such as captopril) tend to be less effective as a single therapy for African-Americans than for Whites with the same treatment regimen. Zhou, Koshakji, Silberstein, et al. (1989) noted that even when body surface area and body weight were considered, Chinese men tend to need only about half as much propranolol as White American men.

Psychotropic drugs are also metabolized differently depending on race. When blood plasma levels of alprazolam (Xanax) were studied in 42 healthy men (14 American-born Asians, 14 foreign-born Asians, and 14 Whites), the Asian clients needed smaller doses to achieve the same blood plasma levels as their White counterparts (Lin, Lau, Smith, et al., 1988). Body heights and weights were not a factor in the study results. Nonetheless, in both Asian groups (American-born and foreign-born), the drug remained in the blood longer (Lin, Lau, Smith, et al., 1988). It is important for the nurse to remember that certain psychotropic drugs can cause higher blood levels in certain individuals by virtue of race (such as Asian Americans). It is essential to modify the dosage of these drugs based not only on body surface area and weight but also on racial considerations.

Lawson (1986) noted that third-world clients are routinely given smaller doses of neuroleptics because some racial groups metabolize drugs more slowly and therefore experience a greater drug effect. For neuroleptic medications, these same variations by race are found in the United States.

In a prospective study of tardive dyskinesia, Glazer, Morgenstern, and Doucette (1993) found that among psychiatric outpatients treated with neuroleptic medications, race was a probable factor for this iatrogenic movement disorder. The data indicated that non-White clients, 97% of whom were African-American, were about twice as likely to develop tardive dyskinesia as their White counterparts. To ensure the accuracy of the results, the researchers controlled for other demographic and clinical risk factors.

In a follow-up study, Glazer, Morgenstern, and Doucette (1994) found that, compared with Whites, non-Whites were younger, less skilled, more likely to be unmarried, and more likely to have a diagnosis of schizophrenia. Non-Whites were also more likely to receive higher doses of neuroleptics, principally because they were frequently given more high-potency depot medications. Despite the control for known tardive dyskinesia factors, the estimated rate of tardive dyskinesia was nearly twice as high for non-Whites as for Whites. According to Glazer, Morgenstern, Doucette, et al. (1994), none of the other demographic, clinical, psychosocial, or general health variables measured in the study appeared to explain the association between race and the propensity for tardive dyskinesia. The correlation between race as biological marker and the development of tardive dyskinesia remains unclear (Glazer, Morgenstern, Doucette, et al., 1994). Habits such as drinking and smoking are known to speed drug metabolism, and thus the fact that some Whites and African-Americans drink significantly more alcohol than some Asian Americans is an important consideration.

Lefley (1990) contends that African-American clients are significantly misdiagnosed as psychotic. Because they are viewed as more violent, they receive more medication and spend more time in seclusion than Whites, Hispanics, or Asians (Lefley, 1990). The higher dose of medication prescribed for African-Americans may result more from staff perception than from a decision based on serum levels and careful observation (Keltner & Folks, 1992).

Gender is another cultural consideration that may have a profound effect on the metabolism of drugs. Yonkers, Kando, Cole, and Blumenthal (1992) suggest that women have the potential for higher blood plasma levels of psychotropic drugs, especially when used with oral contraceptives. In addition, they note that women have greater efficacy of antipsychotic agents and a greater likelihood of adverse reactions, such as hypothyroidism and, in older women, tardive dyskinesia. Although plausible explanations for these differences have been offered, women have traditionally been excluded from clinical trials measuring the efficacy and metabolism of certain drugs.

Electrocardiographic Patterns

A common finding in African-Americans, particularly in African-American men, is the occurrence of inverted T waves in the precordial leads of the electrocardiogram. This aberration is a normal variant in the African-American population but would indicate a pathological condition if found in other racial groups, such as Whites.

Susceptibility to Disease

Another category of differences between racial groups is susceptibility to disease. The increased or decreased incidence of a particular disease may be genetically determined.

Tuberculosis. Historically, some American Indians have had a tuberculosis incidence that is 7 to 15 times that of non-Indians, whereas African-Americans have had a tuberculosis incidence 3 times higher than that of White Americans (Williams, 1975). Urban American Jews have been the most resistant to tuberculosis (Overfield, 1977, 1995). The increased susceptibility of African-Americans to tuberculosis may be a result of their tendency toward overgrowth of connective tissue components concerned with protection against infection because tuberculosis is a granulomatous infection (Polednak, 1971).

At the turn of the twentieth century, tuberculosis was the leading cause of death in the United States. It remained the leading cause of death until the introduction of antituberculosis drug therapy in the 1940s and early 1950s (Phipps, 1993). The case rates for tuberculosis steadily declined from 83,304 reported cases in 1953 to 22,225 reported cases in 1984 (Centers for Disease Control and Prevention [CDC], 1991). Since 1986, there has been a resurgence in the number of reported cases of tuberculosis in the United States (CDC, Tuberculosis Surveillance Report, 2001). The number of reported cases of tuberculosis has steadily increased from 3.0% in 1986 to 7.0% in 1996. Between 1985 and 2001, the highest reported case rates occurred in Miami, Atlanta, San Francisco, Tampa, Newark, and New York City (CDC, Tuberculosis Surveillance Report, 2001). It is postulated that these cities and their states have higher case rates than other cities have because their states also report the highest number of human immunodeficiency virus (HIV)–positive persons, particularly among intravenous drug abusers. In addition, these states have a larger influx of immigrants from countries in which tuberculosis is endemic (CDC, HIV/AIDS Surveillance Report, 2001).

Many persons with HIV infection have organisms that are resistant to most of the chemotherapeutic agents used to treat this type of tuberculosis. When an individual has drug-resistant tuberculosis, he or she may pass the resistant organisms to others. In such cases, effective treatment of this type of tuberculosis becomes nearly impossible (Phipps, 1993).

The number of reported cases of tuberculosis among certain racial groups has changed dramatically over the last several years. For example, in 1988, the incidence of tuberculosis was 7 times higher among African-Americans than among non-Hispanic Whites, 9 times higher among Asians and Pacific Islanders, and 4 times higher among American Indians and Hispanics (CDC, Tuberculosis Surveillance Report, 2001). Ethnic minorities now account for more than two thirds of all the reported cases of tuberculosis in the United States, partly as a result of the increased incidence of tuberculosis among ethnic minorities infected with HIV (CDC, Tuberculosis Surveillance Report, 2001). For example, in 2001, the states reporting the most cases of tuberculosis included (1) California (3332 cases, of which 365 were in Whites, 292 were in Blacks, 1253 were in Hispanics, 15 were in American Indians, and 1400 were in Asians or Pacific Islanders), (2) Florida (1145 cases, of which 289 were in Whites, 533 were in Blacks, 239 were in Hispanics, 2 were in American Indians, and 82 were in Asians or Pacific Islanders), (3) New York (1676 cases, of which 225 were in Whites, 527 were in Blacks, 490 were in Hispanics, 1 was in an American Indian, and 428 were in Asians or Pacific Islanders), and (4) Texas (1643 cases, of which 270 were in Whites, 417 were in Blacks, 780 were in Hispanics, 5 were in American Indians, and 171 were in Asians or Pacific Islanders) (CDC, Tuberculosis Surveillance Report, 2001). It is also interesting to note that of the cases of tuberculosis reported for children, ethnic minorities account for nearly 83% (CDC, Tuberculosis Surveillance Report, 2001).

It is important to remember that susceptibility to disease may also be environmental or a combination of both genetic and environmental factors. The evidence indicates that tuberculosis can occur in response to both socioenvironmental and psychological stress factors. In a classic study of clients in Seattle, Holmes et al. (1957) found that environmental factors appeared to be relevant in relation to the onset of tuberculosis. In this classic study, data in the life experiences of each client were plotted for a 12-year period preceding hospitalization. Analysis of the data revealed that in the majority of clients, there was a gradual increase in experiences that were perceived by the individual as significant and stressful. The combination of stressful life experiences and personal perception resulted in a psychological crisis situation that was evidenced in the 2-year period preceding hospitalization. Further analysis of the data indicated that clients who are poorly equipped to deal with social relationships, especially when a lot of tension is present, may be at risk for tuberculosis.

Blood Groups, Rh Factor, and Disease. Blood groups also differentiate people in certain racial groups. A prevalence for type O blood has been found among American Indians, with some incidence of type A blood and virtually no incidence of type B blood. Almost equal incidences of types A, B, and O blood are found in Japanese and Chinese people, with the AB blood type found in only about 10% of the Japanese and Chinese population. African-Americans and Whites have been found to have equal incidences of A, B, and O blood types. The predominant blood types of African-Americans and Whites are A and O, with fewer incidences of AB and B types (Jick, Slone, Westerhom, et al., 1969; Overfield, 1995).

Statistically, persons with type O blood are at a greater risk for duodenal ulcers, whereas persons with type A blood are more likely to develop cancer of the stomach. In addition, there is some evidence that women with type O blood have a diminished chance of getting thromboembolitic disease, particularly when taking birth control pills, in comparison with women with other ABO blood types (Jick, Slone, Westerhom, et al., 1969; Overfield, 1995).

The Rh-negative factor in blood is most common in Whites, much rarer in other racial groups, and apparently absent in Eskimos (Lewis, 1942). Because there are at least 27 different antigens in the Rh system, this system is complex and difficult to understand. Of clinical significance is the D antigen because it is more immunogenic than any other Rh antigen and is usually the antigen involved in hemolytic disease of the newborn. When antigen D is present, the term *Rh positive* is used. Approximately 85% of persons in the world have Rh-positive blood. The term *Rh negative* is used when antigen D is absent. Persons with the Rh-negative factor who are exposed to Rh-positive blood form Rh antibodies. After continued exposure to Rh-positive blood, the Rh antibody will bind to corresponding antigens on the surface of red blood cells, which contain the Rh antigen. Ordinarily, Rh antibodies do not fix complement. As a result, there is no immediate hemolysis, such as that occurring with ABO incompatibility. Rather, Rh-antigen red blood cells are broken down rapidly by macrophages in the spleen, resulting in a conversion of hemoglobin to bilirubin, which causes jaundice. Thus the multigravida woman with Rh-negative factor who has a Rh-positive mate and has either delivered or aborted a Rh-positive infant will be more likely to have babies who are susceptible to jaundice. This condition can be prevented in subsequent pregnancies if the Rh-negative woman is given RhoGAM immediately after aborting or delivering an Rh-positive infant.

Diabetes. Other conditions that appear to have biocultural or racial prevalence include diabetes mellitus, hypertension, sickle cell anemia, and systemic lupus erythematosus (SLE). Reportedly there is a high incidence of diabetes mellitus in certain American Indian tribes, including the Seminole, Pima, and Papago. However, diabetes is believed to be quite rare among Alaskan Eskimos (Westfall, 1971). Diabetes mellitus is a major health problem in the United States, with an incidence of more than 11.1 million diagnosed cases and more than 5.9 million undiagnosed cases, which accounts for more than 6.2% of the total population in the United States (American Diabetic Association,

2005; CDC, Diabetes Surveillance Report, 2002). Each year more than 800,000 new cases of diabetes are reported in the United States (American Diabetic Association, 2005; CDC, Diabetes Surveillance Report, 2005). In fact, the incidence of diabetes mellitus is so widespread that it is postulated that for every person with diagnosed diabetes, there is another person who remains undiagnosed (Carter Center of Emory University, 1985).

Diabetes is so prevalent in the United States population that it was the seventh leading cause of death in the United States in 2001 (American Diabetic Association, 2005; CDC, Diabetes Surveillance Report, 2005; U.S. Department of Health and Human Services, 2005). Diabetes was reported as the underlying cause for more than 40,000 deaths and a contributory factor in approximately 160,000 other deaths (U.S. Department of Health and Human Services, 2006). Diabetes is so prevalent in U.S. society that it is estimated that some 7.8% (11.4 million) of all non-Hispanic Whites have diabetes, as well as 13.0% (2.8 million) of Blacks and 10.2% (2 million) of Hispanics.

By proportion of the population, American Indians have a disproportionately high incidence of diabetes at 15.1% of their population (105,000), and Alaska Natives have the lowest percentage with diabetes (5.3%). By geographical region, American Indians residing in the Southeastern United States have the greatest incidence of diabetes at 25.7% (American Diabetic Association, 2005). By race, diabetes is ranked as the seventh leading cause of death in the United States among Whites, Blacks, Chinese, and Filipinos. Women in the general U.S. population have a higher mortality associated with diabetes than do their male counterparts. In 2004, the age-adjusted death rate for diabetes by race was as follows: Whites, 22.8; Blacks, 50.1; American Indians or Alaska Natives, 50.3; Asians or Pacific Islanders, 18.4; and Hispanics, 33.6 (U.S. Department of Health and Human Services, Health United States, 2006).

It is important to note that the prevalence of diabetes varies according to race and gender. It increases with age and at all ages is highest among African-American women. In 1999, the prevalence of diabetes for African-American women (50.9 per

1000) was twice as high as the rate for their White counterparts (23.4 per 1000) (Mirsa, 2002).

While the Institute of Medicine's report *Unequal Treatment* (Smedley, Stith, & Nelson, 2003) suggests that ethnic minorities sometimes receive unequal treatment with regard to health care, the report is further illuminating with regard to care for diabetes. Although Blacks, Hispanics, and American Indians have a 50% to 100% higher burden of illness and mortality due to diabetes than their White counterparts, the disease appears to be more profoundly undermanaged among these vulnerable populations. Chin, Zhang, and Merrell (1998) noted that even after adjustment for gender, education, and age, African-Americans were still less likely to undergo measurements of glycosylated hemoglobin, lipid testing, ophthalmologic visits, and influenza vaccinations than their White counterparts. It is even more interesting to note that Blacks with type 2 diabetes are more likely to be treated with insulin as opposed to an oral antihyperglycemic agent than their White or Mexican counterparts (Cowie & Harris, 1997).

There are three types of diabetes: type 1 (formerly referred to as insulin-dependent) diabetes mellitus, type 2 (formerly referred to as non–insulin-dependent diabetes), and gestational diabetes mellitus. Type 1 diabetes has a peak incidence between 10 and 14 years of age, apparently affects boys somewhat more frequently than girls, has a higher incidence in Whites, and accounts for 10% to 20% of cases (Krolewski & Warram, 2005). The incidence of type 2 diabetes dramatically increases with age, is more frequent in women, has a higher incidence in non-White persons (particularly Hispanics and American Indians), and accounts for 80% to 90% of cases (Carter Center, 1985). Gestational diabetes has been reported in 20% of all pregnant women, increases with maternal age, but is not affected by race or culture (Rifkin, 1984).

Hypertension. The incidence of hypertension has been reported to be significantly higher in African-Americans than in White Americans. The onset by age is earlier in African-Americans, and the hypertension is more severe and is associated with a higher mortality in African-Americans. Studies that demonstrated obvious differences in blood pressure between African-Americans and their White counterparts date back to 1932 (Adams, 1932). Since that time, other studies have also clearly indicated a remarkable difference in blood pressure between African-Americans and individuals of other races (Lerner & Kannel, 1986; Stokes, Kannel, Wolf, et al., 1987).

In 1972, the National High Blood Pressure Education Program (NHBPEP), in concert with the National Heart, Lung, and Blood Institute (NHLBI) of the National Institutes of Health, was implemented (Joint National Committee, 1997). Up to now, this program has succeeded in its original mission of increasing awareness, prevention, and treatment of hypertension. The trends in awareness, treatment, and control of hypertension have been positive among U.S. adults from 1976 to 1994 (Burt, Cutler, Higgins, et al., 1995). Data from the Third National Health and Nutrition Examination Survey (NHANES III) (1991–1994) indicate a level of adult public awareness of hypertension that was 68.4% of the total population. Similarly, knowledge of the adult U.S. population regarding treatment of hypertension has increased from 31% (NHANES II, 1976–1980) to 53.6%. Likewise, knowledge of adults in the general U.S. population regarding control of hypertension in that population increased from 10% (NHANES II, 1976–1980) to 27.4% (NHANES III, 1991–1994) (Burt, Cutler, Higgins, et al., 1995).

For many years, it has been postulated that 35% of African-Americans older than 40 years of age are hypertensive (Tipton, 1974). In a study with a random sample of adults 18 to 79 years of age, 9% of non-Blacks and 22% of African-Americans were found to be hypertensive, according to standards set by the World Health Organization, wherein a diastolic blood pressure of 95 mm Hg or greater indicates hypertension (Boyle, 1970). In another study done by the Chicago Health Association, the analysis of the data confirmed previous findings of a higher prevalence of hypertension among African-Americans in all age groups than among White Americans. Further analysis of the data indicated an equal prevalence of hypertension among both sexes in African-Americans and an increased incidence with advancing age (Merck, Sharp, & Dohme, 1974).

However, contrasting opinions indicate that hypertension may occur slightly more often in men than in women (Joint National Committee, 2003).

Data from the 30-year follow-up study to the classic Framingham study indicate that hypertension may be an independent risk factor for coronary heart disease for both men and women between 35 and 64 years of age (Stokes, Kannel, Wolf, et al., 1987). Other data indicate that the prevalence of hypertension may be highest among Black, non-Hispanic women (National Center for Health Statistics, 2006). In the Maryland Statewide Household Survey of 6425 adults 18 years of age and older, 28.2% of the African-American population showed a prevalence of mild to moderate hypertension (a systolic blood pressure greater than 160 mm Hg and a diastolic blood pressure greater than 95 mm Hg) compared with 20.1% of their White counterparts (Saunders, 1985; *State of Maryland Demonstration*, 1977–1983).

Because the traditional terms *mild hypertension* and *moderate hypertension* failed to convey the major influence of high blood pressure as a risk factor for cardiovascular disease (CVD), the Joint National Committee on Detection, Evaluation, and Treatment of High Blood Pressure (2003) attempted to clarify terminology. According to the committee's report, 50 million Americans have elevated blood pressure, which by current definition implies a systolic blood pressure of 140 mm Hg or greater, a diastolic blood pressure of 90 mm Hg or greater, or both (Joint National Committee, 2003). However, the Joint National Committee (2003) also added new guidelines for prehypertensive status that were absent in prior reports. As of May 2003, the new guidelines state that an individual may be considered prehypertensive if the systolic blood pressure is 120–139 mm Hg or the diastolic blood pressure is 80–89 mm Hg. Treatment of prehypertension depends on compelling indications. If there are no compelling indications, the Joint National Committee (2003) suggests no antihypertensive drugs. However, in case of compelling indications, including heart failure, post–myocardial infarction, high risk for coronary heart disease, diabetes, chronic kidney disease, and recurrent stroke prevention, the Joint National Committee suggests that drugs to control these compelling indications should also be considered. The committee concluded that the prevalence of hypertension increases with age, is greater in African-Americans than in Whites, is greater in both races in less educated individuals than in more educated individuals, and is especially prevalent and devastating in lower socioeconomic groups (Joint National Committee, 2003). In addition, the data indicate that in young adulthood and early middle-age, prevalence of high blood pressure is greater in men than in women. However, after middle age the reverse is true (Joint National Committee, 2003; Roccella & Lenfant, 1989). The Seventh Joint National Committee (2003) had been delayed until after the results of the Antihypertensive and Lipid Lowering Treatment to Prevent Heart Attack Trial (ALLHAT) were released; these data were incorporated into the Committee's seventh report (Czlraky, 2002).

On December 18, 2003, the much-anticipated results of ALLHAT were finally released. In this clinical trial, more than 40,000 subjects were enrolled. The primary objective of this study was to compare a diuretic (chlorthalidone), an angiotensin-converting enzyme inhibitor (lisinopril), a calcium-channel blocker (amlodipine), and alpha-blocker (doxazosin). The findings from this study suggest that thiazide diuretics may now be the initial drug of choice for hypertension, primarily because of their benefits in preventing coronary heart disease and their associated low costs (ALLHAT Officers, 2002a, 2002b). In addition, for patients who are already receiving antihypertensives, findings from ALLHAT suggest that diuretics should be considered concomitantly. Moreover, most clients who have hypertension, particularly African-Americans, will require more than one drug to control blood pressure adequately.

The prevalence for hypertension is also greater by geographical region. For example, both African-Americans and Whites residing in the southeastern United States have a greater propensity for hypertension and a greater rate of stroke-related death as a direct result of the condition than do African-Americans and Whites residing in other areas of the country (Roccella & Lenfant, 1989). The new classifications for hypertension as proposed by the Joint National Committee (2003) are shown in Box 7-1. As indicated previously, a diagnosis of hypertension is confirmed when systolic blood pressure is consistently 140 mm Hg or greater and diastolic blood pressure is consistently 90 mm Hg or greater (based on the average of two or more readings). Reportedly, as a result of this definition, hypertension is of concern for approximately 50 to 60 million Americans (Joint National Committee, 2003; Walsh, 1993). It is essential to remember that hypertension should never be diagnosed on the basis of a single measurement except when the systolic blood pressure is 210 mm Hg or greater and the diastolic blood pressure is 120 mm Hg, with average levels of diastolic blood pressure of 90 mm Hg or greater and systolic blood pressure levels of 140 mm Hg or greater (Joint National Committee, 2003).

Many individuals who are hypertensive remain symptom-free for a long time; thus, researchers at the National Heart, Lung, and Blood Institute have estimated that more than 50% of persons with hypertension do not know that they are hypertensive. Hypertension continues to be the major cause of heart failure, kidney failure, aneurysm formation, and congestive heart failure. Primary hypertension is evidenced in 90% of reported cases, whereas only about 10% of reported cases are classified as secondary. The diagnosis for primary hypertension may be supported when the following risk factors are present:
1. Positive family history
2. Increased sensitivity to the renin-angiotensin system

Box 7-1

CLASSIFICATIONS OF HYPERTENSION*

Classification for Blood Pressure	SBP, mm Hg (Treatment Determined by Highest Blood Pressure Category)	DBP, mm Hg (Treatment Determined by Highest Blood Pressure Category)	Drug Therapy Without Compelling Indications	Drug Therapy With Compelling Indications
Normal	<120	And <80	No antihypertensive drugs are indicated in this category	Use drugs for compelling indications
Prehypertension	120–139	Or 80–89	No antihypertensive drugs are indicated in this category	Administer drugs for compelling indications
Stage 1 hypertension	140–159	Or 90–99	Antihypertensive, including thiazide-type diuretics, for most cases May also consider ACE inhibitors or drugs such as beta-blockers and calcium-channel blockers	Administer drugs for compelling indications; also consider other antihypertensives (e.g., diuretics, ACE inhibitors)
Stage 2 hypertension	≥160	Or ≥100	Two-drug combination (using both thiazide-type diuretics and ACE inhibitors or drugs such as beta-blockers and calcium-channel blockers)	Use drugs for competing indications in addition to other antihypertensives

*Excerpted from the Seventh Report of the National Committee on Detection, Evaluation, and Treatment of High Blood Pressure (2003). Bethesda, Md.: National Institutes of Health—National Heart, Lung, and Blood Institute.
ACE = angiotensin-converting enzyme; DBP = diastolic blood pressure; SBP = systolic blood pressure.

3. Obesity
4. Hypercholesterolemia
5. Hyperglycemia
6. Smoking
7. Abnormal sodium and water retention

Secondary hypertension is diagnosed when the following causes are present (Walsh, 1993):

1. Coarctation of the aorta
2. Pheochromocytoma (a catecholamine-secreting tumor)
3. Cushing's disease
4. Chronic glomerulonephritis
5. Toxemia from pregnancy
6. Thyrotoxicosis
7. Effects of certain drugs such as contraceptives
8. Collagen disease

Primary hypertension affects more African-Americans than White Americans. The NHANES researchers indicated that in persons 24 to 34 years of age, 3.6% of non-Black men and 12.5% of African-American men have primary hypertension, as well as 2.3% of non-Black women and 8.6% of African-American women. According to this study, these figures appear to rise steadily with age and at all ages are conspicuously higher in African-Americans. Thus, the overall ratio of incidence of primary hypertension among African-Americans compared with non-Blacks is estimated to be 2:1. In addition, primary hypertension is believed to be more severe for African-Americans regardless of age. The death rate for primary hypertension at all ages up to 85 years is higher in African-Americans than in non-Blacks. It was reported that among men between 24 and 44 years of age, mortality from primary hypertension was 14.8% for African-Americans and 1% for non-Blacks. In this same age group, female mortality from primary hypertension was reported to be 12.3% for African-Americans and 0.8% for non-Blacks (Merck, Sharp, & Dohme, 1974). These data indicate that African-Americans succumb to primary hypertension almost 15 times more often than non-Blacks do. Furthermore, the death rate for hypertension is probably an underestimation. The nurse must be aware of the significant risk factors for hypertension to assist in early detection

and continued maintenance and treatment, which can help reduce mortality.

Data indicate that African-Americans have a higher propensity for hypertension (CDC, 1992b; Joint National Committee, 2003; Lerner & Kannel, 1986; Stokes, Kannel, Wolf, et al., 1987; National Center for Health Statistics, 2006). In fact, the prevalence of hypertension among persons 20 years of age and older was down from 48.1 per 1000 in 1960–1962 to 34.9 from 1988–1994 in African-American males as compared with 39.3 in 1960–1962 and 24.3 in 1988–1994 in their White counterparts (National Center for Health Statistics, 2006). African-American women do not fare any better than their male counterparts. The prevalence among African-American women 20 years of age from 1988–1994 was 30.6, down from 50.5 from 1960–1962; among white women, the prevalence was 20.4 in 1988–1994, a decrease from 34.9 for 1960–1962 (National Center for Health Statistics, 2006). It remains controversial as to whether genetic markers, such as skin color, can be related to hypertension prevalence among African-Americans and other persons with dark skin color (Braithwaite & Taylor, 2002). However, a classic study of African-Americans residing in Charleston, South Carolina, showed a significant association between blood pressure and skin darkness among both men and women (Boyle, 1970). The effect for this study was independent of age but was minimized by consideration of socioeconomic status.

A later but totally different study was done with African-Americans in the population from the same geographical location. Contrary to the earlier study, the data indicated that skin color was not significantly associated with a 15-year incidence of hypertension noted in African-American women over 35 years of age in this geographical location (Keil, 1981). In this study, skin color was measured by a photoelectric reflectometer on the medial aspect of the upper arm. In addition, the effect for the study was independent of socioeconomic status. Both these studies differ remarkably from a study reported by Braithwaite and Taylor (2002) that was conducted in Detroit on African-American men. According to Braithwaite and Taylor (2002), the data from this study indicate that there is a significant relationship between high blood pressure and skin color as measured by subjective coding of skin color of the forehead, between the eyes.

Klag, Whelton, Coresh, et al. (1991), found an association between skin color and systolic and diastolic blood pressures, which were higher in darker-skinned persons than that in lighter-skinned persons. In the study, 457 African-Americans were surveyed in three United States cities by use of a reflectometer to note the intensity of skin color and the correlation with blood pressure. The findings from the study indicate that both systolic and diastolic blood pressures may be higher in darker persons than in lighter ones and increased by 2 mm Hg for every 1–standard deviation increase in skin darkness. However, the association was dependent on socioeconomic status, whether measured by education or on another index consisting of education, occupation, and ethnicity. Significant findings were present only in persons on the lower level of either index (Klag, Whelton, Coresh, et al., 1991). Using multiple linear regression, the researchers found that both systolic and diastolic blood pressures remained significantly associated with darker skin in the lower socioeconomic status, independent of age and body mass index and concentration of blood glucose. The researchers concluded that the findings may be attributed to one of two factors:

1. The inability of such groups to deal with psychosocial stress associated with darker skin or
2. An interaction between the environmental factors associated with low socioeconomic status and a susceptible gene that has a higher prevalence in persons with darker skin (Klag, Whelton, Coresh, et al., 1991).

Regardless of the race of the client, to obtain blood pressure measurements that are representative of the client's usual levels, it is important that the individual be seated with the arm bared, supported, and at heart level. The client should not have smoked or ingested caffeine within 30 minutes before the measurement is taken (Joint National Committee, 1997). If the measurement must be repeated, it should not be taken for at least 5 minutes after the first reading. To ensure an accurate measurement, the appropriate cuff size must be used. In addition, the bladder of the cuff should nearly (at least 80%) or completely encircle the arm (Joint National Committee, 1997).

Sickle Cell Anemia. The most common genetic disorder in the United States is sickle cell anemia, which occurs predominantly in African-Americans. It has been projected that 50,000 African-Americans have sickle cell anemia (Wyngaarden & Smith, 1992). Sickle cell anemia or the trait also occurs in people from Asia Minor, India, the Mediterranean, and the Caribbean area but to a lesser extent than what has been reported in African-Americans. Sickle cell anemia is characterized by chronic hemolytic anemia and is a homozygous recessive disorder. In sickle cell anemia the basic disorder lies within the globin of the hemoglobin (Hb), where a single amino acid (valine) is substituted for another (glutamic acid) in the sixth position of the beta chain. It is believed that this single amino acid substitution profoundly alters the properties of the molecule; Hb S is formed instead of normal Hb A as a result of the intermolecular rearrangement. The normal oxygen-carrying capacity of the blood is found in Hb A. As a result of deoxygenation, however, there is a change in the solubility of protein, which makes the Hb molecules lump together, thereby causing the cell membrane to contract. The result is a sickle cell shape.

The affected cells have a shortened life span of 7 to 20 days, which is profoundly different from the life span of normal cells, which is 105 to 120 days. Hb SA is the heterozygous state and is often an asymptomatic condition referred to as sickle cell trait.

Sickle cell anemia is believed to have occurred for many years in Africa along the Nile River valley as an adaptive disease. In Africa this disorder was believed to produce resistance to malaria transmission by the *Anopheles* mosquito (Williams, 1975). In Africa, sickle cell anemia or the trait affects approximately 10% of the Black population, and the death rate before 21 years of age has been 100% in those affected with the disease. Before full recognition of the clinical significance of sickle cell anemia in the United States, the death rate was almost of the same magnitude as that in Africa.

Today in the United States, as a result of improved and comprehensive care, as well as early recognition of the crisis of the disease, persons with sickle cell anemia may live through their third and fourth decades of life.

A differential diagnosis for sickle cell anemia should be made for all African-American persons who have (1) chronic anemia of undetermined origin, (2) an increased susceptibility to infections, or (3) unexplained attacks of joint, bone, or abdominal pain. Sickle cell anemia is diagnosed in the laboratory through a technique called *hemoglobin electrophoresis.* This method provides a definitive diagnosis. In addition, a complete history, including a physical examination and laboratory database should be done. The laboratory database should include a complete blood cell count (CBC) with a differential and reticulocyte count, electrolytes, blood urea nitrogen (BUN), glucose, direct bilirubin, and urinalysis (Satcher & Pope, 1974). In addition, radiographs of the chest, abdomen, and bones are indicated if there is evidence of pain or fever. However, a bone scan is preferable.

For persons with sickle cell anemia, the indications for prompt admission to a hospital include the following (Leffall, 1974):

1. Vaso-occlusive pain crisis that does not respond to analgesics within 4 hours of administration
2. Aplastic crisis
3. Splenic sequestration, a life-threatening condition that requires immediate admission to the intensive care unit for continuous observation and therapy
4. Hyperhemolytic crisis, which can occur if the hemoglobin and hematocrit levels continue to drop
5. Infections indicated by a temperature greater than 101° F or a white blood cell count greater than 15,000 cells/L (although viral ear, nose, and throat infections may not indicate admission for pediatric clients)
6. Thromboembolic phenomena in the lungs, cerebrum, and long bones
7. Pregnancy, which indicates an increased risk

A common problem associated with sickle cell anemia is drug use and abuse. At the Martin Luther King Jr. Hospital, a team of health professionals working through the National Sickle Cell Center was involved in the care of clients with sickle cell anemia. Their work revealed three kinds of problems (Satcher et al., 1973):

1. Clients with sickle cell anemia were typically stereotyped as drug abusers by many health professionals.
2. The delay in seeking medical care during a sickle cell crisis was caused by the client's desire to tolerate pain and avoid drug dependence.
3. Drug abuse in clients with sickle cell anemia was found in clients with severe and disabling conditions. These clients required drugs so frequently that they often became mentally and physically dependent.

The nurse must be able to identify early signs of sickle cell crisis and teach the client to recognize these symptoms when they occur. The nurse should impress on the client the significance of early recognition and treatment of crisis symptoms. Ongoing surveillance of signs and symptoms of sickle cell crisis can promote appropriate treatment and perhaps prevent early death (Platt, Brambilla, Rosse, et al., 1994).

Systemic Lupus Erythematosus. Systemic lupus erythematosus (SLE) is a chronic disease of unknown cause that affects organs and systems individually or in a variety of combinations. The disease affects women 8 to 10 times more often than it does men. The age distribution for the disease spans 2 to 97 years. SLE was named after the classic butterfly rash, which is erosive and thus "likened to the damage caused by a hungry wolf" (Rodnan & Schumacher, 1983). This disease was once believed to be relatively rare and always fatal. However, with the advent of better techniques for recognition, the disease is now considered fairly common, and its course can be controlled by corticosteroids. Even today, however, some clients do die as a result of lesions that affect major organs or as a result of secondary infections. Although the cause of the disease is still unknown, three major causative factors are being investigated: (1) an aberration of the immune system that causes immune complexes containing antibodies to be deposited in tissue, which in turn causes tissue damage; (2) a viral infection that is caused by or results from some immunological abnormality; (3) the combination of the first two factors. In addition, some drugs are known to induce lupus-like syndromes, including procainamide (Pronestyl), isonicotinic acid hydrazide (INH, isoniazid), and penicillin (Rodnan & Schumacher, 1983).

As previously indicated, SLE was believed to be a very rare disease. However, because of sophisticated detection procedures, researchers now postulate that this is not so—its incidence has been estimated to be 2.6 per 100,000 population. Although it occurs more frequently in African-Americans than in non-Blacks, it is reported to be extremely rare among the Asian population.

The nurse who understands that signs and symptoms of arthritis may indicate SLE, especially when combined with weakness, fatigue, and weight loss, can assist in early detection. In addition, the nurse should look for symptoms of sensitivity to sunlight, including development of a rash or symptoms of fever or arthritis as a result of exposure to sunlight. The butterfly lesions of SLE generally appear over the cheeks and bridge of the nose. These lesions are often bright red and may extend beyond the hairline, thus causing alopecia (loss of hair), particularly above the ears. Lesions may also be noted on the neck and may spread slowly to the mucous membranes and other tissues of the body. These lesions generally do not ulcerate; however, they do cause degeneration and atrophy of tissues. Other clinical findings may also be present, depending on the organs involved, including glomerulonephritis, pleuritis, pericarditis, peritonitis, neuritis, and anemia. The most severe manifestations of SLE are renal and neurological in nature.

Laboratory tests used to diagnose SLE may need to be specific to the organs involved, such as proteinuria, abnormal cerebrospinal fluid, or radiographic evidence of pleural reactions. Before the advent of the lupus erythematosus (LE)-cell preparation, or what is commonly called the LE-cell test, the diagnosis was based on the presentation of the butterfly rash and systemic complications; the disease was generally fatal. However, as a result of the LE-cell test and other sensitive tests, including the antinuclear antibody (ANA) or the antinuclear factor (ANF) test, clients with more varied symptoms have been confirmed earlier. Thus, through early detection, appropriate treatment has been initiated. Client teaching by the nurse should include instructions on the need for appropriate exercise, appropriate balance of rest and activity, and the necessity of avoiding direct exposure to sunlight. As indicated earlier, SLE has a higher prevalence among some racial groups, and the nurse who recognizes the biocultural significance of the disease is more apt to give culturally appropriate nursing care.

AIDS. According to the *Surgeon General's Report* (1987), one fact that is emerging with clarity is the increasing incidence of acquired immunodeficiency syndrome (AIDS) among African-Americans and Hispanics. In the United States, 1 of every 8 Americans is African-American, but among Americans with AIDS, 1 of every 4 is African-American. These numbers reflect the fact that 24% of the total AIDS cases reported thus far involve African-American persons. In the United States, 1 of every 12 Americans is Hispanic, but 1 of every 7 Americans with AIDS is Hispanic (CDC, 2005).

From June 1981 through December 2005, there were 944,306 reported cases of AIDS in the United States (CDC, 2005). Of this number, 749,887 cases have occurred in men, whereas 170,679 have been reported in women.

Of the number of reported cases of AIDS in men, 313,034 were in Whites, 228,499 were in Blacks; 121,198 were in Hispanics; 5345 were in Asian/Pacific Islanders; and 2057 were in American Indians/Alaska Natives. Similarly, of the number of reported AIDS cases among women in the United States through December 2001, 30,854 were in Whites; 84,681 were in Blacks; 28,554 were in Hispanics; 803 were in Asians/Pacific Islanders; and 480 were in American Indians/Alaska Natives (CDC, 2005).

While women represented just 17% of the total AIDS cases, this figure nearly doubles to 28% of all HIV cases. Proportionately, heterosexual women and in particular heterosexual African-American women continued to be the fastest-growing segment of the population to be diagnosed with AIDS. In addition, proportionately by population size, African-Americans continue to be infected by HIV at a disproportionately high rate (CDC, 2002). In fact, over the past decade AIDS has moved ahead of cardiovascular disease to become the leading cause of death among African-Americans 25 to 44 years of age (CDC, 2005).

Of the number of pediatric cases reported in the United States through December 2005 that involve children under 13 years of age, 1579 were in Whites, 5337 were in Blacks, 1876 were in Hispanics, 54 were in Asians, 31 were in American Indians, and 16 were in persons of unknown races (CDC, 2001). Although these numbers are alarming, they do not accurately reflect the full scope of this widespread problem in the United States. It is estimated that the data available on reported cases of AIDS indicate that the prevalence of AIDS in the United States is so widespread that 1 of every 300 Americans has AIDS, representing 0.3% of the total population (CDC, 2001). Yet, by 2000, only 25 states had initiated an integrated name-based reporting system for HIV and AIDS. These states include the following:

Alabama	Minnesota	South Carolina
Arizona	Mississippi	South Dakota
Arkansas	Nevada	Tennessee
Colorado	New Jersey	Utah
Idaho	North Carolina	Virginia
Indiana	North Dakota	West Virginia
Louisiana	Ohio	Wisconsin
Massachusetts	Oklahoma	Wyoming
Michigan		

Since the reporting of these data, three other states have initiated an integrated name-based reporting system for HIV and AIDS: Florida, New Mexico, and Nebraska (CDC, 2005). The top five leading metropolitan areas reporting the highest number of AIDS cases are New York City (126,237), Los Angeles (43,488), Miami (25,357), San Francisco (28,438), and Washington, D.C. (24,844) (CDC, 2005).

From June 1981 through December 2001, 467,910 people succumbed to AIDS or AIDS-related conditions in the United States. This number includes 462,653 adults and adolescents and 9443 children under 13 years of age. Of the total number of patients who died in 2004 alone (15,798), 4501 were White, 8041 were Black, 2882 were Hispanic, 100 were Asian/Pacific Islander, and 70 were American Indian/Alaska Native (CDC, 2005).

Nutritional Preferences and Deficiencies

Another category of differences among cultural groups is nutritional preferences and deficiencies. **Nutritional Preferences.** Nutritional preferences include habits and patterns. When it comes to food choices, people are creatures of habit (Zifferblatt, Wilbur, & Pinsky, 1980). The term *habit* connotes inflexibility, though people do change their habits for many reasons. The term *food patterns* is more descriptive of food choices. Many factors are associated with the formation of food patterns and preferences. Food patterns are developed during childhood as a result of family lifestyle and ethnic or cultural, social, religious, geographical, economic, and psychological components. All of these variables influence an individual's attitudes, feelings, and beliefs about certain foods. However, the paramount factors that seem to determine food choices are cultural and ethnic in nature. Adults in a particular culture set the tone for cultural food patterns, which establish the foundation for a child's lifelong eating customs regarding the timing of meals, the number of meals per day, foods acceptable for specific meals, methods of preparation, dislikes and likes, and table manners. Over time, children develop a sense of stability and security in regard to certain food patterns and attitudes.

Schwerin, Stanton, and Smith (1982) indicated that people exhibit distinct patterns of consuming foods in different combinations or forms and that for the most part these patterns have remained constant over the past decade. For example, many southern Americans would routinely choose grits as a food but would not routinely choose lentils. However, American diets are becoming more homogeneous because of many factors, including transportation, advertising, mobility, economic status, methods of production, and appreciation of other people's cultural heritage (Katz, Hediger, & Valleroy, 1974; Pangborn, 1975; Riggs, 1980; Saldana & Brown, 1984).

Some people, based on their culture, have not been traditionally known to make food choices solely on the basis of the nutritional and health values of food. For example, one of the most nutritious vegetables is broccoli; however, broccoli ranks twenty-first among vegetables consumed in the United States. On the other hand, the tomato, which is the most commonly eaten vegetable in the United States, ranks sixteenth as a source of vitamins and minerals (Farb & Armelagos, 1980).

When people relocate, they carry established food habits to the new location, but these habits are retained only if the foods are available in the new location and are affordable. Foods in various cultures have different prestige or status. For example, beef and certain seafoods, such as lobster, are regarded as high-status foods among people in the United States. Hindus from India consider cows to be sacred and therefore do not eat beef. In seafaring countries, seafoods have no status value because they are common. Foods obtain their status rating from various factors, including religious beliefs, availability, cost, cultural values, and traditions, or because a highly respected individual has endorsed them. Even today, in many cultures men and their opinions regarding food preferences are more highly regarded than women and their opinions. In fact, in certain cultures men are so highly regarded that they are served meals first, before women and children. As a result of this practice, women and children may receive insufficient quantities and fewer varieties of food.

Food also has symbolic meaning, in some cultures, that has nothing to do with nutritional value. In these cultures eating becomes associated with sentiments and assumptions about oneself and the world (Chang, 1974; Farb & Armelagos, 1980). Food becomes symbolic to people not only because of religious connotations but also because it can be used as a reward. For example, a mother who gives a child candy or ice cream as a reward for good behavior may be reinforcing that food as a good food. On the other hand, a mother who serves a particular food (such as broccoli or cabbage) and says she is doing so because of bad behavior may be reinforcing that food as a bad food or punishment.

Food Patterns and Nutrition Among African-Americans. Food patterns among African-Americans are not significantly different from those of non–African-Americans living in the same geographical area. However, distinct differences do exist for African-Americans living and raised in the North as compared with those living and raised in the South. African-Americans, as a cultural group, are in the low socioeconomic groups, which may precipitate nutritional problems. As a result of nutritional deficiencies, African-Americans tend to have medical problems that are somewhat different from those of White Americans. As mentioned earlier, hypertension is a medical problem that is twice as great in African-Americans as in White Americans. Another medical problem, particularly in women, that has been linked to food patterns and selections is obesity. Soul foods, which are generally cooked for long periods and well seasoned, may also contribute to many of the medical problems that African-Americans encounter. Taking their roots from southern African-Americans who saw their preparation as economical, soul foods are listed in Table 7-1.

A cultural pattern that has been established among African-American pregnant women is the consumption of nonfood items (pica), which supposedly originated because of nutritional needs. Another common practice among children under 3 years of age, pregnant women, and some men is the eating of earthy substances such as dirt or clay. This practice is known as geophagy and is practiced mainly in lower socioeconomic groups. For many years in African society, the biological need for calcium, iron, and other minerals, especially by pregnant and lactating women, was partially met by eating clays that were high in nutrients. An analysis of some clays has revealed significant amounts of calcium, magnesium, potassium, copper, zinc, and iron, which are the same substances that have been

Table 7-1	Foods Enjoyed by African-Americans		
Name of Food	**Region**	**Type of Food**	**Description**
Poke salad	Southern U.S.	Cooked young shoots of pokeweed	Prepared with spicy seasoning and fatback
Collard greens	Southern U.S.	Garden raised	Prepared with spicy seasoning and fatback
Fatback	Southern U.S.	Pork fat	Prepared from loin of pig
Chicken wings	Southern U.S.	Chicken	Prepared by frying with spicy seasoning
Chitterlings	Southern U.S.	Meat	Intestines of young pigs that are boiled or fried
Hog maws	Southern U.S.	Meat	Stomach of pig
Grits	Southern U.S.	Grain	Hulled and coarsely ground corn that is boiled and simmered
Hoppin' John	Southern U.S.	Combination	Black-eyed peas and rice
Dandelion	Southern U.S.	Wild greens	Prepared with spicy seasoning and fatback greens
Ribs	Southern U.S.	Pork meat	Prepared with spicy seasoning and slow heat

prescribed for pregnant and lactating women in modern societies (Farb & Armelagos, 1980). Africans who were brought to the United States as slaves continued to eat clay, which is still bought in some areas of the South and shipped to relatives in the North. However, geophagy leads to iron deficiency, mainly because clay inhibits the absorption of iron, potassium, and zinc (Halsted, 1968). It is believed that geophagy is both a cause and a consequence of anemia. In areas where clay is not readily available, laundry starch is sometimes substituted, though it can irritate the stomach and is almost completely lacking in valuable minerals.

There are many clinical implications for the nurse in meeting the nutritional needs of African-Americans, who normally have lower hemoglobin and hematocrit levels than non–African-Americans have (Dalman, Bar, & Allen, 1978; Garn, Ryan, & Abraham, 1980). Although these lower hemoglobin and hematocrit levels are believed to be partially caused by genetics, some studies suggest that nutritional factors may also be responsible (Jackson, Sauberlich, Skala, et al., 1983).

Another clinical implication for the nurse who cares for African-Americans is that of lactose intolerance. Many African-Americans are lactose-intolerant but can tolerate such milk products as buttermilk, yogurt, fermented cheese, and small quantities of milk. In addition, certain nutrients

known to be low in the African-American diet include iron, calcium, and vitamin A.

Another clinical implication for African-Americans is the high incidence of hypertension, which may necessitate a low-sodium diet. Because African-Americans habitually use large amounts of salt and other spicy seasonings, special attention must be given to the importance of seasoning foods to make them acceptable and at the same time limiting the use of salt.

Food Patterns and Nutrition Among Puerto Ricans. Many Puerto Ricans, like persons from other Latin American cultures, subscribe to the theory of "hot" and "cold." The major difference for Puerto Ricans is that they classify diseases as hot and cold and foods and medications as hot, cold, and cool. Both Indian and Spanish influences are reflected in Puerto Rican native dishes (Table 7-2).

The common fare of Puerto Ricans is rice, cooked grainy and dried, and red or white beans stewed with bacon or olive oil, garlic, and onions. Another common fare is *safrito*, which is a tasty mixture of tomatoes, green peppers, sweet chili peppers, onions, garlic, oregano, and fresh coriander cooked in lard or vegetable oil and used as a relish to season foods. Other foods eaten regularly in Puerto Rico include *viandas* (starchy vegetable dish consisting of plantains, sweet potatoes, and green bananas), cassava, breadfruit, acerola, mango,

Table 7-2	Foods Enjoyed by Puerto Ricans	
Name of Food	**Type of Food**	**Description**
Acerola	Fruit	Barbados cherry (*Malpighia* and *Bunchosia* species)
Arroz blanco	Grain	Enriched white rice
Bacalao	Meat	Salted codfish
San cocho	Combination	Soup prepared with meat and viandas
Safrito	Seasoning	Specially treated tomato sauce
Viandas	Vegetable	Starchy tropical vegetable dish that includes plantains, green bananas, and sweet potatoes

avocado, corn, okra, chayotes, and tubers. The acerola, which is also called the West Indian or Barbados cherry, is the highest known source of vitamin C. The acerola contains 1000 mg (1 g) of vitamin C per 100-g portion. Many of the food items that are common in the United States are very expensive because they have to be imported. Chicken, pork, and beef, which are normally fried, are usually limited in the diet because of their cost. Eggs are generally used as the main dish and may be served as omelets. Milk is a very popular food item in Puerto Rico but is seldom drunk as a beverage. The intake of milk is believed to be low in Puerto Rico because of its cost. A popular beverage is *cafe con leche*, which is a combination of coffee with 2 to 5 ounces of milk. This beverage constitutes the largest portion of milk that is consumed. For the most part, foods are cooked for very long periods, or they are fried. Lard and salt pork are commonly used to flavor many dishes. One food item that has an exaggerated reputation for being nutritious and is often given to children and lactating women is malt beer.

There are many clinical implications for the nurse in meeting the nutritional needs of Puerto Ricans. Pregnant Puerto Rican women have a high incidence of megaloblastic anemia and therefore should be instructed to increase their intake of foods high in folic acid (Parker & Bowering, 1976). For the client who needs to control carbohydrate intake, the nurse should instruct the client about the necessity of counting *viandas* as bread exchanges. The nurse must also be aware that the diet of Puerto Ricans who have moved to mainland cities may lack variety because of the inability of some Puerto Ricans to afford the native island foods that they were accustomed to getting previously. Therefore, the nurse and the client should look for acceptable food items that are comparable in health value.

Food Patterns and Nutrition Among Cubans. A major portion of the Cuban diet includes cut-up vegetables, stews, and casseroles that have been flavored with sage, parsley, bay leaves, thyme, cinnamon, curry powder, capers, onions, cloves, garlic, and saffron. An integral part of Cuban food preparation is saffron, which is so heavily used in the Cuban diet that some dishes are considered anemic looking and unpalatable unless they have a deep golden saffron hue. Chicken, fish, or meat soup is served at least once a day, before each major meal. Salad is also served every day, along with fried foods, especially fish, poultry, and eggs. Most Cuban people eat rice and beans of many different varieties. Although fruits and vegetables are plentiful, most Cuban refugees do not consume fruits and vegetables on a regular basis (Gorden, 1982). The typical breakfast of Cuban people consists of coffee and bread. Some Cuban adults drink a lot of strong coffee and rum. Foods enjoyed by Cubans include the following:

Name of Food	Type of Food	Description
Guava	Fruit	Small yellow or red sweet tropical fruit
Plantains	Fruit	Banana-like fruit that tastes like sweet potatoes and is boiled or fried

There are many clinical implications for the nurse in meeting the nutritional needs of Cuban people. The nurse should be aware that in most Cuban diets calcium intake is normally low; therefore, the nurse should instruct the client to incorporate some cheese and milk into the diet. In addition, the nurse should advise the client to replace fried foods with other methods of food preparation, such as boiling or broiling. In addition, the client should be advised that long cooking periods for some foods, such as pork, are beneficial.

Food Patterns and Nutrition Among American Indians. A problem for American Indians living on reservations that is as prevalent today as it was in the past is food scarcity and a lack of food variety. For American Indians, fresh fruits, vegetables, and meats are very expensive, if they are available at all. Traditional foods may vary among tribes; however, the basic diet of American Indians consists of corn, beans, and squash. A status food for most tribes is corn. Chili pepper is widely used among tribes because it adds spice to the diet and is considered to be a good source of vitamin C. On some reservations and particularly among some tribes, diets are considered to be very poor, supplying less than two thirds of the recommended daily allowances for one or more nutrients (Miller, 1981). The diets tend to be inadequate in calories, calcium, iron, iodine, riboflavin, and vitamins A and C (Owens, Garry, Seymore, et al., 1981).

Poor nutrition has been directly related to several leading causes of death among American Indians, including heart disease and cirrhosis of the liver. Diabetes is three times more common among some American Indian tribes than in the general U.S. population (Miller, 1981). American Indians have the highest reported prevalence of type 2 diabetes mellitus. In the Pima tribe, hyperinsulinemia reflects a resistance to insulin action (Nagulesparan, Savage, & Knowler, 1982). Among some American Indian tribes, low hemoglobin values and mild thyroid deficiencies are prevalent (Interdepartmental Commission, 1964) (Table 7-3).

There are many clinical implications for the nurse in meeting the nutritional needs of American Indians. The nurse must recognize that the diets of most American Indian tribes tend to be inadequate in protein, calcium, and vitamins C and A, which may result from unavailability or economics. Another problem found among American Indian tribes is the prevalence of lactose deficiency. The nurse should advise the client to consume nonmilk foods that are high in calcium and riboflavin.

Food Patterns and Nutrition Among the Japanese. Most Japanese dishes are ideally suited for American life because they are economical and nutritious. Japanese people take great pride in the visual effect of foods that they prepare. In the Japanese culture, the arrangement of food, color contrasts, and even shape are considered to be as important as the cooking and seasoning of a particular food. In addition, the rules for picking up chopsticks, holding bowls and teacups, and eating soups are traditions that are well established and regularly observed. These traditional rules of etiquette are as important to the Japanese people as the preparation of the food.

Most of the foods are cooked on a hibachi (a small earthen grill) by broiling, steaming, and stir-frying. It is thought by the Japanese that stir-frying preserves vitamins because the food is cooked only briefly. Meat, which is very expensive in Japan, is stretched with vegetables. Fish is used in some fascinating ways, such as being served raw. Soybean products, which are considered an important source of protein, and tofu are common fare of the Japanese people. In the Japanese culture, salads are rarely served with meals, and bread is often replaced by rice or noodles. The Japanese people have a tendency to use extraordinary flavors when cooking, such as wheat germ powder, which is called *ajino-moto*. Another important seasoning in Japanese cooking is soy sauce. The common beverages included in the Japanese diet among adults are unsweetened green tea (which is the national beverage), beer, and *sake* (rice wine). Milk is often included in the children's diet in the Japanese culture but is rarely used by adults (Table 7-4).

There are many clinical implications for the nurse in meeting the nutritional needs of the Japanese people. A common clinical problem found among the Japanese people is lactose intolerance.

Table 7-3   Foods Enjoyed by American Indians

Name of Food	Type of Food	Description
Acorns (from some oak trees)	Nut	Leached-out paste
Amaranth	Vegetable, cereal	Leaves, seeds
American lotus	Vegetable	Kernels, tuber
Arrowhead (*Sagittaria*)	Vegetable	Tuber
Arrowroot (*Maranta*)	Vegetable	Tuber
Basswood	Cooked vegetable	Buds, flowers
Cattail	Vegetable, salad	Shoots, spikes, pollen
Chicory	Cooked salad	Young leaves
Dandelion	Salad	Leaves
Ginseng (American ginseng)	Vegetable	Roots
Groundnut	Vegetable	Tuber
Jack-in-the-pulpit	Vegetable	Long-term roasted corn
Jerusalem artichoke	Vegetable	Tuber
Jícama	Vegetable	Tuber
Nettle (collected with gloves)	Vegetable	Cooked shoots
Pawpaw	Pie, pudding	Fruit
Pigweed	Vegetable	Tops of leaves
Pine nuts (piñons)	Nuts	Nuts in pinecones of neoza pine, stone pine, and piñon
Pokeweed	Vegetable	Boiled sprouts, boiled roots
Prickly pear (Spanish tuna)	Fruit	Red fruit of cactus
Rose	Salad, jelly	Fruit high in vitamin C
Smartweed (knotweed)	Salad	Leaves
Sorrel	Salad	Leaves
Sumac (smooth sumac)	Beverage	Steeped berries
Violet	Vegetable	Leaves, entire plant
Watercress	Salad	Leaves
Wild ginger	Vegetable	Root
Yucca	Salad, vegetable	Flowers, pods

Table 7-4   Foods Enjoyed by Japanese People

Name of Food	Type of Food	Description
Aji-no-moto	Grain—wheat germ	Wheat germ
Sake	Beverage	Rice wine
Sashimi	Meat	Raw fish
Shoyu	Seasoning	Soy sauce
Tempura	Combination	Deep-fried seafoods and vegetables
Tofu (Chinese *dòfu*)	Vegetable	Soybean curds

In working with a Japanese client, the nurse should advise the client to consume sources of calcium other than milk, such as tofu. The nurse should also advise the client to use enriched rice and to avoid washing the grains before cooking to preserve the nutrient value. When working with a Japanese client who is on a sodium-restricted diet, the nurse should teach the client to measure the amount of soy sauce used and to avoid eating the many types of pickles that are ordinarily eaten. Another important clinical implication the nurse should remember is the high incidence of stomach cancer among

Japanese people, which has been associated with their high intake of raw fish (Qureshi, 1981). Eating raw fish is believed to carry the risk of infestation with fish tapeworms (Goldman, 1985) and has been associated with outbreaks of gastroenteritis (Morse, Guzewich, & Hanrahan, 1986).

Food Patterns and Nutrition Among Koreans. Just as in other Oriental cultures, the main staple of the Korean diet is rice, which is mixed with other grains. Korean people generally mix rice with barley, millet, and red beans because it is believed that a diet consisting of only white rice causes health problems. Most Korean people eat three meals daily, which are of equal proportions. Before cooking, foods are cut into small pieces to facilitate the use of chopsticks. Soups containing seaweed, meat, or fish are always served. One of the most popular condiments in Korea is ginseng; Korean people believe that ginseng has roots resembling the human fetus, is a panacea for curing illnesses regardless of age or sex, and is a supposed aphrodisiac.

Korea is surrounded on three sides by water; thus, fish products are plentiful and account for 85% of the nation's animal protein intake. Almost every conceivable kind of fish is served, whether raw, freshly steamed, or salted and dried. One of the most expensive food items in Korea is eggs because they are scarce. The preferred meat of Koreans is beef, which is prepared by marination, with lots of sugar to provide a crispy coating.

Kimchi involves one of the most nutritious preservative processes available in Korea and does not require refrigeration. *Kimchi* is prepared with chopped vegetables that are highly seasoned, salted, and fermented underground or in a special earthenware container. *Kimchi* can also be prepared from naturally grown vegetables such as cabbage, turnips, cucumbers, and other seasonable vegetables that are soaked in salt water overnight and seasoned the next day with garlic, scallions, ginger, and hot pepper. *Kimchi* is fermented without disturbance for at least 1 month and is best after 2 or 3 months.

Many vegetables are grown in Korea; thus, Koreans serve both fresh vegetables and *kimchi* routinely. Vegetables are never overcooked and are

seasoned with red and black pepper, garlic, sesame seed oil, and soy sauce. Because Korea is surrounded by water on three sides, seaweed is plentiful and is a food item highly prized for its nutritive value. In the Korean culture, seaweed is a must for the expectant mother. Another common fare in Korea is noodles made from rice flour. A Korean diet includes many products made from soybeans, such as soy sauce, soybean paste, bean sprouts, bean curds, and soybean milk. The dairy products of Korea include bean curd and soybean milk. Because Korea is a densely populated country, there is no room for a dairy industry; thus, milk is very expensive and scarce and is served only to children. Because milk is so scarce, babies are often weaned from the breast as late as 2 years of age.

Fresh fruits are readily available in Korea and include apples, peaches, strawberries, pears, watermelons, blackberries, pomegranates, currants, and cherries. Fruit is generally served with each meal. Pastries such as cakes and pies are usually not served with meals; however, they can be found in many small specialty shops.

The national beverage of Korea is made from ginseng; Korea has never been a tea-drinking nation. Another beverage that usually accompanies a Korean meal is barley water, which is served cold in the summer and warm in the winter. Barley water is prepared with grains that stick to the pan after the rice for the meal has been removed. A cup or two of water is added to this rice, and the liquid is allowed to simmer slowly while the meal is being eaten; it is then served after the meal. Foods enjoyed by Korean people include the following:

Name of Food	Type of Food	Description
Barley water	Beverage	Prepared from leftover rice grains
Ginseng	Condiment	Spice
Kimchi	Combination	Vegetables that are highly seasoned, salted, and fermented underground for 1 to 3 months

There are many clinical implications for the nurse in meeting the nutritional needs of Korean people. Up to now, the medicinal properties of ginseng have been poorly researched (Barna, 1985). However, it is believed that the long-term abuse of ginseng may be a contributing factor to hypertension. Less frequent adverse reactions from the long-term abuse of ginseng include nervousness, sleeplessness, skin eruptions, morning diarrhea, edema (Siegel, 1979), and irregularities in blood glucose levels (Ginseng, 1980). The nurse who works with Korean American clients must remember that in the United States rice is not commonly mixed with other grains, as is practiced in Korea. To increase the nutritional value of rice, the client should use whole-grain or enriched rice.

Because Korean people are accustomed to the taste of seaweed, which is expensive, the nurse should encourage the client to substitute stronger-tasting greens such as turnip greens, kale, and mustard greens. Lactose intolerance is a common problem among adults in Korea. Thus, the nurse should encourage the client to substitute other dairy products for fresh milk, such as cottage cheese, yogurt, and aged cheese, as well as the nondairy product tofu. For a diabetic Korean client, a sugar substitute may be dissolved in hot water and poured over meat that is broiled until the crispy texture has been achieved (Maras & Adolphi, 1985). Although *kimchi* is a zesty accompaniment to plain, broiled foods, it is not readily available in the United States; therefore, a Mexican salsa may be used as a substitute (Maras & Adolphi, 1985).

Food Patterns and Nutrition Among Middle Easterners. The Middle East is composed of nine separate countries around the eastern Mediterranean Sea: Greece, Turkey, Lebanon, Syria, Iraq, Iran, Israel, Jordan, and Egypt. These countries are bound together by foods and certain attitudes about foods. The common staples of Middle Eastern people are lamb and goat. Because of the climate and the lack of suitable pasture land, beef is uncommon in the Middle Eastern countries. In most Middle Eastern countries, *dolma*, a very popular meat dish, is often served. *Dolma* is made of ground meat mixed with rice, herbs, and spices and then wrapped in leaves or stuffed in vegetables. Because many of these countries are contiguous to the eastern Mediterranean seaboard, all varieties of saltwater and freshwater fish, shellfish, and roe are served. In some of the Mediterranean countries bound by religious tradition, some foods are restricted. For example, many Muslims avoid eating pork and wild birds; the main dish of the Muslim people is vegetables and legumes.

For most Middle Eastern people, bread is the staple of life; for every mouthful of food, most Middle Easterners eat a mouthful of bread (Valassi, 1962). A meal without bread is unthinkable for most Middle Eastern people. Bread is generally homemade, fresh, and warm, and the more compact dark bread is preferred to refined white bread. *Pilaf* is a festive dish that is served throughout the Middle East. Other common fares of Middle Eastern countries include beans and lentils, which rank directly behind bread and rice.

In the Middle East, boiled beans are served cold with olive oil dressing and lemon juice. In addition, a variety of vegetables, both cooked and raw, are served. Seasonings commonly used by Middle Easterners in food preparation include onions, fresh tomato paste, olive oil, and parsley. There are more than 120 ways of preparing eggplant, which is a favorite of most Middle Easterners.

Baklava is one of the most popular sweets in the Middle East. However, sweets are generally served only on holidays or during social calls. Unlike Americans, Middle Easterners seldom serve sweets as dessert. Instead, a bowl of fresh fruit consisting of cucumbers, guavas, mangos, citrus fruits, dates, figs, pomegranates, or bananas is the usual dessert. Cooking fats used in Middle Eastern cooking include olive and sesame oil, butter, and ghee, which is a clarified butter made from goat's, sheep's, or camel's milk. Middle Easterners use animal fat to cook foods when the dish is to be eaten hot and oils when the dish is to be eaten cold. Meals are not considered tasteful and well prepared unless a large quantity of fat is used. Popular spices in the Middle East include mint, oregano, and cinnamon. The most popular herb is garlic. The exception to this is found in Iran, where garlic is considered vulgar. Olives in many shapes and colors are popular.

Milk is not commonly served to adults; however, it is given to children. Yogurt is considered a supreme health food that cures many ills, confers long life and good looks, prolongs youth, and fortifies the soul. Yogurt is served in many foods; for example, it is mixed with diced cucumbers and is used as a topping for rice, fried vegetables, and desserts. Thin yogurt that has been diluted with water is considered safer, less perishable, and more thirst-quenching than milk. A specialty cheese served by Greek people is feta, a white cheese made from sheep's or goat's milk.

Wine is a forbidden drink in the Muslim faith, Islam. Other than Christians and Jews, many Near Easterners do not drink alcoholic beverages of any kind. Every meal ends with coffee or tea; however, coffee takes precedence most of the time. The exception to this is found in Iran, where the favorite drink is tea served hot and sweet (Table 7-5).

There are many clinical implications for the nurse in working with people from the Middle East. Because fresh milk is not normally consumed by adults from most Middle Eastern countries, the protein and calcium content of the diet must be increased. The nurse should encourage the Middle Eastern client to substitute yogurt for fresh milk because yogurt is a favorite of most Middle Easterners. White cheese, cottage cheese, and aged sharp cheese can also be substituted for fresh milk. For the client on a carbohydrate-restricted diet, the nurse must remember that bread should be restricted or eliminated from the diet because it is high in carbohydrates. The elimination of bread from the diet of persons in cultures where bread is a main staple is difficult. However, the nurse must

stress to the client the importance of reducing carbohydrate intake. Because fat is used in large quantities to add taste to meals, the amount of fat in the diet could pose problems for clients on low-calorie, diabetic, or low-fat diets. For clients using sodium-restricted diets, feta cheese and olives should be eliminated from the diet.

Nutritional Deficiencies. Racially related nutritional deficiencies include lactose intolerance and G-6-PD deficiency. Lactose intolerance, or intolerance to milk, is a relatively common condition considered normal in many ethnic groups. It is found in more than 66% of Mexican Americans and is very common in African-Americans, some American Indian tribes, Asians, and Ashkenazi Jews (Bayless, 1975; Burns & Neubort, 1984; Kisch, 1953). In fact, it has been reported in approximately 90% of adult African Blacks and 79% of African-Americans, American Indians, and Asians. Although lactose intolerance is very common among these racial groups, it is reported to be much less common among Whites of northern European descent; only 5% to 15% of this population have the disorder. Yet the statistical significance reported among Whites of northern European descent indicates that this condition is more than a rare phenomenon.

The cause of lactose intolerance is an insufficient amount of lactase, the enzyme responsible for converting the nonabsorbable milk sugar, lactose, into the absorbable sugars glucose and galactose. With lactase deficiency, any undigested lactose will remain in the small intestine, where, because of its

Table 7-5	Foods Enjoyed by Middle Eastern People		
Name of Food	**Culture**	**Type of Food**	**Description**
Baklava	Greek	Dessert	Layered pastry made with honey
Bulgur	Middle Eastern	Grain	Granular wheat product with nutlike flavor
Dolmades (*dholmadhes*)	Greek	Combination	Grape leaves stuffed with beef
Feta	Greek	Dairy product	Soft, salty, white cheese made from sheep's or goat's milk
Kibbeh	Middle Eastern	Meat	Fresh, raw lamb, ground and seasoned, similar to meat loaf
Moussaka	Greek	Combination	Meat and eggplant casserole
Phyllo	Greek	Grain	Paper-thin pastry for meat, vegetable, cheese, and egg dishes and pastries

osmotic capacity, it draws water. When the lactose reaches the colon, it begins to combine acetic acid and hydrogen gas, which results in the symptoms of lactose intolerance: cramping, flatulence, abdominal bloating, and diarrhea. These symptoms are dose related—they occur only if the person ingests more food containing lactose than the person's supply of available lactase can metabolize. Foods containing large amounts of lactose include milk, yogurt, and milk chocolate. Of these food items, nonfat dry milk contains the most lactose. Foods containing moderate amounts of lactose include cream, cottage cheese, and most cheeses. Even unlikely foods such as dried soup, cookies made from prepared mixes, cold cuts, and bread and butter contain small amounts of lactose (When Patients Can't Drink Milk, 1976).

The nurse must be cognizant of foods that can cause lactose intolerance symptoms, particularly when working with persons who are extremely lactose-intolerant. For most clients, treatment of this condition is usually a matter of restricting lactose-containing foods rather than eliminating them altogether. An adult who is advised to restrict milk and milk products but otherwise eat a well-balanced diet should not need any nutritional supplements. However, for pregnant or lactating women, nutritional supplements (such as calcium tablets) may be necessary. Lactose intolerance does not generally develop until after childhood; children who are deficient in lactose should be encouraged to eat aged cheeses because the aging process changes lactase to lactic acid. In addition, some physicians may recommend a soybean-based milk substitute, as well as vitamins and calcium supplements. Even for the adult lactose-deficient client, the astute nurse can suggest alternatives to milk products, such as cheese aged over 60 days. The nurse should be aware that telling the client to drink milk may not necessarily be good advice for many adults in the world and should give special consideration to the pregnant or lactating woman because most racial groups, except Whites, cannot tolerate milk in adulthood (Bayless, 1975).

Another enzyme deficiency disorder that is more prevalent in certain racial or ethnic groups is G-6-

PD deficiency. Although this disorder is more prevalent in certain groups, these groups may have different forms of the deficiency. Williams (1975) reported that the type A variety, which moves rapidly on starch-gel electrophoresis, is found in 35% of African-Americans who have the deficiency. The slow-moving type B variety is found in 65% of Blacks who have the deficiency and in nearly all non-Blacks who have the deficiency. However, all forms affect males more than females because the genetic inheritance is carried on the X chromosome. The Cantonese Chinese disorder of G-6-PD has been found among the Chinese and the people of Southeast Asia. The incidence of the Cantonese Chinese form ranges from 2% to 5% (Williams, 1975). Still another form of G-6-PD deficiency is the Mediterranean variety, which is the most clinically severe type. This form of G-6-PD deficiency affects up to 50% of male Greeks, Sardinians, and Sephardic Jews.

An enzyme constituent of the red blood cells, G-6-PD is involved in the hexose monophosphate pathway, which accounts for 10% of glucose metabolism of the red blood cells. Under normal circumstances the proportion of glucose metabolized through this pathway may increase greatly if the cells are subjected to oxidants causing metabolic stress. The result is the formation of increased methemoglobin and degradation of hemoglobin. In addition, certain medications tend to overwhelm the protective mechanism, especially when older red blood cells are involved, because of a decline in G-6-PD activity with the aging of these cells. Red blood cells with a genetically determined deficiency of G-6-PD are unable to withstand lesser oxidative stresses, and as a result a hemolytic process ensues that precipitates a significant anemia.

In the presence of certain conditions, G-6-PD–deficient red blood cells hemolyze, resulting in hemolytic anemia. Conditions that precipitate hemolytic anemia in susceptible persons include the administration of certain drugs, such as quinine, aspirin, phenacetin, chloramphenicol, probenecid, sulfonamides, and thiazide diuretics. The presence of infection and the ingestion of fava beans (also called broad beans or horse beans) are also linked to the precipitous onset of hemolytic anemia. The fava bean is a dietary staple in some of the Mediterranean countries, such as Greece, and those of northern Africa. Favism, a condition induced by ingestion of the fava bean, is one of the most severe forms of G-6-PD hemolysis. In addition, G-6-PD deficiency has been related to an adaptive process that prevents malaria. The discerning nurse should assist the client in identifying substances that are likely to precipitate hemolytic episodes. In addition, the client should be taught to exercise caution to prevent serious infections. Until an exposure occurs, G-6-PD deficiency is a condition that remains asymptomatic. The nurse must understand that hemolytic episodes are the result of culturally related nutritional habits and geographical and environmental location.

Psychological Characteristics

Gaitz and Scott (1974) have indicated that although cultural factors may influence mental health scores in research studies, such scores are not indicative of whether one cultural group has more or fewer incidences of mental illness than another. There are many different definitions of mental health, one of which postulates that a person is mentally healthy when there is a balance in the person's internal life and adaptation to reality. Thus it can be determined that normal behavior is relative to a specific culture and that different psychological characteristics are promoted by each culture. Other variables that influence mental health include family relationships, childbearing practices, language, attitudes toward illness, and social and economic status.

Some cultural groups have a low socioeconomic status, which consequently affects mental health. For example, some Mexican Americans have a low socioeconomic status in terms of substandard housing, education, physical health, political influence, communication, and social exclusion. The concept of social exclusion must be considered as a contributing factor in the failure of any particular cultural group to assimilate the culture of the wider society. Broad exposure to other lifestyles, cultures, environments, and ideas facilitates an understanding and flexibility on the part of an individual when dealing with other people or when solving problems. Feelings of insecurity may also be related to cultural background. For example, psychological adjustment may be difficult for an American Indian who has lived on a reservation and goes to a college where there are few other American Indians. The difficulty in adjustment may be attributable to the fact that this person has lived in an isolated environment that has not assimilated into the mainstream of society. Therefore, health care providers must consider both ethnicity and economic factors when assessing mental health status.

There has been no consistent attack on problems of mental illness around the world. While no continent or island area has been immune from mental illness, the study of mental illness in relation to culture has been restricted and often localized. There may have been a hesitancy to study cultures and mental illness because of possible implications of racism (Griffith & Griffith, 1986). Some authorities cite that psychiatrists have also not seriously discussed the possibility that racism may be a manifestation of an individual psychological disorder (Poussaint, 1975). In any case, research on mental illness from a broad world perspective has been seriously lacking.

Although research, for the most part, is lacking, some interesting cultural data and implications are available in the studies that have been reported. Not only do mental illnesses seem to vary among cultures, but treatment does also. In Japan, psychiatric institutions are small; in the United States, they are large. Societies also have differing demands on individuals emerging from the treatment milieu. Not only do hospitals and treatment milieus differ around the world but also the paths into illness show a different pattern in each culture. Variations in class identity or in the pace of acculturation of class segments may produce differences in deviant types. Similarly, personalities seem to vary among persons from different geographical regions. There is some evidence that the cultural backgrounds and forms of illness vary apart from the question of how these illnesses are treated. For example, stresses placed on a traditional Chinese family are different from those placed on Hindus and Malays (Opler, 1959).

Lawson (1986) reported findings suggesting that racial and ethnic differences exist in the clinical presentations of psychiatric disorders. Significant racial differences have been noted among proposed biological markers for various psychiatric disorders, such as serum creatinine phosphokinase, platelet serotonin, and HLA-A2 determinations. Racial and ethnic differences in response to psychotropic medication, such as higher blood levels of the drugs found among Asians, affect dosage requirements and potential side effects. All these developments underline the importance of considering ethnic and racial factors in caring for psychiatric clients.

In the United States, the incidence of mental illness has been found to vary among certain racial groups. For example, posttraumatic stress disorder (PTSD) has been studied among Vietnam veterans. Because of racism in the military and racial and social upheaval in the United States during the Vietnam War years, as well as limited opportunities for African-Americans in the postwar period, African-American veterans of the Vietnam War often have harbored conflicting feelings about their wartime experiences. African-American veterans have been found to suffer PTSD at a higher rate than White veterans have. Diagnosis and treatment of PTSD in African-Americans are complicated by a tendency to misdiagnose African-American clients; by the varied manifestations of PTSD; by clients' frequent alcohol and drug abuse; and by medical, legal, personality, and vocational problems (Allen, 1986).

Also, in the United States there is evidence that schizophrenia has been consistently overdiagnosed and affective disorders underdiagnosed, particularly in African-Americans and low-socioeconomic groups (Gurland, 1976; Taylor & Abrams, 1978; World Health Organization, 1976). General causes of such misdiagnoses include over-reliance on the classic thought disorder symptoms pathognomonic of schizophrenia and, for affective disorders, lack of clearly defined boundaries between normal and abnormal mood, as well as failure to realize that clients with affective illness can manifest cognitive thought processes. In addition, according to Jones and Gray (1986), misdiagnoses among African-

Americans result from such factors as cultural differences in language and mannerisms, difficulties in relating between African-American clients and White therapists and staff, and the myth that African-Americans rarely suffer from affective disorders. The effects of cultural and racial differences on baseline behaviors and symptoms have thus far received little consistent attention. Research is needed to investigate more closely how the general diagnostic problems in psychiatry affect certain racial groups. Research is also needed on how cultural and racial differences may affect diagnosis. Finally, baseline behaviors and symptoms for racial groups must be established.

Meinhardt and Vega (1987) have reported that most studies of use of mental health services by ethnic groups have used parity as a measure of whether members of ethnic groups are receiving a fair share of services. The level of service is assumed to be adequate if the percentage of ethnic group members in the treatment population is the same as the group's percentage in the general population. However, service planning based on achieving parity fails to consider that some groups may have higher levels of need than others. Equitable care among ethnic and racial groups based on need is another issue that mental health professionals are addressing (López, 1981).

A better understanding of the differences among various cultures in the area of mental health and treatment for mental illness will enable culturally appropriate mental health care. Griffith and Griffith (1986) have pointed out that mental health professionals should give more consideration to the fact that cultural issues such as racism can cause psychological injury. It is evident from the increasing quantities of literature on culture and mental health that there is a growing awareness among health professionals that care for clients with mental problems must be culturally appropriate and that cultural factors do affect mental health. Although rice and tea may not be the most potent tools of modern psychiatry, they may play an important role in making psychiatric care acceptable to the acutely disturbed Asian or Pacific Islander psychiatric client (Lu, 1987). It is important for the nurse to study what is available about the population groups being served and consider the important differences that may be required in the care provided. Not only must nurses appreciate that caring for clients from different cultural groups may require different care methods, but they must also assist other mental health workers in being sensitive to differing care needs.

Domestic Violence

In 1998, more than 900,000 women experienced some type of violent offense at the hand of an intimate (Rennison & Welchans, 2000). This figure may be disproportionately low and actually as high as 1.8 million over the course of 1 year (Heise, Ellsberg, & Gottemoeller, 1999). Other data suggest that the percentage of women who experience dating violence, including sexual assault, physical violence, or verbal or emotional abuse may be as high as 65% of all women (Heise, Ellsberg, & Gottemoeller, 1999). According to the U.S. Department of Justice, Bureau of Justice Statistics (Rennison & Welchans, 2000), *domestic violence* is defined as violent crimes by current or former spouses, boyfriends, and girlfriends. These violent crimes include lethal (homicide) and nonlethal (rape, sexual assault, robbery, aggravated assault, and simple assault) offenses (Rennison & Welchans, 2000). It is interesting to note that the Justice Department failed to mention other types of abuse, such as mental or emotional abuse, harassment, or stalking, all of which need to be factored into the equation to more fully understand the incidence of domestic violence (Rennison & Welchans, 2000). Pampel and Williams (2000) note that researchers who use the Justice Department database must recognize the need to address the problem of missing data. They conclude that missing data are typically the result of the failure to file, inconsistent filing of reports to the FBI by local police agencies, or incomplete records about the characteristics of specific incidents of homicide. They further noted that, in particular, information about the perpetrators of the crimes may be missing even when reports of such crimes are filed, and this contributes significantly to skewed and vastly flawed data in many databases (Pampel & Williams, 2000).

By definition, the term *battering* implies that an individual is either physically or emotionally abused (Campbell, 1989; Flitcraft, 1991; Newman, 1993). Although there are reported cases of "male battering" perpetrated by women, the victims of abuse are women in more than 90% of all reported domestic violence cases (Flitcraft, 1991; Newman, 1993). Although battered women syndrome has been heavily documented in the literature (Campbell, 1989; Chez, 1988; Flitcraft, 1991; Newman, 1993; Pampel & Williams, 2000; Rennison & Welchans, 2000), it has not received the adequate attention it has needed as a social concern until recently. Battered women syndrome moved to the forefront of social concerns with the murders of Nicole Brown Simpson (wife of famed running back O.J. Simpson) and her friend Ronald Goldman. Simpson, who pled "no contest" to "wife-beating" in 1989, was later acquitted of the murder of his ex-wife (Brown Simpson) and her friend (Goldman). However, in the civil trial brought by the estate of Nicole Brown Simpson and the father of Ronald Goldman, Simpson was found liable for the murders of Brown Simpson and Goldman. The plaintiffs were awarded an astounding $33 million. At this writing, Simpson continues to appeal this verdict. Nonetheless, because of Simpson's celebrity status, more attention was focused on battered women syndrome.

One in every three adult women experiences at least one physical assault by a partner during their adult lifetime (American Psychological Association, 2002). In fact, nearly 4 million American women will experience a serious physical assault by an intimate partner during a 12-month window (American Psychological Association, 2002). In addition, it is estimated that some 12 million women (25% of all women) will be abused in their lifetime (Pampel & Williams, 2000). Although it remains largely unknown how frequently domestic violence occurs, it has been suggested that it occurs 10 times more frequently than those statistics reported by the Bureau of Justice. Nonetheless, this report does help identify some very interesting trends (Rennison & Welchans, 2000). In addition, the data suggest that there is a difference by race and ethnicity regarding the frequency of domestic violence. For example, Black women and their male counterparts have the highest rate of domestic violence. In fact, Black women experience domestic violence at a rate 35% higher than their White counterparts and 22 times higher than that of women of all other races (Rennison & Welchans, 2000). Domestic violence also appears to be prevalent among women 18 to 24 years of age (Rennison & Welchans, 2000). Additionally, women of lower socio-economic status are significantly more likely to experience domestic violence (Rennison & Welchans, 2000).

In the majority of cases involving "woman battering," the assailants were usually an intimate who was a family member, spouse, or boyfriend. The phenomenon of battered women syndrome has become so widespread that it is believed to be the leading cause of injury among women in the United States (Rennison & Welchans, 2000). Battering accounts for one in every five visits to the hospital emergency room by women in this country (Rennison & Welchans, 2000).

The incidence of battering may have a direct relationship to other violent crimes committed against women, such as rape and homicide. Homicide is the eleventh leading cause of death in the United States (National Center for Health Statistics, Health, United States, 2006). In fact, it is estimated that one of every six homicides in this country involves a family member (U.S. Department of Health and Human Services, 2002). Of the murders of women committed in the United States, about half are committed by a spouse. While the number of people who were murdered by an intimate partner was down from the high in 1976 of 1600 women and 1357 men to 1219 women and 424 men in 1999, the number is still alarming. In addition, about one third of all murdered females are likely to have been killed by intimates, as compared with 4% of male murder victims (Rennison & Welchans, 2000). Although most homicide statistics, by race, are only presented by White or Black racial categories, the data available suggest that homicides of women by intimates are declining. For White women, the number of homicides by an intimate declined from a high of 1600 women in 1976 to a low of 812 women in 1999. Similarly, the homicides of Black women declined from 714 murdered by an intimate in 1976 to a low of 338 women in 1999 (Rennison & Welchans, 2000).

Between 1973 and 1994, approximately 155,000, or 1 in every 600, women were raped. Like the number of actual domestic violence cases, this number is greatly underestimated because 53% of women fail to report a rape (Strickland & Giger, 1994). The incidence of rape varies with race and ethnicity. Women who are raped are likely to be African-American women who have been raped by African-American men. Of the number of rapes, 65% occur at night (between the hours of 8 P.M. and 4 A.M.), 43% occur near the victim's home, and 15% occur at a friend's house. Although a greater number of women report "stranger rape," the incidence of acquaintance rape (date rape) and domestic violence rape is greatly underreported.

Case Study

Sarah Jennings is a 21-year-old African-American married woman and the mother of a 12-month-old daughter. Mrs. Jennings was diagnosed at age 11 as having sickle cell anemia. For the last 3 years, she has remained largely asymptomatic. She is admitted to the hospital in sickle cell crisis. Her admitting complaints include severe joint pains in both the upper and lower extremities, a temperature of 101.8 °F, and shortness of breath. On physical examination, the nurse notes that Mrs. Jennings has coarse rales in the base of both lungs and that her lips are cyanotic and dry. Her nail beds are also cyanotic, and when they are blanched, capillary refill is slow. Initial laboratory examination reveals a hemoglobin level of 8 g/dL. During the nursing history, it is revealed that Mrs. Jennings has also had problems drinking milk and eating certain dairy products for most of her adult life.

✳ STUDY QUESTIONS

1. List at least two contributing factors for Mrs. Jennings's sickle cell anemia that relate to biological variations by race and ethnic heritage.
2. List at least one other racial group with a predisposition for sickle cell crisis.
3. List the basic causes of sickle cell anemia.
4. List at least two other conditions that Mrs. Jennings could be at risk for developing because of her race and ethnic heritage.
5. Describe at least two differences noted when the nurse is assessing the skin color of dark-skinned individuals.

NCLEX-RN REVIEW QUESTIONS

1. Blood groups are said to differentiate people in different racial groups. You have a 29-year-old American Indian client admitted to your unit with diabetes. Based on what you know about American Indians, you might expect your patient's blood type to be which of the following:
   A. Type A
   B. Type B
   C. Type AB
   D. Type O

2. To make a correct nursing diagnosis regarding a rash on a patient, the nurse should

   A. Become familiar with the patient's normal coloring to establish a baseline.
   B. Assess the skin in artificial lighting, not in sunlight.
   C. Assess darkly pigmented areas first, as it is less difficult to note color changes there.
   D. Assess lightly pigmented areas first, as it is less difficult to note color changes there.

3. Mongolian spots are a common finding in which of these groups? Mark all that apply.
   A. Black Americans
   B. White Americans
   C. Asian Americans
   D. American Indians

References

Adams, J. M. (1932). Some racial differences in blood pressures and morbidity in groups of white and colored workmen. *American Journal of Medical Science,* 184, 342–350.

Allen, I. (1986). Posttraumatic stress disorder among Black Vietnam veterans. *Hospital and Community Psychiatry,* 37(1), 55–60.

ALLHAT Officers and Coordinators for the ALLHAT Collaborative Research Group. (2002a). Major outcomes in high-risk hypertensive patients randomized to angiotensin-converting enzyme inhibitor or calcium channel blocker vs. diuretic. *Journal of the American Medical Association,* 288, 2981–2997.

ALLHAT Officers and Coordinators for the ALLHAT Collaborative Research Group. (2002a). Major outcomes in moderately hypercholesterolemic, hypertensive patients randomized to pravastatin vs. usual care. *Journal of the American Medical Association,* 288, 2998–3007.

American Diabetic Association. (2005). *Vital statistics.* Alexandria, Va: American Diabetic Association.

American Psychological Association. (2002). *Facts about family.* Retrieved January 7, 2002, at www.apa.org.

Appel, S., Giger, J. N., & Davidhizar, R. (2005). Opportunity cost: the impact of contextual risk factors on the cardiovascular health on low income southern African American women. *Journal of Cardiovascular Nursing,* 20(50), 315–324.

Atrash, H., & Hunter, M. (2006). Health disparities in the United States: a continuing challenge. In Satcher, D., & Pamies, R. Multicultural medicine and health disparities. New York, McGraw-Hill.

Ayanian, J. Z., Weissman, J. S., Chasan-Taber, S. et al (1999). Quality of care by race and gender for congestive heart failure and pneumonia. *Medical Care,* 37 (12), 1260–1269.

Barker-Cummings, C., McClellan, W., Soucie, J. M. et al (1995). Ethnic differences in the use of peritoneal dialysis as initial treatment for end-stage renal disease. *Journal of the American Medical Association*, 274, 1858–1862.

Barna, P. (1985). Food or drug? The case of ginseng. *Lancet*, 2, 548.

Bayless, T. (1975). Lactose and milk intolerance: clinical implications. *New England Journal of Medicine*, 292 (5), 1156–1159.

Bennett, K. A., Osborne, R. H., & Miller, R. J. (1975). *Biocultural ecology: annual review of anthropology.* Palo Alto, Calif: Annual Reviews.

Boyle, E. (1970). Biological patterns in hypertension by race, sex, body weight, and skin color. *Journal of the American Medical Association*, 213, 1637–1643.

Braithwaite, R., & Taylor, S. (2002). *Health issues in the Black community* (ed. 2) San Francisco: Jossey-Bass.

Branch, M., & Paxton, P. (1976). *Providing safe nursing care for ethnic people of color.* New York: Appleton-Century-Crofts.

Brues, A. M. (1977). *People and race.* New York: Macmillan Publishing Co (Reprinted 1990. Prospect Heights, Ill.: Waveland Press.).

Bulmer, M. (1970). *The biology of twinning in man.* Oxford: Clarendon.

Burns, E., & Neubort, S. (1984). Sodium content of koshered meat [letter]. *Journal of the American Medical Association*, 252(21), 2960.

Burt, C. (1966). The genetic determination of difference in intelligence: a study of monozygote twins reared together and apart. *British Journal of Psychology*, 57, 137–153.

Burt, V. L., Cutler, J. A., Higgins, M. et al (1995). Trends in the prevalence, awareness, treatment, and control of hypertension in the adult U.S. population. *Radiology*, 26(1), 60–69.

Campbell, J. (1989). A test of two exploratory models of women's response to battering. *Nursing Research*, 38 (1), 18–24.

Carter Center of Emory University (1985). Closing the gap: the problem of diabetes mellitus in the United States. *Diabetes Care*, 8, 391–401.

Centers for Disease Control and Prevention. (1991). Nosocomial transmission of multi-drug resistant tuberculosis among HIV-infected persons—Florida and New York, 1988–1991. *Morbidity and Mortality Weekly Report*, 40(34), 585–591.

Centers for Disease Control and Prevention. (1992). Recommendations of the Advisory Council for the reduction of hypertension among minority populations. *Morbidity and Mortality Weekly Report*, 40, 1–7.

Centers for Disease Control. (2001). *Tuberculosis surveillance report*, 13(2). Atlanta, Ga.: U.S. Department of Health and Human Services.

Centers for Disease Control and Prevention. (2002). *Diabetes surveillance report, 2001.* Atlanta, Ga: U.S. Department of Health and Human Services.

Centers for Disease Control and Prevention. (2005). *HIV/AIDS surveillance report: U.S. HIV and AIDS cases reported through December 2004,* (17 Atlanta, Ga: U.S. Department of Health and Human Services.

Chan, A. W. (1986). Racial differences in alcohol sensitivity. *Alcohol & Alcoholism*, 21(1), 93–104.

Chang, B. (1974). Some dietary beliefs in Chinese folk culture. *Journal of the American Diet Association*, 65(4), 436.

Chen, W., Bao, W., Begum, S. et al (2000). Age-related patterns of the clustering of cardiovascular risk variables of metabolic syndrome (syndrome X) from childhood to young adulthood in a population made up of black and white subjects. *Diabetes*, 49, 1042–1048.

Chez, R. (1988). Woman battering. *American Journal of Obstetrics and Gynecology*, 156, 1–4.

Chin, M., Zhang, J., & Merrell, K. (1998). Diabetes in the African-American Medicare population: morbidity, quality of care, and resource utilization. *Diabetes Care*, 21(7), 1090–1095.

Collins, F. (1997). Sequencing the human genome. *Hospital Practice*, 32(1), 35–55.

Cowie, C., & Harris, M. (1997). Ambulatory medical care for non-Hispanic Whites, African-Americans and Mexican-Americans with NIDDM in the U.S. *Diabetes Care*, 20(2), 142–147.

Crawford, P., Story, M., Wang, M., Ritchie, L., & Sabry, Z. (2001). Ethnic issues in the epidemiology of childhood obesity. *Pediatric Clinics of North America*, 48(4), 855–878.

Cummings, S., Kelsey, J., Nevitt, N., & O'Dowd, K. (1985). Epidemiology of osteoporosis and osteoporotic fractures. *Epidemiology Review*, 7, 178–208.

Czlraky, M. (2002, September). BHBPEP: working to reduce death and disability from high blood pressure. *Journal of the American Pharmaceutical Association*, 4296, 886–888.

Dalman, P. R., Bar, G. D., & Allen, C. M. (1978). Hemoglobin concentration in White, Black and Oriental children: is there a need for separate criteria in screening for anemia? *American Journal of Clinical Nutrition*, 31(3), 377.

Davis, S., Northington, L., & Kolar, K. (2000). Cultural considerations for treatment of childhood obesity. *Journal of Cultural Diversity*, 7(4), 128–132.

Divan, D. (1989). Letter to the editor. *New England Journal of Medicine*, 321(4), 259.

Echizen, H., Horai, Y., & Ishizaki, T. (1989). Letter to the editor. *New England Journal of Medicine*, 321(4), 258.

Farb, P., & Armelagos, G. (1980). *Consuming passions: the anthropology of eating*. Boston: Houghton Mifflin.

Flitcraft, A. (1991). Domestic abuse: diagnosing, treating, and understanding its victims. *Clinical Nurse Practitioner*, 9(2), 3–5.

Freis, E. (1986). Antihypertensive agents. In Kalow, W., Goedde, H. W., & Agarwal, D. (Eds.), *Ethnic differences in reactions to drugs and xenobiotics*. New York: Liss.

Gaitz, C., & Scott, J. (1974). Mental health of Mexican Americans: do ethnic factors make a difference? *Geriatrics*, 1(11), 110–113.

Garn, S., Nagy, A., & Sandusky, S. (1972). Differential sex dimorphism in bone diameters of subjects of European and African ancestry. *American Journal of Anthropology*, 37, 127–130.

Garn, S., Ryan, A., & Abraham, S. (1980). The Black-White difference in hemoglobin levels after age, sex, and income matching. *Ecology of Food Nutrition*, 10 (2), 69.

Garn, S., Sullivan, T., & Hawthorne, V. (1989). Educational level, fatness, and fatness differences between husbands and wives. *American Journal of Clinical Nutrition*, 50, 535.

Giger, J., Davidhizar, R., & Wieczorek, S. (1993). Culture and ethnicity. In Bobak, I., & Jensen, M. (Eds.), *Maternity and gynecologic care* (ed. 5) (pp. 43–67). St. Louis: Mosby.

Giger, J., Richardson, J., & Jones, D. (2002). African American children: a precious commodity at risk [editorial]. *Journal of National Black Nurses Association*, 13 (1), vii–viii.

Gilsanz, V., Roe, T., Mora, S. et al (1991). Changes in vertebral bone density in black girls and white girls during childhood and puberty. *New England Journal of Medicine*, 325(23), 1597–1600.

Ginseng (1980). Medical Letter Drugs. *Therapy*, 22(17), 72.

Glazer, W. M., Morgenstern, H., & Doucette, J. T. (1993). Predicting the long-term risk of tardive dyskinesia in outpatients maintained on neuroleptic medications. *Journal of Clinical Psychiatry*, 54(4), 133–139.

Glazer, W. M., Morgenstern, H., & Doucette, J. T. (1994). Race and tardive dyskinesia among outpatients at a CMHC. *Hospital and Community Psychiatry*, 45 (1), 38–45.

Goedde, H. W. (1983). Population genetic studies on aldehyde dehydrogenase isoenzyme deficiency and alcohol sensitivity. *American Journal of Human Genetics*, 35, 769.

Goedde, H. W. (1986). Ethnic differences in reactions to drugs and other xenobiotics: outlook of a geneticist. In Kalow, W., Goedde, H. W., & Agarwal, D. (Eds.), *Ethnic differences in reactions to drugs and xenobiotics* (pp. 9–20). New York: Liss.

Goldman, D. R. (1985). Hold the sushi [letter]. *Journal of the American Medical Association*, 253(17), 2495.

Gorden, A. M. (1982). Nutritional status of Cuban refugees: a field study on the health and nutrition of refugees processed at Opa-Locka, Florida. *American Journal of Clinical Nutrition*, 35(3), 582.

Grant, D., Tang, B. K., & Kalow, W. (1983). Variability in caffeine metabolism. *Clinical Pharmacology Therapy*, 33, 591–602.

Greaves, K., Puhl, J., Baranowski, T. et al (1989). Ethnic differences in anthropometrics characteristics and their parents. *Human Biology*, 61(3), 459.

Griffith, E., & Griffith, E. (1986). Racism, psychological injury, and compensatory damages. *Hospital and Community Psychiatry*, 37(1), 71–75.

Gurland, B. (1976). Aims, organization, and initial studies of the cross-national project. *International Journal of Aging and Human Development*, 7, 283–293.

Haffner, S. M., Stern, M. P., Hazuda, H. P. et al (1986). Upper body and centralized adiposity in Mexican Americans and non-Hispanic Whites: relationship to body mass index and other behavioral and demographic variables. *International Journal of Obesity*, 10, 493.

Halsted, J. A. (1968). Geophagia in man: its nature and nutritional effects. *American Journal of Clinical Nutrition*, 21(12), 1384.

Harper, P. (1993). *Practical genetic counseling*, (ed. 4) Oxford, England: Butterworth-Heinemann.

Heise, L., Ellsberg, M., & Gottemoeller, M. (1999). *Ending violence against women*. Population reports, series L, no. 11, Baltimore: Johns Hopkins University School of Public Health, Population Information Program.

Holmes, T. H. et al (1957). Psychosocial and psychophysiological studies of tuberculosis. *Psychosomatic Medicine*, 19, 134–143.

Interdepartmental Commission on National Defense and Division of Indian Public Health (ICND & DIPH). (1964). *Fort Belknap Indian Reservation: nutrition survey*. Washington, D.C.: U.S. Public Health Service.

Jackson, R. T., Sauberlich, H. S., Skala, J. H. et al (1983). Comparison of hemoglobin values in Black and White male U.S. military personnel. *Journal of Nutrition,* 113(1), 165.

Jarvis, A. (1972). Minor orofacial abnormalities in an Eskimo population. *Oral Surgery,* 33, 417–427.

Jensen, A. R. (1969). How much can we boost IQ and scholastic achievement? *Harvard Education Review,* 29, 1.

Jensen, A. R. (1974). Cumulative deficits: a testable hypothesis? *Developmental Psychology,* 10, 996.

Jensen, A. R. (1977). Cumulative deficit in IQ of Blacks in the rural South. *Developmental Psychology,* 13, 184.

Jick, H., Slone, D., Westerhom, B. et al (1969). Venous thromboembolic disease and ABO blood type. *Lancet,* 1, 539–542.

Joint National Committee. (1997). *The report of the Joint National Committee on Detection, Evaluation and Treatment of High Blood Pressure.* Washington, D.C.: National Institutes of Health, National Heart, Lung, and Blood Institute.

Jones, B., & Gray, B. (1986). Problems in diagnosing schizophrenia and affective disorders among Blacks. *Hospital and Community Psychiatry,* 37(1), 61–65.

Kalow, W. (1972). Pharmacogenetics of drugs used in anesthesia. *Human Genetics,* 60, 415–427.

Kalow, W. (1982). The metabolism of xenobiotics in different populations. *Canadian Journal of Physiological Pharmacology,* 60, 1–19.

Kalow, W. (1986). Outlook of a pharmacologist. In Kalow, W., Goedde, H., & Agarwal, D. (Eds.), *Ethnic differences in reactions to drugs and xenobiotics.* New York: Liss.

Kalow, W. (1989). Race and therapeutic drug response. *New England Journal of Medicine,* 320(9), 588–589.

Kamlin, L. J. (1974). *The science and politics of IQ.* New York: Halstead Press.

Kasiske, B. (1998). Race and socio-economic factors influencing early placement on the kidney transplant waiting list. *Journal of the American Society of Nephrologists,* 9(11), 2142–2147.

Katz, S. H., Hediger, M. L., & Valleroy, L. A. (1974). Traditional maize processing techniques in the New World. *Science,* 184, 765.

Keil, J. (1981). Skin color and education effects on blood pressure. *American Journal of Public Health,* 71, 532–534.

Keltner, N. (1994, October) Personal communication to J.N. Giger.

Keltner, N., & Folks, G. (1992). Psychopharmacology update: culture as a variable in drug therapy. *Perspectives in Psychiatric Nursing,* 28(1), 33–35.

Kisch, B. (1953). Salt poor diet and Jewish dietary laws. *Journal of the American Medical Association,* 153(16), 1472.

Klag, M., Whelton, P., Coresh, J. et al (1991). The association of skin color with blood pressure in U.S. blacks with low socioeconomic status *Journal of the American Medical Association,* 265(5), 599–602.

Krolewski, A., & Warram, G. (2005). Epidemiology of diabetes mellitus. In Joslin, E. P. (Ed.). *Joslin's diabetes mellitus* (ed. 14). Philadelphia: Lippincott Williams & Wilkins.

Kudzma, E. (1992, December) Drug responses: all bodies are not created equal. *American Journal of Nursing,* 92, 48–50.

Kuh, D. L., Power, C., & Rodgers, B. (1991). Secular trends in social class and sex differences in adult height. *International Journal of Epidemiology,* 20(4), 1001–1009.

Laor, A., Seidman, D., & Danon, Y. L. (1991). Changes in body height among selected ethnic groups. *Journal of Epidemiology and Community Health,* 45(2), 169–170.

Lawson, W. (1986). Racial and ethnic factors in psychiatric research. *Hospital and Community Psychiatry,* 37 (1), 50–54.

Leffall, L. D. (1974). Cancer mortality among Blacks. *CA: A Cancer Journal for Clinicians,* 24, 42–46.

Lefley, H. (1990). Culture and chronic mental illness. *Hospital and Community Psychiatry,* 41, 277.

Leininger, M. (1970). *Nursing and anthropology: two worlds to blend.* New York: John Wiley & Sons.

Lerner, D., & Kannel, W. (1986). Patterns of coronary heart disease morbidity and mortality in the sexes: a 26-year follow-up of the Framingham population. *American Heart Journal,* 11, 383–390.

Lewis, J. H. (1942). The biology of the Negro *(Chicago University Monographs in Medicine).* Chicago: University of Chicago Press.

Lewis, R. (2007). *Human genetics: concepts and applications* (ed. 7). Boston: McGraw-Hill Higher Education.

Li, J., Specker, B., Ho, B., & Tsang, R. (1989). Bone mineral content in Black and White children 1 to 6 years of age: early appearance of race and sex differences. *American Journal of Disorders in Children,* 143, 1346–1349.

Lin, K. M., Lau, J. K., Smith, R. et al (1988). Comparison of alprazolam plasma levels in normal Asians and Caucasian male volunteers. *Psychopharmacology,* 96, 365–369.

Lindquist, C., Reynolds, K., & Goran, M. (1999). Sociocultural determinants of physical activity among children. *Preventive Medicine,* 29(4), 305–312.

López, S. (1981). Mexican Americans' usage of mental health facilities: underutilization reconsidered. In Baron, A. (Ed.). *Explorations in Chicano psychology.* New York: Praeger.

Lorton, J., & Lorton, E. (1984). *Human development through the life span.* Belmont, Calif: Brooks/Cole.

Lu, F. (1987). Culturally relevant inpatient care for minority and ethnic patients. *Hospital and Community Psychiatry*, 38(11), 1126–1127.

Luzzato, L. (1986). Glucose-6-phosphate dehydrogenase and other genetic factors interacting with drugs. *Progress in Clinical and Biological Research*, 214, 385.

Maras, M. L., & Adolphi, C. L. (1985). Ethnic tailoring improves dietary compliance. *Diabetes Education*, 11 (4), 47.

Matthews, D., Hosker, J. P., Rudenski, A. et al (1985). Homeostasis and assessment: insulin resistance and beta-cell function from fasting plasma glucose and insulin concentrations in man. *Diabetologia*, 28, 412–429.

Meinhardt, K., & Vega, W. (1987). A method of estimating underutilization of mental health services by ethnic groups. *Hospital and Community Psychiatry*, 38(11), 1186–1190.

Melton, L., & Riggs, B. (2000). Epidemiology of age-related fractures. In Avioli, L. (Ed.). *The osteoporotic syndrome: detection, prevention, and treatment* (ed. 4). San Diego, Calif: Academic Press.

Merck, Sharp, & Dohme Inc. (1974). *Hypertension handbook for clinicians.* Westpoint, Pa: Merck, Sharp, & Dohme Inc.

Miller, M. B. (1981). Supplementing and adding variety to the diets of Indians on a reservation in Minnesota. *Journal of the American Dietetic Association*, 78(6), 626.

Mirsa, D. (2002). *Women's health data book: a profile of women's health in the United States* (ed. 3) (pp. 51–100). Washington, D.C.: Jacob's Institute of Women's Health and the Henry J. Kaiser Family Foundation.

Morse, D. L., Guzewich, J. J., & Hanrahan, J. P. (1986). Widespread outbreaks of clam- and oyster-associated gastroenteritis. *New England Journal of Medicine*, 314 (11), 678.

Moser, M., & Lunn, J. (1982). Responses to captopril and hydrochlorothiazide in black patients with hypertension. *Clinical Pharmacology Therapy*, 32, 307–312.

Nagulesparan, M., Savage, P. J., & Knowler, W. C. (1982). Increased in vivo insulin resistance in nondiabetic Pima Indians compared with Caucasians. *Diabetes*, 31(11), 952.

Najjar, M. (1987). *Anthropometrics reference data and prevalence of overweight, United States 1976–1980.* Vital and Health Statistics Series II, No. 2380.

National Center for Health Statistics. (2006). *Health, United States, 2006 with chartbook on trends in the health of Americans.* Hyattsville, Md.: National Center for Health Statistics.

National Institutes of Health (US). (2002). Strategic plan for addressing health disparities for fiscal years 2002–2006. Available at: http://www.niaid.nih.gov/healthdisparities/NIAD_HD_Plan_Final.pdf.

Newman, K. (1993). Giving up: shelter experience of battered women. *Public Health Nursing*, 10(2), 108–113.

Ogden, C. L., Carroll, M. D., Curtin, L. R., McDowell, M. A., Tabak, C. J., & Flegel, K. M. (2006, April). Prevalence of overweight and obesity in the United States, 1999–2004. *JAMA*, 295(13), 1549–1555.

Opler, M. (Ed) (1959). *Culture and mental health.* New York: Macmillan.

Ortiz, O., Russell, M., Daley, T. L. et al (1992). Differences in skeletal muscle and bone mineral mass between Black and White females and their relevance to estimates of body composition. *American Journal of Clinical Nutrition*, 55(1), 8–13.

Overfield, T. (1977). Biological variations. *Nursing Clinics of North America*, 12(1), 19–27.

Overfield, T. (1995). *Biologic variation in health and illness: race, age and sex differences*, (ed. 2) Boca Raton, Fla: CRC Press.

Owens, G. M., Garry, P. J., Seymore, R. D. et al (1981). Nutrition studies with White Mountain Apache preschool children in 1976 and 1969. *American Journal of Clinical Nutrition*, 34(2), 266.

Pampel, F., & Williams, K. (2000). Intimacy and homicide: compensating for missing data in the SHR. *Criminology*, 32(2), 661–680.

Pangborn, R. M. (1975). Cross-cultural aspects of flavor preferences. *Food Technology*, 29(6), 34.

Parker, S. L., & Bowering, J. (1976). Folacin in diets of Puerto Ricans and Black women in relation to food practices. *Journal of Nutrition Education*, 8(2), 73.

Phipps, W. (1993). The patient with pulmonary problems. In Long, B. C., Phipps, W. J., & Cassmeyer, V. (Eds.), *Medical surgical nursing: concepts and clinical practice* (ed. 4) St. Louis: Mosby–Year Book.

Platt, O., Brambilla, D., Rosse, W. et al (1994). Mortality in sickle cell disease: life expectancy and risk factors for early death. *New England Journal of Medicine*, 330 (23), 1639–1644.

Polednak, A. P. (1971). Connective tissue responses in Negroes in relation to disease. *American Journal of Physical Anthropology*, 41, 49–57.

Pollitzer, W., & Anderson, J. (1990). Ethnic and genetic differences in bone mass: a review with a hereditary vs. environmental perspective. *American Journal of Clinical Nutrition*, 52, 181.

Poussaint, A. F. (1975). Interracial relations. In Freedman, A. M., Kaplan, H. I., & Sandock, B. J. (Eds.), *Comprehensive textbook of psychiatry* (vol. 2. Baltimore: Williams & Wilkins.

Qureshi, B. A. (1981). Nutrition and multi-ethnic groups. *Royal Social Health Journal*, 101(5), 187.

Reid, I. R., Cullen, S., Schooler, B. A. et al (1990). Calcitropic hormone levels in Polynesians: evidence against their role in interracial differences in bone mass. *Journal of Endocrinology Metabolism*, 70(5), 1452–1466.

Rennison, H., & Rifkin, W. (1984). *The physician's guide to type II diabetes (NIDDM): diagnosis and treatment.* New York: The American Diabetes Association.

Rennison, M., & Welchans, W. (2000). *Intimate partner violence* (NCJ178247, revised 1/14/00). Washington, D.C.: U.S. Department of Justice, Office of Justice Programs, Bureau of Justice Statistics.

Riggs, S. (1980). Tastes of America. *Regionality Institutions*, 87(12), 76.

Roccella, E. J., & Lenfant, C. (1989). Regional and racial differences among stroke victims in the United States. *Clinical Cardiology*, 12(4), 1213–1220.

Rodnan, G. P., & Schumacher, H. R. (1983). *Primer on the rheumatic diseases* (ed. 8). Atlanta, Ga.: Arthritis Foundation.

Rouch, L. (1977). Color changes in dark skin. *Nursing*, 7 (1), 48–51.

Saito, S., Okui, K., Tokino, T. et al (1992). Isolation and mapping of 68 RFLP markers on human chromosome 6. *American Journal of Human Genetics*, 50(1), 65–70.

Saldana, G., & Brown, H. E. (1984). Nutritional composition of corn and flour tortillas. *Journal of Food Science*, 49(4), 202.

Satcher, D., & Pope, L. (1974). *Emergency evaluation and management of persons with sickle cell disease.* Bethesda, Md.: National Institutes of Health.

Satcher, D. et al (1973). *Sickle cell counseling: a committee's study and recommendations.* New York: National Foundation–March of Dimes.

Saunders, E. (1985). Special techniques for management of hypertension in Blacks. In Hall, W. D., Saunders, E., & Shulman, N. B. (Eds.), *Hypertension in blacks: epidemiology, pathophysiology, and treatment* (pp. 209–236). St. Louis: Mosby.

Schwerin, H. S., Stanton, J. L., & Smith, J. L. (1982). Food, eating habits, and health: a further examination of the relationships between food eating patterns and nutritional health. *American Clinical Nutrition*, 35(suppl. 5), 1319.

Siegel, R. K. (1979). Ginseng abuse syndrome: problems with the panacea. *Journal of the American Medical Association*, 24(15), 614.

Smedley, B., Stith, A., & Nelson, A. (2003). *Unequal treatment: confronting racial and ethnic disparities in health care.* Institute of Medicine, Washington, D.C.: National Academy Press.

Srinivasan, S., Myers, L., & Berenson, G. (2002). Predictability of childhood adiposity and insulin for developing insulin resistance syndrome (metabolic syndrome [syndrome X]) in young adulthood: The Bogalusa Heart Study. *Diabetes*, 51, 204–209.

State of Maryland demonstration of statewide coordination for the control of high blood pressure (1977–1983, October). (1977). *National Heart, Lung, and Blood Institute Contract No. 1-HV-2986.*

Stewart, S. H. (2002). Racial and ethnic differences in alcohol-associated aspartate amiotransferase and gamma-glutamyltransferase elevation. *Archives of Internal Medicine*, 162(19), 2236–2239.

Stokes, J., Kannel, W., Wolf, P. et al (1987). The relative importance of selected risk factors for various manifestations of cardiovascular disease among men and women from 35 to 64 years old: 30 years of follow-up in the Framingham study. *Circulation*, 75(6), 65–73.

Strauss, R., & Pollack, H. (2001). Epidemic increase in childhood overweight, 1986–1998. *Journal of the American Medical Association*, 286(22), 2845–2848.

Strickland, O., & Giger, J. (1994). Women's health in the decade of the woman. In Strickland, O., & Fishman, D. (Eds.), *Nursing issues in the 1990s* (pp. 362–400). Albany, N. Y.: Delmar.

Surgeon General. (1987, April). *Speech to the media and the nation on AIDS.*

Taylor, M. A., & Abrams, B. (1978). The prevalence of schizophrenia: a reassessment using modern diagnostic criteria. *American Journal of Psychiatry*, 135, 945–948.

Thompson, M., McInnes, R., & Willard, H. (1991). *Thompson and Thompson genetics in medicine*, (ed. 5) Philadelphia: WB Saunders.

Tipton, D. (1974). Physiological assessment of Black people. *Care of black patients* (X428.1), A group of papers presented at a conference on care of the Black patient, sponsored by Continuing Education in Nursing, University of California, San Francisco.

Todd, K. H., Deaton, C., D'adamo, AP. et al (2000). Ethnicity and analgesic practice. *Annals of Emergency Medicine*, 35(1), 11–16.

U.S. Department of Health and Human Services, Healthy People 2000. (2002). *National health promotion and disease prevention objectives.* (DHHS Publication No. PHS 91-50212). Washington, D.C.: U.S.Government Printing Office.

U.S. Department of Health and Human Services. (2000). *Healthy People 2010: Understanding and improving health*, (ed.2). Washington, D.C.: U.S. Government Printing Office.

Valassi, K. V. (1962). Food habits of Greek Americans. *American Journal of Nursing*, 11(3), 240.

Vessell, E. S. (1972). Therapy—pharmacogenetics. *New England Journal of Medicine*, 287(18), 904–909.

Walsh, E. (1993). The patient with peripheral vascular problems. In Long, E., Phipps, B. C., & Cassmeyer, W. J. (Eds.), *Medical surgical nursing: concepts and clinical practice* (ed. 4) St. Louis: Mosby—Year Book.

Weber, W. (1999). Population and genetic polymorphisms. *Molecular Diagnosis*, 4(4), 299–307.

Westfall, D. (1974, November). Diabetes mellitus among the Florida Seminoles. *HSMHA Health Reports*, 86, 1037–1041.

When patients can't drink milk. (1976, August). *Nursing Update*, (pp. 10–12).

Williams, R. A. (Ed.) (1975). *Textbook of Black-related disease*. New York: McGraw-Hill.

Witcop, E. et al (1963). Oral and genetic studies of Chileans, 1960: 1. oral anomalies. *American Journal of Physical Anthropology*, 21, 15–24.

World Health Organization. (1975). *Schizophrenia: a multinational study*. Geneva: World Health Organization Press.

Wyngaarden, J. B., & Smith, L. H. (1992). *Cecil textbook of medicine* (ed. 19). Philadelphia: W.B. Saunders.

Yonkers, K. A., Kando, J. C., Cole, J. O., & Blumenthal, S. (1992). Gender differences in pharmacokinetics and pharmacodynamics of psychotropic medication. *American Journal of Psychiatry*, 149(5), 587–595.

Zhou, H. H., Koshakji, R. P., Silberstein, D. J. et al (1989). Racial differences in drug response: altered sensitivity to and clearance of propranolol in men of Chinese descent as compared with American Whites. *New England Journal of Medicine*, 320, 565–570.

Zifferblatt, S. M., Wilbur, C. S., & Pinsky, J. L. (1980). Understanding food habits. *Journal of American Diet Association*, 76(1), 9.

Application of Assessment and Intervention Techniques to Specific Cultural Groups

CHAPTER 8 African-Americans

Brenda Cherry and Joyce Newman Giger

Behavioral Objectives

After reading this chapter, the nurse will be able to:

1. Identify ways in which the African-American culture influences African-American individuals and their health-seeking behaviors.
2. Recognize the need for an in-depth understanding of variables that are common within and across cultural groups to provide culturally appropriate nursing care when working with African-Americans.
3. Recognize physical and biological variances that exist within and across African-

American groups to provide culturally appropriate nursing care.
4. Develop a sensitivity and an understanding for communication differences evidenced within and across African-American groups to avoid stereotyping and to provide culturally appropriate nursing care.
5. Develop a sensitivity and an understanding for psychological phenomena that influence the functioning of an African-American when providing nursing care.

In a time when people are seeking to become more culturally aware, it is important to note distinctions in terminology regarding cultural groups. This is certainly true of African-Americans. Some African-American individuals and groups are encouraging the use of the term *Black Americans*, whereas others are encouraging the use of the term *African-Americans*. The term *African-Americans* is used to refer to a cultural heritage that is a combination of African and American. On the other hand, the term *Black Americans* is believed to place more focus on biological racial identity than on cultural heritage. The term *African-Americans* is used in this book except in instances where its descriptive characteristic is inappropriate, for example, Black skin, Black race, non-Black, Black English, and Black dialect. We have chosen this term because it is now commonly used in the literature.

OVERVIEW OF AFRICAN-AMERICANS

According to the U.S. Census Bureau, there are approximately 37, 908,341 African-Americans residing in the United States, representing approximately 12.9% of the American population (*Time Almanac with Information Please*, 2007; U.S. Department of Commerce, Bureau of the Census, Summary File 1, 2000). Of the number of African-Americans residing in this country, 54.8% live in the South, 18.8% live in the Midwest, 17.6% live in the Northeast, and 8.8% live in the West (U.S. Department of Commerce, Bureau of the Census, Summary File 1). Although African-Americans live throughout the United States, the states with the greatest number of African-Americans are New York (3,234,165), California (2,513,041), Texas (2,493,057), Florida (2,471,730), and Georgia (2,303,425) (U.S. Department of Commerce, Bureau of the Census, Summary File 1).

The cities with the most African-Americans are metropolitan New York City (2,129,762), Chicago (1,065,000), Detroit (775,772), Philadelphia (655,824), Houston (494,496), Baltimore (418,951), Los Angeles (415,195), Memphis (399,208), and New Orleans (325,947) (U.S. Department of Commerce, Bureau of the Census, Summary File 1; U.S. Department of Commerce, Bureau of the Census, Census 2000 Brief, 2000).

In 2002, African-Americans represented more than 50% of the total population in 10 U.S. cities: Gary, Indiana (84.0%); Detroit (82.8%); Birmingham, Alabama (73.5%); Jackson, Mississippi (70.6%); New Orleans (67.3%); Baltimore (64.3%); Atlanta (61.4%); Memphis (61.4%); Washington, D.C. (60.0%); and Richmond, Virginia (57.2%) (U.S. Department of Commerce, Bureau of the Census, Census 2003 Brief).

The median age of African-Americans residing in the United States is 30.2 years, compared with 35.3 years for the rest of the general population (U.S. Department of Commerce, Bureau of the Census, Summary File 1, 2000). This age is up from 29.2 years of age in 1990. African-American men have a lower mean age than African-American women (28.2 versus 31.7 years). In 2002, only 8.2% of African-Americans were 65 years of age or older, compared with 14% of their White counterparts and 13% of the rest of the general population. The number of African-Americans 65 years of age or older was 2.5 million in 1990 (up from 2.1 million in 1980). It is interesting to note that in 2002 African-American women dominated the older age groups (62% compared with 38% for their male counterparts). It is believed that the disproportionately low number of African-American males 65 years of age or older is a result of the higher mortality for African-American males (U.S. Department of Commerce, Bureau of the Census, Summary File 1, 2000; U.S. Department of Commerce, Bureau of the Census, The Older Population, 2000, 2001.)

In 2000, 77.0% of African-Americans 25 years of age or older held at least a high school diploma, compared with 88% of their White counterparts. In 2000, only 16.4% of African-Americans 25 years of age or older held a bachelor's degree or higher, compared with almost double that percentage (28.0%) for their White counterparts. In 2000, in actual numbers, of the 19,858,095 African-Americans age 25 or older, 8,980,716 were males and 10,877,379 were females. Of the African-American males 25 years of age or older, 742,701 had less than a ninth-grade education; 1,868,068 had less than a high school degree with 9 to 12 years of education; 2,816,161 were high school graduates; 462,861 held an associate degree; 787,036 held a bachelor's degree; and 389,656 held a graduate or professional degree. In contrast, of the African-American females 25 years of age or older, 832,854 had less than a ninth-grade education; 2,064,053 had less than a high school degree with 9 to 12 years of education; 3,093,622 were high school graduates; 682,140 held an associate degree; 1,090,435 held a bachelor's degree; 564,142 held graduate or equivalency or a professional degree, and 2,550,133 had some college education (U.S. Department of Commerce, Bureau of the Census, Summary File 1; U.S. Department of Commerce, Bureau of the Census, 2003; The U.S. Department of Commerce, Bureau of the Census, The Older Population, 2000, 2001).

From the sixteenth to the nineteenth centuries, more than 10 million Africans were brought to the United States and bonded into slavery (Ploski & Williams, 1989). By historical accounts, nearly 600,000 slaves arrived in the United States in the sixteenth century, 2,000,000 in the seventeenth century, 5,000,000 in the eighteenth century, and 3,000,000 in the nineteenth century (Ploski & Williams, 1989). Because of these historical accounts, the perception held by most Americans is that African-Americans may be the only cultural and ethnic group who reside in the United States today who did not immigrate to this country voluntarily. Although this perception has merit, in reality, the history of the arrival of Africans in the United States has become somewhat distorted throughout the years. In actuality, many Europeans (meaning those persons of English, German, and Scotch-Irish ancestry) voluntarily immigrated to the American colonies as laborers and became "indentured servants" (Ploski & Williams, 1989). Many of these people were paupers or debtors who used indentured servitude to gain a better way of life. The first 20 African-Americans to land at Jamestown in 1619 (preceding the *Mayflower*) were accepted into the community as "indentured servants." Although it is true that these 20 African-Americans did not have freedom of choice in the decision to come to the colonies because they were systematically captured against their will, they nonetheless, over the same course of time as European indentured servants (7 years), enjoyed the same liberties and privileges of the "free working class," including the right to own property (Ploski & Williams, 1989).

Two of the most notable African-Americans who arrived in this country as "indentured servants" were Anthony Johnson, who became a "freeman" as early as 1622, and Richard Johnson. Anthony Johnson prospered so well that by 1651, he himself was able to acquire five "indentured servants." Likewise, Richard Johnson, having been given 100 acres of land of his own, acquired two indentured servants by 1654, two of whom were White (Ploski & Williams, 1989). However, it is appropriate to note that both of these men were the exception, not the rule. In fact, a fissure was cracking open, and African-American servitude and White servitude were beginning to be viewed differently. By 1640, African-Americans had ceased to be viewed as servants and were assigned the status of chattel (meaning one who remained a fixed item of personal property for the duration of life).

In 1661, the Virginia House of Burgesses formally recognized the institution of African-American slavery (Ploski & Williams, 1989). Of the 13 original colonies, only Pennsylvania protested the system of slavery. By 1667, Virginia had written into its statutes that even purifying the African-American soul through baptism could not alter the condition of the African-American regarding bondage or freedom. Thus, color became the real cutting edge that separated the African, now American, from the rest of the colonists (Ploski & Williams, 1989).

Even today, the cultural roots of African-Americans are entrenched in the African-American life experience. According to Bloch (1983), it is the African-American life experience that has established what has become known as the African-American view of the external world. The African-American life experience has shaped the internal attitudes and belief systems of African-Americans, and it continues to influence interactions of African-Americans with persons from other cultural groups.

Some of the health problems noted particularly in African-Americans are believed to be the result of varying genetic pools and hereditary immunity. However, many of these problems have been found to be more closely associated with economic status than with race. Three intervening and reinforcing variables are poverty, discrimination, and social and psychological barriers. These variables are regarded as being so profound in their effect on African-Americans that they tend to keep these individuals from using the health care services that are available. These variables may also explain why morbidity and mortality rates are higher among African-Americans than for the rest of the general population. Although underrepresented in the general population, African-Americans remain overrepresented among the health statistics for life-threatening illness.

The life expectancy for African-Americans, 73.3 years, continues to lag behind that for Whites, which is 77.9 years (*Time Almanac with Information Please*, 2007). In 2006, the life expectancy for African-American men was 69.8 as compared with 75.2 for their White counterparts. Similarly, the life expectancy for African-American women was 76.5 compared with 80.4 for their White counterparts (*Time Almanac with Information Please*, 2007).

While overall the infant mortality rate in the United States declined slightly from 7.2 in 1990 to 6.9 in 2000, African-Americans continued to have a higher infant mortality rate (14.1 per 1000 live births in 2000) compared with White Americans (6.9 per 1000 live births in 2000) (National Center for Health Statistics, 2002). Although the average life expectancy for African-Americans at birth edged upward to the low 70s, it is important to note that the life expectancy for African-American male babies born between 1986 and 2000 actually shrank (National Center for Health Statistics, 2002). A portion of the shrinkage is attributable to infant mortality, which is twice as high for African-American babies as for White babies. Yet another portion of the shrinkage is attributable to disparities in health concerns, especially chronic illnesses, that contribute significantly to premature deaths (before 65 years of age) among African-American males. In fact, in 2000, the rate of deaths for African-American males was 55% higher for heart disease, 26% higher for cancer, 180% higher for stroke, and 100% higher for lung disease than for the rest

of the general U.S. population (National Center for Health Statistics, 2002). Perhaps the greatest disparity was the rate of deaths or the potential for life lost for African-American males attributable to homicides, which was 630% higher, compared with White males (National Center for Health Statistics, 2002). In health status disparities, African-American women do not fare much better than their male counterparts. When the life expectancy of White women is compared with the life expectancy of African-American women, African-American women have a shorter life expectancy (75.0 years versus 80.0 years) (National Center for Health Statistics, 2002).

COMMUNICATION

Communication is the matrix for thought and relationship between all people regardless of cultural heritage (Murray & Huelskoetter, 1991). Verbal and nonverbal communication is learned in cultural settings. Difficulties arise if a person does not communicate in the way or manner prescribed by the culture because the individual cannot conform to social expectations. Communication, therefore, is basic to culturally appropriate nursing care.

Dialect

Dialect refers to the variations within a language. African-Americans speak English; however, there are widespread differences in the way English is spoken between African-Americans and other ethnic and cultural groups. Different linguistic norms evolve among groups of people who are socially or geographically separated. Social stratification alters the nature and frequency of intercommunication between groups. When social separation by factors such as ethnic origin or class is responsible for the origin and perpetuation of a particular dialect, the dialect is referred to as a *stratified dialect*. When differences in dialect emerge as a result of geographical separation of people, the dialect is called a *regional*, or *geographical*, dialect.

Origins of African-American Dialect in the United States. Accurate and reliable data concerning the different dialects spoken by most African-Americans are unavailable to the public or to educators

(Turner, 1948). The study of pidgin and Creole language has facilitated an intelligent study of Black English and of the notable differences between Black English and Standard English (Hymes, 1971). Research into the languages of Brazilians of African descent, as well as Haitians, Jamaicans, and the present-day African-American inhabitants off the seacoasts of South Carolina and Georgia, indicates a correlation of structural features of several of the languages spoken in parts of West Africa, as well as a similarity to the English spoken by Whites in the United States (Hymes, 1971).

The first Africans brought to the United States as slaves were systematically separated during transportation, and this separation continued after arrival. As a result, the various African languages combined with the languages of other cultural groups in the New World, such as the Dutch, the French, and the English. This combination of the different African languages with other languages fostered a need for a "common language" for all African-Americans, which ultimately led to the restructuring of grammar of all languages, including English. This process is referred to as "pidginization" and "creolization." Pidgin English is not a language but a dialect. Pidgin tends to be simple in grammar and limited in vocabulary. Typically, in communities where pidgin is spoken, its use is limited to trade purposes, task-oriented activities, and communication between cultural or ethnic groups (Hymes, 1971). When a pidgin dialect undergoes internal expansion and extension of use, the results are creolization. It is from a pidgin dialect that a Creole language was born. In the United States several Creole dialects developed that still exist, particularly in the rural South and in such places as New Orleans, Louisiana; Hattiesburg and Vicksburg, Mississippi; and Mobile, Alabama. Furthermore, the migration of African-Americans from the South saw the development of pidginization and creolization in some northern cities such as New York, Chicago, and Detroit. Evidences of past migration and its effect on dialect and Black English remain obvious even today.

Language Usage. The dialect that is spoken by many African-Americans is sufficiently different from Standard English in pronunciation, grammar, and syntax to be classified as "Black English." The use of Standard English versus Black English varies among African-Americans and in some instances may be related to educational level and socioeconomic status, though this is not always the case. The use of Standard English by African-Americans is important in terms of social and economic mobility. However, the use of Black English has served as a unifying factor for African-Americans in maintaining their cultural and ethnic identity. It is not uncommon for some African-Americans to speak Standard English when serving in a professional capacity or when socializing with Whites and then revert to Black English when interacting in all African-American settings. Some African-Americans who have not mastered Standard English may feel insecure in certain situations where they are required and expected to use Standard English. When confronted with such situations, they may become very quiet, with the result that they may be labeled hostile or submissive.

Pronunciation of Black English

There is a tendency for users of what is often referred to as "Black dialect" to pronounce certain syllables and consonants somewhat differently. For example, *th*, as in *the, these,* or *them,* may be pronounced as *d,* as in *de, des,* and *dem* (Dillard, 1972; Wolfram & Clark, 1971). In Black English there is also a tendency to drop the final *r* or *g* from words; thus *father* and *mother* become *fatha* and *motha.* The words *laughing, talking,* and *going* are pronounced *laughin, talkin,* and *goin.* Speakers of Black English may also place more emphasis on one syllable as opposed to another; for example, *brother* may be pronounced *bro-tha.* In addition, the final *th* of words is pronounced as *f* in Black English; thus *bath, birth, mouth,* and *with* are pronounced *baf, birf, mouf,* and *wif.*

Copula deletion of the verb *to be* is a common omission in some environments; for example, the speaker of Black English might say, "He walking" or "She at work" in contrast to the Standard English "He is walking" or "She is at work." Black English speakers may also use the unconjugated form of the verb *to be* where Standard English speakers would use the conjugated form. An example of this would be "He be working" in contrast to the Standard English "He is working."

In Standard English every verb is in sequence and must be marked as either present or past tense. However, in Black English only past-tense verbs need to be marked. For example, in Black English the *s* marking the present tense may be omitted, thus "He go" or "She love." Attempts to correct this can result in phrases such as "I goes" and "We loves." Speakers of Black English may also omit the possessive suffix. For example, in Black English one might say, "Richard dog bit me" or "Mary dress," in contrast to the Standard English "Richard's dog bit me" or "Mary's dress" (Dillard, 1972).

Speakers of Black English also have some words that are classified as slang. These words are different from slang words used in other dialects and may or may not convey the same meaning. For instance, African-Americans may use the word *chilly* or *chillin* to infer sophistication, whereas a White individual may use the word *cool* or (formerly) *groovy* to convey the same meaning. Some African-Americans may use the verb *to fix* to denote planned actions, for example, "I'm fixin to go home," whereas the user of Standard English would say, "I am getting ready to go home."

The speech of some African-Americans is very colorful and dynamic. For these persons, communication also involves body movement (kinesics). Some African-Americans tend to use a wide range of body movement, such as facial gestures, hand and arm movements, expressive stances, handshakes, and hand signals, along with verbal interaction. This repertoire of body movements can also be seen in sports and in dance, which is the highest communicative form of body language.

Some African-Americans use sounds that are not words to add expression to their conversation or to music, such as *oo-wee* or *uh huh*, which have analogies in some of the West African languages as expressed in the surviving Gullah dialect (Sea Islands, South Carolina) but not in English.

The term *signifying* describes an approach wherein one attempts to chide or correct someone indirectly. For example, one might correct someone who is not dressed properly by saying, "You sure are dressed up today."

Most African-Americans use Black English in a systematic way that can be predictably understood by others; thus Black English cannot and should not be regarded as substandard or ungrammatical. It is estimated that approximately 80% of African-Americans use Black English at least some of the time (Dillard, 1972).

Implications for Nursing Care

The nurse must develop a sensitivity to communication variances as a prerequisite for accurate nursing assessment and intervention in multicultural situations. In all nursing environments the potential for misunderstanding the client is accentuated when the nurse and the client are from different ethnic groups. Perhaps the most significant and obvious barrier occurs when two persons speak different languages. However, the nurse must be cognizant of the fact that barriers to communication exist even when individuals speak the same language. The nurse may have difficulty explaining things to a client in simple, jargon-free language to facilitate the client's understanding. The nurse must develop a familiarity with the language of the client because this is the best way to gain insight into the culture. Every language and dialect is special and has a unique way of looking at the world and at experiences (Kluckhohn, 2003). Every language also has a set of unconscious assumptions about the world and life. According to Kluckhohn (2003), people see and hear what the grammatical system of their language makes them sensitive to perceive.

The nurse who works with African-American clients may find that although the language is the same, the perception of what message is being sent and received by the nurse and the client may be different. Therefore, it is of the highest priority for the nurse who is working with African-Americans, particularly those who speak Black English, to understand as much of the context of the dialect as possible.

The nurse must bear in mind that Black English cannot be viewed as an unacceptable form of

English. Thus it is important for the nurse to avoid labeling and stereotyping the client. The nurse should avoid chiding and correcting the speech of African-Americans because this behavior can result in the client's becoming quiet, passive, and, in some cases, aggressive or hostile. On the other hand, although the nurse should attempt to use words common to the client's vocabulary, mimicking the client's language can be interpreted as dehumanizing. For example, if a nurse were to say *dem* for *them*, or *dese* for *these*, the client may perceive this as ridicule.

When working with persons who speak Black English, the nurse must keep in mind that the client may use slang to convey certain messages. However, slang terms often have different meanings between individuals and especially between cultural groups. For example, an African-American client's response to questioning about a diagnostic test, "It was a real bad experience," may actually mean that it was a unique and yet positive experience. The nurse working with this client will need to clarify the exact meaning of the word *bad*. In Black English the word *bad* is often used for the exact opposite, in other words, "good." In another example, an African-American client who states that the medication has been taken "behind the meal" may mean the medication has been taken "after eating." A nurse may interpret *behind* to mean "before" rather than "after" because the dictionary definition states that *behind* means "still to come." The nurse must be cautious about interpreting particular words each time an African-American uses certain terms.

It is essential that the nurse identify and clarify what is happening psychologically and physiologically to the African-American client. When possible, the nurse should substitute words commonly understood by the African-American client for more sophisticated medical terms. When this is done, the nurse will find that the African-American client is more receptive to instructions and more cooperative. Stokes (1977) offers a list of terms commonly used by nurses and equivalent words used by some African-Americans:

Conditions (Medical/Black English)	Functions (Medical/Black English)
Diabetes/sugar	Constipation/locked bowels
Pain/miseries	Diarrhea/running off, grip
Syphilis/bad blood, pox	Menstruation/red flag, the curse
Anemia/low blood, tired blood	Urinate, urine/pass water, tinkle, peepee
Vomiting/throw up	

The nurse must remember that some African-Americans place a great deal of importance on nonverbal elements of communication and that the verbal pattern of some African-American clients may differ significantly from that of a non–African-American nurse. It is also important for the nurse to keep in mind that words used by some African-American clients may be the same as those used by the nurse but have different, idiosyncratic meanings. When working with African-American clients, the nurse must also remember that eye contact, nodding, and smiling are not necessarily essential or direct correlates that the African-American client is paying attention (Sue, 2003).

SPACE

According to Hall (1990), the degree to which people are sensorially involved with each other, along with how they use time, determines not only at what point they feel crowded or have a perception that their personal space is collapsing inwardly but the methods for alleviating crowding as well. For example, Puerto Ricans and African-Americans are reported to have a much higher involvement ratio than other cultural groups such as German Americans or Scandinavian Americans. It is believed that highly involved people, such as African-Americans, require a higher density than less involved people. However, highly involved people may at the same time require more protection or screening from outsiders than people with a lower level of involvement do.

To understand the variable of space, it is essential to understand time and the way it is handled because the variable of time influences the structuring of space. According to Hall (1990), there are two contrasting ways in which people handle time, monochronic and polychronic, and each affects the way in which an individual perceives space. People with low involvement are generally monochronic because such individuals tend to compartmentalize time; for example, they may schedule one thing at a time and tend to become disoriented if they have to deal with too many things at once. On the other hand, polychronic individuals tend to keep several operations going at once, almost like jugglers, and these individuals tend to be very involved with each other.

Implications for Nursing Care

The nurse who works with Latin Americans, Africans, African-Americans, or Indonesians may feel somewhat uncomfortable because these cultures generally dictate a much closer personal space when personal and social spaces are involved (Sue, 2003). Because some African-Americans are perceived as polychronic individuals, it is important for the nurse to remember that polychronic individuals tend to collect activities.

When polychronic individuals interact with monochronic individuals, some difficulties may be experienced because of the different ways in which these individuals relate to space and to each other. An example of a difficulty encountered between monochronic and polychronic individuals is when monochronic individuals become upset or angry because of the constant interruptions of polychronic individuals.

Some monochronic individuals believe that there must be order to get things done. On the other hand, polychronic individuals, such as some African-Americans, do not believe that order is necessary to get things done. The nurse who works with African-Americans must keep in mind that to reduce polychronic effects, it is necessary to reduce multiple-activity involvements on the part of the client. The nurse can accomplish this by separating activities with as much screening and scrutiny as necessary (Hall, 1990). One goal of nursing intervention should be to help the client structure activities in a ranked order that will produce maximal benefits for the client.

SOCIAL ORGANIZATION

Social organization refers to how a cultural group organizes itself around particular units (such as family, racial or ethnic group, and community or social group). Most African-Americans have been socialized in predominantly African-American environments. Historically, because of legalized segregation, African-Americans were separated or isolated from the mainstream of society. Consequently, African-Americans are the only cultural group in the United States that has not been assimilated into the mainstream society. Even today, African-Americans maintain separate and in most cases unequal lifestyles compared with other Americans. Evidence of the failure to assimilate on the part of African-Americans is seen in the existence of predominantly African-American neighborhoods, churches, colleges and universities, and public elementary and high schools.

Historical Review of Slavery and Discrimination

Patterns of discrimination have existed in the United States since the inception of slavery. With the inception of slavery came the foundations of attitudes and beliefs that were and continue to be the pillars that support the institution of racism. Racism, discriminatory practices, and segregation combined have produced insularity or separatist feelings and attitudes on the part of some African-Americans. As a result, African-Americans are often accused of having more separate and more insular patterns of communication, which have restricted some African-Americans from participating in the wider White society. Thus some African-Americans prefer to maintain themselves within their own group. Accordingly, this insularity has promoted the retention of culturally seeded beliefs that differ from the beliefs held by the dominant culture. Leininger (1978) noted that every cultural group has unique beliefs that influence their attitudes regarding health. These beliefs tend to determine the type of behavior and health care practices that a particular cultural group views as appropriate or inappropriate. In other words, the attitudes and beliefs regarding health and illness vary in the United States between African-Americans and Whites and even among African-Americans themselves.

Attitudes, beliefs, values, and morals are the basic structural units of any culture. Culture is an outward manifestation of a way of life; it is dynamic, fluid, and ever evolving. The family is the basic social unit of most cultures and is the means by which culture is passed down from one generation to the next. The inception of slavery in the United States precipitated the beginning of the destruction of the transplanted African culture. In Africa, Africans had been accustomed to a strictly regulated family life with rigidly enforced moral codes. The family unit was close-knit, well organized, connected with kin and community, and highly functional for the economic, social, psychological, and spiritual well-being of the people (Jones, 1998). The family was the center of African civilization.

The destruction of the African family began with the capture of slaves for transplantation to the New World, which began in 1619. As slaves were captured, the young, healthy men and women and children were forcibly removed from their families and tribes. This separation continued as these slaves journeyed to the New World because they were placed on ships without regard for family unity, tribe, or kinship. On the arrival of the slaves in the United States, this systematic separation of individuals from families persisted.

The cruelest form of emasculation of the Black Africans, now Americans, was the breeding of slaves for sale. Infants and children were taken from their mothers and sold as chattel. Marriage between slaves was not legally sanctioned and generally left to the discretion of the owners. Some slave owners assigned mates when slaves reached breeding age. Others would not permit their slaves to marry a slave from another plantation. Most slave owners sold husbands, wives, and children without consideration for family ties. The children who were produced of the slave union belonged to the slave owner, not to the parents. The African-American family in the United States during slavery lacked autonomy because the family members were someone else's property. The parents were unable to provide security or protection for their children.

Husbands were unable to protect their wives. In a documentary of the lives of 75 African-American women, Angelou (1989) describes the heartbreaking tenderness of African-American women and the majestic strength they needed to survive the subjugation and horror of the slavery experience.

In contrast to this view of the destruction of the African-American family during slavery, Gutman (1976) contends that the African-American family was not disaggregated because of slavery. In fact, Gutman (1976) presents compelling evidence to suggest not only that some African-American families remained intact during slavery but also that many slave marriages were officially documented as the names of their offspring were. Gutman (1976) cautions, however, that no more misleading inference could be drawn from these data than to argue that the data alone show that slaves lived in stable families.

Changing Roles of the African-American Family

Under the system of slavery in the United States, the role of the African-American man as husband and father was obliterated. The African-American man was not the head of the household, nor was he the provider or the protector of his family. Instead, he was someone else's property. Under the system of slavery, the African-American man remained powerless to defend his wife and children from harm, particularly when they were beaten or sexually assaulted by the White overseer or owner or by any other White person. The African-American male slave was often referred to as "boy" until he reached a certain age, at which point he became "uncle." The only crucial function for the African-American man within the African-American family was siring children.

In the United States under the system of slavery, the African-American woman became the dominant force in the family. She was forced to work side-by-side with her male counterpart during the day and additionally had the responsibility of caring for family members at night. The African-American woman was forced to bear children for sale and to care for other children, including those of the slave owner. Some African-American women during slavery were also forced to satisfy the sexual desires of any White man, and any children born out of this union were considered slaves. If the African-American woman had a husband, he was merely her sexual companion and was referred to as her "boy" by the slave owner and by White society in general. The inception of slavery, the division of the African family and subsequently the African-American family, and the subordinate role of the African-American man played a significant part in the establishment of the female-dominated African-American household that exists even today in the United States.

Even after slavery was abolished in the United States, the destructive forces against the African-American family persisted. Today, the residual effects of slavery are still evident in some parts of the country. After slavery was abolished and during the emancipation period and the years that followed, the African-American man was either denied jobs or given tasks that were demeaning and dehumanizing. From the time of the abolition of slavery until the mid-1960s, African-Americans in some parts of the country were attacked, lynched, and murdered. Sexual attacks on African-American women also continued. Such actions further served to drive some African-American men away from their families. Thus there was further weakening of the family and subsequently of the African-American male role (Bullough & Bullough, 1982). Despite the discriminatory practices and the continued hostile attacks against African-Americans, some African-American families nevertheless were able to establish themselves. As these African-American families were increasingly able to develop a secure economic status, they began to establish schools, churches, and other social organizations.

Characteristics of the African-American Family

In the United States there are basically two types of family structures: the male-headed (patriarchal) family structure and the female-headed (matriarchal) family structure. In 2000 the number of African-American female-headed households crept slowly downward. Today, such families constitute 44% of African-American families. In addition, between 1950 and 2000, the number of African-American female-headed householders who had never been married quadrupled, from 9% in 1950 to 42.4% in 2000 (U.S. Department of Commerce, 2002). The fact that approximately half of the African-American families in the United States are female-headed is attributable in part to factors related to and carried over from slavery. For example, the African-American family has not been able to overcome deficits related to education and income. According to the U.S. Department of Commerce, Bureau of the Census (2002), the average income for African-American men, compared with men in other cultural groups with similar skills and educational levels, is significantly lower. African-American males, in particular, have not made significant strides in gaining entry into the workforce since the 1980 census. The annual labor participation rate for African-American males in 2000 remained virtually unchanged from the 1990 data at 65.9%, compared with 70.6% in 1980. In addition, the annual salary for African-American males remains disproportionately low compared with their White counterparts. In 2000, 65.9% of African-American men and 63.4% of African-American women participated in the workforce, compared with 74.3% of White men and 60.3% of White women (U.S. Department of Commerce, Bureau of Census, the Black Population, 2002). Overall, African-Americans are less likely to participate in the workforce than other racial and ethnic groups. While the median household income (which takes into account all sources of income, including full- and part-time jobs and interest income, for a household) for the nation was $41,994, it was only $29,423 for African-Americans; in comparison, for their White counterparts the median income was $44,667. The median earnings figure for African-Americans in general (which takes into account only full-time work status) was only $27,264, as compared with $33,955 for their White counterparts (U.S. Department of Commerce, 2002). In addition, the median earnings figure for

African-American males ($30,000) was disproportionately lower than that of their White counterparts ($39,235). Similarly, African-American women had lower median earnings ($25,589) than their White counterparts ($27,878) (U.S. Department of Commerce, 2002).

Implications for Nursing Care

Even today, the African-American family is often oriented around women; in other words, it is matrifocal. This has implications for the nurse because within the African-American family structure the wife or mother is often charged with the responsibility for protecting the health of the family members. The African-American woman is expected to assist each family member in maintaining good health and in determining treatment if a family member is ill. This responsibility has both positive and negative effects because African-American clients often enter the health care delivery system at the advice of the matriarch of the family. The nurse must recognize the importance of the African-American woman in disseminating information and in assisting the client in making decisions. Although the African-American family may be matrifocal, it is nevertheless essential to include the African-American man in the decision-making process.

Some African-American families are composed of large networks and tend to be very supportive during times of crisis and illness. Large-network groups can have both positive and negative effects on wellness, illness, and recovery behaviors. Jackson, Neighbors, and Gurin (1986) found that network size was positively related to distress: the more informal helpers there were, the higher the distress score on the instrument used in the survey. One conclusion of the study is that network size is not a good measure of perceived social support. According to the findings from the study, the more serious the problem, the more people within the network are consulted for help. But a greater number of people consulted does not necessarily reduce the severity of the problem; rather, an individual with an acute illness may spend so much time seeking assistance within the network that necessary and timely treatment is delayed. The nurse should include all the members of the network in planning and implementing health care because some members of the network may provide advice or care that could be detrimental to the client. For example, an African-American client who is admitted with an electrolyte imbalance and is brought laxatives from home by a relative may have additional electrolyte problems when the laxatives are taken without consulting members of the health care team. In this case the nurse must emphasize the importance of the nurse's role in providing health care. Once the family develops a feeling of trust, the nurse is more likely to be consulted should perceived health needs arise, for example, when the client needs a laxative.

TIME

Time is a concept that is universal and continuous. All emotional and perceptual experiences are interrelated with the concept of time. The perception of time is individual and determined by cultural experience (Hall, 1989). In the United States, time has become the most important organizing principle of the dominant culture (Hall, 1989). The majority of individuals of the dominant culture are time conscious and very future oriented; they make it a common practice to "plan ahead" and "save for a rainy day." Time has become very important and comparable to money in the American society. Doing things efficiently and faster has become the American way.

It is impossible to characterize African-Americans and their perceptions of time as one way or the other because African-Americans, just as individuals from other cultural groups, vary according to social and cultural factors. Some African-Americans who have become assimilated into the dominant culture are very time conscious and take pride in punctuality. These individuals are likely to be future oriented and believe that saving and planning are important. They are likely to be well educated and to hold professional positions, though this is not always the case, because some African-Americans who are not well educated and do not hold professional jobs still value time and have hopes for the future (and are likely to encourage their children to seek higher education and to save for the future) (Poussaint & Atkinson, 1970).

On the other hand, some African-Americans react to the present situation and are not future oriented; it is their belief that planning for the future is hopeless because of their previous experiences and encounters with racism and discrimination. They believe that their future will be the same as their present and their past (Poussaint & Atkinson, 1970). These individuals are likely to be jobless or have low-paying jobs. Educational levels may vary from junior high school to college degrees among persons who share this belief. Such individuals are unlikely to value time; thus they do not value the concept of punctuality and may not keep appointments or arrive much later than the scheduled time. It is the belief of some African-Americans that time is flexible and that events will begin when they arrive. This belief has been translated down through the years to imply an acceptable lateness among some African-Americans of 30 minutes to 1 hour. This perception of time can be traced back to West Africa, where the concept of time was elastic and encompassed events that had already taken place as well as those that would occur immediately (Mbiti, 1990).

Finally, some African-Americans have a future-oriented concept of time because of their strong religious beliefs. These individuals may be from all socioeconomic and educational levels. It is their belief that life on Earth, with all its pain and suffering, is bearable because there will be happiness and lack of pain after death. African-Americans who hold this belief plan their funerals and even purchase their grave plots long before their deaths (Smith, 1976).

Implications for Nursing Care

Because some African-Americans perceive time as flexible and elastic, it is essential for the nurse to include the client and family in the planning and implementation of nursing care. When planning nursing care with the client and family, the nurse should emphasize events that have flexibility where time is concerned, such as morning care and bathing. On the other hand, the nurse must also emphasize events that have no flexibility where time is concerned and where delay in doing something, such as taking time-released medications or medications for certain conditions, would have serious implications for the client's well-being. For example, a client with high blood pressure must be made to understand that the medication must be taken as and when prescribed, not as and when desired. A medication missed today cannot be made up by taking double the amount tomorrow. As another example, a client with type 1 diabetes cannot delay the time between meals.

Some African-Americans are perceived as individuals with present-time orientations. Such persons may have a more flexible adherence to schedules and may believe that immediate concerns are more relevant than future concerns. Because appointment schedules may lack meaning, the nurse must emphasize the importance of adhering to the appointment schedule. If the nurse knows a particular client has a pattern of arriving late, the nurse may advise that client to arrive for scheduled appointments at least half an hour early. For the nurse who works with clients who are focused on the present, it is essential to avoid crisis-oriented nursing and promote preventive nursing (Sue, 2003).

ENVIRONMENTAL CONTROL

Health Care Benefits

In the United States the system of health care beliefs and practices is extremely complex and diverse among cultural groups. Variations in health care beliefs and practices cross ethnic and social boundaries. These variations are evidenced even within families. Culture influences individual expectations and perceptions regarding health, illness, disease, and symptoms related to disease. Accordingly, culture, cultural beliefs, and cultural values influence how one copes when confronted with illness, disease, or stress (Anderson & Bauwens, 1981).

In the United States a distinction between "illness" and "disease" has been made by anthropologists and sociologists (Staples, 1976). *Illness* has been defined as an individual's perception of being sick, which is not necessarily related to the biomedical definition of disease. *Disease* has been defined as a condition that deviates from the norm. Thus illness may exist in the absence of disease and vice versa (Staples, 1976). Norms used to determine a disease condition, by Western standards, have for the most part been taken from studies conducted on White subjects. Thus, when these norms are applied to other cultural groups, such as African-Americans, the norm values may be meaningless and lead to erroneous conclusions. For example, to receive a 2 for color on the Apgar scoring system for newborns, the infant must be completely pink. Another example of a Western norm expectation is that an inverted T wave may be an ominous, pathological finding. However, in the case of African-Americans and particularly African-American men, such a finding should be the expectation, rather than being perceived as ominous and pathological. Also, growth as related to body size and physique is often normed by White Western standards. Thus African-Americans, who mature at an earlier age and typically have larger physiques than those of their White counterparts, may be perceived as being either overweight or oversized when White Western norms are applied.

Health Care Beliefs and the African-American Family

African-Americans in the United States are a highly heterogeneous group; thus, it is impossible to make a collective statement about their health care beliefs and practices. Many health care beliefs that are exhibited by African-Americans in the United States are derived from their African ancestry (Smith, 1976). For example, in West Africa, where most African-Americans originated, man was perceived as a monistic being, that is, a being from which the body and soul could not be separated (Smith, 1976). Man was also perceived as a holistic individual with many complex dimensions. Religion was interwoven into health care beliefs and practices. (West Africans continue even today to believe that illness is a natural occurrence resulting from disharmony and conflict in some area of the individual's life.) Because life was centered on the entire family, illness was perceived as a collective event and subsequently a

disruption of the entire family system. The traditional West African healers always involved the individual's entire family in the healing process, even when the disorder was believed to be somatic. Thus the traditional West African healer based treatment on the premise of wholeness, the necessity for reincorporation of the client into the family system, and involvement of the entire family system in the care and treatment of the individual (Smith, 1976).

Perception of Illness. In the United States some African-Americans perceive illness as a natural occurrence resulting from disharmony and conflict in some aspect of an individual's life. This belief is a cultural value that has been passed down through the generations to African-Americans as a result of West African influences and tends to involve three general areas: (1) environmental hazards, (2) divine punishment, and (3) impaired social relationships (Snow, 1977). An example of an environmental hazard would be injuries as the result of being struck by lightning or bitten by a snake. Divine punishment would include illnesses or diseases that the individual would attribute to sin. Impaired social relationships may be caused by such factors as a spouse leaving or parents disowning a child (Snow, 1977).

Another belief held by some African-Americans is that everything has an opposite. For every birth, there must be a death; for every marriage, there must be a divorce; for every occurrence of illness, someone must be cured (Snow, 1978). Some African-Americans may not be able to distinguish between physical and mental illness and spiritual problems and as a result may present themselves for treatment with a variety or combination of somatic, psychological, and spiritual complaints (Smith, 1976). For example, a client may present real symptoms of an ulcer but relate the symptoms to past sins or grief over a financial loss. The client desires assistance not only for the somatic disorder but also for the psychological and spiritual complaints.

African-Americans who share mainstream attitudes about pain may respond to pain stoically out of a desire to be a perfect client. This means that they tend not to "bother" the nurse by calling for attention or for pain medication. For such clients the nurse must make it clear that the client has a right to relief from pain. On the other hand, some African-American clients exhibit a different form of stoicism. Hard experience has convinced them that trouble and pain are God's will. In this case the nurse needs to help the client understand that pain retards healing and is medically undesirable (LoBiondo-Wood, Zimmerman, & Gatson-Johansson, 1989).

Folk Medicine

Folk medicine is germane to many cultural and ethnic groups. Individuals from all aspects of society may use folk medicine either alone or with a scientifically based medical system. The importance of folk medicine and the level of practice vary among the different ethnic and cultural groups, depending on education and socioeconomic status (Bullough & Bullough, 1982). In contrast to the scientifically based health care system in the United States, folk medicine is characterized by a belief in supernatural forces. From this perspective, health and illness are characterized as natural and unnatural.

According to Snow (1983), it matters whether an African-American person comes from a rural background when it is necessary to select health care providers. Some African-Americans who were reared in the rural South may have grown up being treated by folk practitioners and may not have encountered a physician until they reached adulthood. Therefore, these people are more likely to turn to a neighborhood folk practitioner when they become ill. According to White (1977), folk medicine is still used within the African-American community because of the humiliation encountered in the mainstream health care system, lack of money, and lack of trust in health care workers. Today, some African-Americans go to physicians in order to get prescribed medications, not because they believe the physician is superior in knowledge or training (Murray & Huelskoetter, 1991).

Witchcraft, voodoo, and magic are an integral aspect of folk medicine (McKenzie & Chrisman, 1977). Natural events are those that are in harmony with nature and provide individuals who believe in

and practice folk medicine with a certain degree of predictability in the events of daily living. Unnatural events, on the other hand, represent disharmony with nature, and so the events of day-to-day living cannot be predicted (Snow, 1983). Another aspect of the folk medicine system is a belief in opposing forces—that everything has an opposite. For example, for every birth, there must be a death. Also incorporated into the system of folk medicine is the belief that health is a gift from God, whereas illness is a punishment from God or a retribution for sin and evil (Snow, 1983). This concept is evidenced by the belief held by some African-Americans that if a child is born with a physical handicap, it is a punishment from God for the past wrongdoings of the parents. In this way, sins of the father and mother are passed on for retribution by the children (Snow, 1983). Such beliefs are not limited to African-Americans but are also found among other cultural groups in the United States; for example, some Mexican Americans believe that illness is a punishment for some sin or misdeed (Snow, 1983).

Practice of African-American Folk Medicine. There are still some African-Americans in the rural South and in the urban northern ghettos who practice folk medicine based on spirituality, including witchcraft, voodoo, and magic (McKenzie & Chrisman, 1977). Some of these individuals may also use the orthodox medical system. Historically, such cities as New Orleans and Baton Rouge, Louisiana, were very much voodoo oriented, and such beliefs were held not only by African-Americans but also by members of other cultural groups. Even today, the African-American folk medicine system is practiced by the high-ranking voodoo queen in some Louisiana cities. The Louisiana Voodoo Society is a carryover from a combination of Haitian and French cultural influences (Mitchel, 1978). Voodoo and witchcraft are not restricted to Louisiana and are also practiced in such places as the Georgia sea islands, which are just off the coast of Savannah. Interestingly enough, some of the inhabitants of the Georgia sea islands remain pure-blooded descendants of West African ancestry. Even today, some people there have refused to intermarry with members of other cultural groups, thus maintaining the tradition of "pure-blooded" lineage (Wolfram & Clark, 1971). Pure-blooded descendants of West Africans are also found off the coast of South Carolina. A few of these people still speak Gullah (English with an admixture of various African languages) and tend to isolate themselves when possible from the mainstream of society (Wolfram & Clark, 1971).

African-American Folk Medicine System Defined. In the system of African-American folk medicine, illness is perceived as either a natural or an unnatural occurrence. A natural illness may occur because of exposure to the elements of nature without protection (such as a cold, the flu, or pneumonia). Natural illnesses occur when dangerous elements in the environment enter the body through impurities in food, water, and air. However, the words *natural* and *unnatural* are connoted to mean more or less than the dictionary definitions of these words. For example, cancer, which is linked to such environmental hazards as smog, cigarette smoke, toxic waste, and other chemical irritants, would be considered a natural illness in a professional medical system. However, those persons who share beliefs in African-American folk medicine might view cancer as an unnatural illness, perceiving it as a punishment from God or a spell cast by an evil person doing the work of the devil (Snow, 1974). Such persons may not readily acknowledge the fact that cancer, for example, may be caused by environmental factors such as cigarette smoking; thus they may continue smoking even after being diagnosed with cancer. Unnatural illnesses are perceived as either a punishment from God or the work of the devil. This perception is in contrast to the dictionary definition of illness as an unhealthy condition of the body or mind.

Types of Folk Practitioners. Jordan (1975) identified distinct types of folk practitioners. The first type is the "old lady" or "granny" who acts as a local consultant. This individual is knowledgeable about many different home remedies made from certain spices, herbs, and roots that can be used to treat common illnesses. Another duty of this individual is to give advice and make appropriate referrals to another type of practitioner when an illness

or a particular medical condition extends beyond her practice (Jordan, 1975). The second type of practitioner is the "spiritualist," the most prevalent and diverse type of folk practitioner. This individual attempts to combine rituals, spiritual beliefs, and herbal medicines to effect a cure for certain illnesses or ailments. The third type of practitioner is the voodoo priest or priestess. In some West Indies islands, the voodoo practitioner can be a man, whereas in some rural southern areas of the United States, the voodoo practitioner must be a woman and may inherit this title only by birthright and a perceived special gift (Snow, 1974).

In contrast to the type of voodoo priest or priestess found in some West Indies islands and in some rural or urban southern United States areas is the type of voodoo priest or priestess found in some larger urban areas such as Chicago; Queens or Jamaica, New York; or Los Angeles. In these cities the voodoo folk practitioner may be either male or female, does not have to inherit the right to practice by virtue of bloodline, and does not have to possess significantly powerful gifts (Snow, 1974). Historically, the voodoo priestess found in cities such as New Orleans must possess certain physical characteristics; that is, she must be African-American, and more specifically she must be of mixed ancestry, either an octoroon (a person of one-eighth Black ancestry) or a quadroon (a person of one-fourth Black ancestry) if her powers are to be superior (Snow, 1974).

Even today, some African-Americans still turn to one of these three types of practitioners when seeking medical advice. Educational level or socioeconomic status does not appear to alter or affect how some African-Americans perceive folk practitioners. Similar views are shared by some members of other cultural groups. In the summer of 1988, newspaper articles throughout the United States carried the story that the First Lady of the United States refused to make any moves or to allow her husband, the president of one of the most powerful countries in the world, to make decisions unless an astrologer was consulted.

Witchcraft: An Alternative Form of Folk Medicine. The practice of witchcraft is quite widespread and is not limited to the boundaries of the United States. Various degrees of witchcraft are practiced in countries throughout the world. In addition, the practice of witchcraft is not limited to any one particular cultural group. Persons who believe in witchcraft feel that it can be used not only to cure illness or disease but also to cause illness or disease. For example, strokes, dementia, and some gastrointestinal disorders may be perceived by some persons who believe in witchcraft to be the direct result or influence of witchcraft (Henderson & Primeaux, 1981).

The practice of witchcraft is based on the belief that there are some individuals who possess the ability to mobilize the forces of good and evil. These abilities are based on the principles of sympathetic magic, which underlie many of the beliefs of folk medicine practice. The basic premise of sympathetic magic is that everything in the universe is connected. There is a direct connection between the body and the forces of nature. Interpretation and direction of events are accomplished by understanding these connections. Sympathetic magic is categorized into *contagious* and *imitative magic*. The basic premise of contagious magic is the perception that physically connected objects can never be separated; therefore, any actions against the parts constitute an action against the whole (Henderson & Primeaux, 1981). Individuals who practice witchcraft may use a piece of clothing or nail clippings from someone to cast an "evil" spell or to protect the individual. The basic premise of imitative magic is that like follows like, or that one will imitate what one desires to achieve. For example, a knife placed under the bed will cut pain; an evil charm put on when the moon is waxing will increase the moon.

A recurring theme in the practice of witchcraft is that of animals being in the body. Lizards, toads, snakes, and spiders are believed to be the most common types of intruders. These animals are dead and pulverized and are generally believed to enter the body by means of food or drink. It is not uncommon for persons who believe in witchcraft to refuse to eat or drink food prepared by someone they believe may have put a hex on them. Individuals who believe that such a spell has been cast on them may present themselves at health care facilities with symptoms described as "reptiles crawling over the body or snakes wiggling in their stomach." Some of these individuals may also share the belief that the physician is powerless to help them once they have been "hexed" (Jordan, 1979).

Perceptions Concerning Folk Medicine and Other Alternative Medical Solutions. The prevalence of the belief in and the use of folk medicine remedies and other alternative forms of health care is not fully understood (Jacques, 1976). It is impossible to generalize or postulate how widespread the use of folk medicine remedies is among African-Americans. However, evidence does exist that there are some African-Americans in all areas of the United States who believe in and practice folk medicine as well as other alternative forms of health care, such as witchcraft, voodoo, and spiritualism (Snow, 1983). There is also evidence to support the notion that different levels of folk medicine are practiced (Jacques, 1976). The boundaries of folk healers for some African-Americans may also vary. For example, the "granny" folk healer may possess the skills and knowledge to cure only simple illnesses or ailments. In contrast, a "witch doctor" is believed to possess supernatural powers that allow the "casting out of such things as animal demons" (Jordan, 1979). In addition, African-American folk medicine practitioners may have titles different from those of folk practitioners found in other cultural groups in the United States, such as "conjure doctor," "underworld man," "father divine," the "root doctor," and the "root worker" (Jacques, 1976).

Origins of African-American Folk Medicine. African-American folk medicine practices in the United States can be traced back to regions of West Africa (Smith, 1976). There are also influences on African-American folk medicine that originated in other countries, such as Haiti, Jamaica, and Trinidad (Smith, 1976). Because of slavery, there was a blending of various African tribes, particularly in slave cities and states such as New Orleans, Louisiana, and Savannah, Georgia, with other cultural groups such as the French, the Creoles, and the Indians. Various folk medicine practices found among some African-Americans in the North and the South have been handed down from generation to generation. Even today, the consistent use of some form of African-American folk medicine continues, and such continuity indicates that these practices have withstood the test of time and are presumed to be valid, though no empirical data exist that would indicate the validity or reliability of such practices.

Rationale for the Use of African-American Folk Medicine. Some African-Americans choose to use folk medicine because of tradition, whereas others have made this choice based on previous discriminatory practices and unfair treatments that have existed throughout some regions of the United States. In this regard, the delivery of health care services were not exempt from Jim Crow laws, which were legally sanctioned until the mid-1960s throughout the South. However, the Northern regions of the United States also were not exempt from such discriminatory practices in regard to health care. This is evident in the passage of the Hill-Burton Act in 1946, which was not abolished until 1966 with the passage of the Federal Medicare Act (Bullough & Bullough, 1982).

The Hill-Burton Act, also known as the Hospital Construction Survey Act, provided federal grants for hospitals, both private and public, that admittedly did not serve African-Americans. Under this law, hospitals, whether private or public, were allowed to discriminatorily serve populations based on race. In addition, these same hospitals were allowed to continue these discriminatory practices in regard to hiring and staffing patterns. From such practices were born the all–African-American hospitals, which were found not only in the South but also in the North. Inclusions and exclusions for purposes of rendering health care services to those persons in need were left to the proprietors of the hospital. Thus patterns of admission and service to African-Americans varied throughout the country without regard to regional locale. In some northern and western states, admission to and service by some hospitals remained theoretically open to all races on equal terms, whereas in other states the courts upheld the rights of hospital proprietors to segregate as they saw fit.

This discriminatory practice was dramatically emphasized by the deaths of two famous African-Americans: Bessie Smith, in 1937, and Charles Drew, in 1950. Bessie Smith was a legendary blues singer who was critically injured in an automobile accident while traveling from Jackson, Mississippi, to Memphis, Tennessee. White attendants at the scene of the accident surmised correctly that Smith had a severed right arm and therefore needed immediate medical attention. The attendants took Smith to a hospital designated as "all White," and the administrators at the hospital refused to treat her despite the severity of her injuries. The ambulance attendants were forced to take Smith to Memphis, where she could be treated. On arrival, Smith was in profound shock, having lost a great quantity of blood. It has been said that despite Bessie Smith's obvious fame and the great admiration shown her by millions of fans, both African-American and White, the fact that she was African-American ultimately caused her death (Albertson, 2003).

Charles Drew, a surgeon, discovered blood plasma and developed the procedure for blood plasma transfusion. Even today, people throughout the world, regardless of race, benefit from his discovery. However, despite his profoundly important contribution to the medical field, the discovery of blood plasma was of no benefit to Drew when he, like Smith, was involved in an automobile accident and similarly was refused treatment in an "all-White" hospital. Although Drew was responsible for the technique of blood plasma transfusion, it was not used to save his life because he was taken to a hospital that legally had the right to refuse him treatment.

African-American folk medicine therefore took roots not only as an offshoot of African cultural heritage but also as a necessity when African-Americans could not gain access to the traditional health care delivery system. Furthermore, some African-Americans turned to African-American folk medicine because they either could not afford the cost of medical assistance or were tired of the insensitive treatment by caregivers in the health care delivery system (Bullough & Bullough, 1982).

Today African-Americans have access to the health care delivery system through legal channels. Some African-Americans still refuse to use the system, however, citing reasons such as past experiences, the escalating cost of health care, and the sometimes insensitive treatment on the part of non-Black caregivers in regard to the physiological and psychosocial differences evidenced among African-Americans.

Some African-Americans have a strong religious orientation, and most African-Americans belong to the Protestant faith. Although folk medicine and folk practices are widely documented in the literature as being common practices for the treatment of illnesses among African-Americans, the most common and frequently cited method of treating illness remains prayer (Spector, 2004). According to Snow (1977), many of her informants found it impossible to separate religious beliefs from medical ones.

Death and Dying Rituals

It is important to note that that there are variations in customs regarding death and dying rituals among African-Americans depending on country of origin, religious affiliation, geographic region, economic level, and educational background of each family member (Dowd, Poole, Davidhizar, & Giger, 1998; Perry, 1993). Many African-American families are composed of large networks, and often it is thought that such large networks tend to be very supportive during times of crises, such as during death and the dying process (Dowd, Poole, Davidhizar, & Giger, 1998). Some researchers have suggested that among many African-Americans there are varying ways that emotions are expressed about the death of a love one (Lobar, Youngblut, & Brooten, 2006). For example, while many people believe that African-Americans are quite expressive at the death of a love one, this may not always be the case. For example, some African-Americans cry, whereas others remain silent and stoic (Hines Smith, 2002). It is not unusual to see large gatherings at the time of death and during the burial process (Perry, 1993). Even today, some African-Americans, and particularly those in the rural South, have maintained the tradition of keeping the body of the deceased in the home the evening before the funeral (Perry, 1993). This practice is probably what began the ritual of people coming to a home to help where they could. The church services for the deceased certainly depend on the religious affiliation. But regardless of the religious affiliation, it is not uncommon to see church "nurses" help family members view the body and deal with the stress of a funeral (Perry, 1993). African-Americans view death as a natural part of living, and their strong religious beliefs (which include seeing death as inevitable and a part of God's will, the sure and certain hope that the deceased is in God's hand, and the future hope that they will be reunited in heaven after death with the deceased) helped many of them deal effectively with death (Hines Smith, 1999, 2002). Nonetheless, it is essential for the health care professional to remember that many bereaved African-Americans are more likely to seek help to adjust to the death from their clergy than from a health care professional (Neighbors, Musick, & Williams, 1998).

Implications for Nursing Care

Cultural health practices are often considered efficacious, neutral, or dysfunctional (Pillsbury, 1982). Practices that are considered efficacious are recognized by Western medicine as beneficial to health regardless of whether they are different from scientific practice. Practices the nurse regards as beneficial should be actively encouraged. The nurse should keep in mind that a treatment plan that is congruent with the client's own beliefs has a better chance of being successful. For example, some African-Americans believe that certain herbs and spices are essential in the treatment of certain disequilibriums in the body. In this case an herbal decoction could be used in place of water and might be just as beneficial for the treatment of specific conditions such as dehydration. Neutral practices (such as putting a knife under the bed to cut pain) are considered to be of no significance one way or the other to the health of an individual. However, psychological benefits may have a profound effect on the perception of pain. Dysfunctional health practices are viewed as harmful from a health point of view.

For example, it is considered a dysfunctional health practice in Western medicine to use sugar and overrefined flour excessively. Dysfunctional health practices found among some African-Americans include such practices as using boiled goat's milk and cabbage juice for stomach infection.

Because some African-Americans tend to equate good health with luck or success, an illness may be viewed as undesirable and equated with bad luck, poverty, domestic turmoil, or even unemployment. As indicated previously, illnesses may be classified as natural or unnatural. Natural illnesses occur because a person is affected by natural forces without adequate protection. The nurse may be able to help the client more readily understand how these natural illnesses, such as colds and flu, can be avoided. Unnatural illnesses, which are believed to be the direct result of evil influences, are much more difficult for the nurse to combat. If the nurse has a client who believes that unnatural illness has resulted from witchcraft or voodoo or is a punishment from God, it may be very difficult to convince the client that a treatment can be implemented that will minimize or eliminate the problem. For example, a client may view breast cancer as a punishment from God. In this instance the client should be encouraged to seek medical treatment because unnecessary delay can have serious consequences. Although the nurse may not subscribe to cultural healing beliefs, it is essential that the nurse recognize their existence and their importance for some African-American clients. It is also important for the nurse to remember that effective nursing care cannot be implemented until the nurse acknowledges certain cultural health beliefs that have an effect on the client's behavior and recovery.

Among some African-Americans it is believed that the maintenance of health is strongly associated with the ability to read the signs of nature. Subsumed in this belief is the idea that natural phenomena, such as the phases of the moon, the seasons of the year, and the planetary positions, all either singly or in combination affect the human body and human physiological functioning. Some African-Americans believe that the best days to wean babies, for example, or to have dental or surgical procedures done can be found in the *Old Farmer's Almanac* (Snow, 1974). To the nurse, such beliefs may seem peculiar; however, the nurse must acknowledge the existence of such beliefs before culturally appropriate nursing care can be given. The nurse must also recognize that although some of these beliefs may be helpful, others may be neutral, and still others may be extremely dangerous for the client. The nurse must be able to sort beliefs into these three categories and assist the client in recognizing beliefs that may be dangerous.

Some African-Americans believe that cultural healing remedies help a person psychologically in dealing with discomfort. However, when these things fail, they believe a physician should be consulted. These same African-Americans may also believe that the nurse should recognize these cultural beliefs and use remedies based on these beliefs that prove to be helpful to the client (Bloch, 1976a). When an African-American client does arrive for professional health care, the nurse might assume that the client has tried all the cultural healing remedies known. While doing the initial assessment, the nurse needs to find out what the client has been using at home to minimize illness symptoms. This initial assessment will assist the nurse in determining whether these home remedies will interact or interfere with orthodox medical approaches. If the client has been using harmless home remedies, such remedies may continue to be used in the client's treatment. Other harmless remedies might be added to the client care plan at the client's suggestion (Bloch, 1976a).

Religion for some African-Americans has functioned primarily as an escape mechanism from the harsh realities of life. The African-American church functions to promote self-esteem among its membership. The African-American church also acts as a curator for maintaining the culture of many African-Americans. Therefore, the nurse cannot overlook the importance of the African-American minister and the African-American church in the recovery of the client. If there is no African-American minister within the hospital facility, the nurse should contact the client's own minister. It is essential for the nurse to remember that the African-American minister can essentially bridge the gap between the African-American client and other health care workers because the African-American minister understands the rituals, folkways, and difference in the mores of African-Americans (Smith, 1976).

BIOLOGICAL VARIATIONS

Until recently, the education of health care practitioners was based on the biopsychosocial characteristics of the dominant White culture. The lack of an in-depth understanding of biological and cultural differences resulted in less than optimum health care for persons who were not members of the dominant culture. When providing care to African-American clients, the nurse must realize that racial differences involve more than skin color and hair texture. African-American people have distinctive genotypes and phenotypes that characterize them as a racial group and as different from other racial groups. Moreover, the nurse must understand that African-Americans also have ethnic and cultural differences that distinguish them from other ethnic and cultural groups. It is essential for nurses and other health care providers to understand these biological variations in order to avoid racial and ethnic disparities in health care.

In 2002, a committee under the auspices of the Institute of Medicine released a seminal report titled *Unequal Treatment: Confronting Racial and Ethnic Disparities in Health Care*. The committee unequivocally noted that evidence of racial and ethnic disparities in health care is for the most part consistent regardless of the nature of the illness or the type of health care services rendered (Institute of Medicine, 2002). While it has been previously noted that socioeconomic status plays a major contributory factor in unequal treatment, particularly where African-Americans are concerned, Braithwaite and Taylor (2001) noted that even if income levels were standardized and if all impediments regarding access to care were eliminated, disparities in health outcomes might still exist. They contend that this argument gives credence for the need to eliminate cultural incompetence among health care providers. Seemingly, nurses would not be exempt from this argument, as they must serve as advocates for

culturally competent care for all clients entrusted to their care.

Birth Weight

Data from previous epidemiological reports consistently reveal that there is a difference in the mean birth weight of approximately 200 g between African-American infants and White infants, with White infants weighing more. These differences persist even when socioeconomic status, maternal age, parity, and smoking are controlled for (Hulsey, Levkoff, & Alexander, 1991). Davis, Cutter, Goldenberg, et al. (1993) used ultrasound examinations to compare biparietal diameter (BPD), head circumference (HC), abdominal circumference (AC), and femur length in 5405 African-American and White fetuses. They found no significant difference in the BPD, HC, and AC; however, femurs in African-American fetuses were significantly longer. The birth weights of the infants were also compared, and these data again revealed differences in birth weight between African-American and White infants (3331 versus 3135 g; $P < 0.001$), with White infants being heavier.

It is postulated that birth weight contributes significantly to neonatal mortality among African-American neonates (Braithwaite & Taylor, 2001). It is clear that prematurity, which is defined as a birth weight under 2500 g, is twice as common for African-Americans as it is for Whites (Iyasu, Becerra, Rowley, & Hogue, 1992) and it has been suggested that the definition for prematurity be lowered from 2500 to 2200 g for African-Americans (Morton, 1977). The gestational period for African-Americans tends to be 9 days shorter than that for Whites, and a slowing down of gestational growth occurs in African-American infants after 35 weeks. Before 35 weeks of gestation, African-American infants are usually larger than White infants (Giger, Davidhizar, & Wieczorek, 1993; Pratt, Janus, & Sayal, 1977). The reasons for these differences in birth weights remain vague. Nonetheless, because the death rates for African-American infants are nearly three times the national average, some researchers have suggested that approximately three quarters of the disparity in infant mortality rates are primarily attributable to the larger proportion of babies with low birth weight (LBW) and the very low birth weights (less than 1500 g) among these vulnerable neonates (Braithwaite & Taylor, 2001; Iyasu, Becerra, Rowley, & Hogue, 1992).

Growth and Development

African-American children tend to mature faster than White children. Today African-American children are more mature at birth in both the musculoskeletal and the neurological systems (Falkner & Tanner, 1978). Neurologically, African-American children tend to be more advanced until about 2 or 3 years of age, and in the musculoskeletal system they tend to be more advanced until puberty (Roche, Roberts, & Hamell, 1978). The differences in skeletal maturity are attributed to genetic and environmental factors.

Body size, height, weight, bone length, and body structure of African-Americans and Whites have been extensively studied in the United States. Studies done by Abraham, Clifford, and Najjar (1976) revealed that the average height and weight of African-American and White men 18 to 74 years of age are approximately the same; White men tend to be 0.5 cm taller than African-American men. The average height for African-American and White women is the same; however, African-American women are consistently heavier than White women at every age, and between 35 and 64 years of age they are typically an average of 20 pounds heavier than their White counterparts.

Body Proportion

The body proportions of African-Americans differ from those of Whites, Asians, and American Indians. There are definitive differences in bone length that are obvious on study. African-Americans have shorter trunks than Whites and tend to have longer legs than Whites, Asians, and American Indians. African-American men tend to have wider shoulders and narrower hips than Asians, who tend to have narrow shoulders and wide hips. The long bones of African-Americans are significantly longer and narrower than those of Whites (Farrally & Moore, 1976). The bones of African-Americans are

also denser. African-American men have the densest bones, followed by African-American women, White men, and finally, White women, who have the lowest bone density of the two races. The greater bone density explains why osteoporosis is rare in African-Americans and why White women have a greater incidence of osteoporosis. Bone curvature also varies among the different races. The femurs of African-Americans are quite straight; in comparison, femurs of American Indians are anteriorly convex and those of Whites have intermediate curvature. This characteristic appears to be genetically determined, but weight also seems to be a factor because obese African-Americans and Whites tend to demonstrate more curvature than other individuals do (Gilbert, 1977).

Body Fat

The amount and distribution of body fat is another area where there are pronounced differences by virtue of race and ethnic group. The racial differences are mostly related to socioeconomic status. Persons from the lower socioeconomic class tend to have more body fat than those from the middle class, and persons from the middle class tend to have more body fat than those from the upper class. There is some evidence indicating that fat distribution may vary according to race. African-American people tend to have smaller skin-fold thickness in their arms than Whites have, but the distribution of fat on the trunk is similar for both Whites and African-Americans (Bagan, Robson, & Soderstrom, 1971). Whites have a larger chest volume than African-Americans; hence they have greater vital capacity and forced expiratory volume (Oscherwitz, 1972). African-Americans, on the other hand, have a larger chest volume than American Indians and Asians and thus greater vital capacity and forced expiratory volume than members of these racial groups (Oscherwitz, 1972).

Skin Color

Skin color, or pigmentation, is the most distinguishing physical difference among the various races and is determined by melanin. All people have some melanin, but some racial groups have more melanin than others. The greater the amount of melanin an individual has, the darker the skin pigmentation will be. The skin color of persons who are classified as African-Americans ranges from "white" to very dark brown or perhaps even black. Melanin provides protection from the effects of the sun; thus African-Americans and other dark-skinned individuals have a lower incidence of skin cancer. African-Americans do get sunburned, but not so easily as Whites do (Overfield, 1995).

The skin coloring should be uniform, but areas that are not exposed to the sun may be lighter, such as the buttocks, abdomen, and thorax. The exceptions to this rule for African-American people are the skin folds in the groin, the genitalia, and the nipples, which tend to be darker than the rest of the body. (An old wives' tale suggests that to determine the true color of a newborn infant, one should look at the ears, which tend to be darker at birth than the rest of the body.) Except for the areas just mentioned, hypopigmentation and hyperpigmentation (unless it is a birthmark) are abnormal (Bloch, 1983). Pigmentation of the lips, nail beds, palmar surfaces, creases of the hands, and plantar surfaces and creases of the feet may vary, just as skin coloring does. The range of coloring for the lips of African-Americans may vary from pink to plum. The palmar and plantar surfaces may range from light pink to dark pink to a brown, and the creases may range from dark pink to dark brown, depending on the amount of pigmentation (Bloch, 1976b). The gums may have areas of hyperpigmentation, and the sclerae may have scattered areas of brown pigmentation that appear to be freckles.

Mongolian spots are a common variance found in African-American infants. They are migratory leftovers of melanocytes that have lingered in the lumbosacral region at a greater than normal depth, which accounts for their dark blue-green appearance. Mongolian spots occur in 90% of African-Americans, 80% of Asians and American Indians, and only 9% of Whites (Jacob & Walton, 1976). Normally found on the buttocks, thighs, ankles, and arms, mongolian spots usually disappear in the first year of life and should not be mistaken for a bruise.

Birthmarks appear to be most common in African-American individuals, occurring in 20% of African-Americans, compared with 2% to 3% of Whites, Mexicans, and American Indians. These pigmented marks appear as sharply demarcated macules that vary from light tan to dark brown, depending on the skin color. They may be present anywhere on the body (Overfield, 1995).

Black skin is also more susceptible to an overgrowth of connective tissue in response to injury, or keloid formation. Keloids are raised areas of scar tissue that can result from minor injuries such as skin tears or punctures, from more major injuries such as burn injuries or traumatic lacerations, or from surgical incisions (Rook, 1970).

Normal, healthy skin should be warm, dry, and elastic. There should be a red glow present in Black skin. Color changes associated with abnormal conditions are rashes, which may be difficult or impossible to detect in the individual who is darkly pigmented. Darkly pigmented lips and nail beds with melanin deposits make nursing assessment even more difficult. When possible, the nurse should become familiar with the client's normal coloring to establish a baseline value. The skin assessment should be done in a well-lighted room. Sunlight is the best lighting; if artificial lighting is used, it should be nonglaring (Bloch & Hunter, 1981). When assessing the darkly pigmented individual for specific color changes such as pallor, jaundice, or cyanosis, the nurse should inspect the conjunctivae and oral membranes of the buccal mucosa. Jaundice also appears as a yellowish discoloration of the sclerae if they are not pigmented. The mucous membranes of the buccal mucosa and the palmar and plantar surfaces may also be inspected for yellow discoloration.

The nurse may also rely on palpations and the client's history to detect the presence of bruises in the darkly pigmented client. The nurse should use the dorsal surface of the hand to assess for areas of increased warmth and tenderness. Questioning should include a history of recent trauma. The petechiae cannot be readily visualized on the dark-skinned individual. The nurse should inspect the sclerae for dark blue spots. The client history should include questioning about symptoms of conditions in which petechiae would be present. Palpation and the client history may also be used to detect the presence of a macular rash on the client who is dark skinned (Bloch, 1983).

Genetic Differences

Methylenetetrahydrofolate Reductase (MTHFR). Some researchers have noted that moderate hyperhomocysteinemia is a putative risk for the development of cardiovascular disease (Dilley, Hooper, EI-Jamil, et al., 2002). Hyperhomocysteinemia is an independent risk factor for premature arteriosclerotic vascular disease and venous thrombosis (Clarke, Daly, Robinson, et al., 1991). Mutations in the gene, which code for methylenetetrahydrofolate reductase (MTHFR), account for reduced enzyme levels and elevated plasma homocysteine (Gallagher, Meleady, Shields, et al., 1996; Hugh, Ali, Madira, et al., 1997; Kluitjmans, Lambers, Van der Heuval, et al., 1996; Motulsky, 1996). The heterozygote state results in mild hyperhomocysteinemia, a risk factor for cardiovascular disease. Homocysteine levels are also influenced by diet. Dilley Hooper, EI-Jamil, et al. (2002) attempted to determine whether the mutation C→T677 in the *MTHFR* gene or the TC833/844in68 and G→A919 mutations in the *CBS* gene were associated genetically with myocardial infarctions among African-Americans. The analysis of the data suggested that 15% of the cases analyzed demonstrated that these individuals were heterozygous for C→T677 (*MTHFR*) mutation, whereas 1.8% of the subjects were homozygous. Further findings from this study showed that their controls were 15% heterozygous and 2.1% homozygous and suggested that there was no significant association with myocardial infarction among these African-Americans who participated in the study. Yet, these researchers noted that while no association was noted for T→C833 (*CBS*) among the experimental or controls, and while there was no significant association between this mutation and myocardial infarction, the prevalence of the heterozygous state among African-Americans (15%) was significantly higher than that among their White counterparts (12%).

These researchers concluded that the racial differences of these genes warranted further investigation. **Tumor Necrosis Factor Alpha.** One candidate gene predisposing to type 2 diabetes within the major histocompatibility complex (MHC) region is TNFα, a cytokine. In rats, elevated levels of TNFα have been shown to produce "sustained increase in glucose production, utilization and clearance," as well as an insulin resistance (IR) state (Bendtzen, Morling, Fomsgaard, et al., 1988; Fernandez-Real, Gutierrez, Ricart, et al., 1997; Dilley, Hooper, EI-Jamil, et al., 2002; Gokhan, Hotamisligil, Murray, Choy, & Spiegelman, 1994; Gokhan, Hotamisligi, Armer, et al., 1995; Hotamisligil, Shargill, & Spiegleman, 1993; Jongeneel, Briant, Irina, et al., 1991.) TNFα expression has also been observed in rodent models of obesity and diabetes. When TNFα was neutralized in obese fa/fa rats, a significant increase in peripheral uptake of glucose in response to insulin was observed. Treatment of adipocytes with TNFα resulted in down regulation of GLUT4 messenger RNA. TNFα also interferes with the signaling of insulin and blocks its biological action (Gokhan, Hotamisligil, Murray, Choy, & Spiegelman, 1994; Hotamisligil, Shargill, & Spiegleman, 1993). In humans, abnormal expression of TNFα appears to play a role in obesity-related insulin resistance (Gokhan, Hotamisligil, Murray, Choy, & Spiegelman, 1994; Hotamisligil, Shargill, & Spiegleman, 1993). A polymorphism in the TNFα promoter has been associated with increased levels of basal serum insulin and leptin (Gokhan, Hotamisligil, Murray, Choy, & Spiegelman, 1994; Hotamisligil, Shargill, & Spiegleman, 1993). The differences were greater in women than in men. TNFα has been linked to the development of insulin resistance among African-Americans and is considered to be one of the precursors to the development of metabolic syndrome (syndrome X).

Metabolic syndrome (syndrome X) is a clustering of abnormalities characterized by the primary defect of compensatory insulin resistance, glucose intolerance, dyslipidemia, and centrally distributed obesity (Matthews, Hosker, Rudenski, et al., 1985). Chen, Bao, Begum, et al. (2000) conducted a study to examine the age-related patterns of cardiovascular risk factor clusters relative to the metabolic syndrome (syndrome X) among African-American and White children. The clusters in this study for the metabolic syndrome (syndrome X) included (1) insulin resistance index, (2) body mass index (BMI), (3) triglycerides/HDL cholesterol ratio, and (4) mean arterial pressure. Regardless of age, four mediating factors contribute to the development of coronary heart disease: hyperinsulinemia (syndrome X), hypercholesterolemia, hypertension, and obesity. A sedentary lifestyle, the large percentage of fat consumed per day by African-American children, and the prevalence of obesity all may contribute to the development of metabolic syndrome (syndrome X) even among African-American children (Giger, Richardson, & Jones, 2001). In other words, African-American children are not exempt because of their tender years from developing syndrome X and starting the downward spiral toward diabetes and ultimately coronary heart disease (CHD).

It is interesting to note that findings from the study by Chen, Bao, Begum, et al. (2000) suggest that overall, White children had a higher total of adverse clusters among the four indices measured (9.8; $P < 0.01$) than their African-American counterparts (7.4; $P < 0.01$). These follow-up findings to the Bogalusa Heart Study are interesting. Prior and recent analyses of these data sets suggest that while predictability of childhood adiposity and insulin resistance syndrome is difficult to determine with certainty in children, the contributions of these adverse clusters can provide convincing evidence for the future development of syndrome X, thereby leading to the development of coronary heart disease (CHD) in adulthood (Srinivasan, Myers, & Berenson, 2002). As African-Americans age, the adverse clusters outrank those of their White counterparts, and this ultimately leads to the development of syndrome X and coronary heart disease in adulthood. Srinivasan, Myers, and Berenson (2002) also examined the contributions of childhood adiposity and insulin as a weighed predictor to adulthood risk of developing metabolic syndrome (syndrome X) among African-American and White children with baseline ages of 8 to 17

years. Using a logistic regression model, these researchers noted that childhood BMI and insulin resistance served as significant predictors of adult clustering for metabolic syndrome (syndrome X). In this study, BMI was the strongest indicator, exhibiting a curvilinear relationship. Further findings from this study also suggest that childhood obesity often is a powerful predictor of the development of metabolic syndrome (syndrome X) later in life. These findings suggest that children, and particularly African-American children, can benefit tremendously from programs that underscore the importance of weight control and increased physical activity (Srinivasan, Myers, & Berenson, 2002). Tumor necrosis factor α has also been linked with human leiomyoma, of which African-American women tend to have a disproportionate prevalence (Kurachi, Matsuo, Samoto, & Maruo, 2001). In fact, Kurachi et al. (2001) were among the first researchers to demonstrate increased cellular levels of TNFα in leiomyoma cells.

Apolipoprotein E. Apolipoprotein E (ApoE) is a polymorphic protein involved in the catabolism of chylomicron remnants. Various ApoE phenotypes are related to the development of combined hyperlipidemia and familial combined hyperlipidemia, total and low-density lipoprotein (LDL) cholesterol, and insulin levels and are associated with CHD, stroke, and type 2 diabetes (Dallongeville, Roy, Lebouef et al., 1991; Ferrucci, Guaralnik, Faho, et al., 1995; Imaru, Koga, & Ibayashi, 1988; Margaglione, Seripa, Gravine, et al., 1998; Valdez, Howard, Stern, & Haffner, 1995). The high frequency of the appearance of ApoE supports this gene as a candidate marker for coronary heart disease. It is thought that ApoE (apoE) participates in the receptor-mediated clearance of blood lipids such as cholesterol, which is considered a major risk factor for CHD (Amemiya, Arinami, Kikuchi, et al., 1996). In North America, it has been estimated that the variability of this gene (*apoE* gene locus) accounts for up to 6% of the variation in CHD. The *apoE* locus lies on chromosome 19 and has three common alleles ($_E2$, $_E3$, $_E4$), which are coded for the e isoforms *apoE2*, *apoE3*, and *apoE4*, respectively (Amemiya, Arinami, Kikuchi, et al., 1996).

While the frequencies of these isoforms vary from race to race, it is thought that *apoE3* shows the highest frequencies ($\geq$49%) and *apoE2* the lowest ($\leq$15%). The frequency by population in North America is generally no higher than 6%. Among African-Americans there tends to be a direct correlation between the frequency of this candidate gene and the development of coronary heart disease (Dallongeville, Roy, Lebouef, et al., 1991; Valdez, Howard, Stern, & Haffner, 1995).

Enzymatic Variations

Biochemical variations and their effects on health vary according to race. As with other racial variations, biochemical variations are attributed to genetic factors and environmental influences. Lactose intolerance is a well-known condition that is correlated with race: 90% of African Blacks and 75% of African-Americans have lactose intolerance (Giger, Davidhizar, & Cherry, 1991; McCrackin, 1971). Individuals with lactose intolerance lack the enzyme to convert lactose to glucose and galactose, and as a result, gastrointestinal symptoms of bloating, cramping, and diarrhea occur. The condition is genetically transmitted, though the specific gene has not been identified (Johnson, Cole, & Abner, 1981). There appear to be two periods in life during which symptoms occur: infancy shortly after weaning and the teen years or early twenties. The condition is diagnosed on the basis of signs or symptoms that occur after the ingestion of milk or other products containing lactose. Treatment consists of avoidance of these products, with appropriate substitution of other products. In addition, there are products available on the market that can be taken to help alleviate symptoms associated with this condition. Some people report a degree of success with such products, whereas other people report little benefit from their use. The nursing implications for nurses caring for African-American clients include (1) knowledge of the condition and its prevalence among African-Americans and (2) education of clients with the condition to avoid products containing lactose. The education of these clients should include encouraging them to read labels and make appropriate food substitutions (Bloch, 1974).

Susceptibility to Disease

Cardiovascular Disease. Cardiovascular disease (CVD) has reached pandemic proportions and is now recognized as the leading cause of death worldwide. A major cause for the increased prevalence of cardiovascular disease in developing countries is the Westernization of native cultures (Yusuf et al., 2001). According to the World Health Organization, CVD accounted for 17 million deaths worldwide or 29.2% of the total global mortality (Yusuf et al., 2001). In African countries, CVD accounted for 9.2% of total deaths in 2001, with hypertension, stroke, cardiomyopathies, and rheumatic heart disease identified as the most prevalent causes. In urban areas, the prevalence of most common risk factors for coronary heart disease (CHD), with the exception of hypertension and smoking, is lower among Blacks compared with other racial groups living in Africa, and mortality rates for African Blacks are lower than rates for Whites who live in Africa (Yusuf et al., 2001).

Despite significant progress made in the treatment and prevention of CVD, myocardial infarction, stroke, and other forms of heart disease, CVD continues to be the leading cause of mortality and morbidity in the United States for adults in all demographic groups. Heart disease and stroke are the first and third leading causes of deaths, respectively, in the United States, accounting for nearly 40% of all deaths annually (Heart Disease and Stroke Statistics, 2006). Data from the American Heart Association Heart Disease and Stroke Statistics (2006), indicate that over 70 million adults in the United States have some form of CVD. This statistic includes diseases of the heart, stroke, high blood pressure, congestive heart failure, congenital cardiovascular defects, atherosclerosis, and other circulatory system diseases. Before 72 years of age, the average annual event rate for the first coronary event in men between 35 and 44 years of age is 7 per 1000. With advancing age, this figure rises dramatically to 68 per 1000. For women, rates of death from CVD, while lower, may be perceived as somewhat comparable because of their sheer numbers; however, death tends to occur at a later age (Appel, Moore, &

Giger, 2006; Giger, Strickland, Weaver, Acton, & Taylor, 2005). Recent data from the American Heart Association (2006) and the Third National Health and Nutrition Examination Survey (NHANES) indicate that over the past 3 decades more women have died of CVD than men (2006).

Cardiovascular disease is the number one cause of deaths in African-Americans. In fact, coronary heart disease and stroke together account for more than one third of all deaths in African-Americans (Heart Disease and Stroke Statistics, 2006). It is interesting to note that among African-Americans, 41.1% of men and 44.7% of women have CVD. The percentage of African-Americans with CHD is 9.6%, compared with 12.2% of non-Hispanic Whites. Despite this fact, African-Americans are more likely to die of a myocardial infarction than any other racial or ethnic group (Heart Disease and Stroke Statistics, 2006). The disparity between African-Americans and Whites is partly due to hereditary predisposition for hypertension, type 2 diabetes, and lifestyle choices. Moreover, African-Americans have more CVD risk factors, such as hypertension, type 2 diabetes, and obesity, which places them at an increased risk for heart and cerebral vascular disease. Hypertension is a major independent risk factor for coronary artery disease, stroke, and peripheral arterial disease. The prevalence of hypertension in African-Americans is the highest in the world. It is estimated that 30% of all cardiovascular disease can be attributed to hypertension; therefore, this condition is an extremely important consideration for the African-American in the development of CVD (Heart Disease and Stroke Statistics, 2006).

Since the 1900s, cardiovascular disease has been the number one cause of death every year except 1918. Despite this well-known fact, the general public continues to have a misguided perception about the health risk of heart disease (Blumenthal & Flack, 2003). Most Americans still fear cancer more than heart disease. According to Blumenthal and Flack (2003), women rank breast cancer high on the list of personal health threats when in fact, 1 death in 29 among women is due to breast cancer compared with 1 death in 2.4 due to CVD. In African-American women, the greatest risk for CVD is the high prevalence of hypertension (HTN) and type 2 diabetes. Despite advances in management of CVD, African-American women have a higher prevalence of HTN compared with other ethnic and gender groups (Fongwa et al., 2006). The rate of HTN in African-American women has reached epidemic proportions, with 45% of African-American women affected nationwide compared with 30% of White women (Fongwa et al., 2006). African-American women have greater mortality and morbidity from HTN compared with women from other racial and ethnic groups (Heart Disease and Stroke Statistics, 2006). In 2001, the mortality rate from stroke was 74% in African-American women compared with 54% in White women (Heart Disease and Stroke Statistics, 2006).

Coronary heart disease was once perceived as a disease that most commonly afflicted men. This perception probably developed because the condition strikes men more often in the middle years of life. This perception had been reinforced by the Framingham study, which was initiated in 1948. In this classic study, the data indicated that, on the average, women develop the symptoms of heart disease a decade later than men. Work relative to this study is ongoing, and though earlier data show that the incidence of the disease was disproportionately higher among men than women, current data indicate that coronary heart disease is the number one killer of women and is more prevalent in African-American women than in African-American men (Yusuf et al., 2001).

Of the estimated 71,300,000 American adults with one or more types of CVD, over 25% are age 65 years or older (Heart Disease and Stroke Statistics, 2006). Data from the National Health and Nutrition Examination Survey 1999–2002, reveal that 1 in 2 adult men and women have some form of cardiovascular disease. It is estimated that 2500 Americans die of CVD every day, an average of one death every 35 seconds. The majority of deaths from cardiovascular disease are due to coronary heart disease (CHD). Further, 565,000 new myocardial infarctions and 300,000 recurrent myocardial infarctions occur annually. An additional 175,000 silent myocardial infarctions occur each year (Heart

Disease and Stroke Statistics, 2006). From 1993 to 2003, the overall CVD death rate declined by approximately 4.6%, but African-American men and women continue to show higher rates of death from CVD compared with Whites. According to the American Heart Association Heart Disease and Stroke Statistics Update 2006, the 2003 preliminary mortality rates from CVD were 308.8 per 100,000. Rates of death from CVD were 359.1 per 100,000 for White males compared with 479.6 per 100,000 for African-American males. In White and African-American females the CVD mortality rates were 256.2 and 354.8 per 100,000, respectively. Data from this report also show that African-American women and Mexican women have a higher prevalence of CVD risk factors than White women of comparable socioeconomic backgrounds. In 2003 the overall mortality rate from coronary heart disease was per 162.6 per 100,000, with disproportionately higher rates for African-American males and females. Among African-American males, the CVD mortality rate in 2003 was 241.4. per 100,000 compared with 209.2 per 100,000 for White males (Heart Disease and Stroke Statistics, 2006). Similarly, African-American women did not fare much better than their male counterparts, with a disproportionately higher mortality rate (160.3 per 100,000) compared with their White counterparts (125.1 per 100,000) (Heart Disease and Stroke Statistics, 2006). According to Woods (1998), African-American women tend to develop coronary heart disease much earlier than White women do. Furthermore, the death rate for African-American women under 55 years of age is twice that of White women. Finally, until 75 years of age the mortality from coronary heart disease is higher in African-American women than in women of other racial backgrounds (*Chartbook on Trends in the Health of Americans/Health United States*, 2005).

There are nine easily measured and potentially modifiable risk factors that account for over 90% of the risk of an initial acute myocardial infarction. The pathophysiological effects of the risk factors are seen in both men and women in different racial and ethnic groups. These nine risk factors are cigarette smoking, abnormal blood lipid levels, hypertension, diabetes, abdominal obesity, physical inactivity, poor daily dietary intake of fruits and vegetables, excessive alcohol consumption, and stress. Hypertension, obesity, and dyslipidemia continue to be the major independent risk factors for coronary heart disease and stroke (*Chartbook on Trends in the Health of Americans/Health United States*, 2006). Hypertension is now identified as one of the components of metabolic syndrome and it is recognized as a syndrome of vascular and metabolic disorders that occur along a continuum.

As indicated previously the term *metabolic syndrome* or *dysmetabolic syndrome* is used to describe the constellation of disorders that eventually lead to end-stage vascular disease and metabolic derangements (Dumas, 2003). Clinical findings associated with metabolic syndrome include a waist–hip ratio greater than 0.8 in women and greater than 0.95 in men, a body mass index greater than 24.9 kg/m^2, dyslipidemia (triglycerides > 150 mg/dL, HDL cholesterol < 40 mg/dL in men and <50 mg/dL in women, elevated LDL or total cholesterol), blood pressure greater than 140/90 mm Hg, two elevated fasting glucose values greater than 126 mg/dL, and acanthosis nigricans on the neck or axilla (Dumas, 2003).

Data from the National Health and Nutrition Examination Survey (NHANES) collected between 1999 and 2002 indicated that 39% of women and 24% men between ages 55 and 64 years had at least two or three risk factors for heart disease or stroke. Further findings from this study also revealed that approximately 50% of African-American adults had two or three risk factors, compared with less than one-third of non-Hispanic Whites and Mexican Americans. Data from both the American Heart Association and the National Heart, Lung, and Blood Institute support the strong correlation between the identified risk factors and CVD morbidity and mortality (Heart Disease and Stroke Statistics, 2006).

Hypertension. Hypertension is a major independent risk factor for CVD morbidity and mortality (Heart Disease and Stroke Statistics, 2006). Approximately 50% of individuals with a first myocardial infarction and 60% with a first stroke have blood pressure greater than 160/95 mm Hg (National Heart, Lung, and Blood Institute, 2004). The prevalence of hypertension among African-Americans and Whites in the Southeastern United States is greater and mortality due to myocardial infarction and stroke is greater than in any other region in the country (Yusuf et al., 2001). According to results of NHANES III (1991–2001), the age-adjusted mortality rate from hypertension increased by 36.4%. In 2001, the mortality rate from hypertension in African-Americans was 47.8% for males and 38.9% for females, compared with 13.7% and 13.4% for White males and females, respectively (Heart Disease and Stroke Statistics, 2006). Of the four leading causes of death in African-Americans, hypertension can be associated with at least three of the four disease states: coronary heart disease is the leading cause of death in African-Americans, cerebrovascular accident is listed as third, and diabetes is listed as the fourth (Kloner et al., 2004). Coronary heart disease and cerebrovascular accident can occur as a direct result of sustained hypertension or due to pathological changes that are exacerbated as a result of hypertension. Individuals with diabetes have a higher risk of coronary heart disease and hypertension, and diabetes can accelerate pathophysiological vascular changes, thereby exacerbating both conditions (Lamendola & Mason, 2004).

Approximately 30% of all deaths in hypertensive Black males and 20% of all deaths in hypertensive Black females can be directly attributed to elevated blood pressure (American Heart Association, 2004). African-Americans develop hypertension at an earlier age and have a more severe form of the disease at every age level. The progression of hypertension is more rapid and the incidence of target organ damage is greater than for any other ethnic group. As a result, when compared with Whites, Black Americans have a 1.3 times higher incidence of nonfatal stroke, a 1.8 times higher incidence of fatal stroke, a 1.5 times higher incidence of fatal heart disease, and 4.2 times higher incidence of end-stage renal failure (Heart Disease and Stroke Statistics, 2004). The prevalence of hypertension in Black women is more than 3 times that of White males and females. Compared with White females,

Black females have an 85% higher rate of ambulatory medical visits for hypertension (Heart Disease and Stroke Statistics, 2004).

Serum Cholesterol Levels. Elevated serum lipid levels, another major risk factor, is associated with increased risk for cardiovascular disease. Elevated total cholesterol levels greater than 240 mg/dL have been shown to be an accurate predictor of CVD morbidity and mortality. The mean level of LDL cholesterol for American adults age 20 and older is 127 mg/dL. Levels of 130–159 mg/dL are considered borderline high. Levels of 160–189 mg/dL are classified as high, and levels above 190 mg/dL are very high (NHANES III [1988–1994]). Among non-Hispanic Whites, 20.4% of men and 17% of women have LDL cholesterol levels of 160 mg/dL or greater; in comparison, among non-Hispanic Blacks, 19.3% of men and 18.8% of women have LDL cholesterol levels of 160 mg/dL or higher (NHANES III [1988–1994]). According to data from the American Heart Association Heart Disease and Stroke Statistics (2004), the age-adjusted prevalence of elevated total serum cholesterol levels for persons 20 to 74 years of age was lower in Black American females and males compared with their White counterparts. For total serum cholesterol levels greater than 200 mg/dL, the prevalence was 37.3% for Black males and 46.4% for Black females as compared with 51% and 53.6%, respectively, for their White counterparts. The prevalence of total cholesterol levels of 240 mg/dL or higher was 10.6% for Black males and 17.7 % for Black females compared with 17.8% and 19.9% for White males and females, respectively. Although total serum cholesterol levels tend to be lower in Black adult males and females than in their white counterparts, some data indicate that Black Americans have higher rates of cardiovascular disease due to a greater prevalence of comorbid conditions such as diabetes, obesity, and hypertension (Heart Disease and Stroke Statistics, 2004). For example, in individuals 20 to 74 years of age, the available data suggest that the prevalence of total serum cholesterol levels greater than 240 mg/dL is higher among White males and females (18% and 20%, respectively) than among their Black male and female counterparts (15% and 18%) (Heart Disease and Stroke Statistics, 2006).

It is interesting to note that High Density Lipoprotein cholesterol (HDL) is considered cardioprotective. Higher HDL cholesterol levels are associated with greater protection against CVD. In adults, HDL cholesterol levels less than 40 mg/dL are a known risk factor for CVD. Men and women who have low HDL cholesterol and high total cholesterol levels have the highest risk for myocardial infarction. The mean level of HDL cholesterol in American adults age 20 and older is 50.7 mg/dL (Heart Disease and Stroke Statistics, 2006). Data from the American Heart Association Heart Disease and Stroke Statistics 2004 indicated that 40.5% of White males and 14.5% of White females had HDL cholesterol levels less than 40 mg/dL, compared with 24.3% and 13% of Black males and females and 40.1% and 18% of Mexican American males and females, respectively.

While the proportion of women with cholesterol levels above 240 mg/dL has steadily declined over the past decade, the number of women 20 to 74 years with elevated serum cholesterol levels remains alarmingly high. In fact, in 2001, of the number of women with high serum cholesterol levels, 20.4% were White, 19.4% were Black, and 17.4% were Mexican American (Mirsa, 2001). For African-American women, these numbers become more disconcerting because elevated LDL cholesterol, VLDL cholesterol, and triglyceride levels are positively associated with diabetes and obesity, and African-American women tend to have higher rates of diabetes and obesity. In Blacks, these conditions may negate estrogen's protective mechanism against coronary heart disease (Black, 2002; Fletcher, Gulanick, & Lamendola, 2002).

Smoking. Tobacco use is the leading cause of preventable death and the underlying cause of approximately 5 million premature deaths per year worldwide and just under 500,000 deaths in the United States. Smoking is a powerful risk factor contributing to the development of cardiovascular disease. Smoking has been linked to 30% of deaths from cardiovascular disease (Heart Disease and Stroke Statistics, 2006). Persons who smoke are two to four times more likely to develop CHD than nonsmokers, and they have a higher incidence of sudden cardiac death. Cigarette smokers have twice the risk for stroke and myocardial infarction of nonsmokers. From 1997 to 2001, an estimated 437,902 Americans each year died of smoking-related illnesses; 34.7% of the deaths were due to cardiovascular disease (Centers for Disease Control and Prevention, 2003). Data from the 2006 Heart and Stroke Statistics illuminate the fact that smoking is a prevalent problem among adolescents in high school. In 2003, 30% of male students and 24% of female students in grades 9 to 12 reported current tobacco use; 19.9% of males and 9.4% of females reported current cigar use. Data from the American Heart Association Heart Disease and Stroke Statistics 2006 revealed that more White male and female students reported current cigarette smoking (23.3% and 26.6%, respectively) than Black male and female students (19.3% and 10.8%, respectively). Further, data in this report revealed that White youths age 18 to 24 from families with lower educational attainment had substantially higher rates of smoking than African-American and Mexican American youths with similar educational attainment. Data from the American Heart Association Heart Disease and Stroke Update (2004) indicated that in 2001, the use of any tobacco product was 31.2% for Whites, 27.7% for Blacks, 44.9% for American Indians and Alaska Natives, 28.5% for Native Hawaiians and other Pacific Islanders, 13.6% for Asians, and 22.9 % for Hispanics or Latinos. American Indian/ Native Alaskans have higher rates of smoking (32%) than Black males (27.6%), and American Indian/Native Alaskan females have higher rates of smoking (36.9%) than Black females (18.0%). For all cigarette smokers, there is a 1.5- to 3-fold increase in risk for myocardial infarction (MI). However, in young women who smoke cigarettes, the risk may be increased as much as tenfold (Swank & Fell, 1990). In the adult population, while other racial groups have higher smoking prevalence than do African-Americans, the potential effect of smoking appears to produce more devastating consequences among young premenopausal

African-American women, including lowering HDL2-C, an associated risk for cardiovascular disease and myocardial infarction (Swank & Fell, 1990).

Exposure to environmental smoke is also known to increase the risk for developing CVD and respiratory diseases. An estimated 35,052 nonsmokers die from coronary heart disease each year as a result of exposure to secondhand smoke. Data from NHANES III (1988–1991) show that non-Hispanic Whites have greater environmental exposure to smoke (37.4%) than do Blacks (36.9%). The American Heart Association Heart Disease Stroke Statistics 2004 revealed that smoking rates were substantially higher in families with lower educational attainment. In the same report, data showed that smoking rates were highest among persons living below the poverty level. It is well documented that the percentage of African-Americans who live in poverty is higher than that for other racial and ethnic backgrounds. This may explain why poor African-American women have higher rates of smoking than their White counterparts.

Diabetes. Diabetes is defined as a heterogenous group of chronic metabolic disorders caused by defects in insulin secretion or insulin action. The physical manifestations of diabetes are impaired glucose tolerance, hyperglycemia, and insulin resistance (Zettervall, 2005). In type 1 diabetes, which accounts for 1% to 5% of cases, there is an absolute deficiency of insulin secretion. In type 2 diabetes, which accounts for 90% to 95% of cases, the cause is a combination of resistance to insulin action and inadequate compensatory insulin secretory response (Hohn, Kulkarni, & Seley, 2005). Hypertension is present in 20% to 60% of persons with diabetes. Hypertension often is an initial presenting symptom of insulin resistance and the metabolic syndrome and may be a hallmark for the onset of type 2 diabetes. Diabetes is now an epidemic in the United States, with an estimated 20 million Americans affected. From 1990 to 2000, the percentage of adults with diabetes increased by 48% (Sahebzamani, 2005). Diabetes is diagnosed by a physician in over 14 million Americans, and another 6 million individuals are unaware that they

have the disease. In 2005, 1.5 million new cases were diagnosed, and the number of persons with diabetes is expected to continue to rise over the next decade (American Diabetes Association, 2006). The prevalence of diabetes varies according to race and gender, increases with age, and at all ages is highest among African-Americans (Heart Disease and Stroke Statistics, 2006). In 2001, diabetes was recorded as the seventh leading cause of death in the United States.

More recent data rank diabetes as the fourth leading cause of death (*Chartbook on Trends in the Health of Americans/Health United States*, 2005). In 2003, diabetes was the cause of death for approximately 80,000 people, and it was identified as the contributing cause of death for another 224,100 individuals (*Chartbook on Trends in the Health of Americans/Health United States*, 2005). The prevalence of type 2 diabetes is higher in African-Americans than in Whites, and the overall mortality is 27% higher for African-Americans. African-American, American Indian, and Hispanic women experience the highest diabetes mortality rates (Heart Disease and Stroke Statistics, 2006). In 2003, the overall age-adjusted rate of death from diabetes for African-American males and females was 50.5% and 47.3%, respectively, compared with 26.8% and 20%, respectively, for their White counterparts (Heart Disease and Stoke Statistics, 2006). African-Americans with diabetes have a higher risk for coronary artery disease, stroke, and other major complications of diabetes (such as end-stage renal disease, limb amputations, and blindness) than their White counterparts (American Diabetes Association, 2006).

Obesity and Sedentary Lifestyle. It is a well-documented fact that obesity and inactivity are significant risk factors for cardiovascular disease and diabetes. Obesity is another health condition that has reached pandemic proportions; in the United States, approximately 300,000 deaths per year can be directly attributed to obesity. Central adiposity, one of the components of metabolic syndrome, is associated with an increase in glucose abnormalities, hypertension, and atherosclerosis. Abdominal obesity is an independent risk factor for ischemic stroke in all racial and ethnic groups (Heart Disease and Stroke Statistics, 2006). Overweight in children is defined as a value at or above the 95th percentile of the gender-specific body mass index (BMI) for age growth charts. Obesity among adults is defined as a BMI of 30 kg/m^2 or greater. Approximately 65% of Americans are overweight, including 80% of African-American women over age 40 (Jamerson, 2005). Data from the National Health and Nutrition Examination Survey (NHANES 2003–2004), showed that 17% of American children and adolescents are overweight and that 32.2% of American adults are obese (Ogden, et al., 2006). This change represents a significant increase in the prevalence of overweight children and adolescents and obesity among men. Data from NHANES 2003–2004 revealed that obesity is more prevalent among certain racial and ethnic groups and that gender and age are contributing factors. Results from the 1999–2003 NHIS study of the CDC showed that rates of obesity were higher in African-American women: 36.6% compared with 20.3% for White women and 5.8% for Asian women. Data from the same study showed a direct link between obesity and the development of cardiovascular disease, dyslipidemia, type 2 diabetes, and sleep apnea (Ogden, et al., 2006).

Results from NHANES III revealed a positive correlation between obesity and hypertension in African-Americans. Persons who are overweight or obese have an increased risk of developing hypertension, type 2 diabetes, coronary heart disease, and stroke (Jamerson, 2005). There is a higher prevalence of obesity in women with lower incomes, and African-American women are more likely to be in a lower income bracket than White women (National Center for Health Statistics, 2006). This fact is also supported by recent data from the American Heart Association (2006). This report showed that 77.2% of non-Hispanic Black females and 62.9% of non-Hispanic Black males are overweight, compared with 69.4% of White males and 57.2% of White females. Non-Hispanic Black females also have the highest rate of obesity (49%) compared with non-Hispanic Black males (27.9%), non-Hispanic White males (28.2%), and non-Hispanic White females (30.7%) (American Heart Association 2006; NHANES, 2003–2004). Factors contributing to obesity include excessive dietary intake of calories and fatty foods and physical inactivity (American Heart Association, 2006; NHANES, 2003–2004; National Center for Health Statistics, 2002). Persons with lower incomes and less education typically have poorer dietary habits and are not as physically active as those who have high incomes and are better educated (American Heart Association, 2006; National Center for Health Statistics, 2006; Mirsa, 2001; U.S. Department of Health and Human Services, 2000). African-Americans and Hispanics in general have lower incomes and are more likely to live in poverty than Whites (National Center for Health Statistics, 2006). In fact, 8,146,146 African-Americans live below the poverty index. If being overweight is a common problem in the general U.S. population, it is said to be at epidemic proportions for children in this country (Strauss & Pollack, 2001).

Childhood obesity continues to increase steadily and rapidly among African-American children (Ogden, et al., 2006). Some researchers conclude that childhood obesity often serves as a primary marker for high-risk dietary and physical inactivity practices (Crawford, Story, Wang, Ritchie, & Sabry, 2001). Childhood obesity can also contribute to the development of metabolic syndrome, leading to early onset of CVD and type 2 diabetes.

Stroke. Strokes are the third leading cause of death in the United States. In African-Americans, the rate of death from stroke is almost twice as high as it is for Whites because of a greater prevalence of comorbid conditions, along with an increased severity and a more rapid progression of disease processes. Cardiovascular disease, hypertension, and diabetes, the major risk factors for strokes, are seen in disproportionate numbers of African-Americans. Of the four leading causes of death in African-Americans, hypertension can be associated with at least three of the four disease states: coronary heart disease, the leading cause of death among African-Americans; cerebrovascular accidents, listed as third; and diabetes, listed as fourth. Coronary heart disease and cerebrovascular accidents can occur or are exacerbated as a result of hypertension. Individuals with diabetes have a higher risk of coronary heart disease and hypertension, and both conditions are exacerbated by diabetes (Heart Disease and Stroke Statistics, 2006).

Sudden Cardiac Deaths. Significant differences have been noted in the incidence of sudden cardiac arrest among African-Americans. A 2001 report from the CDC indicated that rate of sudden cardiac death was much higher for young African-Americans than for Whites (Centers for Disease Control and Prevention, 2001b). Not only are African-Americans more likely to experience sudden cardiac arrest, but also they are more likely to succumb to the arrest (American Heart Association, 2002). In fact, among African-Americans in all age groups, both men and women have higher rates of cardiac arrests than their White counterparts have. The survival rate for African-Americans, compared with Whites, was remarkably different (0.8% versus 2.6%). The difference in survival rate can be attributed to the fact that the mortality rate for African-Americans with coronary artery disease, left ventricular hypertrophy, congestive heart failure, and cardiomyopathy is higher than that for Whites (Heart Disease and Stroke Statistics, 2006). Data from a Duke University study on age, sex, racial disparities in heart hospital transfer patterns revealed that older, female, and minority patients rushed to community hospitals with acute myocardial infarctions were less likely to be transferred to larger hospitals offering procedures to restore artery patency. The authors found that women were 16% less likely to be transferred than men; compared with White patients, African-Americans were 31% and Hispanics were 41% less likely to be transferred (Berger, 2006). In another Duke University study, researchers found that hypertrophic cardiomyopathy (HCM), a common cause of sudden cardiac death in young competitive athletes, was an important issue for African-Americans (Maron, et al., 2003). Maron et al. (2003) found a large discrepancy in clinical diagnosis of HCM in African-American compared with White athletes. Of 1986 patients clinically diagnosed with HCM, only 158 (8%) were African-American. Furthermore, among the 286 cardiovascular deaths, most were caused by hypertrophic cardiomyopathy HCM($n = 102$). Results of this study showed that of the 102 athletes who died from HCM, 42 were White (41%) and 56 were African-Americans (55%). The authors concluded that HCM is underdiagnosed in African-American athletes and that the condition is a common cause of sudden death in this population.

Other plausible explanations for the differences between the rates and lethality of sudden cardiac arrest for African-Americans and their White counterparts are as follows: (1) inexperience and lack of familiarity with basic CPR techniques of the persons at the site; (2) response time of the emergency ambulance to the site, particularly in "African-American neighborhoods"; and (3) response time of the hospital emergency team to the African-American client in full cardiac arrest (Becker, Han, Meyer, et al., 1993). Because the findings from this study indicate that the incidence of cardiac arrest is significantly higher among African-Americans in every age group, early intervention and prevention techniques to reduce the chronicity of coronary heart disease appear to be a plausible mechanism to prevent cardiac arrest in this population.

AIDS (HIV) Risk. While cardiovascular diseases have been heralded as the single leading cause of death across all ethnic and racial groups, little attention has been paid to the growing incidence of deaths from AIDS among African-Americans under 35 years of age. HIV/AIDS was once thought of as a disease that primarily affected gay, single White males. However, in 2005, more African-Americans with AIDS were reported than any other ethnic/racial groups residing in the United States (Centers for Disease Control and Prevention, 2005). In fact, 22,030 cases of AIDS were reported among African-Americans. By comparison, in 2005, the rates of HIV/AIDS cases were 72.8 per 100,000 among African-Americans, 28.5 per 100,000 among Hispanics, 10.6 per 100,000 among American Indians and Alaska Natives, 9.0 per 100,000 among Whites, and 7.6 per 100,000 among Asian/Pacific Islanders (Centers for Disease Control and Prevention, 2005). From this figure, nearly 50% of all new cases of AIDS (44,198) reported in 2005 occurred among African-Americans. In 2001, nearly two thirds (64%) of all new cases of AIDS in women were reported in African-Americans. Similarly, in 2001 nearly two thirds (65%) of all new pediatric cases reported were among African-Americans.

In 2005, while by proportion of the population African-American males represented only 13% of U.S. males, they disproportionately represented 47% of all reported cases of AIDS (Centers for Disease Control and Prevention, 2005). Even more astounding is the number of African-American women who had AIDS (84,681) compared with their White counterparts (30,854). In addition, while by proportion of the population African-American women make up only 14% of U.S. females, these individuals disproportionately represent 65% of all reported cases of AIDS in women. In fact, overall, African-Americans now represent approximately 45% of all reported cases of AIDS in the United States to date (Coalition on Urban Renewal and Education, 2002). Moreover, African-Americans between 13 and 24 years of age now account for 35% of reported AIDS cases in that age group (Centers for Disease Control and Prevention, 2005). More importantly, these data also suggest that 1 in 50 African-American men and 1 in 160 African-American women are infected with HIV. In addition, African-Americans between 13 and 24 years of age now account for 57% of all HIV diagnoses (Centers for Disease Control and Prevention, 2005).

Currently, men who have sex with men still represent the largest group of individuals with HIV/AIDS in the United States (Ward & Duchin, 1998). However, since the first reported case in 1981, HIV/AIDS has become a major cause of morbidity and mortality among African-Americans. Ward and Duchin reported in 1998 that for the first time the number of African-Americans with a diagnosis of AIDS was approximately equal to the number of reported cases in Whites. Since 1995, HIV infection has become the leading cause of death in persons 24 to 44 years of age (Centers for Disease Control and Prevention, 2005).

A disproportionate number of individuals with AIDS in this age range (22 to 44) are African-American. According to the CDC (2005), the rate of death from AIDS was about 129% greater for African-American males (178.0 per 100,000) than for White males (138.0 per 100,000). African-American females fare even worse (53 per 100,000), with a death rate 8.833 times greater than that for White females (6 per 100,000) (Centers for Disease Control and Prevention, 2001a). Statistical data from the CDC support the fact that a greater percentage of African-Americans are infected with HIV and are dying of AIDS compared with other races. According to demographic data from the CDC AIDS hotline, a total of 612,078 persons have died of AIDS (Table 8-1).

Moore, Stanton, Gopalan, and Chaisson (1994), researchers at Johns Hopkins University School of Medicine, conducted a study on HIV-positive individuals to determine whether there were notable differences in the administration of antiretroviral drugs among Black and White clients. Findings from this study suggest that Black HIV-positive individuals are less likely than their White counterparts to be given antiretroviral drugs, including medication to prevent *Pneumocystis carinii*

Table 8-1 Cumulative AIDS Mortalities Occurring Through December 2001 in the United States*

Demographic Variable	Male	Female	Pediatric
Non-Hispanic White	197,724	15,466	1002
Non-Hispanic Black	127,450	40,753	2912
Hispanic	67,557	14,236	1224
Asian Pacific Islander	2828	351	37
Native American	1070	216	21
Unknown origin	601	10	16

* From the Centers for Disease Control and Prevention (2001). HIV Surveillance Report. Atlanta: Centers for Disease Control and Prevention, 13(2).

pneumonia (PCP). Of Blacks surveyed, only 58% of those medically eligible received drug therapy, compared with 82% of their White counterparts. Researchers found no significant differences in receipt of drug therapy with respect to such moderating variables as age, gender, mode of HIV transmission, type of insurance, income, education, or place of residence. Similarly, Shapiro, Morton, McCaffrey, et al. (1999) noted that even after adjustment for insurance status, CD4 cell count, sex, age, methods of exposure to HIV, and region of the country, African-Americans, along with their Hispanic counterparts, were 24% less likely than their White counterparts to receive protease inhibitors or nonnucleoside reverse transcriptase inhibitors at the initial assessment by their health care providers.

Guidelines published by the U.S. Public Health Service (PHS) suggest that to effectively treat HIV-infected persons, antiretroviral therapy should begin when the client's CD4 cell count falls to 500 cells/mm^3 or less. These PHS guidelines also suggest that prophylactic treatment for PCP should begin when the CD4 count reaches 200 cells/mm^3 or less. Because CD4 cells are integral to the body's immune defense, reduction in CD4 cells is generally associated with a weakening in the immune system. This reduction, particularly among HIV-positive individuals, generally signals an onset of disease symptoms, including PCP (Moore, Stanton, Gopalan, & Chaisson, 1994). Moore, Stanton, Gopalan, and Chaisson. (1994) also noted that among clients with a CD4 cell count of 500 cells/mm^3 or less, only 48% of Blacks, compared with 68% of Whites, received antiretroviral therapy. Despite the PHS guidelines for administration of prophylactic therapy to all clients with a CD4 cell count of 200 cells/mm^3 or less, researchers found an even greater disparity between Blacks and their White counterparts, with Blacks invariably receiving little intervention when CD4 cell counts dropped to 200 cells/mm^3 or less.

Psychological Characteristics

Some studies depict the pattern of interaction in the African-American family as pathological and unstable. Findings from one study indicate that if there is stability in the African-American family it is attributable to the presence of a controlling, domineering mother. The pathological family interaction that occurs in some African-American families is said to affect the son so profoundly that in later life he is unable to adjust to the role of husband and father. Consequently, in unstable African-American families, the African-American male is unable to form mature, lasting relationships with others (Culture of Poverty Revisited, n.d.). In studies done on African-American male alcoholics, these individuals were found to have the lowest scores on tests of personality integration, with a more passive and compliant coping style than any other ethnic group of male alcoholics (Carroll, Klein, & Santo, 1978). It is believed that this passive and compliant coping style was rooted in the slavery era. During slavery, African-American mothers were forced to teach their male children to be passive if they were to survive the authority of the slave master because to be "uppity" meant possible physical punishment or even death. Today it would seem essential that the African-American male display the same survival skills because the authority figure still remains (police, educators, employers, and so forth).

A study done on African-American boys from father-absent homes found that dependency and a passive coping style were evident among these boys (Barclay & Cusumano, 1967). Other studies suggest that boys from father-absent homes tend to be more dependent on their peer groups, display fewer aggressive behaviors, have lower self-esteem, and are more likely to display overt masculine behavior. In some studies looking at psychological issues of father-absent homes, social class appeared to be an intervening variable. A more deleterious effect on sex-role orientation was found in boys who lived in father-absent homes before 5 years of age (Covell & Turnbull, 1982). Because there is a greater probability of an African-American male being reared in a female-headed household, it has become necessary for African-American mothers to encourage masculine traits in their sons. An earlier study found that mothers who encouraged masculine traits in their sons had more of an effect in father-absent homes than in father-present homes (Biller, 1969).

Some social scientists and health care providers contend that African-Americans are at risk for the development of mental health problems. Corrective steps have been taken to alleviate the development of mental health problems; however, the mental health system continues to struggle to meet the emotional needs of African-Americans (Snowden, 1982; Snowden & Todman, 1982). Bullough and Bullough (1982) reported that rates of admission to mental health hospitals are higher and the hospital stay is longer for African-Americans than for any other ethnic group in the United States. However, when socioeconomic status was carefully controlled for, psychosis rates among Whites and African-Americans appeared similar.

Chemical Abuse. Alcoholism is one of the major health problems in the African-American community, contributing to reduced longevity. Among African-Americans, there are high incidence rates of acute and chronic alcohol-related diseases, such as alcoholic fatty liver; hepatitis; cirrhosis of the liver; heart disease; cancer of the mouth, larynx, tongue, esophagus, and lung; and unintentional injuries and homicide (Ronan, 1987).

Harper and Dawkins (1976) reported that of 16,000 articles on alcohol abuse published from 1944 to 1974, only 77 included references to African-Americans, and only 11 were specifically about African-Americans. King (1982) reported that most studies between 1977 and 1980 dealt only with patterns of alcohol use. Only one study (Stalls, 1978) explored racial differences in patterns of alcohol metabolism. Stalls (1978) found an increasing incidence of alcohol abuse among African-American youth and women, with serious implications for fetal alcohol syndrome. Drinking appeared to peak between 16 and 23 years of age, and, among women, drinking was highest for divorced women younger than 45 years of age. Brisbane (1987) noted that women who drank were typically younger than 45 years of age, were employed, and considered themselves middle class. Williams (1986) noted a contradiction in the high incidence of alcohol-related diseases and drinking patterns reported in African-Americans: when age and socioeconomic levels were controlled, African-Americans actually abstained more, drank less frequently, and consumed less alcohol than their White counterparts. African-American women were the exception, with 11% of African-American women drinking heavily, compared with 4% of White women.

Several causes of alcohol abuse and misuse in African-Americans have been identified in the literature. A primary factor is economics. Many African-American men drink as a result of unemployment, which leads to depression and frustration because of their inability to meet financial commitments. Williams (1986) concluded that unemployment is correlated with a high risk for alcohol problems among African-Americans. Availability is also a factor (Parker & Harman, 1978). Brown and Tooley (2004) have reported that in Los Angeles there are approximately three liquor stores per city block. African-American peer pressure is also reported as a contributing factor; peers expect heavy drinking, and brand names and quantity are often status identifiers. Finally, heavy alcohol use may be related to a desire to escape unpleasant feelings. Sterne and Pittman (1972) have also pointed out themes that seem to be present in African-American alcohol use. They linked being paid on the weekend to Saturday relaxation and thus drinking. A second theme is the prevalence of taverns in the African-American community that serve as social centers. Finally, alcohol appears to be used as an escape from personal problems.

African-Americans are less likely to seek treatment for problem drinking than any other ethnic group in the United States (Lawson & Lawson, 2004). Research indicates that several areas must be addressed to increase the likelihood of successful treatment outcomes. The first step is to get the African-American alcoholic into a treatment program. Programs that are located within the community and are accessible to public transportation are more likely to be used, except by the upwardly mobile African-American person, who is more likely to seek private services outside the community. The African-American church can and in some instances does serve a dual role in this first step because it can provide a facility and at the same time act as a referral source.

Most African-American churches are centrally located within the African-American community, and even as members relocate, they tend to maintain their roots in the African-American church. Also, prayer has been associated with the treatment modality and overall success rate for the recovering alcoholic. The church continues to be the mainstay of the African-American family, and rather than seeking outside help for alcoholism, the family often attempts to resolve problems by going to the minister. Some African-Americans have reported that they stopped drinking before seeking professional help because of their spirituality, which assisted with the transition (Brisbane, 1987; Hudson, 1986; Knox, 1986; Westermeyer, 1984).

When treating the recovering alcoholic, the nurse must remember that the family can often provide assistance in the form of shelter, food, money, or clothing. The extended family may also take on counseling roles that close relatives find too painful (Brisbane & Womble, 1986). The nurse must also have an awareness of the socioeconomic context and its effect on intrapsychic processes. The elimination of stereotypical bias by both the nurse and the client and the inclusion of social values and traditions are necessary to maximize intervention, give culturally appropriate nursing care, and affect recovery rates (Institute of Black Chemical Abuse, 1988).

Posttraumatic Stress Disorder. Many studies indicate that minority Vietnam veterans have experienced a greater degree of maladjustment after the Vietnam War than their White counterparts (Allen, 1986; Laufer, Gallops, & Frey-Wouters, 1984). Some of these studies have given a variety of reasons for this maladjustment, including the fact that minorities felt more conflict about participating in the war because they had less to gain than persons in the dominant culture. Another reason postulated by the researchers was that minorities were more likely to be identified with the enemy, who were also different in skin color from White Americans. Perhaps the most significant reason for posttraumatic stress disorder (PTSD) among minority Vietnam veterans was that the status of minorities declined in the United States during the turbulence of the 1960s

at the same time that African-Americans were fighting for the United States in Vietnam (Allen, 1986; Laufer, Gallops, & Frey-Wouters, 1981).

In a more recent study, Penk, Robinowitz, Black, et al. (1989) also found that among Vietnam combat veterans, African-Americans appeared to be more maladjusted than their White counterparts. One conclusion of this study is that ethnicity emerges as a significant parameter in studies of PTSD, but the exact contributions of ethnicity have not been explained fully by current findings on the subject. Many researchers have postulated that significant increases in PTSD in African-American Vietnam veterans may be attributable in part to the fact that during the Vietnam War years (1964–1975), African-Americans suffered the major loss of a leader (through the assassination of Martin Luther King Jr. in 1968) and experienced the racial conflicts evidenced by rioting in Washington, D.C., Watts (in Los Angeles), and other cities throughout the country (Karnow, 1997).

Other Psychological Characteristics. The psychiatric literature on psychological characteristics of African-Americans and treatment of African-Americans by mental health professionals is controversial. The psychiatric literature has reported increased psychopathological disorders among African-Americans (Pasamanick, 1964). Anatomical, neurological, and endocrinological differences have been cited as signs of African-American inferiority (Thomas & Sillen, 1972; Tobias, 1970). Research has been done on African-Americans that would not have been considered for other ethnic groups. For example, in the Tuskegee project, African-American men with syphilis were intentionally denied treatment without being informed of their disease (Cave, 1975; Jones, 1993). Research on IQs has been used to support statements of genetic inferiority and justify social policies such as selective immigration laws and school segregation (Hirsch, 1981). Such psychological research has added to racial stereotyping and bias among some mental health professionals.

According to Meyers and Weissman (1980–1981), some differences in phobias have been found between African-Americans and Whites. Robins,

Helzer, Croughan, and Ratcliff (1981) noted that the lifetime prevalence of acrophobia was significantly higher for African-Americans than for Whites. Vernon and Roberts (1982) found that African-Americans, compared with Whites, had a significantly lower lifetime rate of both major and minor depression but had a rate of bipolar depression that was twice that of Whites. A possible explanation for the discrepancy in findings is the lack of national data on racial differences in diagnostic analogs. It is now widely accepted that on the Minnesota Multiphasic Personality Inventory (MMPI) African-Americans tend to score higher on the paranoia and schizophrenia scales than Whites because the instrument was not standardized on an African-American population (Bell & Mehta, 1981; Gynther, 1981; Jones, Gray, & Parson, 1981). When standardized diagnostic systems are used today, African-Americans do not differ from Whites in the prevalence of most psychiatric disorders. Robins, Helzer, Croughan, and Ratcliff (1981) and Meyers and Weissman (1980–1981) have reported finding no significant race differences for schizophrenia or affective disorders (Adebimpe, 1981; Lawson & Lawson, 2004; Mukherjee, Shukla, & Woodle, 1983; Spurlock, 1985).

Snow (1978) found that a belief in witchcraft was shared by a third of the African-American clients who were treated at a Southern psychiatric center. African-Americans who believe they have a folk illness may use the services of a root worker, reader, spiritualist, or voodoo priest. It is important for the nurse to know that the client may have used the services of a folk practitioner before or with scientific mental health therapy. Wintrob (1973) has promoted the idea that individuals who believe in folk remedies such as root work or obeah (Black ritual) may regard scientific treatment only as palliative because curing the total condition requires neutralization by a specially skilled folk healer. Wintrob (1973), Kreisman (1975), Weclew (1975), and Sandoval (1977) have suggested that mental health professionals should attempt to complement use of scientific medicine with folk practices for clients who believe mental disorders are attributed to folk causes.

Implications for Nursing Care

The best reason for including the concept of biological variations in nursing practice is that knowledge of scientific facts aids the nurse in giving culturally appropriate care. It is also essential for the nurse who cares for people from other cultures to know certain biological concepts not only to give culturally appropriate nursing care but also to give nonharmful nursing care.

Important biological variations that the nurse should be aware of are related to body size, birth weight, and body proportion. It is important for the nurse who works with African-American children to remember that at birth African-American children tend to weigh less and be shorter than their White counterparts and that these variations may be attributable in part to socioeconomic status. Therefore, the nurse, whether in a hospital or in a clinic setting, must carefully evaluate growth status in terms of height and weight for African-American children. Some nurses believe that because growth charts are White normed, data gleaned from these charts lack implications in regard to African-American children. It is important for the nurse to recognize that even for African-American children serious growth deviation can have implications for intervention for nutritional deficiencies. These variations between African-American and White children may continue as the child grows. For example, African-American preschoolers are neurologically more advanced than their White counterparts. In addition, African-American children tend to have less subcutaneous fat than White children but are taller and heavier by 2 years of age (Owen & Lubin, 1973). The fact that African-American preschoolers are taller and heavier may indicate a need for appropriate client teaching about nutritional needs of the growing child.

Because the average weight for an African-American woman is consistently higher than that for her White counterpart at every age, the nurse must teach African-American clients the value of serving nutritiously sound meals. In addition, the nurse must emphasize the importance of exercise, not only to maintain ideal weight but also for cardiovascular purposes.

It is essential that the nurse develop a sensitivity for and familiarity with physical features that are common to African-Americans, as well as with African-American–related illnesses and diseases. If the nurse is unable to develop a familiarity with physical features common to African-Americans and with African-American illnesses or diseases, the nurse cannot possibly hope to recognize or diagnose conditions that may cause disequilibrium in the body. In addition, the nurse must be prepared to deal promptly, efficiently, and appropriately with clinical variables that are common to all African-American clients and yet have significant variability in some African-American clients, such as hypertension or sickle cell anemia. Some researchers assert that there is no clear correlation between hypertension and obesity in African-Americans as there is with other ethnic groups such as Whites. On the other hand, there appears to be a direct correlation between the amount of skin pigmentation and the frequency of hypertension. Therefore, because it has been suggested that there is a direct relationship between skin pigmentation and hypertension, the nurse should emphasize the need for the African-American client to undergo hypertension screening (Boyle, 1970).

Because G-6-PD deficiency is a hematological problem that is present in 35% of African-Americans, it is essential that the nurse stress the importance of the fluorescent spot test as a screening tool in diagnosing this deficiency. The nurse can serve as a client advocate and insist or mandate that this test be a routine part of laboratory testing for all African-American clients. Also, precautions should be taken to eliminate the transfusion of G-6-PD–deficient blood, particularly in transfusions for infants (Beutler, 1983). In addition, the nurse should exercise caution when planning diets for African-American clients, particularly African-American infants, because they may be lactose intolerant. In these cases the nurse should plan diets that allow substituting more compatible products with the same nutritional value for milk and milk products (Bloch, 1981).

SUMMARY

Some researchers contend that the disproportionate morbidity and mortality rates in the African-American population are directly attributed to discriminatory practices in health care and to inequalities in social, economic, and educational opportunities rather than biological variations and genetics (Geronimus, Bound, Waidmann, Colen, & Steffick, 2001). It is a well-known fact that a greater percentage of African-Americans are more likely to live in poverty and have lower educational achievement than other racial and ethnic groups in the United States (U.S. Department of Commerce, Bureau of the Census, Summary File 3, 2002). It is plausible to assume that inequalities in income and education underlie many health disparities in the United States. Population groups that experience the worst health problems are also those that have the highest poverty rates and the least education (U.S. Department of Health and Human Services, 2000). In addition, because disparities in income and educational levels are often associated with differences in rates of illness and death, including heart disease, diabetes, and obesity, it is conceivable that an overriding theme with health disparities may logically rest with socioeconomic status.

Educational achievement for African-Americans continues to lag behind that for Whites, Asians, and Pacific Islanders. Higher educational levels are associated with a greater likelihood of obtaining and comprehending the health-related information that is needed to develop health-promoting behaviors and beliefs in prevention. When educated, individuals are more likely to make informed choices regarding health promotion behaviors. Furthermore, educated individuals are more likely to have knowledge of disease symptoms and to comprehend the seriousness of the symptoms. Access to health care, delays in treatment, and inappropriate treatment contribute to increased morbidity and mortality for minorities, women, and the poor (Institute of Medicine, 2002; Richards, Funk, & Milner, 2000). These practices place a tremendous economic burden on society and contribute to the perpetuation of poverty, despair, and separation from mainstream society.

Braithwaite and Taylor (2001) conclude that even when holding socioeconomic status, access to care, and poverty rates constant, health disparities tend to remain constant along racial lines, particularly among African-Americans. Thus, it is plausible to assume that changing variables related to socioeconomic status and educational attainment, while admirable and laudable, by themselves with no attention to unequal treatment, cultural incompetence on the part of health care providers, and lack of knowledge about culture, cultural heritage, and biological variations will contribute only modestly to changing health outcomes and thereby eliminating health disparities.

In caring for the African-American client, the nurse must recognize and acknowledge the client's racial, cultural, and ethnic background because it is in these areas that the client's experiences occur. It is important not only for the nurse to consider necessary adjustments in client care when the client is from a different racial origin but also that the racial origin of the nurse be considered. In a classic and innovative study by Remington and DaCosta (1989), the effects of ethnocultural differences between supervisor and caregiver are dramatically illustrated. The nurse who denies or does not believe race is a factor denies a significant part of the client's being. It is important that nurses recognize the cultural, economic, and social barriers that inhibit the client's ability to articulate and comprehend the relevant symptoms. All aspects of care provided must be adapted to the client's cultural experiences and educational and socioeconomic background. As a client advocate, it is imperative that the nurse perform an accurate, culturally competent assessment, document findings, and clearly articulate data to other health care providers.

Case Study

Initial Presentation

Mrs. Betty Perry, a 45-year-old African-American female, resides with her husband and two children in a small city in the Midwest. Mrs. Perry teaches high school math. Her husband works as an insurance agent. Mrs. Perry saw her primary care physician 1 week ago for her annual physical exam.

History

Mrs. Perry reports that she has been in good health. Her past medical history is unremarkable with the exception of a "weight problem." Mrs. Perry reports that she has been overweight since the birth of her last child, 15 years ago.

Prior history includes a tonsillectomy at age 10 and two cesarean sections. Mrs. Perry has a positive family history of type 2 diabetes (both parents), coronary heart disease (father and brother), and hypertension (both parents). Mrs. Perry does not smoke or drink. She admits to eating fast foods 3 or 4 times a week because of her hectic schedule, and she very rarely exercises.

Physical Examination

Vital signs: blood pressure, 140/88 mm Hg right arm, 140/90 mm Hg left arm; heart rate, 80 beats/min; temperature, 98.7 °F; respirations, 18 breaths/min. Height, 5′ 5″; weight, 180 lbs; body mass index, 30.

PU: lungs clear throughout.

COR: RRR, S1S2 heart sounds, ø murmurs, capillary refill < 3 seconds.

GI: abdomen soft, protuberant; active bowel sounds all 4 quadrants.

GU: normal female genitalia.

Integument: warm dry, normal hair distribution.

(Continued)

Laboratory and Diagnostic Tests
ECG and chest x-ray: normal.
Blood glucose: 342 mg/dL.
Urinalysis: negative for protein, RBC, WBC.

Mrs. Perry was instructed to return in 1 week for follow-up evaluation and for the results of the chemistry profile, lipid profile, and hemoglobin A_{1c}, PT, and PTT.

Mrs. Perry returned the following week for follow-up evaluation and for results of lab values.

The results were as follows: hemoglobin A_{1c}, 12%; fasting blood glucose, 240 mg/dL; creatinine, 1.9 mg/dL; sodium, 137 mEq/L; BUN 30 mg/dL; LDL cholesterol, 288 mg/dL; HDL cholesterol, 42 mg/dL; triglycerides, 239 mg/dL. Her blood pressure on this visit was 140/90 right arm and 140/88 left arm. Mrs. Perry was diagnosed with type 2 diabetes and obesity. In addition, her blood pressure remained in the high normal range (140/90). She was given a prescription for metformin, 500 mg bid, and scheduled for a follow-up appointment in 2 weeks. Because of the concerns regarding Mrs. Perry's blood pressure and weight, she was given a referral for diabetic education, a weight reduction program, and an exercise program.

CARE PLAN

❋ *Nursing Diagnosis: Nutrition, imbalanced: more than body requirements related to excessive caloric intake and lack of exercise*

Client Outcomes
1. Client will verbalize importance of complying with prescribed exercise program.
2. Client will verbalize importance of complying with prescribed diet.

Nursing Interventions
1. Assess client knowledge of diabetes and therapeutic regimen.
2. Assess client's usual dietary intake.
3. Review prescribed diet with client.
4. Assess client barriers to exercise.
5. Explain the importance of regular exercise for weight loss and blood sugar control.

❋ *Nursing Diagnosis: Ineffective health maintenance related to inability to make thoughtful judgments about management of diabetes*

Client Outcome
1. Client and family will verbalize understanding of pathological condition, complications, and importance of lifelong management of diabetes.

Nursing Interventions
1. Assess client knowledge level and readiness to learn.
2. Teach client and family the symptoms that require immediate medical attention.
3. Teach client correct method of glucose testing and recording values.
4. Review sick day care.
5. Discuss the complications of uncontrolled diabetes.
6. Explain pathophysiology of diabetes.
7. Explain the risk factors for developing type 2 diabetes.
8. Explain to client that there is no cure for type 2 diabetes.
9. Explain the actions and indications of antihyperglycemic medication.
10. Review the symptoms of hyperglycemia and hypoglycemia.

❋ Nursing Diagnosis: Risk for injury related to adverse effects of the antihyperglycemic drug

Client Outcome

1. Client will verbalize understanding the side effects of oral antihyperglycemic medications and the importance of notifying physician of symptoms rather than stopping medication.

Nursing Interventions

1. Assess client knowledge of prescribed drug.
2. Provide client with information related to adverse effects of metformin, such as headache, dizziness, fatigue, nausea, abdominal pain, diarrhea, anorexia.
3. Stress the importance of notifying the physician of side effects rather than stopping the medication abruptly.

❋ Nursing Diagnosis: Anxiety related to change in health status (therapeutic regimen, lifestyle changes, lack of control of condition, and potential complications of diabetes)

Client Outcome

1. Client will identify methods to promote physiological and emotional comfort and a sense of well-being.

Nursing Interventions

1. Explore client's perception of type 2 diabetes and related lifestyle changes.
2. Ask client and family to discuss how type 2 diabetes has affected their lifestyle.
3. Assess stressors in client's life and effective coping mechanisms.
4. Assess family resources and support systems.
5. Involve client and family in goals to reduce anxiety and to develop effective coping methods.

❋ Nursing Diagnosis: Knowledge deficit related to unfamiliarity with pathophysiological state and therapeutic regimen for diabetes

Client Outcome

1. Client will be able to define type 2 diabetes; state the complications of type 2 diabetes; explain the actions, indications, and side effects of medications and the necessity for lifelong compliance with therapy.

Nursing Interventions

1. Assess client's knowledge of type 2 diabetes.
2. Assess client's knowledge of the therapeutic regimen for type 2 diabetes.
3. Provide oral and written instructions related to type 2 diabetes, including therapeutic management.
4. Discuss the possibility of hyperglycemia if the prescribed medication, dietary restrictions, and exercise program are not adhered to.
5. Discuss the complications of uncontrolled type 2 diabetes.
6. Elicit client and family input in measures to achieve compliance with lifelong therapy.

❋ STUDY QUESTIONS

1. Explain how obesity, physical inactivity, and poor dietary habits contribute to the development of type 2 diabetes.
2. Explain how persistent elevation of blood glucose levels leads to the development of cardiovascular disease.
3. List the complications of uncontrolled type 2 diabetes.
4. Explain why it is important for the nurse to get a detailed health history from Mrs. Perry.
5. Based on the information in the care plan, identify factors that place Mrs. Perry at high risk for developing cardiovascular disease.
6. Identify measures for the nurse to use to help Mrs. Perry verbalize concerns related to noncompliance with medication, diet, weight reduction, and lifestyle changes.
7. List several strategies that may help health care providers develop and use culturally appropriate communication techniques for African-Americans.

8. Describe ways in which health care providers may show sensitivity and acceptance of African-American folk health care practices.
9. Compare and contrast the social organization of African-Americans from diverse social and economic backgrounds.
10. List several practices from ancient African ancestry that are a part of modern nursing philosophy.

NCLEX-RN REVIEW QUESTIONS

1. When providing care for an African-American client, it is important for the nurse to remember that African-Americans are perceived as being:
   A. Polychronic
   B. Monochronic
   C. Polymorphic
   D. Monomorphic

2. To reduce polychronic effects while caring for an African-American client, the nurse should:
   A. Permit the client to have frequent, constant interruptions.
   B. Allow the client to keep the perception of the need for order.
   C. Allow the client to structure activities in a ranked order that will produce maximal benefit.
   D. Assist the client to structure activities in a ranked order that will produce maximal benefits.

11. Describe the importance of folk medicine practices and folk healers to African-Americans in the rural setting.
12. Describe the significance of the Institute of Medicine report on unequal treatment to the development of culturally competent care.
13. List several strategies that assist in organization of time as a method of assisting in the adherence to treatment and medication regimens.

3. You are taking care of an African-American female who recently had a cerebrovascular accident, leaving her unable to talk. As you attempt to give her medications with her milk on her tray, she resists. After explaining the importance of taking her medications, and on time, your client reluctantly takes the medications with milk. Later she has a large diarrhea stool. What biological variation should have been considered with this client?
   A. Lactose intolerance is high among African-Americans.
   B. Hypertension is high among African-Americans.
   C. Tuberculosis is high among African-Americans.
   D. Dietary variations may cause diarrhea in African-Americans.

References

Abraham, S. J., Clifford, L., & Najjar, M. F. (1976, November). Height and weight of adults 18–74 years of age in the United States. *Advance Data*, 3, 1–18.

Adebimpe, V. (1981). Overview: White norms and psychiatric diagnosis of Black patients. *American Journal of Psychiatry*, 138, 279–285.

Albertson, C. (2003). *Bessie*. New Haven: Yale University Press.

Allen, I. M. (1986). Post-traumatic stress disorder among Black Vietnam veterans. *Hospital and Community Psychiatry*, 37, 55–61.

Amemiya, H., Arinami, T., Kikuchi, S., et al. (1996). Apolipoprotein(a) and pentanucleotide repeat polymorphisms are associated with the degree of atherosclerosis in coronary heart disease. *Atherosclerosis*, 123(1–2), 181–191.

American Diabetes Association (2006). Total prevalence of diabetes and pre diabetes. Available at http://www.diabetes.org/diabetes-statistics/prevalence.jsp. Accessed: May 24, 2006.

American Heart Association (2002). *Heart and stroke statistical update*. Dallas: American Heart Association.

American Heart Association (2004). *Heart disease and stroke statistics.* Dallas: American Heart Association.

American Heart Association (2006). *Heart disease and stroke statistics.* Dallas: American Heart Association.

Anderson, S. V., & Bauwens, E. E. (1981). *Chronic health problems: concepts and application.* St. Louis: Mosby.

Angelou, M. (1989). Maya Angelou (personal interview and portrait). In Lanker, B. (Ed.), *I dream a world: portraits of Black women who changed America.* New York: Stewart, Tabori, & Chang.

Appel, S., Moore, T. M., & Giger, J. N. (2006 Dec). An overview and update on the metabolic syndrome: implications for identifying cardiometabolic risk among African-American women. *Journal of National Black Nurses Association,* 17(2), 47–62.

Bagan, M., Robson, J., & Soderstrom, R. (1971). Ethnic differences in skin fold thickness. *American Journal of Clinical Nutrition,* 24, 864–868.

Barclay, A., & Cusumano, D. R. (1967). Father absence, cross sex identity, and field-dependent behavior of male adolescents. *Child Development,* 38, 343–350.

Becker, L., Han, B., Meyer, P., et al. & CPR Chicago Project (1993). Racial difference in the incidence of cardiac arrest and subsequent survival. *New England Journal of Medicine,* 329(9), 600–607.

Bell, C., & Mehta, H. (1981). The misdiagnosis of Black patients with manic depressive illness: second in a series. *Journal of the National Medical Association,* 73, 101–107.

Bendtzen, K., Morling, N., Fomsgaard, A., et al. (1988). Association between HLA-DR2 and production of tumor necrosis factor α and interleukin 1 by mononuclear cells activated by lipopolysaccharide. *Scandinavian Journal of Immunology,* 28, 599–606.

Berger, J. (2006, March). Age, sex, racial disparities in heart attack transfer pattens. In *Duke Med News.*

Beutler, E. H. (1983). Glucose-6-phosphate dehydrogenase deficiency. In Williams, W. J. (Ed.), *Hematology* (ed. 3). New York: McGraw-Hill.

Biller, H. B. (1969). Father absence, maternal encouragement, and sex role development in kindergarten boys. *Child Development,* 40, 539–546.

Black, S. (2002, April) Diabetes, diversity, and disparity. What do we do with the evidence? *American Journal of Public Health,* 543–551.

Bloch, B. (1974, May 3–4). A look at nursing intervention and Black patient care. In Bloch, B. (Coordinator), *Care of the Black patient on the job: an on the job look at health care needs of the Black patient.* Conference presented by Continuing Education in Nursing, University of California, San Francisco, School of Nursing.

Bloch, B. (1976a). *Health care from a minority viewpoint.* Unpublished study, University of California, San Francisco, School of Nursing.

Bloch, B. (1976b). Nursing intervention in Black patient care. In Luckraft, D. (Ed.), *Black awareness: implications for Black patient care* (pp. 27–35). New York: American Journal of Nursing Company.

Bloch, B. (1981). Black Americans and cross-cultural counseling experiences. In Marsella, A. J., & Pedersen, P. B. (Eds.), *Cross cultural counseling and psychotherapy.* New York: Pergamon Press.

Bloch, B. (1983). Bloch's assessment guide for ethnic/cultural variations. In Orque, M. S., Bloch, B., & Monrroy, L. S. A. (Eds.), *Ethnic nursing care: a multicultural approach* (pp. 49–75). St. Louis: Mosby.

Bloch, B., & Hunter, M. (1981). Teaching physiological assessment of Black persons. *Nurse Educator,* 6, 24–27.

Blumenthal, R., Flack, J. (2003). Establishing cardiovascular risk. In Blumenthal, R., & Flack, J., *Managing cardiovascular disease: a focus on hypertension and dyslipidemia.* (pp. 1–16). Cleveland: Advanstar Medical Economics.

Boyle, E., Jr. (1970). Biological pattern in hypertension by race, sex, body weight, and skin color. *Journal of the American Medical Association,* 213, 1637–1643.

Braithwaite, R., & Taylor, S. (2001). *Health issues in the Black community* (ed. 2). San Francisco: Jossey-Bass.

Brisbane, F. L. (1987). Divided feeling of Black alcoholic daughters. *Alcohol Health and Research World,* 12, 48–50.

Brisbane, F. L., & Womble, M. (1986). Afterthoughts and recommendations. *Alcoholism Treatment Quarterly,* 2(3–4), 249–270.

Brown, F., & Tooley, J. (2004). Alcoholism in the Black community. In Lawson, G., & Lawson, A. (Eds.), *Alcohol and substance abuse in special populations.* Austin, Tex.: Pro-Ed.

Bullough, V. L., & Bullough, B. (1982). *Health care for the other Americans.* East Norwalk, Conn.: Appleton-Century-Crofts.

Burt, V., Whelton, P., Rocella, E., et al. (1995). Prevalence of hypertension in the U.S. adult population: results from the third National Health and Nutrition Examination Survey (NHANES III), 1988–1991. *Hypertension,* 25(3), 305–313.

Carroll, J. F., Klein, M. I., & Santo, Y. (1978). Comparison of the similarities and differences in the self-concepts of male alcoholics and addicts. *Journal of Consulting Clinical Psychology,* 46, 575–576.

Cave, V. (1975). Proper uses and abuses of the health care delivery system for minorities with special reference to the Tuskegee syphilis study. *Journal of the National Medical Association, 67,* 82–84.

Centers for Disease Control and Prevention (2001a). *HIV/AIDS Surveillance Report,* 13(2). Atlanta: Centers for Disease Control and Prevention.

Centers for Disease Control and Prevention (2001b). Sudden death in US young adults: 1989–96 Centers for Disease Control AIDS hotline (1997). *National Center for Health Statistics monthly vital statistics report (1996),* 45(3), 10 (DHHS Publication No. PHS 3, 10). Hyattsville, Md.: Public Health Services.

Centers for Disease Control and Prevention (2003). (CDC) Racial/ethnic and socioeconomic disparities in multiple risk factors for heart disease and stroke—United States. *Morbidity and Mortality Weekly Report,* 54, 113–117.

Centers for Disease Control and Prevention (2005). *HIV/AIDS Surveillance Report,* 17(2). Atlanta, Ga.: Centers for Disease Control and Prevention.

Centers for Disease Control and Prevention. National Health and Nutrition Examination Survey. Available at:http://www.cdc.gov/nchs/about/major/nhanes/datalink.htm. Accessed: May 15, 2006.

Chartbook on trends in the health of Americans/Health United States. (2005). Atlanta: National Center for Health Statistics.

Chen, W., Bao, W., Begum, S., et al. (2000). Age-related patterns of the clustering of cardiovascular risk variables of syndrome X from childhood to young adulthood in a population made up of black and white subjects. *Diabetes,* 49, 1042–1048.

Clarke, R., Daly, L., Robinson, K., et al. (1991, April). Hyperhomocysteinemia: an independent risk factor for vascular disease. *New England Journal of Medicine,* 324, 1749–1755.

Coalition on Urban Renewal and Education. (2002). *African-Americans and AIDS.* Los Angeles: Coalition on Urban Renewal.

Covell, K., & Turnbull, W. (1982). The long-term effects of father absence in childhood on male university students' sex-role identity and personal adjustment. *Journal of Genetic Psychology,* 141, 271–276.

Crawford, P., Story, M., Wang, M., Ritchie, L., & Sabry, Z. (2001). Ethnic issues in the epidemiology of childhood. *Cultural Diversity,* 7(4), 128–132.

Culture of poverty revisited. New York: Mental Health Committee against Racism.

Dallongeville, J., Roy, M., Lebouef, N., et al. (1991). Apolipoprotein E polymorphism association with lipoprotein profile in endogenous hypertriglyceridemia and familial hypercholesterolemia. *Arteriosclerosis and Thrombosis,* 11, 272–278, March–April, 1991.

Davis, R. O., Cutter, G. R., Goldenberg, R. L., et al. (1993). Fetal biparietal diameter, head circumference, abdominal circumference and femur length: a comparison by race and sex. *Journal of Reproductive Medicine,* 38, 201–206.

Dillard, J. L. (1972). *Black English: its history and usage in the United States.* New York: Random House.

Dilley, A., Hooper, W. C., El-Jamil, M., et al. (2002, July). Mutations in the genes regulating methylene tetrahydrofolate reductase (MTHFR C∅T677) and cystathione beta-synthase (CBS G∅A919, CBS T∅c833) are not associated with myocardial infarction in African Americans. *Thrombosis Research,* 103(2), 109–115.

Dowd, S., Poole, V., Davidhizar, R., & Giger, J. N. (1998). Death, dying and grief in a transcultural context: application of the Giger and Davidhizar model. *The Hospice Journal,* 13(4), 33–56.

Dumas, M. (2003, July). Reversing the tide of metabolic syndrome. A guide to women's health. *Nursing,* 7(10), 2–5.

Falkner, F., & Tanner, J. (1978). *Human growth I: principles and prenatal growth.* New York: Plenum Press.

Farrally, M., & Moore, W. (1976). Anatomical differences in the femur and tibia between Negroids and Caucasians. *American Journal of Physiology and Anthropology,* 43(1), 63–69.

Fernandez-Real, JM., Gutierrez, C., Ricart, W., et al. (1997, September). The TNA-α gene Nco 1 polymorphism influences the relationship among insulin resistance, percent body fat, and increased serum leptin levels. *Diabetes,* 46(9), 1469–1472.

Ferrucci, L., Guaralnik, J., Faho, M., et al. (1995, December). Apolipoprotein E epsilon Z allele and risk of stroke in the older population. *Stroke: A Journal of Cerebral Circulation,* 28(12), 2410–2416.

Fletcher, B., Gulanick, M., & Lamendola, C. (2002). Risk factors for type 2 diabetes mellitus. *The Journal of Cardiovascular Nursing,* 16(2), 17–23.

Fongwa, M., Evangelista, S., Doering, L. (2006, May/June). Adherence to treatment factors in hypertensive African-American women. *The Journal of Cardiovascular Nursing,* 21(3), 201–206.

Gallagher, P., Meleady, R., Shields, D., et al. (1996, November). Prevention of cardiovascular disease: homocysteine and risk of premature coronary heart disease. Evidence for common gene mutation. *Circulation*, 94(9), 2154–2158.

Geronimus, A., Bound, J., Waidmann, T., Colen, C., & Steffick, D. (2001, May). Inequality in life expectancy, functional status, and active life expectancy across selected Black and White population in the United States. *Demography*, 38(2), 227–251.

Giger, J., Davidhizar, R., & Cherry, B. (1991, April–May). Biological variations in the Black patient. *Imprint*, 38(2), 95, 97–98.

Giger, J., Davidhizar, R., & Wieczorek, S. (1993). Culture and ethnicity. In Bobak, I., & Jensen, M. (Eds.), *Maternity and gynecologic care* (ed. 5) (pp. 42–67). St. Louis: Mosby.

Giger, J., Richardson, J., & Jones, D. (2001). African-American children: a precious commodity at risk, *Journal of National Black Nurses Association*, 13(1).

Giger, J. N., Strickland, O. L., Weaver, M., Taylor, H., & Acton, R. T. (2005 Spring). Genetic predictors of coronary heart disease risk factors in pre-menopausal African-American women. *Ethnicity and Disease*, 15(2), 221–232.

Gilbert, B. M. (1977). Anterior femoral curvature: its probable basis and utility as a criterion for racial assessment. *American Journal of Physical Anthropology*, 45(3), 601–604.

Gokhan, S., Hotamisligil, G., Armer, P., et al. (1995, May). Increased adipose tissue expression of tumor necrosis factor-α in human obesity and insulin resistance. *Journal of Clinical Investigation*, 95, 2409–2415.

Gokhan, S., Hotamisligil, G., Murray, D., Choy, L., & Spiegelman, B. (1994, May). Tumor necrosis factor inhibits signaling from the insulin receptor. *Proceedings of the National Academy of Science*, 911, 4854–4858.

Gutman, H. (1976). *The Black family in slavery and freedom: 1750–1925*. New York: Vintage Books.

Gynther, M. (1981). Is the MMPI an appropriate assessment device for Blacks? *Journal of Black Psychology*, 7, 67–75.

Hall, E. T. (1990). *The hidden dimension*. New York: Anchor Books.

Hall, E. T. (1989). *Beyond culture*. New York: Anchor Books.

Harper, F., & Dawkins, M. (1976). Alcohol and Blacks: survey of periodical literature. *British Journal of Addiction*, 71, 327–334.

Henderson, G., & Primeaux, M. (1981). *Transcultural health care*. Reading, Mass.: Addison-Wesley.

Hines Smith, S. (1999). Now that mom is in the Lord's arms, I just have to live the way she taught me: Reflections on an elderly African American mother's death. *Journal of Gerontological Social Work*, 32, 41–51.

Hirsch, J. (1981). To "unfrock the charlatans." *Sage Race Relations Abstracts*, 6, 1–65.

Hohn, S., Kulkarni, K., Seley, J. (2005). In *Enhancing patient care in type 2 diabetes: a CE Monograph*. Thompson.

Hotamisligil, G., Shargill, N., & Spiegleman, B. (1993). Adipose expression of tumor necrosis factor-α: direct role in obesity-linked insulin resistance. *Science*, 259, 87–91.

Hudson, H. L. (1986). How and why Alcoholics Anonymous works for Blacks. *Alcoholism Treatment Quarterly*, 2(314), 11–29.

Hugh, M., Ali, D., Madira, M., et al. (1997, September). A common polymorphism in the methylenetetrahydrofolate reductase gene homocysteine, and ischemic cerebrovascular disease, *Biochemical Society Transaction*, 25(3), 386S.

Hulsey, T. C., Levkoff, A. H., & Alexander, G. R. (1991). Birth weight of infants of Black and White mothers without pregnancy complications. *American Journal of Obstetrics and Gynecology*, 164, 1299–1302.

Hymes, D. (Ed.) (1971). *Pidginization and creolization of languages*. London: Cambridge University Press.

Imaru, Y., Koga, S., & Ibayashi, H. (1988, December). Phenotypes of apolipoprotein E and abnormalities in lipid metabolism in patients with non-insulin dependent diabetes mellitus. *Metabolism*, 37(12), 1134–1138.

Institute of Black Chemical Abuse (1988). Annual report. Minneapolis: Institute of Black Chemical Abuse.

Institute of Medicine (2002). *Unequal treatment: confronting racial and ethnic disparities in health care*. Washington, D.C.: National Academy Press.

Iyasu, S., Becerra, J. E., Rowley, D. H., Houge, C. J. (1992, Sep–Oct). Impact of very low birthweight on the black-white infant mortality gap, *American Journal of Preventive Medicine*, 8(5), 271–277.

Jackson, J., Neighbors, H., & Gurin, G. (1986). Findings from a national survey on Black mental health: implications for practice and training. In *National Institute of Mental Health: Mental health research and practice in minority communities*. Rockville, Md.: U.S. Department of Health and Human Services.

Jacob, A. H., & Walton, R. G. (1976). Incidence of birthmarks in the neonate. *Pediatrics*, 58, 218–222.

Jacques, G. (1976). Cultural health traditions: a Black perspective. In Branch, M. F., & Paxton, P. P. (Eds.), *Providing safe nursing care for ethnic people of color*. East Norwalk, Conn.: Appleton-Century-Crofts.

Jamerson, K. (2005, May). What are the consequences of obesity on CV risk? *Type 2 Diabetes Digest*, 9(2), 4.

Johnson, R., Cole, R., & Abner, F. (1981). Genetic interpretation of social/ethnic differences in lactose absorption and tolerance. *Human Biology*, 53(1), 1–3.

Jones, L. (1993). *Bad blood: the Tuskegee syphilis experiment*. New York: Free Press.

Jones, L. (1998). *Home: social essays*. Hopewell, N.J.: Ecco Press.

Jones, B., Gray, B., & Parson, E. (1981). Manic-depressive illness among poor urban Blacks. *Journal of the National Medical Association*, 72, 141–145.

Jongeneel, V., Briant, L., Irina, A., et al. (1991, November). Extensive genetic polymorphism in the human tumor necrosis factor α region and relation to extended HLA haplotypes immunology. *Proceedings of National Academy of Sciences of the United States of America*, 88, 9717–9721.

Jordan, W. C. (1975). Voodoo medicine. In Williams, R. A. (Ed.), *Textbook of Black-related diseases* (pp. 115–138). New York: McGraw-Hill.

Jordan, W. C. (1979). The roots and practice of voodoo medicine in America. *Urban Health*, 8, 38–48.

Karnow, S. (1997). *Vietnam: a history* (ed. 2). New York: Penguin Books.

King, L. M. (1982). Alcoholism—studies regarding Black Americans: 1979–1980. Alcohol and Health Monograph 4: Special Population Issues, 385–407.

Kloner, R., Grimm, R, Flack, J. et al. (2004, October). Managing hypertension: the value of optimal blood pressure control. *Clinical Advisor*, 2–19.

Kluckhohn, C. (2003). The gifts of tongues. In Samovar, L. A., & Porter, R. E. (Eds.), *Intercultural communication: a reader* (ed. 10). Belmont, Calif: Wadsworth/Thomson Learning.

Kluitjmans, L., Lambers, P., Van der Heuval, G., et al. (1996). Hyperhomocysteinemia: a common mutation in the methylenetetrahydrofolate reductase gene is a genetic risk factor for cardiovascular disease. *American Journal of Human Genetics*, 58, 35–41.

Knox, D. H. (1986). Spirituality: a tool in the assessment and treatment of Black alcoholics and their families. *Alcoholism Treatment Quarterly*, 2(3–4), 313–343.

Kreisman, J. (1975). The curandero's apprentice: a therapeutic integration of folk and medical healing. *American Journal of Psychiatry*, 132, 81.

Kurachi, O., Matsuo, H., Samoto, T., Maruo, T. (2001, May). Tumor necrosis factor-alpha expression in human uterine leiomyoma and its down-regulation by progesterone. *Journal of Clinical Endocrinology & Metabolism*, 86(5), 2275–2280.

Laufer, R. S., Gallops, M. S., & Frey-Wouters, E. (1981). War stress and trauma: the Vietnam veteran experience. *Journal of Health and Social Behavior*, 25, 65–85.

Lawson, G., & Lawson, A. (2004). *Alcoholism and substance abuse in special populations*. Austin, Tex.: Pro-Ed.

Leininger, M. (1978). *Transcultural nursing*. New York: John Wiley & Sons.

Lobar, S. L., Youngblut, J., Brooten, D. (2006, January–February). Cross-cultural beliefs, ceremonies, and rituals surrounding death of a loved one. *Pediatric Nursing*, 32(1), 44–50.

LoBiondo-Wood, G., Zimmerman, L. M., & Gatson-Johansson, F. J. (1989, April 2). Pain descriptors selected by different ethnic groups, Paper presented at the thirteenth annual Midwest Nursing Research Society Conference, Cincinnati, Ohio.

Margaglione, M., Seripa, D., Gravine, C., et al. (1998, February). Prevalence of apolipoprotein E alleles in healthy subjects and survivors of ischemic stroke: an Italian case-control study. *Stroke: A Journal of Cerebral Circulation*, 29(2), 399–403.

Maron, B. J., Carney, K. P., Lever, H. M., et al. (2003, March). Relationship of race to sudden cardiac death in competitive athletes with hypertrophic cardiomyopathy. *Journal of the American College of Cardiology*, 41(6), 974–980.

Matthews, D., Hosker, L., Rudenski, A., et al. (1985). Homeostasis and assessment: insulin resistance and β-cell function from fasting plasma glucose and insulin concentrations in man. *Diabetologia*, 28, 412–419.

Mbiti, J. (1990). *African religions and philosophies* (ed. 2). Portsmouth, N.H: Heinemann.

McCrackin, R. (1971). Lactose deficiency: an example of dietary evaluation. *Current Anthropology*, 12(4–5), 479–517.

McKenzie, J., & Chrisman, N. (1977). Healing herbs, gods, and magic. *Nursing Outlook*, 25(5), 325–327.

Meyers, J., & Weissman, M. (1980–1981). The prevalence of psychiatric disorders (DSM-III in the community: 1980–1981). Unpublished manuscript.

Mirsa, D. (Ed.) (2001). *Women's health data book: a profile of women's health in the United States*. (ed. 3). Washington, D.C.: Jacobs Institute of Women's Health and the Henry J. Kaiser Family Foundation.

Mitchel, F. (1978). *Voodoo medicine: Sea Islands herbal remedies*. Berkeley, Calif.: Reed, Cannon, & Johnson.

Moore, R., Stanton, D., Gopalan, R., & Chaisson, R. (1994). Racial differences in the use of drug therapy for HIV disease in the urban community. *New England Journal of Medicine,* 330(11), 763–768.

Morton, N. E. (1977). Genetic aspects of prematurity. In Reed, D. M., & Stanley, F. J. (Eds.), *Epidemiology of prematurity.* Baltimore: Urban & Schwarzenberg.

Motulsky, A. (1996). Nutritional ecogenetics: homocysteine-related: arteriosclerotic vascular disease, neural tube defects, and folic acid. *American Journal Human Genetics,* 58, 17–20.

Mukherjee, S., Shukla, S., & Woodle, J. (1983). Misdiagnosis of schizophrenia in bipolar patients: a multiethnic comparison. *American Journal of Psychiatry,* 140, 1571–1574.

Murray, R. B., & Huelskoetter, M. W. (1991). *Psychiatric/mental health nursing.* (ed. 3). East Norwalk, Conn.: Appleton & Lange.

National Center for Health Statistics. (2002). Health, United States, 2002, with urban and rural chartbook. Hyattsville, Md.: National Center for Health Statistics.

National Center for Health Statistics, Healthy People 2000 Review (2002). Health, United States, 2002 (DHHS Publication No. PHS 93-1232). Hyattsville, Md.: Public Health Services.

National Institutes of Health, National Heart, Lung and Blood Institute (2004). *Morbidity and Mortality Chart Book on Cardiovascular, Lung and Blood Diseases.* Bethesda, Md.: National Heart, Lung, and Blood Institute.

Neighbors, H. W., Musick, M. A., Williams, D. R. (1998, December). The African American minister as a source of help for serious personal crises: bridge or barrier to mental health? *Health Education Behavior,* 25(50), 759–767.

Ogden, C., Carroll, M. D., Curtin, L. R., et al. (2006, April). Prevalence of overweight and obesity in the United States, 1999-2004. *Journal of the American Medical Association,* 295(13), 1559–1565.

Oscherwitz, M. (1972). Differences in pulmonary function in various racial groups. *American Journal of Epidemiology,* 96(5), 319–327.

Overfield, R. T. (1995). *Biologic variations in health and illness: race, age and sex differences.* (ed. 2). Reading, Mass.: Addison-Wesley.

Owen, G. M., & Lubin, A. (1973). Anthropometric differences between Black and White preschool children. *American Journal of Diseases in Children,* 126, 168.

Parker, D., & Harman, M. (1978). The distribution of consumption model of prevention of alcoholic problems: a critical assessment. *Journal of the Study of Alcohol,* 39, 377–399.

Pasamanick, B. (1964). Myths regarding prevalence of mental disease in the Negro. *Journal of the National Medical Association,* 58, 6–17.

Penk, W. E., Robinowitz, R., Black, J., et al. (1989). Ethnicity: post-traumatic stress disorder (PTSD) differences among black, white, and Hispanic veterans who differ in degrees of exposure to combat in Vietnam. *Journal of Clinical Psychology,* 45(5), 729–735.

Perry, H. L. (1993). Mourning and funeral customs of African Americans. In Irish, D. P., Lundquist, K. F., & Nelson, V. J. (Eds.), *Ethnic variations in dying, death, and grief.* Washington, DC: Taylor & Francis.

Pillsbury, B. (1982). Doing the month: confinement and convalescence of Chinese women after childbirth. In Kay, M. (Ed.), *Anthropology of human birth.* Philadelphia: F.A.Davis.

Ploski, H., & Williams, J. (1989). *The Negro almanac: a reference work on the African-American.* (ed. 5). Detroit: Gale Research.

Poussaint, A., & Atkinson, C. (1970). Black youth and motivation. *Black Scholar,* 1, 43–51.

Pratt, M. W., Janus, Z. L., & Sayal, N. C. (1977). National variations in prematurity (1973 and 1974). In Reed, D. M., & Stanley, F. J. (Eds.), *The epidemiology of prematurity* (pp. 53–74). Baltimore: Urban & Schwarzenberg.

Remington, G., & DaCosta, G. (1989). Ethnocultural factors in resident supervision: black and white supervisors. *American Journal of Psychotherapy,* 43(3), 343–355.

Richards, S., Funk, M., & Milner, K. (2000). Differences between blacks and whites with coronary heart disease in initial symptoms and delay in seeking care. *American Journal of Critical Care,* 9(4), 237–244.

Robins, L. N., Helzer, J. E., Croughan, J., & Ratcliff, K. S. (1981). National Institutes of Mental Health Diagnostic Interview Schedule: its history, characteristics, and validity. *Archives of General Psychiatry,* 38, 381–389.

Roche, A. F., Roberts, J., & Hamell, P. V. (1978). Skeletal maturity of youths 12–17 years of age: racial, geographic and socioeconomic disproportions. *National Health,* 11(167), 1–98.

Ronan, L. (1987). Alcohol-related health risks among Black Americans. *Alcohol Health and Research World,* 12, 36–39.

Rook, A. (1970). *Racial and other genetic factors in dermatology.* Philadelphia: F.A. Davis.

Sahebzamani, F. (2005, April). Improving outcomes for your patients with diabetes [editorial]. *CE Today for Nurse Practitioners*, 4(3), 7.

Sandoval, M. (1977). Santería: Afro-Cuban concepts of disease and its treatment in Miami. *Journal of Operational Psychiatry*, 8(52), 48–53.

Shapiro, M. F., Morton, S. C., McCaffrey, D. F., et al. (1999, June). Variations in the care of HIV-infected adults in the United States: results from the HIV cost and services utilization study. *JAMA*, 28(24), 2305–2315.

Smith, J. A. (1976). The role of the Black clergy as allied health care professionals in working with Black patients. In Luckraft, D. (Ed.), *Black awareness: implications for Black care* (pp. 12–15). New York: The American Journal of Nursing Company.

Snow, L. E. (1974). Folk medical beliefs and their implications for care of patients: a review based on studies among Black Americans. *Annals of Internal Medicine*, 81, 82–96.

Snow, L. E. (1977). Popular medicine in a Black neighborhood. In Spicer, E. H. (Ed.), *Ethnic medicine in the Southwest*. Tucson: University of Arizona Press.

Snow, L. E. (1978). Sorcerers, saints, and charlatans: Black folk healers in urban America. *Culture, Medicine, and Psychiatry*, 2, 69.

Snow, L. E. (1983). Traditional health beliefs and practice among lower class Black Americans. *Western Journal of Medicine*, 139(6), 820–828.

Snowden, L. (1982). *Reaching the underserved: mental health needs of neglected populations*. Newbury Park, Calif.: Sage Publications.

Snowden, L., & Todman, P. A. (1982). The psychological assessment of Blacks: new and needed developments. In Johns, E. E., & Korchin, S. J. (Eds.), *Minority mental health* (pp. 193–226). New York: Praeger.

Spector, R. E. (2004). *Cultural diversity in health and illness* (ed. 6). Upper Saddle River, N.J.: Pearson Prentice Hall.

Spurlock, J. (1985). Psychiatric states. In Williams, R. A. (Ed.), *Textbook of Black-related diseases*. New York: McGraw-Hill.

Srinivasan, S., Myers, L., & Berenson, G. (2002). Predictability of childhood adiposity and insulin for developing insulin resistance syndrome (syndrome X) in young adulthood. *Diabetes*, 51, 204–209.

Stalls, F. A. (1978). Racial differences in alcohol metabolism. *Alcohol Clinical and Experimental Research*, 2(1), 10.

Staples, R. (1976). *Introduction to Black sociology*. New York: McGraw-Hill.

Sterne, M., & Pittman, D. J. (1972). *Drinking practices in the ghetto*. St. Louis: Washington University Social Science Institute.

Stokes, L. G. (1977). Delivering health services in a Black community. In Reinhardt, A. M., & Quinn, M. B. (Eds.), *Current practice in family-centered community nursing* (pp. 51–65). St. Louis: Mosby.

Strauss, R., & Pollack, H. (2001). Epidemic increase in childhood overweight, 1986–1998. *Journal of the American Medical Association*, 286(22), 2845–2848.

Sue, D. (2003). *Counseling the culturally diverse: theory and practice* (ed. 4). New York: J. Wiley.

Swank, A. M., & Fell, R. D. (1990). Effects of acute smoking and exercise on high-density lipoprotein-cholesterol and subfractions in Black female smokers. *Metabolism*, 39, 343–349.

Thomas, A., & Sillen, S. (1972). *Racism and psychiatry*. New York: Brunner/Mazel.

Time almanac with information please. (2007). Boston: Information Please, Inc.

Tobias, P. (1970). Brain-size, grey matter, and race: fact or fiction. *American Journal of Physical Anthropology*, 32, 3–26.

Turner, L. (1948, April). *Problems confronting the investigation of Gullah*. American Dialect Society Publications, 9, 78–84.

U.S. Department of Commerce, Bureau of the Census (2000). Population and housing data by race and Hispanic origin, Summary File 1. Washington, D.C.: U.S. Government Printing Office.

U.S. Department of Commerce. Bureau of the Census (2000). *The older population in the United States, 2000*. U.S. Government Printing Office.

U.S. Department of Commerce. Bureau of the Census (2001). *The 65 years and older population: 2000*. Washington, D.C., U.S. Government Printing Office.

U.S. Department of Commerce, Bureau of the Census (2002). *Population profiles by age, sex, race, and Hispanic origin, Summary File 3*. Washington, D.C., U.S. Government Printing Office.

U.S. Department of Commerce, Bureau of the Census (2003). *The Black population in the United States: March 2002*. U.S. Government Printing Office Washington, D.C.

U.S. Department of Health and Human Services. (2000). *Healthy People 2010: Understanding and improving health* (ed. 2). Washington, D.C.: U.S. Government Printing Office.

Valdez, R. Howard, B., Stern, M., & Haffner, S. (1995, July). Apolipoprotein E polymorphism and insulin levels in biethnic populations. *Diabetes Care*, 18(7), 992–1000.

Vernon, S., & Roberts, R. (1982). *Use of the SAD-RDC in a triethnic community survey.* Springfield, Mass.: Merriam-Webster.

Ward, J., & Duchin, J. (1998). US epidemiology of HIV and AIDS. In Volberding, P.A, & Jacobson, M. A. (Eds.), *AIDS clinical review* (pp. 10–32). New York: Marcel Dekker Publications.

Weclew, R. (1975). The nature, prevalence, and level of awareness of curanderismo and some of its implications for community health. *Community Mental Health Journal*, 11, 145.

Westermeyer, J. (1984). The role of ethnicity in substance abuse. In Stimmel, B. (Ed.), *Cultural and sociological aspects of alcoholism and substance abuse* (pp. 9–18). New York: Haworth Press.

White, E. H. (1977). Giving health care to minority patients. *Nursing Clinics in North America*, 12, 27–40.

Williams, M. (1986). Alcohol and ethnic minorities: Native Americans—an update. *Alcohol Health and Research Works*, 11(2), 5–6.

Wintrob, R. (1973). The influences of others: witchcraft and rootwork as explanations of behavior disturbances. *Journal of Nervous and Mental Disorders*, 156, 318.

Wolfram, W. A., & Clark, H. (Eds.) (1971). *Black-White speech relationships.* Washington, D.C.: Center for Applied Linguistics.

Woods, S. (1998). Can aspirin prevent heart disease in women? *Women's Health in Primary Care*, 1, 210–214.

Yusuf, S., Reddy, S., Ounpuu, S., Anand, S. (2001). Clinical cardiology: global burden of cardiovascular diseases part II: Variations in cardiovascular disease by specific ethnic groups and geographic regions and prevention strategies. *Circulation* 1004, 2855–2864.

Zettervall, D. (2005). A pragmatic approach to the management of diabetes and its complications. *CE Today for Nurse Practitioners*, 4(3), 17–27.

CHAPTER 9

Mexican Americans

Elizabeth W. Gonzalez, Donna C. Owen, and M. Christina R. Esperat

Behavioral Objectives

After reading this chapter, the nurse will be able to:

1. Discuss the influence of Spanish-language usage by Mexican Americans in adapting to the mainstream U.S. culture.
2. Explain the distance and intimacy behaviors of Mexican Americans.
3. Describe the organization of the Mexican American family unit.
4. Explain the Mexican American orientation to time.
5. Describe the impact of locus of control on Mexican Americans' perceptions of the environment and their ability to control it.
6. Describe how the "hot–cold" beliefs of Mexican Americans influence their health and illness beliefs.
7. Identify the biological variations of Mexican Americans.

OVERVIEW OF MEXICO

Mexico, or what is officially referred to as the United Mexican States (*Estados Unidos Mexicanos*), is a country in the southern part of North America. Mexico consists of 31 states and a federal district. The boundaries of Mexico extend southward from the United States to Guatemala and Belize in Central America. The western coast of Mexico borders on the Pacific Ocean, which includes the Gulf of California and the Gulf of Tehuantepec. The eastern coast of Mexico fronts on the Caribbean Sea and the Gulf of Mexico, which includes the Bay of Campeche. Mexico, which includes several outlying islands, has a total area of 761,604 square miles and is the third largest Latin American nation after Brazil and Argentina. Mexico is about a fifth the size of the United States.

Most Mexicans are *mestizos*, that is, of mixed Spanish and Indian descent (Guarnero, 2005). They trace their native heritage back to Indian groups that built great civilizations in Mexico long before the Spanish explorers arrived in the 1500s (Falicov, 2005). When the Spaniards came to Mexico in 1519, they found Indians who were skilled in writing, mathematics, astronomy, painting, sculpture, and architecture. Indian pottery, metalwork, and textiles were very highly developed for the time period. Many Spaniards married women from the native Indian population. Spain's discovery and eventual conquest of Mexico marked the start of the destruction of many elements of existing civilizations (Villarruel & Leininger, 2004). Missionaries were sent to convert the Indians to Christianity. Many of the riches of the land were carried back to Spain.

After centuries of Spanish rule, the people rose and a republic was declared in 1823. After numerous conflicts and the U.S.–Mexican War (1846–1848), Mexico lost the lands north of the Rio Grande to the United States. French invasions were also repulsed. However, internal conflict continued, with years of rebellion and factional fighting. A new constitution in 1917 finally brought social reform, as the Institutional Revolutionary Party (IRP) assumed control and dominated politics from 1929 to the late 1990s. During 1983 and 1984, Mexico suffered its worst financial crisis in 50 years, leading to critically high unemployment and an inability to pay its foreign debt. The collapse of oil prices in 1986 cut into Mexico's export earnings and worsened the situation. Political and governmental conflict resulted in an unstable situation that contributed to many Mexicans seeking economic gain in the United States. Although the value of the peso fell drastically, an austerity plan and assistance from the United States saved Mexico's currency from complete collapse in 1995. In 1996 the Popular Revolutionary Army guerrillas began attacks on the Mexican government. When the IRP failed to win a congressional majority in 1997 and again in 2000, the winner, opposition candidate Vicente Fox Quesada, took office. Fox's National Action Party suffered a setback in midterm elections in July 2003 that resulted in a 2005 law allowing an estimated 11 million emigrants, mostly to the U.S., to vote by mail-in ballots in the 2006 election (*Time Almanac with Information Please*, 2007).

In 2005, the population of Mexico was 106,202,903 (World Almanac, 2007). The average annual rate of natural increase was estimated at 1.2% (2005 estimate) (*Time Almanac with Information Please*, 2007). The birth rate of Mexico is 21.00 births per 1000 persons, whereas the infant mortality is estimated to be 20.9 (*Time Almanac with Information Please*, 2006). Over the past four decades, the life expectancy at birth has increased from 35 to 72.4 years for males and 78.1 years for females (*Time Almanac with Information Please*, 2007). Approximately 50% to 75% of the Mexican population suffer from malnutrition, making it one of the leading causes of death among children. The problem of malnutrition in Mexico is primarily economic, although lack of education is a contributing factor. The gross domestic product (2004 estimate) is $1 trillion, with a per capita income of $6900 (*Time Almanac with Information Please*, 2007).

MEXICAN AMERICANS

The southwest region of the United States was settled by Spaniards in 1598 in what is today New Mexico. Later, citizens of the United States began settling in what was then Mexican territory. Mexicans helped establish many southwestern cities and taught the settlers skills in mining, farming, and ranching. After the U.S.–Mexican War, which separated Mexico, a treaty provided those of Mexican descent land and cultural rights. Unfortunately, these rights were never fully honored, and Mexican Americans living in these areas have tended to become an economically segregated working-class group (Moore & Pachon, 1985).

Over the years numerous socioeconomic and political conditions in Mexico and the demand for cheap agricultural and industrial labor in the United States have contributed to the movement of Mexicans to the United States (Camarota, 2006; Villarruel & Leininger, 2004). Because of the geographical closeness of Mexico and the United States and the permeability of the border, some Mexicans move back and forth between Mexico and the United States legally and some illegally. It is estimated that at least one third of the undocumented aliens in the United States are from Mexico (Hudson, 1995). The movement back and forth across the border allows them to remain in contact with their families and native customs while at the same time seek economic opportunities in the United States. Lack of citizenship may present a significant barrier to psychosocial and physical health and to gaining education, skills, stable jobs, decent living conditions, and government benefits. Mexican Americans who are illegal aliens frequently experience tension regarding discovery and deportation back to Mexico. Preoccupation with possible discovery and deportation for illegal aliens serves to further augment the symptoms of posttraumatic stress disorder (PTSD) (Cervantes, Snyder, & Padilla, 1989). The plight of the illegal alien has worsened since enactment of the Immigration Reform and Control Act of 1986 (Gelfand & Bialik-Gilad, 1989). In an attempt to control illegal immigration to the United States, employers are now required to verify citizenship status within 24 hours after hiring an employee. Thus, undocumented aliens are often forced into low-paying day labor jobs.

Mexican Americans who have immigrated have tended to move into the southwestern section of the United States, where the majority reside in Texas and California. Most Mexican Americans have rural agricultural backgrounds (U.S. Department of Commerce, Bureau of the Census, 1993). However, it is difficult to generalize about geographical location and the occupational background of people in this ethnic group. The diversity in Mexican Americans ranges from rural villagers in New Mexico and Colorado (Saunders, 1954; Weaver, 1970), to agricultural laborers in Texas (Rubel, 1966), to low-income residents in Arizona, and to urban low-class individuals in California (Clark, 1970). Some 56.8% of Mexican Americans live in the West while 32.6% live in the South (U.S. Department of Commerce, Bureau of the Census, 2002). The remaining 12.6% are scattered throughout the United States. Just as the people are diverse, studies often represent specific populations of Mexicans and offer differing definitions of Mexican Americans. Discussion of Mexican Americans is complicated by the diversity of this population (Davidhizar, 2001; Bollenbacher, Heck, & Davidhizar, 2000). Because of this, making general conclusions about Mexican Americans as a result of individual studies must be done with great caution.

The Hispanic American population is growing rapidly in the United States. In fact, in 2000 the number of Hispanics exceeded the number of African-Americans, escalating this group to the largest ethnic minority group in the United States. In 2000, the number of Hispanic Americans was 35,305,818. Between 1990 and 2000, the Hispanic population increased 58% and now represents 12.5% of the total U.S. population (U.S. Department of Commerce, Bureau of the Census, 2000). As in the past, in the 2000 census, people of Hispanic origins, including Mexican Americans, Puerto Ricans, Cubans, and persons from Central or South America, could identify themselves as Hispanic (U.S. Department of Commerce, Bureau of the Census, 2000). However, in the 2000 census, the term *Latinos* was used for the first time on the census form (U.S. Department of Commerce, Bureau of the Census, 2000). The terms *Hispanic* or *Latinos* may be used interchangeably. In fact, these terms now reflect new terminology set forth in standards issued by the Office of Management and Budget in 1997. The final implementation of the standards for use of these terms took effect in 2003 (U.S. Department of Commerce, Bureau of the Census, 2003).

The Mexican American population has been rapidly growing. According to the U.S. Department of Commerce, Bureau of the Census (2002), the Mexican American population nearly doubled between 1970 and 1980. Between 1980 and 2000, the number of Mexican Americans residing in the United States doubled again. Today there are 20,640,711 Mexican Americans residing in the United States, 7.3% of the general U.S. population (*Time Almanac with Information Please*, 2007; U.S. Department of Commerce, Bureau of the Census, 2000, 2002). Mexican Americans, or Chicanos, are also the largest Hispanic group residing in the United States. In fact, Mexican Americans represent 58.5% (20,640,711) of the Hispanic population, followed by Puerto Ricans (9.6%; 3,406,175), Cubans (3.5%; 1,241,685), Central Americans (4.8%; 1,686,937), South Americans (3.8%; 1,353,562), Dominicans (2.2%; 765.945), and other Hispanic and Latinos (17.3%; 6,211,800) (U.S. Department of Commerce, Bureau of the Census, 2000).

The proximity of Mexico to the United States has resulted in a noteworthy amount of drug trafficking. The practice of smoking cannabis leaves came to the United States with Mexican immigrants who came north during the 1920s (Musto, 1991). Much of the cocaine that reaches the United States from Colombia comes by way of Mexico (Booth, 1996). Along with the drugs has come an increase in violence for border cities, creating problems for the judicial system by packing jail cells, and for the health care system, which is often unprepared for the influx of health and socially related problems (Camarota, 2006).

Use of the health care system in America has been problematic for many Mexican Americans because of lack of insurance (Hahn, 1995). Ross (1995) noted that job-based insurance covers 63% of Whites in the United States, 57% of Asians, 46% of Blacks, but only 37% of Hispanics.

Explanations for lack of insurance are partly related to communication difficulties and to lack of understanding that insurance is needed. Lack of health insurance is also related to culture, because most Hispanics who have recently immigrated do not understand the competitive health care market and that they need insurance, and many still place their trust in traditional herbal remedies (Ross, 1995; Villarruel & Leininger, 2004). Health care agencies are not eager to treat uninsured, indigent people since undocumented aliens do not qualify for Medicare or Medicaid funds. Angel, Angel, and Markides (2002) noted that most of Mexican Americans who were uninsured are younger, female, poor, and foreign. These persons report fewer health care visits, are less likely to have a usual source of care, and more often receive care in Mexico. Additionally complicating the use of the health care system is that many Mexican Americans live in crowded substandard city housing, which has limited access to high-quality health care facilities (Ross, 1995). When comparing Mexican American, African-American, and White American low-income women, Keenan, Marshall, and Eve (2002) noted that while psychosocial variables were significant predictors for health care use, for Mexican American women, psychosocial vulnerability was mediated by barriers that affected utilization in a more complex way. Borders, Xu, Rohree, and Warner (2002) studied rural Mexican Americans living in Texas and noted that psychosocial variables including part-time employment, lack of continuous health insurance coverage, and poor health status could be related to levels of satisfaction with health care.

Immigration of Mexicans to the United States has created difficulties in schools, such as the special needs of teaching children who do not have English-speaking skills (Serrano, 1997). Yet another problem can be noted in California, where funds are not provided for educating children who are illegal aliens. The educational achievement of Mexican Americans is steadily rising. For example, in the early 1970s, 27% had completed high school; in the 1980s, 37.6% had completed high school; in 1990, 44% had completed high school; and by

2000, 51% had at least a high school education (U.S. Department of Commerce, Bureau of the Census, 2000). Illegal and legal immigrants from Mexico present other problems for the United States since many immigrant have relatives who are citizens and who participate in the debate about deportation and obstruction to the path to citizenship (Campo-Flores, 2006).

In general, it is estimated that Hispanic Aericans have less formal education than the national average. In fact, only 56% of Hispanic Americans over 25 years of age have graduated from high school, and only 11% of Hispanic Americans have graduated from college. These figures are compared with national averages of 83% and 25%, respectively, for all racial groups in the United States (U.S. Department of Commerce, Bureau of the Census, 2002). Moreover, in 1999, only 44% of foreign-born Hispanics 25 years of age or older were high school graduates, as compared with 70% of their U.S.-born Hispanic counterparts (U.S. Department of Commerce, Bureau of the Census, 2002).

Increased education has resulted in a decrease in problems related to poor housing, jobs, and discrimination. However, many customs in the United States, including needing a driver's license and insurance to avoid problems with the police, being quiet in the evening in a conservative neighborhood, and exhibiting polite behavior toward women are part of the socialization process that must be learned in order to adapt to most communities in the United States (Woodbury, 2000). While some Mexican Americans are positive about the socialization process, many Mexican Americans try to retain a cultural identity within the dominant population (Chávez, 1986).

"Cultural uniqueness" is not academic nomenclature for Mexican Americans. The phrase is used to describe physical, emotional, and behavioral distinctions unique to many Mexican Americans (Chávez, 1986). Unlike European immigrants, who often hasten to absorb the culture found in the United States, many Mexican Americans have not. In *Megatrends*, John Naisbitt (1982) states that "none of the new groups individually can begin to match the numbers and the potential influence of

Spanish-speaking Americans." Concepts such as *machismo* (manliness), *confianza* (confidence), *respeto* (respect), *vergüenza* (shame), and *orgullo* (pride) predominate in the culture, and traditional gender and family roles continue to be part of the heritage that separates Mexican Americans from other cultural groups. Unfortunately, and perhaps because of the desire to retain cultural identity, many Mexican Americans have experienced discrimination in education, jobs, and housing. Skin color, language differences, and Spanish surnames have all contributed to discrimination (Camarota, 2006).

In 2000, 70.2% of Mexican American families were married couple families, 8.8% were single male householder families, and 21.0% were female-headed households. In addition, in 2000, 31% of Hispanic households had five or more people, compared with 12% among non-Hispanic Whites. This increase in persons per household partly accounts for the rapid growth of the Hispanic population. Hispanics are a younger population; 35.7% of Hispanics are 18 years or younger compared with 23.5% of non-Hispanic Whites (U.S. Department of Commerce, Bureau of the Census, 2000). The mean age for Hispanics is 25.8 years. Mexican Americans are the youngest group among all Hispanics (U.S. Department of Commerce, Bureau of the Census, 2000).

Of the total number of Hispanic males in the workforce, 28.1% held jobs as operators, fabricators, and laborers; 19.7% held jobs in precision, production, craft, and repair; 16.1% held jobs in services; 16.7% held jobs in technical, sales, and administrative support; 12.0% held jobs in managerial and professional specialties; and 7.4% held jobs in farming, forestry, and fishing (U.S. Department of Commerce, Bureau of the Census, 2002). Despite the shift from jobs related to agriculture for the general population of Hispanics residing in the United States, in 2000 the median income for Hispanics in general was only $23,859, as compared with $33,955 for their White counterparts. The median income for Hispanic men was only $25,400 as compared with $39,955 for their White counterparts. Similarly, the median income for

Hispanic women was disproportionately low ($21,634) as compared with $27,878 for their White counterparts. Among all Hispanics at all ages, 7,797,847 live below the federally defined poverty level (U.S. Department of Commerce, Bureau of the Census, 2002).

While Mexican Americans are merging into the general labor force, other than seasonal work, Kissam (1993) reported that except for southern Florida, 80% to 90% of all the migrant and seasonal labor force were foreign born and almost all were of Mexican origin (Mines, Gabbard, & Samardick, 1992). Kissam reported the following developments in the migrant Mexican labor force: (1) diffusion into other geographical areas of the United States, (2) greater ethnic and linguistic diversity than earlier workers, (3) increasing numbers of unaccompanied males supporting families who remain at home, (4) changing characteristics of reunited families settling in the United States after the father had migrated for 5 to 10 years (children of these families transfer to U.S. schools after years of school in Mexico, rather than having K–12 schooling in the United States, and these families experience a high level of stress in assimilating as a united family and as immigrants), (5) increasing numbers of very young and very old migrant workers, and (6) growing numbers of female-headed households. The changing demographics of Mexican migrant farmworkers present many challenges to U.S. agencies in adequately meeting their needs.

COMMUNICATION

Spanish, the primary language for many Mexican Americans, is the fourth most commonly used language in the world and one of the six languages used by the United Nations (Gordon, 2005).

Dialect

The Spanish language is spoken in many dialects; Mexican Americans who have an Indian heritage may speak one of more than 50 Spanish dialects. Fortunately, however, most of the words spoken have the same meaning (Zoucha & Purnell, 2003). Differences in dialect may be found in certain communities. Dialects may also be identified by their proximity to the Mexican border. In the nineteenth century, the dominant language in the barrios and rural settlements was that of Mexico, though some Tejanos also attained facility in English and thus became bilingual. Various linguistic codes characterize oral communications in present-day enclaves, however, because of continued emigration from Mexico, racial separation, and exposure to American mass culture. Some Texas Mexicans speak formal Spanish only, just as there are those who communicate strictly in formal English. More common are those Spanish speakers using English loanwords as they borrow from the lexicon of mainstream society. Another form of expression, referred to as *codeswitching*, involves the systematic mixing of the English and Spanish languages. Another mode of communication is *caló*, a hip code composed of innovative terminology and codeswitching used primarily by boys in their own groups (Rodolfo, 2007). This southwestern regional form of dialogue, now used across subculture groups of Mexican American teens, is also used to a lesser extent by older Mexican Americans (Cummings, 2003).

Touch

Adult Mexican Americans can be characterized as tactile in their relationships. Embracing or holding hands while walking is common among close friends of the same gender. Although female Mexican Americans may initiate more tactile behavior in communicating, there is a contradiction where modesty is concerned. Mexican American women have been taught to highly value female modesty and to not expose their bodies to men or even other women. Nakedness is avoided and will cause embarrassment, even among close family members. Consequently, being touched by health care providers is often a source of embarrassment (Lagana & Gonzalez-Ramirez, 2003). Women will generally prefer to receive care from a female health care provider, and adolescent girls may desire to have their mother or female relative present for pelvic examinations and other intimate aspects of a physical exam. Although religious beliefs may explain lack of birth control, discomfort with certain areas of the body may also explain why some Mexican American women avoid the use of a diaphragm. Men also have strong feelings about modesty and may feel threatened if expected to have a complete physical examination (Murillo, 1978). While this modesty may explain the reluctance of some Mexican American men to use condoms, this reluctance may also reflect the imbalance of power between men and women. Increasingly, women in committed relationships are being included in contraceptive decision making (Harvey, Beckman, Browner, & Sherman, 2002). Consideration of the Mexican American client's need for modesty suggests approaches for nurses doing physical assessments. During the exam, care should be taken to uncover only the body part being examined and to allow only persons essential to the exam in the exam room (Davidhizar, Bechtel, & Giger, 1998).

Some Mexican Americans avoid touching even their own genitalia (Clark, 1970). Breast self-examinations are embarrassing but are done by women who are more acculturated (Borrayo & Jenkins, 2003). Education about breast health is often better accepted by Mexican American women when breast models and videotapes are used (Lagana & Gonzalez-Ramirez, 2003).

Context

When being interviewed, Mexican Americans may engage in small talk before approaching the business of the interview. It is important for the nurse to remember that small talk will often facilitate accomplishing nursing objectives for the interview and is therefore not a waste of time.

Traditionally, in communicating with others, Mexican Americans have used diplomacy and tactfulness. There is also pride in verbal expression, which is likely to be elaborate and indirect. Direct confrontation and arguments are considered rude and disrespectful. Self-disclosure is reserved for those whom the individual knows well. The Mexican American may appear agreeable on the surface regarding an issue because of the value of courtesy. However, the nurse may later be surprised and disappointed because agreements are not being carried out. Kidding is seen as rude, deprecating, and offensive and

is likely to generate a negative response (Zoucha & Purnell, 2003). In communicating, Mexican Americans use all the physiological senses: smelling, tasting, touching, feeling, and hearing.

Kinesics

Eye behavior is important to Mexican Americans, especially when children are involved. *Mal ojo* ("evil eye") is a folk illness described as a condition that affects infants and children (Dorsey & Jackson, 1976) and occurs because an individual who is believed to possess a special power voluntarily or involuntarily injures a child by looking at and admiring but not touching the child (Foster, 1978). With this condition the child cries, develops a fever, vomits, and loses his or her appetite. This disorder may be prevented by touching or patting a child when admiring the child. The spell is broken when the individual who has given the "evil eye" touches the child. Therefore, the nurse should touch the child when giving care because in the minds of Mexican Americans this action can both prevent and treat the illness.

English as a Second Language

Most Mexican Americans can also speak some English. However, the inability to speak English fluently has led to a high failure rate for school-aged Mexican Americans. Lack of language fluency has also limited the ability to improve job status and, in turn, the quality of life. Laosa (1975) reported that the longer Mexican immigrants stay in the United States, the less likely they are to retain the mother language, which probably is most directly attributable to the fact that English is the language used in schools and at work. Increasing attention is being given to the need for bilingual education for Mexican American students, and as a result, more Mexican Americans are becoming bilingual. However, a reverse problem is sometimes encountered when young Mexican children learn English as their primary language and then are not able to communicate with older relatives who speak only Spanish (Gonzales, 1997).

Communication by Mexican Americans is also complicated because many Mexican Americans learn a language that blends English and Spanish. Mexican American adults use this blended form of language more often than children do. Consequently, a nurse who may know both English and Spanish may still have difficulty understanding this blended language.

Some Mexican Americans still use English selectively. In an extensive study on language loyalty among various ethnic groups residing in the United States, it was found that Spanish remains the most persistent of all foreign languages. Thus, because of its persistent use, Spanish seemingly has the greatest prospects of survival (Fishman, 1967). Although other ethnic groups have become disillusioned with the use of their mother tongue, Mexican Americans have been more likely to retain their mother language in succeeding generations in the United States. Even today, some fluency in Spanish characterizes most Mexican Americans at all income levels. Another reason for the persistence of Spanish among Mexican Americans is that in the United States the mass media for information and entertainment are permeated with Spanish. Today, Spanish accounts for approximately 66% of the total foreign-language broadcasting in the United States. The demand for more Spanish-language media has led to the development of two national Spanish-language television networks. During the 1980s, 200 U.S. radio stations broadcast in Spanish. There has been a dramatic increase in Spanish-language newspapers, magazines, and journals (Galván, 1993). This is significant for the provision of improved health care for these people.

It is not uncommon for people who speak different languages to use each language in different contexts or for different purposes. Perhaps the most frequent situation is that of Mexican Americans who use English in their work and Spanish at home or with their friends (Marcos, 1988). There are several rather isolated villages in northern New Mexico where the only English spoken is for official occasions, such as conferring with a government agency. Because of the remoteness of these communities, these Mexican Americans may retain Spanish as their principal language.

Implications for Nursing Care

Because some Mexican Americans rely on Spanish to communicate with other people, it may be very frightening for them to participate in the American health care system, and it is frustrating for the nurses giving them care. In a qualitative study, nurses caring for clients who did not speak English described the need to develop and use their own strategies to communicate with these clients (Kirkham, 1998). Having a translator present was not sufficient for nurses to connect with their Mexican American clients. Friendly facial expressions, facing the client, and talking directly to the client even when using the services of an interpreter were found to be important. Hahn (1995) noted that some White Americans are ethnocentric, and although they work with Mexican Americans, they may think that it is unimportant to learn the language. Schillinger and colleagues (2003) conducted a study of primary care physicians speaking with diabetics and reported that patients with low literacy in the primary language of the physician received less interactive communication about their disease process. Thus, while efforts should be increased to recruit Mexican Americans into the health professions and to encourage students and professionals to study Spanish in order to communicate with clients, attention to the social features of how people speak when languages differ is needed (Street, 2002). The way people use language to motivate health behavior or persuade one another is affected by cultural differences (Pope, 2005). When professional staff cannot speak Spanish, interpretation services must be obtained in order to provide culturally competent care. Based on the recommendations of the Office of Minority Health National Standards for Culturally and Linguistically Appropriate Services in Health Care (CLAS Standards), family and friends should not be used as interpreters. Using children as translators should be avoided since children lack understanding of medical conditions and, as with other untrained interpreters, conflict of interest is likely to arise. Bilingual hospital staff members have as high as 50% inaccuracy when interpreting

(Elderkin-Thompson, Silver, & Waitzkin, 2001). The CLAS Standards recommend asking individuals to rate their primary language and capacity in English, and to use qualified institutional interpreters (Pope, 2005).

It is important for the nurse to remember that language is a cultural factor that influences health care practices (Villarruel, 2000). Zoucha (1998) reported findings from a qualitative study of registered nurses, Mexican American clients receiving care in an outpatient clinic, and friends and family members who had come with the client to the clinic. In this study, Mexican American clients viewed nurses who attempted to speak some Spanish as caring and respectful. It is uncommon for Mexican Americans to be aggressive or assertive when interacting with health care providers. Direct conflict or disagreement with a health care provider generally does not occur; rather, the Mexican American client will be silent or not adhere to the prescribed treatment plan. The nurse who works with bilingual Mexican Americans must remember that when under stress, these persons often may revert to their first language, Spanish. The nurse should explain that the nurse can be more helpful if the client communicates in the language that both the nurse and the client understand. When this is impossible because of high levels of stress on the part of the client, the nurse should find a translator. Understanding the profound effect of bilingualism on the client also requires appreciation of the dimension of language independence—the capacity to acquire, maintain, and use two separate language codes, each with its own lexical, syntactic, phonetic, semantic, and ideational components. Many Mexican Americans who are proficient in both Spanish and English operate parallel language codes, each with its own associations between message words and events in their ideational system (Marcos & Alpert, 1976). A good example of language compartmentalization can be found in the saying of Emperor Charles V: "To God I speak in Spanish, to women in Italian, to men in French, and to my horse in German" (*Oxford Dictionary of Quotations*, 1980). In certain situations a client may speak to his or her family in Spanish, to the nurse in English, and, when extremely stressed, to both family and nurse in a combination of both English and Spanish (Sobralske & Katz, 2005).

It is also important for the nurse to keep in mind that Mexican Americans tend to describe emotional problems by using dramatic body language. In addition, research has shown that when Mexican Americans are interviewed in English, or across their language barrier, they are usually judged by experienced clinicians as showing more severe symptoms than when they are interviewed in their mother tongue (Favazza, 1983; Marcos, Alpert, Urcuyo, & Kesselman, 1973). The nurse should keep in mind that nonverbal communication differs between cultures; thus, it is important to work closely with the client and family in order to evaluate symptoms from a variety of perspectives.

The nurse must guard against the use of idioms and abstractions when dealing with clients who do not completely understand the language. The nurse should also avoid responding to the client in a joking manner. Jokes are easily misinterpreted, frequently based on nuances of communication or language, and for the most part are lost in translation. When working with a Mexican American client who lacks understanding of the language, statements using slang or colloquialisms should be avoided because they may be interpreted literally.

One of the most important roles of the nurse in caring for the Mexican American client is that of teacher. Teaching should begin with an assessment of the client's ability to communicate and understand, which will guide the nurse in deciding which other family members should be included in the teaching process. The home situation must be carefully evaluated to adapt care to the reality of the living situation. Instruction should include all aspects of the client's condition and treatment and should be communicated in simple, concrete terms with ample opportunity allowed to raise questions and validate understanding. There should be continuous evaluation of learning by questioning and return demonstrations, and problem solving should be encouraged. Throughout this process, the nurse must continue to build a trusting relationship with the client so that follow-up care will be maintained, helping to ensure that the client will seek medical care before future situations get out of control.

SPACE

Kluckhohn (1976) categorized people and the modalities of relationships as individualistic, collateral, or lineal. Some Mexican Americans are categorized as both collateral and lineal, implying that there may be a patron–peon system, such as a boss–worker relationship, or a family-versus-individual relationship.

Mexican Americans value physical presence, including that of extended family members. It is important for Mexican Americans to see relatives face to face, embrace, touch, and just be with each other (Keefe, 1984). Mexican Americans as a group demonstrate a great need for group togetherness. Some Mexican Americans think of Anglos as distant because they require more personal space during conversation than Mexican Americans (Juckett, 2005). Ford and Graves (1977) found that when Mexican American second-graders related to others, there was closer interpersonal distance and more touching among girls. Touching was of longer duration when spatial distances were closer. Boys tended to be less tactile when relating to others. It is believed that this pattern of socialization begins with the parent–child relationship and continues into adulthood. During the early years, the parents are permissive, warm, and caring with all their children. However, in later years, the girls remain much closer to home and are protected and guarded in their contacts. In contrast, the boys are allowed to be with other boys in informal social groups, where they develop their machismo (Murillo, 1978). Gorek and colleagues (2002) described issues encountered by Mexican American families trying to adapt to the placement of an older adult in long-term care settings and the concern for staff to create a living space for their parents that respected their cultural heritage and routines.

Implications for Nursing Care

Despite the fact that Mexican Americans like consistent, close relationships and physical touching, female nurses should always assist a male physician in examining a female client and guard against exposing body parts other than those that are the focus of the examination (Murillo-Rohde, 1977). Male clients may refuse to allow a complete examination because of their modesty. Females will seek out female providers so as not to be seen by a male.

The nurse who plans care delivery for Mexican American clients must keep in mind that Mexican Americans may resist care provided by those perceived as being different or from a different ethnic background (Monrroy, 1983). Some Mexican Americans may also have cultural biases that prohibit care being administered by persons of the opposite sex. For example, a male student nurse was assigned to a Mexican American client in labor. This assignment precipitated problems because the client, husband, and family were all very uncomfortable because "only her husband should see her like that." It was necessary to change the assignment in order to provide care. However, while same-sex health care providers are preferred, a health care provider of the opposite sex is usually acceptable by Mexican Americans as long as the care provider is sensitive to the modesty needs of the client (Lagana & Gonzalez-Ramirez, 2003).

SOCIAL ORGANIZATION

Within the Mexican culture, the family is the most valued institution and the main focus of social identification. Most Mexican Americans have nuclear families that live separately, though some extended family or other relatives often live in the same household (Glick, 1999). According to Chávez (1986), new immigrants (especially those who are undocumented) tend to live in a multiple-family arrangement, which offers the advantages of social and economic support. As the length of residency increases and the family becomes more financially independent, the nuclear family tends to find a singular arrangement for its household.

Traditional females display subdued qualities, while males have been the authority figure in the family, assuming responsibility for being head of the household and the decision maker (Monrroy, 1983). For the male family member, there is a strong sense of machismo that is incompatible with the loss of self-esteem or authority. The male is considered the decision maker (Bonder, Martin, & Miracle, 2002). The mother of the family has the primary role of keeping the family cohesive. Although the mother may influence family decisions, she does not have a dominant role in the family. Increasing numbers of Mexican American women are finding work outside the home. Women who live in a rural setting often help with the family farming activities. Divorce is uncommon, but stable out-of-wedlock relationships are common in the lower socioeconomic levels. Meleis, Douglas, Eribes, et al. (1996) reported that when a group of employed, low-income Mexican women who worked in urban hospitals were studied, role overload and stress were experienced. There appeared to be difficulty reconciling the traditional cultural expectations of a woman's role in the changing society, which added the role of working outside the home.

Families are usually large, consisting of the parents and four or more children. Parent–child connectedness and respect for parental authority are valued over the husband–wife bond emphasized by the Western nuclear family. It is generally believed that Mexican Americans are familistic. *Familismo* or family interdependence is valued in the Mexican American culture. *Familismo* involves sharing by extended family members the responsibilities to nurture and discipline children, provide financial aid, provide companionship for lonely or isolated members, and engage in problem-solving. There is low reliance on institutions and outsiders. Mexican families value behavior in children that denotes respect, responsibility, and compliance and being "well brought up" (Arcia & Johnson, 1998; Reese, Balzano, Gallimore, & Goldenberg, 1995). For some Mexican Americans, *familism* has been perceived as curtailing mobility by sustaining emotional attachment to people, places, and things. In the Mexican American culture, *familism* has been identified as the prime cause not only of low mobility but also of resistance to changes of all kinds. For Mexican Americans, *familism*, along with the specially assigned male role, is a source of collective pride. Nevertheless, Mexican Americans are

believed to be deterred from collective and individual progress because of *familism.*

The major dominating theme of the traditional Mexican American family is the need for collective achievement of the family as a group. The collective needs of family supersede the needs of individual members. Also, any dishonor or shame that may occur for an individual member is considered a reflection on the entire family. The Mexican American family takes pride in family endeavors and generally does not seek help from outsiders to solve problems or meet needs. Mexican American families highly value having many relatives live nearby. The local extended family is tightly integrated, has frequent face-to-face encounters, and provides members with mutual aid (Glick, 1999). Lantican and Corona (1989) reported that Mexican Americans have a mean network size of 5.78, which may include in-laws, grandparents, and a substantial number of other relatives, with some 69% of those studied reporting that most of their support was provided by immediate family members. Villarruel and Denyes (1997) reported that the importance and obligation of Mexican Americans in meeting the needs of others indicate that there may be a higher priority placed on promoting and supporting the development of abilities to care for others than on abilities to care for self. Two other patterns, the "accepted obligation to perform roles within the family" and the "willingness to bear the burden so as not to cause pain for others" further indicate that caring for others is both expected and rewarded (Villarruel & Denyes, 1997; Villarruel & Leininger, 2004).

There is a high incidence of teenage pregnancy among Mexican Americans. Fitzpatrick, Fujii, Shragg, et al. (1990) found that, among U.S. teenage girls, Mexican Americans have the highest teenage pregnancy rate. In 2000, the birth rate for Mexican American women under 18 years of age was 6.3 per 1000 population, compared with 7.48 per 1000 for African-American women and 3.5 per 1000 for White women (National Center for Health Statistics, 2002). Likewise, the teenage pregnancy rate in 2000 for Mexican Americans 18 to 19 years of age was 10.4, compared with 11.9 for

African-Americans and 7.1 for Whites (National Center for Health Statistics, 2002).

The entire family may contribute to the financial welfare of the family. Parental control in Mexican American families is strong. Older children contribute by caring for younger family members or animals or by helping with the production of food or other family enterprises. Children in migrant families often earn money by working along with other family members.

Children also assume other responsibilities in the family. For example, Valenzuela (1999) found that older children of immigrant families served multiple roles in assisting their parents learn certain skills or activities that ranged from filing taxes to understanding difficult-to-read manuals, and intervening or advocating on behalf of their parents or their household on complicated transactions. The elderly are respected and live with married children if they are not self-sufficient. The elderly also pass down cultural and folk medicine beliefs. Elder care among Mexican Americans is greatly influenced by the belief that the family is the most important and main source of assistance, thus, Mexican American elders turn to their children and other family members for assistance before seeking out any services in the community.

Váldez (1980) found that Mexican American families of a lower socioeconomic class tended to show more ethnic identification than those of a higher socioeconomic class. This phenomenon served to provide support for Mexican Americans of lower socioeconomic classes and a more positive adaptation to the mainstream U.S. culture. Smith (2002) investigated gender and academic success among Mexican Americans. The findings indicated that Mexican American females in New York City choose high schools that ensure academic success in spite of the expectation that they return home after school to care for their younger siblings and help with housework. On the contrary, males took little time in selecting a high school and after school had no responsibility, giving them unstructured time that often led to gang activity and eventually dropping out of high school. Smith noted that whereas this enabled Mexican women to be

upwardly mobile, the opposite effect was noted in men.

An important institution in the Mexican heritage is the Catholic practice of *compadrazgo*, or coparenthood (godparenthood), which was introduced to Mexico by the Spaniards. Godparents, *compadrazgos*, accept coresponsibilities for a child along with the parents. This kinship begins with the baptism of the child and continues throughout the child's life; it is used for religious purposes and becomes an important resource for coping with the stresses of life (Kemper, 1982). Frequently, a godparent is chosen from a higher socioeconomic level, which enables the child to have social resources that are more extensive than what the family could provide.

Another important tradition for many Mexican American families is the way in which holidays are celebrated with Mexican traditions. Others continue to celebrate Mexican holidays. During the celebration of the Mexican Christmas, called *Las Posadas*, the children are fond of breaking a *piñata*, a papier-mâché container filled with candy and gifts. Other important holidays are Cinco de Mayo (May 5) and Guadalupe Day (December 12), which is Mexico's most important religious holiday. Affluent Mexican Americans often spend significant amounts of money on special food and drink, decorations, and fireworks for a holiday festival. Holidays provide an opportunity for Mexican Americans to share with others.

Beliefs and Practices in Death and Dying

Many Mexican Americans believe that whatever the cause of death, it is the will of God, often referred to as fatalism (Beutter & Davidhizar, 1999). For example, Kalish and Reynolds (1981) found that 72% of Mexican Americans believed that accidental death was attributable to divine will, as compared with 56% of Anglo Americans. Kalish and Reynolds (1981) also found that 27% of Mexican Americans thought of their own death daily, compared with 13% of Anglo Americans. Whereas none of the Anglo Americans believed that individuals should be allowed to die when they feel unproductive or unhappy, 3% of Mexican Americans reported they believed this should be allowed. Seventy-six percent of the Mexican Americans in this study reported that they are likely to touch the body of a deceased family member compared with 51% of Anglo Americans. Additionally, 59% reported they would be likely to kiss the body of the deceased, compared with 33% of Anglo Americans. In addition, 59% of Mexican Americans believe that a person should visit the grave of his or her spouse at least six times during the first year, compared with 35% of Anglo Americans. Gelfand and associates (2001) reported that Mexican Americans do not use hospice care because they are a close-knit community who prefer to take care of their own. On the other hand, Iwashyna and Chang (2002) examined differences in place of death among Whites, Mexican Americans, and Blacks that could not be explained by age, sex, income, education, and cause of death. After an inpatient stay, 56% of Mexican Americans died, compared with 50% of blacks and 43% of whites. Twenty-two percent of Mexican Americans died in a nursing home compared with 18% of Blacks and 20% of Whites. Only 9% of Mexican Americans died in a private residence, compared with 18% of Blacks and 22% of Whites.

Because of strong family ties among Mexican Americans, the idea of truth telling and decision making during the end of life may have to be viewed differently from the traditional Western lens of individual autonomy, and broadened to integrate the needs of the family. Religion and faith, and the role of the clergy, are important components of life in Mexican American families, and these components become intensified in the death and dying experience. Spiritual beliefs, the role of prayer, and the role of family in caregiving were predominant aspects in the end-of-life experience investigated in a sample of Mexican Americans (Gelfand et al., 2001). The study validated the need to focus on the role of religious institutions in Mexican American culture, where spirituality and religion are strong influences in the life experience. Pain and suffering are common aspects in the experience of death and dying. If the nurse and other health care providers do not understand Hispanic values about causes of pain, illness, and suffering, these experiences may go unrecognized or untreated (Valente, 2004). Differences in the expression of pain and suffering may exist even in the same culture. Hispanic males tend to be stoic and uncomplaining (Kemp, 2005), while among the women, moaning and crying are accepted means of expression of discomfort and pain.

Implications for Nursing Care

Of primary importance for the nurse caring for Mexican American clients is the concept that family values and roles are paramount in the client's treatment and recovery. The nurse should remember that the male head of the family should be consulted in health care decision making for other family members. It is also important that the nurse include the entire family, both immediate and extended members, in the assessment, planning, and implementation of nursing care if treatment is to be effective (Hough, 1985). Rather than viewing a large family who wishes to be with the client as an annoyance and frustration to staff, the nurse should discuss with the family how visits can be planned so that care can still be delivered and the client can obtain needed rest.

Murillo-Rohde (1977) has suggested that nurses use the family to help with the client's care. She says the family could feed, bathe, or walk the client, thus decreasing the anxiety and guilt of the family and the client. In addition, the nurse could be relieved of some of the workload. Allowing the family to participate in the client's care builds trust and respect and encourages compliance and support for discharge planning and teaching. However, the nurse should be aware that in one study by researchers at the University of California, only two thirds (65%) of the Mexican Americans in the study believed that the patient should be told if there was a diagnosis of metastatic cancer. The other respondents believed that the giving of information and the decision-making responsibility and information should rest with the family (Ethics, 1995). Thus, Mexican clients and families may not agree on who has the right to have medical information.

When the nurse is experiencing difficulty in getting a client to follow a particular medical regimen, the nurse may suggest that the client solicit the opinions of other family members regarding proposed actions. Suggesting family consultation will demonstrate that the nurse understands the importance of the family in regard to health matters. Nurses can encourage Mexican American clients to use health-promoting behaviors, with the rationale that the family cares about their health and will support them in meeting their goals (Kerr & Ritchey, 1990). Furthermore, the nurse's actions should help to build a relationship of trust between the nurse and the client. Burk, Wieser, and Keegan (1995) note that to facilitate provision of culturally sensitive care to Mexican Americans at a birthing center on the Mexican border, prospective certified nurse-midwives (CNMs) are evaluated for their understanding of and desire to work with this particular population. New staff are required to read culture-specific information and are encouraged to attend Spanish classes to develop a familiarity with the language. Knowledge of the client's culture has been found to be a positive dimension in the client–provider process and important in providing culturally appropriate care.

TIME

Mexican Americans are usually characterized as having a present orientation of time and as being unable or reluctant to incorporate the future into their plans. An example of this orientation is that some Mexican Americans may spend several years' savings on an important religious festival. Also, the Mexican custom of the siesta in some ways represents the belief that rest (or the present) has a priority over continued work that could produce monies to safeguard the future. Individuals with this present orientation of time may appear to lack practical concern about the future or the need for deferring gratification to a future time. Many investigators believe that this orientation restrains Mexican Americans from upward social mobility. In addition, some regard the present orientation of time as a barrier to assimilation and integration into the mainstream of American culture. However, of particular significance in terms of time orientation is the fact that Mexican Americans place more

value on the quality of interpersonal relationships than on the length of time in which they take place (Marin & Marin, 1991).

Khoury and Thurmond (1978) found few differences in the time perceptions of Mexican American and White American college students, despite the fact that the Mexican American students in the study were still maintaining cultural ties with the Mexican American culture. However, these findings cannot be generalized to Mexican Americans who are more immersed in their culture and less educated.

Implications for Nursing Care

Flexibility and creativity may be needed in order to work with differences in time orientation. It is important for the nurse to remember that personal ethnocentric attitudes toward time may negatively affect the planning of care for clients with a different time orientation. In the Western culture, health care settings tend to be future oriented, with weekly appointments, long-term treatment goals, and strict adherence to schedules. Scheduling can pose a barrier because patients and their families may not be able to leave work during the day to attend regular appointments. Because health care scheduling tends to be fixed and rigid, and traditional Hispanic culture time orientation tends to be more present oriented, Mexican American patients may encounter difficulties when trying to work within the time schedules of the medical setting. A Mexican American client may be late for an appointment not because of reluctance or lack of respect but because the client may be more concerned with a current activity than with the activity of planning ahead to be on time. This concept, known as *elasticity*, implies that future-oriented activities can be recovered but present-oriented activities cannot.

Because Mexican Americans are likely to be present-time oriented, the nurse may experience difficulties in planning and implementing health care measures such as long-term planning. In addition, the nurse may experience difficulties in explaining why and when medications should be taken. When working with a client who has a condition such as hypertension, it is important for the nurse to emphasize the effects of this condition, as well as short-term problems that can occur if the medication is not taken on time. Emphasis on short-term problems is more likely to be beneficial because it is more likely to get results. Because Mexican Americans are present-time oriented, their perceptions and understanding of acute and chronic illness may be affected.

ENVIRONMENTAL CONTROL

Locus of Control

Many Mexican Americans have an external locus of control, believing that external forces operate in many social and individual circumstances. Some Mexican Americans perceive life as being under the constant influence of the divine will. There is also a fatalistic belief that one is at the mercy of the environment and has little control over what happens. Associated with this view is the belief that personal efforts are unlikely to influence the outcome of a situation; thus, some Mexican Americans do not believe that they are personally responsible for present or future successes or failures. This belief may precipitate feelings of hopelessness regarding the future and positive change. The effect of this fatalistic belief was noted in Sennott-Miller's (1994) study of Hispanic women who had difficulty maintaining cancer-prevention activities.

Effect on Personal Control. Data from transcultural studies have found that people with a belief in external control can be expected to have more distress as an outcome of this view (Hough, 1985). On the other hand, Mirowsky and Ross (1984) noted that distress was not observed in the Mexican culture as an outcome of a belief in an external locus of control. They also suggested that although distress can result from strong family ties, it is offset by the family's strong support and responsibility to the individual. A consequence of strong family ties is that the individual may have a greater feeling of personal control, which in turn deters anxiety. When Mexican Americans experience pain, they value stoicism and self-control. Calvillo and Flaskerud (1991) suggest that crying and moaning in these clients may serve the purpose of relieving pain rather than communicating that the pain is intolerable and intervention is desired.

Research has shown that health practices among Mexican-Americans are influenced by psychosocial variables hypothesized in various models of health beliefs and behavior. Duffy, Rossow, and Hernandez (1996) reported that when the Health-Promoting Lifestyle Profile (HPLP) was administered, Mexican women had the highest total scores of all minority groups but lower scores than all predominantly White groups. HPLP self-actualization and interpersonal support were the highest subscale scores. Although Mexican American women in this study tended to practice more health-promoting lifestyle behaviors than other minority groups, it was also noted that a high number of the women worked in professional health care–related fields. However, their scores were lower than those reported for predominantly White groups, an indication that Mexican American women may lag substantially behind their White counterparts in the practice of "heart-healthy" lifestyles, even when the influence of socioeconomic status (SES) was removed. The exercise subscale was the lowest score for all groups, including minorities. Age, education, self-efficacy, health locus of control (internal and powerful others), and current health status made statistically significant contributions to the HPLP subscale scores. The Theory of Reasoned Action was tested by Poss (2000) in Mexican farmworkers; this study revealed that certain constructs in the model predicted participation in health screenings for tuberculosis, for which this group is at risk because of recent immigration history and exposure. Friedman-Koss, Crespo, Bellantoni, and Anderson (2002) noted that whereas the number of all women over 60 using hormone replacement therapy is 37%, the number of Mexican American women is 24%. On the other hand, Borrell, Lynch, Neighbors, Burt, and Gillespie (2002) conducted a study of prevalence and predictors of periodontitis. In a study of African-Americans, Mexican Americans, and non-Hispanic Whites, Mexican Americans had periodontal health profiles closer to those of non-Hispanic Whites than did African-Americans. These findings have significant implications for health professionals in terms of education related to health-promotion activities for Mexican Americans.

Skaff et al. (2003) studied a sample of 74 Latino Americans and 115 European Americans with type 2 diabetes to determine if a sense of control was related to health. A model of control beliefs, disease-management behaviors, and health indicators was tested with two measures of control beliefs, one diabetes-specific (diabetes self-efficacy) and one global (mastery), which were used to examine effects on management behaviors (diet and exercise) and on health (hemoglobin A_{1c} and general health). Results indicated that the relationship between control and management behaviors varied by measure of control and by group. For Latino participants, global mastery was related to management behaviors, whereas self-efficacy was related to such behaviors among European Americans. This study provides support for a diversified approach to control, behavior, and health, particularly in dealing with minority populations.

Health Care Beliefs

Health care beliefs are determined by several factors inherent in an individual's history, environments, cultural norms and patterns, mores and folkways. In turn, health behaviors are influenced by these health beliefs and determine how they respond to interventions designed to improve health behaviors. Keller and Fleury (2006) reviewed literature on physical activity in Hispanic women and found that factors such as individual, social, and cultural influences can serve as promoting as well as hindering factors to physical activity among this group. For instance, self-efficacy and social support tend to be positively related to increased physical activity among Mexican American women; however, the likelihood of engaging in physical activity may be modulated by traditional values that considers this inappropriate for older women. This review supported the notion that ethnic groups cannot be considered heterogenous based upon a common language and that socioeconomic factors influence health behaviors significantly (Keller & Fleury, 2006).

The cultural belief in external locus of control influences the manner in which some Mexican Americans view health. Some Mexican Americans believe that health may be the result of good luck or a reward from God for good behavior. For some Mexican Americans, health represents a state of equilibrium in the universe wherein the forces of "hot," "cold," "wet," and "dry" must be balanced. This concept is believed to have originated with the early Hippocratic theory of health and the four humors. According to the Hippocratic theory, the body humors—blood, phlegm, black bile, and yellow bile—vary in both temperature and moisture (Harwood, 1971). Persons who subscribe to this theory believe that health exists only when these four humors are in balance. Thus health can be maintained by diet and other practices that keep the four humors in balance. Illness, on the other hand, is believed to be misfortune or bad luck, a punishment from God for evil thoughts or actions, or a result of the imbalance of hot and cold or wet and dry. Cox (1986) found that a large number of elderly Hispanics attributed their health problems to old age and therefore did not seek any type of intervention.

Theory of Hot and Cold and Perception of Illness. One category of disease is hot and cold imbalance, in which illness is believed to be caused by prolonged exposure to hot or cold. To cure the illness, the opposite quality of the causative agent is applied to assimilate the hot or cold. Included in this category are illnesses that, rather than being caused by temperature itself, are associated with hot or cold aspects of substances found in medicines, elements, air, food, and bodily organs (Richardson, 1982). Treatment is focused on such things as suggestions, practical advice, prayers, or indigenous herbs, with the goal of reestablishing balance (Ruiz, 1985).

Although cold is believed to harm the body from without, excesses of heat developed from within the body itself and extending outward are believed to be related to such diseases as cancer, rheumatism, tuberculosis, and paralysis (Wilson & Kneisl, 1996) (Box 9-1). The focus of heat in the body is the stomach, whereas the head, arms, and legs are believed to be cool. Hot illnesses, such as skin ailments and fever, may be visible to the outside

Box 9-1

HOT-COLD CONDITIONS AND THEIR CORRESPONDING TREATMENT

Hot conditions	Cold conditions
Fever	Cancer
Infections	neumonia
Diarrhea	Malaria
Kidney problems	Joint pain
Rashes	Menstrual period
Skin ailments	Teething
Sore throat	Earache
Liver problems	Rheumatism
Ulcers	Tuberculosis
Constipation	Colds
Hot foods	Headache
Chocolate	Paralysis
Cheese	Stomach cramps
Temperate-zone fruits	**Cold foods**
Eggs	Fresh vegetables
Peas	Tropical fruits
Onions	Dairy products
Aromatic beverages	Meats such as goat, fish,
Hard liquor	chicken
Oils	Honey
Meats such as beef, waterfowl,	Cod
mutton	Raisins
Goat's milk	Bottled milk
Cereal grains	Barley water
Chili peppers	**Cold medicines and**
Hot medicines and herbs	**herbs**
Penicillin	Orange flower water
Tobacco	Linden
Ginger root	Sage
Garlic	Milk of magnesia
Cinnamon	Bicarbonate of soda
Anise	
Vitamins	
Iron preparations	
Cod-liver oil	
Castor oil	
Aspirin	

Adapted from Wilson, H., & Kneisl, C. (1992). *Psychiatric nursing*. Reading, Mass.: Addison-Wesley.

world. Many of the disorders caused by hot and cold imbalances are digestive in nature, which is related to the fact that an imbalance of hot and cold foods is believed to be damaging and suggests that to ensure good health, both hot and cold foods

must be taken into the body (Currier, 1966). The quality of the food eaten determines whether diarrhea is a hot or cold condition. If the stool is green or yellow, then the diarrhea is hot and the remedy is cold tea, whereas if the stool is white, then the diarrhea is cold and the remedy is hot tea.

Hot and cold are also associated with other aspects of life. Symbolically, cold is related to things that menace the individual, whereas hot is related to warmth and reassurance. In addition to air, water is seen as a source for cold. If an individual has participated in an activity that is considered hot, this person will not go near water because of its association with death. (At death, blood is believed to be turned into water.) The effort to balance hot and cold forces in the Mexican American belief system reflects the relationship between the individual and the environment. It is a symbolic attempt to attain a social order that is equitable (Ingham, 1970).

Theory of Hot and Cold and Effects on Growth and Development. Hot and cold have symbolic significance for the nature and process of reproduction. During pregnancy, a woman may be advised not to eat hot foods. On the other hand, during menstruation or after childbirth, a woman might be told to avoid cold foods or taking a bath. Infertility is associated with a "cold" womb, lack of intimacy, and rejection. A pregnant woman is believed to have an especially warm body, and to dissipate the warmth, she should bathe often and take short walks (Currier, 1966). The idea that warmth relates to intimacy follows in the relationship of mother and child. If a mother rejects her child, she is subject to an emotionally based disease called *bilis*, which can cause the infant to have chronic headaches and permanent injury. This belief indicates that the child may display chronic malnutrition, which Currier (1966) relates to a lack of affection and support. Nursing of the child is also related to hot and cold characteristics. A diminished milk flow is believed to result from coldness, whereas warmth is believed to increase the flow. An excess of warmth causes the child to become ill because the milk curdles and becomes indigestible.

During the first year of life, a child is kept physically close to the mother, either by being wrapped in her shawl or by sleeping in a bed next to her. When the child is weaned and starts walking, the mother deprives the child of this physical contact, and when the child experiences the cold floors and lack of physical attachment, he or she may experience rage and depression. This condition is related to a lack of support and physical warmth (Currier, 1966).

Folk Medicine

Use of folk medicine and folk practitioners is considered one of the most important variables leading to the underutilization of Western medicine by Mexican Americans (Tajalli, 1984; Beecham, 1995; Ericksen, 2006). The belief that health is a matter of chance and controlled by forces in nature is the basis of folk medicine. Folk medicine as practiced by Mexican Americans combines elements of the European Roman Catholic view and the view of the original Indians of Mexico. These beliefs have led to unique ways of accounting for physical and mental illnesses and their consequences and to unique methods of dealing with illnesses. This belief and practice system regarding health care is indigenous to the Mexican American community and is known as *curanderismo* (Rivera & Wanderer, 1986). Within this folk medicine system, illness is viewed from a religious and social context rather than the medical-scientific perspective of the dominant Western society (Applewhite, 1995).

Types of Folk Practitioners. Operating within the *curanderismo* folklore system of beliefs and practices are several levels of healers. The first healer sought out is a member of the family; if the case is or becomes more complicated, healers within the community are sought out. Several levels of folk healers are described here, beginning with the lowest level, the family healer.

Family Folk Healer. The first person to be consulted at the time of illness is a key family member who is respected for her knowledge of folk medicine. This individual may be a wife, mother, grandmother, or other revered elderly relative. The healing practices are passed down in the family from mother to

daughter. If the client does not improve, an intermediary person usually directs the client to the *curandero*.

Yerbero. The *yerbero* (or *herbero*) is a folk healer who specializes in using herbs and spices for preventive and curative purposes. This person grows and distributes herbs and spices and explains how to use them effectively (Richardson, 1982).

Curandero and Curandera. The more serious physical and mental or emotional illnesses are brought to the *curandero*. If the practitioner is a woman, she is referred to as a *curandera*. The *curandero* perceives life as being under the consistent influence of the divine will. People are believed to be born as sinners, with death being the result of their sins. The central focus of these healers' treatment is relieving clients of their sins. Suffering is seen as a component of illness, and death is seen as failure to be cured of sin (Ruiz, 1985). The *curandero* believes that water, food, and air are important to the maintenance of health. Imbalance of these elements, imbalance between God and man, and imbalance between hot and cold are believed to contribute to illness.

Weclew (1975) and Ness and Wintrob (1981) have reported that *curanderos* see clients with a wide range of both physical and psychological symptoms, such as gastrointestinal distress, back pain, headache, fever, depression, anxiety, irritability, fatigue, hostility, shame, guilt, sexual problems, alcoholism, and the common folk diseases. The diagnosis is made after a thorough assessment of all aspects of the client's life, including the family and even the supernatural. The treatment is provided in a room in the *curandero's* home that is decorated with much religious paraphernalia. Treatments used include massage, diet, rest, suggestions, practical advice, indigenous herbs, prayers, magic, and supernatural rituals. Although *curanderos* generally use white magic, there are times when they may resort to black magic because the cure is difficult.

The *curandero*, who is believed to have the "God-given" gift of healing and is a full-time specialist, is often consulted before medical contact is made or may be consulted concomitantly with a medical contact. The effectiveness of *curanderos* seems to be in their ability to use their personality and healing regalia to encourage hope and trust on the part of the client. The beliefs and practices of this healer are supported by the family and the community, which tends to strengthen the client's sense of control over the situation. *Curanderos* are often preferred over the medical community because they are personal, are less dehumanizing, know the family, and are an integral part of the Mexican American community. *Curanderos* in most cases are thought to have power over witches because they are believed to heal through the power of God (Burk, Wieser, & Keegan, 1995).

Brujos and Brujas (Witches). The level of healers called witches may not be sought out until other forms of healing have been tried. The practitioners of witchcraft utilize several kinds of magic. Black magic is practiced by both male witches (*brujos*) and female witches (*brujas*), and red magic and green magic are believed to empower a witch to solve love problems by assuming an animal form. As mentioned previously, white magic is practiced by a *curandero*, is considered good magic, and is used in folk healing (Wanderer & Rivera, 1986). A motive for witchcraft may be hatred, jealousy, or envy. To cure, witches may use food or drink, imitative magic (such as dolls), evil air, or animal metamorphosis to bewitch (Wanderer & Rivera, 1986). There are many superstitions adhered to in this healing mode; for example, keeping black animals protects against witchcraft.

Among adult Mexican Americans, recourse to traditional healers are commonly encountered along with the use of Western medicine. The strongest predictors of use of traditional healers is limited English proficiency and dissatisfaction with medical practice. Treatments involve traditional rituals, social reintegration, and penance (Kaiser Permanente, 2001). The following are common folk illnesses observed among Mexican-Americans.

Folk-related Illnesses. Concepts of disease among Mexican Americans relate to the negative effects of intensely emotional states experiences, dislocation or malfunctions of organs or body parts, infant susceptibility, and magical thinking. Common childhood folk illnesses include *empacho, mal de ojo*, and *mollera caída* (Kaiser Permanente, 2001). Folk illnesses have been linked to morbidity and mortality (Baer, Weller, Garcia, Glazer, Trotter, Pachter, & Klien, 2003; APA, 1994).

Caída de la Mollera. *Caída de la mollera* refers to a fallen fontanel in infants caused by a fall, by bouncing the child roughly, or by removal of the nipple from the baby's mouth with too much force. This condition is viewed as an imbalance between the fontanel and the palate that blocks the passage of foods and liquids. Associated with *caída de la mollera* are the symptoms of inability to suck or grasp the nipple, vomiting, diarrhea, fever, restlessness, and crying spells.

Before seeking out a physician, mothers often seek out older women in the community who seem to know how to treat this problem. The following remedies have been noted by Ruiz (1985): pressing against the palate from inside the mouth, praying, applying eggs to the head and then pulling hairs, and holding the child with the head down. Reinert (1986) has noted that this condition is usually caused by severe dehydration and that correct medical treatment with intravenous fluids is essential.

Mal Ojo (Evil Eye). As mentioned earlier, *mal ojo* occurs when an individual who is believed to possess a special power admires or covets the child of another and looks at but does not touch the child. *Mal ojo* at times is associated with witchcraft and black magic. This condition is characterized by headaches, high fever, crying, diarrhea, restlessness, irritability, loss of weight and sleep, and sunken eyes (Rivera & Wanderer, 1986; Ruiz, 1985). The cure for the problem is to mix a hen's egg with water and place this under the head of the child's bed, which supposedly drives the bad influence out of the child's body. Another remedy is to have the person believed to be the source of the evil eye touch the afflicted individual. It is believed that the child will deteriorate, with severe coughing and vomiting, and possibly die if not treated. Families are known not to bring children with this problem to physicians because they fear the physician will misdiagnose the child and the child's condition will worsen.

Empacho. Children suffering from *empacho* ("obstacle") are believed to have a chunk of food that they are unable to pass, causing a lot of abdominal pain. They are taken to an older woman who possesses the knowledge to treat this problem. To diagnose the illness, the client is held face down by the skin of the back. During this procedure, if a crack is heard, the diagnosis is *empacho*, and the following treatment is instituted: body massages around the back and waist are given to restore the body's balance of hot and cold, which, in turn, allows the food chunk to pass through the intestine (Ruiz, 1985).

Susto (Magical Fright). *Susto* is commonly observed among adults experiencing stress. It is caused by a frightening experience or event and leads to the temporary loss of one's spirit from the body. This condition may even affect an unborn child if the mother is frightened. *Susto* is associated with childhood epilepsy, is seen more often in females, and if left untreated is believed to develop into tuberculosis or even death. Symptoms of *susto* include crying, insomnia, anorexia, restlessness, nightmares, stomachache, diarrhea, high fever, and involuntary tics. Treatment for *susto* involves holding a ceremony known as "*barrida*," in which a curandero sweeps the body with fresh herbs while the healer recites ritual prayers. A more severe form of susto is *espanto*. Studies have shown that individuals who suffer *espanto* long term have higher mortality and morbidity indices than those who suffer the less severe form (Kaiser Permanente, 2001).

Nervios. *Nervios* refers to restlessness, insomnia, loss of appetite, headaches, and nonspecific aches and pains. This is linked to chronic experience of negative life circumstances, particularly revolving around interpersonal relationships (Kaiser Permanente, 2001). *Nervios* is now noted in the *Diagnostic and Statistical Manual of Mental Disorders*, fourth edition (DSM-IV) (APA, 1994). There is evidence that Mexican Americans would seek a medical provider for *nervios* but would seek folk healers or use

home remedies for *susto* (Baer, Weller, Garcia, Glazer, Trotter, Pachter, & Kleine, 2003).

Religious Views. Roman Catholicism is the predominant religion practiced by Mexican Americans. Common religious practices are baptism, confirmation, communion, weddings, and funerals. During times of crisis, Mexican Americans may rely on the priest and family for prayers. When a family member is ill, rituals that are practiced include making promises, lighting candles, visiting shrines, and offering prayers (Logan & Semmes, 1986).

Roman Catholic Mexican Americans may have beliefs that are influenced by ancient Indian practices of witchcraft and voodoo. As a result, some Mexican Americans may believe in demons. Incorporated in this system is a belief in witchcraft practices to manipulate evil forces (Wanderer & Rivera, 1986). Wanderer and Rivera (1986) have noted that in the Mexican American community witchcraft is called *brujería* and is seen as a magical or supernatural illness and occasionally as an emotional illness. *Brujería* has no scientific basis and is believed to be precipitated by opponents using the evil forces of hexes and spells. Symptoms of *brujería* include paranoia, delusions, hallucinations, feelings of being controlled by another person, mania, perverted and fitful behavior, depression, suspicion, and anxiety. Motives for witchcraft include envy, vengeance, hatred, and jealousy (Kiev, 1968; Madsen & Madsen, 1969).

Implications for Nursing Care

It is important for the nurse to be aware that use of alternative therapies from Mexico is very prevalent among Mexican Americans. Keegan (1996) reported that 44% of Mexican Americans in a study in the Texas Rio Grande Valley reported using alternative practitioners one or more times during the previous year. The most commonly sought therapies were herbal medicine, spiritual healing and prayer, massage, relaxation techniques, chiropractic, and visits to a Mexican folk healer, or *curandero*. The majority (66%) indicated that they never reported visits to alternative practitioners to their established primary health care provider.

The belief held by many Mexican Americans that external forces control the outcome of circumstances can influence adherence with medical or health care recommendations. This perspective may influence the practice of wellness programs in the U.S. health care system, such as smoking cessation, addiction programs, prenatal care, health-promotion activities, and chronic disease treatment by Mexican Americans. Because the traditional healing system of *curanderismo* incorporates religious beliefs, some Mexican Americans may also believe that they are more in touch with the divine will, and therefore the origin and healing of illness, when they enter the health care system. The nurse should understand that Mexican Americans will have more respect for the caregiver who accepts the spiritual and folk basis of their health beliefs.

The nurse should observe how the client is implementing health management; in particular, client self-management in chronic disease is key to the success of care. In cases of nonadherence to the management protocol, the nurse should discuss any issues with the client and family to determine if the basis for nonadherence is folk beliefs. For instance, beliefs regarding hot and cold characteristics will affect how the client accepts some of the treatment plan. The nurse might inquire if the condition is considered a hot or cold disease. The client may have some definite beliefs about this and about whether the medical treatment can restore the hot–cold balance within the body. If the treatment is incongruent with folk beliefs, the nurse should attempt to find compromises or solutions that will resolve the incongruence, and allow the client to maintain his or her belief system, while at the same time adhere to the prescribed medical or health care management. One can expect the older client or first-generation immigrant to be more attached to these beliefs; therefore, focusing health teaching on younger family members may be more useful in establishing adherence. Communication between the nurse and client enhances adherence (Miller & Davidhizar, 2001).

The healers in the folk medicine system are people with whom the Mexican Americans have established relationships and with whom they can easily communicate. These healers know and can treat the folk illnesses that the uninitiated health care worker may not recognize. It is helpful for the nurse to understand the respect this culture has for the *curandero*, who is often consulted simultaneously with the physician or nurse. The long-term goal of a nurse working in a Mexican American community should be to understand the folk medicine beliefs and to try to establish a relationship with the *curandero* in the hope of influencing acceptance and understanding of the rationale for modern health care practices and thereby gaining the community's confidence.

The nurse should recognize that the *curandero* is involved in relieving people of their sins so that they can experience healing and that a spiritual perspective is usually an integral part of the U.S. health care system. One might compare the healer's influence in this ethnic group to that of the clergy in the dominant U.S. society, wherein mutual cooperation is focused on meeting clients' spiritual and physical needs. Mexican American clients also need to be encouraged to practice their religious beliefs and to receive supportive visits from the clergy. Acknowledging the client's reliance on the folk health care system as well as on his or her religious beliefs and medical assistance will promote a more holistic focus for nursing care.

It is important to recognize the strong influence of hot and cold imbalance in folk beliefs. Some of these healing beliefs and practices are practical, such as massage, prayer, listening, or the application of cold for a fever. However, some practices can lead to missed clues for serious conditions that do not respond to these remedies, such as prolonged diarrhea, vomiting, dehydration, parasites, or malnutrition in children. For example, the nurse should suspect that malnutrition in a 1-year-old child may be caused by the practice of separating the child from the mother at the time of weaning. Teaching the mother about the child's physical and emotional needs may improve the malnutrition. When dealing with children, Leininger (2002) warns the nurse to touch the children so that if the parents fear the evil eye, the cultural remedy of touch will cure the condition.

In dealing with folk-related diseases, the nurse needs to understand perceived causes for these conditions, for example, environmental influences, such as *caída de la mollera* or *empacho*, or evil influences, such as *mal ojo* or *susto*. Because these diseases are considered indigenous to the culture, they are usually seen and treated first by the *curandero*. Patients coming to the nurse's attention with these conditions probably have had these symptoms for a while and have already been treated unsuccessfully by the *curandero*. The nurse's physical assessment needs to be thorough. Cultural variables should be included in the assessment. In managing pain, Calvillo and Flaskerud (1991) believe that the important variables to assess are cultural, psychological, and social factors that affect attitudes and responses to pain and how pain is reported. Rather than showing disrespect for the folk healer, the nurse should develop the relationship with the client in such a way as to maintain the support of the folk healer. Respect should also be shown for amulets that the client might wear to protect against the evil eye or evil spirits. For example, the *mano milagroso* ("miraculous hand") is worn by many people of Mexican origin for luck and the prevention of evil. The *mano milagroso* is worn by some people of Mexican background to ward off evil. Amulets worn by persons from Mexico may have red yarn attached (Spector, 2004). The nurse should allow the client to continue to wear the amulet rather than attempting to take it away. The nurse should appreciate that eating eggs and bread, drinking tea, and sleeping are methods that some persons from Mexico believe are effective to maintain health, and these beliefs should be respected (Spector, 2004).

BIOLOGICAL VARIATIONS

Skin Color

The skin color of Mexican Americans can vary from a natural tan to dark brown. Persons with lighter color have more Spanish ancestry, whereas darker-skinned persons have more Indian ancestry. It is more difficult to recognize vasodilatation or vasoconstriction in the darker-skinned client, in whom vasoconstriction and anemia are manifested as an ashen color rather than a bluish coloration. The mongolian spots (areas of darker skin found on the sacral area) found on infants usually disappear by 4 years of age. The hair of Mexican Americans is usually dark and may be curly and woolly, straight, or wavy (Monrroy, 1983).

Susceptibility to Disease

Diabetes. Diabetes affects 8.9% of the adults in New Mexico (New Mexico Department of Health, 2000). Approximately 17% of people aged 40 and over in New Mexico have diabetes (C.A.R.E.S, 2003). Diabetes tends to be more severe in Hispanics than non-Hispanic Whites. Diabetes occurs at a younger age, more often requires insulin to be controlled, results in more limb amputations, contributes to eye disease, is responsible for six times higher incidence of kidney failure, and results in a death rate two to four times the rate for non-Hispanic Whites (Vásquez, 1997; Otiniano, Black, Ray, Du, & Markides, 2002). The adverse impact of uncontrolled diabetes is compounded by lack of access to primary care and preventive services and by education of less than 12 years (Philis-Tsimikas et al., 2004; Otiniano, Black, Ray, Du, & Markides, 2002). In a study of the impact of diabetes on employment and earnings outcomes of middle-aged and older Mexican Americans in the Southwest, Bastida and Pagan (2002) found men had a lower probability of employment but no effect on earnings, whereas women had lowered productivity and earnings but no significant change in their probability of employment. In a study by Luyas (1989), low-income Mexican American women with type 2 diabetes explained diabetes onset in terms of economic and family problems. Eid and Kraemer (1998) interviewed Mexican Americans with type 2 diabetes residing in California. Concerns about the cost were particularly expressed by the uninsured. Subjects tended to blend the treatment plan of conventional medicine with native customs. Mexican Americans with diabetes who had less than 12 years of education were more likely to report diabetic complications than those with more education. Both Philis-Tsimikas et al. (2004) and Davidson (2003) report the effectiveness of nurse-managed care for diabetic Hispanic patients in California.

Hypertension. Hypertension is also found with increased prevalence among Mexican Americans (National Center for Health Statistics, 2002). Mexican Americans are slightly more likely to have high blood pressure than non-Hispanic Whites (29% vs. 27%) and slightly less likely to have high-risk cholesterol than their non-Hispanic White counterparts (18% vs. 21%) (Stewart & Silverstein, 2002). Nelson, Norris, & Mangione (2002) found that even when Mexican Americans were diagnosed with high cholesterol requiring medication, they were less likely than their White counterparts to take cholesterol-lowering agents. In a study using census figures from 1969 to 1971 and 1979 to 1981, Stern, Bradshaw, Eifler, et al. (1987) reported less decline in the death rates of Mexican American men from total ischemic heart disease and myocardial infarction than in the death rates of other men.

Pernicious Anemia. Pernicious anemia, most often seen in the elderly, has been shown to occur in those of Latin American origin at a younger age than in White patients (Carmel, Johnson, & Weiner, 1987). There is evidence that a low SES has a strong effect on hemoglobin and hematocrit levels and that, given similar socioeconomic conditions, Mexican Americans tend to have higher hematocrit levels than their White counterparts have (Overfield, 1995). Hispanics in the Southwest were found to have a poorer prognosis with melanoma because such melanoma arose from the palms, sublingual regions, mucous membranes, and soles; were more advanced in stage; occurred in older people; and metastasized (Black, Goldhahn, & Wiggins, 1987).

Communicable Diseases. Approximately 85% of the health problems common to Mexican Americans involve communicable diseases (National Center for Health Statistics, 2002) including respiratory tract infections, diarrhea, skin disorders, nutritional problems (particularly during the first year of life), macroscopic parasitosis, and amebiasis. One of the most severe medical problems facing nations throughout the world is tuberculosis, which is believed to occur in areas where there are crowded living conditions, low income, substandard housing, and inadequate health care, such as that which existed for many in Mexico. In the United States, the population that is most at risk for the incidence and transmittal of tuberculosis is newly arrived immigrants, including Mexicans (Hood & Jackson, 1989; Phipps, 1993). Because there is a high prevalence of tuberculosis in Mexico, it is believed that Mexican Americans may have a predisposition to a higher prevalence of tuberculosis than other Americans have (Phipps, 1993). Findings from a study of 845 African-American, Mexican American, and White adolescents in San Diego indicate that, among the subjects surveyed, Mexican American adolescents had a higher rate of positive tuberculin tests, necessitating treatment (Fitzpatrick, Fujii, Shragg, et al., 1990). McQuillan, Kruszon-Moran, Deforest, Chu, and Wharton (2002) noted that adult Mexican Americans were slightly less likely than other Americans to have protective levels of antibody to diphtheria and tetanus.

Hepatitis C. Hepatitis C has also been found to occur at a higher rate among Mexican Americans. Although the rate among Whites in the United States is 1.5%, among Mexican Americans it is 2.1% (Cronin, 1997). Although an estimated 3.9 million persons in the United States have hepatitis C virus, this blood-borne virus, which can kill, was not identified until 1989. Since blood banks began screening for hepatitis C in 1990, the rate of new infections has declined. Although half of those who obtained the disease before 1990 are believed to have received it from blood, the other half probably did so by sharing needles or straws to inject drugs (Cronin, 1997). It is estimated that more people could die from the complications of hepatitis C than from AIDS (Cronin, 1997). Some 70% of the cases result in liver damage that leads to death. Once the disorder is diagnosed, lifestyle changes, such as avoiding alcohol, can prolong length and quality of life.

Childhood Obesity. There is a growing incidence of childhood obesity noted among Mexican Americans. Alexander and Blank (1988) suggest that the increasing incidence of obesity in Mexican American children may be a result of mothers believing that a fat baby is a healthy baby. The mothers in this study had a greater body mass index than mothers in a control group did. These subjects also had "pushier" feeding practices with their children. To prevent the complications of adult obesity stemming from childhood obesity, nurses should identify mothers and their children who are at risk for obesity and encourage a weight-reduction program. The nurse should make an assessment of the potential need for nutritional education among Mexican American clients. Hispanic women may have cultural dietary variations prenatally. For example, antepartal cravings, including that for clay, are not denied. In the postpartum period, warm tea, broth, and corn gruel are acceptable foods, whereas citrus fruits, port (a wine), and tomatoes are avoided. It is believed harmful to eat and breastfeed simultaneously. The mother may believe stress and anger makes bad milk, which makes a breastfeeding infant ill. Some Hispanics neutralize the bowel when weaning from breast to bottle by feeding only anise tea for 24 hours (White, Linhart, & Medley, 1996). Twenty-nine percent of Mexican Americans are more likely to be obese, compared with 21% in the general population (Carter-Pokras, 2000).

HIV/AIDS. Nationwide, AIDS cases among Hispanics are occurring at triple the rate among non-Hispanics (Caudle, 1993). For Hispanic people, the cumulative total of deaths reported from January 1999 through December 2001 was 81,793. The number of deaths has steadily risen in this vulnerable group. Among Hispanic men the cumulative total of deaths through December 2001 was 67,557. For Hispanic males age 15 to 24, the number of deaths reported was 1373. For Hispanic women at all ages, the number of cumulative deaths reported through December 2001 was 14,236. The number of Hispanic women in the age range between 15 and 24 years of age was 7, as compared with only 8 for Whites (National Center for Health Statistics, 2002). Mexican Americans are not listed separately. Because of the

unsanitary working and housing conditions of migrant farmworkers and their limited opportunity to protect themselves, the opportunity for higher risk for HIV infection exists (Aplemis, 1996). Marin (2003) reports an HIV prevention program in an American Hispanic community in which factors including marginalization, homophobia, poverty, and racism were addressed to increase feelings of empowerment.

Psychological Characteristics

According to Reinert (1986), Mexican Americans often encounter serious health problems resulting from the stress of coping with poverty. The harsh socioeconomic conditions and discrimination in the United States have been suggested as a possible reason that some Latino men psychologically react by adapting rigid macho behaviors (Sugihara & Warner, 2002). Alcohol and drug comorbidity poses a particular challenge for Mexican-Americans because of barriers to health and mental health care, language problems, and low educational attainment (Vega & Lopez, 2001). Because of their belief that alcohol consumption is a way of celebrating life, alcohol is consumed in all aspects of life and contributes to the increased incidence of accidents, violence, homicide, unintentional injuries, and other lifestyle diseases (Bechtel, Davidhizar, & Tiller, 1998). For Mexican Americans, alcoholism is the most crucial health problem (Arrendondo, Weddige, Justice, & Fitz, 1987; Vega, Scribney, & Achara-Abrahams, 2003). Research on substance abuse among Hispanics indicates that alcohol is the most frequently abused intoxicant. Vega and associates (2003) examined co-occurrence of comorbid alcohol, drug, and non–substance use psychiatric disorders in a population sample of Mexican-origin adults for rural and urban areas of central California. They found that alcohol abuse or dependence with co-occurring psychiatric disorders is a primary disorder among Mexican-origin adult males with 7.5% lifetime prevalence. The co-occurring lifetime rates of alcohol and other drug disorders with non–substance use psychiatric disorders, or both, were 8.3% for men and 5.5% for women and were

12.3% for the U.S.-born and 3.5% for immigrants. Specifically, among male immigrants, dual diagnoses consist primarily of an alcohol disorder and a non–substance use disorder. Among U.S.-born males, dual diagnoses consist of alcohol abuse or dependence, an illicit drug abuse or dependence disorder, and an additional non–substance use disorder. Mexican American U.S.-born women have dual diagnosis rates similar to those of Mexican American U.S.-born males, and these rates are higher among either immigrant males or immigrant females. Comorbidity among immigrant women is not primarily a dual diagnosis but rather a mood disorder co-occurring with anxiety disorder. Men are most often affected because the male role may be correlated with being able to ingest large amounts of alcohol. Accelerating risk for alcohol and drug abuse or dependence disorders associated with either immigrant acculturation suggests that the prevalence of comorbidity involving alcohol and other drug disorders in the Mexican population will increase over time. Some research has reported that children who have alcoholic parents or grandparents are at higher risk for alcoholism because of their physiological relationship (Vega, Scribney, & Achara-Abrahams, 2003). Arrendondo, Weddige, Justice, and Fitz (1987) noted that Mexican Americans have a higher death rate from illnesses related to chronic alcohol consumption, such as cirrhosis of the liver.

In a study on the prevalence of psychiatric disorders, Grant, Stinson, Hasin, Dawson, Chou, & Anderson (2004) found that foreign-born Mexican Americans and foreign-born non-Hispanic whites were at significantly lower risk of DSM-IV substance use and mood and anxiety disorders compared with U.S.-born counterparts. Specifically, the prevalence of alcohol use disorder, mood disorder, and anxiety disorder among U.S.-born Mexican American and non-Hispanic Whites were twice as large as foreign-born rates. The rate of drug use disorder among U.S. born Mexican Americans was 8.3 times greater than for foreign-born Mexican Americans, while for the non-Hispanic Whites the ratio was about 2:4:10. Other research has found, however, that when rates of substance abuse are

considered among Mexican Americans, marijuana is the second most abused drug, with heroin and cocaine ranking third and fourth (Eden & Aguilar, 2004). Inhalants are also frequently abused among young Hispanics (Eden & Aguilar, 2004). Using a subset sample derived from an epidemiologic survey in the Mexican American Prevalence and Services Survey (MAPSS) that examined the effects of immigration status on mental health status, Ortega and associates (2000) found that U.S.-born Mexican Americans had higher rates of any psychiatric disorder and posttraumatic stress disorder than their foreign counterparts.

There is evidence that family structure and family functioning are important protective and risks factors for the Latinos. In Mexican American families, the family may serve as a buffering mechanism that encourages individual members to share, thereby reducing anxiety and stressful situations. For example, Bray and associates (2001) surveyed adolescent children in a 3-year longitudinal study to determine the influence of family cohesion, family conflict, and family separation on alcohol usage. They found that family cohesion was related to decrease in alcohol use while family separation and conflict increase alcohol use. Murguia et al. (1998) found that family warmth had a direct effect in preventing association with drug-using peers in adolescent Mexican Americans. While others have found that family cohesiveness and warmth in Mexican American family is a protective factor for pregnancy (Balcazar, Krull, & Peterson, 1997). The Mexican American's view of the world also enables some Mexican Americans to blame external forces for failures, thereby reducing guilt. Mexican Americans are unlikely to seek treatment (Katerndahl & Realini, 1998), and they have low rates of service utilization for mental health problems (Peifer, Hu, & Vega, 2000). Mexican American women have been found to have slightly more dysthymic disorders, panic disorders, and phobias than other women (Murillo, 1978). Heilemann, Lee, and Kury (2002) found that women who spent all of their childhood years in Mexico before coming to the United States have a lower level of depressive symptoms and more satisfaction with life than women who were exposed to the United States in childhood. However, there is growing evidence that Mexican American adolescents may be at risk for depressive symptoms (Joiner, Perez, Wagner, Berenson, & Marquina, 2001; Romero & Roberts, 2003). Mexican American elders are also at risk for depression, and depression has been linked to chronic financial strain, being a woman, and presence of health problems (Chiriboga, Black, Aranda, & Markides, 2002).

Social and cultural differences between the Mexican American and the dominant American society appear to be a recurring theme among Mexican American clients with symptoms of psychological disorders. Feelings of social isolation may serve to increase personal feelings of isolation. For some Mexican Americans, feelings of isolation, persecution, and discrimination have resulted in acute paranoid reactions and posttraumatic stress disorder (PTSD) (Cervantes, Snyder, & Padilla, 1989; Murphy, Giger, & Davidhizar, 1994; Rivera, 1978). In a classic study evaluating the role of discrimination and acculturation stress on Mexican-origin adults, Finch, Hummer, Kolody, and Vega (2001) noted a clear association between discrimination and poorer physical health. They found the effect of job market stress on self-rated health analogous to a nearly 8-point increase in one's depression score. It is important for the nurse to be aware of self-image problems that are socially created and those that are personal. Knowledge of these factors will assist the nurse in making the diagnosis and planning nursing care that will help lower the client's psychological risk.

Implications for Nursing Care

In providing health care education for the Mexican American, the nurse must remember to address cultural differences such as health values, ethnic care practices, family life patterns, dietary practices, the presence of insurance, and a usual source of care. It is also important to communicate the necessity of commitment by the whole family to making lifestyle changes if they are to be successful.

Hispanic Americans in the San Antonio Heart Study were found to be less knowledgeable about preventing heart attacks and not engaging in risk-reducing behaviors as often as non-Hispanic Whites (Hazuda, Stern, Gaskill, et al., 1983). Derenowski (1990) noted that cardiovascular risk reduction and changes in lifestyle are necessary components of education for some Mexican Americans.

It is important for the nurse to recognize that the informal health care system in Mexico is generally composed of several elements, one of which is self-medication. In the early 1980s in Mexico, just as in the United States, prescriptions were required for all medications, such as antibiotics and steroids. However, during this time the sale of drugs in Mexico was uncontrolled, except for narcotics, barbiturates, and other addictive drugs. The pharmacist was, in effect, the chief physician's surrogate, and many Mexican American immigrants have been accustomed to receiving medication from a pharmacist without a prescription. In addition, some Mexican Americans consider medication to be always necessary and may not believe that their illness is being treated unless a particular medication is ordered.

The massive scale to which self-medication is practiced in Mexico is potentially dangerous (Anthony-Tkach, 1981). To illustrate this point, in 1974 an outbreak of typhoid fever that was considered the worst in the century occurred in and around Mexico City. The causative agent was identified as chloramphenicol-resistant *Salmonella typhi*. Health officials in Mexico City believed that the indiscriminate use of antibiotics may have caused the organism to become resistant to the effects of chloramphenicol. It is important for the nurse to assess whether a Mexican American client with a communicable disease is practicing self-medication for treatment. The assessment of the potential for self-medication as well as close follow-up study may be beneficial in reducing the drug-resistant causative organisms that can ensue from self-medication. The nurse who works with Mexican American clients with communicable diseases needs to emphasize that communicable diseases are preventable and that prompt care is essential to reducing exposure to, as well as morbidity from, communicable diseases.

Public health concerns are present in all ethnic minority groups, particularly those with recent immigration histories. This is particularly true among Mexican migrant farmworkers in the United States, who, because of their highly mobile existence, may have difficulty accessing screening services for certain health conditions (Poss, 2000). In the US population 25% of all tuberculosis (TB) cases among are Latinos; however, they account for 13% of the total population. The increased incidence of TB among Latinos has been attributed to the increasing number of Latino immigrants from the developing world, where TB is endemic (Ailinger et al., 2004). Because of the rise in tuberculosis, syphilis, and AIDS in Hispanic migrant workers, nurses should assess for these diseases and urge appropriate follow-up care. Nurses should be aware that the initial use of folk remedies can allow these diseases to spread and cause the delay of medical treatment.

Treatment of chemical dependency among Mexican Americans is a major challenge because of three central factors that inhibit treatment: integration of alcohol consumption within the Hispanic culture, the psychology of the Hispanic culture, and the family dynamics of the traditional Hispanic. Markides and Coreil (1998) use the term "fiesta drinking," referring to the consumption of large amounts of alcohol on special occasions. Drinking behavior is so ingrained in the Mexican culture that social functions ranging from baptisms to funerals generally include alcoholic beverages (Arrendondo, Weddige, Justice, & Fitz, 1987). Drinking occurs among Mexican Americans when the individual is coping with negative feelings, as well as when the individual is experiencing positive feelings. Although drinking and driving has substantially declined in the United States in the past two decades, this trend has not been seen among Hispanic drivers. Higher rates of driving while impaired, arrests, and alcohol-related crashes are particularly noted among Mexican Americans. In a study by Ferguson, Burns, Fiorentino, Williams,

and Garcia (2002), Mexican Americans vastly overestimated the number of drinks that would make them unsafe drivers (8 to 10 drinks). The nurse must remember that the fatalistic element of Hispanic psychology helps to incorporate and at the same time augment drinking problems among Mexican Americans. When a drinking problem is described by a Mexican American in an intake interview, it may be followed by the client saying, "That's life" or "This is our cross to bear." For the most part, this external locus of control serves to block the identified alcoholic, and the family as well, from assuming a more active role in the recovery process.

Rather than seeking outside professional help for the treatment of alcohol abuse, Mexican Americans may collaborate with the *curandero* in treating the alcoholism or may try self-medication. The nurse must assess whether the client who is a substance abuser is using a *curandero* or is self-medicating with other drugs because these factors may further intensify the problem. The nurse must also assess carefully whether a client with a drug-abuse problem would be best suited for individual, group, or family therapy. This determination can be made only after a thorough intake interview. Because the Mexican American family is built on a system of family orientation, it is believed that perhaps the best mode of treatment for Mexican Americans is family therapy. The initial purpose of family therapy for Mexican American substance abusers should be to evaluate the family's influence on the client's chemical dependency problems. The nurse should incorporate both the nuclear and the extended family in the evaluation. Preventive interventions among youths, adults, and families may offer the best hope of preventing first use or progression of drug dependence and secondary substance disorders among individuals with signs of mood and anxiety disorders. Additionally, more school- and community-based programs are needed in English and Spanish that can reach the Mexican American population with effective intervention strategies, limit alcohol access to adolescents, and reduce social marketing to this population. Treatment interventions that communicate knowledge and promote skills to assist immigrant parents to counteract the health risks trends of acculturation on substance use.

To plan safe, effective, individualized nursing care for members of the Mexican American community that is appropriate and congruent with their lifestyles and cultural beliefs, nurses must know and understand the cultural patterns and belief systems of this ethnic group (Murillo-Rohde, 1977). Conway and Carmona (1990) caution nurses that Mexican American beliefs in traditional health and home remedies are often perceived by Mexican Americans as a wealth of options that decreases their need for using the modern health care system.

Mexican American farmworkers face many health problems because of their alienation, poverty, and ongoing seasonal mobility. O'Brien (1983) relates that if they have worked as migrants since childhood, they frequently experience debilitating back pain and arthritis. In addition to other chronic health problems, short-term illnesses present problems (such as hemorrhaging after childbirth or abortion, dental problems), and nutritional illnesses occur because of inadequate food supplies. Nurses should be aware of local migrant programs that can assist in meeting their various health needs.

Kerr and Ritchey (1990) suggest that Mexican American migrant farm workers have the following potential needs for improved health: improved access to health resources, improved knowledge of health-promoting behaviors, and fewer language barriers. Taking portable equipment (such as cholesterol screening equipment) to the migrant camps would improve accessibility. Health-promoting behaviors could be improved by assessment of the migrants for their current knowledge and healthful practices. Language barriers could be decreased if English classes were taught and if nutritional labeling in Spanish were instituted.

It is important for the nurse to remember that Mexican Americans differ from other cultural groups in their expression of symptoms and in how the ill person is perceived and treated by others. For example, in the Mexican American culture, epilepsy carries far less social stigma than in other ethnic and cultural groups.

SUMMARY

To provide appropriate health care for the Mexican American population, it is crucial for nurses to be aware of the stereotypes that commonly are held in viewing minority groups. This is especially true for Mexican Americans, who are often stereotyped as "Hispanic" despite the fact that there are many Hispanic subgroups with their own demographic characteristics and beliefs (Hahn, 1995). It is critical for the culturally sensitive nurse to evaluate each client as a unique individual despite the client's cultural group. It is also essential to consider that Mexican Americans are one of the major ethnic groups in the United States in which health disparities exist and contribute to chronic health conditions and death (Esperat, Feng, Owen, & Green, 2005).

Mexican American immigrants present many special needs and potential problems in adjustment. There are many males who have left their families in Mexico and face the difficulty of separation. Some families are reunited after separation but experience difficulty in readjusting as a family and in negotiating the U.S. educational system, health care system, and other aspects of the new American culture. The Mexican American community in the United States is rich in cultural beliefs and values. This group has adhered to traditional beliefs and values more than other minority groups have. Because this group is growing rapidly in size and now is gradually moving to areas of the country other than the Southwest, more nurses will be coming into contact with Mexican Americans through community and health care systems and need to respond to the challenges this presents. Nurses who do not understand the culture of their clients are likely to be negative and consequently less effective. By understanding the cultural diversity unique to Mexican Americans and accepting beliefs that affect health care, nurses can plan effective, culturally appropriate care.

Case Study

George García, a 23-year-old migrant farm worker, and his wife, Anita, age 20, bring their 4-month-old daughter to the emergency room of a small community hospital. They speak only broken English. They have another small child with them, as well as two older women. They are very worried about the infant, who they say has been unable to retain feedings of diluted cow's milk. Now, because of poor sucking and increased sleeping, the infant has not had anything by mouth for the past 24 hours. When asked, the parents indicate that the infant has had only three wet diapers since yesterday. The nurse notices that the infant's eyes are sunken, she is listless, and her fontanels are depressed. When asked, the parents say the infant has been sick for 3 or 4 days. One of the older women makes a pushing-up motion with her hand as she points to the infant's mouth. Further assessment reveals a rectal temperature of 103 °F. The family has not taken the temperature at all in the past 3 to 4 days. Skin turgor is good; mucous membranes are tacky. There has been no diarrhea. The infant's heart rate is 120 and regular, but thready. Respirations are 12 per minute at rest. The infant does not cry during rectal temperature taking or when touched with a cold stethoscope.

CARE PLAN*

✳ **Nursing Diagnosis: Fluid-volume deficit related to active fluid loss (vomiting and no intake for 24 hours)**

Client Outcome
1. Infant will exhibit signs of adequate hydration.

Nursing Interventions
Offer appropriate fluids as tolerated. Maintain accurate record of intake.
Weigh daily.
Assess all parameters (such as vital signs, skin character) for hydration.
Apply urine collection device if indicated.
Measure urine volume and specific gravity.

✳ **Nursing Diagnosis: Imbalanced nutrition, less than body requirements related to inability to ingest nutrients**

Client Outcome
1. Infant will consume and retain appropriate number of calories per weight per day.

Nursing Interventions
Gradually reintroduce foods as indicated, clear liquids then formula (give samples) or breast milk.
Determine family's source of water and refrigeration for milk products.
Determine if mother had been breastfeeding prior to giving diluted cow's milk.
Encourage her to resume breastfeeding.
Observe infant while feeding.
If unable to suck, consult physician for intravenous order.

(Continued)

---

*Stacie Hitt, RN, MSN, assisted in developing this case study and care plan.

CARE PLAN — CONT'D

✳ *Nursing Diagnosis: Ineffective infant feeding pattern related to neurological impairment as evidenced by listlessness*

Client Outcome	Nursing Interventions
1. Infant will progress to normal feeding pattern.	Assess infant's oral reflexes (root, gag, suck, swallow).
	Record intervals of sleep and wakefulness; observe infant's level of activity when awake.
	Provide pacifier to encourage sucking if infant must receive hyperalimentation.
	Assess ease of arousal.
	Encourage family to participate in holding, caring for, and talking with client.

✳ *Nursing Diagnosis: Communication, impaired verbally, related to cultural differences (foreign-language barriers)*

Client Outcome	Nursing Interventions
1. Family will be able to communicate basic needs and understanding of infant's condition and care	Assess language spoken best by family.
	Assess family's ability to comprehend English.
	Talk slower than normal to family.
	Use gestures or drawings for clarity.
	Be careful to touch children after looking directly at them.
	Make a conscious effort to address father when explaining care.
	Show respect to older women.
	Obtain a fluent, consistent translator.

✳ *Nursing Diagnosis: Health maintenance, ineffective related to inability to make thoughtful judgments in regards to health of infant*

Client Outcome	Nursing Interventions
1. Family will demonstrate understanding and ability to perform skills necessary for care of infant at home.	1. Determine information family needs.
	2. Determine folklore beliefs related to health care. Initiate the teaching.
	3. Determine influence older women have on family's health care beliefs.
	4. Determine equipment needed for home care.
	5. Seek social service referral.
	6. Seek assistance from agencies.

✳ STUDY QUESTIONS

1. Which family member is likely to make the decision about whether to allow the infant to be hospitalized?
2. What might the nurse do to encourage the best communication with this family?
3. What kinds of data should be obtained in the history?
4. What folk disease does the family probably believe the infant has?
5. How should the nurse explain to the family why the infant needs to be hospitalized?
6. Why would it be advantageous for the nurse to touch both the infant and the other child while relating to them?
7. How could the nurse show acceptance of the folk remedies that may have already been tried with the infant?

8. The infant is admitted to the hospital. What could be expected in terms of family visitation?

NCLEX-RN REVIEW QUESTIONS

1. Mexican Americans tend to subscribe to which of following beliefs?
   A. Smooth and dark
   B. Yin and yang and light and dark
   C. Hot and cold and wet and dry
   D. Black and white

2. Mrs. M., a Mexican-American who just gave birth, tells the nurse not to include certain foods on her meal tray because her mother told her to avoid those foods while breastfeeding. The nurse tells her that she doesn't have to avoid any foods and should eat whatever she desires. This demonstrates:

9. What teaching goals should the nurse have for this family?

   A. Cultural relativism
   B. Ethnocentrism
   C. Assimilation
   D. Subculture

3. To plan effective care, the nurse needs to understand that the family characteristic reflecting the world-view of a Hispanic American family that will most affect how decisions are made about care is:
   A. The mother as head of the household.
   B. The father as the authority figure.
   C. Giving considerable freedom to women.
   D. Using emotional communication styles.

References

Ailinger, R., Armstrong, R., Nguyen, N., & Lasus, H. (2004). Latino immigrants' knowledge of tuberculosis. *Public Health Nursing*, 21(6), 519–523.

Alexander, M., & Blank, J. (1988). Factors related to obesity in Mexican American preschool children. *Image: Journal of Nursing Scholarship*, 20(2), 79–82.

American Psychiatric Association (1994). *Diagnostic and statistical manual of mental disorders* (ed. 4) Washington, D.C.: American Psychiatric Association.

Angel, R., Angel, J., & Markides, K. (2002). Stability and change in health insurance among older Mexican Americans. *American Journal of Public Health*, 92, 1264–1271.

Anthony-Tkach, C. (1981). Care of the Mexican American patient. *Nursing and Health Care*, 24, 24–427.

Aplemis, L. (1996, Fall). Migrant health care: creativity in primary care. *Advanced Practice Nursing Quarterly*, 45–49.

Applewhite, S. (1995). Curanderismo: demystifying the health beliefs and practices of elderly Mexican Americans. *National Association of Social Workers*, 20, 247–253.

Arcia, E., & Johnson, A. (1998). When respect means to obey: Immigrant Mexican mothers' values for their children. *Journal of Child and Family Studies*, 7, 79–95.

Arrendondo, R., Weddige, R., Justice, C., & Fitz, J. (1987). Alcoholism in Mexican Americans: intervention and treatment. *Hospital and Community Psychiatry*, 38(2), 180–183.

Baer, R., Weller, S., Garcia de Alba Garcia, J., Galzer, M., Trotter, R., Pachter, L. & Kelin, R. (2003). A cross-cultural approach to the study of folk illness nervios. *Culture, Medicine and Psychiatry*, 27, 315–337.

Balcazar, H., Krull, J., & Peterson, G. (1997). Acculturation and family cohesiveness in Mexican American pregnant women: social and health implications. *Family Community Health*, 20(3), 16–31.

Balcazar, H., Krull, J., & Peterson, G. (2001). Acculturation and family functioning are related to health risks among pregnant Mexican American women. *Behavioral Medicine*, 27, 62–70.

Bastida, E., & Pagan, J. (2002, July). The impact of diabetes on adult employment and earnings of Mexican Americans: findings from a community based study. *Health Economics*, 11(5), 403–413.

Bechtel, G., Davidhizar, R., & Tiller, C. (1998). Patterns of mental health care among Mexican Americans. *Journal of Psychosocial Nursing*, 36(11), 20–27.

Beecham, M. (1995). Maria: developing a culturally sensitive treatment plan in pre-hospice south Texas. *The Hospice Journal*, 10(2), 19–34.

Beutter, M., & Davidhizar, R. (1999, September). A home care provider's challenge: caring for the Hispanic client in the home. *Journal of Practical Nursing*, 49(3), 26–36.

Black, W., Goldhahn, R., & Wiggins, C. (1987). Melanoma within a southwestern Hispanic population. *Archives of Internal Medicine*, 123(10), 1331–1334.

Bollenbacher, L., Heck, J., & Davidhizar, R. (2000, Fall). Maternity nurse's attitudes towards Mexican-American clients. *Journal of Practical Nursing*, 50(3), 14–16.

Bonder, B., Martin, L., & Miracle, A. (2002). *Culture in clinical care*. Thorofare, N.J.: Slack Inc.

Booth, C. (1996, February 26). Caribbean blizzard. *Time*, 46–48.

Borders, T., Xu, K., Rohree, J., & Warner, R. (2002, Winter). Are rural residents and Hispanics less satisfied with medical care? Evidence from the Permian Basin. *Journal of Rural Health*, 18(1), 84–92.

Borrayo, E. A., & Jenkins, S. R. (2003). Feeling frugal: socioeconomic status, acculturation, and cultural health beliefs among women of Mexican descent. *Cultural Diversity and Ethnic Minority Psychology*, 9, 197–206.

Borrell, L., Lynch, J., Neighbors, H., Burt, B., & Gillespie, B. (2002, Winter). *Ethnicity and Disease*, 12(1), 97–110.

Bray, J., Adams, G., Getz, G., & Baer, P. (2001). Development, family, and ethnic influences on adolescent alcohol usage: a growth curve approach. *Journal of Family Psychology*, 15(2), 301–314.

Burk, M. E., Wieser, P. C., & Keegan, L. (1995). Cultural beliefs and health behaviors of pregnant Mexican-American women: implications for primary care. *Advances in Nursing Science*, 17(4), 37–52.

Calvillo, E., & Flaskerud, J. (1991). Review of literature on culture and pain of adults with focus on Mexican-Americans. *Journal of Transcultural Nursing*, 2(2), 16–23.

Camarota, S. (2006). *Immigration from Mexico*. Retrieved from: http://www.cis.org/articles/2001/mexico/toc.html. Accessed on July 1, 2006.

Campo-Flores, A. (2006, April). Immigration. *Newsweek*, 28–32.

C.A.R.E.S. Needs Assessment (2003). *Community actions resource enhancement strategies community wide needs assessment in Taos County*, Taos, N.M.: Community coalition, Taos County.

Carmel, R., Johnson, C., & Weiner, J. (1987). Pernicious anemia in Latin Americans is not a disease of the elderly. *Ethnology*, 147(11), 1995–1996.

Carter-Pokras, O. (2000). Toward a healthy Hispanic population: Healthy People 2010. In *Crossing borders in Hispanic health care*. Arlington, Tex.: University of Texas at Arlington.

Caudle, P. (1993). Providing culturally sensitive health care to Hispanic patients. *Nurse Practitioner*, 18(12), 40–51.

Cervantes, R., Snyder, S., & Padilla, A. (1989). Posttraumatic stress in immigrants from Central America and Mexico. *Hospital and Community Psychiatry*, 40(6), 615–619.

Chávez, N. (1986). Mental health services delivery to minority populations: Hispanics—a perspective. In Miranda, M., & Kitano, H. (Eds.), *Mental health research and practice in minority communities*. Rockville, Md.: National Institute of Mental Health.

Chiriboga, D., Black, S., Aranda, M., & Markides, K. (2002). Stress and depressive symptoms among Mexican American elders. *The Journal of Gerontology*, 57B(6), 559–568.

Clark, M. (1970). *Health in the Mexican American culture*. Berkeley: University of California Press.

Conway, R. & Carmona, P. (1990). Cultural complexity: the hidden stressors. *Journal of Advanced Medical-Surgical Nursing*, 1(4), 65–72.

Cox, C. (1986). Physician utilization by three groups of ethnic elderly. *Medical Care*, 24(8), 667–676.

Cronin, M. (1997, July 30). Billboard campaign spotlights growing hepatitis C epidemic. *The Seattle Times*, A1.

Cummings, L. (2003). Cloth-wrapped people, trouble, and power: Pachuco culture in the greater southwest. *Journal of the Southwest*, 45.

Currier, R. (1966). The hot-cold syndrome and symbolic medicine. *Ethnology*, 5(3), 251–263.

Davidhizar, R. (2001, Spring). So your patient is Latino. *Journal of Practical Nursing*, 51(1), 18–20.

Davidhizar, R., Bechtel, G., & Giger, J. N. (1998, November/December). When your client in the surgical suite is Mexican American. *Today's Surgical Nurse*, 29–35.

Davidson, M. Effect of nurse-directed diabetes care in a minority population. *Diabetes Care*, 26(8), 2281–2287.

Derenowski, J. (1990). Coronary artery disease in Hispanics. *Cardiovascular Nursing*, 4(4), 13–21.

Dorsey, P., & Jackson, H. (1976). Cultural health traditions: the Latino-Chicano perspective. In Branch, M. F., & Paxton, P. P. (Eds.), *Providing safe nursing care for ethnic people of color* (pp. 41–80). Norwalk, Conn.: Appleton-Century-Crofts.

Duffy, M., Rossow, R., & Hernandez, M. (1996). Correlates of health-promotion activities in employed Mexican American women. *Nursing Research*, 45(1), 18–24.

Eden, S., & Aguilar, R. (2004). The Hispanic chemically dependent client: considerations for diagnosis and treatment. In Lawson, G., & Lawson, A. (Eds.). *Alcoholism and substance abuse in special populations*. Austin, Tex.: Pro-Ed.

Eid, J., & Kraemer, H. (1998, Fall). Mexican-Americans experience with diabetes. *Image: Journal of Nursing Scholarship*, 30(4), 393.

Elderkin-Thompson, V., Silver, R. & Waitzkin, H. (2001). When nurses double as interpreters: a study of Spanish-speaking patients in a US primary care setting. *Social Science & Medicine*, 52, 1343–1358.

Ericksen, A. (2006, January). Hispanic healthcare. *Healthcare traveler*, 15–21.

Esperat, MC., Feng, D., Owen, D., & Green, A. (2005). Transformation for health: a framework for health disparities research. *Nursing Outlook*, 53, 113–120.

Ethics. (1995, November). Cultures diverge on patient autonomy. *American Journal of Nursing*, 95, 10.

Falicov, C. (2005). Mexican families. In McGoldrick, M., Pearce, J. K., & Giordano, J. (Eds.), *Ethnicity and family therapy* (ed. 3). New York: Guilford Press.

Favazza, A. (1983). Cultural factors in diagnosis and treatment. In *ACP Psychiatric Update*. New York: Medical Information Systems.

Ferguson, S., Burns, M., Fiorentino, D., Williams, A., & Garcia, J. (2002, July). Drinking and driving among Mexican American and non-Hispanic white males in Long Beach, California. *Accident, Analysis and Prevention*, 34(4), 429–437.

Finch, B., Hummer, R., Kolody, B., & Vega, W. (2001). The role of discrimination and acculturative stress in the physical health of Mexican-origin adults. *Hispanic Journal of Behavioral Sciences*, 23(4), 399–429.

Fishman, J. (1967, April). Bilingualism with and without diglossia: diglossia with and without bilingualism. *Journal of Social Issues*, 23, 29–38.

Fitzpatrick, S. B., Fujii, C., & Shragg, G. P., et al. (1990). Do health care needs of indigent Mexican American, Black, and White adolescents differ? *Journal of Adolescent Health Care*, 11(3), 128–132.

Ford, J., & Graves, J. (1977). Differences between Mexican American and White children in interpersonal distance and social touching. *Perceptual and Motor Skills*, 45(3), 779–785.

Foster, G. (1978). Relationship between Spanish and Spanish American folk medicine. In Martínez, R. A. (Ed.), *Hispanic culture and health care: fact, fiction, folklore* (pp. 183–202). St. Louis: Mosby.

Friedman-Koss, D., Crespo, C., Bellantoni, M., & Anderson, R. (2002, July-August). The relationship of race/ethnicity and social class to hormone replacement therapy. *Menopause: The Journal of the North American Menopause Society*, 9(4), 264–272.

Galván, M. (1993). Hispanic Americans. *World Book Encyclopedia*, (pp. 244–259). Chicago: World Book.

Gelfand, D., Balcazar, H., Parzuchowski, J., Lenox, S. (2001). Mexicans and care for the terminally ill: family, hospice and the church. *American Journal of Hospice and Palliative Care*. 18(6): 391–396.

Gelfand, D., & Bialik-Gilad, R. (1989). Immigration reform and social work. *Social Work*, 34(1), 23–27.

Glick, J. (1999). Economic support from and to extended kin: a comparison of Mexican Americans and Mexican immigrants. *Internation Migration Review*, 33(3), 745–765.

Gonzales, J. (1997, May 26). Relearning a lost language. *Los Angeles Times*, A-1.

Gordon,R. G., Jr. (Ed.). (2005). *Ethnologue: languages of the world* (ed. 15). Dallas, Tex.: SIL International. Online version.

Gorek, B., Martin, J., White, N., Peters, D., & Hummel, F. (2002). Culturally competent care for Latino elders in long-term care settings, *Geriatric Nursing*, 23, 272–275.

Grant, B., Stinson, F., Hasin, D., Dawson, D., Chou, S., & Anderson, D. (2004). Immigration and lifetime prevalence of DSM-IV psychiatric disorders among Mexican Americans and non-Hispanic whites in the United States. *Archives of General Psychiatry*, 61, 1226–1233.

Guarnero, P. (2005). Mexican Americans. In Lipson, J., Dibble, S., & Minarik, P. (Eds.), *Culture and clinical care*. San Francisco, Calif.: UCSF Nursing Press.

Hahn, M. (1995, November). Providing health care in a culturally complex world. *Advance for Nurse Practitioners*, 3, 43–45.

Harvey, S. M., Beckman, L. J., Browner, C. H., & Sherman, C. A. (2002). Relationship power, decision making, and sexual relations: an exploratory study with couples of Mexican origin. *Journal of Sex Research*, 39, 284–291.

Harwood, A. (1971). The hot-cold theory of disease. *Journal of the American Medical Association*, 216(7), 1153–1158.

Hazuda, H. P., Stern, M. P., Gaskill, S., et al. (1983). Ethnic differences in health knowledge and behaviors related to the prevention and treatment of coronary heart disease. *American Journal of Epidemiology*, 117, 717–728.

Heilemann, M. V., Lee, K. A., & Kury, F. S. (2002, May-June). Strengths and vulnerabilities of women of Mexican descent in relation to depressive symptoms. *Nursing Research.* 51(3), 175–182.

HIV infection, syphilis, and tuberculosis screening among migrant farm workers—Florida. (1992).*Morbidity and Mortality Weekly Report*, 41, 39.

Hood, L., & Jackson, N. (1989). Caring for the patient with TB. *Advancing Clinical Care*, 4(4), 14–18.

Hough, R. (1985). Life events and stress in Mexican-American culture. *Stress and Hispanic mental health: relating research to service delivery* (pp. 110–146). Rockville, Md.: U.S. Government Printing Office.

Hudson, T. (1995). Cutting of care. *Hospitals and Health Networks*, 69(12), 36–40.

Ingham, J. (1970). On Mexican folk medicine. *American Anthropologist*, 72(1), 76–87.

Iwashyna, T., & Chang, V. (2002, June). Racial and ethnic differences in place of death: United States, 1993. *Journal of the American Geriatrics Society*, 50(6), 1113–1117.

Joiner, T., Perez, M., Wagner, K., Berenson, A., & Marquina, G. (2001). On fatalism, pessimism, and depressive symptoms among Mexican-American and other adolescents attending an obstetrics-gynecology clinic. *Behaviour Research and Therapy*, 39, 887–896.

Juckett, G., (2005). Cross-cultural medicine. *American Family Physician*, 72, 2267–2274.

Kaiser Permanente. (2001). *A provider's handbook on culturally competent care. Latino population*–(ed. 2.) Kaiser Permanente National Diversity Council and the Kaiser Permanente National Diversity Department.

Kalish, R., & Reynolds, D. (1981). *Death and ethnicity: a psychocultural study.* Los Angeles: USC.

Katerndahl, D., & Realini, J. (1998). Panic disorder in Hispanic patient. *Family Medicine*, 30(3), 210–214.

Keefe, S. (1984). Real and ideal extended familism among Mexican Americans and Anglo Americans: on the meaning of "close" family ties. *Human Organization*, 43(1), 65–70.

Keegan, L. (1996, December). Use of alternative therapies among Mexican Americans in the Texas Rio Grande Valley. *Journal of Holistic Nursing*, 14(4), 277–294.

Keenan, L., Marshall, L., & Eve, S. (2002, Winter). Extension of the behavioral model of healthcare utilization with ethnically diverse, low-income women. *Ethnicity and Disease*, 12(1), 111–123.

Keller, C., & Fleury, J. (2006). Factors related to physical activity in Hispanic women. *Journal of Cardiovascular Nursing*, 21(2), 142–145.

Kemp, C. (2005). Cultural issues in palliative care. *Seminars in Oncology Nursing*, 21(1), 44–52.

Kemper, R. (1982). The compadrazgo in urban Mexico. *Anthropological Quarterly*, 55(1), 17–30.

Kerr, M., & Richey, D. (1990). Health-promoting lifestyles of English-speaking and Spanish-speaking Mexican-American migrant farm workers. *Public Health Nursing*, 7(2), 80–87.

Khoury, R., & Thurmond, G. (1978). Ethnic differences in time perception: a comparison of Anglo and Mexican Americans. *Perceptual and Motor Skills*, 47(3), 1183–1188.

Kiev, A. (1968). *Curanderismo: Mexican American folk psychiatry.* New York: Free Press.

Kirkham, S. R. (1998). Nurses' descriptions of caring for culturally diverse clients. *Clinical Nursing Research*, 7, 125–146.

Kissam, R. (1993, May 11). *Everyday realities and effective public policy: the case of migrant and seasonal farmworkers.* Paper presented at the meeting of the National Conference on Migrant and Seasonal Farmworkers, Denver, Colorado.

Kluckhohn, F. (1976). Dominant and variant value orientations. In Brink, P. J. (Ed.), *Transcultural nursing: a book of readings* (pp. 63–81). Englewood Cliffs, N.J.: Prentice Hall.

Lagana, K., & Gonzalez-Ramirez (2003). Mexican Americans (pp. 218–235). In St. Hill, P. F., Lipson, J. G., & Meleis, A. I. (Eds.), *Caring for women cross-culturally.* Philadelphia: F.A. Davis Company.

Lantican, L., & Corona, D. (1989, November 14). A comparison of the social support networks of Filipino and Mexican American primigravidas, Paper presented at the Sigma Theta Tau International Conference, Indianapolis, Indiana.

Laosa, L. M. (1975). Bilingualism in three United States Hispanic groups: contextual use of language by children and adults and their families. *Journal of Educational Psychology*, 67(5), 617–627.

Lawson, L. (1990). Culturally sensitive support for grieving parents. *Journal of Maternal Child Nursing*, 15(2), 76–79.

Leininger, M. (2002). *Transcultural nursing: concept, theories, research and practice* (ed. 3). New York: McGraw-Hill.

Logan, B., & Semmes, C. (1986). Culture and ethnicity. In Logan, B., & Dawkins, C. (Eds.), *Family centered nursing in the community* (pp. 112–113). Reading, Mass.: Addison-Wesley.

Luyas, G. (1989, November 14). An explanatory model of diabetes by Mexican American women. Paper presented at the Sigma Theta Tau International Conference, Indianapolis, Indian.

Madsen, W., & Madsen, C. (1969). *A guide to Mexican witchcraft*. Mexico: D.F. Minutiae.

Marcos, L. R. (1988). Understanding ethnicity in psychotherapy with Hispanic patients. *American Journal of Psychoanalysis*, 48(1), 35–42.

Marcos, L. R., & Alpert, M. (1976). Strategies and risks in psychotherapy with bilingual patients: the phenomenon of language independence. *American Journal of Psychiatry*, 133, 1275–1278.

Marcos, L. R., Alpert, M., Urcuyo, L., & Kesselman, M. (1973). The effect of interview language on the evaluation of psychopathology in Spanish-American schizophrenic patients. *American Journal of Psychiatry*, 130, 549–553.

Marin, B. (2003, July). HIV prevention in the Hispanic community: sex, culture, and empowerment. *Journal of Transcultural Nursing*, 14(3), 186–192.

Marin, G., & Marin, B. (1991). *Research with Hispanic populations*. Newbury Park: Sage Publications.

Markides, K., & Coreil, J. (1998). The health of Southwestern Hispanics: an epidemiologic paradox. *Public Health Reports*, 101, 253–265.

McQuillan, G., Kruszon-Moran, D., Deforest, A., Chu, S., & Wharton, M. (2002, May 7). Serologic immunity to diphtheria and tetanus in the United States. *Annals of Internal Medicine*, 136(9), 660–666.

Meleis, A., Douglas, M., & Eribes, C., et al. (1996). Employed Mexican women as mothers and partners: valued, empowered, and overloaded. *Journal of Advanced Nursing*, 23(1), 82–90.

Miller, S., & Davidhizar, R. (2001, June). Sociocultural aspects of adherence to medical regimens for Mexican Americans. *Care Management*, 44–48.

Mines, R., Gabbard, S., & Samardick, R. (1992, September). *Harvest worker analysis*. Los Angeles: Commission on Agricultural Workers.

Mirowsky, J., & Ross, C. (1984). Mexican culture and its emotional contradictions. *Journal of Health and Social Behavior*, 25(1), 2–13.

Monrroy, L. S. A. (1983). Nursing care of Raza/Latina patients. In Orque, M. S., Block, B., & Monrroy, L. S. A. (Eds.). *Ethnic nursing care: a multicultural approach* (pp. 115–148). St. Louis: Mosby.

Moore, J., & Pachon, H. (1985). *Hispanics in the United States*. Englewood Cliffs, N.J.: Prentice Hall.

Murguia, E., Chen, Z., & Kaplan, H. (1998). A comparison of causal factors in drug use among Mexican Americans and non-Hispanic whites. *Social Science Quarterly*, 79(2), 341–360.

Murillo, N. (1978). The Mexican American family. In Hernández, C. A., Haug, M. J., & Wagner, N. N. (Eds.). *Chicanos: social and psychological perspectives* (pp. 15–25) (ed. 2). St. Louis: Mosby.

Murillo-Rohde, I. (1977). Care for all colors. *Imprint*, 24 (4), 29–32, 50.

Murphy, J., Giger, J. N., & Davidhizar, R. (1994). Strategies for designing culturally relevant client education materials. *American Society for Healthcare Education and Training of the American Hospital Association*, 8(3), 8–12.

Musto, D. (1991, July). Opium, cocaine and marijuana in American history. *Scientific American*, 40–47.

Naisbitt, J. (1984). *Megatrends*. New York: Warner Books.

National Center for Health Statistics. (2002). *Health United States, 2002 with urban and rural chartbook*. Hyattsville, Md.: National Center for Health Statistics.

Nelson, K., Norris, K., & Mangione, C. (2002, April 22). Disparities in the diagnosis and pharmacologic treatment of high serum cholesterol by race and ethnicity data from the Third National Health and Nutrition Examination Survey. *Archives of Internal Medicine*, 162 (8), 929–935.

Ness, R., & Wintrob, R. (1981). Folk healing: a description and synthesis. *American Journal of Psychiatry*, 138(11), 1477–1481.

New Mexico Department of Health (2000). *Statistics on New Mexico Health Issues*.

O'Brien, E. (1983). Reaching the migrant worker. *American Journal of Nursing*, 83a(6), 895–897.

Ortega, A., Rosencheck, R., Alegria, M., & Desai, R. (2000). Acculturation and the lifetime risk of psychiatric and substance use disorder among Hispanics. *Journal of Nervous & Mental Disorder*, 188, 728–735.

Otiniano, M., Black, S., Ray, L., Du, X., & Markides, K. (2002, Spring). Correlates of diabetic complications in Mexican-American elders, *Ethnicity and Disease*, 12(2), 252–258.

Overfield, T. (1995). *Biologic variations in health and illness: race, age, and sex differences* (ed. 2). New York: CRC Press.

Oxford dictionary of quotations. (1980). New York: Oxford University Press.

Peifer, K., Hu, T., & Vega, W. (2000). Help-seeking by persons of Mexican origin with functional impairments. *Psychiatric Services*, 51(10), 1293–1298.

Philis-Tsimikas, A., Walker, C., Rivard, L., Talavera, G., Reimann, J., Salmon, M., & Araujo, R. (2004). Improvement in diabetes care of underinsured patients enrolled in Project Dulce. *Diabetes Care*, 27(1), 110–115.

Phipps, W. (1993). The patient with pulmonary problems. In Long, B. C., Phipps, W. J., & Cassmeyer, V. (Eds.). *Medical surgical nursing: concepts and clinical practice* (ed. 3). St. Louis: Mosby.

Pope, C. (2005). Addressing limited English proficiency and disparities for Hispanic postpartum women. *Journal of Obstetric, Gynecologic, and Neonatal Nursing*, 34, 512–520.

Poss, J. (2000). Factors associated with participation by Mexican migrant farmworkers in a tuberculosis screening program. *Nursing Research*, 49(1), 20–28.

Reese, L., Balzano, S., Gallimore, R., & Goldenberg, C. (1995). The concept of education: Latino family values and American schooling. *International Journal of Educational Research*, 23(1), 57–81.

Reinert, B. (1986). The healthcare beliefs and values of Mexican Americans. *Home Healthcare Nurse*, 4(5), 23–27, 29–31.

Richardson, L. (1982). Caring through understanding: part 2. Folk medicine in the Hispanic population. *Imprint*, 29(2), 21, 72–77.

Rivera, G. K., & Wanderer, J. (1986). Curanderismo and childhood illnesses. *The Social Science Journal*, 23(3), 361–372.

Rivera, J. (1978). *The new faces of racism: the Chicano case.* Report to the Association for Humanist Sociology, New York, N.Y.

Rodolfo, A. (2007). *Occupied American: a history of Chicanos* (ed. 6). New York: Pearson Longman.

Romero, A. & Roberts, T. (2003). Stress within a bicultural context for adolescents of Mexican Descent. *Cultural Diversity and Ethnic Minority Psychology*, 9(2), 171–184.

Ross, J. (1995, October 5). Who are they, where are they and how do we talk to them? Hispanic Americans. *Hospitals and Health Networks*, 69(19), 65.

Rubel, A. (1966). *Across the tracks: Mexican Americans in a Texas city.* Austin, Tex.: University of Texas Press.

Ruiz, P. (1985). Cultural barriers to effective medical care among Hispanic-American patients. *Annual Review of Medicine*, 36, 63–71.

Saunders, L. (1954). *Cultural difference and medical care.* New York: Russell Sage Foundation.

Schillinger, D., Piette, J., Grumbach, K., Wang, F., Wilson, C., Daher, C., et al. (2003). Closing the loop: physician communication with diabetic patients who have low health literacy. *Archives of Internal Medicine*, 163, 83–90.

Sennott-Miller, L. (1994, November). Using theory to plan appropriate interventions: cancer prevention for older Hispanic and non-Hispanic White women. *Journal of Advanced Nursing*, 20(5), 809–814.

Serrano, B. (1997, June 1). A lesson in inequality: districts in wealthy areas, where school levies are common, often have better schools. *The Seattle Times*, A-1.

Skaff, M., Mullan, J., Fisher, L., & Chesla, C. (2003). A contextual model of control beliefs, behavior and health: Latinos and European Americans with Type 2 diabetes. *Psychology & Health*, 18(3), 295–312.

Smith, R. (2002). Barnard study links gender, academic success among Mexican-Americans. *Black Issues in Higher Education*, 19(8), 16.

Sobralske, M., & Katz, J. (2005). Culturally competent care of patients with acute chest pain. *Journal of the American Academy of Nurse Practitioners*, 173, 42–349.

Spector, R. (2004). *Cultural diversity in health and illness*, (ed. 6) Englewood Cliffs, N.J.: Prentice Hall Health.

Statistical abstracts of the United States. (1988). Washington, D.C.: U.S. Department of Commerce, Bureau of the Census.

Stern, M. P., Bradshaw, B., & Eifler, C. W., et al. (1987). Secular decline in death rates due to ischemic heart disease in Mexican Americans and non-Hispanic Whites in Texas, 1970–1980. *Circulation*, 76(6), 1245–1250.

Stewart, S., & Silverstein, M. (2002, June). Racial and ethnic disparity in blood pressure and cholesterol measurement. *Journal of General Internal Medicine*, 17(6), 405–411.

Street, R. (2002). Gender differences in health care provider–patient communication: are they due to style, stereotypes or accommodation? *Patient Education and Counseling*, 48, 201–208.

Sugihara, Y., & Warner, J. (2002). Dominance and domestic abuse among Mexican Americans: Gender differences in the etiology of violence in intimate relationships. *Journal of Family Violence*, 17(4), 315–330.

Tajalli, I. Q. (1984). *Selected cultural, organizational, economic factors related to prenatal care utilization by middle-income Hispanic Women.* University of Illinois at Urbana Champaign. Ann Arbor, Mich.: U.M. I. Dissertation Service.

Time almanac with information please. (2006). Boston: Information Please, Inc.

U.S. Department of Commerce, Bureau of the Census. (1993, November). *We the Americans . . . Hispanic people*, Washington, D.C.: U.S. Government Printing Office.

U.S. Department of Commerce, Bureau of the Census. (2000). *Hispanic Americans: census brief 2000.* Hyattsville, Md.: U.S. Government Printing Office.

U.S. Department of Commerce, Bureau of the Census. (2002). *Population profiles by age, sex, race, and Hispanic origin*, Summary File 3, Hyattsville, Md.: U.S. Government Printing Office.

U.S. Department of Commerce, Bureau of the Census. (2003). *Population profiles*, Summary File 4, 2000. Hyattsville, Md.: U.S. Government Printing Office.

Váldez, A. (1980). *Ethnic maintenance among Mexicans and Puerto Ricans.* Report to Southwestern Sociological Association, Waco, Texas.

Valente, S. (2004). End of life and ethnicity. *Journal for Nurses in Staff Development.* 20(6), 285–293.

Valenzuela, A. (1999). Gender roles and settlement activities among children and their immigrant families. *The American Behavioral Scientist.* 42(4), 720–742.

Vásquez, S. (1997, May 20). Diabetes alert: high-fat, genetics make Hispanics prone to the disease. *Rocky Mountain News*, 3d.

Vega, W., & Lopez, S. (2001). Priority issues in Latino mental health research. *Mental Health Service Research*, 3, 189–200.

Vega, W., Scribney, W., & Achara-Abrahams, L. (2003). Co-occurring alcohol, drug, and other psychiatric disorders among Mexican-origin people in the United States. *American Journal of Public Health*, 93(7), 1057–1064.

Villarruel, A. (2000). The challenge of linguistic competence. *Crossing borders in Hispanic health care.* Arlington, Tex.: The University of Texas at Arlington.

Villarruel, A., & Leininger, M. (2004). Culture care of Mexican Americans. In Leininger, M. (Ed.), *Transcultural nursing* (ed. 3). New York: McGraw-Hill.

Villarruel, A., & Denyes, M. (1997). Testing Orem's theory with Mexican American's. *Image: Journal of Nursing Scholarship*, 29(3), 283–288.

Wanderer, J., & Rivera, G. (1986). Black magic beliefs and white magic practice: the common structures of intimacy, tradition and power. *The Social Science Journal*, 23(4), 419–430.

Weaver, T. (1970). Use of hypothetical situations in a study of Spanish-American illness referral systems. *Human Organisms*, 29, 140.

Weclew, R. (1975). The nature, prevalence, and level of awareness of "curanderismo" and some of its implications for community mental health. *Community Mental Health Journal*, 11(2), 145–154.

Wilson, H., & Kneisl, C. (1996). *Psychiatric nursing*, (ed. 5) Menlo Park, Calif.: Addison-Wesley.

White, J., Linhart, J., & Medley, L. (1996, September). Culture, diet and the maternity. *Advance for Nurse Practitioners*, 4, 26–28.

Woodbury, R. (2000, May 1). A class for strangers in a strange land. *Time*, 8.

World almanac. (2006). New York: World Almanac Books.

Zoucha, R.D (1998). The experiences of Mexican Americans receiving professional nursing care: an ethnographic study. *Journal of Transcultural Nursing*, 9, 34–44.

Zoucha, R., & Purnell, L. D. (2003). People of Mexican Heritage. In Purnell, L. D., & Paulanka, B. J. (Eds.), *Transcultural Health Care* (pp. 264–278). Philadelphia: F.A. Davis Company.

CHAPTER 10 Navajos

Catherine E. Hanley

Behavioral Objectives

After reading this chapter, the nurse will be able to:

1. Identify ways in which the Navajo culture influences Navajo individuals and health-seeking behaviors.
2. Recognize physical and biological variances that exist in and across Navajo groups to provide culturally appropriate care.
3. Develop a sensitivity and understanding for communication differences as evidenced within and across Navajo groups to avoid stereotyping and to provide culturally appropriate nursing care.
4. Develop a sensitivity and understanding for psychological phenomena that influence the functioning of a Navajo when nursing care is being provided.
5. Describe the influence of traditional Navajo folk medicine and the relationship to health-seeking behaviors.

OVERVIEW OF THE NAVAJOS

Archeological evidence places Navajos in the Gobernador Canyon area of northwestern New Mexico by the late 1400s or early 1500s. By the early 1600s, some Navajos had migrated as far as the Black Mesa country of northern Arizona (Iverson, 1990). The first written historical observations of the Navajos have been attributed to Arate Salmerón (1626) and Father Benavides (1630).

According to Iverson (1990), the various Pueblo peoples exerted a tremendous influence on the evolution of the Navajo culture in the new region. There is historical evidence indicating that the Navajos and Pueblos were at times foes. However, Brugge (1968) suggested a number of instances when Navajo and Pueblo villages allied themselves against the Spanish and other outside groups. Young (1961) concluded that the Navajos and the Pueblos existed together in a more peaceful than hostile relationship. Regardless of whether the Pueblos and the Navajos lived peacefully, the Pueblos probably did influence change in the Navajo lifestyle in some critical ways. For example, the Navajos have a matrilineal clan system that still exists today and dictates that a Navajo inherits the clan and thus the lineage from the mother (Iverson, 1990). The implication is that people from the same clan are considered relatives with varying responsibilities to one another.

For the western Pueblos the clan traditions were strong, and it is probable that they influenced the Navajos in the direction of clan formation (Iverson, 1990). In addition, the Pueblo people were very sedentary and had agricultural ways that undoubtedly also had some effect on the Navajos. As a consequence of these influences, the Navajos gradually adopted a way of life that was significantly less nomadic, with less emphasis on hunting than that of other Apachean groups. Seemingly, the Navajos learned trades such as weaving, pottery making, silversmithing, and agriculture from the Pueblo people en route to the Southwest. According to Iverson (1990), the Navajos credit "Spiderwoman" with their instruction in weaving. Differences existed in that Pueblo men traditionally were weavers, whereas Navajo men very rarely became weavers.

During the sixteenth, seventeenth, and eighteenth centuries, the Navajo people underwent tremendous expansion, cultural acquisition, and social change. According to Young (1961), the Navajos have always had a great capacity to absorb and elaborate on cultural traits adopted from other people. For example, the Pueblo weaving tradition is responsible for producing the Navajo blanket, which is unmistakably the product of the *Diné* (the Navajo word for "people"). The language, though distinctively Navajo (from the entirely different Athapaskan family of languages), was learned by other Indians; however, few Navajos attempted to master a foreign tongue (Young, 1961). The Navajo people lived freely on the land of their forefathers, located between the four sacred mountains: Mount Blanca (Colorado) to the East, Mount Taylor (New Mexico) to the South, San Francisco Peak (Arizona) to the West, and Mount Hesperus (Colorado) to the North. Four directional colors were associated with the four sacred mountains: white with Mount Blanca, blue with Mount Taylor, yellow with San Francisco Peak, and black with Mount Hesperus. To understand the history of the Navajo people, it is important to understand the significance of the four sacred mountains, which historically were considered the cardinal boundary peaks surrounding the Navajo country. Even today, Navajo people believe that the four sacred mountains were gifts from the "Holy People" (*diyín dine'é*, or *haashch'ééh dine'é*); therefore, traditions, prayers, songs, and sacred trust are embodied in these mountains (Navajo Health Systems Agency, 1985).

Perhaps one of the most significant periods of Navajo history occurred during 1864, when more than 9000 Navajo people were captured in what is now Arizona and forced to journey to Fort Sumner on the Bosque Redondo Reservation in what is now New Mexico. During this long journey (known in Navajo history as the "long walk") and internment at Fort Sumner, more than 2000 Navajo men, women, and children died of respiratory tract diseases, gastrointestinal disorders, and exhaustion.

During May 1868, the fourth year of their forced internment, the Navajos' elected leader, Chief Barboncito, said to a Washington delegation appointed by President Andrew Johnson, "I hope to God you will not ask me to go to any other country except my own." In speaking these words, Chief Barboncito expressed the feelings, beliefs, traditions, and desires of the Navajo people. On May 28, 1868, the United States of America and the Navajo tribe entered into a treaty that was ratified on August 12, 1868, by President Andrew Johnson (Treaty, 1973).

After the signing of the 1868 treaty, the Navajos moved progressively in the direction of the Four Sacred Mountains. Gradual as it might have seemed, the call from the Four Sacred Mountains for the return to Navajo ways reflected the futuristic response of self-determination, self-governance, and self-actualization (Hanley, 1987). Although the treaty signed at Fort Sumner was not the first treaty but the eighth treaty made between the Navajo people and the United States in 22 years, it was historically significant because it led to their release from Fort Sumner and to the establishment of their first reservation at Fort Defiance, Arizona. (At that time Arizona was a separate territory; it became the forty-eighth state in 1912.) After the Navajo people were released from their internment at Fort Sumner, they began to develop a diversified economy. For the Navajo, raising livestock was an important element of the economy but not the only element. From early and later historical accounts, it appears that the Navajos have always been perceived as great farmers. A reemerging question about the Navajo people concerns why they traditionally needed such a diverse economy; another reemerging question concerns why livestock took on a more essential role within the Navajo economy. The answers to these questions seemingly overlap and are mutually reinforcing: for the Navajo people, a diversified economy made more thorough and efficient use of the different opportunities provided by various soils, altitudes, and vegetations.

Three different climatic zones exist in the area in which the Navajo people live. The humid, or mountain, zones account for roughly 8% of the total Navajo area; the mesas and high plains, with their intermediate steppe climate, account for roughly 37% of the Navajo area; and the comparatively warm desert regions account for roughly 55% of the Navajo area. Winter temperatures in these regions range from an average minimum of 4° to 15° F in the humid zone, to 10° to 25° F in the steppe zone, to 11° to 30° F in the desert zone. Summer temperatures in these regions range from an average maximum of 70° to 80° F in the humid zone, to 80° to 88° F in the steppe zone, to 100° F or higher in the desert. The average rainfall in all three areas is concentrated in the late summer period, which extends from July to September, with great variation in amount within each zone. The desert and humid zones each receive an additional 41% of precipitation in the form of winter snow.

The soils in the Navajo region may be classified as excellent, good, or fair in terms of runoff, grass-producing ability, and erosion. Only about a third of the area is considered excellent or good in terms of soil productivity, and about 15% of the soil is unproductive, with little vegetation cover. The vegetation includes grassland, meadows, sagebrush, browse (shrub), and woodland (which is inaccessible and barren in some places). More Navajo land is covered with coniferous timber than with sagebrush (Young, 1961).

It was believed that the conflicts between the Navajos and their neighbors were contributing factors to their economic diversification. For example, historical accounts suggest that as raiding by and against the Navajo people grew in intensity, it consequently complicated agricultural pursuits and led to an increased need for mobility. In addition, the steady growth of the Navajo population figured greatly in the economic diversification: as the Navajo tribe grew in number, so did the quantity of livestock. Two principal periods of growth occurred in the Navajo tribe. The first period came in the last years of the eighteenth century and in the early years of the nineteenth century, before the White American campaign against the Navajos. The second principal period of growth followed the Navajo return from Bosque Redondo. It was during the first period of expansion that livestock was established as an economically important commodity (Brugge, 1964).

The spectacular growth of the Navajo population began during the post–Fort Sumner era. In 1870 the Navajo population numbered 15,000 (Boyce, 1942). By 1900 the Navajo population had grown to 21,000, and by 1935 the population had grown to 35,500. The population has grown steadily ever since. In 1981 there were approximately 151,000 Navajo Indians, who resided primarily in rural areas on or near the 27,000-square-mile reservation that is located in Arizona, New Mexico, Colorado, and Utah (U.S. Department of Commerce, Bureau of the Census, 2002). By 1986 the Navajo population had grown to 171,097, making the Navajo tribe the largest Indian tribe in the continental United States. Today, however, the Navajo are the second largest tribe in the United States, with a population of 269,202 (U.S. Department of Commerce, Bureau of the Census, 2002), with the first being Cherokees at about 281,069. These new figures represent an increase of 516,772 or 26% between 1990 and 2000 for the American Indian population alone (not in conjunction with Alaska Natives) (U.S. Department of Commerce, Bureau of the Census, 2002). If the American Indian population was used in conjunction with other races, for example, Alaska Natives, the 2000 census data suggest that there was an increase in that population by as many as 2.2 million people or 110% (U.S. Department of Commerce, Bureau of the Census, 2002).

Today, there are approximately 500 Indian tribes (2,423,457 people) residing in 26 states, with most American Indians residing in the western part of the United States as a consequence of the forced western migration of the tribes (U.S. Department of Commerce, Bureau of the Census, 2002). In fact, according to the Census Bureau, in 2000, 43% of American Indians reported living in the West, 31% lived in the South, 17% lived in the Midwest, and 9% lived in the Northeast (U.S. Department of Commerce, Bureau of the Census, 2000).

It should be noted that there is a clear distinction between American Indian (AI) and the Alaska Natives (AN). The term *Native American* is intended to imply tribes residing in the continental United States (in contrast to Native Canadians). Today, although many American Indians remain on reservations and in rural areas, an equal number reside in cities, especially in Oklahoma, California, New Mexico, and Alaska (Henderson & Primeaux, 1981; U.S. Department of Commerce, Bureau of the Census, 2002).

In 2000, the median family income for the American Indians was $26,039, as compared with $33,956 for the U.S. White population (U.S. Department of Commerce, Bureau of the Census, 2002). American Indian women fared worse than their White American counterparts, with a median income of $22,834 compared with $27,878, respectively. American Indian men barely made more than White women and made considerably less than their White American counterparts, with a median income of $28,919, compared with $39,235, respectively (U.S. Department of Commerce, Bureau of the Census, 2002). The Navajo tribe derives revenue from oil, coal, uranium, and federal grants and contracts. Nevertheless, high unemployment rates continue to be a major problem among the Navajos (Heraldson, 1988).

COMMUNICATION

Dialect and Style

The Navajo language is classified as Athapaskan because historically it has been shown to be derived from the languages used by the people of Lake Athabasca in northwestern Canada. The Navajo language is also similar to the languages spoken by some peoples living in Alaska, some on the northern coast of the Pacific Ocean, and some in northern California (such as the Hupas). In addition, Navajo and the 12 groups of Apache dialects form a dialect continuum of one single language. These separate groups speaking a language similar to the Navajo language are referred to as Athapaskans.

The language of the Navajo people involves tonal speech in which pitch is of great importance. Every vowel and consonant is fully sounded, regardless of how many times they are doubled or tripled in the same word. Vowels are often interchanged, creating several variations and meanings of the same word.

The Navajo language is believed to reflect a concept of the universe that is constantly in motion. In the Navajo language, position is defined as a withdrawal from motion. For example, a person speaking

English says "on," whereas a Navajo person says something directly opposite in meaning for the word on: the Navajo speaker says "at rest." Whereas an English speaker says, "I dressed" or "One dresses," the Navajo speaker says, "I moved into my clothes" or "One moves into clothes." The language directly parallels mythological thought in that not only is the language in motion, but so too are cultural and spiritual heroes (Sobralske, 1985).

When Navajo people speak, most of the sentences contain the concept *good*. For some Navajo people, the concept good may be defined as a favorable or desirable quality that promotes prosperity and happiness. Therefore the word *good* is synonymous with other words, such as *agreeable, attractive*, or *beautiful* (*nizhóni*). The concept of goodness is directly related to the ideology of health and is even found in the Blessingway healing ceremony. This ceremony is viewed by the Navajos as a "good" event because it promotes everlasting harmony or perfection.

Even today the majority of Navajo people still speak the native language. Although many Navajo Indians are fluent in both the Navajo language and the English language, there are also many who do not speak English and therefore require the assistance of a Navajo interpreter when seeking or receiving health care. The Navajo language does not always have an equivalent single word for an English word; instead, the language uses a description of all occurrences affecting what is being said.

Until recently the Navajo language was unwritten. In World War II, a special branch of the U.S. Marine Corps was developed for Navajos who served as Navajo code talkers. It has been estimated that this highly esteemed group saved millions of lives because the enemy was unable to understand the Navajo language or infiltrate its code.

Touch

Instead of shaking hands on meeting another person, as it is practiced in the dominant U.S. culture, Navajos extend a hand and lightly touch the hand of the person they are greeting. Other examples of the use of touch in the Navajo culture include the tradition of massaging a newborn baby as a bonding experience between mother and baby and the tradition of giving a small gift and preparing a small feast for the family when the baby laughs for the first time because this token of esteem touches the heart of all the people around the baby. Another example is the taboo against touching a dead person or an animal killed by lightning, which is extended to touching articles associated with the deceased individual or animal. This taboo is not extended to animals whose death resulted from the other natural causes.

Use of Silence and the Importance of Names

On initially meeting strangers, Navajo people may appear silent and reserved. Once the Navajo individual becomes familiar with the other person, warm behavior is usually demonstrated. In addition, when introducing themselves by name, Navajos give honor to ancestors by stating the clan and the location of the home.

Kinesics

Kinesics practiced within the Navajo culture includes the avoidance of eye contact. In dominant cultures in the United States, eye contact is considered important and if not present may cause suspicion. However, the opposite is true in the Navajo culture, where eye contact is considered a sign of disrespect.

In earlier days, Navajo people frowned on pointing anything at another person because pointing was considered insulting. Some Navajos believed that an object being passed to another person should be held upright so that an end would not point at the other person.

Language Lateralization

In a study of language lateralization in Navajo reservation children, one group of Navajo children was tested by a researcher who spoke only Navajo (McKeever, Hunt, Wells, & Yazzie, 1989). Another group of Navajo and White children was tested by a researcher who spoke only English. Findings from the study indicate that there appeared to be a strong right-ear advantage for the White children tested by the English-speaking researcher. A similar right-ear advantage was found in the Navajo children when they were tested by the Navajo-speaking researcher, whereas the Navajo children tested by the English-speaking researcher revealed minimal, nonsignificant right-ear advantage. Most of the previous research has suggested that Navajos and other Native Americans have an absence of right-ear advantage. The results of this study were found to be inconsistent with the view that Navajos and other Native Americans are right-brain-hemisphere dominant and thus have a left-ear advantage as a function of the appositional mode of language and thought (McKeever, Hunt, Wells, & Yazzie, 1989).

Implications for Nursing Care

Because the Navajo language does not always have one single word that is similar to one English word in meaning, to do a nursing assessment and develop a nursing diagnosis, goals, and interventions, the nurse must remember that what is being said must be interpreted by approximation. Because some Navajo people do not speak English, it may be necessary to provide a person who is fluent in the Navajo language. When a Navajo interpreter is utilized, this person must be knowledgeable about medical terminology as well as the cultural aspects of the Navajo lifestyle.

It is also important to remember that the first encounter is not always made to deal with official matters. It is meant to provide an opportunity for the nurse to become acquainted with the family and vice versa. Future rapport with the family is based on this consideration.

Navajo individuals who enter the profession of nursing may experience a cultural shock when care must be provided for a dying patient because of the taboo against touching a dead or dying person and items associated with death. Because of the taboos associated with death, some Navajo nurses may have a healing ceremony performed after contact with a dead person.

SPACE

Time and space are bound to each other; therefore, it must be remembered that the elimination of time alters spatial concepts (Hall, 1990). For some Navajo people there is no such thing as imaginary space. Space is so real a concept that it may not be located in any dimension other than real space. For example, space may not be located in the realm of thought; there is no abstract space. For the Navajo Indian, a space such as that found in a room or a house is the same as a small universe (Hall, 1990).

For the Navajo people, personal living space, or that of the traditional Navajo dwelling (*hooghan*, "*hogan*"), is surrounded with many traditions and superstitions or taboos. The *hogan* is a round, open room with distinct functional areas. Many Navajo people believe that shared space provides a spiritual security and a sense of trust. Sheepskins, with the head facing the fire, are used for sleeping. A wood-burning stove, situated center front with the vent pipe extending through the ceiling, provides a means of cooking food. Taboos associated with death in a *hogan* include the need to seal the entry, warning other Navajos to stay away, and frequently the need to abandon or burn the *hogan* when a death has occurred. Another event that renders a *hogan* unusable is lightning striking in proximity; even wood from such a *hogan* is never used for any purpose by a Navajo, except for a Navajo medicine man in relation to ceremonies. Before a new *hogan* is occupied, it is usually blessed by a hired Navajo medicine man, who either strews pollen along the cardinal points or performs a formal ceremony. The *hogan* is so important to the Navajo culture that all Navajo ceremonies are performed in it. Although the *hogan* is often crowded with members of both nuclear and extended families, the Navajo need for extension of space is demonstrated by the fact that miles often separate one *hogan* from another or one camp from another.

Implications for Nursing Care

Because personal space is so important and has no imaginary boundaries, it is important for the nurse to remember that some Navajo clients may have difficulty adapting to situations that place them in spaces that are not familiar. It is important for the nurse to familiarize the client with the space provided during hospitalization and when personal space is limited during health care administration. The nurse should be sensitive to the fact that a hospital might be unfamiliar to some Navajo people, with new things and experiences, such as different types of food, different buildings and equipment, different varieties of uniforms, different types of health professionals and support staff, and different types of communication. This situation is particularly true when Navajo clients are hospitalized off the reservation, where Navajo interpreters are unavailable, or when great distances from their home prevent visitation from their extended family.

The nurse may encounter other health concerns and problems related to life in the cramped environment of a *hogan*, such as infectious diseases from the lack of indoor plumbing and water supply and burns related to the indoor stoves. Lack of food and food storage may contribute to nutritional deficiencies. In addition, the distance between *hogans* has a public health implication because isolation from the mainstream creates barriers in the delivery of health care. One main barrier is the lack of public transportation. Non–Navajo-speaking public health nurses cope with this barrier with the assistance of Navajo interpreters traveling as a team in a four-wheel-drive vehicle over treacherous terrain and unpaved roads.

SOCIAL ORGANIZATION

Family

The Navajo culture is extremely family oriented, but the term *family* has a much broader meaning than just referring to the nuclear family of father, mother, and children. The biological family is the center of social organization and includes all members of the extended family. The Navajo people are traditionally a matriarchal society, which means that when a couple marry, the husband makes his home with his wife's relatives, and his family becomes one of several units that live in a group of adjacent hogans or other types of dwellings.

There is no set number or type of relatives limiting the extended family, and their focus is to help one another grow, to collaborate on resources that will provide an adequate livelihood, and to participate in daily life occurrences. Assistance with ceremonies, particularly those associated with birth, death, marriage, or sickness, is shared and has great importance. Usually a male family member looked on as having the greatest amount of prestige will rise as leader for the extended family and provide necessary direction. However, in settling issues, all sides are listened to and the entire group determines the outcome.

The family is considered so important in the Navajo culture that to be without relatives is to be really poor; children learn from infancy that the family and the tribe are of paramount importance. In the Navajo culture, being available for a family member is extremely important, and it is common practice for many members of the extended family to come to the hospital and stay with the client or in proximity to the client until discharge. This situation is particularly true of mothers who have a child in the pediatric unit. All efforts should be made to provide overnight accommodations for the mother in the same room with the child if this is not medically contraindicated.

Family Roles and Structure

In the traditional nuclear family, the mother is responsible for the domestic duties associated with the home. The father, on the other hand, is responsible for any outside work necessary to maintain the family and the home. Children are responsible for assisting both parents (Roessel, 1981). Within Navajo families, children are viewed as assets, not liabilities. Navajo Indian children are rarely told they cannot do something but instead are frequently told of the consequences of doing a particular thing (Primeaux, 1977). Children are encouraged by their parents and members of the extended family to live and learn by their decisions. Because the Navajo traditions are passed down by the elderly, Navajo children are taught to respect tradition and to honor wisdom (Primeaux, 1977).

Marriage

Even today, some Navajo marriages are still arranged. In any case, marriage and the family are considered the foundation of Navajo life. In Navajo society, women are expected not to excel or achieve more success than their husbands (Roessel, 1981). This is even the case among some Navajo nurses, who may be cautious about excelling in the profession at the risk of their marriage. In earlier times, divorce among traditional Navajos occurred when the wife placed her husband's belongings outside the *hogan* (Roessel, 1981).

Traditional Navajo Dress

The dress of traditional Navajo women has been adapted from the dress of the Spaniards encountered during the internment of the Navajo people at Fort Sumner. The dress usually consists of long, gathered calico skirts and brightly colored velveteen blouses. Because of the harsh terrain and great amount of walking done by Navajo women to get from one place to the other, sneakers and socks are the primary type of footwear.

Traditional Navajo men have adapted the western type of garb, which includes jeans, cotton western shirts, boots, and wide-brimmed hats. Both men and women commonly carry woolen blankets and wear large amounts of turquoise, coral, and silver jewelry as well as ornate buttons and belts. Also, both men and women traditionally wear their long hair tied in a knot behind their head; the knot is covered with rows of white woolen yarn.

Religion

Historically the Navajo people have been guided by sacred myths and legends that describe the tribe's evolution from inception to the present. Supernatural beings portrayed in these stories symbolize the Navajo culture, in which religion and healing practices are blended. Values and beliefs intrinsic to their culture and religion form the Navajo day-to-day living experiences.

Implications for Nursing Care

It is important for the nurse to remember that both the nuclear family and the extended family are of paramount importance to the Navajo client. Because Navajo people believe that family members are responsible for each other, it is not uncommon for many relatives to come to the hospital to care for the Navajo client. Restrictive hospital rules that allow only two visitors at a time or only immediate relatives have no meaning for some Navajo people. The nurse and other members of the health care team should be sensitive to the reality that *hogans* and camps are at times located a great distance from one another and that visiting a sick relative in the hospital may necessitate travel for many miles, with other family sacrifices needed to obtain funding for this journey. Referral to appropriate available resources will have a positive influence on family-centered care. The presence of family members also provides an ideal opportunity for their inclusion in discharge-planning sessions. Flexibility in scheduling follow-up clinic appointments should also be considered.

Because the Indian kinship or clan system is unfamiliar to most nurses in the United States, it is important for the nurse to develop a sensitivity to and an understanding of the significance of Indian clanships. For example, not only does one inherit lineage from one's mother but also it is not uncommon for a Navajo child to have several sets of grandparents, uncles, cousins, brothers, and sisters. Among the Navajo people first cousins may be treated as brothers and sisters, and great aunts and uncles as grandparents. The whole system of clanship may prove to be thoroughly confusing to the nurse because several sets of grandparents, brothers, sisters, uncles, and aunts may show up at the hospital, all claiming close relationship to the client.

TIME

The cultural interpretation of time has a temporal focus that views human life as existing in a three-point range that includes past, present, and future (Kluckhohn & Strodtbeck, 1973). Navajo Indians are viewed as being primarily present-time oriented. However, it should be noted that some Navajo Indians are perceived as being both past- and present-time oriented. The common orientation regarding the man–nature theme is a mixed perception that espouses that man is subjugated to nature and at the same time is suggestive that man should learn to live in harmony with nature. In a classic study by Kluckhohn and Strodtbeck

(1973), it was noted that the present-time orientation was the preferred mode of time orientation for the population of Rimrock Navajos sampled. The findings of the study also suggested that past-time orientation was somewhat more preferable than future-time orientation but that the difference in preference was not statistically significant. In the study it was also noted that although some of the respondents preferred to be perceived as being subjugated to nature, the one significant preference was a perception of being in harmony with nature.

Implications for Nursing Care

Most people in the dominant culture in the United States are regulated by clocks and are therefore very time conscious. Future-oriented individuals may have a great deal of difficulty with some Navajo people because of their present-time orientation. It is important for the nurse to remember that because Navajo Indians are perceived as being present-time oriented, time is viewed as being on a continuum, with no beginning and no end (Primeaux, 1977). In some Navajo homes there are no clocks because Navajo time is casual, present-time oriented, and relative to present needs that must be accomplished in a present-time frame. Because certain tasks are associated with present needs, it may be difficult for the nurse to counsel and advise a Navajo client about crucial future events, such as taking medications. The present-time orientation of a Navajo client may cause this person to eat two meals today, four meals tomorrow, no meals the next day, and three meals the day after. This becomes an important nursing implication if a client is told to take the medicine with meals, particularly if the medication is to be taken three times a day. Another indication of the Navajo present-time orientation is related to the failure to keep clinical appointments.

ENVIRONMENTAL CONTROL

Some Navajo Indians are perceived as having an external locus of control; although they believe that man is not subjugated to the effects of nature, they also believe that it is essential for man to live in harmony with nature and its elements. As mentioned earlier, Kluckhohn and Strodtbeck (1973) noted that the Rimrock Navajos sampled preferred the orientation theme of "man in harmony with nature." One conclusion from the study was that some Navajo Indians had a mixed locus of control that was suggestive of both a "being"-oriented and a "doing"-oriented culture.

In the past, self-esteem and a health-oriented locus of control have been postulated as predictors of attitudes and behaviors directly related to children's health. Lamarine (1987) conducted a study to measure the relationship between self-esteem, a health-oriented locus of control, and health attitudes of Navajo children in the fourth to sixth grades. The analysis of the data indicates that there is a statistically significant relationship between self-esteem and positive attitudes toward health. In addition, the study found that self-esteem was a modest predictor of health attitudes and health behavior intentions among Navajo and Pueblo children.

A craniofacial team at the University of New Mexico Medical Center at Albuquerque has been successful in the treatment of a large population of Navajos because of team awareness of the Navajo concept of health (Smoot, Kucan, Cope, & Asse, 1988). This understanding of the Navajo concept of health, in which man is viewed as being in balance with the environment (and therefore an understanding of the Navajo concerns with ghosts, "skinwalkers," and rules for orderly living), allowed team members to integrate the family, as well as the Navajo medicine man, into the care and treatment of children with craniofacial diseases. In addition, to provide culturally appropriate care, the craniofacial team had to develop an understanding of traditional Navajo healing ceremonies and the need for special handling of disposed body parts during surgery.

Illness and Wellness Behaviors

Traditional Navajo concepts espouse the need for the Navajo people to be in harmony with the surrounding environment and with the family. Some Navajo Indians have a perception of health that is not limited to the physical body but encompasses congruency with the family, environment, livestock, supernatural forces, and community. To maintain spiritual health, some Navajo people believe that it is essential to be in harmony with supernatural forces. Iverson (1990) concluded that health and religion cannot be separated in the Navajo world; rather, the link between traditional religion and healing ceremonies found among Navajo Indians is obvious.

Traditional Navajo concepts of health and disease have a fundamental place in the Navajo concept of man and his place in the universe. Native healing ceremonies encompass traditional Navajo medicine and general native healing practices and form the foundation of Navajo culture. These ceremonies are central to the attitudes, beliefs, values, and perceptions of the Navajo people.

Blessingway is the main philosophy from which more than 35 major and minor ceremonial variations are derived. This Navajo practice attempts to remove ill health by means of stories, songs, rituals, prayers, symbols, and sand paintings (Sobralske, 1985). In the Blessingway ceremony, the importance of family and clan members is emphasized in the healing process. The mother is considered particularly important because she can relate prenatal incidents of ill nature that affect health.

Native Healers

Navajo medicine men and medicine women spend many years learning their skills and serving as apprentices. There are several types of medicine men and women:

1. Diagnosticians, or those who diagnose illness or the cause of disharmony. Their title may be "crystal gazer" or "hand trembler," depending on the method used in diagnosing the patient.
2. Singers (*hataaii*, an undifferentiated singular-plural noun), or those who perform and direct the elaborate and complex healing ceremonies.
3. Herbalists, or those specialized practitioners who use herbs to treat patients and who may also diagnose illness and causes of ailments.

Medicine men and medicine women have *jish*, or medicine bundles, containing symbolic and sacred items, including corn pollen, feathers, stones,

arrowheads, and other instruments used for healing and blessing. Many of these sacred objects and plants are found on the sacred mountains that border the Navajo reservation and are gathered by medicine people only (Navajo Health Systems Agency, 1985).

There is great effort on the part of the Indian Health Service and the traditional Navajo healers to work together in a collaborative and cooperative way. It is not uncommon to observe a medicine man or medicine woman in the hospital speaking with a physician regarding the care of a client. When medically indicated, clients may also receive passes to participate in a healing ceremony held outside the hospital. There has been a continued and sustained mutual respect on the part of these two groups for the expertise of the other (Navajo Health Systems Agency, 1985).

In 1984 the Navajo Health Systems Agency conducted a research study to investigate the types of traditional healing services being provided and the types of cultural orientation to traditional healing practices being provided for newly hired Indian Health Service care providers. The conclusions of the survey reiterated the need for continued and improved collaboration and cooperation between traditional medicine people and Western physicians. For example, serious cases of injury and illness are often referred to the hospital by medicine people, and physicians have sent clients to medicine people when deemed appropriate, particularly in cases of psychological or behavioral disorders (Navajo Health Systems Agency, 1985).

Death and Dying Rituals

The Navajo are considered to be a traditional people. They have often been characterized as being very respectful of death and the dead (Kluckhohn & Leighton, 1974; Lewis & Bourne, 1989). Yet it is essential to remember that the beliefs held by the Navajo depend on personal experience, the level of acculturation into traditional U.S. society, beliefs in traditional religion, Christianity, and/or in the Native American Church. Traditional Navajo are so respectful of the dead that they do not touch the body (Braun, Pietsch, & Blanchette,

2005). In fact, when a Navajo dies, it is suggested by tradition that other Navajo not touch the body (Braun, Pietsch, & Blanchette, 2005). It is thought that if a Navajo touches the body of the dead, then the spirit of the deceased might possibly contaminate them and thus the individual would require what is known as a "cleansing ceremony" (Braun, Pietsch, & Blanchette, 2005). Some Navajo believe that the Ghost of the dead might possibly return to their home, so traditional Navajo may build a temporary home or *hogan* away from the main home and move the dying person to this new structure (Braun, Pietsch, & Blanchette, 2005). It is essential to remember that even traditional Navajo may send terminally ill Navajo to the hospital. The dead are usually quickly buried by the Navajo (Braun, Pietsch, & Blanchette, 2005). The Navajo tend to often avoid discussion of death and dying as it is a revered experience, and the name of the dead is not spoken out loud (Braun, Pietsch, & Blanchette, 2005). Some researchers contend that while the Navajo believe in the afterlife, it is perceived as only as very "shadowy and uninviting phenomenon" (Braun, Pietsch, & Blanchette, 2005; Kluckhohn & Leighton, 1974). The afterlife for most Navajo is not necessarily equated with reward, good behavior, or a quality of one's life (Braun, Pietsch, & Blanchette, 2005). For Navajos who commit suicide, it is believed that such an individual is destined to carry the object used to commit the suicide in the afterlife (Braun, Pietsch, & Blanchette, 2005). The Navajo have been slow to embrace the concept of advance directives, or truth in disclosure of terminal illness. For example, Carrese and Rhodes (1995) found that because the Navajo believe that thought and language shape reality, discussions of negative information such as the disclosure of risk in informed consent, truth in telling about terminal illness, and advance directives for future illness may all possibly be a violation of traditional Navajo values.

Implications for Nursing Care

To a Navajo Indian the concept of being is a fundamental concept; as mentioned earlier, Navajos are considered more "being" oriented than achievement oriented. Individuals are perceived as being more important than possessions, wealth, or other material things. If something is perceived as good, it is only as good as its value to other people. It is important, therefore, for the nurse to remember that some Navajo Indians believe that goodness is found only when one is in complete harmony with the surrounding environment. The nurse should also keep in mind that if a Navajo is to have the perception of being in harmony with the environment, the environment must be structured in such a way that harmony is promoted. If a nurse were to deny or not allow the client the opportunity to achieve harmony with other people, animals, plants, nature, weather, and supernatural forces, the client would not be able to obtain a sense of assuredness in relation to physical, social, psychological, and spiritual health.

It is important for the nurse to determine which cultural health practices are beneficial, neutral, or harmful to the client to provide culturally appropriate care. If a cultural practice is considered either beneficial or neutral, the practice should be incorporated into the plan of care. However, if a cultural practice is considered harmful, the nurse should devise a teaching strategy that will assist the client in developing an understanding of the implications of the practice on continued health maintenance. For example, after delivery the umbilical cord is taken from the newborn, dried, and buried near an object or place that symbolizes what the parents want for the child's future. Burial close to the home of the infant signifies the continued tie or relationship with the child's home and Mother Earth. Because this neutral practice does not negatively affect health care, it should be acknowledged, accepted, and incorporated into the plan of care. Also, to provide culturally appropriate nursing care, it is essential that the nurse respect the need for Navajo people to maintain traditional rituals even when hospitalized. For example, it would not be uncommon for a Navajo individual to sprinkle certain foods, such as corn and cornmeal, around the bedside during a curative ritualistic ceremony. The nurse who comes in the room and finds cornmeal around the bedside may initially be disturbed and insist that it be removed. However, the nurse should keep in mind that this cornmeal (as well as other rituals) is extremely important in the ritual and that, because it does not have any negative health-related implications, it should be left at the bedside until the client and the family desire its removal (Primeaux, 1977).

The U.S. government has passed numerous acts and implemented numerous programs specifically to address health-related issues among the Navajo people and their involvement in the determination of their health care. The 1975 Indian Self-Determination Act provides that any federal program serving the health needs of Navajo people may be either self-determined or contracted for by the Navajo tribe or its designee. Services contracted for must be comparable to or exceed existing services under the direction of federally operated programs, such as the Indian Health Service. Through collaborative efforts, the commitment to improve the health status of the Navajo population and to increase tribal involvement in health care management has been enhanced, reconfirmed, and extended to other components of health care (Hanley, 1987).

The basic authority for health care for American Indians and Alaskans is provided by the Snyder Act of 1921. The Bureau of Indian Affairs assumed responsibility as a federal branch for providing health care services for the Navajo people until 1954. At that time, the responsibility was transferred to the Indian Health Service as a result of the U.S. Transfer Act of 1954. In 1967 the Navajo area of the Indian Health Service was established to address the health care needs of Navajos. Today, the Navajo area is one of 12 areas within the Indian Health Service and has its administrative location in Window Rock, Arizona.

BIOLOGICAL VARIATIONS

Many American Indians are faced with a number of health-related problems. Some of the contributing factors include the fact that many of the old ways of diagnosing and treating illness have not outlasted the migration and changing ways of most American Indians. It has been estimated that at least one third of all American Indians live in a state of absolute poverty. As a direct result of this poverty, the compounded problems of lost skills and economic endeavors, and the increased complexity of disease entities, many American Indians are in a health-related crisis. In addition, as a result of poverty, many illnesses and diseases are related to such factors as poor living conditions and malnutrition. American Indians are believed to be at risk for tuberculosis, maternal and infant deaths, diabetes, and malnutrition.

In the past, American Indians continuously had the highest infant mortality in the United States. While it is true that the infant mortality rate for American Indians declined from an average of 13.9 per 1000 live births from 1983 to 1985, to an average of 12.6 per 1000 live births during the period from 1989 to 1991, to 10.2 per 1000 live births in 2003, these rate are all disproportionately high compared with the national average of 7.2 in 2002. (Henderson, Lickerman, & Flynn, 2002; U.S. Department of Health and Human Services, Health, United States, 2006). The infant, child, and youth death rates also remain disproportionately high for American Indians, led only by African-Americans. In 2003, the infant mortality rate for children younger than 1 year of age was 730 per 100,000, as compared with 573.1 for their White counterparts. Similarly, the death rate for American Indian children 1 to 4 years of age was 55.8 per 100,000, as compared with 27.9 for their White counterparts. In addition, the death rate for American Indian children 5 to 14 years of age was 24.0 per 100,000, as compared with 17.2 for their White counterparts. The rate for deaths for American Indians adolescents 15 to 19 years of age was also disproportionately high at 105.2 per 100,000 population, as compared with 63.3 per 100,000 for their White counterparts (Child Trends Data Bank, 2002).

In 1999, the age-adjusted death rate for all causes of death for the American Indian population was 716.1 per 100,000 population (U.S. Department of Health and Human Services, Health, United States, 2002). The life expectancy at birth for American Indian males is 69.1 years and 77.5 for females, which is an increase of at least 6 years from 1990

(U. S. Department of Health and Human Services, Indian Health Service, 2002).

However, although American Indians have had an increase in life expectancy, their life expectancy still lags behind that for all other races in the United States (U.S. Department of Health and Human Services, Health, United States, 2002). From 1990 to 1999, the leading causes of death in the American Indian population included (1) diseases of the heart, (2) cerebrovascular disease, (3) malignant neoplasms, (4) chronic lower respiratory diseases, (5) influenza, (6) chronic liver disease and cirrhosis, (7) diabetes mellitus, (8) HIV, (9) external causes (accidents and other unintentional injuries), and (10) suicide and assaults (U.S. Department of Health and Human Services, Health, United States, 2002).

The leading causes of death and the figures change dramatically when American Indian data are reviewed by gender and by age. For example, in 2000, the leading cause of death for American Indian males 25 to 44 years of age in ranked order were (1) accidents (with 172 deaths per 100,000 population representing 42.0% of total deaths and a death rate of 89.1 per 100,000 population); (2) intentional self-harm (with 59 deaths per 100,000 population representing 14.4% of total deaths and a death rate of 30.6 per 100,000 population); (3) assault (with 46 deaths per 100,000 population representing 11.2% of total deaths with a death rate of 23.8 per 100,000 population); (4) chronic liver disease and cirrhosis (with 23 deaths per 100,000 population representing 5.6% of total deaths with a death rate of 11.9 per 100,000 population); and (5) diseases of the heart with 16 deaths per 100,000 population representing 3.9% of total deaths) (U.S. Department of Health and Human Services, HIV/AIDS Surveillance Report, 2002). In 2000, the leading cause of deaths for American Indian females 25 to 34 and 35 to 44 years of age in ranked order were (1) accidents (with 67 deaths per 100,000 population representing 36.0% of total deaths and a death rate of 36.6 per 100,000 population); (2) intentional self-harm (with 19 deaths per 100,000 population representing 10.0% of total deaths); (3) chronic liver disease (with 16 deaths

per 100,000 population representing 8.6% of total deaths); (4) malignant neoplasms (with 13 deaths per 100,000 population representing 7.0% of total deaths); (5) assault (homicide) (tied for fourth with 13 deaths per 100,000 population representing 7.0% of total deaths); and (6) diseases of the heart (with 8.0 deaths per 100,000 population representing 4.3% of total deaths) (U.S. Department of Health and Human Services, HIV/AIDS Surveillance Report, 2002).

Body Size and Structure

Navajo children tend to have low length-for-age and high weight-for-length measures. These reference indicators suggest a suboptimal nutritional status among Navajo Indians. Navajo children with birth weights of less than 2500 g tend to be shorter, lighter, and thinner than children with birth weights of over 2500 g. In a study by Peck, Marks, Kibley, et al. (1988), the analysis of the data indicates that much of the nutritional risk, as indicated by growth abnormality among Navajo infants, is most directly attributable to the persistent effects of intrauterine growth retardation and low birth weights.

There is documented evidence of a high prevalence of obesity in American Indian children. For example, Lohman and associates (1999) found a high prevalence of obesity among American Indian children representing six different Indian nations. Similarly, White et al. (1997) noted that weight, body mass index (BMI), skin folds, and waist circumference were greatest among participants 40 to 59 years of age and lowest in participants 60 years of age and older. Among American Indian men who participated in the study, the prevalence of overweight was 37% among those 20 to 39 years of age. Similarly, it was 50% among male American Indians 30 to 59 years of age but was only 15% for male American Indians over 60 years of age (White, Ballew, Gilber, et al., 1997).

Skin Color

Skin color is perhaps the most recognizable way in which people are categorized. Although other surface characteristics subtly add to this categorization, skin color is perhaps one of the most obvious ways in which people vary across ethnic and cultural barriers. Skin-color variability is caused by a pigment that is produced by the melanocytes located in the epidermal layer of the skin. According to Wasserman (1974), the melanocytes originate in the neural crest, which is near the embryonic central nervous system, and seemingly migrate into the fetal epidermis. This origin explains the significance of pigmentation. Mongolian spots are therefore leftovers that somehow linger in the lumbosacral region at a somewhat greater than ordinary depth and cause the bluish effect seen on the skin surface. Mongolian spots are obvious in 90% of Blacks, 80% of Asians and American Indians, and 9% of Whites (Jacobs & Walton, 1976). Mongolian spots are commonly found on the buttocks and back and occasionally on the abdomen, thighs, and arms. Mongolian spots appear so ominous on inspection that a nurse who is unfamiliar with this type of discoloration may easily mistake them for child abuse. The neural origin of melanocytes explains the shape. Mongolian spots resemble neurons with dendritic appendages that insert themselves well up into the epidermal cells. These appendages inject melanosome granules containing melanin pigments into the epidermal cells (Szabó, 1975).

Dark-skinned individuals are seemingly protected from the effects of sunlight to a greater degree than light-skinned individuals are. One reason for this may be the dispersal of the melanosomes from the basal cells directly to the stratum granulosum. Therefore, when inspecting the skin of Whites, Asians, and American Indians, the nurse will find that melanosomes are incorporated singly (Szabó, Gerald, Pathak, & Fitzpatrick, 1969).

Other Visible Physical Characteristics

One visible physical difference that appears to be a startling finding for the nurse is the cleft uvula, wherein the uvula may be separated at the tip, thereby giving it a fishtail appearance. Although this is the most common variation, the separation can also occur as a complete division into two uvulas (Meskin, Gorlin, & Isaacson, 1964). Although this condition is rare in Blacks and Whites, it occurs in about 10% of Asians and as many as 18% of American Indians (Schaumann, Peagler, & Gorlin, 1970).

Another visible physical difference is associated with age-related increases in earlobe creasing. A study of Eskimos, Navajos, and Whites by Overfield and Call (1983) found no differences among the groups in the frequency of age-related earlobe creasing. However, findings from the study did indicate a difference in relation to age and onset of earlobe creasing across ethnic and cultural barriers. Whites were found to have earlobe creases at least a decade earlier than Navajos were.

Enzymatic Variations

Lactose intolerance occurs among the majority of the populations of the world. In fact, it affects 94% of Asians, 90% of African Blacks, 79% of American Indians, 75% of American Blacks, 50% of Mexican Americans, and 17% of White Americans (Bose & Welsh, 1973; Leichter & Lee, 1971; McCracken, 1971; Sowers & Winterfeldt, 1975).

Susceptibility to Disease

Tuberculosis. The role of socioeconomic factors in the incidence of tuberculosis, which includes conditions such as overcrowding and poor nutrition, cannot be disregarded. However, ethnicity also appears to be an important factor in the incidence of tuberculosis. Numerous studies suggest a high incidence of tuberculosis among American Indians (Delien, 1951; Heath, 1980). The incidence of tuberculosis varies among tribes, from a low of 2% for Apaches to 4.6% for Navajos (Reifel, 1949). In the 1980s the previously high incidence of tuberculosis among American Indians was greatly decreased, but the incidence is still considered high compared with the general population.

Type 2 Diabetes. Type 2 diabetes mellitus is a major health problem for American Indians, occurring as early as the teens or early twenties. The earlier onset has led to an earlier onset of complications, as well as excessive mortality in the early and middle adult years. Age-specific death rates for diabetes appear to be 2.6 times higher for American Indians between 25 and 54 years of age compared with the rest of the general U.S. population (U.S. Department of Health and Human Services, Health, United States, 2002). The age-adjusted death rate for diabetes as the single underlying cause among American Indians was 34.8, as compared with 19.5 for White Americans, 26.9 for Hispanics, and 13.1 for Asian Americans (U.S. Department of Health and Human Services, Diabetes surveillance report, 2002). In addition, the complications from diabetes among American Indians are appearing with distressing frequency. The National Diabetes Advisory Board noted in 2002 that complications such as amputations have a rate of occurrence 2 to 3 times that of the general U.S. population and a renal failure rate 20 times that of the general U.S. population. In a recent study of the Ute Indians, the prevalence of diabetes among this tribe was noted to be 4 times the statewide rate and that the rate of diabetic neuropathy is at least 43 times that of the diabetic population in the general Utah population.

According to the U.S. Department of Health and Human Services (2000), 45% of outpatient visits in some facilities for Indian health services are for diabetes-related problems. In addition, in some Indian tribes the rate of newly diagnosed diabetes is as high as 25%. (It is interesting to note, however, that before the 1940s, the occurrence of diabetes among Indians was rare [Tom-Orme, 1984]). The highest prevalence rates of diabetes among American Indians are found among the Pimas of Arizona, the Senecas of Oklahoma, and the Cherokees of North Carolina; the lowest rates are found in the Navajos, Hopis, and Apaches (Tom-Orme, 1984).

It is uncertain as to why diabetes mellitus is so prevalent among American Indians. One hypothesis suggests that some American Indians have a genetic predisposition for diabetes that is seemingly triggered by changes in dietary practices and increasing obesity (Neel, 1962). Another hypothesis, called the "thrifty-gene" hypothesis, suggests that during the centuries when American Indians lived a migratory life characterized by periods of feast and famine, a "thrifty gene" developed as a result of natural selection. It has been proposed that this gene might have possibly affected carbohydrate metabolism and storage so that during times when food was readily available, carbohydrates could be more readily stored in the body to be used during periods of scarcity. This theory proposes that, even today, some American Indians continue to store carbohydrates in excess, but because periods of food scarcities or famine no longer occur as they once did, American Indians tend to become obese, which ultimately leads to the development of diabetes (Andrews & Boyle, 2003).

Numerous studies support the idea that American Indians have a predisposition for diabetes mellitus. In a study by Sugarman (1989), 177 cases of gestational diabetes and 13 cases of preexisting diabetes were identified in a retrospective analysis of 4094 deliveries among Navajo women. The findings of the study therefore suggest a prevalence of 4.6% for gestational diabetes. The study also noted that when women with preexisting diabetes or previously documented gestational diabetes were excluded, the prevalence of gestational diabetes was 3.4%. Although each data source independently failed to identify 20% to 40% of diabetic pregnancies, more than 97% of cases were identified when the data sources were used collectively (Sugarman, 1989).

In a similar study, 181 pregnant Navajo women were screened for gestational diabetes (Massion, O'Connor, Gorab, et al., 1987). The findings of this study indicated that the 50-g oral glucose screening test was greater than 7.2 mmol/L or 130 mg/dL in 44 of the subjects, or approximately 24.3% of the women. In addition, the test was greater than 8.3 mmol/L or 150 mg/dL in 23 of the subjects, or approximately 12.7%. With use of standard oral glucose tolerance testing, the incidence of gestational diabetes in the study population was 6.1%. Therefore, the study concluded that universal screening of gestational diabetes is recommended among Navajo women because they are perceived as a high-risk population (Massion, O'Connor, Gorab, et al., 1987).

Sugarman and Percy (1989) noted an age- and sex-adjusted prevalence of type 2 diabetes of 10.2% among the approximately 76% of Navajo adults living on reservations. This figure was approximately 60% greater than the estimated prevalence of 6.4% for the general U.S. population. In addition, findings from the study suggest that Navajo people are more overweight than the general U.S. population (Sugarman & Percy, 1989).

O'Connor, Fragneto, Coulehan, and Crabtree (1987) conducted a cross-sectional study to assess the association of various demographics and medical care variables with metabolic outcomes in Navajos with type 2 diabetes. In the study, the dependent variable was identified as metabolic control and was measured as the mean of all random plasma glucose values obtained at scheduled clinic visits for diabetes over a 2-year period. Using multivariate analysis, the researchers noted that better metabolic control was most strongly associated with compliance with appointments. In addition, the study noted an association between the mode of treatment and metabolic control.

More recently, researchers have begun to examine the relationship between the use of select oral contraceptives and the development of diabetes among American Indian women. For example, Kim, Seidel, Begier, and Kwok (2001) found that American Indian women who use depot medroxyprogesterone are more likely to develop diabetes than patients who had used combination estrogen-progestin oral contraceptives (odds ratio, 3.8; confidence interval, 1.8–1.9). Further findings suggest that even after adjustment for body mass index, the excess risk for the development of diabetes by these women persisted (Kim, Seidel, Begier, & Kwok, 2001).

It is postulated that Navajos with diabetes mellitus are at great risk to develop other life-threatening illnesses. For example, Donahue and Orchard (1992) noted that, as with all other racial populations, Navajos with diabetes mellitus are at a high risk to develop atherosclerotic macrovascular complications. Hoy, Light, and McGill (1995) noted that that about one fourth of all the Navajos enrolled in their study over 20 years of age who attended an Indian Health Service clinic had cardiac disease. Further findings from this study suggest that this figure represented more than five times the prevalence for heart disease in their age-matched counterparts without diabetes.

O'Connor, Crabtree, and Nakamura (1997) found that there is a greater incidence in mortality experiences of Navajos with type 1 diabetes mellitus. Findings from this study suggest that among the Navajos enrolled in the study, there were 30 deaths among the 154 study subjects (39%) from the diabetic groups, as compared with 13 (17%) from their age-matched controls (O'Connor, Crabtree, & Nakamura, 1997).

Hypertension. Hypertension is rapidly becoming an increasingly important health problem among American Indians and in particular the Navajos. Percy, Freedman, Gilbert, et al. (1997) conducted a community-based study in 1991 and 1992 that included three standardized measurements of blood pressure on the Navajo reservation. Findings from this study indicated that the overall age-standardized prevalence of hypertension among the 780 adults examined (systolic >140 mm Hg; diastolic >90 mm Hg) was 19%, with a 24% prevalence noted among men and a 15% prevalence noted among women. Further findings from this study suggest that among the subjects surveyed the prevalence of hypertension increased with age and relative weight, was more prevalent among men, and was associated with diabetes mellitus (Percy, Freedman, Gilbert, et al., 1997).

Shigella. The resistance to trimethoprim-sulfamethoxazole (TMP-SMX) emerged among *Shigella* isolates from the Navajo reservation in the southwestern United States in 1985 and consequently was of paramount importance to health care workers (Griffin, Tauxe, Redd, et al., 1989). In 1983 TMP-SMX resistance was noted at a rate of 3%; however, by 1985 this rate had increased significantly to 21%. The findings of the study indicated that all the respondents who were studied and examined were resistant to ampicillin and streptomycin and had minimal inhibitory concentrations resistant to sulfamethoxazole. The findings also indicated that polyclonal, highly TMP-SMX–resistant *Shigella* emerged through transfer of trimethoprim-resistant genes from aerobic bowel flora to endemic *Shigella* strains. Therefore, the findings indicated that the use of antimicrobials can lead to symptomatic shigellosis.

Myocardial Infarction. Klain, Coulehan, Arena, and Janett (1988) noted that the myocardial infarction rate for Navajo men had more than doubled in comparison with an earlier study by the researchers. In addition, they noted that there was a gradual increase in myocardial infarctions among Navajo women. The study concluded that the majority of the Navajos who sustained acute myocardial infarctions were hypertensive (51%), diabetic (50%), or both (31%). However, it was noted that very few of the respondents in the study admitted that they smoked cigarettes.

Arthritis. There appears to be a high prevalence of arthritis, including rheumatoid arthritis, among selected American Indian tribes as compared with non-Indian populations (Hill & Robinson, 1969; Rosenberg, Petty, Oen, & Schroeder, 1982). Rheumatoid arthritis was found at a rate of 6.8% in Chippewa Indians, and Willkens, Hansen, Malmgren, et al. (1982) noted in a study on Yakima Indians in Washington State that Chippewa women had an arthritis incidence of 3.4%. Although it has been suggested that Navajo Indians have a unique form of arthritis, the findings of one study suggest that Navajos have the same type of arthritis as that of the rest of the U.S. population (Rate, Morse, Bonnell, & Kuberski, 1980). Nurses should also be aware that there have been notable findings of arthritis in the presence of negative blood studies in the Navajo population. Although it has been suggested that geographical location is one major contributing factor to the problem of arthritis, tribes that reside in one location and then move to another do not exhibit any changes in prevalence rates (Overfield, 1995).

HIV and AIDS. American Indians and Alaska Natives in a 13-state area had twice the reported gonorrhea and syphilis morbidity than the rest of the general population. In addition, in some states, they also had the highest incidence of hepatitis B. Among these populations, there was also an increase in epidemic intravenous methamphetamine use in one rural American Indian–Alaska Native community. The number of persons who are HIV seropositive is reported to be low in these groups. However, it is believed that this low number is somewhat distorted because of the racial misclassification of these individuals (U.S. Department of Health and Human Services, Indian Health Service, 2002). From 1999 to 2000, the total number of American Indians and Alaska Natives reported to have succumbed to AIDS was 1286. Of this number, 1070 were male and 216 were female. It is important to remember, however, that although there has been a relatively lower number of cumulative AIDS cases among American Indians and Alaska Natives, the incidence of AIDS is steadily increasing among this population (U.S. Department of Health and Human Services, 2001, 2002).

Nutritional Preferences

Because there are more than 500 different American Indian tribes, American Indian dietary practices vary widely. However, it should be noted that contemporary American Indian diets combine foods indigenous to the areas with modern processed foods. Food practices are also influenced by tribal beliefs and practices, geographical area, and local availability of selected foods. In certain tribal areas where game and fish are plentiful, these foods are important food sources in the diet. Although fruits, berries, roots, and wild greens are perceived to have important nutritional value, they are scarce in many federally defined Indian geographical regions. They are also scarce in urban centers such as large cities, except when found in season in supermarkets (Andrews & Boyle, 2003; U.S. Department of Agriculture, Food, and Nutrition Service, 1984).

Foods preferred by many Navajos include meat and blue cornmeal. Milk, on the other hand, is usually not listed by Navajo people as a preferred food, and this lack of preference for milk has contributed to protein malnutrition among Navajos. One study reporting protein malnutrition among elderly Navajo clients indicates that protein malnutrition is present and is more common in males, hospitalized clients, and the elderly (Williams & Boyce, 1989). The importance of cultural dietary preferences among Navajos in relation to client teaching has been identified by Koehler, Harris, and Davis (1989). According to these researchers, dietitians and nutritionists should be aware of the rich ethnic diversity among American Indians and use this knowledge accordingly in nutritional counseling.

After 6 months of ethnographic research, Wolfe and Sanjur (1988) conducted a study on 107 Navajo women who for the most part were in the food assistance program. With its primary purpose being to describe and evaluate the contemporary Navajo diet, the study was done on the basis of a 1-day dietary recall. Using data from this 1-day dietary recall, mean nutrient intakes were found to be below the recommended daily allowances for calcium, phosphorus, iron, and vitamin A. Analysis of the data also suggested that 63% of the women in the sample were overweight or obese. Although overall percentages of energy from fat, carbohydrates, and protein were closer to those recommended in the dietary allowances than the percentages found in the general U.S. population were, the fat intake appeared to be primarily saturated, and fiber intake was lower than the average for the rest of the general U.S. population. In addition, among the Navajo women sampled in the study, traditional foods were infrequently consumed. Another significant finding indicated that women with higher incomes tended to have better diets. The study also noted that commodity foods supplied by the U.S. Department of Agriculture's food distribution program provided approximately 43% of caloric intake and 37% to 57% of the intake of all nutrients except for fat and vitamin C for 72% of the population sampled. Thus a significant finding of the study was the important contribution that the food distribution program makes to the contemporary Navajo diet.

Alcohol Metabolism

For many years behavioral scientists have been searching for the biological reason why certain racial or ethnic groups such as Asians and American Indians react to alcohol differently than the way other racial or ethnic groups do, and they have noted that alcohol metabolism varies as a result of ethnic heritage. For example, some Asians and American Indians have reported physical symptoms, such as profound facial flushing and other vasomotor symptoms, after drinking alcohol. Wolff (1973) noted that most Whites do not experience similar symptoms. It has also been suggested that a high incidence of alcoholism is found in some ethnic groups, such as American Indians, Blacks, and Whites (Klatsky, Friedman, Siegelaub, & Gérard, 1977).

As indicated in Chapter 7, there are two different enzymes involved in alcohol metabolism, both of which are variations of alcohol dehydrogenase (ADH): a high-activity type of ADH, which converts alcohol to acetaldehyde rapidly, and a low-activity variant, which converts it slowly (Kalow, 1982, 1986, 1989; Stamatoyannopoulos, Chen, & Fukui, 1975). The enzyme involved in metabolism of acetaldehyde to acetic acid also has several varieties, including acetaldehyde dehydrogenase 1 through 4. Acetaldehyde dehydrogenase 1 (ALDH-1) is considered "normal" other types are considered "deficient" in their ability to metabolize acetaldehyde (Goedde, 1983, 1986; Keltner, 1994).

In Whites, alcohol is metabolized "fairly efficiently" by the liver enzyme alcohol dehydrogenase, whereas in American Indians and Asians it is metabolized by acetaldehyde dehydrogenase, which works faster, often causing circulatory and unpleasant effects such as facial flushing and palpitations (Kudzma, 1992). Studies have indicated that American Indians and Asians experience noticeable facial flushing and other vasomotor symptoms after ingesting alcohol as compared with their White and African-American counterparts, who experience less severe reactions.

Although attempts have been made to explain biological variations of metabolic absorption of alcohol in different racial or ethnic groups, it is not meant in this context to explain the causes of alcoholism. Alcoholism exists among American Indians in very high percentages.

Psychological Characteristics

There appears to be one interesting racial difference in brain development in regard to cerebral speech-lateralization differences noted among Asians, American Indians, and other races. It has been suggested that Hopi, Navajo, and Japanese individuals either process linguistic information in both hemispheres or have right-hemisphere dominance

(Overfield, 1995; Scott, 1979). Among Navajos this finding is very demonstrable, particularly when one is given a dichotic listening task. Navajos appear to have a left-ear advantage, which is suggestive of right-cerebral-hemisphere dominance, as opposed to their White counterparts, who have the usual right-ear advantage suggestive of left-cerebral-hemisphere dominance. For the nurse who is working with an aphasic client, possible racial differences in cerebral dominance cannot be overlooked (Overfield, 1995).

Implications for Nursing Care

It is important for the nurse to remember that although many researchers have implicated socioeconomic factors as a causative agent in tuberculosis, other researchers have related ethnicity to the high incidence of tuberculosis. Regardless of the causation, nurses need to assist Navajo people in learning about the significance of tuberculosis. Teaching should be clear and attempt to clarify any misunderstandings about tuberculosis. The nurse should use straightforward and easy-to-understand language. For example, the nurse might teach the client and the family how tuberculosis is spread and demonstrate how the organism can actually be seen through a microscope. The nurse should also make every effort to explain the symptoms of tuberculosis in simple terms so that the client and the family develop an understanding of the condition. For example, the nurse might begin by telling the client and the family that the symptoms begin with the client losing weight, then developing

a cough, and then starting to spit up blood. In addition, the nurse might lessen the anxiety created by the need for radiographs by saying that the taking of radiographs is just like the taking of photographs (Wauneka, 1962).

Harris, Davis, Ford, and Tso (1988) designed and tested a cardiovascular health education curriculum using 215 fifth-grade students from rural New Mexico, including Navajo, Pueblo, and Hispanic children. The teaching effort of the program was augmented by materials, examples, and exercises relevant to these particular cultures. The findings of the study suggested a significant increase in knowledge among these students about the cardiovascular system, obesity, tobacco use, and the need for exercise, nutrition, and habit change. The study concluded that a culturally oriented program can be valuable in promoting a healthful lifestyle in minority children.

SUMMARY

Today, the Navajo nation is a culture in transition. As changes occur in educational levels, employment, and environment, the Navajo people find themselves assimilating more with the dominant culture of the United States. The need to be able to blend their traditional culture with the dominant culture of the United States is creating conflict for some Navajo people. When providing health care to Navajo clients, nurses are being challenged to seek ways to bridge the gap between traditional cultural practices and Western medical practices to provide culturally appropriate nursing care.

Case Study

Mary Littlejohn, a 20-year-old Navajo Indian, is admitted to the hospital for a high-risk pregnancy related to gestational diabetes. This is Mrs. Littlejohn's second pregnancy. She is married and has a 2-year-old daughter at home. She lives in a *hogan* with her daughter, husband, mother, father, and two aunts. There is no running water, electricity, or plumbing in the home. When Mrs. Littlejohn arrives at the hospital for admission, 12 of her family members are with her. Once she has been admitted to her room and is in bed, her grandmother sprinkles cornmeal around her bed. When the nurse takes the client's history, Mrs. Littlejohn relates that she had the same problem the last time she was pregnant. Mrs. Littlejohn also relates to the nurse that she has felt tired and very weak, has had some spots before her eyes, and has had headaches. In addition, she has had to urinate very frequently at night and does not appear to be able to get enough water or food. The nurse notes on examination that the client's blood pressure is 140/88, her temperature is 99.8° F, her pulse is 102, and her tongue appears coated. The laboratory test done at Mrs. Littlejohn's last clinic visit 1 week ago revealed that her serum glucose level was 160 mg/dL.

CARE PLAN

❋ *Nursing Diagnosis: Health maintenance, ineffective, related to inability to make thoughtful judgments regarding a high-risk pregnancy*

Client Outcomes

Client and family will verbalize a desire to learn more about high-risk pregnancies, diabetes, gestational diabetes, and appropriate techniques to reduce symptoms.

Client and family will verbalize a willingness to comply with a medical therapeutic regimen to control gestational diabetes.

Client and family will verbalize an understanding of the need to comply with routine, scheduled follow-up care to prevent an at-risk delivery.

Nursing Interventions

Identify with client and family sociocultural factors that influence health-seeking behaviors.

Determine client's and family's knowledge level about diabetes, gestational diabetes, and implications for high-risk pregnancies.

❋ *Nursing Diagnosis: Communication, impaired verbal, related to cultural difference*

Client Outcomes

Family will be able to communicate personal and family-related needs to health care personnel.

Family will be able to communicate feelings about diabetes, gestational diabetes, and treatment regimen.

Each family member will be able to send precise, understandable messages to one another through appropriate verbal and nonverbal communication.

Nursing Interventions

Assist family in developing adequate communication techniques to communicate feelings and anxieties to one another and to health care personnel.

Assist family in developing the ability to determine discrepancies in communicated verbal and nonverbal behavior.

Assist family in developing appropriate language skills and nonverbal perception to decrease the possibility of faulty perception.

❋ *Family processes interrupted, related to shift in health status of family member because of gestational diabetes and high-risk pregnancy*

Client Outcome

Family will participate in care and maintenance of client.

Family will assist nurse in helping client return to a high level of wellness.

Family will verbalize difficulties encountered in seeking appropriate external resources.

Nursing Interventions

Determine family's understanding of client's condition.

Determine support systems available to family from external resources.

Determine with family supportive networks of friends and extended family members. Involve family in care and management of client.

Encourage family to verbalize fears and anxieties.

❋ STUDY QUESTIONS

1. List several factors that may contribute to diabetes among Navajos.

2. Identify at least one reason why Mrs. Littlejohn's grandmother sprinkled cornmeal around the client's bed.

3. Describe at least two communication barriers encountered by nurses in the dominant society when providing care to Navajo clients.

4. Describe at least one health practice that Mrs. Littlejohn may adhere to that may be perceived as negative.

5. Describe the structure of the traditional Navajo family and the relationship to health-seeking behaviors.

6. Identify the possible negative effects of the environment and spatial relationships in a *hogan* on health and health-seeking behaviors.

NCLEX-RN REVIEW QUESTIONS

1. John Ahiga, a Navajo, often arrives late when medications are being dispensed on a psychiatric unit. As his nurse you understand that this patient is
   A. Receiving hallucinogenic drugs.
   B. Demonstrating present-time orientation.
   C. Demonstrating past-time orientation.
   D. Demonstrating future-time orientation.

2. The style of communication that would be most effective for a culturally competent nurse to adopt during an assessment interview with a 30-year-old Navajo client would be:
   A. The frequent use of nonverbal behaviors such as gesturing, smiling, and making wry faces.
   B. A loud voice, unbroken eye contact, minimal gesturing, and straight-to-the-point questions.
   C. To be open and friendly, ask direct questions, and touch the client's arm or hand occasionally for reassurance.
   D. A soft voice, avoiding eye contact, with general leads and reflective techniques.

3. When providing nursing care for someone of the Navajo Indian culture, the nurse should remember:
   A. To make frequent eye contact.
   B. To avoid eye contact
   C. To shake hands firmly
   D. To use pointing to assist with communication

References

Andrews, M. M., & Boyle, J. S. (2003). *Transcultural concepts in nursing care* (ed. 4), Philadelphia: Lippincott, Williams & Wilkins.

Bose, D. P., & Welsh, J. D. (1973). Lactose malabsorption in Oklahoma Indians. *American Journal of Clinical Nutrition*, 26, 1320–1322.

Boyce, G. (1942). *A primer of Navajo economic problems.* Mimeographed material. Window Rock, Ariz: Navajo Service, Bureau of Indian Affairs.

Braun, K.L., Pietsch, J.H., & Blanchette, P.L. (2005). *Cultural Issues in End-of-Life Decision Making.* Thousand Oaks, California: Sage Publication.

Brugge, D. (1964). Navajo land usage: a study in progressive diversification. In Knowlton, C.S. (Ed.), *Indian and Spanish adjustments to arid and semiarid environments*, Lubbock, Tex.: Texas Technological College Committee on Desert and Arid Zone Research, Contribution No. 7.

Brugge, D. (1968, Spring). Pueblo factionalism and external relations. *Ethnohistory*, 191–200.

Carrese, J.A., & Rhodes, L.A. (1995). Western bioethics on the Navajo reservation. *Journal of the American Medical Association*, 274, 826–829.

Child Trends Data Bank. Infant, child, and youth mortality. Retrieved January 1, 2002, from www.childtrends databank.org.

Delien, H. (1951). Continuity of program—a necessity of tuberculosis control among American Indians. *Lancet*, 71(4), 136–137.

Donahue, R., & Orchard, T. (1992). Diabetes mellitus and macrovascular complications. *Diabetes Care*, 15, 1141–1155.

Goedde, H. (1983). Population genetic studies on aldehyde dehydrogenase isozyme deficiency and alcohol sensitivity. *American Journal of Human Genetics*, 35, 769–772.

Goedde, H. (1986). Ethnic differences in reactions to drugs and other xenobiotics: outlook of a geneticist. In Kalow, W., Goedde, H.W., & Agarwal, D.P. (Eds.),

Ethnic differences in reactions to drug and xenobiotics (pp. 9–20). New York: Alan R. Liss.

Griffin, P.M., Tauxe, R.V., Redd, S.C., et al. (1989). Emergence of highly trimethoprim-sulfamethoxazole-resistant *Shigella* in a Native American population: an epidemiologic study. *American Journal of Epidemiology*, 129(5), 1042–1051.

Hall, E. (1990). *The hidden dimension*. New York: Anchor Books.

Hanley, C.E. (1987, April). *Changing patterns of health care on the Western Navajo reservation*. Unpublished thesis, Chicago: American College of Healthcare.

Harris, M.B., Davis, S.M., Ford, V.L., & Tso, H. (1988). The checkerboard cardiovascular curriculum: a culturally oriented program. *Journal of School Health*, 58(3), 104–107.

Heath, C. (1980). *A descriptive and evaluative study of the tuberculosis occurring in American Indians residing in Shannon and Washabaugh Counties, South Dakota, 1970 through 1978*. Master's thesis, Houston: University of Texas, Houston.

Henderson, G., & Primeaux, M. (1981). *Transcultural health care*. Reading, Mass: Addison-Wesley.

Henderson, H., Lickerman, J., & Flynn, P. (2002, February). Health indicators: infant mortality in the U.S.A., 1983–1998; updated February 2002. Retrieved June 14, 2007, from www.calvert-henderson.com.

Heraldson, S.S. (1988). Health and health services among the Navajo Indians. *Journal of Community Health*, 13(3), 129–142.

Hill, R.H., & Robinson, H.S. (1969). Rheumatoid arthritis and ankylosing spondylitis in British Columbia Indians. *Canadian Medical Association Journal*, 100, 509–511.

Hoy, W., Light, A., & McGill, D. (1995). Cardiovascular disease in Navajo Indians with type II diabetes. *Public Health REP*, (110), 87–94.

Iverson, P. (1990). *The Navajos*. New York: Chelsea House Publishers.

Jacobs, A.H., & Walton, R.G. (1976). Incidence of birthmarks in the neonate. *Pediatrics*, 58, 218–222.

Kalow, W. (1982). The metabolism of xenobiotics in different populations. *Canadian Journal of Physiological Pharmacology*, 60, 1–19.

Kalow, W. (1986). Outlook of a pharmacologist. In Kalow, W., Goedde, H.W., & Agarwal, D.P. (Eds.), *Ethnic differences in reactions to drugs and xenobiotics*. New York: Liss.

Kalow, W. (1989, March). Race and therapeutic drug response. *New England Journal of Medicine*, 320(9), 588–589.

Keltner, N. (1994, November). Personal communication with J. Giger.

Kim, C., Seidel, K., Begier, E., & Kwok, Y. (2001). Diabetes and depot medroxyprogesterone contraception in Navajo women. *Archives of Internal Medicine*, 161(14), 1766–1771.

Klain, M., Coulehan, J.L., Arena, V.C., & Janett, R. (1988). More frequent diagnosis of acute myocardial infarction among Navajo Indians. *American Journal of Public Health*, 78(10), 1351–1352.

Klatsky, A.L., Friedman, G.D., Siegelaub, A.B., & Gérard, M.J. (1977). Alcohol consumption among White, Black, or Oriental men and women: Kaiser-Permanente multiphasic health examination data. *American Journal of Epidemiology*, 105(4), 311–323.

Kluckhohn, C., & Leighton, D. (1974). *The Navaho*. Cambridge, Mass.: Harvard University Press.

Kluckhohn, F., & Strodtbeck, F. (1973). *Variations in value orientations*. Westport, Conn: Greenwood Press.

Koehler, K.M., Harris, M.B., & Davis, S.M. (1989). Core, secondary, and peripheral foods in the diets of Hispanic, Navajo, and Jemez Indian children. *Journal of American Dietary Association*, 89(4), 638–640.

Kudzma, E. (1992, December). Drug responses: all bodies are not created equal. *American Journal of Nursing*, 92, 48–50.

Lamarine, R.J. (1987). Self-esteem, health locus of control, and health attitudes among Native American children. *Journal of School Nursing*, 57(9), 371–374.

Leichter, J., & Lee, M. (1971). Lactose intolerance in Canadian West Coast Indians. *Journal of Digestive Diseases*, 16(9), 809–813.

Lewis, E., & Bourne, S. (1989 Dec). Perinatal death. *Baillière's Clinical Obstetrics and Gynaecology*, 13(4), 935–953.

Lohman, T., Caballero, B., & Himes, J., et al. (1999). Body composition assessment in American Indian children. *The American Journal of Clinical Nutrition*, 69(4), 764S–766S.

Massion, C., O'Connor, P., Gorab, R., et al. (1987). Screening for gestational diabetes in a high-risk population. *Journal of Family Practice*, 25(6), 569–575.

McCracken, R. (1971). Lactase deficiency: an example of dietary evolution. *Curriculum Anthropology*, 12(4–5), 479–517.

McKeever, W.F., Hunt, L.J., Wells, S., & Yazzie, C. (1989). Language laterality in Navajo reservation children: dichotic test results depend on the language context of the testing. *Brain Language*, 36(1), 148–158.

Meskin, L.H., Gorlin, R.J., & Isaacson, R.J. (1964). Abnormal morphology of the soft palate: the prevalence of cleft uvula. *Cleft Palate Journal*, 1, 342–346.

Navajo Health Systems Agency. (1985). *Report on traditional medicine survey.* Window Rock, Ariz.: Navajo Health Systems Agency.

Neel, J.V. (1962). Diabetes mellitus: a "thrifty" genotype rendered detrimental by progress. *American Journal of Human Genetics,* 14, 353–362.

O'Connor, P., Crabtree, B., & Nakamura, R. (1997). Mortality experiences of Navajo with type 2 diabetes mellitus. *Ethnic Health,* 2(3), 155–162.

O'Connor, P.J., Fragneto, R., Coulehan, J., & Crabtree, B. F. (1987). Metabolic control in non–insulin-dependent diabetes mellitus: factors associated with patient outcomes. *Diabetes Care,* 10(6), 697–701.

Overfield, T. (1995). *Biologic variation in health and illness* (ed. 2). Reading, Mass.: Addison-Wesley.

Overfield, T., & Call, E.B. (1983). Earlobe type, race, and age: effects on earlobe creasing. *Journal of American Geriatric Society,* 31(8), 479–481.

Peck, R., Marks, J., Kibley, M., et al. (1988). Birth weight and subsequent growth among Navajo children. *Public Health Reports,* 33, 88.

Percy, C., Freedman, D.S., Gilbert, T.J., et al. (1997). Prevalence of hypertension among Navajo Indians. *Journal of Nutrition,* 127(10 suppl.), 2114S–2119S.

Primeaux, M. (1977). Caring for the American Indian patient. *American Journal of Nursing,* 77(1), 91–94.

Rate, R.G., Morse, H.G., Bonnell, M.D., & Kuberski, T.T. (1980). Navajo arthritis reconsidered: relationship to HLA-B27. *Arthritis Rheumatism,* 23(11), 1299–1302.

Reifel, A. (1949). Tuberculosis among Indians of the United States. *Diseases of the Chest,* 16, 234–249.

Roessel, R. (1981). *Women in Navajo society.* Rough Rock, Navajo Nation, Ariz.: Navajo Resources Center.

Rosenberg, A.M., Petty, R.E., Oen, K.G., & Schroeder, M.L. (1982). Rheumatic diseases in western Canadian Indian children. *Journal of Rheumatology,* 9(4), 589–592.

Schaumann, B.F., Peagler, F.D. & Gorlin, R.J. (1970). Minor orofacial anomalies among a Negro population. *Oral Surgery,* 29(4), 566–575.

Scott, S. (1979). Cerebral speech lateralization in the Native American Navajo. *Neuropsychologia,* 17(1), 89–92.

Smoot, E.C., Kucan, J.O., Cope, J.S., & Asse, J.M. (1988). The craniofacial team and the Navajo patient. *Cleft Palate Journal,* 25(4), 395–402.

Sobralske, M. (1985). Perceptions of health: Navajo Indians. *Topics in Clinical Nursing,* 7(3), 32–39.

Sowers, M., & Winterfeldt, E. (1975). Lactose intolerance among Mexican Americans. *American Journal of Clinical Nutrition,* 28, 704–705.

Stamatoyannopoulos, G., Chen, S., & Fukui, M. (1975). Liver alcohol dehydrogenase in Japanese: high population frequency of atypical form and its possible role in alcohol sensitivity. *American Journal of Human Genetics,* 27, 789–796.

Sugarman, J.R. (1989). Incidence of gestational diabetes in a Navajo Indian community. *Western Journal of Medicine,* 150(5), 648–651.

Sugarman, J.R., & Percy, C. (1989). Prevalence of diabetes in a Navajo Indian community. *American Journal of Public Health,* 79(4), 511–513.

Szabó, G. (1975). The human skin as an adaptive organ. In Damon, A. (Ed.), *Physiological anthropology.* New York: Oxford University Press.

Szabó, G., Gerald, A.B., Pathak, M.A., & Fitzpatrick, T.B. (1969). Racial differences in the fate of melanosomes in human epidermis. *Nature,* 222, 1081–1082.

Tom-Orme, L. (1984). Diabetes intervention on the Uintah-Ouray reservation. In Carter, M. (Ed.), *Proceedings of the ninth annual Transcultural Nursing Conference.* Salt Lake City, Utah: Transcultural Nursing Society.

Treaty between the United States of America and the Navajo tribe of Indians. (1973). Las Vegas: KC Publications.

U.S. Department of Agriculture, Food and Nutrition Service. (1984). *American Indians: a guide for nutrition educators.* Washington, D.C.: U.S. Government Printing Office.

U.S. Department of Health and Human Services, Indian Health Services. *Trends in Indian Health: 1998–1999.* Washington, D.C. U.S.: Government Printing Office.

U.S. Department of Commerce, Bureau of the Census. (2000). The American Indians and Alaska Native population, 2000 census brief. Washington, D.C.: U.S. Government Printing Office.

U.S. Department of Commerce, Bureau of the Census. (2002). Population profiles by age, sex, race and Hispanic origin, Summary File 3. Hyattsville, Md.: U.S. Government Printing Office.

U.S. Department of Health and Human Services, (2002). *Health, United States, 2002, Urban and rural health chartbook.* Hyattsville, Md.: National Center for Health Statistics.

U.S. Department of Health and Human Services, Centers for Disease Control and Prevention. (2001, December). Persons reported to be living with HIV infection and AIDS, as of December 2001. Centers for Disease Control and Prevention.

U.S. Department of Health and Human Services, Centers for Disease Control and Prevention. (2002, December). HIV/AIDS surveillance supplemental report: deaths among persons with AIDS through December 2000, 13(2). Centers for Disease Control and Prevention.

U.S. Department of Health and Human Services, Centers for Disease Control and Prevention. (2002). Diabetes surveillance report. Atlanta: Centers for Disease Control and Prevention, U.S. Department of Health and Human Services.

U.S. Department of Health and Human Services, Indian Health Service. (2002). Comprehensive health care program for American Indians and Alaska's natives. Retrieved January 3, 2003, from www.hhs.gov/non-medical programs.

Wasserman, H.P. (1974). *Ethnic pigmentation: historical, physiological and chemical aspects.* New York: Elsevier.

Wauneka, A. (1962). Helping a people to understand. *American Journal of Nursing,* 62(2), 88–96.

White, L.M., Ballew, C., Gilber, T., et al. (1997). Weight, body image, and weight control practices of Navajo Indians: findings from the Navajo Health and Nutrition Survey. *The Journal of Nutrition,* 127(10), 2094s–2098s.

Williams, R., & Boyce, W.T. (1989). Protein malnutrition in elderly Navajo patients. *Journal of American Geriatrics and Sociology,* 37(5), 397–406.

Willkens, R.F., Hansen, J.A., Malmgren, J.A., et al. (1982). HLA antigens in Yakima Indians with rheumatoid arthritis. *Arthritis and Rheumatism,* 25(12), 1435–1439.

Wolfe, W.S., & Sanjur, D. (1988). Contemporary diet and body weight of Navajo women receiving food assistance: an ethnographic and nutritional investigation. *Journal of American Dietary Association,* 88(7), 822–827.

Wolff, P. (1973). Dietary habits and cancer epidemiology. *Cancer,* 43, 1955–1961.

Young, R. (1961). The origin and development of Navajo tribal government. In Young, R.W. (Ed.), *The Navajo yearbook* (vol. 8, pp. 371–411). Window Rock, Ariz.: Bureau of Indian Affairs.

CHAPTER 11 Appalachians

Toni Tripp-Reimer, Lisa Skemp Kelley, and Cynthia C. Small

Behavioral Objectives

After reading this chapter, the nurse will be able to:

1. Describe the history of the Appalachian region.
2. Describe Appalachian communication patterns.
3. Describe the Appalachian orientation to time and space.
4. Explain values related to family that may be held by persons with Appalachian heritage.
5. Describe the Appalachian traditional health care system, including folk beliefs, herbal remedies, and lay practitioners.
6. Describe factors affecting Appalachian use of biomedical health services.
7. Discuss illnesses that tend to have higher mortality among Appalachians.

OVERVIEW OF APPALACHIA

In 1964 the President's Appalachian Regional Commission report concluded that "Appalachia is a region apart—geographically and statistically" (PARC, 1963, p. xvii). The basis for this distinction in socioeconomic terms was Appalachia's poverty, deficits in living standards and education, and lack of urbanization. Over the past 38 years, dramatic changes have occurred in economic development, resulting in associated social and cultural transitions. Yet Appalachians, especially in the central region, are characterized by unique features.

Approximately 27 million people live in the federally defined Appalachian region, which is nearly 200,000 square miles across 410 counties in 13 states, including all of West Virginia and selected counties in Alabama, Georgia, Kentucky, Maryland, Mississippi, New York, North Carolina, Ohio, Pennsylvania, South Carolina, Tennessee, and Virginia (U.S. Department of Commerce, Bureau of the Census, Summary File 3, 2002; Appalachian Regional Commission, available at www.arc.gov/research/resmain.htm). Originally, the Appalachian region was defined as 360 counties in 11 states in a bill enacted by the U.S. Congress in 1965, titled the Appalachian Regional Act, and subsequently revised. Today, data on the Appalachian region are collected with federal authority by the Appalachian Regional Commission (U.S. Department of Commerce, Bureau of the Census, Summary File 3, 2002).

The Appalachian area has three subregions: Northern, Central, and Southern Appalachia. Northern Appalachia is the largest region and consists of portions of New York, Pennsylvania, Ohio, and Maryland and most of West Virginia. It is the most urbanized, populated, and relatively economically advantaged of the three subregions. Southern Appalachia includes counties in Southern Virginia, Eastern Alabama, Georgia, Tennessee, Mississippi, and North and South Carolina. Of the 13 states, West Virginia is the most rural and the only state residing entirely within the Appalachian region.

Central Appalachia includes parts of Kentucky, Tennessee, Virginia, and the southern area of West Virginia. It is the smallest and poorest of the three areas, is predominantly rural, and has a coal mining economic base. Central Appalachia, particularly the rural areas, stands out most distinctly as a severely distressed economic area, along with particular areas of Northern Appalachia (the rest of West Virginia and portions of Ohio) and Southern Appalachia (clusters of counties in northern Mississippi and Alabama) (Cushing & Rogers, 1996). In 2000 the Appalachian Regional Commission identified nine Appalachian states as having distressed counties, that is, counties with immediate concerns because of the high infant mortality rate, poverty, unemployment, and low income.

Originally home to American Indian tribes such as the Cherokee, the Appalachian area is now populated overwhelmingly by non-Hispanic Whites, with only 1% of the population American Indian and 8% African-American. Most African-American Appalachians reside in the urban areas or in the rural counties in Southern Appalachia. However, the population is experiencing rapid demographic change, with an increase of nearly 50% in the minority population in the last decadal census, with increases of 239.3% for the Hispanic population and 18.7% for the African-American population. Minority population growth surpassed that of Whites for all Appalachian states, and was particularly high for children with persons of younger working ages (18–43 years) (Pollard, 2004)

For the most part, the Appalachian region is classified as a rural, nonfarming area, although some large cities are encompassed in the area, including Pittsburgh, Pennsylvania; Charleston, West Virginia; Knoxville and Chattanooga, Tennessee; and Birmingham and Montgomery, Alabama. Many Appalachians live in and around the rocky, mountainous terrain, and the roads to their small homes are long, rough, steep, narrow, and often difficult to navigate. Because of the terrain, many communities have only recently been able to support public utilities, such as municipal heating, water, and sewage systems. Only since the 1980s have paved primary highways, telephones, electricity, and running water become widely accessible.

Because of the isolation, lack of distinguishing physical characteristics, and low visibility of the people, Appalachians have been relatively overlooked as an American ethnic minority. Although the Appalachian region is federally designated, the Appalachian people are not awarded the status of a federally defined ethnic/minority group. Further, Appalachians don't generally identify themselves as being "Appalachian" or "mountaineers" or any other ethnic designation. Yet this designation may be useful to providers because of the shared history, core values, beliefs, and behavioral patterns that have been identified for this group. Although persons who are considered Appalachian generally reside in the Appalachian region, some have migrated to other parts of the United States. On the other hand, some Americans from other areas have migrated to Appalachia; however, migration to the region does not in itself result in classification as an Appalachian.

History

In 1749, Thomas Walker was the first known European American to penetrate the Appalachian maze of hogback ridges and deep valleys. Some 20 years later Daniel Boone blazed the Wilderness Trail through the Cumberland Gap, soon to be followed by more than 100,000 settlers (MacAvoy & Lippman, 2001). The forefathers of the new settlers came from Northern European countries such as England, Wales, Scotland, Germany, and France, often seeking religious or personal freedom and available land (Tripp-Reimer, 1982). Life in the rural wilderness areas and the continuing isolation of Appalachians, particularly the central and southern mountaineers, has distinguished Appalachians from the mainstream of American society (Simon, 1987).

Historically, like many ethnic groups, Appalachians have borne the brunt of discriminatory characterizations. As with much labeling of minority groups, this stereotyping has emphasized negative behaviors and serves as a barrier to our understanding the health needs, core values, beliefs, and behaviors that the Anglo-Celtic rural mountain-dwelling people may share. This holds not only for those

who live in Appalachia but also for the approximately 4 million Appalachian people who migrated to major urban areas of the North Central United States beginning in the late 1950s and peaking in the 1980s (Obermiller & Malong, 1994). Early migrants from the Appalachian region to urban areas such as Cincinnati, Columbus, Detroit, and Cleveland often remained at the poverty level and often congregated with other persons from Appalachia (Tripp-Reimer, 1982); more recently, they are increasingly absorbed into working-class and middle-class neighborhoods because of their increased access to employment and education.

Economy

Historically, Appalachia was a rural, agricultural area. Then beginning in the late 1800s, the economic base and the landscape were changed by the dominant industries of mining, lumber, and textiles. The local communities were often not advantaged by these industries. Generally, the wealth that was generated was not reinvested in the region, but exported to the urban areas, largely in the East. This resulted in a low tax base and high rates of poverty (Barnett, Halverson, Elmes, & Braham, 2000). Often there was corporate ownership of the resource-rich land; in some counties in West Virginia, coal companies and railroads own up to 90% of the surface land. As a result, much of the usable land was unavailable to the local Appalachians. In addition, health services, schools, and other public services were underfunded because of the lack of a solid tax base (resulting from incentives given to the corporations) (Burkhardt, 1991).

In general, rural populations across the United States tend to be poorer, older, less educated, and more likely to be uninsured. Rural residents generally have poorer overall health status, less access to care, and difficulty with paying for services (even if they have insurance), and they participate in fewer health promotion activities (Appalachian Regional Commission, available at www.arc.gov/research/resmain.htm; Friedell, Rubio, Maretzki, et al., 2001; Huttlinger, Schaller-Ayers, & Lawson, 2004; Huttlinger, Schaller-Ayers, Kenny, & Ayers, 2004). In contrast, metropolitan areas have more public utilities and better health infrastructure, the population is generally better educated, and more are employed at higher-paying jobs (Barnett, Halverson, Elmes, & Braham, 2000).

In 2000, the per capita income of those persons residing in the federally defined Appalachian regions was approximately $4000 less than the per capita income for the rest of the general United States (Appalachian Regional Commission, available at www.arc.gov/research/resmain.htm) Yet taken at face value, these figures are somewhat misleading. Appalachia is characterized by extremes of wealth and poverty. Because the per capita income is slightly lower than the national average, the poverty rate is at least twice the national average at 15.3%. In 2000, the unemployment figure for persons identified as rural Appalachian was 4.8% as compared with 4.5% for the rest of the general U.S. population (Barnett, Halverson, Elmes, & Braham, 2000; Muratova, Islam, Demerath, Minor, & Neal, 2001; U.S. Department of Labor, 2002; Appalachian Regional Commission, available at www.arc.gov/research/resmain.htm). With increasing environmental concerns and international competition, there has been a loss of mining and textile jobs.

Education

In 1970 the proportion of the adult population that completed high school in the Appalachian region was 27% in the rural areas and 52% in the metropolitan areas; by 2000, this proportion had risen to 53% and 79%, respectively (Appalachian Regional Commission, available at www.arc.gov/research/resmain. htm). Currently, in all of Appalachia, 11.4% of persons 25 years of age or older have less than an eighth-grade education; 35.4% have some high school education but no diploma; 69.4% hold a high school diploma or GED; and 15.0% hold a 4-year college degree or higher (Appalachian Regional Commission, available at www.arc.gov/research/resmain.htm). Although more Appalachian children now graduate from high school, the 17% dropout rate is still higher than that for children of other ethnic groups (Appalachian Regional Commission, available at www.arc.gov/research/resmain.htm; Obermiller & Maloney, 1990; Penn, Borman, &

Hoeweler, 1994). While education is increasingly seen as important, school attendance may also tax a family's meager resources. Denham (1999a) noted that the need for new clothing, transportation, homework, and peer conflicts placed additional burdens on many families.

Public Services

In the 1960s, 39% of persons in all of Appalachia (and 63% in rural areas) lived in houses without complete indoor plumbing, yet by 1990, this figure had transitioned to only 2%. Even in the rural areas of Central Appalachia, only 5% of homes today are without complete indoor plumbing (Isserman, 1997). Similarly, the proportion of households with telephones has now risen, so that only 10% to 15% of occupied housing units currently lack phones (Cushing & Rogers, 1996). In Central Appalachia, 14% of occupied homes do not have a vehicle or any available means of public transportation (Cushing & Rogers, 1996).

Core Cultural Patterns

Four interacting core cultural patterns provide the underlying structure of much that will be discussed throughout this chapter, but first, two caveats: The intention here is not to provide a rigid stereotype of Appalachians but to identify patterns that may serve as guides to understanding. Furthermore, cultural value patterns are identified for aggregates and, as such, are not directly transferable to individuals (Dreher & MacNaughton, 2002; Tripp-Reimer & Fox, 2001). Rather, these patterns provide a contextual understanding by which health care providers may assess an individual's unique health care abilities and needs.

In the classic work of Tripp-Reimer (1980) four interacting Appalachian cultural patterns were identified: independence, the ethic of neutrality, familism, and personalism. Independence developed out of a history of escaping religious persecution and as a survival mechanism. There is a pride in self-sufficiency (Blakeney, 1987). At a time when most people hire others to fix their cars or build their homes, Appalachians take pride in doing things for themselves. This helps explain the difficulty encountered by many Appalachians when it is necessary to ask for financial help or welfare. However, this pattern is context specific and may not apply in unfamiliar clinical settings, particularly in a crisis. For example, while Appalachian nurses wanted to promote more decisional control for hospitalized patients, Appalachian patients reported a desire for much less control (Rosswurm, Dent, Armstrong-Persily, Woodburn, & Davis, 1996). Hunsucker, Frank, and Flannery (1999) found that interdependence, not independence, characterized rural Southern Appalachian family members who had a member in the intensive care unit. Other rural Appalachian family member needs that were different from urban families included a preference for informal support systems (family, friends, and religious) over formal systems, close personal relationships and a desire for frequent communication with professionals, flexible visiting hours, permission for emotions, and provision for time alone.

In his early ethnographic work, Hicks (1976) reported that Appalachians demonstrate what he termed an ethic of neutrality. This is evidenced in four behavioral imperatives: (1) avoiding aggression or assertiveness, (2) not interfering in another person's business unless requested to do so, (3) avoiding domination over other people, and (4) avoiding arguments and seeking agreement. Consequently, there may be low tolerance for paternalistic or prescriptive behavior patterns. Rather than messages attacking an organization or individual, politeness is valued (Denham, Meyer, Toborg, & Mande, 2004). For example, according to Blakeney (1987), an occupational therapist and native of Appalachia, "It is more important to get along with others than to make conflicting true feelings known" (p. 62).

Familism emphasizes the importance of relationships with consanguineous nuclear and extended family members rather than self-actualization through individual accomplishments (Tripp-Reimer, 1980). The high reliance on family may influence choice of employment, religious affiliation, marriage partners, and health care practices. A sense of family is central to the Appalachian sense of self, which in turn is intricately linked with the land, homestead, and trusted neighbors (Blakeney, 1987; Rowles, 1991). Appalachians who have migrated elsewhere often strongly continue to value their connection to the "hills" and homeland and go to great lengths to maintain those connections (Blakeney, 1987).

While trust is extended cautiously, it may be built through a personal orientation in contrast to a bureaucratic or service-oriented relationship (Tripp-Reimer, 1980). In health interactions, a person-focused rather than disease-focused approach is preferred. This preference for a personal orientation may explain why nursing care has been noted to be preferred to medical-based cure modalities (Blakeney, 1987).

COMMUNICATION

Appalachians are English-speaking people; however, they have several idiomatic differences in the meanings of specific words. Throughout the Appalachian region, there are various dialects with high concentrations of words of Scottish or Elizabethan English heritage (Dial, 1975). Thus phrases used by some Appalachians may be interpreted entirely differently by non-Appalachians. For example, an Appalachian person may say "running off," which may be interpreted by a non-Appalachian as leaving home or running away but may actually mean diarrhea. These examples of stylistic differences represent generally rare opportunities for miscommunication. On the other hand, the Appalachians' use of folk categories of illness may be the basis for greater misunderstanding. As will be described in greater detail in the folk belief section, several illnesses sound like, but are conceptually distinct from, the biomedical terms. For example, *high blood pressure* and *hypertension* are two folk illness categories in the Appalachian region that are distinct from the biomedical category of hypertension.

Variations in meta-communication patterns are generally more important than the idiomatic differences just described. Meta-communication patterns include mode, style, strategy, explanation, problem exposure, and orientation. Hall (1989, 2006) typified cultures on the basis of high- or low-context communication. For high-context cultures

Table 11-1	Comparison of How High- and Low-Context Cultures Differ in Negotiations	
	Low-Context Cultures	**High-Context Cultures**
Mode	Direct	Indirect
Style	Control/confrontation	Accommodation/avoidance
Strategy	Competition	Collaboration
Explanation	Linear, analysis	Nonlinear, synthesis
Problem exposure	Direct/confrontational	Indirect/nonconfrontational
Orientation	Action and solution focused	Relationship oriented and process focused

(HCCs), most of the meaning of a communication comes from the context; it is unspoken. For low-context cultures (LCCs), most of the meaning comes from the actual words used. Gudykunst and Ting-Toomey (1988) provide a framework for comparing how high- and low-context cultures differ in their approach to negotiation (see Table 11-1). Because the dominant communication mode for Appalachians is high context and that for health providers is low context, opportunities for misunderstandings are maximized.

Nonverbal communication patterns may also vary. Although common among many groups, direct eye contact is often viewed by Appalachians as impolite or lacking good manners (Hicks, 1976; Mullen & Phillips, 1998) or even as aggressive or hostile behavior (Helton, 1995; Murray & Huelskoetter, 1991). Many Appalachians use a verbal pattern that is much more concrete than the patterns displayed by middle-class Americans, who tend to be more abstract. For example, in health education materials politeness, succinct facts presented without "sugar coating it" or "getting preachy," and "Talk. Just like one-on-one" was preferred (Denham, Meyer, Toborg, & Mande, 2004, p. 299).

Implications for Nursing Care

As the textile, mining, and lumber industries began to grow in the Appalachian regions, many Appalachian persons were stripped of their land and other natural resources. Company towns controlled the stores, educational systems, and financial capital, exploiting the people and the land. This historical context fostered mistrust of outsiders. Positive interactions between an Appalachian person and an outsider often require that a trusting relationship first be established. Strategies to improve communication include making the time to listen and talk about matters that are important to the individual and the family. It may be helpful to use a direct approach, giving the facts, discussing within the context of prior family experiences, and soliciting the opinion and advice of family members before making recommendations.

Again, the nurse should be aware that some Appalachians, because of the ethic of neutrality, might wish to avoid confrontation and tell nurses what they believe the nurse wants to hear. The nurse can diminish this possibility by adopting a high-context communication style: speaking indirectly, emphasizing collaboration, avoiding confrontation, and developing the relationship (Lewis, Messner, & McDowell, 1985; Tripp-Reimer, 1980). Finally, because many Appalachian folk illnesses sound like biomedical disease categories, nurses need to take special care to understand what clients truly mean in their use of illness categories.

SPACE

Personal space is very important to Appalachians, evident in maintaining a personal distance when interacting (Purnell & Counts, 2003). As addressed earlier, familism and the sense of self are intimately linked to the land and homestead (Blakeney, 1987; Rosswurm, Dent, Armstrong-Persily, Woodburn, & Davis, 1996; Rowles, 1991). Appalachians love the land, and some prefer to live apart from the rest of society, nestled in the privacy of the hollows and hills. Appalachians are considered present-oriented (Blakeney, 1987) and focused on "being" rather than "doing" (Lewis, Messner, & McDowell, 1985; Purnell & Counts, 2003; Rowles, 1991, 2000; Tripp-Reimer, 1982). They have been described as believing that because tomorrow is not promised, they must live for today. While this has been interpreted as fatalism, it may also be interpreted as a realistic understanding of life circumstances. Poverty, harsh living conditions, rudimentary municipal supports, and isolation may make "unhurried" adaptive patterns of behavior necessary to conserve energy and accomplish the everyday work necessary to meet basic needs for survival.

Implications for Nursing Care

In contrast to the typical behavioral characteristics of Appalachians, which is to be family oriented and concerned with the well-being of others, when an Appalachian is ill, personal space collapses inwardly (Simpkins, 1979), meaning that the Appalachian person expects to be waited on and cared for by others. Thus the focus of both the individual and the members of the family is on the ill person. In a hospital setting, this may create obstacles to planning and executing nursing care because it is not unusual for a large number of family members to arrive with the client and to expect to maintain proximity with the client throughout the duration of the hospitalization. This desire for proximity is also evidenced when a client is scheduled for a clinic appointment, even if the condition is perceived by the health care professionals as minor.

SOCIAL ORGANIZATION

Family

The major unit of Appalachian social organization and group identity is generally the family rather than the community or Appalachian region (Blakeney, 1987). The nuclear and extended families are both very important. Some Appalachians are so intensely loyal that they feel a personal responsibility for in-laws, nieces, and nephews, as well as other distant family members. Appalachians tend to place a greater importance on the extended family than do most middle-class Americans; the extended

family is considered important regardless of the social, educational, or economic level of the individual. Thus relatives are sought for advice, validation, and support on many matters, particularly those pertaining to health and illness (Culture of Poverty Revisited, 1977; LaFargue, 1980). Kinship groups are the major social organizing force in the region (Tripp-Reimer & Friedl, 1977) on which to build community-level involvement. The dedication to family is of such paramount importance to most Appalachians that Purnell and Counts (2003) note most Appalachians rarely move more than 30 miles from their families.

The extensive ties to the nuclear and extended family are evident when a family member becomes ill or dies, in that members of the entire family may take leave from their jobs to be with the ill or dying relative for the duration of the crisis. This tendency to miss work for a family illness may have negative job consequences. If a family member is chronically ill, continued employment may be sacrificed for the "good" of the family (Jones, 1983). This intense loyalty for being with ill family members may remain long after an Appalachian person migrates from the region (Helton, 1995). This loyalty is also carried over into housing in northern areas; a landlord may find a property deserted, with all personal belongings intact, because the tenant had returned to the Appalachian region to be with a sick relative.

The Appalachian family is basically patriarchal (Murdock, 1982; Tripp-Reimer, 1982), but mothers and grandmothers make most health decisions (Denham, Meyer, Toborg, & Mande, 2004). Denham (1999a, 2002) conducted three ethnographic studies over a 5-year period in two southeastern Ohio counties. She found that most families focused on present rather than future health. The concept of "family health routines" involves multiple interacting individuals that constitute a family perspective. She notes that for the Appalachian families studied, mothers assume primary roles in establishing the behaviors viewed as important for children's health needs. Mothers are the main health care teachers and decision makers and are pragmatic in caring for family health. For example, mothers are more likely to encourage family members to incorporate health information into family routines when it is viewed as meaningful, aligned with family values, and applicable to members' needs and when adequate resources or supports are available (Denham, 2002). Determination of need for medical care was made after a "wait and see" time period, upon the counsel of close friends and family, and based on the mother's judgment (Denham, 1999b).

Children are viewed as security for the future (Tripp-Reimer, 1982). While marriage before childbirth is preferred, in the case of an early pregnancy, the family tends to become more cohesive, providing love and security to the expectant mother. The grandparents often care for grandchildren, particularly if both parents work. The children appear to have a sense of who they are and a greater sense of belonging. In recent years, the desired family size has decreased dramatically; the norm is now two to three children (Murray & Huelskoetter, 1991).

Elderly family members are generally respected and often reside with their children or nearby. The attitude among Appalachians toward elders is reported to be one of honor, attributable to the elders' role in cultural transmission to later generations. Rowles (1983) found that spatial separation of elders from their adult children when they relocated generated critical dilemmas for the Appalachian elders. It was difficult to reconcile their fear of leaving the familiar environment (with its physical, social, and emotional support) with their desire to be close to the family. The study was based on a 4-year observation of elderly persons in a rural northern Appalachian community and was intended primarily to explore the tensions between factors that reinforced locational stability and factors that encouraged relocating to the homes of children residing outside the Appalachian region.

Religion

Initially on arrival in the United States, many Appalachian persons were Presbyterians, Episcopalians, or members of some other formally organized denomination. However, these churches required educated clergy and a centralized organization, both of which proved to be impractical in the wilderness (Burkhardt, 1991). As a result, in rural areas locally autonomous nondenominational churches emerged throughout the Appalachian region. For the most part, these individualistic churches stress the centrality of grace, authority of the Bible, religious experience, a call to preach, and local church governance (Simpson & King, 1999). While some social reformers have viewed the local churches as a hindrance to social progress, others recognize their adaptive features, making life worth living in grim situations (Jones, 1983). Mainstream denominations, particularly Southern Baptist and United Methodist, are more prevalent in the urban areas of Appalachia and generally attended by more economically advantaged congregations.

Simpson and King (1999) explored health-related and religious activities in the local autonomous churches to include prayer requests, anointing, and testimony. They proposed that religious health partnerships could provide a channel for health promotion effects in rural Appalachia. On the other hand, churches differ in their willingness to engage in progress that is "of the world"—not inspired by God.

Implications for Nursing Care

Rather than an individualist experience, health and illness are a family affair, negotiated and understood within a family context and often under the purview of women, especially mothers. In health care, family members' involvement may include consultation regarding etiology, severity, and treatment options. Integration of concrete examples of risk behavior, health problems, and treatments within the experiences of the nuclear and extended family system may be an effective health care strategy for providers (Denham, Meyer, Toborg, & Mande, 2004).

In contrast to the well Appalachians' emphasis on independence, ill Appalachian interdependence is emphasized. The family surrounds the person and often provides needed care (Hunsucker, Frank, & Flannery, 1999; Rosswurm, Dent, Armstrong-Persily, Woodburn, & Davis, 1996). In a hospital or clinic setting, it is not unusual for a large number of family members to arrive with the client and expect to maintain proximity with the client throughout the duration of the hospitalization. Consequently, mechanisms for family involvement need to be incorporated in the plan of care and hospital policies.

Familism, the ethic of neutrality, and poverty may influence health behaviors. Because Appalachians tend to be family oriented, it may be important to elicit family opinions in regard to health care. If the family's ideas and opinions are not incorporated into the plan of care, the family and client may not accept the health care recommendations or services. It may be helpful to blend the informal and formal systems (Ramey, 1993) or recruit family members or other trusted care providers as care brokers.

It may be helpful to develop mechanisms for supporting and encouraging family involvement in care (Maas, Reed, Specht, et al., 2001; Specht, Kelley, Manion, et al., 2000). Minimally, the nurse must recognize that changes in health behaviors affect the entire family system, and consequently the nurse should incorporate family members in health education. For example, if a person is admitted to the hospital for diabetes, not only should the client be given instructions on diabetes care but also the family members should be given the same level of instruction. Instruction must take into account the resources the family has in the home, including the informal care network and assets such as running water, finances to purchase supplies, and refrigeration.

Additionally, since the family context, health beliefs, practices, and religion are often intertwined, it is important that an assessment of these be done on admission to the health care system. For example, a study done with Appalachian women found that premature birth is associated with a woman's negative feelings about pregnancy, low self-esteem, and depression (Jesse, Seaver, & Wallace, 2003). On the other hand, Appalachian pregnant women who had a greater sense of spirituality and lower levels of personal stress were found to participate in fewer risky health behaviors (for example, smoking) (Jesse & Reed, 2004). As such, integrating stress

reduction and spirituality in prenatal health care promotion visits may be helpful. This may be particularly important for Medicaid-supported pregnant women who were found to have an increased incidence of smoking, depressive symptoms, and physical abuse than private-pay pregnant women (Jesse, 2003). Confusion regarding professional stereotyping of fatalism for clients' lack of personal resources of time, money, or access to health care beliefs must be recognized and avoided. Finally, church-health partnerships may be useful in the delivery of health promotion information.

TIME

Tripp-Reimer (1982) found a strong difference in interpretations of time perceptions between Appalachians and non-Appalachian health care providers. Non-Appalachian health care professionals interpreted missed appointments negatively and were judgmental in their characterization of Appalachians as not having skills for long-term planning. On the other hand, the Appalachian professionals understood that Appalachians focus on the present to meet overwhelming needs and the uncertainty of what tomorrow will bring. Furthermore, Appalachian professionals understood that Appalachian persons may miss appointments or be late because they are working to meet everyday needs, may lack transportation, or are concerned about being fired if they take off from work.

The way in which rural Appalachians structure time differs from the urban population. Blakeney (1987) explains that the Appalachians

View modern man as having lost the technique of enjoying time for itself, the art of "sitting for a spell" to visit with another person or to cherish a moment in solitude. An isolated self-sufficient lifestyle still requires hard work and offers few modern conveniences. However, those people in Appalachia who continue this lifestyle achieve a self-directed balance in their lives and establish their own individualized patterns of work, leisure, self-care, and rest. (pp. 65–66)

Implications for Nursing Care

Because of Appalachians' perspectives on time, they may live at a pace that facilitates an awareness of body rhythms as opposed to clock time. Because some Appalachians are present-time oriented, it is best and often necessary for the nurse to assess kinesthetic needs and gently access personal and emotional space by visiting with the client before an examination or treatment is performed. Another consideration is that it is common for some Appalachian clients to arrive for an appointment at a time that is different from when the appointment is scheduled. If they are turned away, they may not access those services again. There are a number of alternative methods for delivery of health services that are being explored and tested. Modes of health care delivery to facilitate community-level and client access to health care include family involvement in care planning, teleconferencing and telehealth, assistance with transportation, flexible scheduling and extended clinic hours, open walk-in clinics, outreach clinics close to clients' homes, home visits, parish nursing, and clinics done in association with churches and other sites of congregation (Calico, 1996; Edwards, Lenz, & East-Odom, 1993; Friedell, Rubio, Maretzki, et al., 2001; Hurley, Turner, & Floyd, 2000; Hunsucker, Frank, & Flannery, 1999; Simpson & King, 1999; Wallace, Tuck, Boland, & Witucki, 2002).

ENVIRONMENTAL CONTROL

Environmental Health Threats

Factors contributing to the Appalachians' having health status lower than U.S. average include low-paying jobs, lack of employment, lack of health insurance, environmental toxins, noise, and numerous occupational health hazards. Workers in the textile mills were often exposed to high levels of cotton, flax, or hemp dust, leading to the highest rates of "brown lung disease" in the country. Brown lung disease or *byssinosis* is irreversible and characterized by shortness of breath, coughing, and wheezing (Levenstein, Delaurier, & Dunn, 2002). Analogously, between 1950 and 1970, the mines were locations where "black choking death was accepted as normal and inevitable" (Caudill, 1976, p. 145). The high-impact machines created inches of dust on the tunnel floors that covered the miners' bodies. Lung disease incapacitated the miners.

Black lung disease (*pneumoconiosis*) is a progressive incurable condition that is characterized by extreme shortness of breath. Additionally, approximately 90% of coal miners over the age of 54 report hearing problems (Murray-Johnson et al., 2004). While coal miners identified that hearing loss is a serious concern and voiced the importance of protective devices, they also reported a greater need for unencumbered hearing while in the mine. It was perceived to be important to remain aware of "roof talk" or noises that warn of the mine ceiling caving in (Murray-Johnson et al., 2004, p. 748). In addition to decreasing noise from the machinery, miners recommended that information be given to miners about decibel noise exposure throughout the mine, ongoing hearing screening services, and public campaigns to increase awareness about the problems and need for prevention to decrease hearing loss.

Death, Dying, and Death Rituals

While there is increasing and considerable diversity, Appalachian death rituals have been well characterized by Crissman (1994) and Sherrod (2005). When death is imminent, a vigil sometimes called a "death watch" is held by family and friends either in the home or, more commonly today, in the hospital. Participants in the vigil often observe for signs of impending death, such as premonitions, visions, and the death rattle. Usually the evening before the funeral, a wake or visitation period is often held at a funeral home or church; this is a time for paying respects to the dead and his or her family and to view the deceased. Funeral services are generally held in funeral homes or churches; these often include prayer, music, scriptural reading, and a sermon or eulogy. Following the funeral service, close mourners may process to the site of internment—sometimes on foot, but more often by car. Today, graves are typically dug by service workers rather than friends. Before the casket is lowered, ministers may preside over a committal service. Graves are often marked with headstones with chiseled writing (name, birth/death dates, and sometimes an epitaph) and sometimes a picture (Crissman, 1994; Sherrod, 2005).

Barriers to Care

Lack of available services; ethnocentric providers; difficult terrain; geographic isolation; cost; and lack of transportation, insurance, and telephones are common barriers to utilization of health care services by Appalachians (Beck, Jijon, & Edwards, 1996; Elnicki, Douglas, Morris, & Shockcor, 1995; Hall, Uhler, Coughlin, & Miller, 2002; Hansen & Resick, 1990).

In rural areas of Appalachia, 67% of the counties are federally designated shortage areas; the proportion of primary care physicians per population is less than half that in the rest of the United States (Barnett, Halverson, Elmes, & Braham, 2000; Friedell, Rubio, Maretzki, et al., 2001). Rural clinic offices are often staffed by single providers with no laboratory support (Hesselgrave, 2001). In one study, most family members indicated they were unable to access primary care physicians because few providers accepted medical cards (Medicaid/Medicare) as payment; further, 80% had no or unreliable transportation (Denham, 1999b). Additionally, the ethnocentrism of many providers and the higher proportion of foreign-trained physicians in underserved areas may deter Appalachians from returning for services (Tripp-Reimer, 1982).

Locus of Control

Appalachians' locus of control has been characterized as fatalistic, with strong roots in fundamentalist religion. Many Appalachians believe that God has control over their lives and that however things turn out, it is the "Lord's will." While most middle-class Americans believe that science can most often control events and health, many Appalachians do not believe that they have control over their future or their health. However, this idea of fatalism is more complex than usually described and may not be related to lack of health efforts. Several studies report that while Appalachians may believe they can't prevent an illness, they have strong self-determination about coping with and managing an illness (Ford, 1967; Hansen & Resick, 1990; Hunsucker, Flannery, & Frank, 2000; Rosswurm, Dent, Armstrong-Persily, Woodburn, & Davis, 1996). This has been termed by Rosswurm et al. (1996) as "adaptive acceptance"

(p. 456). This interpretation fits well with other research indicating a strong sense of self-reliance and inner strength among Appalachians (Burkhardt, 1993).

While Appalachians may not believe they are capable of maintaining their health without God's help, many believe they may be to blame for many chronic illnesses (such as diabetes). Smith and Tessaro (2005) documented that diabetes is often perceived by Appalachians as a self-induced illness, indicating a moral weakness and brought on by "laziness and lack of self discipline" (p. 295). Sometimes, if they believe that nothing can be done about a serious health condition, Appalachians may prefer not be told the diagnosis (Sortet & Banks, 1997). Finally, when hospitalized, Appalachian patients may desire less decisional control than what nurses view as ideal (notably, in this study, physicians and patients preferred about the same level of patient decisional control) (Rosswurm, Dent, Armstrong-Persily, Woodburn, & Davis, 1996).

Additionally, we see variations in reports related to the coping styles of the Appalachians when confronted with critical illnesses of family members. In a study of the critical care coping styles of 30 family members of critically ill patients in two rural Appalachian hospitals, dominant coping styles were supportive, optimistic, confrontive, and self-reliant, with fatalism and evasive styles being ranked much lower (Hunsucker, Flannery, & Frank, 2000). Supportive strategies emphasizing the importance of close personal contacts were key. Action-focused coping centered on seeking information about the problem, handling things one step at a time, and keeping busy.

In contrast to middle-class America's "doing" activity orientation, Appalachians are considered "being" oriented, which means they focus more on interpersonal relationships than on personal accomplishments. In contrast with middle-class individualistic emphasis, Appalachian culture emphasizes the lineal-collateral orientation, indicating that an individual's most significant relationships are with family-related groups, kinship groups, or close neighbors. Many middle-class Americans seek self-actualization through individual accomplishments and autonomously set goals, whereas Appalachians tend to seek fulfillment through kin and neighbor interactions.

The "being" and lineal-collateral orientations, coupled with the present-time orientation, may influence health care practices, promoting a reactive rather than proactive stance. A nurse's initial encounter with an Appalachian client may be an emergency situation, such as a birth.

Appalachian Folk Health System

The Appalachian folk health system encompasses traditional beliefs about how to maintain health; the definition, nature, cause, and treatment of illnesses; traditional remedies; and lay health specialists. Again, many of these elements are in transition.

Beliefs. Illnesses are thought to result from the "will of God," a natural imbalance, or the body's response to personal habits, specific situations, or external exposures, particularly cold weather or "the cold" in general. Lack of "personal care" is an additional cause of illness. It includes (1) keeping the body strong, (2) eating right, and (3) taking fluids (Hansen & Resick, 1990). There are several Appalachian folk illnesses; three are discussed in more detail next.

High Blood. One of the major health concerns of the Appalachian region is the state of the blood. The characteristics of the blood at issue may include whether it is thick or thin, good or bad, and high or low. Among Appalachians, the characteristic of *high* or *low blood* is a measure of blood viscosity and/or increased blood volume rushing to the head. High blood can be caused by diet, particularly pork and rich meats, fatty foods, and salt. These foods increase the viscosity of the blood by thickening it (pork and rich foods) or drying it up (salt). Many believe that emotions (anger, nervousness, stress) contribute to the etiology. Leading symptoms include dizziness, followed by headaches, visual disturbances, red or hot face, nausea, and nervousness.

Treatment focuses on restoring the proper balance so the blood is the right consistency. Keeping calm is thought to prevent a future attack. Some report an astringent (pickle brine, vinegar, Epson salts, garlic) may be an effective treatment; others do not find that (Nations, Camino, & Walker, 1985; Snow, 1976). High blood is distinguished from hypertension, which is a high "tension" or stress state (Nations, Camino, & Walker, 1985).

Nerves. A lay idiom of distress, *nerves* is most often characterized by stressful social situations or events. Symptoms may include disturbed sleep patterns (falling and staying asleep), nervousness, tiredness, abdominal pain, shortness of breath, and anxiety attacks. (Nations, Camino, & Walker, 1985).

Sugar or Sweet Blood. The disorder of *sugar* or *sweet blood* results from the accumulation of sugar particles in the blood through one's life from eating sweet foods. Symptoms include dizziness, visual disturbances, and aching feet. The hazy vision is believed to be caused by the accumulation of sugar particles in the blood, which eventually settle in the eyes. Lay diagnostic signs include bruises that don't heal and having ants attracted to one's urine. Bitter herbs and foods (vinegar, gentian, Cerasee, or aloe teas) may be used to temporarily restore balance (Nations, Camino, & Walker, 1985).

Knowledge of Biomedical Diseases. Particularly in rural Central Appalachia, the level of biomedical health information and knowledge is often very low (Hansen & Resick, 1990). There may be little knowledge of the biomedical explanations for how persons become ill, the complication of pregnancy, or how to prevent cardiovascular illness or diabetes. This unfamiliarity with the biomedical system may explain what has been termed "lack of interest" in the specifics of a biomedical diagnosis or interpreted as "denial" (Hansen & Resick, 1990; Lewis, Messner, & McDowell, 1985; Messner, Lewis, & Webb, 1984).

Medicinal Plants. Herbal remedies used in Appalachia are an integration of remedies derived from three primary sources: (1) American Indians, (2) nineteenth-century standard medical practice, and (3) ancestral practices rooted in Northern Europe. The text *Medicinal Plants and Home Remedies of Appalachia* is an extensive resource. In this book, Boylard (1981) details the medicinal use of 90 plants in Central Appalachia and compares uses of each plant there with use by American Indians, nineteenth-century medical practitioners, and Appalachians in the Southern region. For example, Lycoperdaceae (puffball, devil's puff) spores are used as a hemostat to stop bleeding in all groups. Phytolaccaceae (pokeweed) is used to treat rheumatism by all groups and as a spring tonic in Central and Southern Appalachia. Other common remedies include white pine as an antiseptic, black pine as a cough medicine, ginseng for infant colic and general health, windroot for pleurisy, may apple root for rheumatism, elderberry as a disinfectant, and boneset (fever wort) tea for rheumatism or the flu, all of which have been shown to have some medicinal value (Boylard, 1981). However, the strength of the drugs that are used in home remedies is more variable than that of the drugs used in pharmaceutical preparations (Lewis, Messner, & McDowell, 1985). Herbs and over-the-counter medications may also be used in combination or sequentially.

In this domain, as in most other ethnic communities across the country, there is a shift from home remedies and use of wild medicinal herbs to over-the-counter remedies. This pattern was reported in the research of Denham (1999b), Mullen and Phillips (1998), and Rosswurm, Dent, Armstrong-Persily, Woodburn, & Davis, (1996). Importantly, in the study of ethnomedical beliefs and clinic visits for folk illnesses, over-the-counter therapies were the most commonly used treatment (40%) prior to coming to the clinic. Further, the patients with ethnomedical conditions did not use home remedies or self-treat more than the others who presented only with biomedicine conditions (Nations, Camino, & Walker, 1985).

Chronic illness management often integrates financial exigencies; norms of self-reliance; a preference for "natural" foods, herbs, and vitamins over processed substances such as prescription medications (Smith & Tessaro, 2005). Noted are chromium, garlic, and vitamins to control blood glucose levels.

Lay Practitioners. The Appalachian folk medicine system had a tradition of folk healers commonly referred to as "granny women" and "herb doctors." These folk healers were commonly used because they were accessible, familiar with the culture, and well known to the family; lived in close proximity;

used personalized interactions; and provided accepted remedies. However, lay practitioners are used much less frequently today. In a group of clinic patients in which nearly half reported ethnomedical complaints, only 4% reported consulting a faith healer or other alternative practitioner prior to their clinic visit (Nations, Camino, & Walker, 1985).

Illness and Wellness Behaviors

Risk Behaviors. There are several lifestyle factors that place Appalachians at risk for health problems. These include a diet that is high in fats and carbohydrates, higher use of tobacco, lack of a regular exercise program, low use of seat belts, coal mining–associated hearing loss, and the poorest oral health in the U.S., with the highest rate of toothlessness among elders (Maine Nurse, 2004; Murray-Johnson, Witte, Patel, Orrego, Zuckerman, Maxfield, & Thimons, 2004; Reed, Wineman, & Bechtel, 1995). For example, smoking is initiated earlier and more widely than in the general U.S. population. Although aware of the antismoking lung cancer health campaigns, some Appalachians ignore this information because of personal experiences. They know neighbors who have "smoked all their lives" and do not have lung cancer, and others who never smoked but died of lung cancer or other lung ailments. A higher than United States proportion of Appalachian smokers are in the "Precontemplation" Stage of the transtheoretical model (TTM) of behavior change (Macnee & McCabe, 2004). Recent research by Denham, Meyer, and Toborg (2004) investigated patterns of smoking among Appalachian adolescents in Ohio, Tennessee, and Virginia. They found that (1) the social community in tobacco-growing communities is a significant influence in tobacco use; (2) the family is important among young people in tobacco-growing communities and influences cessation positively and negatively; (3) parental smoking was an influence to smoking; (4) while some parents condone and even facilitate tobacco use by their children, others actively discourage use; and (5) concern for the health of younger brothers and sisters elicits a strongly protective reaction from youth in discussions of health risks related to secondhand smoke (p. 170). Further, smoking is often used to relieve stress and is viewed as positive for weight control and alleviating boredom (Ahijevych, Kuun, Christman, Wood, Browning, & Wewers, 2003). Thus, the benefits of smoking may be perceived to outweigh future health risks (Denham, 1999b).

Health Screening. Appalachian providers and consumers participate less often in preventive health screening programs. In a focus group study of rural Appalachian primary care providers, the perceived barriers to performing cancer screening were as follows (1) provider-perceived patient barriers, including patients' fatalistic view of cancer; religious beliefs; low educational attainment; lack of cancer knowledge; a present, day-to-day orientation; and patients' not considering screening and health prevention a priority, and (2) provider-driven barriers, including a lack of time, lack of screening as part of the regular routine, a lack of provider continuity, and conflicting guidelines. Conversely, consumers' reasons for low participation in accessing preventive and routine health care include a lack of primary and/or specialty care providers, geographic or financial accessibility, long waiting periods for appointments, and level of health knowledge (Denham, 1999b; Elnicki, Douglas, Morris, & Shockcor, et al., 1995; Huttlinger, Schaller-Ayers, & Lawson, 2004). Additionally, a recent study reported considerable knowledge deficits for breast cancer screening and personal risk factors among even well-educated Appalachian women (Leslie et al., 2003).

Another perspective on cancer screening comes from studies reporting high rates of participation by low-income Appalachian women in preventive screening programs (cervical, breast, and rectal screens) when resources (clinics) were geographically and financially available (Reed, Wineman, & Bechtel, 1995). Further, the lack of mammography screening (less than half of the other screens) was largely attributed to lack of availability of those services at the same facilities. Innovative practice settings have demonstrated that Appalachians will use preventive services if they are available, accessible, and affordable (Edwards, Lenz, & East-Odom, 1993). Recent structures, such as Community Coalitions (Garland et al., 2004) and The Appalachian Cancer Network (Lengerich et al., 2004), show particular promise.

Illness Behaviors. When ill, Appalachians expect and receive aid from family members (Hansen & Resick, 1990). In a study of 257 randomly selected rural and urban Appalachian patients in eight hospitals in West Virginia, a significantly larger proportion of rural Appalachians reported that family help would be available at home for recovery. In follow-up interviews, there was generally at least one adult child who was available to assist a parent (Rosswurm, Dent, Armstrong-Persily, Woodburn, & Davis, 1996).

Nations, Camino, and Walker (1985) conducted a study to determine if ethnomedical beliefs and practices play an important role in primary care. In their study, 33 of 73 clients from a rural Appalachian area who presented themselves at a university primary care internal medicine program had 54 ethnomedical complaints. Of the ethnomedical complaints presented, 24.1% were of high blood pressure, 22.2% were of feeling weak and dizzy, 16.7% were of "nerves," 5.6% were of "sugar," and 3.7% were of "falling out." These 33 clients also reported biomedical complaints; the remaining 40 clients had biomedical complaints only, without evidence of ethnomedical complaints. No clients presented ethnomedical complaints alone. In the study, approximately two thirds of the clients consulted laypersons, primarily family members and friends, for their complaints, and at least 70% engaged in self-treatment before any clinical consultation. About 4% consulted a lay specialist. Approximately 130 biomedical complaints were presented and recorded by the clients' physicians; however, none of the 54 ethnomedical complaints was formally recorded. The high incidence of ethnomedical complaints among Appalachians and the failure of physicians to recognize these complaints indicate the need for providers to improve their history-taking skills, particularly regarding ethnomedical illnesses.

Mullen and Phillips (1998) used Giger and Davidhizar's Transcultural Assessment Model to identify six cultural phenomena of interest among Appalachians in southern Ohio. Results indicated that these participants had some characteristics commonly identified as Appalachian, such as strong character, stoic, nonassertive, and strong belief in a Supreme Being. However, they also were found to communicate more openly, have a greater internal locus of control, be more future oriented, use no significant home remedies, be more time-conscientious about appointments, and be more likely to follow medical protocols than the stereotypic view of Appalachians. These findings may reflect the rapid transition occurring in the Appalachian region and provide a caution to practitioners not to forget about the dynamic nature of culture.

Implications for Nursing Care

The traditional Appalachian folk health system is in transition. While some traditional practices remain, others are diminishing. The health beliefs and any herbal therapies should be explored in depth in relation to the current clinical situation. Appalachians have a high need for health information and actively seek information resources. Aiding the client to find an appropriate level of health information is a central function of the nursing role. Folk therapies that are neutral or beneficial should be encouraged. In the case where folk therapies or over-the-counter combinations may prove harmful, the nurse should provide health information in a clear, nonjudgmental manner.

BIOLOGICAL VARIATIONS

Health Disparities

Appalachia is one of the areas in the United States with excess mortality, morbidity, and disability (Geronimus, Bound, Waidmann, Colen, & Steffick, 2001); it has the highest concentration of regional Social Security Administration Disability claims and Supplemental Security Income (SSI) for persons age 18 to 64 (McCoy, Davis, & Hudson, 1994). The disability rates are high largely because of dangerous or toxic occupations, such as mining and textiles; poverty; and insufficient insurance coverage to screen and treat depression, as well as dental, vision, and hearing problems (Huttlinger, Schaller-Ayers, & Lawson, 2004).

Traumatic Injuries. In rural Appalachian Kentucky, males across all age groups have a higher risk for death from traumatic injury (Kerney, 2000). For children in rural Appalachian Kentucky, burns and child abuse were the most frequent cause for traumatic death for children under the age of 1, while motor vehicle accidents accounted for most of the injuries over the age of 1 (Svenson, Spurlock, & Nypaver, 1996). The higher rural death rate was attributed to factors such as decreased access to prehospital care, delayed acute care because of geographic isolation, and the need for provider training in pediatric advanced life support.

Respiratory Tract Diseases. Mortality from tuberculosis among Appalachians is 50% higher than the national average (National Center for Health Statistics, 1993). High-risk occupations, such as in the mining, timber, and textile industries, increase the number of respiratory and other disabling physical health problems. These diseases, such as black lung, are incurable, progressive, and debilitating (Carroll, 1999), contributing to disabilities that are far greater than the national average (McCoy, Davis, & Hudson, 1994). Additionally, tobacco, a local industry, is widely used and contributes to lung disease (Ramey, 1993).

Coronary Artery and Coronary Heart Disease. The incidence of coronary artery disease, coronary heart disease, and mortality from heart disease and stroke among Appalachians exceeds the national average (www.cdc.gov/mmwr/preview/mmwrhtml/055774.htm, retrieved July 22, 2002; Halverson, Barnett & Casper, 2002), especially in the Central and Southern regions of Appalachia (Dzik, 1997; Huttlinger, Schaller-Ayers, & Lawson, 2004; Neal, Demerath, Gonzales, et al., 2001). Ramsey and Glenn (1998) investigated medical records in one poor, underserved, rural Appalachian county in Tennessee. This county of approximately 7000 residents was found to have the highest poverty level in the state, with an unadjusted mortality rate for heart disease of 531.9 per 100,000, compared with the state mean of 318.1 per 100,000. The findings indicated that excessive smoking, lack of exercise, a high-fat diet, and abnormal serum lipid levels were key risk factors associated with heart disease. This supported an earlier study of middle-aged Appalachian women in an isolated county in northeast Tennessee, which identified that past or present smoking, history of lung disease, physical inactivity, obesity, and hypercholesterolemia were health risk factors leading to mortality (Edwards, Shuman, & Glenn, 1996). A relationship was found between the risk factors and low formal education levels, poverty, and limited access to health care. Thus, a better understanding of risk factors through education, more access to health care, and increased resources for adequate diet must all be addressed if heart disease is to be decreased among Appalachians. Neal and colleagues (2001) discuss the Coronary Artery Risk Detection in Appalachian Communities (CARDIAC) and Rural Health Education Partnerships (WVRHEP) currently under development in West Virginia as community-level screening and school-based health promotion programs to influence both children and parental health behavior.

Cancer. While breast cancer rates are lower than the national average, cervical cancer remains higher for both Black and White Appalachian women (Hall, Rogers, Weir, Miller, & Uhler, 2000; Hopenhayn, Bush, Christian, & Shelton, 2005). White women in Appalachia have twice the incidence of cervical cancer than the national average, approaching the national rate for Black women (Erikson, 2001). African-American Appalachians (Newell-Withrow, 2000) were found to be actively engaged in health promotion and prevention. In particular, Fisher and Page (1987) found that women participated in Pap smear health screening if it was convenient, required, or requested. Recently, Huttlinger, Schaller-Ayers, and Lawson (2004) found that a major barrier is the cost that insurance plans will not cover for health screening.

Infant Mortality

The high infant mortality rate, which is 9.3% (U.S. Department of Commerce, Bureau of the Census, 1997), corresponds closely to the level of poverty. Spurlock, Moser, and Flynn (1989) conducted a study to examine differences in postnatal mortalities between the Appalachian portions of Kentucky and the remainder of the state. A key factor related to increased infant mortality in the Appalachian region was maternal education. Three types of postnatal deaths were disproportionately high among infants in the Appalachian region: sudden infant death syndrome, congenital malformations, and infections.

Nutrition

Food patterns in the Appalachian region have been described as "unpretentious, solid, and filling" (Flasher, 2002). Consequently, obesity is a considerable problem among all ages (Demerath et al., 2003). The Appalachian diet tends to be high in fats, carbohydrates, and salt. A wide variety of domestic and wild meats are eaten, and bread is generally served at each meal. Cornbread, biscuits and gravy, fried potatoes, and beans are staple food items (Flasher, 2002; Tribe & Oliveri, 2000).

While little work has been conducted on the provision of nutritional advice to children who are overweight/obese, Demerath et al. (2003) describe the promise and potential of school-based obesity screening and nutritional counseling program—The Coronary Artery Risk Detection in Appalachian Communities (CARDIAC).

SUMMARY

Although access to health care remains problematic, there are community intervention programs and practice models being developed to help address this problem (Baker, McKenzie, & Harrison, 2005; Glisson & Schoenwald, 2005; Huttlinger, Schaller-Ayers, Kenny, & Ayers, 2004). One example of a successful community-based project to increase awareness of remote rural Appalachian health needs and provide access to health care services is the collaborative Remote Area Medical (RAM) project (Huttlinger, Schaller-Ayers, Kenny, & Ayers, 2004). This collaborative project provided primary, dental, and vision health care services to 3310 persons during July and October 2002 in the Wise, Virginia, and Mountain City, Tennessee, areas. Participants reported high satisfaction with each of the events, after driving 1.5–250 miles (Wise attendees) and 0.5–240 miles (Mountain City attendees) to attend. While most of the participants had health insurance, this did not assure affordability of health care. The events did demonstrate the desire and drive to acquire and provide culturally appropriate, consumer-based health care services.

The Appalachian people have a rich heritage, but one that has been in dramatic transition over the past half-century. For generations these beliefs and values were passed down and have persevered. In recent years, some Appalachians, especially the young, have moved to urban areas, and health providers are now more likely to come into contact with Appalachian people through the conventional medical system. When working with persons from the Appalachian region, the nurse can build on some of the positive aspects inherent in the people, such as strength, independence, interdependence, sensitivity, and faith, to foster a therapeutic nurse–client relationship. In addition, knowledge of the traditional health care beliefs and the importance of the family can aid the nurse in giving culturally sensitive, individualized nursing care.

Case Study

Sarah James, an 89-year-old widow who lives alone next door to one of her sons in Sweetwater, Tennessee, is seen at the clinic by the family clinical nurse specialist because she "feels bad." She arrives at the clinic with her three sons and their families, who are concerned because Sarah has been "running off" several times a day and will not eat. The clinical nurse specialist visits "for a spell" and then begins to take a health history. When the clinical nurse specialist asks what has brought Mrs. James to the clinic, the eldest son reveals that Sarah has "run off" six or seven times since yesterday and cannot drink her tea. Also, according to the eldest son, Mrs. James has not recently traveled out of Sweetwater, does not have proper refrigeration, and has recently eaten some "tater" salad that had sat out all day in the hot weather. It is determined that the diarrhea is watery, brown, and nonodorous. Mrs. James has also had dry heaves but has not vomited and does not verbalize symptoms of pain.

Further assessment by the clinical nurse specialist reveals that Mrs. James has generalized weakness, poor skin turgor, dark circles around the eyes, sticky mucous membranes, pale skin, rectal temperature of 101° F, generalized abdominal tenderness, hyperactive bowel sounds, thready but regular heart rate of 100, blood pressure of 110/60 mm Hg, respirations of 24, and weight of 110 pounds.

After a complete physical examination, the clinical nurse specialist orders a stool culture, electrolytes, and a complete blood cell count. After collaboration with the clinic physician, the eldest son approves Mrs. James's admission to the hospital with her entire family in attendance. Mrs. James is crying as she enters the hospital. A diagnosis of dehydration and *Salmonella* poisoning is made. Arrangements are made for follow-up examination after discharge from the hospital.

CARE PLAN

✳ *Nursing Diagnosis: Diarrhea related to infectious processes (salmonella) as a result of inadequate refrigeration of food, as evidenced by six to seven watery brown stools per day*

Client Outcomes
1. Client will exhibit signs of adequate hydration within 24 hours
2. Client will resume normal elimination and peristaltic action within the next 24 to 48 hours.

Nursing Interventions
1. Measure daily weight.
2. Record amount, character, and volume of stools.
3. Record intake and output.
4. Obtain stool culture.
5. Assess pain status.
6. Explain specific reason for problem (that is, lack of refrigeration of potato salad and other foods that need refrigeration).
7. Note results of complete blood count and electrolytes.

✳ Nursing Diagnosis: Communication, impaired verbal, related to cultural differences

Client Outcome

1. Communication will be established between client, nurse, and family to understand health condition and needs.

Nursing Interventions

1. Determine meaning of verbal and nonverbal cues.
2. Establish rapport with client and family.
3. Be aware of cultural factors, such as avoiding eye contact.
4. Communicate with client in an unhurried manner.
5. Communicate in specific terms.
6. Ask client and family for their advice.
7. Avoid criticism and spend extra time with client.
8. Communicate on a first-name basis.

✳ Nursing Diagnosis: Anxiety related to perceived threat of death

Client Outcome

1. Client will show signs of decreased anxiety.

Nursing Interventions

1. Involve family in nursing care.
2. Provide arrangement for one family member to stay during the night.
3. Exhibit a calm and unhurried manner.
4. Reassure client.
5. Be flexible in visiting regulations.
6. Be accepting of client's cultural differences.
7. Explain procedures to client in specific terms.
8. Arrange for a social service worker to visit for planning financial issues.

✳ Nursing Diagnosis: Nutrition, altered: less than body requirements, related to inability to absorb nutrients (diarrhea), as evidenced by absence of food intake for the past 48 hours

Client Outcome

1. Client will consume a balanced diet for body size and maintain present weight before discharge.

Nursing Interventions

1. Monitor weight.
2. Provide nutritionally balanced diet at times client feels like eating.
3. Document food intake.
4. Explain necessity for proper diet in specific terms.
5. Determine what foods she prefers to eat.
6. Encourage rest.

✳STUDY QUESTIONS

1. List some strategies that may help the nurse communicate with an Appalachian family.
2. Describe the significance of the extended family and the roles within the Appalachian family structure.
3. Compare and contrast the differences in illness beliefs between middle-class Americans and Appalachians.
4. Describe the possible importance of home remedies to persons from Appalachian regions.
5. Identify three major barriers to health screening by rural Appalachians.
6. Describe how nurses can aid Appalachian patients in obtaining health information.
7. Indicate resources that health care providers can use to facilitate wellness.
8. List at least three major conditions for which Appalachians are at greater risk than the general U.S. population.

NCLEX-RN REVIEW QUESTIONS

1. While taking a history on an Appalachian patient, Mrs. Brown tells the nurse that she has had "high blood." The competent nurse interprets this to mean the patient has a history of:
   A. Increased low density lipoproteins
   B. Hypercholesterolemia
   C. Hypertension
   D. Hemodilution

2. When an Appalachian client is ill, personal space collapses inwardly. For the nurse providing nursing care, this means:
   A. The person will try to be independent and self sufficient.
   B. The person expects to be waited on and cared for by others.
   C. The person wants to be cared for by the family only.
   D. The person expects that health care decisions will be made by the family.

3. In planning health care screening for rural Appalachians, which of the following would be of least concern for the nurse?
   A. Tuberculosis
   B. Coronary heart disease
   C. Cervical cancer
   D. Breast cancer

References

Ahijevych, I., Kuun, P., Christman, S., Wood, T., Browning, K., & Wewers, M. (2003). Beliefs about tobacco among Appalachian current and former users. *Applied Nursing Research*, 16(2), 93–102.

Appalachian Regional Commission. (2002). *Annual report 1992*. Washington, D.C.: Appalachian Regional Commission.

Baker, G., McKenzie, a., & Harrison, P. (2005). Local physicians caring for their communities: an innovative model to meeting the needs of the uninsured. *North Carolina Medical Journal*, 66(2), 130–133.

Barnett, E., Halverson, J. A., Elmes, G. A., & Braham, V. E. (2000). Metropolitan and non-metropolitan trends in coronary heart disease mortality within Appalachia, 1980–1997. *Annual Epidemiology*, 10, 370–379.

Beck, R. W., Jijon, C. R., & Edwards, J. B. (1996). The relationships among gender, perceived financial barriers to care, and health status in a rural population. *The Journal of Rural Health*, 12(3), 188–196.

Blakeney, A. B. (1987). Appalachian values: implications for occupational therapists. *Occupational Therapy in Health Care*, 4(1), 57–72.

Boylard, J. L. (1981). *Medicinal plants and home remedies of Appalachia*. Springfield, Ill.: Charles Thomas.

Burkhardt, M. (1991). *Exploring understandings of spirituality among women in Appalachia*. Dissertation. Ann Arbor, Mich.: University Microfilms International.

Burkhardt, M. (1993). Characteristics of spirituality in the lives of women in a rural Appalachian community. *Journal of Transcultural Nursing*, 4(2), 12–18.

Calico, F. (1996, October). Home health moving toward "high touch, high tech": Appalachian regional health-care pioneers homecare technology. *Health Management Technology*, 17(11), 22–25, 27.

Carroll, M. (1999). Viewpoint: Appalachian coal miners mutual help and advocacy. *Public Health Reports*, 114, 326–327.

Caudill, H. M. (1976). *The watches of the night*. Boston: Little, Brown.

Crissman, J. K. (1994). *Death and dying in central Appalachia: changing attitudes and practices*. Chicago: University of Illinois Press.

Culture of poverty revisited: a critique by the Mental Health Committee against Racism. (1977). New York: Mental Health Committee against Racism.

Cushing, B. J., & Rogers, C. (1996). *Income and poverty in Appalachia: a report to the Appalachian Regional Commission*. Regional research paper 9511. Morgantown, W.V.: West Virginia University, Regional Research Institute.

Demerath, E., Muratova, V., Spangler, E., Li, J., Minor, V. E., & Neal, W. A. (2003). School-based obesity screening in rural Appalachia. *Preventive Medicine*, 37, 553–560.

Denham, S. (1999a). Epilogue: summary of three studies on family health with Appalachian families. *Journal of Family Nursing*, 5(2), 214.

Denham, S. (1999b). Part III: family health in an economically disadvantaged population. *Journal of Family Nursing*, 5(2), 184–213.

Denham, S. (2002). Family routines: a structural perspective for viewing family health. *Advances of Nursing Science*, 24(4), 60–74.

Denham, S. A., Meyer, M. G., & Toborg, M. A. (2004). Tobacco cessation in adolescent females in Appalachian communities. *Family & Community Health*, 27(2), 170–181.

Denham, S. A., Meyer, M. G., Toborg, M. A., & Mande, M. J. (2004). Providing health education to Appalachia populations. *Holistic Nursing Practice*, 18(6), 293–301.

Dial, W. (1975). The dialect of the Appalachian people. In Maurer, B. (Ed.). *Mountain heritage*. Ripley, W.V.: Mountain State Art and Craft Fair.

Dreher, M., & MacNaughton, N. (2002). Cultural competence in nursing: foundation or fallacy? *Nursing Outlook*, 50(5), 181–186.

Dzik, A. J. (1997). Looking for dangerous places: some aspects of medical geography and disease mapping. *West Virginia Medical Journal*, 93(5), 250–253.

Edwards, J. B., Lenz, C. L., & East-Odom, J. (1993). Nurse-managed primary care: serving a rural Appalachian population. *Family Community Health*, 16(2), 50–56.

Edwards, J. B., Shuman, P., & Glenn, L. L. (1996). Relationships among health risk factors and objective physical findings in well rural Appalachian women. *Family Community Health*, 18(4), 67–80.

Elnicki, D., Douglas, K., Morris, M., & Shockcor, W. (1995). Patient-perceived barriers to preventive health care among indigent, rural Appalachian patients. *Archives of Internal Medicine*, 155(4), 421–424.

Erikson, J. (2001). Cervical cancer in Appalachia focus of study by new NCI Center. *Oncology Times*, 23(5), 46, 51.

Fisher, S., & Page, A. I. (1987). Women and preventive health care: an exploratory study of the use of pap smears in a potentially high-risk Appalachian population. *Women's Health*, 11(3/4), 83–99.

Flasher, W. C. (2002). *Cultural diversity: eating in America*. Columbus: Ohio State University Extension Office.

Ford, T. (1967). The passing of provincialism. In Ford, T. (Ed.). *The southern Appalachian region*. Lexington, Ky.: University of Kentucky Press.

Friedell, G. H., Rubio, A., & Maretzki, A., et al. (2001). Community cancer control in a rural, underserved population: the Appalachian leadership initiative on cancer project. *Journal of Health Care for the Poor and Underserved*, 12(1), 5–19.

Garland, B., Crane, M., Marino, C., Stone-Wiggins, B., Ward, A., & Friedell, G. (2004). Effect of community coalition structure and preparation on the subsequent implementation of cancer control activities. *American Journal of Health Promotion*, 18(6), 424–434.

Geronimus, A. T., Bound, J., Waidmann, T. A., Colen, C. G., & Steffick, D. (2001). Inequality in life expectancy, functional status, and active life expectancy across selected black and white populations in the United States. *Demography*, 38(2), 227–251.

Glisson, C., & Schoenwald, S. (2005). The ARC organizational and community intervention strategy for implementing evidence-based children's mental health treatments. *Mental Health Services Research*, 7(4), 243–259.

Gudykunst, W., & Ting-Toomey, S. (1988). *Culture and interpersonal communication*. Newbury Park, Calif.: Sage.

Hall, E. T. (1989). *Beyond culture*. New York: Anchor Books.

Hall, E. T. (2006). Context and meaning. In Samovar, L., Porter, K., & McDaniel, E. (Eds.), *Intercultural communication: a reader* (pp. 60–70) (ed. 7). Belmont, Calif.: Thomson/Wadsworth.

Hall, H. I., Rogers, J. D., Weir, H. K., Miller, D. S., & Uhler, R. J. (2000). Breast and cervical carcinoma mortality among women in the Appalachian region of the U.S., *Cancer*, 89(7), 1593–1602.

Hall, H. I., Uhler, R. J., Coughlin, S. S., & Miller, D. S. (2002). Breast and cervical cancer screening among Appalachian women. *Cancer Epidemiology, Biomarkers and Prevention*, 11, 137–142.

Halverson, J. A., Barnett, E., & Casper, M. (2002). Geographic disparities in heart disease and stroke mortality among black and white populations in the Appalachian region. *Ethnicity & Disease*, 12(4), S3, 82–91.

Hansen, M. M., & Resick, L. K. (1990). Health beliefs, health care, and rural Appalachian subcultures from an ethnographic perspective. *Family Community Health*, 13(1), 1–10.

Helton, L. (1995, Winter). Intervention with Appalachians: strategies for a culturally specific practice. *Journal of Cultural Diversity*, 2(1), 20–26.

Hesselgrave, B. (2001). Polypharmacy. *Managed Care Quarterly*, 9(4), 9–15.

Hicks, G. (1976). *Appalachian valley*. New York: Holt, Rinehart, & Winston.

Hopenhayn, C., Bush, H., Christian, A., Shelton, B. (2005). Comparative analysis of invasive cervical cancer incidence rates in three Appalachian states. *Preventive Medicine*, 41, 859–864.

Hunsucker, S., Flannery, J., & Frank, D. (2000). Coping strategies of rural families of critically ill patients. *Journal of the American Academy of Nurse Practitioners*, 12(4), 123–127.

Hunsucker, S., Frank, D., & Flannery, J. (1999). Meeting the needs of rural families during critical illness: the APN's role. *Dimensions of Critical Care Nursing*, 18(3), 24–32.

Hurley, J., Turner, S., & Floyd, D. (2000). Development of a health service at a rural community college in Appalachia. *Journal of American College Health*, 48, 181–185.

Huttlinger, K., Schaller-Ayers, J., Kenny, B., & Ayers, J. (2004). Research and collaboration in rural community health. *Online Journal of Rural Nursing and Health Care*, 4(1), [Online]. Retrieved June 15, 2007, from http://www.rno.org/journal/issues/Vol-4/issue-1/Huttlinger_article.htm.

Huttlinger, K, Schaller-Ayers, J, & Lawson, T (2004). Health care in Appalachia: a population-based approach. *Public Health Nursing*, 21(2), 103–110.

Isserman, A. M. (1997). Appalachia then and now: an update of "the realities of deprivation" reported to the President in 1964. *Journal of Appalachian Studies*, 3(4), 43–73.

Jesse, D. E. (2003). Prenatal psychosocial needs: differences between a TennCare group and a privately insured group in Appalachia. *Journal of Health Care for the Poor and Underserved*, 14(4), 535–549.

Jesse, D. E., & Reed, P. G. (2004). Effects of spirituality and psychosocial well-being on health risk behaviors in Appalachian pregnant women. *Journal of Obstetric, Gynecologic, & Neonatal Nursing*, 33(6), 739–747.

Jesse, D. E, Seaver, W., & Wallace, D. (2003). Maternal psychosocial risks predict preterm birth in a group of women from Appalachia. *Midwifery*, 19, 191–202.

Jones, L. (1983). Appalachian values. In Whisnant, D. (Ed.). *All that is native and fine: the politics of culture in an American region*. Chapel Hill: University of North Carolina Press.

Kerney, K. B. (2000). Appalachia: the place, the people, and home care. *Home Health Care Management and Practice*, 12(6), 56–61.

LaFargue, J. P. (1980). A survival strategy: kinship networks. *American Journal of Nursing*, 80(9), 1636–1640.

Lengerich, E. J., Wyatt, S. W., Rubio, A., Beaulieu, J. E., Coyne, C. A., Fleisher, L., Ward, A. J., & Brown, P. K. (2004). The Appalachia Cancer Network: cancer control research among a rural, medically underserved population. *The Journal of Rural Health*, 20(2), 181–187.

Leslie, N. S., Deiriggi, P., Gross, S., DuRant, M. E., Smith, C., & Veshnesky, J. G. (2003). Knowledge, attitudes, and practices surrounding breast cancer screening in educated Appalachian women. *Oncology Nursing Forum*, 30(4), 659–667.

Levenstein, C., DeLaurier, G. F., & Dunn, M. L. (2002). *The cotton dust papers: science, politics, and power in the "discovery" of byssinosis in the U. S..* Amityville, N.Y.: Baywood.

Lewis, S., Messner, R., & McDowell, W. (1985). An unchanging culture. *Journal of Gerontological Nursing*, 11(8), 20–26.

Maas, M. L., Reed, D., & Specht, J. P., et al. (2001). Family involvement in care: negotiated family-staff partnerships in special care units for persons with dementia. In Funk, S. G., Tornquist, E. M., Leeman, J., Miles, M. S., & Harrell, J. S. (Eds.), *Key aspects of preventing and managing chronic illness* (pp. 330–345). New York: Springer Publishing.

MacAvoy, S., & Lippman, D. (2001, July). Teaching culturally competent care: nursing students experience rural Appalachia. *Journal of Transcultural Nursing*, 12(3), 221–227.

Macnee, C. L., & McCabe, S. (2004). The transtheoretical model of behavior change and smokers in Southern Appalachia. *Nursing Research*, 53(4), 243–250.

McCoy, J. L., Davis, M., & Hudson, R. E. (1994). Geographic patterns of disability in the United States. *Social Security Bulletin*, 57(1), 25–26.

Messner, R., Lewis, S., & Webb, D. D. (1984). Unique problems and approaches in Appalachian patients with Crohn's disease. *The Society of Gastrointestinal Assistants Journal*, 7, 38–46.

Mullen, S., & Phillips, C. (1998, April 29–30). Cultural beliefs of southeastern Ohio Appalachians. Proceedings of the fourth Interdisciplinary Health Research Symposium, *1998 Health Care and Culture*, Morgantown, W.V.

Muratova, V. N., Islam, S. S., Demerath, E. W., Minor, V. E., & Neal, W. A. (2001). *Preventive Medicine*, 33, 1–6.

Murdock, G. (1982). *Outline of cultural materials* (ed. 5). New Haven, Conn.: Human Relations Area Files.

Murray, R. B., & Huelskoetter, M. W. (1991). *Psychiatric/ mental health nursing* (ed. 3). East Norwalk, Conn.: Appleton & Lange.

Murray-Johnson, L, Witte, K., Patel, D., Orrego, V., Zuckerman, C, Maxfield, A. M., & Thimons, E. (2004). Using the extended parallel process model to prevent noise-induced hearing loss among coal miners in Appalachia. *Health Education & Behavior*, 31(6), 741–755.

National Center for Health Statistics, Healthy People 2000 Review. (1993). *Health, United States, 1992*. Hyattsville, Md.: U.S. Public Health Service.

Nations, M. K., Camino, L. A., & Walker, F. B. (1985). "Hidden" popular illnesses in primary care: resident's recognition and clinical implications. *Culture, Medicine, and Psychiatry*, 9(3), 223–240.

Neal, W. A., Demerath, E., & Gonzales, E., et al. (2001). Coronary artery risk detection in Appalachian communities (CARDIAC): preliminary findings. *The West Virginia Medical Journal*, 97, 102–105.

Newell-Withrow, C. (2000). Health protecting and health promoting behaviors of African Americans living in Appalachia. *Public Health Nursing*, 17(5), 392–397.

Obermiller, P., & Malong, M. (1994). Living city, feeling country: the current status and future prospects of urban Appalachians. In Borman, K. M., & Obermiller, P. J. (Eds.), *From mountain to metropolis: Appalachian migrants in American cities* (pp. 3–12). Westport, Conn.: Greenwood.

Obermiller, P. J., & Maloney, M. (1990, December). The current status and future prospects of urban Appalachians. *Urban Advocate*, 7.

Penn, E. M., Borman, K. M., & Hoeweler, F. (1994). Echoes from the hill: urban Appalachian youths and educational reform. In Borman, K. M., & Obermiller, P. J. (Eds.), *From mountain to metropolis: Appalachian migrants in American cities* (pp. 83–92). Westport, Conn.: Bergin & Garvey.

Pollard, K. M. (2004). The 1990s: An era of increasing diversity within Appalachia. In Pollard, K. M. (ed.), *A "New Diversity": Race and ethnicity in the Appalachian region* (pp. 5–15). Washington, D.C.: Population Reference Bureau.

President's Appalachian Regional Commission (PARC). (1963). *Appalachia: a report by the President's Appalachian Regional Commission*. Washington, D.C.: U.S. Government Printing Office.

Purnell, L., & Counts, M. (2003). Appalachians. In Purnell, L., & Paulanka, B. (Eds.), *Transcultural health care: a culturally competent approach* (ed. 2). Philadelphia: F. A. Davis.

Ramey, R. (1993, November–December). COPD in rural Appalachia: a model for pulmonary rehabilitation. *Tar Heel Nurse*, 32–35.

Ramsey, P. W., & Glenn, L. L. (1998). Risk factors for heart disease in rural Appalachia. *Family Community Health*, 20(4), 71–82.

Reed, B. W., Wineman, J., & Bechtel, G. A. (1995). Using a health risk appraisal to determine an Appalachian community's health care needs. *Journal of Cultural Diversity*, 2(4), 131–135.

Rosswurm, M., Dent, D., Armstrong-Persily, C., Woodburn, P., & Davis, B. (1996). Illness experiences and health recovery behaviors of patients in Southern Appalachia. *Western Journal of Nursing Research*, 18(4), 441–459.

Rowles, G. D. (1983). Between worlds: a relocation dilemma for the Appalachian elderly. *International Journal of Aging Human Development*, 17(4), 301–314.

Rowles, G. D. (1991). Beyond performance: being in place as a component of occupational therapy. *The American Journal of Occupational Therapy*, 45(3), 265–271.

Rowles, G. D. (2000). Habituation and being in place. *The Occupational Therapy Journal of Research*, 20, 52S–67S.

Sherrod, M. (2005). Remembering the dead, comforting the living: adapting Christian ministry to Appalachian death practices. In Keefe, S. E. (Ed.), *Appalachian cultural competency: a guide for medical, mental health, and social service professionals* (pp. 89–113). Knoxville, Tenn.: The University of Tennessee Press.

Simon, J. M. (1987). Health care of the elderly in Appalachia. *Journal of Gerontological Nursing*, 13(7), 32–35.

Simpkins, O. (1979). Appalachian culture. In Maurer, B. (Ed.). *Rural and Appalachian health* Springfield, Ill.: Charles C. Thomas, Publisher.

Simpson, M. R., & King, M. G. (1999). "God brought all these churches together": issues in developing religion-health partnerships in an Appalachian community. *Public Health Nursing*, 16(1), 41–49.

Smith, S. L., & Tessaro, I. A. (2005). Cultural perspectives on diabetes in an Appalachian population. *American Journal of Health Behavior*, 29(4), 291–301.

Snow, L. (1976). High blood is not high blood pressure. *Urban Health*, 5, 4–55.

Sortet, J. P., & Banks, S. R. (1997). Health beliefs of rural Appalachian women and the practice of breast self-examination. *Cancer Nursing*, 20(4), 231–235.

Specht, J. P., Kelley, L. S., Manion, P., et al. (2000). Who's the boss? Family/staff partnership in care of persons with dementia. *Nursing Administration Quarterly*, 24 (3), 64–77.

Spurlock, C. W., Moser, M., & Flynn, L. J. (1989). Regional differences in death rates among postneonatal infants in Kentucky, 1982–1985. *Journal of the Kentucky Medical Association*, 87(3), 119.

Svenson, J. E., Spurlock, C., & Nypaver, M. (1996). Factors associated with the higher traumatic death rate among rural children. *Annals of Emergency Medicine*, 27(5), 625–632.

Tribe, D. I., & Oliveri, C. S. (2000). *Changing Appalachian foodways: perceived changes and rationale for food habits of Appalachian Ohioans*. Columbus: Ohio State University Extension Office.

Tripp-Reimer, T. (1980). Appalachian health care: from research to practice. *Transcultural Nursing Care*, 5, 48–59.

Tripp-Reimer, T. (1982). Barriers to health care: variations in interpretation of Appalachian client behavior by Appalachian and non-Appalachian health professionals. *Western Journal of Nursing Research*, 4(2), 179–191.

Tripp-Reimer, T., & Fox, S. S. (2001). Beyond the concept of culture: or, how knowing the cultural formula does not predict clinical success. In McCloskey, J., & Grace, H. (Eds.), *Current issues in nursing* (ed. 6) St. Louis: Mosby.

Tripp-Reimer, T., & Friedl, M. C. (1977). Appalachians: a neglected minority. *Nursing Clinics of North America*, 12(1), 41–54.

U.S. Department of Commerce, Bureau of Census. (2002). *Population profiles by age, sex, race, and Hispanic origin, Summary File 3*. Washington, D.C.: U.S. Government Printing Office.

U.S. Department of Labor. (2002). *Labor profiles of the United States: 2001*. Washington, D.C.: U.S. Government Printing Office.

Wallace, D. C., Tuck, I., Boland, C. S., & Witucki, J. M. (2002). Client perceptions of parish nursing. *Public Health Nursing*, 19(2), 128–135.

CHAPTER 12 American Eskimos: The Yup'ik and Inupiat

Ruth Elaine Davidhizar and Tina D. DeLapp

Behavioral Objectives

After reading this chapter, the nurse will be able to:

1. Understand verbal and nonverbal communication barriers that may affect health care for the Yup'ik and Inupiat.
2. Describe values related to space that may be found among the Yup'ik and Inupiat.
3. Discuss the value and role of elders for the Yup'ik and Inupiat.
4. Explain how traditional time orientation may affect compliance with a health regimen for the Yup'ik and Inupiat.
5. Discuss attitudes and beliefs of the Yup'ik and Inupiat that relate to health and illness.
6. Identify the shift in health and illness patterns as persons of Eskimo descent have adopted the Western diet and lifestyle.

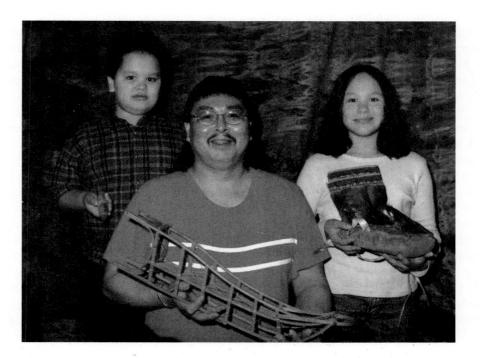

Acknowledgment

Special appreciation is noted to Dolly Lefever and Dr. Nancy Sanders for their contributions to this chapter.

Settlements of Eskimos are found in diverse locations, including the northern territories of Canada, Alaska, Russia, and Greenland. Although Eskimos may be found throughout the world, this chapter focuses on Alaskan Yup'ik and Inupiat who have remained in their native land and those who have migrated to the mainland United States. To provide culturally appropriate nursing care, it is necessary for the nurse to understand the culture and heritage of the Eskimo people.

OVERVIEW OF ALASKA

The Land

Alaska is often described in superlatives. One fifth the size of the continental United States, Alaska has more coastline than the other 49 states combined and is by far the largest state in the continental United States. With a land area of 570,374 square miles, it is more than twice the size of Texas. Everything in Alaska appears to be on a grand scale. It is the home of the largest mountain in North America, Mount Denali (Mount McKinley), which rises to a height of 20,320 feet and is joined by six other peaks that are over 14,500 feet high. Furthermore, Alaska also is the home of Malaspina, a great glacier that is larger than Rhode Island. There are more than 100,000 glaciers in Alaska, and these generally cover more than 28,000 square feet each, providing Alaska with 125 times more glacier area than the rest of the United States combined (*World Almanac and Book of Facts*, 2006). Alaska is a land where great brown bears, polar bears, and other wild animals roam relatively undisturbed (Castagno, 2005).

The chief influences on the climate in Alaska are its northern latitude, its large landmass, and its coastal waters. In the southern part of Alaska, the climate is temperate and damp because of the influence of the warm marine currents. The resulting spruce rain forests can be found on Kodiak Island and in the southern panhandle of Alaska. On the Aleutian Islands, where the climate is also temperate, grasses and shrubs predominate.

The interior of Alaska is bordered on the north by the Brooks Range, on the south by the Alaska Range, and on the west by Arctic environment of the coast. The boreal forests of the interior consist of "relatively small specimens of white and black spruce, alder, birch and aspen that covers most of the rolling hills" (Langdon, 1987, p. 6). The river drainages are marshy and flat. They attract many species of waterfowl important to the Athapaskans who live in this area. The temperature in the interior of Alaska varies dramatically from lows of $-50°$ F in the winter to greater than $90°$ F in the summer.

The area along the western coast of Alaska from Bristol Bay to the border of Alaska and Canada in a 200-mile-wide band is the Arctic region (Langdon, 1987). This area is also drained by the Yukon and Kuskokwim rivers and their tributaries. It is in this area that Eskimos live. The Inupiats live in the northern section from the Seward Peninsula north to the Canadian border. Yup'iks live south of the Seward Peninsula to Bristol Bay in southwestern Alaska, both along the coast and inland along the Yukon and Kuskokwim Rivers. Winters in this area are long, and summers are short and cool.

Because of its northern latitude, an unusual feature of Alaska's terrain is permafrost, or permanently frozen ground. In the Arctic region, continuous permafrost underlies surface dirt in depths of about 2000 feet. Some buildings and highways have been erected on permafrost. This has created some problems because, as the permafrost thaws, the structures may sink. In regions where there is permafrost, aboveground cemeteries are commonplace.

Annual snowfall over most of the subarctic is light, often no more than 4 to 6 inches, and actual snowstorms are rare. Ground blizzards frequently occur in coastal areas, however, where most settlements are located. High winds and a furious swirling of dry snow already on the ground often persist for days and are commonly referred to as a *blizzard*. The windchill factor, $-1°$ F for every 1 mph in winter, causes rapid skin freezing (Morris, 1985).

Alaska has 33,000 miles of coastline (*Time Almanac with Information Please*, 2006; Langdon, 1987). Migratory marine mammals (walrus, seals, and whales), fish (particularly salmon), and birds return to Alaska in the summer to give birth to their offspring. The Bering Sea, the Yukon and Kuskokwim Rivers and their tributaries, and the migratory bird nesting areas make the hunting and fishing resources an important source of subsistence food for the Alaskan Native population, including the Yup'ik and the Inupiat Eskimos (Langdon, 1987). In many smaller rural villages, few income-generating opportunities exist and subsistence activities are crucial for survival.

For many years the Eskimos have claimed that certain lands belong to them. Nevertheless, these claims were ignored. In the former Soviet Union, Eskimo communities near and on the Bering Strait were moved inland to limit contact with the communities in Alaska. In the late 1980s, as relationships improved between the United States and the Soviet Union, friends and relatives across the Bering Sea were reunited and visits have continued (Garrett, 1988). In Alaska the American government has recognized the right of Eskimos to their traditional lifestyle, and a part of the Alaska Native Land Settlement was set aside for them. Today in Alaska 16 villages are united in the Bering Strait Native Corporation. The Inupiat Eskimos, who currently hold title to 92,000 acres of land in Alaska's Arctic National Wildlife Refuge (ANWR), are actively involved in lobbying against environmental groups for oil exploration, which is estimated would create more than 735,000 jobs across the United States. Environmentalists argue that while other Alaskan oil projects have not harmed the region's polar bears and caribou, this project could threaten the species (Freddoso, 2002).

OVERVIEW OF THE PEOPLE

Archeologists believe that the ancestors of the Eskimos came across the Bering Strait from Asia about 30,000 years ago (Haggett, 2002). A genetic study of Eskimos of five populations by Schanfield, Crawford, Dossetor, and Gershowitz (1990) suggests that at least four separate migrant groups crossed the Bering Strait at various times. For centuries, the native people of Alaska lived in isolated regions and were undisturbed by outside cultures.

Archeologists have estimated that during the period from 1750 to 1800, 48,000 Eskimos lived along the Arctic region of North America. Nearly one half (26,000) lived in the area now known as Alaska. Approximately two fifths of these early Alaskans spoke Yup'ik. These Eskimos lived in southwestern Alaska, with the Yukon River as the natural dividing line between this group and the more northern coastal Inupiat (Milan, 1980). In the eighteenth century, certain areas of Alaska were among the most densely populated in the New World, and it is estimated that the Eskimo population numbered 100,000 (Morris, 1985).

With the purchase of Alaska from Russia by the United States in 1867, the population began to undergo significant change. Beginning in 1883, missionaries began to convert the Alaska Native population to Christianity and introduced limited health services (Nord, 1995). In the early 1900s, outsiders discovered the wealth of Alaska's natural resources, and the long-undisturbed culture of the natives in the rural areas came face to face with elements of the Western culture brought by Alaska's new occupants, the "outsiders." Not only did the outsiders bring Western culture but also they brought exposure to diseases, including smallpox, influenza, hepatitis, and measles, to which the native people had no immunity (Morris, 1985). Epidemics killed thousands of the native people.

The gold rushes in the early 1900s brought miners and their families. In the 1940s and 1950s, military personnel came to Alaska because of its strategic geographical location. Between 1941 and 1945 over $1 billion was pumped into Alaska by the federal government to develop transportation systems: the railroad, highways, airfields, docks, and breakwaters. The most recent influx of Westerners arrived after 1968, when a large oil and gas reservoir estimated to be twice as large of any other oil field in North America was found near Anchorage, Alaska. The 800-mile Trans-Alaskan pipeline was completed in 1977 at a cost of $7.7 million (*Time Almanac with Information Please*, 2007). The pipeline is so revered in the northern state that some Alaskans even refer to it as America's Great Wall of China (Brown, 1997).

Today, Alaska has a diverse population. The 2000 Census found 634,892 people residing in Alaska (U.S. Department of Commerce, Bureau of the Census, 2002). Of this number, 69.3% were White, 3.5% were Black, 15.6% were Alaska Native or American Indian, 4.5% were Asian or Pacific Islander, and 4.1% were Hispanic (U.S. Department of Commerce, Bureau of the Census, Summary File 3, 2002). In 2000, Eskimo was the largest Alaska Native tribal grouping reported in the census (U.S. Department of Commerce, Bureau of the Census, 2002). A distinction between Inupiat Eskimos and Yup'ik Eskimos, however, was not made on the census form. According to the 2000 Census, the number of Alaska Natives in Alaska was 85,698 (15.6% of the Alaskan population) (U.S. Department of Commerce, Bureau of the Census, Summary File 3, 2002). The indigenous population, who are often referred to as *Alaska Natives*, is divided culturally and linguistically into five major groupings: Interior Indians (Athapascans), Aleuts, Southeast Coastal Indians (Tlingit and Haida), Northern Eskimos (Inupiat), and Southern Eskimos (Yup'ik) (*Time Almanac with Information Please*, 2006; Langdon, 1987). The median age for all Alaska Natives as of 2002 was 23.6 years, compared with the median age of the Alaska population of 32.4 years and the U.S. median age of 35.3 years for all races (Indian Health Service, 2002). Although Alaska Natives are a young population, their life expectancy at birth is 69.2 years, compared with 76.7 years for U.S. people of all races and 74.7 years for all Alaskans (Indian Health Service, 2002).

Unemployment in Alaska in February 2006 was 7%, ranking number 1 in the nation (U.S. Department of Labor, 2006). Further, among Alaska Native males and females over 16 years of age, 27.3% and 16.1%, respectively, are unemployed. Thus, adult Alaska Native males experience unemployment rates that are four times higher than the national average of 6.4% among females, the proportion of unemployed adults is more than two and a half times the national average of 6.2% (Indian Health Service, 1996). A total of 24% of Alaska Natives live below the poverty level (1.8 times the overall national average of 13.1%). In Alaska, there are 103.2 males to every 100 females, with the rate among the native population being about 50% (*World Almanac and Book of Facts*, 2006).

CULTURE AND HERITAGE OF THE ESKIMOS

The word Eskimo is from the French *esquimau(x)*, possibly from *eskimot*, an Algonquian word meaning "eater of raw flesh," but this word has now been found to have been first applied to the Algonquian Micmacs of the Gaspé Peninsula because it meant "speaking the language of a foreign land" (Mailhot, 1978) or possibly "snowshoe-netter" (*Random House Dictionary of the English Language*, 1987). Some Eskimos believe the "eaters of raw flesh" attribution puts them in a poor light with modern audiences and prefer that "Yup'ip" and "Inupiat" be used instead (American Native Heritage Center, 2006; Chance, 1990).

Although some customs, traditions, and heritage are shared among Alaska Native groups, these groups have traditionally been enemies. Disputes over territorial rights to land or game resulted in the development of an animosity that has been carried on through the generations. For example, it has been reported that some Eskimo parents caution their children to stay near their village to avoid being "carried off by the Indians" (Holderman, 2006). These superstitions are kept alive through the retelling of tales, and when things are missing from an Eskimo village, "the Indians" are blamed (Damas, 1984; Hall, 1975; Holderman, 1960; Morris, 1985).

The Eskimo people, more than any other native Alaskans, have managed to preserve artifacts as well as many interesting and unique native customs. Artifacts of the Eskimo can be found in various museums, such as a museum outside Ketchikan at the White Salmon Falls Resort. The public can see a 1300-piece collection that includes Native basketry, Native trade beads, ivory, miniature kayaks, moccasins, 3-foot canoes, masks, furs, totems, and a Chilkat blanket from the early 1800s (Saari, 1997). However, the traditional way of life is changing for the Eskimo as they become assimilated into the dominant culture, take on mechanical trades, and move away from reliance on the land. Young Eskimos are leaving the villages to go away to school and are returning with new knowledge of the outside world. Some do not return (Hinsley, 2001).

The Eskimo people have lived in the harsh and frigid regions of western and southwestern Alaska. Until recently, parkas and footgear (*mukluks*) made of animal skins were worn to survive the temperature, wind, and blizzards (Gall, 1998). To survive in this frozen, non–crop-producing region, the Eskimos have hunted, fished, trapped, and gathered food on the tundra. Thus the dietary mainstay of the people traditionally consisted mainly of wild meat, such as caribou, and seafood, such as seal, fish, and whale. A century ago the government brought reindeer to Alaska from Russia and Scandinavia in an effort to improve the meat supply. Only the Eskimos were allowed to own reindeer, and it proved a successful addition to the local diet (Loshbaugh, 1996). However, commercial ranching has remained small. Today, there are only eight reindeer herders and a couple of Native corporations that own herds (Loshbaugh, 1996).

Traditionally, dog teams were used for traveling, but this is no longer common. When dog teams were used, they had to be chained to reduce the risk of catching rabies from Arctic foxes. One tradition that remains from dogsled days is the annual Iditarod Trail sled dog race across Alaska to Nome. However, this is one tradition of the Natives that has almost entirely been taken over by non-Natives who can afford to pay the high cost of competition, estimated to be at least $30,000 (Rosen, 1997). Although animal rights activists annually oppose the race, it is a special event for many Alaskans and is promoted around the world as a tourist attraction (Giblin, 1997; Rosen, 1997). Today, many Eskimos use "snow machines" for transportation, especially in rural areas. Dogs are slower than snow machines, but they run on cheap fish rather than expensive gasoline, and in a crisis an Eskimo could eat a dog. Dogs will always get you there; snow machines break down. On the other hand, snow machines travel up to 40 miles per hour and require no driver's license. Unfortunately, when children drive snow machines, accidents often occur

(Holderman, 2006). Also frequently used throughout rural Alaska are all-terrain vehicles (ATVs), commonly know as three- or four-wheelers. ATVs are usable year-round and have been implicated in the causation of many deaths and serious injuries of children and young adults.

Traditionally, kayaking served as water transportation, and whaling was an important component of the economy for most Eskimos who lived near the ocean (Lubbock, 1937; Newberg, 1997; Stefansson, 1969). Today, whaling can still be found along the northern coastlines. Some Yup'ik Eskimos in the Delta region subsist on salmon, seal, migratory birds, and eggs. The popular Eskimo "blanket toss game" originated from the lofting of a member of the tribe as high as possible above flat terrain to look seaward to spot whales. When a whale was spotted, open sealskin boats called *umiaks* were outfitted with paddles, bailers, and harpoons and launched from the shore. Great knowledge and skill were required to harpoon a whale and tow it back to shore, where the entire village participated in butchering the beast. Today *umiaks* have been replaced with outboard motorboats. Life jackets are not used because the sea temperature is near freezing and causes rapid death by fibrillation. The benefit of wearing a life jacket is that it aids efforts to find the body later. Eskimos usually do not know how to swim because the water is too cold for learning purposes (Holderman, 2006).

Eskimos traditionally have been noted for their honesty. For example, if a piece of driftwood were turned in a position in which it would not have washed ashore, others would know it had been claimed and would not take it (Holderman, 2006). The concept of sharing is deeply ingrained among American Indians, who hold it in greater esteem than the White American ethic of saving (Lange, 1988; Lewis & Ho, 1975). In the Northwest culture area, primarily among Indians, the *potlatch*, a festive gathering of friends and neighbors, would involve sharing not only food but also blankets and other useful items (Jilek-Aall, 1981).

It is a popular misconception that most Eskimos live in dome-shaped ice-block shelters called igloos. In fact, these shelters were used primarily as emergency bivouacs by the Canadian Eskimos. The early Alaskan Eskimos lived in dwellings that were partially underground and covered with sod. Both the ice igloo and the sod huts had long, dipped tunnels as entrances so that the cold air, which is heavier, was caught in a natural trap, thus permitting the interior of the hut to be heated more easily. However with the passage of the Alaska Native Claims Settlement act (ANCSA) in 1971, rapid and continuing change has occurred in many Alaskan Native villages (Wind, Sickle, & Wright, 2004). Today, houses are constructed of wood frames in small villages that are scattered widely along the coast and major river systems (Pollick, 1997). Houses are heated with fuel oil or wood and may have water storage tanks that allow running water as well as sewage storage tanks; both require regular servicing, with water tanks being filled periodically and sewage tanks being emptied at regular intervals.

Originally, "honeybuckets" were used for sewage disposal. Later, honeybuckets became black polyethylene bags that, when full, were tied and thrown outside the door to be collected and transported to a dump outside the village (Fienup-Riordan, 2001). Today, because of government projects, many of the larger villages have a sewage treatment plant that includes a piping system where central water tanks supply water to houses by plastic pipe, and raw sewage is piped out to sewage holding and treatment areas. Some houses even have flush toilets. However, winter temperatures play havoc with such systems because of frozen lines. Consequently, during the winter months the old honeybucket system may still be found in larger villages. In the Yukon Delta regions, where it is extremely cold, the honeybucket collection is still an important part of village life. Permanent villages range in population from 20 to 1000 persons, with an average of 400 persons. Most of these villages share community water supplies, electricity, churches, stores, and irregular mail service by airplane.

The social disorganization and cultural conflict that accompanied the rapid changes among Eskimos contributed to increased health risks for all ages of Eskimos, just as living in remote areas, severe climate, harsh terrain, subsistence, and

primitive lifestyle have (Taylor, 1988). According to the Indian Health Service, from 1994 to 1996 the three leading causes of death among Alaska Natives (all groups) were accidents (18.3%), heart disease (18%), and cancer (17.9%). Nationally, in 1995 accidents accounted for only 4% of deaths, whereas heart disease (31.9%) and cancer (23.3%) were the two leading causes of death (Regional Differences in Indian Health, 1998–1999).

Nationwide, one of three children has had a serious injury. The average figure for Alaska is higher than this. Injuries are the major cause of hospitalization within the Alaska Area Native Health Services Unit (Taylor, 1988). Jackson (2000) noted that American Indians and Alaska Natives have the highest rate of reported disability of any racial or ethnic group in the United States. In 1998–1999, 63% of American Indians and Alaska Natives age 65 and older reported having a disability, with 52% reporting a severe disability. This compares with 52.5% of the general population of that age and 33.4% who report severe disability (U.S. Department of Commerce, Bureau of the Census, Summary File 3, 2002). Alaska Native elders constitute a major risk group for poor health, chronic disease, high medical expenditures, and institutionalization (National Center for Health Statistics, 2002; Jackson, 2000). Death by violence has increased significantly among Alaska Natives, whose rate of suicide, frequently related to alcohol and self-inflicted gunshot wounds, is three times that of the general U.S. population (Kost-Grant, 1983; National Center for Health Statistics, 2002; U.S. Department of Health and Human Services, Indian Health Services, 2000a and 2000b). American Indian–Alaska Native adolescents show high rates of health-compromising behaviors and risk factors related to unintentional injury, substance use, poor self-assessed health status, and emotional distress (Blum, 1992). Even infants have an unusually high death rate in Alaska; from 1994 to 1996, the infant death rate among Alaska Natives was 9.1 per 1000 lives births, compared with a U.S. rate of 7.6 (Regional Differences in Indian Health, 1998–1999). Rates of sudden infant death syndrome, accidents and injuries, fetal alcohol syndrome, and infectious disease exceed those for the United States (Fleshman, 1992; Regional Differences in Indian Health, 1998–1999).

Over the years the Indian Health Service has targeted specific health problems, such as the high rate of maternal and child health problems, with specific programs. In 1984, Alaska was one of 10 states to receive a Child and Adolescent Service System Program to improve state services for troubled youth (VanDenberg & Minton, 1987). An Indian Health Service work group on aging was established in 1991 to plan strategies for helping aging Alaska Natives through the year 2000 (National Center for Health Statistics, 1993). The Indian Health Service (IHS) has endeavored to bring general health services to the small villages. For many years, because of the remoteness of the villages, the Indian Health Service Bureau has sponsored regular clinics in each village, which were staffed by a community health nurse who traveled to the villages by air or dogsled. In 1999, a total of 170 Alaskan village health clinics were identified, as well as an increasing number of dental services (U.S. Department of Health and Human Services, Indian Health Services, 2001b). Areas not served by clinics with on-site staff have field nurses who make rounds by airplane and have replaced the former system. In some places, teachers from the lower 49 states and native, trained health aides were the only health service available to give antibiotics, pull teeth, deliver babies, and handle both major and minor medical emergencies (Holderman, 1962, 1993; Lancaster, 1990; Ross, 1989; U.S. Department of Health and Human Services, Indian Health Services, 1992; 2000a and 2000b). The level of care provided by the village health aides, in consultation with physicians located in regional field hospitals, has increased substantially in recent years; most recently telemedicine technology has been used with success throughout the regions occupied by Yup'iks and Inupiats. In fact, injury rates declined from 1979 to 1998 (Day & Lanier, 2003).

Until recently, medical care was provided to Yup'iks and Inupiats by the United States IHS, as a treaty right. Doctors assigned to the IHS hospitals in Bethel, Nome, Kotzebue, and Barrow, and the Alaska Native Medical Center in Anchorage provided in-patient and outpatient care. The doctors also traveled at least one time per year to the villages where most Yup'ik and Inupiat people live to provide medical care. After the Alaska Native Claims Settlement Act (ANCSA), nonprofit health corporations of the regional (for-profit) Native corporations established programs to work on many health concerns (Dixon, 1998, 2001; Wiggins, 1996). In 1999, the health care of Alaska Natives came under the control of the health corporations. This was accomplished through the Alaska Tribal Health Compact, a self-governance agreement with the Indian Health Service (Alaska Native Tribal Health Consortium). In the rural areas, the regional hospitals and clinics are managed by the health corporations. In Anchorage, the Alaska Native Tribal Health Consortium, a body of tribal organizations, manages the Alaska Native Medical Center, a new state-of-the-art comprehensive medical facility. In this way, decisions about how to allocate funds are made by the Alaska Native recipients, which allows direct input into the prioritization of health concerns to be addressed.

In addition, the State of Alaska provides preventive health services by means of public health nurses who travel to each village at least two times per year. Over time, a system of health care using indigenous residents located in each village was instituted by the Indian Health Service. These "health aides" work in conjunction with the IHS doctors through the regional hospitals by using standing orders and consulting with the doctors via telephone. All of these approaches to the provision of health care are within the Western biomedical paradigm.

COMMUNICATION

Language

Although some authorities have related the language of persons native to the Arctic to the Athapaskan or Algonquian language groups (Szathmary, 1984), others have found the Eskimo language or Eskimoan to be a unique language. Eskimoan is a difficult language because one word is often used to express a whole sentence. Originally the Eskimo language had no written forms; thus the recounting of events in story form and in dance provided the only record of Eskimo life. Today a phonetically written form of the Eskimo language that was developed by missionaries exists and is being refined at the Alaska Native Language Center on the University of Alaska Fairbanks campus. The early missionaries and educators demanded that the Eskimo people learn English, which has now become the primary language of the younger generation of Eskimos. A few school systems have initiated bilingual study programs as a direct result of the desire of Eskimos to preserve the Eskimo heritage.

In the oral language spoken by Eskimos, present-time oriented actions are communicated with the Eskimos referring to themselves, as well as others, in the third person. For example, when referring to himself or herself, an Eskimo person would say, "Someone is going hunting" or "Someone is hungry." There is no terminology recognizing the future or vocabulary to discuss abstract concepts; language is used to describe action occurring in the present (Vaudrin, 1974). Unlike children learning English, who learn the passive structure of the language later, children learning *Inuktitut* (one dialect of the Eskimo language) learn a simple and complex form of passive vocabulary very early in language development (Allen & Crago, 1996).

In the past, each person in the Eskimo culture had a defined role in the group; therefore, the anticipation of each person's action required little verbal communication. With the desire to be accepted by incoming Westerners, the Eskimo people learned to speak simple English. Idioms, abstract ideas, and double-meaning phrases were not understood in early acculturation (Vaudrin,1974). However, with English as a primary language of the young people and with the exposure to the world by means of satellite television and education, idioms and abstract ideas have begun to have meaning. Still, the nurse who cares for Eskimo clients from the bush or remote areas should avoid the extensive use of idioms, such as "a bull in a china shop," "out in left field," or "robbing Peter to pay Paul," because such idioms may lack meaning.

The language of the Eskimo people reflects their dominant concerns and interests. Certain words take on a more significant meaning than other words do. Because Alaska for the most part is a land of snow and ice, these words take on a more significant meaning. For example, there are three different words for snow for which there are no single-word equivalents in the English language. Different words are used for falling snow, soft snow on the ground, and drifting snow. Another important word for the Eskimo is ice. Again, different words describe freshwater ice, saltwater ice, and icebergs because ice also serves different and important purposes in these cultures (Armstrong, Roberts, & Swithinbank, 1973; Holderman, 2006).

For the older generation, English is the second language. Thus, when one is speaking to an older person, comprehension can be facilitated by speaking slowly and in literal terms. Children who know only English may have trouble communicating with their grandparents who know only Eskimo (Taylor, 1988). Translators may be helpful, but it is important to remember that the Eskimo language has no translation for the future or for abstract ideas. When providing care to an Eskimo client, the nurse should provide an explanation about specific therapeutic interventions both in English and, if a translator is available, in Eskimo (Glassetter, 1989). The need for a trained medical translator fluent in the Eskimo language of the patient cannot be overemphasized, especially when working with elders.

Use of Silence

Eskimos tolerate periods of silence more easily than people in Western society do (Kleinfeld, 1971). In fact, it is considered rude to fill silences with chatter because such chatter only prevents one from having the space to express viewpoints. The perceived Western intolerance of silence serves to increase the Eskimo's feelings of being dominated and inferior (Kleinfeld, 1971; Vaudrin, 1974). Traditionally in Eskimo culture, each adult is given the opportunity to express a viewpoint without a time limit. For example, an Eskimo may go to see a White person for some reason and just sit in silence for many minutes before saying why he or she has come (Holderman, 2006). However, individuals in Western society may be insensitive to this mode of communication and interpret silence as nonparticipation or passive acceptance. Generally, Eskimos are a polite people who are unlikely to criticize other people's opinions and actions unless such actions cause a threat to the social group. There appears to be a proscription against verbal expression of negative effect (Kost-Grant, 1983). In dealing with people in Western society, the younger generation of Eskimos has for the most part adopted Western ways, which includes becoming more verbal.

Touch

There is a wide range of acceptable open demonstration of affection displayed in public among various subgroups in the Eskimo culture. However, the handshake is considered universally acceptable and a mandatory politeness. Hugging is an acceptable greeting between family members and between women friends. Eskimo men are more reserved in their expressions of affection, using a handshake with only one movement, not up and down, as a common way to greet friends and family (Glassetter, 1989).

Traditional Eskimos are very modest about exposing the body, and it is often difficult to persuade older Eskimo people to undergo complete physical examinations, particularly for diagnostic purposes. The nurse who cares for Eskimo clients needs to establish a trust relationship before diagnostic examinations will be allowed. In the presence of pain and illness, however, there is less resistance to physical examination (Schaefer, 1973).

The late Eskimo healer Della Keats healed many people through the use of manipulation, bloodletting, and love (Book, Dixon, & Kirchner, 1983; Dixon & Kirchner, 1982; Juul, 1979; Keats, 1985). According to Keats, she inherited the skill of her hands and learned the use of herbs for healing from her mother and other Eskimo elders. Through love, touch, and a combination of old and new medicines, Keats reportedly healed her people (Pender, 1987). The older Eskimo people give credence to the power of touch as a direct result of a shaman's healing powers (Glassetter, 1989). Shamanism, a belief that a person holds supernatural powers, still exists among the Inupiat and Yup'ik of Alaska but is not openly discussed, especially with non-Eskimos.

Kinesics

Eskimos use nonverbal communication extensively through body posture and facial expression (Albert, 1988; Boas, 1983). Years of watching animal behavior for survival needs have made the Eskimo people experts in the interpretation of nonverbal language. The nurse who understands the Eskimo culture will look for nonverbal clues, such as watching the face for raised eyebrows or blinking (indicating "yes") or a wrinkled nose (indicating "no"). Eskimos seldom disagree publicly with others. Although smiles and head nods in the Western culture may indicate agreement, in the Eskimo culture they may simply acknowledge the other person's words. Among Eskimos, actual agreement is determined by action. Insincerity and deceptiveness are quickly perceived through body talk and lead to distrust and eventually to social ostracism. Thus others are evaluated by body language, and this evaluation is nonverbally communicated back by inclusion or exclusion of the person in future activities. The nurse who lives and works among the Eskimo people will eventually understand the nonverbal language of Eskimos and its significance.

Implications for Nursing Care

For effective communication to occur, the nurse must develop a trust relationship with the client that in time will give rise to acceptance of the nurse. When the nurse works in an Alaskan village, the villagers may appraise the nurse not on skills but on the nurse's endorsement of the community. Some villagers may perceive acceptance in terms of the nurse's willingness to visit in homes, to take time to have a cup of coffee, and to participate in village activities. It is important for the nurse to recognize that some Eskimos have a need to know they are accepted as individuals and as a community. Thus insincerity and discrepancy between nonverbal and verbal language will cause mistrust and block communication. When dealing with Eskimo clients, whether in villages or in an integrated mainland U.S. society, the nurse should be assertive but not aggressive and use a suggestive rather than a direct approach (Davidhizar & Giger, 2000). Time should be provided for a slower pace of communication with Eskimo clients. The nurse should be aware that Eskimos are sensitive to comments that indicate lack of respect and that Eskimos report feelings of racism and lack of respect by health care workers (Whalen, 1999).

Some Eskimos respect the right of personal choice and self-determination as long as these actions do not affect the welfare of the family or community. Above all, the nurse must avoid direct orders because they tend to be viewed as being "bossy." When working with some Eskimo clients, it is best for the nurse to approach the situation in a roundabout way. For example, a public health nurse, while making a home visit, may notice a baby's bottle rolling around on a dirty floor. Later the nurse may see the toddler pick the bottle up, take a few sips, and throw it back on the floor. If the nurse corrects the mother about failure to protect the child from the dangers of unrefrigerated milk and bottle-mouth syndrome, that mother may not come to the clinic or allow the nurse in the house again. However, the advice may be more readily accepted if the nurse waits until the mother brings the child in for health care, where teaching can be implemented and emphasis placed on the importance of refrigerated milk and the prevention of bottle-mouth syndrome.

Eskimos are very sensitive to the power of the dominant culture and will withdraw from any form of judgment implied by health care providers. For example, it is of little value to lecture about alcohol use, chewing tobacco, or dipping or pinching snuff. (Yup'ik women may "chew" up to 6 to 10 times daily.) The development of trust and acceptance is the best form of demonstrating support for the community. This approach will allow the village community to educate itself and seek to change unhealthy lifestyles of community members. Health care providers should not fall into the trap of thinking that they alone can effect change, which is a collaborative interaction of support and nonjudgment between providers and the community.

When providing health teaching for a client who lacks English-language skills, the nurse must use educational material that can be understood. Many educational materials available for children in English do not address the specific kinds of injuries encountered in Alaska. The Emergency Medical Services program at the Yukon-Kuskokwim Health Corporation has developed four educational curricula with specific focus on safety and first-aid issues appropriate for the Alaskan Eskimos. Two sets of books were created, one written in English and the other in Yup'ik, thus making culturally and linguistically appropriate materials available (Taylor, 1988).

It is also important for the nurse to be aware that some Eskimos have been found to have chronic otitis media, which has impaired their ability to learn. Services are being developed to provide hearing aids for students and audiological services to the Eskimos (Baxter, 1980; Baxter, Katsarkas, Ling, & Carson, 1979; Crago & Tremblay, 1991; Goodbody & Stubbing, 1991; Ling, 1976). Problems in service have often been the product of two very different cultures coming together, and they include attitudes toward hearing-aid service, noise exposure, and adequate audiovisual materials (Ilecki & Baxter, 1981). Providing services in remote areas of Alaska is often difficult because of the availability of health personnel and because of weather conditions.

SPACE

In the Eskimo culture, individual space is often shared with family members (Lange, 1988; Roberts & Ross, 1979). What is perceived as crowded living conditions by individuals in Western society may be viewed by the Eskimo as living in the warmth and security of the family group. The Western cultural need to be territorial by owning private space was not a traditional value of the Eskimo people. Instead, the Eskimo people valued sharing and perceived it as a preferable norm. Acculturation has weakened this particular value system, but family rights still take precedence over individual rights.

For example, if a family member desires the privacy of a room for a few hours, this request may be accepted as a personal need. However, if this same individual demands such privacy continuously in a two-room house with five members, ridicule and accusations of selfishness may result. As the need for individual space arises, individual family members may go on hunting, fishing, or camping trips to meet privacy needs as well as to return to nature.

A handshake distance between two people is considered the acceptable space for socialization on a daily basis. Closer approaches without permission are perceived as threatening, whereas greater distances are perceived as rude. An outsider who desires input from the Eskimos in a public meeting must recognize the decision-making process of the people and the effect that spatial requirements have on the decision-making process. The public zone for communication incorporates an intimate physical space where people sit in a circle, without a leader dominating the group. Some Eskimos view Westerners as masters of the savior attitude, which can serve to block communication with an impenetrable wall (Damas, 1984).

Implications for Nursing Care

The nurse who cares for Eskimo clients must remember that certain requirements for spatial distances must be observed. Requirements for space must take into account that the client may have unique beliefs about space and may be disturbed when a nurse ventures into personal space to do such routine procedures as give a bed bath or provide oral care, especially if a trust relationship has not been established. The nurse must determine how much self-care can be implemented by the client and how much must be implemented by the nurse. When self-care is threatened, clients who are protective of space may become withdrawn, overly aggressive, or overly passive. The nurse must be careful to allow the client to make decisions about care, and thorough explanations should be given when the nurse must venture into the intimate or personal zone without blocking communication.

SOCIAL ORGANIZATION

Family

The family unit, with its kinship ties, was paramount to survival in the harsh Arctic environment. The survival of the group traditionally was considered more important than the survival of the individual members. Several family units would band together in a migrating social group. These social groups were not permanent because families could disband and join other groups during a lifetime. However, the roles for individuals and for families within a social group were clearly delineated, so that the groups were not weakened by the shifting of members (Nida, 1954). In fact, this shifting may have strengthened the culture by extending kinships. Extended families consisted of parents, their children (from a current or previous marriage or from adoption), grandparents, and single blood relatives. The husband was the head of the family, but the responsibility of bonding the family into a strong unit belonged to the mother. Thus, if the family was unsuccessful, the blame was placed on the woman. The woman's role for family bonding was continued into the modern cultural adaptation. However, the role is continued despite lack of male support. The male members of the Eskimo society find themselves at a loss with the depletion of the role of hunter and subsistence gatherer. Inactivity and lack of jobs for men have led to alcoholism and family dysfunction.

The role of Eskimo elders in the family had been one of respect, honor, and inclusion in the family unit. Branch (2002) notes that when Eskimo elders are relocated to nursing or assisted living homes, this results in considerable stress on the family as well as the elder. Branch (2002) describes a *Marrulet Eniit* (Yup'ik for "Grandmother's house"), which opened in Dillingham, Alaska, in February 2000 and has provided a model for other such assisted living facilities in Alaska.

Kinships were vital social relationships when Eskimos lived in isolated areas. Kinship boundaries extended beyond blood relations through such practices as wife sharing, hunting partnerships, and the adoption of children. The code of behavior between kin was as binding as that between blood relatives. These extensive kinship relationships were partially responsible for the cultural similarities in Eskimos that spread across the vast Arctic regions (Williamson, 1974). History has recorded incidents of lost Eskimo hunters who crossed paths with another Eskimo band and were killed if the lost person could not prove kinship to a member of the new group (Williamson, 1974).

In Eskimo culture today, the extended family plays a very important role (Gallinek, 2006). Survival no longer depends on kinships, but these relationships are far from dead. There still is a linking of families, which is evidenced by the sharing of Native foods or the formation of business partnerships. These ties go beyond simple friendship considerations. Eskimos feel that "to be really poor is to be without relatives" (Holderman, 2006). Eskimo villages have multigeneration families living in the same household or in a household in close approximation. Conflict has begun to occur because of the impact of the members of the younger generation adopting dominant culture views toward elders instead of maintaining the strong influence of the views of elders in guiding family functioning.

The extended family involves the informal adoption of babies between families. If someone finds it impossible to care for a baby, adoption is an accepted practice. In the past, adoptions were frequently carried out with little or no litigation. Over the past decades, the informal process has been replaced with a more formal process. In addition, the Indian Child Welfare Act strictly limits adoption of Alaska Native babies by non-Natives (Legal Information Institute, nd). An adopted child is fully incorporated into the extended family. Because of close family ties, the child is often related to the adoptive parents.

The rapid entry of the Eskimo into the American cash economy and value system has led to the restructuring of the Eskimo social and economic system. The nurse who interacts with persons from these cultures must recognize that partially accepted Western values may be superimposed over Eskimo values that may still be practiced. The new elite class in Eskimo society is based on the ability to earn money without regard for old, established kinships and extended families, and a disregard for and severance of family and kinship ties underlie conflicts that may be found in villages today (Klausner & Foulks, 1982).

Individual Freedom Exists Within the Family or Group. These cultures maintain respect for individual thought and personal freedom for behavior and decisions. At times, this individual freedom appears extreme because others in the society take on a noninterference attitude. For example, a husband may beat his wife without anyone lifting a finger to stop the beating, or a person may drink to oblivion day after day, and no one will take the bottle away (Roberts & Ross, 1979). The value of individual choice of behavior is honored so long as the integrity of the group is not in jeopardy. However, the Eskimos have decided as a group that alcoholism is destroying the fabric of their culture. A sobriety movement, headed by an Eskimo, that urges Natives to become and stay sober has become widespread across the region.

Social Status Within the Family Structure. Formerly, social status was attained by successful hunters who could provide food and skins not only for their own families but also for others. Successful hunters soon were recognized as leaders in the social group by the members. The opinions of successful hunters were given precedence over the opinions of others. A woman's status was secondary to her husband's and was gained through her own skills in keeping her family well fed and clothed. Each family member had an expected role to play. Grandparents were the primary educators of the children and imparted knowledge and skills required for survival. Children learned skills through play activities that also contributed to family needs, such as finding birds' nests for the eggs or challenging a playmate in picking the most berries (Holderman, 2006).

Some Eskimo parents do not punish or even correct their small children because tradition says that the spirits of a deceased relative guide each youngster. In the Eskimo cultures the spirit of the deceased relative was considered so paramount to the survival of the young child that while a woman was in labor an old woman was brought to the bedside to recite the names of the child's dead relatives. The name that was uttered at the time the child became visible was regarded as the appropriate name, and thereafter that deceased ancestor was believed to become the guardian spirit of the child (Holderman, 2006; Nida, 1954; Polk, 1987). Although this is not practiced today, many Eskimos still believe that the essence of a dead relative is found in children born around the time of the death of a relative. For this reason many new babies may have the same name of a recently deceased family member.

For the Eskimo child, praise from parents and grandparents provides a positive learning experience and a strong self-concept (Polk, 1987). In Eskimo culture undesirable behavior traditionally was ignored, and if the behavior continued, the child was shamed through teasing and ridicule. Social controls within the community followed a similar pattern. There were no rigid rules. If a social standard was broken, it was assumed that the individual had a valid reason for the breach of conduct. Behavior was kept in control through teasing, gossip, and ridicule. If the behavior threatened group survival, the person was ostracized. To be isolated from the group meant certain death because an individual could not survive alone for long in the Arctic. The traditional Eskimo society is an example of a society that bases status on sharing and contributing to the well-being of the group and can thus establish a positive feedback system to control its members (Gove, 1982; Williamson, 1974).

Traditional Eskimos did not have any formal recognition of puberty (Polk, 1987). This was in strong contrast to other primitive societies wherein formal rituals frequently marked the coming of age. Boys are recognized by a feast at the first kill and share with all the family. In traditional Yup'ik Eskimo culture, girls were recognized when they danced with the older women for the first time.

For the nurse to give culturally appropriate nursing care to the client whose cultural makeup encompasses traditional values regarding social status, it is necessary for the nurse to appreciate traditional family roles. In most cases, it is also necessary to involve both nuclear and extended family members in the planning, implementation, and evaluation of nursing care.

Political Structure

The political development of Eskimos has evolved out of the development of councils, native corporations, and health care corporations. The Native Land Claims Act of 1971 spurred a political development pattern similar to the political system in other states. Where once each community had an informal social structure that revolved around family and kin, now most villages have a decision-making council headed by an elected spokesperson (U.S. Department of Health and Human Services, Indian Health Services, 1991a).

Implications for Nursing Care

Extended family ties can be used to encourage noncompliant clients into following recommended therapy. These ties can also be used to find reasons for noncompliance because the client may not feel free to contradict the nurse. In Eskimo culture it is considered impolite to openly disagree with others. Cooperation, patience, and nonaggression are important values. Attempts to persuade or counsel another person, even to keep that person from doing something dangerous or foolish, are considered rude and are not tolerated. When health care staff attempt to "help" through advising and counseling, they are seen as meddling and will encounter interference (Lange, 1988). The nurse may need to resolve a difficult situation by asking other family members for guidance. With the increased educational levels of the younger people and with the help of the nurse as an advocate, some Eskimos are beginning to assume more autonomy in questioning medical therapy and social programs. It is essential that the nurse encourage the Eskimo client to take personal responsibility for health or illness in consultation with the appropriate family members. As appropriate, the nurse should directly involve the client in planning health care and in activities that pursue solutions to health needs.

There are a mixture of childrearing practices in the Eskimo culture today (MacDonald-Clark &

Boffman, 1995). Eskimo parents tend to use more positive reinforcements, praising desired behavior and ignoring undesired actions. Children are considered individuals as soon as they learn to express themselves. What this means for the nurse is that a child is given the right to refuse or accept health-related care. Some parents will not force a child to do something that the child refuses to do. For example, a parent may make a statement such as "I tell Sam to brush his teeth, but he won't do it" or "JoJo won't let me put drops in her ear." The parent may tease, shame, or ridicule the child in an attempt to persuade the child, but the parent will seldom demand the appropriate behavior. The nurse needs to emphasize that certain health care behaviors or techniques, such as brushing teeth or appropriately using medications, are important because they may prevent more overriding problems, such as dental cavities and otitis media. However, the implementation of these health-related practices is difficult because of the present-time orientation and the cultural childrearing practices.

It is also important for the nurse to be aware that according to a 2000 IHS survey of dental patients, more than 80% of Alaska Native children 2 to 4 years of age experience dental decay in their primary teeth (Indian Health Service, 2000). This is commonly caused by giving a child a bottle containing carbohydrates at naptime or bedtime and by bottle-feeding past the age of 12 months. This high prevalence of dental caries results in increased cost of treatment and requires community-based intervention (Bruerd, 1997).

TIME

The Arctic Circle marks the point at which there is no sunrise on December 21, which is considered the winter solstice (or the shortest day of the year), and no sunset on June 21, the summer solstice (or the longest day of the year). This factor gives rise to a unique phenomenon that occurs in the northernmost part of North America. When the sun rises on May 10 in Barrow, Alaska, which is North America's northernmost city, it does not set again until August 2. As a result, there are 84 days of continuous sunlight. When the sun sets on November 18 in Barrow, it does not rise again until January 24. Therefore, Barrow residents have 67 days of continuous semidarkness. There is daylight even though the sun does not rise over the horizon. However, the daylight is very short, for example, from 3 to 5 hours.

The extended periods of daylight and darkness give rise to seasonal, geographically related behavior. For example, it is not uncommon to see small children playing outside in the summer at 2 o'clock in the morning (Gottberg, 1988). Also during the summer months, the extended hours of daylight are used for fishing. Likewise, because of the extended periods of darkness in the winter, northerners tend to sleep late. Although most northerners have rearranged their lives in recent times to synchronize themselves with the Western day–night rhythm, some Eskimos remain on "Eskimo time," which is a result of both the unusual daylight pattern and a present-time orientation. Rather than being structured by the clock, time is cyclical, based on naturally recurring phenomena: sunrise, sunset, days, nights, moons (months), and seasons (Lewis & Ho, 1975). Use of "Eskimo time" may prompt Eskimo families to keep their children out of school and in fish camp several weeks after school officially opens. Some Eskimos believe that fish camp, a present-time oriented activity, is a time to be enjoyed, whereas school, a future-time oriented activity, prepares children for future goals. Committing to year-round jobs on a 9-to-5 schedule is difficult for some Eskimos because of the strong tradition of spending summer and fall in fish camps.

The present-time orientation of culture is sometimes reflected in the ways in which money is spent. There is an emphasis on consumable things that give immediate benefit. Budgeting and investing for the future may not be motivating concepts. Some Eskimos who have been away from the village and have earned a large sum of money during a season may come home and blow it in one spending spree for the family. This action exemplifies two values: sharing what you have with others and living for today because tomorrow will take care of itself.

Use of "Eskimo time" requires readjustment by the nurse for such things as scheduling appointments for health care because some Eskimos prefer to come in when they feel like it. Consequently, a nurse who works in a remote area of Alaska should seldom schedule a clinic appointment before 9 or 10 AM and should be prepared to work late into the evening. A visiting nurse may be on a tight schedule and insist that the villagers accept a Western time frame. This insistence causes such comments as "You are always rushed" or "You must not like our village because you are always in a hurry to leave."

Implications for Nursing Care

It is important for the nurse to remember that a village may have a different time orientation than that of health care providers from the majority culture. For example, some people may stay up late and sleep late. During the summer, when it is daylight most of the time, villagers may sleep only when they are tired, and children may stay up very late. This may present real challenges for the nurse, whether in a clinic or in a hospital setting, because the lack of a definitive schedule interferes with the nurse's obtaining medical histories and the client's keeping appointments and taking medications on time and correctly. The public health nurse learns to take medical histories by village events and seasons. On the other hand, the hospital nurse must emphasize in simple terms the necessity for the medical history. In either case, it is important to know a little about the client's daily routine if nursing care is to be implemented and effective. Because schedules are flexible and time is relative, the nurse needs to inquire about daily schedules before requiring medication to be taken at a certain time. Many families do not eat meals together. Therefore, telling a client to take a pill at mealtime may have no meaning.

ENVIRONMENTAL CONTROL

The early Eskimos believed that the individual had three parts: body, soul, and name. All of these were considered of equal importance and combined to make the whole person. Early Eskimos also believed that everything, such as earth, wind, flowers, animals, and birds, had a spirit. In Yup'ik culture, a set of rules for living guided individual action (Sanders, 2000). Each family inherited a specific taboo system, and each person had a guiding spirit to help him or her during his or her lifetime. When a girl married, she had to abide by both families' taboos (Gove, 1982). The spiritual leader, called a *shaman*, had the vital role of keeping the group healthy by persuading the spiritual world to continue smiling on the people. When famine struck or illness occurred, the shaman communicated with the spiritual world during trances to learn what taboo had been broken and who needed to appease the spirits. Appeasement often meant that the guilty person confessed to breaking the taboo and suffered humiliation. It is interesting to understand that the shaman was not blamed if the shaman failed to find the cause for negative events. The people accepted their situation as a matter of fate (Blodgett, 1978; Lantis, 1986; Mitchell & Patch, 1986). Famine, bad luck, and failure in hunting meant the spirits were displeased with the Eskimo people, whereas successful hunting and times of plenty meant the spirits were pleased. Consequently, each Eskimo perceived his or her relationship with nature as being in harmony or out of harmony with the spiritual world. Today shamanism has been largely replaced by Christianity, except for various remote areas of Alaska (Blodgett, 1978).

Today it is common for Eskimos to be Christian, depending on the denomination of the missionaries in a particular part of Alaska. Examples include the Catholic, Moravian, Russian Orthodox, and Presbyterian religions. Death is accepted as a part of life, which makes an enormous difference in attitudes about suffering, stress, and even acculturation. In the past, Eskimos were buried in wooden boxes above the ground because of the difficulty in digging graves; people are now buried in graves dug with jackhammers. Whereas wood was once at a premium and one cross contained many names, imported wood is now readily available (Morris, 1985).

Illness and Wellness Behaviors

Early Eskimos believed that each person had a spiritual healer who could be offended by the person breaking a taboo. A broken taboo was manifested by the person becoming ill. Possession by harmful spirits was recognized as a cause of illness. For example, it was considered taboo to eat polar bear liver, and any Eskimo who offended the bear spirit in this manner became ill or died. Studies in the 1940s indicated that vitamin A toxicity, rather than the ill effects of the broken taboo, was the cause of illnesses associated with eating polar bear liver (Rodahl, 1964). Regardless, the taboo protected the people by discouraging consumption of polar bear liver.

Written information on shamanism is limited because of the prohibition of this religion by early missionaries. Folklore indicates that the shaman had predicted the coming of the strangers who would cause the death of the Eskimo; thus, when nearly one half of the Eskimos died of diseases brought by the early traders, whalers, and missionaries (Fortuine, 1989), the prophecy was fulfilled. Unfortunately, while the Westerners brought medicine, they also brought new diseases to which the Eskimo people were not immune (Fortuine, 1989). With the influx of Westerners, the lifestyle of the Eskimos changed, as they moved into permanent settlements to take advantage of schools, churches, and medical care. The spread of communicable disease became rampant among the people, who now lived in permanent houses occupied by many people in close proximity. Before the influx of Westerners, the constant moving of living sites prevented the hygiene problems that were now incurred by permanent villages. Over the years, the Eskimos have learned about the physical causes of illness and the appropriate techniques necessary to prevent the spread of disease.

Shamanism lost face with the people as they turned to the magic of medicine brought by the Westerners to cure the devastating infectious diseases. Many of the medical people were missionaries who implied that illness was related to the people's sinfulness and that the cure depended partly on their confession and acceptance of Western religion. The early Eskimos did not oppose the switch to the new religion because it seemed similar to shamanism. Medical treatment by Westerners was often restricted to the Eskimos whose names appeared on the church roster.

In the Eskimo cultures, there is a generation gap in health and illness concepts. An older person may have a more holistic view of health and believe that a happy person is less likely to develop physical ills, whereas a younger person may assign illness to direct physical causes. For example, in the case of suicidal behavior, a young person may blame alcohol, stating that if the person did not drink he or she would not commit suicide. Therefore, the treatment for the prevention of suicide is to take the alcohol away. On the other hand, older Eskimos may see suicidal behavior as an illness of the spirit that creates a disharmony, leading to the choice of drinking. The cure is to heal the spirit; then the need for alcohol will disappear.

Implications for Nursing Care

When giving culturally appropriate nursing care to Eskimo clients, whether in remote areas of Alaska or in the mainland United States, the nurse must realize that an individual's feelings of environmental control are an important factor in the nursing assessment of client status. Illness and wellness behaviors among some Eskimo clients may be attributable to past belief systems and a belief in supernatural powers. The nurse may need to combat some superstitious beliefs because of the delay in medical treatment. It is also important for the nurse to appreciate that lifestyle changes, social change, and changes in society and the environment are all major determinants of health among the Inuit (Bjerregaard, Young, Dewailly, & Ebbesseon, 2004).

Because some Eskimos tend to view nature as an entity that can be in equilibrium or disequilibrium, the nurse can build on this concept and teach the client that certain conditions in the body can also be in equilibrium or disequilibrium. Coupling the theory of equilibrium or disequilibrium with supernatural beliefs, the nurse may be able to adequately explain an illness in terms that are acceptable to the patient.

BIOLOGICAL VARIATIONS
Body Size and Structure

Ancestors of the Indians and Eskimos originated from the Asian race (Bank, 1956; Zegura, 1985). Anthropologists believe that there was a land bridge between Asia and Alaska that was crossed by the early Native people. Genetic studies have related the origin of Eskimos to a population of Asiatic Beringia (Szathmary, 1984). The Mongolian racial traits seen in the Eskimos include a short muscular body, large oblong skull with a definite occipital protuberance, well-developed lower jaw and maxillary bone, epicanthal folds, little or no body hair, dark-pigmented skin, and lumbar mongolian spots (Bank, 1956; Chance, 1966; Mann & Scott, 1962). The head shape and jaw structure have been attributed to the evolutionary process from prehistoric man and have little significance in the Eskimo culture today (Carpenter, 1973; Chance, 1966).

Early medical research noted the short stature and heavier weight per height of Eskimos, which was greatly different from that of Europeans and other circumpolar people, such as Icelanders and Finns (Milan, 1980). Three theories were proposed to explain this difference: (1) a genetic inheritance, (2) a combination of genetic inheritance and environmental adaptation, and (3) a condition of long-term nutritional deficiency. Part of this weight difference was attributed to the Eskimo's thicker bony skeleton and muscular chest and arms (Hrdlicka, 1930, 1941; Milan, 1980). Researchers demonstrated by the use of triceps and body skinfold measurements that the extra weight was not caused by an extra layer of fat, negating the adaptation theory that Eskimos carried extra fat to protect the body from the cold (Hrdlicka, 1941). Muscular development resulting from an active lifestyle and genetic inheritance contributed to the early Eskimo's body structure.

The birth weights and heights of today's Eskimos are statistically similar to those of their White counterparts (Heller, 1947; Johnston, Laughlin, Harper, & Ensroth, 1982; Mann & Scott, 1962; U.S. Department of Health and Human Services, Indian Health Services, 1991b). By 11 months of age, Eskimo infants fall within the 5% range for height on Faulkner's growth charts, whereas their weight is in the 50% range. By 18 months of age, Eskimo children are consistently heavier than their White counterparts. This pattern of growth continues until 6 years of age, when Eskimo children become lighter in terms of weight than White children. The average height of Eskimo children remains shorter throughout life. This pattern may be a genetic trait, though in the past three decades the Eskimos have had a growth (height) increase pattern of greater than 1 cm per decade (Milan, 1980). Some researchers believe that the growth increase is indirectly related to a decrease in hibernation. However, in 1970, Schaefer presented some convincing data directly linking the growth rate to sugar consumption. The pattern seen in Eskimos discredits the supposition that growth increase is a result of a high-protein diet. Since the Eskimo diet changed from an almost total protein intake to the current high-sugar, high-carbohydrate diet, their growth pattern has increased (Bells, Draper, & Bergan, 1973). Unfortunately, obesity is now a problem.

When using the Faulkner growth chart in health assessments of Eskimo children, the nurse must remember that the chart is based on White averages. Sequential growth patterns are needed in health and nutrition assessment. For example, it is easy to identify Eskimo children born with fetal alcohol syndrome by following the sequential growth pattern on the standard growth charts.

Skin Color

Eskimos have a "tanned" complexion that becomes deep brown to black with continuous exposure to the sun. This pigmentation is part of their Mongoloid heritage. However, evolutionary selection may also explain this feature. Skin cancer research indicates that deeply pigmented skin has some natural protection from the ultraviolet rays of the sun. Therefore, the evolutionary conclusion is that Eskimos are more protected from skin cancer because of their deep skin pigmentation (Young, 1986).

Other Visible Physical Characteristics

Mongoloid heritage among Alaskan Eskimos is reflected in the lumbar pigmented spots and the epicanthal eye folds. However, neither of these characteristics gives rise to significant health problems. The nurse who cares for Eskimo children needs to be able to distinguish between mongolian spots and those bruises that might be associated with child abuse. Child abuse may be reported to health care providers by well-meaning Westerners who notice "bruises" on an infant's arms and buttocks when these are only mongolian spots. However, during physical assessment it is important for the nurse to remember to document unusual placement of mongolian spots on areas such as the wrist, legs, and chest.

Enzymatic Variations

Enzyme deficiencies in lactase and sucrose have been documented in Eskimos. When given a lactose load equivalent to 3 to 4 cups of milk, 80% of Eskimo adults and 70% of Eskimo children demonstrated intolerance symptoms of flatulence and diarrhea (Bells, Draper, & Bergan, 1973; Duncan & Scott, 1972). However, most of them could tolerate a daily glass of milk without symptoms. In the past, Eskimos had no dietary source of milk after being weaned from the breast, and nutritional analysis of traditional foods indicates that the diet of adult Eskimos remains quite low in calcium. Research is needed to determine if there is a genetic protective factor for calcium metabolism or if this population is at risk for osteoporosis from calcium-deficient diets. It is essential for the nurse who works with Eskimo clients to encourage using alternative forms of milk, such as cheese, yogurt, and powdered milk. The nurse should note that Eskimos rarely like milk products; however, cheese is an exception. The nurse must also remember that another source of calcium that is readily available to Eskimos is fish bones that are canned with the flesh.

A few Alaskan (approximately 5%) and Greenland Eskimos (approximately 10%) are intolerant of sucrose. Some classic research studies indicate that a can of soda or a piece of cake can cause debilitating diarrhea in some Eskimos (Bells, Draper, & Bergan, 1973; Shephard, 1974).

Friedrich and Ferrell (1985) found that the alpha-keto acid reductase locus is monomorphic in most cultural groups, despite earlier studies that suggested its existence as a genetic polymorphism. Thus the Eskimo population is no more prone to having an alpha-keto acid reductase locus than any other cultural group.

Susceptibility to Disease

The isolation of Eskimos from outsiders caused them to be susceptible to the devastating effects of infections brought to Alaska. Eskimos who lacked exposure to certain diseases had no antibodies to these diseases. It has been documented that Eskimos develop antibodies to antigens as well as their Western counterparts do. Thus the rapid spread of disease among Eskimos is believed to have occurred because of the short incubation time of the organisms (Fortuine, 1989) and because of a lack of knowledge about hygiene techniques necessary to stop the spread of communicable disease, not because of failure to develop antibodies to antigens (Young, 1986).

Communicable Disease. Today, increased incidences of communicable diseases are still being reported among some populations of Eskimos. For example, in an epidemiological study of streptococcal disease that affected 706 Alaskan Eskimo children, throat cultures were obtained during a long-term surveillance program (Brant, Bender, & Marnell, 1982). In this study a binary-variable, multiple-regression model was used to study the association between streptococcal colonization of the children and the following six potential risk factors: age, sex, number of children in the household, region, health aide rating, and colonization rate for the child from the previous year. The factors significantly associated with streptococcal colonization among the Eskimo children included age, past colonization, competence of the local health aide in providing care, and region in which the care was provided. However, the number of children in overcrowded homes and the child's sex were not factors important to the incidence of streptococcal colonization (Brant, Bender, & Marnell, 1982). Holman, Curns, Cheek, Bresee, Singleton, Carver, and Anderson (2004) reported that while respiratory syncytial virus (RSV) infection is one of the leading causes of hospitalization among all infants in the U.S., Alaskan native infants have an unusually high hospitalization rate of 34.4 per 1000 infants.

In some remote villages in Alaska, hygiene techniques remain a nursing priority. When working with Eskimos, the nurse must implement teaching programs emphasizing hygienic practices and medical asepsis. Because some villages are extremely crowded and lack running water and proper sanitation systems, susceptibility to disease is augmented; thus the nurse must also emphasize hygienic practices with these individuals. Lum, Knutson, Hall, et al. (1986) reported the significant effect that improved immunization programs, prenatal care, and improved health care have had on infant mortality. Deaths from infectious diseases, measles, and pertussis were dramatically reduced as health care was improved among southwestern Alaskan Eskimos between 1960 and 1980. Still another problem for Eskimo infants is increased exposure to *Haemophilus influenzae* type B (Hib) disease (Hall, Lum, Knutson, et al., 1987). Alaskan Eskimos have the greatest known endemic risk for this disease, which seems to have genetic factors that contribute to susceptibility (Petersen, Silimperi, Rotter, et al., 1987; Ward, Lum, Hall, et al., 1986). In 1990, effective Hib vaccines were licensed for infants, and over the next year infants in the Yukon–Kuskokwim Delta and Bristol Bay areas of Alaska were immunized. Vaccination for Hib has continued with positive results. In 2000, there were only 11 cases in the area of Alaska where Yup'ik and Inupiat Eskimos reside (State of Alaska, Section of Epidemiology, 2001c). Petersen, Silimperi, Chiu, and Ward (1991) noted that living in extended families at the time of disease onset was significantly associated with Hib disease. In a classic study on the effect of immunization, Singleton (1992) reported that infant immunization with Hib vaccine resulted in a drop from 18 cases per year for the periods from 1980 to 1989 in the Bristol and Delta Bay areas of Alaska to no deaths in 1992. Bijlmer (1991) investigated *Haemophilus influenzae* meningitis in nonindustrialized versus industrialized areas of the world and concluded that, rather than industrialization, accessibility of health care facilities was related to the case fatality rate.

Tuberculosis. Tuberculosis has a long history in Alaska. Fortuine (1989), a physician and historian, classifies tuberculosis as an introduced disease. Some of the earliest written references to symptoms of tuberculosis are from the late 1700s and early 1800s, after the Russian explorers and fur traders had contact with the Alaska Native population.

It is difficult to quantify the extent of tuberculosis in the Yup'ik and Inupiat population because the data are reported for Alaska Natives, not specifically Yup'iks and Inupiats. There is, however, historical evidence that the incidence of tuberculosis was greatest in the southwestern and northern regions of the state, the areas where Yup'iks and Inupiats live. In 1952 there were 1853 cases of tuberculosis per 100,000 Alaska Natives, resulting in a huge impact on the Alaska Native population. By 2002, the rate was 8.4 per 100,000 population, almost 6 times the rate for non-Hispanic Whites (Schneider, 2005). It is an illness that is 5 to 10 times more prevalent among Yup'iks and Inupiats than in the general Alaskan population (State of Alaska, Department of Health and Social Services, 2001a).

The incidence of tuberculosis is related to environmental and socioeconomic issues, such as houses that are cramped because of the cold temperature, poor availability of clean water (Stevenson, 1984), and poor nutrition. Effective intervention includes both prevention and curtailment of possible spread once a case is present. Health education is essential and must include not only direct information on tuberculosis but also information on predisposing factors, such as hygiene, overcrowding, alcohol abuse, and nutrition. Butler and colleagues (2001) stated that tuberculosis is an example of a disease that has reemerged but is now in decline. Regardless, the annual incidence for Native Americans (including Alaska Natives) is twice as high as for the U.S. population overall. Causes for these cases of tuberculosis that were identified as preventable were noncompliance, intravenous drug use, HIV infection, and tuberculosis in correctional institutions (Snider, Salinas, & Kelly, 1989). Additional reasons include crowded living conditions, high rates of type 2 diabetes mellitus, and deterioration of the public health infrastructure (Butler, Crengle, Cheek, et al., 2001). Denny, Holtzman, Goins, and Croft (2005) conducted telephone surveys to compare chronic disease risk factors and health status among

Alaskan natives elders. They concluded that for all health behavior and status measures, Alaskan Natives reported greater risks than Whites, thus emphasizing the importance of addressing risk factors to eliminate health disparities.

STDs. Sexually transmitted diseases (STDs) have unusually high prevalence among Alaska Natives. From 1984 through 1988, Alaska Natives had five times the reported gonorrhea and syphilis morbidity of non-Native Alaskans (Toomey, Oberschelp, & Greenspan, 1989). In Canada, data from Manitoba in the early 1980s indicated that Natives were affected three times more often than non-Natives (Lee, Brunham, Sherman, & Harding, 1987). The State of Alaska, Department of Health and Social Services, Division of Public Health, Section of Epidemiology (2000), in an epidemiology bulletin on HIV infection in Alaska 1999, reported that Alaska Natives (as a whole, not just Yup'ik and Inupiat Eskimos) are slightly overrepresented in cases of HIV, although this difference is not statistically significant. Alaska Natives account for 19% of the HIV cases (including AIDS cases), while they account for 17% of the population. Alaska Native women are "over-represented relative to their percentages in the population" (p. 9). American Indian/Alaska Native females account for 35% of the female HIV cases (including AIDS). There is some concern that there is the potential for an increase in HIV/AIDS cases among Alaska Natives because of alcohol and drug use, effects of long-term unemployment and poverty, and lack of prevention activities. Chlamydiosis, which is now a reportable disease in Alaska, has a very high incidence rate. The symptoms caused by *Chlamydia* bacteria allow for a possible entrance for HIV. Thus there is concern that such a possibility is high among teenagers whose *Chlamydia* rate is higher than that of the general individual.

Glaucoma. Eskimos are susceptible to primary narrow-angle glaucoma. In persons with primary narrow-angle glaucoma, the eyes have a shallow chamber angle and a thicker lens, both of which are factors that contribute to glaucoma. It is believed that the sex and increasing age of the person, particularly in the case of women, are associated factors as well. Both genetic and environmental components appear to play a major role in the development of primary narrow-angle glaucoma (Schaefer, 1973; Van Rens, Arkell, Charlton, & Doesburg, 1988).

Diabetes Mellitus. In Alaska, the prevalence of diabetes is higher among Alaska Natives than among the population as a whole, and it is increasing rapidly: "Over the past 20 years, the prevalence of diabetes in the Alaska Native population has increased 89%" (State of Alaska, Department of Health and Social Services, Division of Public Health, Section of Epidemiology, 2001b). The largest increase in diabetes in the Alaska Native population is among Eskimos (110%) (State of Alaska, Department of Health and Human Services, Division of Public Health, Section of Epidemiology, 2001b). Although some classic research studies suggest that a normal glucose response is found among Eskimos (Mouratoff, Carrol, & Scott, 1967; Scott & Griffin, 1956), with each passing decade there is an increasing number of glucose-intolerant Eskimos. There are many Eskimos of mixed heritage who are listed as being full-blooded Eskimos, and this could be a factor in the discrepancy.

The risk factors for diabetes are yet to be completely understood. There is strong evidence that the shift from a traditional subsistence diet to a Western diet and the decrease in physical exercise because of a decline in subsistence activities contribute to the increase in the number of cases of diabetes. Over the past decade, obesity among Eskimos has increased, and it is not uncommon for Eskimos (particularly women) to be as much as 50 to 100 pounds over their ideal weight. In Canada, Schaefer (1970) noted that the incidence of diabetes was higher in the Arctic, where Eskimos have had a longer contact with a high-sugar diet. In this classic study, Schaefer concluded that the increase in known diabetes incidence among Alaskan Eskimos follows Campbell's rule, which states that diabetes morbidity generally trails 20 to 30 years behind the introduction of a Western diet. Although Eskimos are not reported to have an increased incidence of glucose intolerance, it is essential for the nurse to keep in mind that some

Eskimos have a prevalence of obesity and a high sugar intake, both of which can be contributory factors in the development of diabetes mellitus. In light of this fact, the nurse must implement teaching techniques that emphasize the importance of exercise and eating right. In addition, the nurse must remember that, if Campbell's rule is correct, an increase in glucose intolerance will be evident among the Eskimo people. The key to control of glucose intolerance is prevention.

Cardiovascular Disease. Fifty years ago, non-Natives died from cardiovascular disease at a rate three times higher than for Alaska Natives. At that time, the major cause of death for Alaska Natives was infectious diseases. By the early 1990s, the rate of death from cardiovascular disease (heart disease and stroke) among Alaska Natives (all groups) was higher than that of non-Natives (Alaska Division of Public Health, Section of Community Health and Emergency Medical Services, 1998; State of Alaska, Section of Epidemiology, 1997).

Dyerberg and Bang (1978) first reported a lower incidence of coronary disease in the Greenland Eskimos. This finding was attributed to their diet, which was rich in fat from whale, fish, and seals. Further analysis revealed that the Eskimos had lower levels of plasma cholesterol and triglycerides and high plasma concentrations of certain polyunsaturated fatty acids (Sipperly, 1989). It remains unclear whether genetic factors protect this population from a high incidence of cardiac disease. However, the nurse must remember that the diet and lifestyle of the Eskimo people have changed dramatically in the last few decades, and those factors have had a profound effect on their cardiovascular health (Young, 1986). The Western world has done extensive research on arteriosclerosis and heart disease in a search for preventive clues. As a result, Americans are encouraged to eat foods that are low in fat (less than 30% of daily caloric intake), limit their red meat and egg yolk intake, and do aerobic exercises. Traditionally, the Eskimo people subsisted on a diet that was 44% protein (sea and land animals, fish, and birds), 47% fat (polyunsaturated), and 8% carbohydrates (berries, beach greens, and roots). More recently, analysis of the dietary intake of Eskimos

indicated protein intake of 26%, fat intake of 37%, and carbohydrate intake of 37% (Mann & Scott, 1962). Although protein and fat intake decreased significantly, carbohydrate intake increased significantly. For some Eskimos the significant increase in carbohydrates is attributable to high intake of sugar.

In certain seasons the early Eskimos ate foods that were high in cholesterol. In other seasons their diet was devoid of cholesterol. Some studies suggest that the body uses stored cholesterol when there is no cholesterol intake (Feldman, Ho, Lewis, et al., 1972). If this is correct, seasonal food variations among Eskimos have provided a protection against heart and blood vessel disease. Today, fewer Eskimos continue to follow a seasonal pattern of dietary habits. Regardless of whether the body uses stored cholesterol, the nurse needs to caution against excessive cholesterol intake.

Although medical knowledge regarding cardiovascular disease in the pre–Western-contact Eskimo is limited, arteriosclerotic plaquing was noted in the blood vessels of mummified bodies that were dated back to 1460. The oldest body had significantly greater evidence of vascular changes (Zimmerman & Aufderheide, 1984).

In a study involving a Bering Strait Eskimo population, similar heart rates and heart-rate rhythmicity and almost identical acrophases were found in the Eskimo, the Aymara Indian, and the French populations. The study also found that Alaskan Eskimos had heart-rate means that varied by approximately 15 beats per minute (Rode & Shephard, 1984). This variation can have serious implications for the nurse who is monitoring the rhythmicity of the heart because of the variation in beats. When monitoring the pulse rate of an Eskimo client, the nurse should, when possible, take an apical rather than a radial pulse and count the heart rate for 1 full minute.

Anemia. Anemia, especially in infants and children, seems to be a direct result of a nutritional deficiency resulting from iron-poor food choices. Hereditary predisposition was eliminated as a possibility for anemia in one epidemiological study (Nobmann, 1984). For the Eskimos who live along the

Kuskokwim and Yukon Rivers, there is a tendency to have a diet high in fish and to store items that are relatively iron poor. A typical meal includes fish soup, "pilot" bread (so named because it was originally brought in by pilots) with shortening, and black, sugared tea. Even preschoolers drink black tea in these areas, and it is believed that the tannic acid in tea interferes with iron absorption (Nobmann, 1984). Thus the diet is considered to be iron poor and additionally has an agent (tannic acid) that prohibits absorption. Sea mammals are an excellent iron source, but with the decrease in subsistence living and the easy access to store-bought foods, even the coastal people succumb to anemia.

It is believed that anemia is one of the factors that contribute to morbidity in infants and children under 3 years of age (Nobmann, 1984). Lactating mothers should be taught nutritional education by the nurse who works in infant programs and should be given vitamin and iron supplements. Infant iron-fortified formulas can now be found even in remote areas in Alaska and should be used instead of canned milk when a mother does not breastfeed. Women, Infants, and Children (WIC) and Aid to Families with Dependent Children (AFDC) programs have been established in areas throughout Alaska and provide money to purchase high-cost formula. Studies done by WIC suggest that its programs have caused a decrease in anemia (Nobmann, 1984).

Cancer. The incidence of cancer in Eskimos is not significantly different from that in the rest of the American population. However, the pattern of cancer is unique. Among Eskimo men, lung, colorectal, nasopharynx, stomach, and liver cancers are the most common. In fact, lung cancer is the most rapidly increasing cancer among Alaska Native people and other indigenous populations in the Arctic (Lanier, Bulkow, Novotny, et al., 1990). High rates of cigarette use occur among Alaska Native children as well as adults. Within Alaska, the prevalence of smoking is higher among Alaska Natives (39% to 50%) than among non-Natives (25%) (Behavioral Risk Factor Surveillance, 1991, 1992). Among Eskimo women, colorectal, breast, lung, and gallbladder cancers are more common (Young, 1986). Data on 239 verified cases of malignant disease in

the western and central Canadian Arctic were studied by Hildes and Schaefer (1984), who found Eskimos to be less prone to developing cancer of the skin, prostate, pancreas, and stomach. Cervical cancer is on the increase, but the cause for the rise is unclear (Toomey, Rafferty, & Stamm, 1987). Apart from risk factors such as smoking and diet, there is considerable interest in the role that infectious agents play as carcinogens. For example, hepatitis B virus (HBV) is the causative agent for hepatocellular carcinoma (McMahon, Heyward, Templin, et al., 1989). Children infected at an earlier age are at a greater risk for becoming HBV carriers, and once a carrier, a child has a 40% chance of developing liver cancer by 40 years of age (Lanier, Bender, Talbert, et al., 1980). Lanier, Holck, Day, and Key (2003) found that Alaskan Native children has a similar rate to that of U.S. whites when all cancers were concerned.

The Epstein-Barr virus (EBV) has been implicated in the development of nasopharyngeal cancers. It has been found in more than 90% of cases of Burkitt's lymphoma in endemic regions, though only 15% of cases in nonendemic regions show evidence of infection (Gaffey & Weiss, 1990). It is suspected that the transmission of viral agents may require a susceptible genotype or other promotional events (Lynch, Schuelke, & O'Hara, 1984). It has been reported that Greenland Eskimos have the highest documented EBV titers in the world (Young, 1986). In Alaskan Eskimos a distinct variant of EBV type 2 was found in nasopharyngeal carcinoma and carcinoma of the parotid gland (Abdel-Hamid, Chen, Constantine, Massound, & Raab-Traub, 1992). Other risk factors associated with this type of cancer include the widespread lifestyle habits of smoking, alcohol, and chewing tobacco. Alaska Native hospitals have reported a significant rise in nasopharyngeal cancer among teenagers and young adults (Young, 1986), and epidemiologists have attributed this increase in nasopharyngeal cancer to tobacco habits (snuff and cigarettes) that begin in preschool-aged groups rather than to the Epstein-Barr virus.

Dietary habits such as the consumption of heavily smoked fish and fermented, salted foods may also add some carcinogenic risks. Insufficient data currently exist to determine whether genetic factors contribute to the cancer patterns of the Eskimo people. Wilson, Rausch, McMahon, and Schantz (1992) noted that chemotherapy effectively treated alveolar hydatid disease in Alaskan Eskimos.

Hepatitis B Virus (HBV). In the 1970s and 1980s, serologic surveys demonstrated that Alaskan Eskimos, Canadian Inuit, and Greenland Inuit had a high prevalence of HBV. More recently a relationship has been noted between hepatocellular carcinoma (HCC) and hepatitis B virus infections among Alaskan Eskimos (Key & Marble, 1999). These researchers noted that Alaska Natives chronically infected with HBV have a relative risk of HCC of 148 compared with Alaska Natives not chronically infected.

Arthritis. According to a study reported in the *Morbidity and Mortality Weekly* (1996), the American Indian and Alaska Native elders have the highest estimated age- and sex-adjusted annual prevalence of arthritis of groups, including Asians, Pacific Islanders, Hispanics, and Blacks. This group reported the highest activity limitation of any group (4.2%).

Asthma. Wind, Sickle, and Wright (2004) examined the asthma perceptions of Yup'ik parents of asthmatic children using data from semistructured ethnographic interviews conducted in five villages and one town of the Yukon-Kuskokwin delta of southwest Alaska. Two interpretations of the increase in asthma among Yup'ik children were presented: (1) that there is a weakening of the collective physical body due to cold air, physical exertion, and dust and (2) that the Yup'ik consider asthma an embodiment of the degradation of the environment in which they live. The fact that childhood asthma is seen as having a multiplicity of causes rather than being linked to a single source of environmental pollution suggests that community consensus about the relationship between locale and chronic disease for the Yup'ik may remain elusive.

Blood Variations

Eskimos as an ethnic group have a distinctive blood group variation; specifically, Rh-negative blood is absent in Eskimos (Overfield, 1977, 1995). The occasional Rh-negative factor turns up in some Eskimos of mixed race. The nurse who counsels a woman during a spontaneous abortion must be alert to her Rh factor. Complacency to the importance of preventable measures can have dire consequences. As the number of mixed-race Eskimos rises, so does this risk.

Nutritional and Lifestyle Preferences

After the control of infectious diseases among Alaskan Eskimos, the health–illness pattern shifted to reflect an increase in chronic disease. This increase in chronic disease may be attributable to the fact that the Eskimo diet and lifestyle changed as people assimilated many of the Western culture's bad habits, such as a sedentary lifestyle and a diet high in sugar, salt, and fat. Many Eskimos now use some form of locomotion, such as four-wheelers or snow machine, to get around villages that are less than a mile long or wide, minimizing needed exercise.

Clean water is sometimes a difficult commodity to obtain in Alaska. In some villages on the ocean, drinking water must be brought in as ice from several miles up the river. In the process of being brought to the village, the chunks of ice are often handled by many people and must then be melted, boiled, and cooled. Yet another concern for Inuits is that departure from the traditional Inuit diet lowers iodine intake. Urinary iodine excretion may be a useful biomarker of traditional Inuit food frequency (Andersen, Hvingel, Kleinschmidt, Jorgensen, and Laurberg, 2005).

Psychological Characteristics

"The suicide epidemic in Bush Alaska continues..." is a headline frequently seen in Alaskan newspapers. The mental health status of Eskimos is complicated by the pressures created by traditional cultural demands, attempts at assimilation of Western values, and the harsh geographic region. Alcohol and drug abuse are the major causes of injury, accidents, and death among Alaskan Eskimos. Suicide is associated with alcohol abuse, which in turn is a symptom of a people attempting to assimilate in a rapidly changing society (Albert, 1988; Travis, 1983; VanDenberg & Minton, 1987).

The suicidal behavior in Eskimo populations is believed to have changed in pattern and quantity over the last decade. The rate of attempted suicide among Eskimos has more than quadrupled, and the incidence of completed suicides among young people has increased. To understand the psychological makeup and characteristics of the Eskimo people, the nurse needs to have an awareness of their history, its relationship to self-destructive behavior as evidenced among some Eskimos, and their present stress of acculturation.

For many Eskimos the rapid breakdown of traditional values, religion, lifestyle, and social relationships has led to an inability to find a meaningful role in the modern world (Albert, 1988). For example, a young Eskimo villager who is a student in a modern school, works on computers, and studies world events may become disillusioned at home, where the old roles and lack of employment may still exist. In this situation the parents may feel inadequate because they are unable to relate to the child as a result of the knowledge that the child has acquired at school. On the other hand, the child may see little importance in subsistence skills, such as fishing or hunting, in which the parents excel. After high school, the student may leave the village to attend college or trade school. However, the student may be unable to tolerate living away from the village or family and thus may return to the village after several months or years. Inadequate education and village schools do not prepare Eskimo children for the modern world. When the adolescent returns to the village, there is a difficult reacceptance of village life. The village's subsistence activities give rise to disillusionment, depression, and self-destructive behavior. Because they find that their own views and values have changed as a result of the outside experience, village life becomes stifling for many. Also, the trade or occupation learned while at school (such as computer science) often has little relevance to life in the village. The result of all of this is that the village now has a frustrated, angry individual who has not readapted to village life and who does not have the emotional ability to survive away from home and family. These contributory factors may lead to depression and hence to

alcohol and drug use (Albert, 1988; Chance, 1966; Seltzer, 1980).

There is a high incidence of suicide among Eskimo males. During the 1980s, 86% of the suicide victims were male. The rate of suicide in men between the ages of 20 and 24 was in excess of 30 times the national rate for all age groups combined (Institute for Social and Economic Research, 1998). Many Eskimo women, on the other hand, attach meaning and purpose to life through the possibility of motherhood. Thus, Eskimo women are less likely than their male counterparts to become severely depressed. However, for Eskimo men, life is perceived as purposeless because of their detachment from the family. In many instances, Eskimo women exist primarily for their children (Albert, 1988).

In a study that compared 567 Alaska Native criminal offenders referred to mental health professionals with 939 White offenders, it was found that alcohol abuse, which is the dominant social problem for some Alaska Natives, is not clearly associated with the degree of sociocultural change. Living in larger communities and higher educational achievement are associated with greater psychosocial maladjustment than the incidence of alcohol abuse is. The region of residence has a stronger influence on the rate and type of maladjustment than the ethnic group (that is, Eskimo, Indian, or Aleut) or the ethnic density of the community of residence (that is, the proportion of Alaska Natives in the population) does (Phillips & Inui, 1986).

For some Eskimos, alcohol use has become an acceptable way to escape. Binge drinking has been related to the stress of acculturation (Mala, 1984) and is characteristic for some Alaska Natives (Albert, 1988). Because binge drinking is directly related to morbidity and mortality in Alaska, programs have been set up to deal with this problem. However, programs such as Alcoholics Anonymous have been relatively unsuccessful in Eskimo treatment, just as other forms of treatment designed for and by White people have (Lange, 1988). Culturally relevant programs have proved to be much more effective and frequently involve resolution of the conflicts created by Westernization (Albert, 1988).

Some reports have identified a biological predisposition of some Canadian Eskimos to be more susceptible to the deleterious effects of alcohol (Seltzer & Langford, 1984). Canadian Eskimos are extremely rapid acetylators, as tested with isoniazid (Schaefer, 1986). Eskimos also tend to clear phenytoin rapidly, as proved in Greenland Eskimos and supported by clinical observations in Canadian Eskimos. Schaefer (1986) also found that metabolism is significantly slower in Canadian Eskimos than in Whites. Although the work with biological predisposition and alcohol metabolism has been done with Canadian Eskimos, these data can easily be generalized to the Alaskan Eskimos in a more westerly area of the Arctic.

Implications for Nursing Care

Seltzer (1983) has reported three interesting cases of Eskimos who claimed to be possessed by spirits. The spirits appeared to represent culture-bound defense mechanisms and attempts at problem solving in Eskimos who had unresolved cultural conflicts. Although reports of spiritual possession are uncommon among mental health professionals in Alaska, Seltzer's report does emphasize the importance of knowledge of myths and customs, as well as culturally significant methods of healing, on the part of health care providers. Napoleon (1991) asserts that as a result of the large number of deaths and displacements due to epidemics of influenza, tuberculosis, and other communicable diseases in the early twentieth century and the resulting rapid cultural change, Yup'iks suffer from a form of posttraumatic stress disorder.

Eschiti (2004) postulates that holistic nursing presents an ideal framework to foster promotion and maintenance of health for Alaskan Natives. Understanding cultural differences will allow the nurse to relate in a positive way to persons from varied cultural backgrounds. If nursing interventions are to be successful, they must not oppose a particular cultural practice. On the other hand, if the cultural practice is detrimental to the health status of the people, the nurse must devise a teaching plan and alternative strategies to combat the negative practice. If the nurse is to use time and energy efficiently, nursing care measures must be planned and implemented cooperatively with the client and family so that it is perceived as being culturally relevant (Overfield, 1995). Community efforts are also important. For example, the Alaska Native Community Suicide Prevention Center is an example of a community-based program that has shown promising results in reducing suicides among young adults (DeBruyn, Wilkins, Stetter-Burns, & Nelson, 1997).

The nurse who works with Eskimo clients must know certain biological concepts that are germane to the Eskimo people in order to give not only adequate care but also nonharmful care. As the Western culture influences Eskimo people, behaviors have changed. For example, Eskimos are consuming large quantities of carbohydrates, bottle-feeding instead of breastfeeding their infants, consuming large quantities of alcohol, increasing their tobacco use, and assuming a more sedentary lifestyle. As behaviors and health care needs of these individuals change, the nurse must modify approaches to client care accordingly.

SUMMARY

Despite the apparent Westernization of Eskimos, they have retained many of their traditional perceptions and responses to life situations. Whether in an Alaskan village or in a clinic or hospital in the mainland United States, the nurse who encounters an Eskimo client must incorporate a theoretical framework that encompasses knowledge of communication, spatial requirements, social organization, time, environmental control, and biological variations to enhance quality nursing care.

Case Study

This case study focuses on a 6-year-old Eskimo girl with chronic otitis media, anemia, poor dietary habits, noncompliance with prescribed medication, and low self-esteem, resulting in failure to adjust to school. The mother brings the child to the village clinic for treatment. When taking the history from the mother, the nurse notes that the child has six siblings and comes from a home where the father is frequently absent and when present is often drunk. The nurse observes that the mother provides inconsistent direction and resorts to threats and ridicule when attempting to correct or change the child's behavior. For example, when the child does not sit still, the mother states, "You be good, or the nurse will give you a shot." The nurse notes that both the child's ears have a gluelike discharge, which the mother states is being treated with eardrops given at the clinic 2 weeks earlier. However, the mother also states that the child refuses to allow the eardrops to be instilled because they "hurt" her ears. The nurse notes that only a small amount of the bottle has been used.

This is the second clinic visit. At the first visit, when asked about what the child ate, the mother responded that most food items came from hunting or fishing or the village store and that they usually had fish soup, pilot bread with shortening, and black, sugared tea. With a hemoglobinometer, the nurse now determines that the child's hemoglobin remains at the same low level as at the previous visit. The iron-supplement tablets given at the last visit have not been taken. When questioned about whether she eats the school lunch provided by the public lunch program, the child replies that no one likes her and that the other children take her food, and so she does not get much.

On examination of the child, the nurse finds a pale mucous membrane and poor muscle tone with decreased muscle activity. The child's temperature is 102° F, her pulse is 75, her blood pressure is 100/66 mm Hg, and her respirations are 22. The nurse notes that the child complains of a sharp, constant pain in both ears and frequently pulls or tugs at both ears, seemingly in an attempt to gain relief. On examination of the ears, the nurse notes that the external canal is free of wax and that the mastoid process behind the ear is not tender to touch. However, the tympanic membrane appears inflamed.

CARE PLAN

✳ Nursing Diagnosis: Nutrition altered, less than body requirements

Client Outcomes

1. Client will have increased iron level.
2. Mother will understand safety measures.
3. Parental knowledge of illness will be increased.
4. Client will have adequate dietary intake.
5. Mother and client will describe causative factors related to inadequate nutrition.
6. Client will experience adequate nutrition through oral intake.

Nursing Interventions

1. Educate mother and client about iron-rich foods, including eggs, dates, and raisins.
2. Do a 24-hour recall dietary history.
3. Obtain height and weight measurements and plot on a standard chart that has been normed for Eskimo children.
4. Involve mother in designing a medication reminder sheet.
5. Reinforce with mother and client the need for taking appropriate does of iron supplements.
6. Teach mother and client about the need to eat a nutritionally balanced diet.
7. Instruct mother to be certain to put iron supplements in a safe place so that other children cannot take the medication indiscriminately, thus avoiding iron toxicity.
8. Teach mother about importance of good nutrition for a child.
9. Use an easy to understand nutrition brochure to illustrate how to make health food choices.
10. Encourage mother to seek additional assistance for dietary requirements, such as the WIC program.
11. Call the school and talk with teachers about lunch time intake.

✳ *Nursing Diagnosis: Management of therapeutic regimen related to decisional conflicts, as evidenced by mother stating that child refuses to use eardrops because they hurt her ears*

Client Outcomes

1. Client will have increased comfort.
2. Measures will be taken to prevent recurrence.
3. Parental knowledge about condition will be increased.
4. Measures will be taken to prevent the possibility of a tympanic membrane rupture.
5. Mother and client will learn value of washing hands and not placing foreign bodies into the ear.
6. Mother and client will learn value of taking prescribed antibiotic for the full amount of time.

Nursing Interventions

1. Teach mother and client to seek early medical care for pharyngitis to prevent spread of infection through eustachian tube to middle ear.
2. Teach mother and child to wash hands to prevent illness.
3. Teach mother and client to not put hard or sharp things into the ear.
4. Assess for hearing impairment or loss.
5. Examine external auditory canal and tympanic membrane.
6. Teach mother and client that antibiotic must be taken as prescribed.
7. Teach mother and client signs and symptoms of tympanic membrane rupture, which include sudden relief of pain, and to call the clinic.
8. Teach mother and client the value of soft and liquid foods when chewing is extremely painful because of movement of the eustachian tube.

✳ *Nursing Diagnosis: Coping, ineffective individual (mother and child)*

1. Related to complex self-care regimens
2. As evidenced by nonassertive response patterns, allows child to refuse medications, allows child to be taken advantage

Client Outcomes

1. Client will describe experiences that cause her to alter prescribed behavior.
2. Mother will develop an appropriate alternative for previous plan for medication administration.

Nursing Interventions

1. Assess causative or contributing factors for noncompliance with prescribed therapy.
2. Assess client's rationale for noncompliance with medication.
3. Teach mother and client how to administer eardrops (room temperature)
4. Watch as mother administers eardrops.
5. Observe mother-child interactions.
6. Explain if modifications needed.
7. Praise mother and child when medications are administered correctly.

✳ *Nursing Diagnosis: Self-esteem disturbance*

Client Outcomes

1. Client will verbalize positive feelings about self.
2. Client will take part in activities with other children in a confident manner.
3. Client will achieve grade-level objectives of school age.

Nursing Interventions

1. Encourage client to express both positive and negative feelings.
2. Encourage mother to set limits on problematic behavior, such as poor hygiene, noncompliance with medication, and other negative behaviors.
3. Accept silence of client, but let her know that the nurse is there for support.

✳ *Nursing Diagnosis: Family process, altered; alcoholism coping, ineffective family: disabling related to impaired ability to constructively manage stressors secondary to alcoholism of father, as evidenced by actions that are detrimental to family well-being, child allowed to be taken advantage of at school, child not treated with ear medications*

Client Outcome

1. Mother relates expectations for what she will do in regard to child not being allowed to eat lunch at school, going to Al-Anon meetings.

Nursing Interventions

1. Explore with the mother and the 6-year-old how their behavior has negatively affected the physical well-being of the 6-year-old girl (refusing ear treatment, allowing others to take away lunch).
2. Explore characteristics of families affected by alcoholism.
3. Provide information on community resources, such as Al-Anon, Alcoholics Anonymous, family therapy.

STUDY QUESTIONS

1. Identify why otitis media may be a common illness among Eskimo children.
2. Identify cultural factors that affect the treatment of otitis media in Eskimo children.
3. List factors that predispose Eskimos to risk as a direct result of regular consumption of tea.
4. List factors that predispose Eskimos to risk as a result of consumption of large quantities of sugar.

5. Using Campbell's rule, can you distinguish whether this cultural group is at risk for glucose intolerance?
6. List several contributing factors related to alcoholism among Alaskan Eskimos.
7. Formerly, tuberculosis was a disease condition to which Eskimos were believed to have inherited susceptibility. Today, however, this is considered untrue. List two factors cited that do have contributing significance.

NCLEX-RN REVIEW QUESTIONS

1. The nurse is caring for a family in which five family members have tuberculosis. The family describes its health belief to the nurse, which included shamanic healing. The nurse knows the patient will be more compliant if she includes use of antituberculin medication as well as:
   A. Services of a folk healer
   B. Behavior therapy
   C. Acupuncture
   D. Yoga

2. A nurse caring for an Eskimo child observes dark spots in the lumbar area as well as other dark areas on the body. The nurse should:
   A. Have the parents investigated for child abuse.
   B. Assess the areas to determine if they are mongolian spots.

   C. Recognize these areas being related to coining.
   D. Ignore the difference in color.

3. As you explain your patient's condition to her husband, you notice that he is leaning toward you and raising his eyebrows. Knowing that he is an Eskimo, your most appropriate response to this behavior is to:
   A. Tell him that you understand his need to be alone.
   B. Ask whether he has any questions.
   C. Ask whether he would prefer to speak to the physician.
   D. Understand he is agreeing.

References

Abdel-Hamid, M., Chen, J., Constantine, N., Massound, M., & Raab-Traub, N. (1992, September). EBV strain variation: geographical distribution and relation to disease state. *Virology*, 190(1), 168–175.

Alaska Division of Public Health, Section of Community Health and Emergency Medical Services. (1998). Take heart Alaska: a cardiovascular disease prevention plan for Alaska, 1(1), Retrieved September 9, 2002, from www.epi.hss.state.ak.us/programs/chronic/cardio/tha.pdf.

Alaska Native Tribal Health Consortium, Office of Human Resources. Anchorage, Alaska. Alaska Native Tribal Health Consortium.

Albert, D. (1988). Impact of acculturation of Alaskan natives, Paper presented at the Ob-Gyn Update 1988 conference, Anchorage, Alaska.

Allen, E., & Crago, M. (1996, February). Early passive acquisition in Inuktitut. *Journal of Child Language*, 23(1), 129–155.

American Native Heritage Center. (2000). Retrieved at http://www.alaskanative.net/35.asp. Date retrieved: April 1, 2006.

Andersen, S., Hvingel, B., Kleinschmidt, K., Jorgensen, T., & Laurberg, P. (2005, March). Changes in iodine excretion in 50–69 y old denizens of an Arctic society in transition and iodine excretion as a biomarker of the frequency of consumption of traditional Inuit foods. *American Journal of Clinical Nutrition*, 81(3), 656–663.

Armstrong, T., Roberts, B., & Swithinbank, C. (Eds.). (1973). *Illustrated glossary of snow and ice*. Cambridge, England: Scott Polar Research Institute.

Bank, T. (1956). *Birthplace of the wind*. New York: Crowell.

Baxter, J. (1980). My experience with the Canadian Inuit. *Journal of Otolaryngology*, 9(1), 63–66.

Baxter, J., Katsarkas, A., Ling, D., & Carson, R. (1979, June). The Nakasuk project: the conservative treatment of chronic otitis media in Inuit elementary school children. *Journal of Otolaryngology*, 8(3), 201–209.

Behavioral Risk Factor Surveillance, 1991. (1992). Fairbanks: Office of Health Promotion, Alaska Division of Public Health.

Bells, R., Draper, H., & Bergan, J. (1973). Sucrose, lactose, and glucose tolerance in northern Alaskan Eskimos. *American Journal of Clinical Nutrition*, 26, 1185–1190.

Bijlmer, H. (1991, June). World-wide epidemiology of *Haemophilus influenzae* meningitis: industrialized versus non-industrialized countries. *Vaccine*, S5–S9.

Bjerregaard, P., Young, T., Dewailly, E., & Ebbesson, S. (2004). Indigenous health in the Arctic, an overview of the circumpolar Inuit population. *Scandinavian Journal of Public Health*, 32(5), 390–395.

Blodgett, J. (1978). *The coming and going of shaman: Eskimo shamanism and art*. Winnipeg, Manitoba: Winnipeg Art Gallery.

Blum, R. (1992, August). American Indians and Alaska Native youths. *The IHS Primary Care Provider*, 17(8), 137–145.

Boas, F. (1983). *The mind of primitive man*. Westport, Conn: Greenwood Press.

Book, P. A., Dixon, M., & Kirchner, S. (1983). Native health in Alaska: report from Serpentine Hot Springs. In Cross-cultural medicine. *Western Journal of Medicine*, 139, 923–927.

Branch, K. (2002, May). Rural affordable assisted living in Dillingham, Alaska. *The IHS Primary Care Provider*, 27 (5), 1–3.

Brant, L. J., Bender, T. R., & Marnell, R. W. (1982). Factors affecting streptococcal colonization among children in selected areas of Alaska. *Public Health Reports*, 97(5), 460–464.

Brown, S. (1997, July 27). Alaskan oil. *Tulsa World*, E1.

Bruerd, B. (1997, March). Preventing baby bottle tooth decay and early childhood caries among AI/AN infants and children. *The IHS Primary Care Provider*, 22(3), 37–39.

Butler, J. C., Crengle, S., Cheek, J. E., & Leach, A. J., et al. (2001). Emerging infectious diseases among indigenous peoples. CDC supplement, 7(3). Retrieved September 9, 2002, from www.cdc.gov/ncidod/eid/vol7no3_supp;butler.htm.

Carpenter, E. (1973). *Eskimo realities*. New York: Holt, Rinehart, & Winston.

Castagno, J. (2005). *Lands and people* (vol. 6). Danbury, Conn.: Scholastic Library Publishing.

Centers for Disease Control and Prevention. (1996). Prevalence and impact of arthritis by race and ethnicity B United States, 1989–1991. *Morbidity and Mortality Weekly Report*, 45(18), 373–378.

Chance, N. (1966). *Eskimo of north Alaska*. New York: Holt, Rinehart, & Winston.

Chance, N. (1990). The Inupiat of arctic Alaska. Harcourt Brace. Retrieved April 1, 2006, from http://arcticcircle.ucon.edu/CulturalViability/Inupiat/1800s.html.

Crago, M., & Tremblay, C. (1991). Obstacles, challenges, and solutions: evolution in audiological service delivery to the hearing-impaired Inuit of northern Quebec. *Arctic Medical Research, Suppl.*, 633–638.

Damas, D. (1984). *Arctic: handbook of North American Indians*, (vol. 5). Washington, D.C.: Smithsonian Institution.

Davidhizar, R., & Giger, J. (2000, January–February). Culture and care: profiling Alaskan Eskimos. *Health Traveler*, 7(4), 12 43–47.

Day, G., & Lanier, A. (2003). Alaska native mortality. *Public Health Reports*, 118(6), 518–530.

DeBruyn, L., Wilkins, B., Stetter-Burns, M., & Nelson, S. (1997). Violence and violence prevention. *The IHS Primary Care Provider*, 22(4), 58–60.

Denny, C., Holtzman, D., Goins, R., & Croft, J. (2005). Disparities in chronic disease risk factors and health status between American Indian/Alaska Native and white elders: findings from a telephone survey, 2001 and 2002. *American Journal of Public Health*, 95(5), 825–827.

Dixon, M. (1998). Managed care in American Indian and Alaska Native communities. *Etudes/Inuit/Studies*, 6(2), American Public Health Association.

Dixon, M. (2001). *Promises to keep: public health policy for American Indians and Alaska Natives in the 21st century*. Washington, D.C.: American Public Health Association.

Dixon, M., & Kirchner, S. (1982). "Poking," an Eskimo medical practice in northwest Alaska. *Etudes/Inuit/Studies*, 6(2), 109–125.

Duncan, I., & Scott, E. (1972). Lactose intolerance in Alaska Indian and Eskimo. *American Journal of Clinical Nutrition*, 25, 867–868.

Dyerberg, J., & Bang, H. (1978). Eicosapentaenoic acid and prevention of thrombosis and atherosclerosis. *Lancet*, 2, 117–119.

Eschiti, V. (2004). Holistic approach to resolving American Indian/Alaska Native health care disparities. *Journal of Holistic Nursing*, 22(3), 201–208.

Feldman, S. A., Ho, K. J., Lewis, L. A., et al. (1972, July). Lipid and cholesterol metabolism in Alaskan Eskimos. *Arctic Pathology*, 94(1), 42–58.

Fienup-Riordan, A. (2001). A guest on the table: ecology from the Yup'ik Eskimo point of view. In J. Grim, (Ed.)., *Indigenous traditions and ecology: the interbeing of cosmology and community* (pp. 541–558). Cambridge: Harvard University Press for the Center for the Study of World Religions, Harvard Divinity School.

Fleshman, C. (1992, October). Injury and deaths among American Indians and Alaska Native infants. *The IHS Primary Care Provider*, 17(10), 186–190.

Fortuine, R. (1989). *Chills and fever: health and disease in the early history of Alaska*. Fairbanks: University of Alaska Press.

Freddoso, D. (2002, March 4). Unions support Bush on Alaska drilling. *Human Events*, 58(9), 5.

Friedrich, C. A., & Ferrell, R. E. (1985, May). A population study of alpha-keto acid reductase. *Annuals of Human Genetics*, 49(Pt. 2), 111–114.

Gaffey, M. J., & Weiss, L. M. (1990, November). Viral oncogenesis: Epstein-Barr virus. *American Journal of Otolaryngology*, 11(6), 375–381.

Gall, T. (1998). *Worldmark encyclopedia of cultures and daily life*. Cleveland, OH: Eastwood Publications Department.

Gallinek, P. (2006, January). Communities of compassion. *Healthcare traveler*, 7(1), 33–37.

Garrett, W. (1988, October). Air bridge to Siberia. *National Geographic*, 174(4), 504.

Giblin, P. (1997). Cooler than cactus. *The Dallas Morning News*, 1A.

Glassetter, M. (1989, February 8). Personal interview with Dolly Lefever concerning Inupiat values.

Goodbody, M., & Stubbing, P. (1991). A study on cost effectiveness of audiology services, Baffin region, N.W.T. *Arctic Medical Research, Suppl.*, 646–647.

Gottberg, J. (1988). *Frommer's dollarwise guide to Alaska*. Englewood Cliffs, N.J.: Prentice Hall.

Gove, C. (1982). *The conflict between cultural persistence and acculturation as it affects individual behavior of northwestern Alaskan Eskimo*. Dissertation presented to graduate faculty of the School of Human Behavior, U.S. International University, San Diego, California.

Haggett, P. (2002). *Encyclopedia of world geography, United States I*. New York: Marshall Cavendish.

Hall, D. B., Lum, M. K., Knutson, L. R., et al. (1987). Pharyngeal carriage and acquisition of anticapsular antibody to Haemophilus influenzae type b in a high risk population in southwestern Alaska. *American Journal of Epidemiology*, 126(6), 1190–1197.

Hall, E. (1975). *The Eskimo storyteller: folktales from Noatak, Alaska*. Knoxville, Tn.: University of Tennessee Press.

Heller, C. A. (1947). *Alaska nutrition survey report*. Juneau, Alaska: Territorial Department of Health.

Hildes, J. A., & Schaefer, O. (1984). The changing picture of neoplastic disease in the western and central Canadian Arctic. *Canadian Medical Association Journal*, 130 (1), 25–32.

Hinsley, K. (2001). *Give me my father's body: the Life of Minik, the New York Eskimo*. New York: Pocket Books.

Holderman, N. (1960, March). The little men. *Alaska Call*, p. 16.

Holderman, N. (1962). Personal correspondence about life as an Alaska Native Service teacher's wife.

Holderman, R. (1993, May 15). Personal correspondence regarding Alaska Native Service teaching experience in the 1950s and the 1960s in Deering and Shungnak, Alaska.

Holderman, R. (2006, August 9). Personal correspondence regarding Alaska Native Service teaching experiences in the 1950s and 1960s in Deering and Shungnak, Alaska.

Holman, R., Curns, A., Cheek, J., Bresee, J., Singleton, R., Carver, K., & Anderson, L. (2004, October). Respiratory syncytial virus hospitalizations among American Indian and Alaska Native infants and the general United States infant population. *Pediatrics*, 114(4), e437–444.

Hrdlicka, A. (1930). Anthropological survey in Alaska (46th annual report). Washington, D.C.: U.S. Department of Commerce, Bureau of Ethnology.

Hrdlicka, A. (1941). Height and weight of Eskimo children. *American Journal of Physical Anthropology*, 28, 331.

Ilecki, H. J., & Baxter, J. D. (1981). Arctic audiology: trials, tribulations, and occasional successes. *Journal of Otolaryngology*, 10(4), 294–298.

Indian Health Service (1998–1999). Regional Differences in Indian Health 1998–99. Retrieved at http://www.ihs.gov. Date retrieved: March 27, 2006.

Indian Health Service. (2000). 2000 Survey Dental Services. Indian Health Services. Rockville, Md.: Indian Health Services.

Indian Health Service. (2002). Alaska Natives: key facts. Retrieved at http://www2.ihs.gov. Date retrieved: September 2, 2002.

Institute for Social and Economic Research, University of Alaska, Anchorage. (1998). Physical and behavioral health statistics from the Alaska Natives Commission. Retrieved at http://www.alaskool.org/resources/anc/anc06.htm. Date retrieved: September 9, 2002.

Jackson, M. (2000, May). Healthy people 2010: Reaching American Indian/Alaska Native Elders. *The IHS Primary Care Provider*, 25(5), 1–2.

Jilek-Aall, L. (1981). Acculturation, alcoholism, and Indian-style Alcoholics Anonymous. *Journal of Studies on Alcohol*, 9, 143–158.

Johnston, F. E., Laughlin, W. S., Harper, A. B., & Ensroth, A. E. (1982). Physical growth of St. Lawrence Island Eskimos: body size, proportion, and composition. *American Journal of Physical Anthropology*, 58(4), 397–401.

Juul, S. (1979). Portrait of an Eskimo tribal health doctor. *Alaska Medicine*, 21(6), 66–71.

Keats, D. (1985). Della Keats: Eskimo healer (Video). Kotzebue, Alaska: Manillnaq.

Key, S., & Marble, M. (1999, April 12). Liver cancer linked to HBV in Eskimos. *Cancer Weekly Plus*, 14.

Klausner, A., & Foulks, E. F. (1982). *Eskimo capitalists: oil, politics, and alcohol.* Englewood Cliffs, N.J.: Prentice Hall.

Kleinfeld, J. S. (1971). *Some instructional strategies for the cross-cultural classroom.* Juneau: Alaska Department of Education.

Kost-Grant, B. (1983). Self-inflicted gunshot wounds among Alaska Natives. *Public Health Reports*, 98(1), 72–78.

Lancaster, M. (1990). Botulism: north to Alaska. *American Journal of Nursing*, 90(1), 60–62.

Langdon, S. J. (1987). *The Native people of Alaska.* Anchorage, Alaska: Greatland Graphics.

Lange, B. (1988). Ethnographic interview: an occupational therapy needs assessment tool for American Indian and Alaska Native alcoholics. *Occupational Therapy in Mental Health*, 8(2), 61–80.

Lanier, A., Bender, T., Talbert, M., et al. (1980). Nasopharyngeal carcinoma in Alaskan Eskimos, Indians, and Aleuts: a review of cases and study of Epstein-Barr virus, HLA, and environmental risk factors. *Cancer*, 46(9), 2100–2106.

Lanier, A. P., Bulkow, L. R., & Novotny, T. E., et al. (1990). Tobacco use and its consequences in northern populations. *Arctic Medical Research*, 49(suppl. 2), 17–22.

Lanier, A, Holck, P., Day, G., & Key, C. (2003, November). Childhood cancer among Alaskan natives. *Pediatrics*, 112(5), 396–403.

Lantis, M. (1986). *Eskimo childhood and interpersonal relationships.* New York: AMS Press.

Lee, C., Brunham, R., Sherman, E., & Harding, G. (1987). Epidemiology of an outbreak of infectious syphilis in Manitoba. *American Journal of Epidemiology*, 125, 277–283.

Legal Information Institute. (nd). U.S. code collection, title 25, chapter 21, section 1915. Retrieved September 8, 2002, from http://www4.law.cornell.edu/uscode/25/1915.html.

Lewis, D., & Ho, M. (1975). Social work with Native Americans. *Social Work*, 20, 379–382.

Ling, D. (1976, July 6). Audiological problems of the Eskimo population in the Baffin zone. In Shepherd, R. J., & Itoh, S. (Eds.), *Circumpolar health* (pp. 409–412). Toronto: University of Toronto Press.

Loshbaugh, D. (1996, December 23). *Rudolph's secret.* Peninsula Clarion, Kenai, Alaska.

Lubbock, B. (1937). *The Arctic whalers.* Glasgow, Scotland: Brown, Son & Ferguson.

Lum, M. K., Knutson, L. R., & Hall, D. B., et al. (1986). Decline in infant mortality of Alaskan Yupik Eskimos from 1960 to 1980. *Public Health Reports*, 101(3), 309–314.

Lynch, H., Schuelke, G., & O'Hara, M. (1984, June). Is cancer communicable? *Medical Hypotheses*, 14(2), 181–198.

MacDonald-Clark, N., & Boffman, J. (1995, June). Mother-child interaction among the Alaskan Eskimos. *Journal of Obstetric, Gynecologic, and Neonatal Nursing*, 24(5), 450–457.

Mailhot, J. (1978). L'étymologie de "Esquimau" revue et corrigée. *Etudes Inuit–Inuit Studies*, 2, 59–69.

Mala, A. (1984). Circumpolar health, 1984: an Alaskan perspective. *Alaska Medicine*, 26(4), 108–111.

Mann, G. V., & Scott, E. (1962, July). The health and nutritional status of Alaskan Eskimos. *American Journal of Clinical Nutrition*, 2, 31–76.

McMahon, B. J., Heyward, W. K., & Templin, D. W., et al. (1989). Hepatitis B–associated polyarteritis nodosa in Alaska: clinical and epidemiologic features and long-term follow-up. *Hepatology*, 9(1), 97–101.

Milan, F. A. (Ed.). (1980). *The human biology of circumpolar populations*. Cambridge: Cambridge University Press.

Mitchell, W., & Patch, K. (1986). Religion, spiritualism, and the recovery of Native American Alcoholics. *The IHS Primary Care Provider*, 11, 129.

Morris, J. (1985). Caribou and ketchup—health implications. *Nursing Practice*, 1(2), 98–101.

Mouratoff, G., Carrol, N., & Scott, E. (1967). Diabetes mellitus in Eskimos. *Journal of the American Medical Association*, 199(13), 107–122.

Napoleon, H. (1991). *Yuuyaraq: the way of the human being*. Fairbanks, Alaska: University of Alaska, Fairbanks.

National Center for Health Statistics. (2002). Health, United States, 2002 with urban and rural chartbook. Washington, D.C: U.S. Government Printing.

National Center for Health Statistics, Healthy People 2000 Review. (1993). Health, United States 1992. Hyattsville, Md.: Public Health Service.

Newberg, J. (1997, April 10). Paddle power on the water. *The Arizona Republic*, OT1.

Nida, E. (1954). *Customs and cultures*. New York: Harper & Brothers.

Nobmann, E. (1984). *Dietary factors and iron deficiency*. Anchorage: Alaska Native Medical Center.

Nord, E. (1995, August). Evolution of a public health nursing program, Yukon Kuskokwim Delta, Alaska, 1893–1993. *Public Health Nursing*, 12(4), 249–255.

Overfield, T. (1977). Biological variations. *Nursing Clinics of North America*, 12(1), 19–27.

Overfield, T. (1995). *Biologic variation in health and illness* (ed. 2). Reading, Mass.: Addison-Wesley.

Pender, J. (1987, March). Little Pinch: memoir of a healer. *Anchorage Daily News Magazine*, p. 3.

Petersen, G. M., Silimperi, D. R., Chiu, C. Y., & Ward, J. I. (1991, November 15). *American Journal of Epidemiology*, 134(10), 1212–1221.

Petersen, G. M., Silimperi, D. R., & Rotter, J. I., et al. (1987). Genetic factors in *Haemophilus influenzae* type B disease susceptibility and antibody acquisition. *Journal of Pediatrics*, 110(2), 228–233.

Phillips, M. R., & Inui, T. S. (1986). The interaction of mental illness, criminal behavior and culture: Native Alaskan mentally ill criminal offenders. *Culture, Medicine, and Psychiatry*, 10(2), 123–149.

Polk, S. (1987, September–October). Helping our children. *Children Today*, pp. 19–20.

Pollick, S. (1997, June 16). Inuit life harsh, often brutal. *The Blade*. Toledo, Ohio.

The Random House dictionary of the English language. (1987). New York: Random House.

Roberts, L., & Ross, C. (1979). Nursing north of sixty. *Canadian Nurse*, 75(5), 26–29.

Rodahl, K. (1964). *Between two worlds*. London: Heinemann.

Rode, A., & Shephard, R. J. (1984). Ten years of "civilization": fitness of Canadian Inuit. *Journal of Physiology*, 56(6), 1472–1477.

Rosen, Y. (1997, February 28). Iditarod trail leads to more pros, fewer native racers. *Christian Science Monitor*, 1.

Ross, D. (1989). Nursing up north. *Canadian Nurse*, 85(1), 22–24.

Saari, M. (1997, June 7). Native art unearthed for all. *Ketchikan Daily News*, 1.

Sanders, N. (2000). The relationship of spirituality and health among the Yup'ik of southwestern Alaska: an exploratory study. Doctoral dissertation. Detroit: Wayne State University.

Schaefer, O. (1970). Pre- and postnatal growth acceleration and increased sugar consumption in Canadian Eskimos. *Canadian Medical Association Journal*, 103(10), 1059–1068.

Schaefer, O. (1973). The changing health picture in the Canadian north. *Canadian Journal of Ophthalmology*, 8, 196–204.

Schaefer, O. (1986). Adverse reactions to drugs and metabolic problems perceived in northern Canadian Indians and Eskimos. *Progress in Clinical and Biological Research*, 214, 77–83.

Schanfield, M., Crawford, M., Dossetor, J., & Gershowitz, H. (1990, December). Immunoglobulin allotypes in several North American Eskimo populations. *Human Biology: An International Record of Research*, 62(6), 773–789.

Schneider, E. (2005, May). Tuberculosis among American Indians and Alaska Natives in the United States. *American Journal of Public Health*, 95(5), 873–880.

Scott, E. M., & Griffin, I. (1956). *Diabetes mellitus in Eskimos*. Anchorage, Alaska: Arctic Research Center.

Seltzer, A. (1980). Acculturation and mental disorders in the Inuit. *Canadian Journal of Psychiatry*, 25(2), 173–181.

Seltzer, A. (1983). Psychodynamics of spirit possession among the Inuit. *Canadian Journal of Psychiatry*, 28(1), 52–56.

Seltzer, A., & Langford, J. A. (1984). Forensic psychiatric assessments in the Northwest Territories. *Canadian Journal of Psychiatry*, 29(8), 665–668.

Shephard, R. J. (Ed.). (1974). *Circumpolar Health: third international symposium.* Yellow Knife, Northwest Territory, Canada.

Singleton, R. (1992). *Haemophilus influenzae* type B infections in the Yukon Kuskokwim Delta and Bristol Bay area of Alaska. *The IHS Primary Care Provider*, 17(8), 123.

Sipperly, M. (1989). Marine lipids and coronary angioplasty: benefit. *Progress in Cardiovascular Nursing*, 4 (4), 119–123.

Snider, D., Salinas, L., & Kelly, G. (1989). Tuberculosis: an increasing problem among minorities in the United States. *Public Health Reports*, 104(6), 646–653.

State of Alaska, Department of Health and Social Services, Division of Public Health, Section of Epidemiology. (2000). HIV infection in Alaska 1999. 4(2). Retrieved at http://www.epi.hss.state.ak.us. Date retrieved: September 9, 2002.

State of Alaska, Department of Health and Social Services, Division of Public Health, Section of Epidemiology. (2001a). Tuberculosis control in Alaska. Juneau, Alaska: State of Alaska, Department of Health and Social Services, Division of Public Health, Section of Epidemiology. Retrieved June 15, 2007, from http://www.hss.state.ak.us.

State of Alaska, Department of Health and Social Services, Division of Public Health, Section of Epidemiology. (2001b). Diabetes in Alaska, 1991–2000: results from the Behavioral Risk Factor Surveillance System (BRFSS). 5(4), 1–5. Retrieved at http://www.epi.hss.state.ak.us. Date retrieved: September 9, 2002.

State of Alaska, Department of Health and Social Services, Division of Public Health, Section of Epidemiology. (2001c). 2000 Annual (January–December) infectious disease report: number of cases by region. Bulletin No. 4. Retrieved at http://www.epi.hss.state.ak.us. Date retrieved: September 8, 2002.

State of Alaska, Section of Epidemiology. (1997). *Cardiovascular disease in Alaska, bulletin no. 3.* Retrieved at http://www.epi.hss.state.ak.us. Date retrieved: September 9, 2002.

Stefansson, V. (1969). *The friendly Arctic.* New York: Greenwood Press.

Stevenson, M. (1984). Tuberculosis in the North: a lifestyle issue. *Canadian Nurse*, 80(1), 41–43.

Szathmary, E. J. (1984). Peopling of northern North America: clues from genetic studies. *Acta Anthropologenetica*, 8(1–2), 79–109.

Taylor, C. (1988). Trauma prevention in rural Alaska. *Journal of Emergency Nursing*, 14(5), 36A–39A.

Time almanac with information please. (2006). Boston: Information Please, Inc.

Toomey, K. E., Oberschelp, A. G., & Greenspan, J. R. (1989). Sexually transmitted diseases and Native Americans: trends in reported gonorrhea and syphilis morbidity, 1984–1988. *Public Health Reports*, 104(6), 566–572.

Toomey, K. E., Rafferty, M. P., & Stamm, W. E. (1987). Unrecognized high prevalence of Chlamydia trachomatis cervical infection in an isolated Alaskan Eskimo population. *Journal of the American Medical Association*, 258(1), 53–56.

Travis, R. (1983). Suicide in northwest Alaska. *White Cloud Journal*, 3(1), 23–30.

U.S. Department of Health and Human Services, Indian Health Services. (1992). Injury deaths among American Indian and Alaska Native infants. *The IHS Primary Care Provider*, 17(10), 186–190.

U.S. Department of Health and Human Services, Indian Health Services. (2000a). Follow-up to the DRI Health Survey for the Indian Health Services. Washington, D.C.: U.S. Government Printing Office.

U.S. Department of Health and Human Services, Indian Health Services. (2000b). Trends in Indian Health 1998–1999. Washington, D.C.: U.S. Government Printing Office.

U.S. Department of Commerce, Bureau of the Census. (2002). Population profiles by age, sex, race, and Hispanic origin, Summary File 3. Hyattsville, Md.: U.S. Government Printing Office.

U.S. Department of Commerce, Bureau of the Census. (2002). The American Indian and Alaska Native population: 2000. Census 2000 brief. Washington, D.C.: U.S. Department of Commerce, Bureau of the Census. Retrieved April 1, 2006, from http://www.census.gov/population/www/cen2000/briefs.html.

U.S. Department of Labor 200. Bureau of labor statistics. Retrieved April 1, 2006, from http://bls.gov/lau.home.htm.

VanDenberg, J., & Minton, B. (1987). Alaska native youth. *Children Today*, 16(5), 15–18.

Van Rens, G. H., Arkell, S. M., Charlton, W., & Doesburg, W. (1988). Primary angle-closure glaucoma among Alaskan Eskimos. *Documenta Ophthalmologica*, 70 (2–3), 265–276.

Vaudrin, R. (1974). Native/non-Native communication: creating a two-way flow. In Orvik, J., & Barnhardt, R. (Eds.), *Cultural influences in Alaska Native education* (pp. 71–83). Fairbanks, Alaska: UAF Press.

Ward, J. I., Lum, M. K., & Hall, D. B., et al. (1986). Invasive *Haemophilus influenzae* type B disease in Alaska: background epidemiology for a vaccine efficacy trial. *Journal of Infectious Diseases*, 153 (1), 17–26.

Whalen, D. (1999, October). Cultural sensitivity: a matter of respect. *Canadian Nurse*, 43–44.

Wiggins, C. (1996, June). A business plan for the IHS. *The IHB Primary Care Provider*, 21(6), 1–4.

Williamson, R. (1974). Eskimo underground socialcultural change in the Canadian central Arctic. Occasional papers (vol. 2). Uppsala, Sweden: Institutet för Allmän och Jämförande, Etnografi, Uppsala University.

Wilson, J., Rausch, R., McMahon, B., & Schantz, P. (1992, August). Parasiticidal effect of chemotherapy in alveolar hydatic disease: review of experience with mebendazone and albendazole in Alaskan Eskimos. *Clinical Infectious Diseases*, 15(2), 234–249.

Wind, S., Sickle, D., & Wright, A. (2004). Health, place and childhood asthma in southwest Alaska. *Social Science & Medicine*, 58(1), 75–88.

World almanac and book of facts (2006). New York: Times Almanac.

Young, T. K. (1986). Epidemiology and control of chronic disease in circumpolar Eskimos/Inuit populations. *Arctic Medical Research*, 42, 25–47.

Zegura, S. L. (1985). The initial peopling of the Americas: an overview from the perspective of physical anthropology. *Acta Anthropogenetica*, 8(1–2), 1–21.

Zimmerman, M. R., & Aufderheide, A. C. (1984). Frozen family of Utqiavik: autopsy findings. *Arctic Anthropology*, 21(1), 531–564.

CHAPTER 13 Japanese Americans

Dawn Liam Doutrich and Yoshiko Colclough

Behavioral Objectives

After reading this chapter, the nurse will be able to do the following:

1. Describe the influence of acculturation on Japanese Americans.
2. Develop a sensitivity and an understanding for the communication styles within and across the Japanese American culture to avoid stereotyping and to provide culturally appropriate care.
3. Describe the time orientation of some Japanese American people and its influence on wellness and illness behavior.
4. Discuss the spatial needs and implications for culturally appropriate care for the Japanese American client.
5. Discuss the influence of family and social organization on behavior.
6. Explain the health care beliefs, folk beliefs, and folk practices of Japanese Americans and their influence on health-seeking behaviors.
7. Recognize physical, biological, and psychological variances that exist within and across the Japanese American culture to provide culturally appropriate care.

OVERVIEW OF JAPAN

Japan is a chain of islands that stretches in an arc more than 1860 miles (2995 km) long from the twenty-fourth parallel, off Taiwan, north to the forty-fifth parallel, just below Sakhalin Island (*Time Almanac with Information Please*, 2007). Japan lies just east of the Asian mainland. The Ryukyu chain, which lies southwest, was once United States–occupied territory. Similarly, the Kuriles, which are northwest, are Russian occupied. The Tsushima Strait separates Japan from Korea.

Japan is composed of four large, closely grouped islands—Hokkaido, Honshu, Shikoku, Kyushu—and 4000 smaller islands. In landmass, Japan is 145,882 square miles. The four main islands constitute approximately 98% of the total landmass of the country. By comparison, Japan is just slightly smaller than California (*Time Almanac with Information Please*, 2007; *World Almanac*, 2007). The habitable and uninhabitable terrain of Japan roughly composes 0.3% of the world's total landmass, yet the population of this country accounts for 3% of the world's population. In 2005, Japan had the seventh largest population in the world, with 127,417,244, people (*Time Almanac with Information Please*, 2007; *World Almanac*, 2007). This number was expected to reach 131 million people by the year 2009. Of the number of people residing in Japan, three fourths live in cities (*Time Almanac with Information Please*, 2007; *World Almanac*, 2007). Because the Japanese landscape is mountainous with angled slopes, only 15% of the total land area is habitable (*Time Almanac with Information Please*, 2007), which accounts for the density of the population in certain regions of the country. In fact, the population of Japan is so dense that there are 873 people per square mile (320 square kilometers). If the uninhabitable areas of Japan were excluded from this equation, a more realistic figure of 3885 people for every 1500 square yards (1760 yards equals a mile) would emerge (*Time Almanac with Information Please*, 2007; *World Almanac*, 2007).

The population explosion of Japan is attributed to industrialization; the population reached 65 million by 1930. After World War II, the Japanese government initiated a population policy to lower the rate of increase. Since the mid-1950s, the population growth rate has corresponded to those in Western European countries (*Time Almanac with Information Please*, 2007). In 2005, the birth rate for Japan was reported to be 9.5 per 1000 and the infant mortality, 3.4 per 1000 live births. In 2005, the average life expectancy at birth was 78.64 for males and 85.59 for females (*World Almanac*, 2007). A declining rate of population growth, coupled with an increased average life expectancy, has resulted in the Japanese population becoming the most rapidly aging population in the world (*Time Almanac with Information Please*, 2007). This has prompted the Japanese government to explore incentives for child-bearing and to look carefully at current exclusionary immigration policies (Onishi, 2005; McNeill, 2006).

The capital of Japan is Tokyo, and with population of 8,483,050 (city proper) and 31,139,900 in the urban surrounding areas, Tokyo is the eleventh largest city in the world (*Time Alamanc with Information Please*, 2006). In addition, with the surrounding metropolitan areas of Yokohama and Kawasaki, Tokyo is the largest city in Japan, followed by Osaka (2,597,000), Yokohama (a part of the Tokyo metro area; 3,494,900), Nagoya (2,189,700), Sapporo (1,848,000), Kobe (part of the Osaka metro area; 1,501,000), Kyoto (part of the metro area of Osaka), Fukuoka (1,368,900), Kawasaki (part of the metro area of Tokyo, 1,276,200), and Hiroshima (1,132,700) (*Time Almanac with Information Please*, 2007). Although Tokyo–Yokohama is a densely populated city, it sprawls over only 800 square miles (2000 square kilometers) (*Time Almanac with Information Please*, 2007; *World Almanac*, 2007). Tokyo is largely industrial and is the home of the Tokyo Stock Exchange (the Nikkei counterpart to the New York Stock Exchange), which is a barometer for the economic climate throughout the world.

Hokkaido is the least populated island in Japan. Although it was once a haven for outcasts, it is now an industrial site where agriculture, leisure activities, and brew-making dominate the economy.

Honshu is the island on which approximately 80% of the Japanese people reside, with the majority concentrated in the plains of Kanto (Tokyo) and Kansai (Kyoto-Osaka). Honshu is known for its distinctive business culture, major ports, and multiple airports (*Time Almanac with Information Please*, 2007; *World Almanac*, 2007).

Shikoku is a comparative backwater devoted primarily to agriculture. Shikoku is not a major attraction for foreign visitors. It is a subtropical island, and the people are reputedly the most outgoing of all Japanese. There is bullet train service to Hakata, which is near Fukuoka, a town that has a major airport.

The Ryukyu chain of islands was occupied by the United States from World War II until 1972 and is perhaps the poorest of all the regions in Japan. These islands are noted for their hybrid population. Several of the islands in the Ryukyus are uninhabited. Okinawa is one of the major islands in the Ryukyus and a major staging base for the U.S. Air Force and Army (*Time Almanac with Information Please*, 2007; *The Economist Business Traveller's Guides*, 2006).

In Japan, there are approximately 60 active volcanoes. In addition, Japan sustains approximately 1000 earthquakes a year, although most result only in minor damage (*Time Almanac with Information Please*, 2007). Two significant exceptions are the Great Kanto Earthquake of 1923, which killed over 100,000 people in the Tokyo and Yokahama area. More recently the Great Hanshin Earthquake of 1995 killed 6000 and injured 415,000 people in the Kobe area (*Time Almanac with Information Please*, 2007). Climatic conditions are favorable, with sufficient warmth and humidity in the summer for cultivation. Winters are cool and dry, unlike the subtropical and tropical winters of much of the rest of Asia. Significant seasonal changes vary with the direction of the prevailing wind, like much of monsoon Asia (*Time Almanac with Information Please*, 2007).

Although more than 67% of the total land area of Japan is forested, not all forests have commercial value because soil erosion is a problem. The sea provides the major portion of protein in the Japanese diet. Both the Japan Sea and the Pacific Ocean are rich fishing grounds. Japan's fishing catch has been the world's largest since 1972. Japan has few mineral resources and depends on imports of raw materials and fuel (*Time Almanac with Information Please*, 2007).

Historically, Japan has primarily had an agriculture-based economy. The economy has changed rapidly since the late nineteenth century with industrialization, especially after World War II. Today, Japan is considered the most urbanized country in Asia.

The *Ainu*, whose name means "human," are known to be the original inhabitants of Japan. Although they once occupied the whole country (Wikipedia, 2006), it is believed that today only 15,000 Ainu remain on the islands of Sakhalin and Hokkaido (*Webster's Dictionary*, 1991). The ancestors of the Japanese are believed to have come from mainland Asia, crossing over from Korea. These early settlers moved eastward from Kyushu and settled in the Kansai Plain (Kyoto–Osaka regions). Eventually, they established an ordered society under chieftains who were dedicated to the cult of the sun. Buddhism was later introduced in the sixth century. The ethics of Confucianism were added to the practice of sun worship and animism (*Shinto*) (Storry, 1993). Today, the Ainu maintain a culture and language that are distinctively different from the rest of the Japanese; however, the Ainu language is now almost extinct. Except for the Ainu, however, the Japanese population tends to perceive itself as ethnically and linguistically homogeneous (Wikipedia, 2007). Yet there are significant numbers of long-term resident foreigners now living in Japan—2 million as of 2006. There are also many Korean descendants, an estimated 1 million in 2005 (Kakuchi, 2005), Japanese-Brazilians, and Japanese-Peruvians, (about 329,000 in 2003; Nakamura, 2005). The foreign-born labor force in Japan is estimated at 800,000, many of whom work illegally (McNeill, 2006). While this is not a large percentage of the population, it does suggest the homogenous label may be misleading.

IMMIGRATION

Today the ability of Japanese Americans to identify with Japanese culture depends largely on when they arrived or whether they were born in the United

States, where they live, and how much acculturation and assimilation have occurred. Before the 1890s a few Japanese scholars and businessmen came to the United States and settled along the East Coast. Because of their small numbers and desire to be acculturated and assimilated into the mainstream society in the United States, they were more readily accepted than later immigrants.

The large influx of Japanese immigrants between 1890 and 1924 settled primarily along the West Coast and in Hawaii. Because of the prejudice they experienced, their lack of knowledge about the new country, and the language barrier, they kept to themselves and formed relatively self-sufficient communities where they were able to retain familiar cultural values. *Nisei*, second-generation Japanese Americans, were largely influenced by the values and norms of their parents. However, third- and fourth-generation Japanese Americans may be less familiar with the Japanese language and customs. This particularly affected Japanese Americans from internment camps, who were dispersed and forced to settle in the Midwest following their release. Many lacked ethnic communities to assist in maintaining their cultural heritage (Adler, 1998). Since the mid-1980s, in some areas, for example, Los Angeles County, Japanese Americans have married outside the Japanese ethnic group at rates as high as 51%, promoting further assimilation into the mainstream American culture (Kitano, Fujino, & Takahashi, 1998).

The Japanese American people are the only immigrant group to identify themselves by the generation in which they were born, and these generation groups are distinguishable by the individual's age, experience, language, and values. The generation groups are the *issei*, the first generation to live in the United States; the *nisei*, the second generation; the *sansei*, the third generation; the *yonsei*, the fourth generation; the *gosei*, the fifth generation; and the *rokusei*, the sixth generation (Hashizume & Takano, 1983). These generational categories provide a framework for understanding family-related cultural values. For the *issei*, the family provided the anchor for the values and traditions of Japan. Today the family remains one of the most important

factors in the lives of the Japanese people. The *issei* withstood extreme hardships and made personal sacrifices for the benefit of their children.

Before the 1890s, the majority of the Japanese persons who immigrated to the United States were men. Generally speaking, it often took many years before a Japanese man was able to afford a wife or family. These men might have been 30 or 40 years of age before they looked back to Japan to find their brides through the exchange of photographs and letters. Thus these Japanese women were often 10 to 20 years younger than their husbands, and even today elderly Japanese men often have much younger wives. For the *issei* descendants, there was a strong, stable family support system. The exclusion law of 1924 prevented some of the early Japanese male immigrants from finding a spouse, which resulted in a group of single elderly men who continue to reside in the United States without the support of a family.

In 1965, with the lifting of the immigration restrictions based on race, creed, and nationality, Japanese immigrants were able to reestablish the continuity of family life (Kobata, 1979). Japanese Americans who immigrated after WWII may be called *shin-issei*, which means "new first generation." Many *shin-issei* came as brides of servicemen after World War II, the Korean Conflict, or the Vietnam War. Others immigrated more recently and some married U.S. citizens. Since these individuals grew up in Japan, their lives, values, and beliefs tend to differ somewhat from those of the descendants of the original *issei* (Fugita & O'Brien, 1991).

Among the various ethnic groups in the U.S, a clear generational distinction among Japanese American groups is not only unique but also meaningful (Fugita & O'Brian, 1991). This distinction highlights different characteristics of Japanese Americans, including values and beliefs the immigrants from Japan brought with them, what they retained and passed on to their offspring, and the impact of historical events and laws on their experience and acculturation. Ethnic community organizations, such as long-term care services established and expanded by the *nisei* and maintained by the *sansei*, are examples of ways that traditional

Japanese values and culture are expressed (Young, McCormick, & Vitaliano, 2002). Increased intermarriage among *sansei*, 50% among men and 60% among women (Fugita & O'Brian, 1991), and dispersed residency, however, suggest that it might be difficult to pass on aspects of Japanese tradition and ethnicity to future generations. Moreover, many of the early *issei* immigrants have died and most *nisei* are between 69 and 80 years of age (Austin, 2002), with some in their 90s (Colclough, 2005). Of significance is the fact that the Japanese American population decreased by 53,000 from 1990 to 2000, in part because of mortality among its aging members (U.S. Bureau of the Census, 2000; Perot & Youdelman, 2001).

Intergenerational relations are close among most Japanese Americans. There continues to be a flow of goods, money, and services between the generations. The general pattern of the Japanese family is the vertical family structure, with the father and other male members in the topmost position. Many of the activities in the Japanese family occur in both the nuclear family and the extended family. Problems are handled within the structure, and the achievement or accomplishment of the individual member is a reflection on the entire family (Kitano, 1976). The younger generation continues to be willing to assist and give more than what is requested and expected by the older generation (Osaka, 1979). Yet despite a long-standing tradition of family connection and caregiving, Japanese American families face challenges similar to other populations—aging parents and "fewer available caregivers owing to greater workforce participation and geographic mobility" (McCormick, Imai, & Rubenstein, 1995; Young et al., 2002). Nonetheless, the *issei* descendants continue to emphasize the importance of caring for their elderly parents. However, it is important to remember that the *issei* generation rarely experienced caring for their own parents because in most cases their parents were in Japan. Today the tradition of caring for aged parents is seen in the *issei* descendants, wherein aged parents continue to maintain separate but close residences and regular communication occurs. Generally one child, often the oldest son or an unmarried child, assumes full responsibility for the care of elderly parents

(Kobata, 1979). As indicated, family contacts are frequent among the elderly. In a study done in Chicago, researchers found that 65% of the elderly Japanese Americans surveyed indicated that they had at least daily contact with at least one child, 30% had contact once a week, and the remaining 5% lived with their children (Osaka, 1979). Similar studies that have been conducted support these findings (Kiefer, 1974; Modell, 1968). Seemingly, reliance on the family structure has resulted in less dependence on outside individual agencies and organizations.

The *nisei* were born in the United States during the pre–World War II period. Although this generation had a higher educational level and was more fluent in English than their parents, they still faced intense racial discrimination in housing and employment (Sato & Takano, 1983). Hostile feelings on the part of many U.S. citizens intensified in 1942 with the declaration of the war with Japan. This sentiment climaxed with the evacuation and internment of Japanese Americans when President Roosevelt signed executive orders 9066 and 9102. Although restrictions applied to Japanese, German, and Italian aliens on the West Coast, only the Japanese, both alien and U.S.-born, were removed from their homes in California, Washington, Oregon, Arizona, and Hawaii and forcibly placed in internment camps (Daniels, Taylor, & Kitano, 1991; Strazar & Fisher, 1996). More than 120,000 persons were imprisoned. The experiences of those who survived are well documented (Yoo, 2000; Spickard, 1996; Daniels, Taylor, & Kitano, 1991; Houston & Houston, 2002; Reid, 1993). What is missing, however, are the accounts by those who did not survive or whose lives were broken and warped by this experience. During the internment, 6485 Japanese Americans were born in camps. Unfortunately, 1990 Japanese Americans died in internment camps (Daniels, Taylor, & Kitano, 1991).

The evacuation and internment of the Japanese in U.S. camps have been described as the most dehumanizing experience for Japanese Americans since their immigration to the United States. It not only disrupted their families and way of life but also had enormous financial implications that were largely created from the loss of their homes and businesses.

To prove their loyalty as Americans and combat the racism that confronted them, an overwhelming number of *nisei* volunteered for the all-*nisei* 100th Infantry Battalion and its larger unit of Japanese Americans, the 442nd Regimental Combat Team (Kakesako, 1993; Yoshishige, 1993). These volunteers, who came from Hawaii and mainland internment camps, emerged as the most decorated unit for its size and duration of service (Chang, 1993).

After the war, the employment and cultural expectations of Japanese Americans from the *nisei* became more aligned with their American background. As this new generation became more acculturated, they began to rely less on the economic sanction of their *issei* fathers. These individuals sought a better way of life and upward mobility. The GI Bill offered many veterans a chance at a first-class education. Japanese Americans have been extremely successful in the assimilation process, particularly in certain states. In Hawaii, successful inroads have been made, particularly in the political arena (Burris, 1993). Succeeding generations of Japanese Americans have benefited tremendously from the efforts of these earlier immigrants. Recognition of Japanese American rights and political power occurred when the U.S. Congress passed the Civil Liberties Act of 1988 to make redress payments of $20,000 to each survivor who had been incarcerated during World War II (Daniels, 1991). In 2005, a U.S. Congressional bill allocating $38 million to memorialize the internment camps of World War II was passed by the House (Epstein, 2005). The bill was sent on to the Senate in 2006 and returned with mark-ups from the Senate to the House (Epstein, 2006). As of July 2007, no further information is available on this bill. It is important to remember that the history of forced internment is a primary difference between early Japanese Americans and their descendants and recent Japanese immigrants.

Life in the United States

According to 2000 census data, there are 796,720 Japanese Americans (designated as Asian alone on the census) residing in the United States (U.S. Department of Commerce, Bureau of the Census, Summary File 3, 2002; *Time Almanac with Information Please,*

2007). This number represents a 0.3% increase in the population of Japanese Americans since the 1990 census. When Japanese and one other Asian group are reported, there are 1,148,932 people who designated themselves in the 2000 census as Japanese. Overall, Japanese Americans represent 12.3% of the total Asian American population. Of the number of Japanese Americans residing in the United States, 75.9% live in the West, 7.9% live in the South, 7.5% live in the Midwest, and 10.2% live in the Northeast. By states, the largest populations of Japanese Americans are found in California (312,989), Hawaii (247,486), New York (35,861), and Washington (43,799) (U.S. Department of Commerce, Bureau of the Census, Summary File 1, 2000).

Whereas the median age of Asian Americans is 32.7 years, it is approximately 36.3 years for Japanese Americans. In the United States, Japanese Americans are the oldest group of Asians by median age. In fact, even when compared with the national median age for all ethnic and racial groups (33 years), Japanese Americans have a higher median age. Of the number of Japanese Americans residing in the United States between 1980 and 2000, 20% were foreign born, compared to 12.4% of Japanese Americans living in the United States before 1975. These data suggest that immigration has played a major role in the increase in numbers of Japanese Americans in the United States (U.S. Department of Commerce, Bureau of the Census, Summary File 3, 2002).

Asian Americans tend to have larger families than other ethnic and racial groups. Japanese Americans may be the exception to this statistical fact. Japanese Americans, on the average, have 3.1 persons per family, compared with the national average of 3.2 persons per family. This number is in stark contrast to other Asian groups. At the higher end of the spectrum are Hmongs, with 6.6 persons per family; Cambodians, with 5.0 persons per family; Laotians, with 5.0 persons per family; and Vietnamese, with 4.4 persons per family (U.S. Department of Commerce, Bureau of the Census, Summary File 3, 2002).

In 2000, the median earnings for Asian Americans were $36,051, as compared with $33,955 for their White counterparts. Similarly, Asian Americans, in terms of income, fare better than their other racial and ethnic counterparts regarding median individual income. In 2000, the median income for Asian American women was $31,049, as compared with $27,878 for their White counterparts. Likewise, the median individual income for Asian American men was $40,650, as compared with $39,235 for their White counterparts (U.S. Department of Commerce, Bureau of the Census, Summary File 1, 2000).

Asian Americans enjoy the longest life expectancy as compared with any other racial and ethnic group residing in the United States. The life expectancy of Asian Americans regardless of gender is 83.0 years. By subpopulations, the life expectancy for Asian Americans is 86.0 for Chinese Americans, 85.0 for Filipino Americans, and 85.0 for Japanese Americans (National Center for Health Statistics, Health, United States, 2002).

COMMUNICATION

Communication and Culture

The official language in Japan, which is spoken by some 190 million inhabitants, is Japanese. There are three systems (glyphs) that are used concurrently to communicate in writing in Japanese. In the Japanese language, one system includes the *kanji*, or *honji*, ideographic or pictographic characters borrowed from the Chinese and used to express chief meanings of words, such as substantive and root meanings of verbs and adjectives (Wikipedia, 2006). *Kanji* characters may have concepts embedded. For example, the *kanji* for human, *hito*, implies "an individual who is supported by another" (Minami, 1985). The *kanji* is composed of two sticks leaning inward against each other; without one, the other falls, pictographically signifying the interconnectedness of the Japanese self. In addition to *kanji*, there are two syllabic scripts, *hiragana* and *katakana* (Wikipedia, 2006). *Hirigana* is the phonetic "alphabet" used to represent Japanese words, while *katakana* is used as the phonetic representation of foreign words. The *katakana* are also used in official documents and advertisements. Today, "Romaji," from the Latin alphabet, is often used in modern Japanese, particularly for such things as company names and advertising, and especially for inputting Japanese into the computer. Western style arabic numbers are more commonly used for numbers, while traditional Chinese/Japanese numberings are more commonplace in the Japanese language (Wikipedia, 2006).

Of the number of Japanese Americans residing in the United States, 42.8% speak an Asian or a Pacific Islander language at home, 57.7% do not speak English well, and 33.0% are linguistically isolated (U.S. Department of Commerce, Bureau of the Census, Summary File 3, 2002).

Style. Japanese characteristics in language and behavior reflect characteristics of some of the values inherent in this ethnic group. The Japanese culture is known as the "culture of anticipatory perception" or "culture of consideration" because of the importance of empathizing with the speaker (Lebra, 1976). A concept central to the issue of communication is "empathic identification." The speaker identifies with and views the listener from the listener's point of view. The expectation is that the listener will also empathize with the speaker. Thus, verbal communication can be held to a minimum. For some Japanese Americans, constant verbal communication is seen as unnecessary. Many Japanese Americans value communication that is implicit, nonverbal, and intuitive over explicit, verbal, and rational (Hsu, Tseng, Ashton, McDermott, & Char, 1985). Therefore communication may be seen by outsiders as less direct, somewhat vague, and somewhat concealing. A talkative person is considered a "show-off" or insincere (Rogers & Izutsu, 1980). There is an underlying assumption that when true connected caring/communication is happening, there is little need for words (Doutrich, 2000).

When communication occurs with someone who is not Japanese, many Japanese people do not expect to have a personal position understood without strong assertions. During these times, it may be necessary for some Japanese Americans to establish their viewpoints before the listener has appropriately comprehended the message.

Behavior and communication are defined by role expectancy and status and by an attempt to preassess the listener's feelings or wishes. According to Schon and Ja (2005), the content of communication depends on the characteristics of the persons involved. Factors such as age, sex, education, social status, family background, and marital status often influence specific behaviors. Behaviors that may be seen as negative or resistive in Western culture may, in fact, be reflective of proper upbringing for some Japanese Americans. Openness may be construed as a sign of immaturity or lack of self-control, which may bring shame to the family.

Context. In a high-context culture such as the Japanese, implicit nonverbal messages are of central importance; in multiethnic low-context cultures, explicit verbal messages are emphasized (Hall, 1976). Behaviors of individuals in a high-context culture reflect the value of thinking before speaking, of modesty in acts and speech. In this sense, context is also viewed as intuitive. This concept is related to the context of empathy, with its value on sensitivity and responsiveness. It is essential for the speaker to avoid superficiality and poor subtleties of speech if intuitive understanding is to occur (Lebra, 1976). In addition, in a high-context culture, esthetic refinement and sophistication are evident in nonverbal, indirect, implicit, subtle messages. Thus it is not surprising that some Japanese Americans may be threatened by or avoid ambiguous situations (Matsumoto, 1989).

Linguistics. The grammatical structure of a language frequently reflects the major theme of a culture (Johnson, Marsella, & Johnson, 1974). Four themes relating to verbal behaviors in Japanese Americans govern interactions: (1) a strong sense of gender differences, (2) a concern for hierarchy and status that manifests itself as deference toward authority, (3) an emphasis on self-effacement, and (4) a focus on nonverbal communication. These themes can be seen in the primacy of hierarchical status in the Japanese culture, where themes of the Meiji-era (post-1868) Japan and Confucian doctrines still dominate social behavior among many Japanese Americans.

Oral Language. The Japanese culture stresses nonverbal communication, and for many Japanese Americans there is a general mistrust of spoken words (Leong, 1986). Lebra (1976) attributes this characteristic to a belief held by some Japanese Americans that indicates that the *ma-gokoro* ("true-heart," thus the innermost self) is incapable of being adequately or sincerely expressed through an outer part of the body such as the mouth, which is inclined toward deception. Directly related to the *ma-gokoro* is the importance of personal self as the monitor of self-identity. Again, words are perceived as a poor substitute for the adequate expression of sincere feelings.

Self-abasement, modesty, and apology used by Japanese Americans when communicating are viewed by some health care professionals as self-effacing behaviors. Many health care professionals believe that this type of behavior is open to misunderstanding. Yet the complex meanings behind these attitudes and behaviors can be understood by the concept of *enryo*, which directs Japanese Americans to be modest, to defer to others, to play down personal accomplishments and achievements, and to direct attention away from oneself (Adler, 1998; Akimoto & Sanbonmatsu, 1999). *Enryo* by near translation means "restraint," "holding back," or "hesitancy" (Doi, 1973). It also may be thought of as "ritualized verbal self-depreciation used to maintain group harmony" (Gudykunst & Nishida, 1994). For some Japanese Americans, self-praise or the acceptance of praise is considered poor manners, resulting in denying, ignoring, or negating another trait or behavior. To many Westerners, this behavior may be interpreted as lack of self-esteem or belittling (Chang, 1981).

The concept of hierarchy and status also dictates communication patterns. For some Japanese Americans, it is considered impolite to disagree publicly with a person of higher status for fear of making this individual lose face. In traditional Japanese society, gender differences are reflected by males tending to be more economical in speech, particularly in public situations, and more direct in their delivery of opinions or ideas than their female counterparts (Johnson, Marsella, & Johnson, 1974). Some Japanese American males tend not to give an opinion, especially on mundane matters. Japanese American women are relatively soft spoken and are more loquacious than their male counterparts. Japanese American women are viewed as pleasant individuals who not only are cooperative but also have less assertive, aggressive, or loud verbal behaviors (Johnson, Marsella, & Johnson, 1974). Overt conflict is minimized both inside and outside the Japanese American home for both women and men.

Oral expression is focused on increasing harmony and avoiding conflict (Chang, 1981; Fisher, 1996). Therefore, answering "yes" to questions may be a way of avoiding embarrassment or shame and does not necessarily imply that communication is agreed with, clear, or understood (Fisher, 1996). Leong (1986) concluded that Asian Americans are more likely to avoid having to express themselves verbally.

In studying communication apprehension among individuals in Japan, Korea, and the United States, Klopf, Cambra, and Ishii (1981) found that the Japanese frequently expressed feelings of nervousness and anxiousness. In some instances, these feelings made some of these individuals generally awkward and unsociable when communicating with strangers, particularly persons from different cultures. Furthermore, when some Japanese Americans become distressed, their communication is often by metaphors and idioms (Marsella, 1993).

Voice Quality. Vocal qualifiers include intensity, volume, pitch, and rate or speed (Ishii, 1987). In general, Japanese speak in a high-pitched voice, which may relate to the love of traditional folk songs (*minyo*) and sentimental nostalgic songs (*enka*), which call for high-pitched voices. Gender differences are also manifested in the manner in which women are expected to speak.

Nonverbal Communication

The Japanese culture is a relatively non–eye contact culture, and this is quite noticeable in public speaking and in the communication process (Ishii, 1987). Most Asian Americans consider it disrespectful to look someone directly in the eyes, especially if that person is in a superior position (Galanti, 1997). In nonverbal communication, integral quality and explicitness of feelings are involved in the process itself and are communicated paraverbally rather than directly. High awareness of nonverbal gestures and facial mimetic nuances exist among Japanese Americans (Johnson, Marsella, & Johnson, 1974). For some Japanese Americans, emotional

expression of anger is unusual, and a stoic reaction is often manifested as a response to pain. *Gaman* is a Japanese concept that stems from the verb *gama-nsuru,* which translates as "to bear, to endure, to tolerate" and which has to do with self-control and endurance (Katada, 1991). It is also considered a valuable social skill to be learned in childhood and used later in life when facing hardships, such as when in pain. Related to the development of *gaman*, Katada (1991) also noted that nonverbal communication is an emphasized Japanese socialization pattern. Bearing up with quiet self-control is valued and expected to be learned at a young age. In a study of preschool Japanese children, Katada found that some Japanese as young as four could verbalize the need for *gaman*. In this study, one child was able to suggest strategies (for example, adequate information about what to expect with surgery) that would have aided him in his struggle to achieve *gaman*. Thus, there is cultural value placed on "bearing up" or doing *gaman,* which can be described as stoicism in the face of hardships such as pain and uncertainty. Japanese behavior patterns require that an individual be trained to recognize subtle cues of nonverbal communications and finely nuanced choices of words. While cultural values for *gaman* and expectations for highly acute nonverbal perception are based upon traditional Japanese values, these values have meaning for many Japanese Americans.

Kinesics. Mehrabian (1968) estimates that, for Japanese Americans, communication of feelings and attitudes is 5% verbal, 38% vocal, and 55% facial expression. Thus, facial expression plays a crucial role in communicating emotions and attitudes. Some Westerners have noted the inscrutability of the Japanese face. It is essential to remember, however, that the traditional behavior of some Japanese Americans is to control emotions, especially in formal and public situations. This value is believed to have originated in *heijo-shin* ("ordinary state of mind") in Zen Buddhism, which advocates controlling emotions and maintaining a neutral presence. An inappropriate smile may sometimes be seen as an unconscious and reflective attempt to avoid troubling others by showing one's true feelings.

Touch. Japanese culture is viewed as a nontouch culture. There is close contact with infants but less touch or physical contact among adults (Ishii, 1987). Barnlund (1989) found that Japanese Americans touch family members less frequently than people in other cultures do. Physical contact may be perceived negatively and introduce tension into relationships (Marsella, 1993).

Silence. The ideal and ultimate pattern of communication in Japanese society is silent communication. Some Japanese Americans do not appreciate aggressive or spoken forms of communication and instead place a premium on intuitive understanding of what is being communicated (Doutrich, 2000; Marsella, 1993). Findings from several studies are suggestive that Japanese adults spend only half as much time in conversation per weekday as their U.S. counterparts (Ishii, 1987; Klopf & Ishii, 1976). The data further suggested that Japanese couples, especially those who had been married for some time and were happy in the relationship, usually remained silent with each other because they had developed *sasshi* ("guesswork" or "intuitive sensitivity"). In other words, they understand each other without speaking. *Sasshi* is also highly appreciated in other situations.

Implications for Nursing Care

Because it is impolite to think of personal needs, some Japanese Americans, when asked if they want something to eat or drink, are likely to respond negatively. In such instances, if the nurse does not try to persuade the client to eat or drink, the nurse may be perceived as insensitive. The nurse should offer at least two to three times, even after receiving a negative reply.

The nurse can learn to anticipate needs and accurately assess discomforts by relying on astute interpretation of the meaning of nonverbal expressions and behaviors. It is essential to remember that subtle facial expressions and gestures are expected to be understood. Japanese American clients may wait silently rather than ask questions because they believe health care providers know best and will meet their needs without being asked (Sato & Takano, 1983). This relates to a high regard for "anticipatory care" and the concept of *omakase*

(Wenger, 1991). For the Japanese, "health professionals are authority figures and are to be trusted" (Suzuki, Kirschling, & Inoue, 1993). Although there is recent evidence that this attitude has changed (Tarn et al., 2005). In this sense, some Japanese are recognizing that patients are recipients of care rather than consumers (Suzuki et al., 1993). *Omakase* refers to a coping style that allows the patient to place his or her trust in the physician or nurse and therefore, the health provider carries the burden for the patient. While Suzuki et al. (1993) identified concepts specific to Japan, there are values embedded in the concepts that have migrated with the Japanese Americans. These include a value for hierarchy and trusting authority, an expectation that one will be cared for, and an expectation that one will not have to ask verbally for what one needs but that it will be anticipated by a caring other (Doutrich, 2000; 2001).

Because direct expression of negative feelings is an unusual behavior for some Japanese Americans, indirect messages should not be mistaken for agreement. For example, rather than verbalize to the staff their discontent with the health care, the client may have the family request a unit change. Nurses who expect clients to express their feelings through direct action may be surprised when they encounter a Japanese American client who is withdrawn and silent. For the nurse who is unfamiliar with the cultural behaviors of the Japanese American, behaviors in ambiguous, embarrassing, or anxiety-producing situations may be difficult to understand, and the client may be labeled as passive or nonresponsive. For some Japanese Americans, it is extremely important to control expressions of anger or pain. The nurse should be aware of situations that may cause discomfort, such as the exclusion of the family from the plan of care. The nurse must also remember that some Japanese Americans consider it insulting to be addressed by their first names, especially the first generation, who follow strict hierarchical rules of deference and respect.

SPACE

Although there are variations in spatial requirements among individuals, Japanese Americans tend to have a higher tolerance for crowding in public spaces than other Americans (Watson, 1980). Families of several generations often reside under one roof, depending on available resources. Even in relative proximity, a personal space can be created. Time and attention is given to the organization of their living space and perception by the senses (Hall, 1976). Privacy is generally maintained by family members by respecting the privacy of others and by limiting self-disclosure to persons in binding or trusting relationships (Baker, 1993). For some Japanese Americans, well-manicured gardens can provide a degree of tranquility and peace that tends to expand personal spatial boundaries.

Japanese Americans, like other Asian Americans, tend to use less physical contact when interacting. They may also appear reserved and formal in new situations as they maintain their social zones. However, a recent study found that while Asian Americans compared with White Americans differ in the way they perceive crowding, all suffer similar negative psychological distress at high-density housing, independent of household income (Evans, Lepore, & Allen, 2000).

Implications for Nursing Care

Nurses should not misinterpret the reserved and formal behavior manifested by some Japanese Americans as a dysfunctional sign. The nurse should remember that these clients need to establish a caring, trusting relationship before they engage in self-disclosure. Japanese Americans may feel uncomfortable with the overuse of physical contact or the invasion of personal space when interacting. When some Japanese Americans are hospitalized, the nurse can help the client by identifying territorial boundaries within the room. Identification of these territorial boundaries may reduce conflicts created from the invasion of privacy of others, particularly when more than one client shares a room.

SOCIAL ORGANIZATION

Effect of Immigration on Social Organization

Most Japanese immigrants who remained in the United States eventually brought their families to the United States. As their numbers increased, many Japanese immigrants experienced increased racial prejudice. Their fairly self-sufficient subcommunities often served as a buffer and provided for their needs and social support. The traditional Japanese value system places emphasis on the family, group orientation, harmony, and mutual aid (Fugita & O'Brien, 1991; Yoo, 2000). This value system has allowed the families and communities to survive, particularly during and after the World War II experience. Japanese behaviors and values, such as not imposing on others or standing out, preserving harmony, controlling emotions, persevering, and respecting authority, have allowed them to acculturate rapidly (Adler, 1998). For many Japanese Americans, interdependence and dependence on each other is perceived as very important (Doi, 1973).

As increasing numbers of the *nisei* generation entered adulthood, they sought ways to overcome the personal, economic, and legal barriers that their parents endured. For example, Japanese Americans were frequently prevented from buying homes in desirable parts of town, using public swimming pools, and entering many professions (Kitano & Daniels, 2001.) The *nisei*, some of them recent college graduates but most still teenagers, wanted to prove their loyalty as Americans and thus combat anti-Japanese sentiment. Citizen organizations sprang up in various West Coast cities in the early 1920s. In 1930, the Japanese-American Citizens League became a national organization (Hosokawa, 2002). Some of the political clout of these organizations can be seen in the successful enactment of an amendment to the Cable Act to permit *nisei* girls who married alien Japanese to regain their citizenship. In addition, a bill was passed to allow foreign-born Asian men who served in the U.S. armed forces in World War I to be granted citizenship. The passage of this bill enabled 700 *issei* to become naturalized citizens (Hosokawa, 2002). More recently, Congress has passed laws that specifically address reparations and repatriation of Japanese Americans interned during World War II (Daniels, 1991).

Family Systems

The general structure of the Japanese family is vertical, with the father and other male members in the topmost positions. "Vertical" social structure means that relationships are clearly defined to those above or below a clearly determined line of social status (Padilla, Wagatsuma, & Lindholm, 1985). In contrast, social structures in the United States have been described as more "horizontal," implying less differentiation among social classes. Many of the activities in the Japanese American family occur in both the nuclear family and the extended family. Problems are handled within the structure, and the achievement or accomplishment of the individual member is a reflection on the entire family (Kitano, 1976).

For some Japanese Americans, the self is viewed as part of a set of interpersonal relationships, of which the family system is the central core (Fugita, Ito, Abe, & Takeuchi, 1991). In this sense, the self is subordinate to the family social unit, and consequently most Japanese Americans find it difficult to stand out publicly as individuals. This difficulty is evidenced by the reluctance of some Japanese Americans to give speeches, talk about themselves in casual conversations, or engage in self-serving behaviors.

The Japanese emphasize collectivity, as evidenced by cooperative family effectiveness rather than by intrafamily lineal authority or filial piety (Caudill & Scarr, 1962). Fostering of *amae*, or "interdependency," is also seen as a method of enhancing group solidarity and social relationships. This concept is also based on preservation of harmony and the suppression of conflict (Fugita, Ito, Abe, & Takeuchi, 1991). *Amae* ("passive love"), as defined by Doi (1962), means "to depend and presume upon the benevolence of others" and is often associated with the Japanese word for "sweet" (*amai*). This relationship may also exist between two people. Some data indicate that this concept is significant for Japanese American families living in the United States (Adler, 1998; Ching, McDermott, Fukunaga, et al., 1995; Kobayashi-Winata & Powers, 1989). In traditional U.S. society, assertiveness is seen by Americans as a characteristic of well-behaved children. For some Japanese American parents, assertiveness is a characteristic of the poorly behaved child (Kobayashi-Winata & Powers, 1989).

The family is one of the most important factors in the lives of most Japanese Americans. The phrase *kodomo no tame ni* ("for the sake of the children") reflects the sacrifices and hardships families would endure to ensure the success of the next generation. Intergenerational relations are close, as evidenced by the flow of food, money, help, and goods between generations. In Japanese American families, contact with other family members occurs frequently.

On (a sense of obligation within the Japanese hierarchy) forms the basis of reciprocal relationships among peers and within social networks (Fugita, Ito, Abe, & Takeuchi, 1991). Intervention and assistance are taken for granted within the family, but casual help from strangers is usually avoided because of the concern of becoming entwined in reciprocal relationships with outsiders. The reluctance to receive help from social service agencies may reflect this value. Within the Japanese American family, *on* is seen as a sacrifice of individual needs and personal goals for the sake of others in the family. Examples of this sacrifice are when a child cares for a parent or other elderly relative to the point of sacrificing financial security, career, or social stability and when the eldest child foregoes school to work in order to send the younger children to college.

According to Kitano (1969), Japanese families traditionally value authoritarian styles of leadership, where the father makes unilateral family decisions. Sue (2004) described the family lifestyle of Chinese and Japanese Americans as patriarchal, with authority and communication exercised from the top down. Sue (2004) also noted that within these families there is a need for interdependent roles, strict adherence to traditional norms, and minimization of conflict by suppression of overt emotion. In a study comparing Japanese and White American couples, Japanese American couples tended to make more unilateral decisions and showed more restraint and less self-disclosure (Hsu, Tseng, Ashton, McDermott, & Char, 1985). The concepts or values related to guilt and shame may be used to control family members. For some Japanese American families, family obligations take precedence over individual desires. Problems are generally handled within the family, and negative behaviors, such as delinquency, school failure, unemployment, or mental illness, are considered family failures that disrupt the desired harmony of family life and reflect badly on the family. Japanese American individuals exhibit close contact among the generations. The care of the elderly is generally the responsibility of the oldest son or an unmarried child. Yet there is a rapidly changing context for elderly care in Japan based on the changing demographics and the economic requirement that women work outside the home. Moreover, according to a study by Young et al. (2002), there is a concomitant evolution of the underlying core values related to caretaking among generations of Japanese Americans.

Active discouragement of verbal communication, avoidance of discussion of personal problems, and limited expression of emotion have also been noted as common patterns in the traditional Japanese family (Hsu, Tseng, Ashton, McDermott, & Char, 1985; McDermott, Tseng, & Maretzki, 1980). However, a number of other studies (Kobayashi-Winata & Powers, 1989; Morris, 1990) have found that a process of cultural change in family norms is becoming more prevalent across generations of Japanese Americans. There is a tendency to adopt more White American family norms and behaviors. **Parent–Child Interaction.** Methods of child care are inextricably linked, not only to the tradition and customs of a culture but also to its systems of values. These methods appear to persist from generation to generation despite the acculturation process. For both the *issei* and the *nisei*, parent–child relationships tended to be intense, with no open expressions of emotion displayed. For these generational groups, there was much tolerance and permissiveness for the child until 5 or 6 years of age, at which time parents began to place emphasis on having the child learn emotional reserve and control.

While third-generation Japanese Americans have appeared to adopt childrearing practices and attitudes of the contemporary American middle class (Kiefer, 1974: Strazar & Fisher, 1996), this may not be completely true. A study of Midwestern Japanese American women of multiple generations revealed that though the women did not always identify the Japanese concepts by name, they transferred important traditional Japanese concepts to their children. The Japanese concepts of *amae, gambare* ("effort, self-motivation"), *gaman* ("endurance, perseverance"), and role perfectionism were reinterpreted and transformed in the Japanese American childrearing practices to teach morality, encourage understanding of social contexts, inculcate work habits, and instill a desire to be an intelligent, educated individual. These Midwestern Japanese American women had very little ethnic community support, compared with those on the West Coast and in Hawaii (Adler, 1998).

In a classic study, Caudill and Frost (1974) compared the maternal and child care habits of Japanese Americans with those of Japanese nationals and White Americans to determine the effect on infant behavior. Findings from the study suggest that Japanese American mothers have a closer behavioral style to other Americans than to their Japanese national counterparts. The data also indicate that certain patterns of behavior from their Japanese cultural heritage were nevertheless retained by these Japanese American mothers and babies. Nonetheless, in contrast to their Japanese counterparts, Japanese American mothers tended to play with their babies for longer times, held their babies more often, and sang to their babies more often (Caudill & Frost, 1974). Further findings from this study also suggested that Japanese American babies did less finger sucking than White American babies and spent less time playing alone (Caudill & Frost, 1974).

In another classic study, in interviews conducted with Japanese Americans in California, Connor (1974) found that the *sansei* were more likely to have a sense of closer family ties; a greater sense of duty, obligation, and deference; less need to dominate; a greater tendency to affiliate; less aggressiveness; a greater need for succor and order; and a greater fear of failure in social role performance than other Americans. These individuals also valued the importance of family and the preservation of the *ie*, which, translated literally, means "household."

However, it can also imply a continuum from past to future members (including the present generation, the dead, and the unborn, with a hierarchical structure with the father as head). Higa (1974) found that Japanese American mothers who were born in the United States were more restrictive in childrearing behaviors than immigrant Japanese Americans were. In addition, Japanese American-born individuals tended to want their children to be obedient to authority rather than independent and aggressive.

Notable differences were found in childrearing practices between Japanese and American parents (Kobayashi-Winata & Powers, 1989). The respondents in the study were Japanese businessmen who lived in Houston. Findings from the study were suggestive that Japanese parents were less likely than their American counterparts to report the use of external types of punishment, such as time-out or physically and socially punishing the child. A plausible explanation for these differences is the assimilation of American cultural values that place emphasis on independence and individuality. It is believed that insistence on individuality makes it necessary to use powerful, external techniques to ensure compliance in some situations (Kobayashi-Winata & Powers, 1989). In a summary of the current literature on the grandparent caregiving role in ethnically diverse families, Kataoka-Yahiro, Ceria, and Caulfied (2004) reviewed grandparents as caregivers in three broad ethnic categories: African-American, Hispanic, and Asian American. They summarized results from 22 articles and 3 chapters published from 1980 to 2003 and state that approximately 6 million grandparents are living with their grandchildren. While clearly this role is on the rise in many populations, information on Asian grandparents giving care was limited to one study of Chinese Americans. Research on Japanese American grandparent caregivers was notable for its absence.

Strazar and Fisher (1996) note that, among Japanese Americans, abortion is not generally condoned but may not be uncommon for numerous reasons. First, some Japanese believe that an unwed mother brings great shame to the family. Second, in Japan there is a great emphasis on population control, and this value has been carried over into the

Japanese American culture. Third, adoption has become more common in recent times, and often some Japanese Americans will adopt a boy to carry on the family name (Strazar & Fisher, 1996).

Family Role in Education Attainment

The model-minority thesis surfaced in the mid-1960s because of publicity regarding high educational attainment levels, high median family incomes, low crime rates, and absence of juvenile delinquency and mental health problems among Asian Americans (Petersen, 1966). Asian Americans have been portrayed as extraordinary achievers. Based on U.S. census data, Sue and Okazaki (1990) found Asian and Pacific-Islander Americans exceeded the national average for high school and college graduates, with high rates of graduation from colleges and universities.

The popular cultural view that Asian American family values and socialization account for educational attainment is supported primarily by anecdotal and observational evidence rather than by empirical findings (Sue & Okazaki, 1990). Mordkowitz and Ginsberg (1987) found that Japanese Americans often reported that their families emphasized educational accomplishment. As a result, these students held high expectations of themselves. More important, they were able to control their behavior because of the direct relationship between appropriate behavior and personal achievement.

Dornbusch, Ritter, Leiderman, et al. (1987) found that Asian American students came from families who exhibited strong authoritarian behaviors and permissiveness and weak authoritative characteristics, which was directly opposite of the family environments of White students. Asian American parents were also reported to have a lower level of parental involvement than White parents. Findings from the study are suggestive that authoritarianism and permissiveness were inversely related, whereas parental involvement was directly related to academic achievements. Also, Asian American responses were not significantly different from those of other groups regarding the value of working hard, parental pressures for academic achievement, need for students to make their parents proud of them, and, most important, avoiding embarrassment to the family. Significant group differences were noted in only one area. Asian Americans were more likely to believe that success in life depends on what is studied in school, which was directly related to the grades they received in high school. According to Sue and Okazaki (1990), a plausible explanation for this behavior is the belief held by some Asian Americans that educational attainment provides opportunities for upward mobility. To the extent that upward mobility is limited in noneducational avenues, education becomes increasingly important as a means for advancement. In addition, education is perceived by some Japanese Americans as a feasible means for mobility in view of limitations for success in other areas. Sue and Okazaki (1990) concluded that the effects of culture have been confused with the consequences of society, while continuing to play an important role in achievement.

Many Asian immigrants came to the United States to obtain a better education for their children. For many Asian Americans, immigration was a great sacrifice because of downward occupational mobility (Chan, 1991). Nonetheless, the sacrifice was considered necessary because many Asian Americans generally think in terms of the family and not of the individual. In this context, they are often willing to sacrifice their own socioeconomic standing in exchange for giving the next generation a better chance to make it or be successful in the world.

Religion

Some of the ingrained cultural values evident in Japanese Americans are derived from Zen Buddhism, Confucianism, and Shintoism. Today, these values are seemingly manifested in Japanese Americans whether they practice Catholicism, Buddhism, Protestantism, or another religion. From the earliest immigrants, who came from mostly Buddhist backgrounds, the Japanese tended to adopt the religion of the area in which they lived, which resulted in divergent religious beliefs and practices among Japanese Americans in different locales. Religion

and the church have both played an important role in acculturating the Japanese within their communities (Adler, 1998; Sato & Takano, 1983).

Implications for Nursing Care

Because many Japanese Americans place a high value on the family system, the nurse should be aware of the significant role the family plays in providing support, interdependence, and the fulfillment of duties. Respect is also greatly valued, and the linear relationship apparent in families and in casual relationships should be maintained and supported when providing care for the Japanese American client and family support system. Although these values are the strength of the Japanese American family, they can create stress and disharmony not only for the client but also for the family unit. It is essential for the nurse to remember that some Japanese American families may want to provide support to the hospitalized family member by keeping a bedside vigil, especially if the individual is elderly and doing poorly. Married men, especially *nisei* and *issei* Japanese Americans, may expect their wives to serve in the traditional caretaker role. Therefore, the wife (or daughter) may be expected to be available at the bedside so that the client does not have to bother the nurses, especially with intimate care or requests for assistance. The nurse must be alert to the overextension and lack of self-care of family members in providing for the client. The nurse should make every effort to assist the family to identify resources, both financial and human, to reduce the stress created when a family member is ill. In addition, the family should be assured that they are not alone. The nurse should not be discouraged if the family initially refuses outside help but rather realize that timing is important. In a study of attitudes toward community-based services among Japanese American families, Young et al. (2002) found that timing and pacing of the resource information was a facilitating factor for Japanese Americans in considering services. Moreover, they found that health care providers could play a more active role in assisting families with service identification, information, and evaluation. Because family name and honor are important for this group, the nurse should be especially cognizant of the issue of confidentiality and respect. Information should not be shared with outsiders, even with extended family members who may appear close to the client. Information concerning illness is often kept within the immediate family.

Shintoism and Buddhism are subscribed to by more than 80% of the Japanese culture. Christianity is also well established in Japan. In the United States, a great number of Japanese Americans are Christians. Nonetheless, funerals for some Japanese Americans, despite this Christian orientation, are likely to be Buddhist, particularly for the *issei* and the *nisei*. *Obon*, an important Buddhist observance honoring the ancestors, is celebrated by many Japanese American communities and has spiritual, cultural, and community significance (Nakao, 2005). In addition, for some Japanese Americans, births and marriages are often colored by Shinto rituals but to a lesser extent for *yonsei* and *gosei* (Strazar & Fisher, 1996).

TIME

In a classic 1962 study, Caudill and Scarr examined Kluckhohn's value orientations in Tokyo-area high schools and concluded that time orientations differed by context, with a future focus in technology and a present focus in social relations. The greatest number of generational changes in these values occurred in political considerations, whereas the smallest number occurred in the religious area. In contrast, Chang (1981) believed that this future orientation originated from a religious, philosophical view of life. Buddhism teaches that death in all living things is inevitable. People are instructed not to make plans in this world without reckoning with death. According to Sato and Takano (1983), time is considered valuable and must be used wisely. The *issei* use the term "waste time" to describe inefficiency or trivial matters. Hard work in the present is seen as important for future successes (Adler, 1998). For Japanese Americans, the time-person perspective with regard to past, present, and future is perceived in terms of generational distance from Japan. This is reflected in the geo-generational grouping of *issei, nisei*, and so forth (Lyman,

1994). Gudykunst and Nishida (1994) noted that in the U.S. monochronic time predominates, which places emphasis on meeting deadlines, making plans, being prompt. Polychronic time is associated with doing many things at once and is concerned with relationship rather than task completion. They suggest that the Japanese tend to use monochronic time when dealing with outsiders but polychronic time in their interpersonal relations.

Decisions are not necessarily made in relation to individual needs or benefits. Sato and Takano (1983) state that the *issei* perception of time was related to death, in which death is seen as continuous and suprapersonal. This view is in stark contrast to the Western view of death as personal and discontinuous. Depending on the degree of acculturation, the *nisei* also accept death more readily than the *sansei* and the *yonsei*, who are more like Americans in their attitudes toward death and time.

Implications for Nursing Care

Because Japanese Americans are both present and future oriented, the nurse must consider the context of the current situation. The Japanese American client is usually prompt and adheres to fixed schedules. However, Japanese American clients tend to be more prompt with persons they hold in high regard such as physicians than with persons not held in high regard. They generally follow directions regarding medications and treatments. Because of future orientation regarding their children, care must be taken regarding their diet and health. Japanese Americans will work hard with little regard for their health in the hope that future generations will have a better life.

ENVIRONMENTAL CONTROL

Locus of Control

Locus of control refers to the extent to which persons ascribe their successes or failures to internal or external causes. Because Japanese Americans tend to place more importance on relationships and familial commitments. As such, they tend to also be more externally influenced than persons from Western cultures (Yeh & Huang, 1996).

Takemura (2007) noted that the concept of the individual is culturally bound and as such needs to be understood from an emic or cultural insider's perspective. In the classic work of Hofstede (1984), cultural interpretations using distinct dichotomies such as "individualism-collectivism" and perhaps the internal/external dichotomies of locus of control may assume a Western concept of individualism (consisting of autonomous individuals) as the starting point for the self. Takemura (2005) observed that for the Japanese are often portrayed in the greater society as "soldier ants" or "worker bees" who will willingly sacrifice their interests as individuals to contribute to the group. Takemura (2007) cautions against interpreting culture based upon false dichotomies and quotes Hamaguchi (1977) who notes that the concept of the "individual" is not universal. The Japanese self is defined in relation to nature and other persons. In this sense, the Japanese culture is contextual, situational, relational, rather than collectivistic (Takemura, 2005). In Japanese, the word for "individualism" (*kojin-shugi*) is an ambivalent word, one "suggesting selfishness rather than personal responsibility" (Reischauer, 1977). Tweed, White, and Lehman (2004) findings are consistent with this notion. They explored internal and externally targeted control strategies cross culturally. Japanese sojourner students in Canada were more likely to use internal control strategies to accommodate the self in adapting to the demands of the environment whereas those students from Western backgrounds were more likely to use strategies to attempt to alter or change the environment. In contrast to these views, Padilla, Wagatsuma, and Lindholm (1985) found that *issei* Japanese American students believe that they have an external locus of control. In contrast, *sansei* and later-generation students indicated an internal locus of control. *Nisei* students were in between an external and an internal locus of control. Ho (1976) noted that the external locus of control in the Japanese American population was fatalistic, which allowed them equanimity and acceptance without question of life as it unfolds. A study with Asian Americans in general found they were more likely than non-Asians to endorse superstitious beliefs about luck (Drake & Freedman, 1997).

Illness and Wellness Behaviors and Folk Medicine

Major beliefs that have contributed to medicine in Japan influence the Japanese American person's view of health and illness. In the Shinto religion, people are seen as inherently good. Evil is caused by outside spirits who cause humans to succumb to temptation and harm, which can be alleviated through purification rites. Disease is believed to be caused by contact with polluting agents, such as blood, corpses, and skin diseases, which accounts for the emphasis on cleanliness (Strazar & Fisher, 1996; Sato & Takano, 1983).

Another important belief held by some Japanese Americans is based on the traditional Chinese concept of harmony and balance among oneself, society, and the universe. Some Japanese Americans believe disharmony (with society or family) or imbalance (as from lack of sleep or exercise or because of poor diet) can cause disease. Therefore, restoration of balance should be the major focus of treatment. In addition, some Japanese Americans believe that illness may cause energy to slow or stop along the meridians of the body. Thus acupuncture, acupressure, massage, or moxibustion may be used to restore the flow of energy (Sato & Takano, 1983).

The *kampo* ("Chinese medicine") medical system was developed around the belief that forces of the universe affect an individual's body processes and activities. Health depends on maintaining a harmonious relationship with the universe. *Kampo* practitioners believe that dietary precautions and preventive measures help resist illness (Ishihara, 1962; Strazar & Fisher, 1996).

Certain foods have special symbolic meaning for Japanese Americans. Special foods, such as soft boiled rice and miso soup (a soup made with fermented soybean paste), may be eaten during illness as well as to promote good health. Traditionally, on their most important holiday, New Year's Day, most Japanese Americans eat special foods that have symbolic meaning for good health, prosperity, and happiness. Such foods include *kazu-no-ko* (dried herring roe) for fertility, *mochi* (steamed rice cake) for longevity and prosperity, *soba* (buckwheat needles) served in clear broth for longevity and prosperity, and *kuromame* (black beans) for good health (Corum, 2000; Engle, 1993). Other symbolic foods include *ozoni* (a clear soup with *mochi* and vegetables) for prosperity; *gobo* (burdock), symbolic of deep family roots; and *tai* (sea bream, a large red fish served whole) for happy occasions.

Although Asian medical traditions recently have regained popularity with the holistic and preventive health movement, most Japanese Americans tend to rely on Western medicine. Some use both Oriental and Western medicine, depending on the illness and the efficacy of Western medicine. Yet for those who still subscribe to the Old World traditional health care practices brought with them from Japan, the basis for health practices may include a mixture of traditional medical practices (*kampo*) brought to Japan from China, Shinto beliefs, and Western medical practices (Strazar & Fisher, 1996). It is important for the health provider to inquire about alternative therapy use (Flaherty, 2001).

Death, Dying, Death Rituals, and Customs Observed

Meaning of Death, the Afterlife. Many Asian Americans believe death is a natural part of the life cycle; thus death cannot be overcome through human intervention (Bowman & Singer, 2001; Braun & Nichols, 1997). This is a fundamental Buddhist belief. According to Tsuchida (1998), traditionally the Japanese have an animistic reverence; nature, *shizen*, means "a force that transcends human control and follows its own course of changes or processes." In this sense, for many Japanese, mechanical interventions to prolong life may be difficult to accept. Likewise the acceptance, or recognition, of brain death without an arrested heart may be problematic. In Japan, unlike in the U.S., cardiopulmonary resuscitation (CPR) is not commonly performed out of the hospital or by lay persons. Some Japanese make pilgrimages to Buddhist temples, which are associated with the belief that prayers made at the specific temples will assist the pilgrim in procuring a sudden death. The

Japanese preference for a quick death is desired not only because there is less suffering involved but also because a prolonged illness may be a burden to the family, either financially or physically.

The concept of *karma* or reincarnation is based on the premise that one's conduct in a previous life affects the condition of the present life. This is also a part of the belief system of some Asian Americans (Braun & Nichols, 1997). For Japanese Americans, an individual's identity and the interpretation of the meaning of life are closely tied to their belief in their ancestors' spirit (Tsuchida, 1998). Therefore, because death is viewed as a natural phenomenon, some Japanese Americans may be better able to accept it when it comes. The Samurai ethos expects one to maintain an attitude of indifference to the minutiae of daily life. Thus, bravery and silent endurance are typical Japanese virtues (Ohara, 2000). Coupled with this is the notion that the bereaved should understand the dying person's last true wishes without there being verbal expression. Because of a strong feeling of connection to offspring consistent with an interdependent self, implicit rather than explicit expression has more weight and value. A strong interrelated society makes it possible to let the dying go without knowing his/her wishes. Moreover, Japanese American family members may accept the challenge of understanding the wishes of a dying person without explicit discussion since it is viewed as evidence of the closeness of their relationship. *Ishin denshin* (mind to mind communication or thought transference) is then put into practice.

Dying Process. Traditionally, the Japanese are willing to discuss death and dying while they are healthy. However, once someone becomes seriously ill, such discussion is taboo. Additionally, anything relating to the numbers four (which has the same pronunciation, *shi*, as the Japanese word for death) and the number nine (pronounced *ku*, -which also means suffering) should be avoided. While fresh flowers are acceptable to give to the dying or the bereaved, a plant gift is considered taboo and is associated with long-term illness. This may be so because for the Japanese, the word for root, *nezuku*, is similar to the word that means "lie down in the bed." Visiting of the sick by a religious leader is accepted in the U.S., but may indicate bad luck for some Buddhist Japanese because Buddhist monks are associated with death or funeral rituals. Whether Japanese Americans know their illness and prognosis depends greatly on their own and their family's acculturation level (Matsumura et al., 2002; Colclough, 2005).

Colclough (2005), in a qualitative study of 16 Japanese Americans, found that although most Japanese Americans preferred family decision making, the older family members tended to share implicit understanding with the ill patient about his or her end-of-life wishes. In contrast, the younger members tended to discuss end-of-life wishes explicitly. Further findings from this study suggest that there are times when the Japanese American patients kept their diagnosis or poor prognosis from their family. Recently, Japanese Americans on the West Coast have options for culturally sensitive long-term care and assisted living facilities (with Japanese language and culturally sensitive providers), and there has been an increased use of these types of care among the Japanese American population. Today, more hospice care is being used among this population (McCormick et al., 1996; Young, McCormick, & Vitaliano, 2002b). A possible issue for Japanese and Japanese American families is the practice of *diagnostic disclosure*, the discussion of a terminal diagnosis or poor prognosis with the patient. In the U.S., diagnostic truthtelling is based upon a concept wherein the patient is considered an autonomous individual and is a key aspect of informed consent. In Japan, where the self is more relationally defined, the family is usually informed first, and they may decide how and when or if the diagnosis is revealed to the patient (Wros, Doutrich, & Izumi, 2004).

Death Rituals. For traditional Japanese in the prefuneral period just after death, the body is bathed, dressed, and laid out with the deceased's head pointed toward the North without a pillow. A monk recites *sutras* (Buddhist prayers) at the bedside and gives the deceased a posthumous Buddhist name. This name is later inscribed on the tombstone and on the family's memorial tablet, which is kept in the home in a Buddhist alter. An overnight vigil is held at the home or a funeral site.

During the vigil it is important to keep incense burning, and visitors reminisce about the deceased. Acquaintances visit the site with "incense money" and offer incense. Usually, a funeral lasts two hours. Cremation occurs right after the funeral and a reception is held during the cremation. Then immediate family members go back to the crematorium to collect pieces of bones, which are placed into a small jar and are put under the tombstone or kept in an altar. Weekly ceremonies occur up to the 7th week and an annual ceremony takes place up to the 50th year (not every year). The celebrations occur on the death date, equinox days, and the summer *Obon* festival and are meant to celebrate the ancestors. The extent to which Japanese Americans follow the traditional rituals depends on their level of religious practice and connections with traditional Japanese culture.

Implications for Nursing Care

Because some Japanese Americans hold traditional value orientations regarding fatalism, they often are perceived as having an external locus of control. The nurse must also remember that some Japanese Americans value self-control, particularly in areas they believe may reflect weakness or inadequacy. The loss of "face" and dignity should be especially considered in procedures and treatment. The desire to *gaman* may affect the Japanese American's willingness to request pain medications. Nurses can offer their time and practice attentive listening skills. Nurses also can make sure the patients and their families understand that it is expected that they express concerns and feelings.

The nurse should inquire about treatments the client is using at home and what measures are most helpful. Special foods, tea, or herbal decoctions may be important for the client to have if there are no contraindications. It is very common for family or friends to bring fruit or special Japanese food when visiting. The client and family are likely to show hospitality by offering food to the nurse and visitors. Although it is unusual for the family and the client to hold special religious ceremonies at the bedside, privacy will be needed if such ceremonies are held.

BIOLOGICAL VARIATIONS

Body Size

Body size and body composition between Japanese Americans and Japanese nationals were compared in the 1980s. The body fat of males and females in both groups was similar; however, Japanese Americans had significantly greater body weight, fat-free mass, and body mass index (BMI) than Japanese nationals (Tahara, Moji, Muraki, Honda, & Aoyagi, 2003). Japanese Americans tend to be of smaller stature than their Euro American counterparts. However, rapid Westernization has brought major changes in diet and lifestyle in Japan. As a result, the height of the average Japanese male has increased 4 inches over the last 30 years, with an average height of 5 feet, 7 inches (Ministry of Health, Labour, and Welfare, 2006). Likewise, the height of the average Japanese female has increased 2.7 inches over the last 30 years. In body proportions, Japanese, like other Asian Americans, tend to have longer trunks and shorter limbs than White Americans. They also tend to have wide hips and narrow shoulders (Overfield, 1995). According to the results of a U.S. national health survey, Asian Americans, compared with other ethnic/racial groups in the U.S., have the lowest rates of obesity (4.8% versus 21.2% to 34.8%), the lowest BMI (24.0 kg/m^2 ± 0.2), and have the highest percentages in the normal weight range (62.4% versus 25.8% to 39.8%) (National Center for Health Statistics, 2005). These data are aggregated Asian American data and do not separate the Japanese American population. While the percentage of Asian Americans with obesity is low, it appears that the more years a foreign-born Asian American spends in the United States, the higher the risk for being overweight or obese. Among U.S. born Asian Americans, Japanese Americans are significantly more likely to be obese or overweight than foreign-born Asian Americans (Lauderdale & Rathouz, 2000). These higher incidences may be a result of a combination of diet and lifestyle.

Skin Color

Skin color varies among Japanese Americans. Some Japanese Americans have more yellow tone than others. One can assess jaundice by looking at the sclerae of the eyes. The amount of sun exposure can make a noticeable difference in the skin color of the same individual.

Other Visible Physical Characteristics

Mongolian spots (bluish pigment from fetal migratory melanocytes), found generally in the lumbosacral region, are present in 80% of Asian infants at birth. They can often be mistaken for bruises (Jacobs & Walton, 1976; Overfield, 1995). Other areas of the skin, such as nipples, areolae, scrotum, and labia majora, are affected by hormones and as a result are often darker in Asian groups than in Whites (Overfield, 1995). Keloid formation varies among Japanese Americans but is greater in this group than in White Americans. Keloid formations can be cause for concern in highly visible areas.

Eye Shape and Mouth and Teeth

Japanese Americans are at higher risk for certain types of glaucoma (Aghaian, Choe, Lin, & Stamper, 2004). The central corneal thickness (CCT) varies among Asian subpopulations, and Japanese Americans have significantly thinner corneas (531.7 micrometers) than Chinese, Filipinos, Caucasians, and Hispanics. Japanese Americans have a higher incidence of cleft lip and cleft palate than the general U.S. population (Chung & Myrianthopoulos, 1968; Erickson, 1976). When the nurse provides care for a Japanese American with these anomalies, it is essential to remember that these conditions require additional attention through culturally appropriate assessment, teaching, and risk-reduction strategies. In particular, for pregnant women or women of childbearing age, the nurse will want to counsel about the addition of folic acid to the diet to reduce the risk of these and other congenital anomalies (Eichholzer, Tonz, & Zimmermann, 2006). Endo (2006) reported a marked prevalence of hypodontia (fewer than the regular number of teeth) among the Japanese population (8.5% of the prevalence; 10.1% of the prevalence of advanced hypodontia) compared with other populations.

Enzymatic and Genetic Variations

Lactose intolerance occurs in a majority of the population of the world. In fact, it affects 94% of Asians, 74% of American Blacks, and 79% of American Indians, compared with only 17% of White Americans (Bose & Welsh, 1973; Duncan & Scott, 1972; McCracken, 1971; Overfield, 1995). The time when symptoms are first noted and the ability to consume or tolerate different amounts of milk or milk products can vary (Caskey, Payne-Bose, Welsh, et al., 1977; Lebenthal, Antonowicz, & Schwachman, 1975; Simoons, 1969). Some dietary strategies for individuals who have low levels of the lactase enzyme have been suggested by Jarvis and Miller (2002) to meet calcium recommendations. These include drinking milk with a meal or snack and eating yogurt; cheese low in lactose, such as cheddar, Swiss, and Parmesan; and whole milk and chocolate milk rather than low-fat or unflavored milks, which may be less tolerated.

Drug Interactions and Metabolism

In tuberculosis therapy involving isoniazid, 85% to 90% of Asians rapidly inactivate the drug, compared with 40% of White Americans and 60% of American Blacks (Overfield, 1995; Vessell, 1972). It is important to remember that the gene *N*-acetyltransferase 2 (*NAT2*), slow acetylation type, may cause adverse drug reactions in some Asian Americans (Hiratsuka et al., 2002). Asian clients must be carefully monitored while they are taking this drug to determine its efficacy. Additionally, related to tuberculosis prevention, Japanese public health policy requires bacillus Calmette-Guérin (BCG) inoculation. Because BCG is contraindicated when screening for tuberculosis, especially when a purified protein derivative test as it may result in a heightened reaction. X-ray may be a preferable screen for individuals who have experienced intense reactions.

Succinylcholine, a muscle relaxant used during surgery, is inactivated by the enzyme pseudocholinesterase. Asians are at risk for having pseudocholinesterase deficiency and thus may suffer prolonged muscle paralysis and inability to breathe after administration of the drug (Kalow, 1972; Overfield, 1995).

Genetic and physiological studies have found that Asian clients display more side effects to antipsychotic medication than their White American or American Black counterparts (Binder & Levy, 1981). In addition, they require significantly lower doses of antipsychotic medication to control symptoms (Lin & Finder, 1983; Yamamoto, Fung, Lo, & Reece, 1979). Difficulty in achieving steady-state haloperidol level–dose ratios on Japanese patients has been reported, especially among those patients who required associated antiepileptic or antiparkinsonian medication (Yukawa et al., 2003). Although lower dosages of psychotropic drugs are needed, some Japanese Americans are at risk for extrapyramidal symptoms because the drugs remain in the blood longer (Kalow, 1986; Lin & Finder; Lin et al., 1989). Factors that may be responsible are a group of drug-metabolizing enzymes called *cytochrome P-450 isozymes* that play a crucial role in psychotropic metabolism (Lin & Cheung, 1999).

Another notable finding concerns flushing after ingesting alcohol. Fifty percent of Asian Americans, including Japanese, have a deficiency of the low-K_m mitochondrial aldehyde dehydrogenase 2 (ALDH2) isoenzyme, which is responsible for metabolizing acetaldehyde. This deficiency is an inherited mutant allele that causes flushing, and in particular facial flushing, after alcohol ingestion (Wall, Peterson, Peterson, et al., 1997). There is some evidence to suggest that other physiological changes among some Asian Americans after the ingestion of alcohol include faster metabolism, differences in pulse pressure, and an increase in heart rate (Sue, 1987). Because of discrepancies noted in the findings relative to the influence of genetic and physiological factors on alcohol consumption, their roles cannot be accurately assessed at this time (Sue, 1987). These unpleasant effects tend to limit drinking and lower alcohol-related disorders for some Asian Americans.

Susceptibility to Disease

There are equal incidences of blood types A, B, and O found among Japanese Americans, with type AB found in only about 10% of Japanese Americans. Statistically, persons with type O blood are at greater risk for duodenal ulcers, whereas persons with type A blood are more likely to develop cancer of the stomach (Overfield, 1995).

Cancer of the stomach, colon, rectum, and liver occurs more frequently among Japanese Americans than among their White counterparts according to the Surveillance, Epidemiology and End Results Program (SEER) data (Miller, Kolonel, Berstein, et al., 1996). A possible cause of stomach cancer is believed to be chronic gastritis. Additionally, salt-cured food (such as dried salty fish), diets high in nitrates, tobacco smoking, and *Helicobacter pylori* (a problem for 80% of Japanese over the age of 40–50 years) are also considered possible causes (National Cancer Center, 2006; Nomura et al., 2002). Not only have diets high in salt-cured foods been associated with stomach cancer, but use of nitrites and the intake of diets poor in vitamin C have also been commonly associated with greater incidence of stomach cancer. In recent years Japanese Americans have experienced an increased incidence of breast, prostate, and colorectal cancer (National Cancer Center, 2004; Nomura et al., 2002; Flood, Weiss, Cook, et al., 2000; Miller, Kolonel, Berstein, et al., 1996), which has been suggested to be related to the adoption of a more Western diet and lifestyle. While having increasing rates of these cancers, Japanese American women are more likely to receive diagnosis at an early stage and have better survival rates than Chinese, Japanese, Filipino, and White women (Lin, Clarke, Prehn, et al., 2002; Pineda, White, Kristal, & Taylor, 2001). Akaza et al. (2004) found that men who have the ability to produce equol (a metabolite of soy products produced in the intestine) have a lower incidence of prostate cancer. This finding suggests that research exploring dietary interventions based on soybean isoflavones in the prevention of prostate cancer would be useful.

In an age-specific comparison of hip fracture incidence, Japanese Americans had approximately half the rate of their White counterparts. Further research is needed to pinpoint the reasons for this significant difference (Greendale, et al., 2002; Lauderdale, Jocobsen, Furner, et al., 1997; Ross, Horimatsu, Davis, et al., 1991). Despite having lower bone mineral density at most bone sites than White American women, Japanese American women had lower rates of hip and vertebral fractures (Rice, Larson, LaCroix, Hutchinson, & Drinkwater, 2001). The risk for injury when Japanese Americans fell, however, was not less than that reported for White Americans (Davis, Ross, Nevitt, & Wasnich, 1997). There are differences in the prevalence of osteoporosis at the same skeletal region for Chinese, Japanese, and Caucasian women 50 years of age and older. The prevalence of osteoporosis in Japanese women is lower (11.6% to 16.8%) compared with the prevalence of osteoporosis in Caucasian women (13.0% to 20.0%) (Greendale et al., 2002).

Kawasaki syndrome, or mucocutaneous lymph node syndrome, a disease first described in Japan and later in Hawaii, has been observed primarily in children of Japanese ancestry. Kawasaki syndrome (KS) is "an acute self-limited vasculitis of childhood that is characterized by fever, bilateral nonexudative conjunctivitis, erythema of the lips and oral mucosa, changes in the extremities, rash, and cervical lymphadenopathy" (Newburger et al., 2004). Coronary artery aneurysms or ectasia develop in approximately 15% to 25% of untreated children. It has been observed in higher rates for children younger than 1 year of age than for those 1 to 4 years of age (74.3 and 37.5 per 100,000). The KS incidence for Asian and Pacific Islander children is twice that of White children (70.9 vs 35.3 per 100,000), and is highest among Japanese American children living in Hawaii (197.7 per 100,000). This incidence is higher than that of children living in Japan (Holman et al., 2005). This condition has been managed by medications but is often accompanied by a variety of complications of the cardiovascular system (Newburger et al., 2004). It is the leading cause of acquired heart disease in children in North America and Japan. Though the cause remains unknown, increasing evidence has supported involvement of an infectious agent or multiple infectious agents (Freeman & Shulman, 2001; Gedalia, 2002).

While the percentage of Asian Americans with obesity is low, seemingly the more years a foreign-born Asian American spends in the United States, the higher the risk for being overweight or obese. The U.S. born Asian Americans, of which Japanese Americans are proportionally the highest number, among Asian groups, are significantly more likely to be obese or overweight than foreign-born Asian Americans (Lauderdale & Rathouz, 2000). These higher incidences may be a result of a combination of diet and lifestyle.

Japanese Americans have a higher prevalence of type 2 diabetes than their counterparts in Japan (Fujimoto, Bergstrom, Boyko, et al., 2000). A study with Japanese immigrants suggests the possible interaction of gene–environment in the development of type 2 diabetes (Nemoto, Sasaki, Deeb, Fujimoto, & Tajima, 2002). Research also suggests that the causative factors may be a Westernized lifestyle (higher intake of saturated fat) and reduced activity. In an intervention study with diet and endurance exercises, BMI, body composition, and body fat distribution improved. Thus, these interventions may delay or prevent type 2 diabetes in Japanese Americans with impaired glucose tolerance (IGT) (Liao et al., 2002). Prevention strategies need to target decreased insulin sensitivity (associated with diet and activity) and beta-cell function (Torréns et al., 2004). It is interesting to note that lifestyle modifications decreased weight and central adiposity and improved insulin sensitivity in Japanese Americans with IGT. However, Carr and colleagues (2005) found that such changes did not improve beta-cell function, suggesting that this degree of lifestyle modification may be limited over the long term. A Hawaiian study noted reduced prevalence of diabetes among men who retained a more Japanese lifestyle, with a higher level of physical activity and consumption of more carbohydrates and less fat and animal protein in their diets (Huang et al., 1996). Other research suggests that the causative factors may be Westernized lifestyle (higher intake of saturated fat) and reduced activity. A Hawaiian study noted reduced prevalence of diabetes among men who retained a more Japanese lifestyle, with a higher level of physical activity and consumption of more carbohydrates and less fat and animal protein in their diets (Huang et al., 1996).

Longitudinal research noting the incidence of coronary heart disease has been conducted on the Japanese in Japan, in Hawaii, and on the U.S. mainland. The mortality from coronary heart disease (as well as breast and colon cancer) has been attributed to variations in diets and lifestyles of Asian, Hawaiian, and mainland Japanese. Coronary artery disease mortality is lowest in Japan, intermediate in Hawaii, and highest on the U.S. mainland (Reed, McGee, Cohen, et al., 1982; Yano, Reed, & McGee, 1984). In a Seattle study, visceral adiposity, blood pressure, and plasma glucose were important independent risk factors for the incidence of coronary artery disease in diabetic and nondiabetic Japanese American men (Fujimoto et al., 1999). In another study, elderly Japanese American men with impaired glucose tolerance and undiagnosed or known diabetes were highly prevalent and associated with adverse cardiovascular factor profiles (Rodriguez, Curb, Burchfiel, et al., 1996). For coronary heart disease, low levels of high-density lipoprotein cholesterol (HDL-C), hypertension, IGT, and high triglyceride levels, which represent the state of the metabolic syndrome, were important predictors of acute myocardial infarction for Japanese living in Japan. And it was suggested that low HDL-C plays a pivotal role in a population whose total cholesterol level is not high (Oyama et al., 2006). The Honolulu Heart Project concluded that proteinuria detected at urine dipstick screening independently predicted increased risk for incident stroke and incident coronary heart disease over 27 years in this cohort (Madison et al., 2006). In a study looking at the relationship between alcohol intake and blood pressure, 3 weeks of alcohol restriction (about one third of the amount) produced reductions in ambulatory systolic blood pressure, heart rate, and the index of sympathovagal balance, and augmentations of parasympathetic indices of heart rate variability in Japanese young adult male drinkers (Minami et al., 2002). Another study supports the positive relationships between decreasing alcohol intake and decreasing systolic blood pressure, heart rate, and other variables (Okubo, Suwazono, Kobayashi, & Nogawa, 2001).

Cerebrovascular disease is the third leading cause of death in Japan (MIAC, 2006a). There are a higher incidence in Japan, an intermediate incidence in Hawaii (less than half of Japan's), and the lowest incidence on the U.S. mainland (Rodriguez, D'Agostino, Abbott, et al., 2002; Syme, Marmot, Kagun, et al., 1975; Yano, Reed, & Kagan, 1985). In a Hawaiian study, while stroke increased significantly with increasing age in Japanese American men, the age-related risk of thromboembolic and hemorrhagic strokes among normotensive men resulted in a decreased percentage of strokes attributable to hypertension, 50% in those aged 45 to 54 years to 18% in those aged 65 or older (Curb et al., 1996). Other unidentified factors may have an increased role in stroke causation with advancing age (Curb, Abbott, MacLean, et al., 1996). In comparing White men in the Framingham Study with the Honolulu Heart Program Japanese Americans, White men had a 40% excess of thromboembolic stroke compared with Japanese men, though the incidence of hemorrhagic stroke was nearly identical. The difference in stroke incidence rates cannot be explained by traditional risk factors. Further studies are needed to identify factors that protect Japanese American men from thromboembolic strokes. (Rodriguez, D'Agostino, Abbott, et al., 2002).

Nutritional Preferences and Deficiencies

The Japanese place great importance on the presentation of food. For these individuals, food should be visually appealing. Color, contrast, and shapes of food are considered as important as the cooking and seasoning of a particular food. Unlike American meals that center on one main dish, Japanese meals usually consist of several small dishes (Corum, 2000; Giger & Davidhizar, 1990). A Japanese American family that has been acculturated may serve a mixture of American and Japanese dishes.

Traditionally, food was cooked on a small grill by broiling, steaming, frying, or simmering. Food was cut so that it cooked quickly and evenly, preserving vitamins. Meat, which is expensive in Japan, is frequently eaten with vegetables. Traditionally, the main sources of protein were fish and soybeans. Tofu, a soybean product, is used extensively as a dish by itself or mixed with other dishes. In a study conducted in Seattle, the soy foods most commonly consumed among Japanese American women 65 years of age or older were tofu (soybean curd), *miso* (fermented soybean paste), and *abura-age* (fried thin soybean curd) (Rice, Larson, LaCroix, Hutchinson, & Drinkwater, 2001). Findings from this study suggest that the mean intake of dietary soy isoflavones was approximately a quarter to a half that of previously published estimates in Japanese samples. Dietary intake of soy isoflavones was positively associated with speaking Japanese, the consumption of traditional Japanese dishes (*kamaboko, manju,* and *mochi*), consumption of low-fat/nonfat milk and yellow/red vegetables, vitamin E supplement use, and walking several blocks each day. Dietary intake of soy isoflavones was negatively associated with the consumption of butter.

The main source of carbohydrate is rice or noodles. A seasoning used extensively is soy sauce, which is high in sodium. Pickled vegetables and unsweetened green tea complete a meal. Sake, or rice wine, is sometimes served. Milk is often included in the diet of children but less often for adults, a finding that may be related to the high incidence of lactose intolerance in the population. The traditional diet is nutritious and low in fat but tends to be high in sodium. In Hawaii, Japanese dishes tend to be sweetened more than they are in Japan. Most Japanese Americans also consume popular American foods, such as pizza, tacos, and hamburgers. A recent study indicated that the *sansei* ate fewer meals per day than the *nisei*. Further findings from this study also suggested that among men, the frequency of takeout foods and eating out was higher in the *sansei* than the *nisei* (Kudo, Falciglia, & Couch, 2000).

Psychological Characteristics

Cultural Values Related to Self. A study of four Asian American groups found that the Japanese Americans tended to score higher on most of the Asian value dimensions than the other three groups. These values were collectivism, conformity to norms, emotional self-control, and family recognition through achievement and filial piety (Kim, Yang, Atkinson, Wolfe, & Hong, 2001). Although furthest removed from immigration, this group demonstrates that generation status is not related to adherence to Asian cultural values, which has implications for acculturation/enculturation theories (Kim, Yang, Atkinson, Wolfe, & Hong, 2001). The Asian sense of self is interdependent and is part of a larger social system. This feature is based on the collective, public self and attributes (Yeh & Huang, 1996). *Enryo* emphasizes modesty, respect, and deference toward others. *Enryo* is related to *hazukashii*, the implicit fear of being ridiculed, which results in feelings of embarrassment and reticence. *Hige* is the concept of denigration of self and others (Kitano, 1970). These concepts emphasize conformity to group norms and minimization of accomplishments (Fugita, Ito, Abe, & Takeuchi, 1991). *Gaman* refers to internalization and suppression of anger and emotion. Avoidance of confrontation and acceptance of the results of negative social interactions can be related to *gaman*. In contrast to earlier studies, ethnic identification with their traditional culture is still strong in fourth-generation (*yonsei*) Japanese Americans, similar to the levels of previous generations (Marsella, Johnson, Johnson, & Brennan, 1998). On the other hand, the more acculturated Asian American men became, the less gender-role conflict was related to restrictive emotionality (Kim, O'Neil, & Owen, 1996). These findings suggest a dynamic interplay of factors that influence ethnic identity and do not follow linear assimilation across generations for Japanese Americans.

Doutrich (2001) conducted a study of Japanese nurse scholars working on their masters or doctoral degrees in the U.S. In total, 42 interviews were completed. Interpretive analysis revealed a prevailing theme related to a change in the self. One participant described the Japanese self and touched on the changes that occur during acculturation: "The way we think is always thinking of the other person's feelings and thinking. If I cannot predict what you think, what you feel, I am lost completely . . . ." The flow of concern from the other is a foundation of self-definition in the Japanese psyche, and language and cultural values reinforce and support this notion. The Japanese nurse scholars in this study did adapt and were able to achieve a level of bicultural fluency, but some described a new "tougher" self unfolding in the process of acculturation. Likewise, the participants in a study of Japanese immigrant youth in the U.S. described feeling conflicted living in two cultures (Yeh et al., 2003). To a lesser degree, depending on the degree of acculturation, Japanese Americans may feel this bicultural conflict and contextually shifting sense of self.

Leong (1986) found that Asian Americans have a lower tolerance for ambiguity. Findings from this study also indicate that Asian Americans are more likely to prefer structured situations. They tend to want practical and immediate solutions to their problems (Leong, 1986). This study indicates that Asian Americans are more likely to show respect for authority figures and are less likely to express their emotions.

Emotional and Behavioral Manifestation of Stress. The length of residence in a new environment and generational status of an individual are important factors in determining levels of stress perceived by an ethnic group undergoing acculturation (Padilla, Wagatsuma, & Lindholm, 1985). Examining variables such as generational status, acculturation level, and personality variables, Padilla, Wagatsuma, and Lindholm (1985) found that *issei* Japanese immigrants (likely *shin-issei*) reported the most stress and were the most externally controlled. A plausible reason for acculturation stress is the disparity noted between culture and expected individual behavior. It is interesting to note that *sansei* and later-generation students scored lower on stress, higher on self-esteem, and higher on internal locus of control. Differences in scores also indicated that *nisei* individuals may be in transition from traditional values held by their parents to values held by some Japanese Americans belonging to *sansei* or later generations.

Mental Health. According to Lin and Cheung (1999), there is considerable evidence to indicate that Asian Americans utilize mental health services less frequently than White Americans. Those who do use mental health services drop out at a significantly higher rate than White American clients (Sue, 1987). Kozuki and Kennedy (2004) explored the "cultural incommensurabilty" that results when Western models of diagnosis and treatment are applied to Japanese and Japanese American clients. Cultural incommensurability refers to the lack of a standard of common measure or fundamental cultural differences between Western and Japanese traditions in mental health. The purpose of the study was to examine how this might influence treatment outcomes. These researchers also found that the most benign consequences were ineffective treatment. The worst consequences resulted in misdiagnoses, labeling, and further damage to the patient's sense of self.

Regarding type of effective counselors, Atkinson and Matsushita (1991) found that *sansei* and *yonsei* Japanese Americans rated Japanese American counselors as more attractive than White American counselors when portraying a directive counseling style but less attractive when portraying a nondirective counseling style. This theory supports an earlier study (Atkinson, Maruyama, & Matsui, 1978) that found that Asian Americans demonstrated a preference for an ethnically similar counselor and a directive counseling style.

Internment Trauma. For Japanese Americans, the imprisonment of more than 120,000 men, women, and children in internment camps by the U.S. government during World War II represents the most traumatic and salient episode of the past (Nagata, 1991). More than 60% of those persons incarcerated were U.S. citizens. No formal charges were ever brought against them, yet they had no opportunity for a trial. In many cases, they were given less than a week's notice to move and to sell their businesses, personal property, and other possessions. In many instances, they were unable to sell these items or were forced to sell them for much less than their actual value, which resulted in severe economic hardship. Many were forced to move twice, first to temporary assembly centers in animal stalls at horse tracks and fairgrounds and later to internment camps in isolated areas. They lived 2 to 3 years in camps enclosed by barbed wire and armed guards,

with the psychological degradation associated with being accused of disloyalty (Nagata, 1991). Nonetheless, many of the individuals interned believed they were victimized and rejected by their own country of citizenship (Nagata, 1991). Even today, transgenerational effects of victimization are evident in *sansei* descendants of individuals who suffered through this ordeal (Nagata, 1991). Many of these individuals reported that their parents maintained a silence about their experience in the camps. For many of these individuals, the results were a loss of self-esteem (Nagata & Takeshita, 2002) and a heightened sense of vulnerability and fear that their rights as U.S. citizens might be violated again (Nagata, 1991). For some, the post-9/11 climate, with military tribunals and "enemy combatant status," is an all too familiar echo from the past, and some among the Japanese American community cautioned against targeting Muslim immigrants (Wood, 2005).

Somatization and Folk Traditions. According to Fujii, Fukushima, and Yamamoto (1993), folk healing is often used to treat physical ailments because Asians tend to express emotional illness or distress through physical symptoms. Being "ill" is a legitimate, socially acceptable manner of receiving care. For some Japanese Americans, complaints are usually physical (Marsella, 1993). Kitano (1969) noted that Japanese people tend to worry needlessly about body functions and are usually obsessed about a potential problem related to their blood pressure.

Tracey, Leong, and Glidden (1986) found that Asian American students appear to find it more acceptable to react to emotional difficulties by focusing on academic and vocational concerns. When counseling was sought, Japanese American students tended to focus more on academic difficulties than on emotional conflict.

For some Canadian Japanese, there was a stigma associated with mental illness. Many believed that mental illness was inherited, contagious, or incurable. These individuals viewed the psychiatrist as someone who treated only severe mental illnesses. For many of these individuals, very little interest was taken in psychotherapy and psychodynamics (Isomura, Fine, & Lin, 1987). Biological treatment methods were viewed as being more helpful than psychiatric intervention (Isomura, Fine, & Lin, 1987).

Degree of acculturation and somatization of symptoms by the Japanese were investigated by Tanaka-Matsumi and Marsella (1976). They found that among Japanese nationals the word *headache* was associated with depression, whereas Japanese Americans and White Americans associated the word *loneliness* with depression.

Psychopharmacology. Recent literature indicates Asians respond to substantially lower doses of psychotropics than Caucasians (Lin & Cheung, 1999). Several studies have suggested that Japanese Americans do well with lower dosages of psychotropic medication for depression or mania (Lin & Cheung, 1999; Yamamoto, 1982) and need significantly lower maintenance dosages (Roseblat & Tang, 1987). Evidence also indicates that Japanese Americans need lower maximum and stabilizing dosages for chlorpromazine. Although lower dosages of psychotropic drugs are needed, some Japanese Americans are at risk for extrapyramidal symptoms because the drugs remain in the blood longer (Kalow, 1986; Lin & Finder, 1983; Lin, Poland, Nuccio, et al., 1989). Factors that may be responsible are a group of drug-metabolizing enzymes called cytochrome P-450 isozymes that play a crucial role in psychotropic metabolism (Lin & Cheung, 1999).

Alcohol Use. Japanese Americans appear to have lower rates of alcoholism than the rest of the U.S. population. Some researchers believe that these lower rates may be attributed to a variety of factors, such as (1) being shielded by their families, (2) seeking treatment only during the late stages of alcoholism, (3) seeking assistance from other sources rather than state mental health facilities (Kotani, 1982), and (4) being protected by *ALDH1* deficiency, the fast flushing response (Nakawatase, Yamamoto, & Toshiaki, 1993). Because of these factors, it is extremely difficult to determine an accurate rate for alcoholism in this ethnic group. The untreated case method would give a better estimate of the severity of alcohol abuse in this group. This method is based on obtaining information on patterns of use among the general population.

In a survey of untreated case methods, Sue (1987) concluded that Asian Americans are less likely than other groups to seek treatment for alcoholism. Findings from other studies also indicate that although Japanese Americans are more likely to abstain from alcohol use than other ethnic and racial groups, among those who drink heavily, Japanese American men tend to drink more than their female counterparts do (Sue, 1987) and younger respondents drink more than older respondents (Higuchi, Parrish, Dufour, Towle, & Harford, 1994).

Implications for Nursing Care

It is important for the nurse to teach and counsel clients about diseases common among Japanese Americans. In addition, preventive health care techniques should be emphasized. To provide culturally appropriate and competent care, the nurse must engage the support of other family members. To reduce chronicity and severity of hypertension, the nurse must stress to the client and the family the importance of limiting use of soy sauce, salt-cured fish, and pickles. Because somatization is often used among some Japanese Americans, the nurse must recognize that frequent physical ailments may be possible signs of underlying stress. Meaning must be attached to behavior if the client is to receive optimal care. It is also essential to identify previous successful strategies in order to help the client develop and refine coping strategies. To reduce stress, the nurse might suggest exercise because it may be perceived by the client as a nonconfrontational form of release. Health promotion should also include reminding women of childbearing age to add folic acid to their diets.

It is essential for the nurse to remember that some Japanese Americans generally do not seek or delay seeking professional help for mental health problems. Of those individuals who do seek treatment, many generally do not complete treatment (Leong, 1986). Kitano (1969) speculated that the reluctance to seek treatment may be a result of several factors, including (1) strength of the family and community and the family's ability to control and hide problem behaviors, (2) different cultural styles of expressing problems, (3) inappropriateness of current therapeutic organizations, and (4) lack of relevant connections to the therapeutic community. Another factor may be related to the inability of the therapist to provide culturally responsive forms of treatment (Sue, 1987). Additionally, some Japanese Americans will look first to their families when they have emotional problems, in order to maintain family honor (Atkinson & Matsushita, 1991; Leong, 1986). Therefore, the major goal of nursing care should be aimed at developing a trusting relationship between the nurse and the client by using a more structured and directive approach that emphasizes collectivism, harmony, and acceptance over individualistic ascendancy (Marsella, 1993).

SUMMARY

Japanese Americans vary in their degree of acculturation. Because of this variability, Japanese Americans may present in the clinical setting with a variety of behaviors, depending on factors such as generational, regional, and individual differences. The nurse must assess the unique needs of each individual and the extent to which the information presented applies to that person or family. The importance of establishing a trusting relationship based on respect and open communication with the client and the family cannot be underestimated.

Case Study

Mr. Robert Kiyoshi Yamamoto, a 71-year-old retired *nisei* electrician, was admitted to the hospital with complaints of nausea and difficulty keeping food down that were related to recurrent colon cancer with liver metastasis. For the past few weeks, Mr. Yamamoto's appetite has been steadily decreasing. His wife of 50 years states that he has been unable to keep any solid foods down but has been able to drink some fluids.

After a few days of nasogastric decompression, Mr. Yamamoto's bowel function begins to return. He is able to eat small amounts of soft foods. Because the tumor has spread despite chemotherapy, Mr. Yamamoto has decided against further chemotherapy. As he becomes weaker and weaker, Mr. Yamamoto insists that his wife remain at his bedside so that he "doesn't have to bother the nurses for little things." Mrs. Yamamoto has kept a bedside vigil and rarely leaves except to go home to shower while one of their three daughters stays with her father. The nurse notices that Mrs. Yamamoto is looking tired and appears to be losing weight. Her daughters have tried to relieve their mother at night so that she can rest at home, but she insists that "Dad is restless and calls out in the night for me." Mr. Yamamoto insists that she bathe him and assist him to the bathroom. One daughter flew in from out of town to assist indefinitely if needed. All daughters take turns in keeping their mother company or relieving her when she goes home to shower or cook special foods for her husband.

Although he never says he is having pain, Mr. Yamamoto has family members constantly massaging his back and legs. He moves cautiously and winces with each movement. Mr. Yamamoto does not talk much to the staff. He lets his family talk for him. He denies pain when asked by the nurse but tells his family otherwise. He does not sleep well. Mr. Yamamoto's current treatment is primarily supportive care. He is constantly requesting special Japanese foods such as sushi and miso soup, which the family brings in daily. Generally, he just tastes it. The hospital staff has brought up the possibility of hospice care. A family meeting to discuss discharge plans was called by his son. Mr. Yamamoto has stated he wants to go home.

CARE PLAN

✳ *Nursing Diagnosis: Altered family processes, related to situational crisis*

Client Outcomes

1. Family will devise a specific rotation plan to meet each other's need for rest and caring for their father.
2. Family will demonstrate mutual support and cohesion.

Nursing Interventions

1. Provide empathy and support for the immediate family members who need to be at the bedside by providing family with liberal visitation, adequate space for members who stay overnight, and privacy.
2. Keep family abreast of current treatments and nature of illness to dispel any misunderstandings and to keep lines of communication open between family and staff.
3. Assess family members for signs of fatigue or overextension.
4. Explore with family members other possible family members or friends who would be willing and be accepted by client to keep him company or support his wife.

✳ *Nursing Diagnosis: Pain, related to cancer metastasis*

Client Outcomes

1. Client will indicate to family that the pain is tolerable.
2. Client will be able to sleep 4 hours at a time at night.

Nursing Interventions

1. Observe nonverbal behaviors that indicate pain, such as wincing with movement and restlessness at night.
2. Check with family about how much pain client is having with the current treatment.
3. Give analgesic on a regular schedule without waiting for him to ask (unless refused), especially before sleep.

✳ *Nursing Diagnosis: Risk for ineffective family coping, related to deteriorating course of disease of a family member*

Client Outcomes

1. Family unit will use own resources and explore outside resources.
2. Family will devise realistic expectations of roles of members.
3. Open communication will be maintained among family members.
4. Family members will perform care without compromising their own physical and emotional health.

Nursing Interventions

1. Develop trusting and respectful relationships with client and family.
2. Encourage the son to call family meetings as needed to discuss realistic plans and expectations of members, using health care providers as needed.
3. Assist and encourage family explore outside resources as well as family resources to assist in dealing with the crisis.
4. Assess if basic physical and emotional needs of client and family members are being met.
5. Encourage family members to support each other, especially Mrs. Yamamoto, and devise a schedule that does not compromise their physical and emotional health.
6. Continue to monitor ability of family members to carry out treatment regimen and care.
7. Discuss management of emotional outbursts, personality changes, and mood swings with family members or those providing care.
8. Encourage realistic expectations of role performance, especially by Mrs. Yamamoto.
9. Teach coping strategies to manage tension and strain if previous techniques are no longer effective.
10. Help with identification of current stressors and strain.

✳ STUDY QUESTIONS

1. List the important cultural values that determine health-seeking and health-practice behaviors in this cultural group.
2. Identify three interventions that incorporate these values in treating the Japanese American client.
3. Analyze different strategies useful in communicating with the Japanese American family.
4. Discuss the importance of understanding generational, geographical, and acculturation issues in working with the Japanese American client.
5. Describe appropriate interventions by health care providers for clients who do not verbally express pain, discomfort, or stress.

NCLEX-RN REVIEW QUESTIONS

1. In the treatment of hypertension for a Japanese client, the nurse needs to stress to the family and client the importance of limiting:
   A. Pepper
   B. Soy sauce
   C. Tofu
   D. Milk

2. When seeking counseling, in assessing a Japanese American student in the mental health center, the nurse is aware that this client is more apt to seek counseling for:

   A. Academic difficulties
   B. Emotional conflict
   C. Family problems
   D. Loss of self esteem

3. The majority of communication of feelings and attitudes among Japanese Americans is:
   A. Verbal
   B. Vocal
   C. Facial expression
   D. Touch

References

Adler, S. M. (1998). *Mothering, education, and ethnicity: the transformation of Japanese American culture.* New York: Garland.

Aghaian, E., Choe, J. E., Lin, S., & Stamper, R. L. (2004). Central corneal thickness of Caucasians, Chinese, Hispanics, Filipinos, African Americans, and Japanese in a glaucoma clinic [abstract]. *Ophthalmology,* 111(12), 2211–2219.

Akaza, H, Miyanaga, N, Takashima, N, Naito, S, Hirao, Y, & Tsukamoto, T, et al, (2004). Comparisons of percent equol producers between prostate cancer patients and controls: case-controlled studies of isoflavones in Japanese, Korean and American residents [abstract]. *Japanese Journal of Clinical Oncology,* 34(2), 86–89.

Akimoto, S. A., & Sanbonmatsu, D. M. (1999). Differences in self-effacing behavior between European and Japanese Americans: effect on competence evaluations. *Journal of Cross-Cultural Psychology,* 30(2), 159–177.

Atkinson, D. R., Maruyama, M., & Matsui, S. (1978). The effects of counselor race and counseling approach on Asian Americans' perceptions of counselor credibility and utility. *Journal of Counseling Psychology,* 25, 76–83.

Atkinson, D. R., & Matsushita, Y. (1991). Japanese American acculturation, counseling style, counselor ethnicity, and perceived counselor credibility. *Journal of Counseling Psychology,* 38, 473–478.

Austin, M. A. (2002). Ethical issues in human genome epidemiology: a case study based on the Japanese American family study in Seattle, Washington. *American Journal of Epidemiology,* 155(7), 585–592.

Baker, J. (1993). Perceptions of privacy in Japan and America, Paper presented at the East West Center, Honolulu, Hawaii.

Barnlund, D. C. (1989). Public-private self in communication with Japan. *Business Horizons,* 32, 32–35.

Binder, R. L., & Levy, R. (1981). Extrapyramidal reactions in Asians. *American Journal of Psychiatry,* 138(9), 1243–1244.

Bose, D., & Welsh, J. (1973). Lactose malabsorption in Oklahoma Indians. *American Journal of Clinical Nutrition,* 26, 1320–1322.

Bowman, K. W., & Singer, P. A. (2001). Chinese seniors' perspectives on end-of-life decisions. *Social Science & Medicine*, 53(4), 455–464.

Braun, K. L., & Nichols, R. (1997). Death and dying in four Asian American cultures: a descriptive study. *Death Studies*, 21(4), 327–359.

Burris, J. (1993, March 21). 442nd vets "shared a tent" in battle, in politics. *The Honolulu Advertiser*, B-1.

Carr, D. B., Utzschneider, K. M., Boyko, E. J., Asberry, P. J., Hull, R. L., & Kodama, K., et al, (2005). A reduced-fat diet and aerobic exercise in Japanese Americans with impaired glucose tolerance decreases intra-abdominal fat and improves insulin sensitivity but not beta-cell function [abstract]. *Diabetes*, 54(2), 340–347.

Caskey, D. A., Payne-Bose, D., & Welsh, J. D., et al, (1977). Effects of age on lactose malabsorption in Oklahoma Native Americans as determined by breath H_2 analysis. *American Journal of Digestive Disease*, 22 (2), 113–116.

Caudill, W., & Frost, L. (1974). A comparison of maternal care and infant behavior in Japanese American, American, and Japanese families. In Lebra, W. P. (Ed.), *Youth, socialization and mental health: mental health research in Asia and the Pacific* (vol. 3). Honolulu: University of Hawaii Press.

Caudill, W., & Scarr, H. A. (1962). Japanese value orientations and culture change. *Ethnology*, 1, 53–91.

Chan, S. (1991). *Asian Americans: an interpretive history.* Boston: Twayne Publishers.

Chang, B. (1981). Asian American patient care. In Henderson, G., & Primeaux, M. (Eds.), *Transcultural health care* Menlo Park, Calif: Addison-Wesley.

Chang, T. (1993, March 21). A legacy of bravery: the 442nd comes home. *The Honolulu Advertiser*, 442nd Special Section.

Ching, J. W. J., McDermott, J. F., & Fukunaga, C., et al, (1995). Perceptions of family values and roles among Japanese Americans: clinical considerations. *American Journal of Orthopsychiatry*, 65(2), 216–224.

Chung, C. S., & Myrianthopoulos, N. C. (1968). Racial and prenatal factors in major congenital malformations. *American Journal of Human Genetics*, 20, 44–60.

Colclough, Y. Y. (2005). *An exploration of end-of-life decision making within Japanese-American families.* Portland, Ore: Oregon Health & Science University, Unpublished doctoral dissertation.

Connor, J. (1974). Acculturation and family continuity in three generations of Japanese Americans. *Journal of Marriage and Family*, 36, 159–168.

Corum, A. K. (2000). *Ethnic foods of Hawaii.* (revised ed.) Honolulu: Bess Press.

Curb, J. D., Abbott, R. D., & MacLean, C. J., et al, (1996). Age-related changes in stroke risk in men with hypertension and normal blood pressure. *Stroke*, 27(5), 819–824.

Daniels, R. (1991). Redressed achieved, 1983–1990. In Daniels, R., Taylor, S. C., & Kitano, H. H. L. (Eds.), *Japanese Americans: from relocation to redress* (pp. 219–223). Seattle: University of Washington Press.

Daniels, R., Taylor, S. C., & Kitano, H. H. L. (Eds.). (1991). *Japanese Americans: from relocation to redress.* Seattle: University of Washington Press.

Davis, J. W., Ross, P. D., Nevitt, M. C., & Wasnich, R. D. (1997). Incidence rates of falls among Japanese men and women living in Hawaii. *Journal of Clinical Epidemiology*, 50(5), 589–594.

Doi, L. T. (1962). Amae: a key concept for understanding Japanese personality structure. In Smith, R. J., & Beardsley, R. K. (Eds.), *Japanese culture: its development and characteristics* Chicago: Aldine Publishing.

Doi, L. T. (1973). *The anatomy of dependence.* New York: Kodansha International.

Dornbusch, S. M., Ritter, P. L., & Leiderman, P. H., et al. (1987). The relation of parenting style to adolescent school performance. *Child Development*, 55, 1244–1257.

Doutrich, D. (2000). Cultural fluency, marginality, and the sense of self. In Riggenbach, H. (Ed.) *Perspectives on fluency* (pp. 141–159). Ann Arbor, Mich.: University of Michigan Press.

Doutrich, D. (2001). Experience of Japanese nurse scholars: insights for U.S. faculty. *Journal of Nursing Education*, 40(5), 210–215.

Drake, P. R., & Freedman, J. L. (1997). The belief in good luck scale. *Journal of Research in Personality*, 31(4), 486–511.

Duncan, I., & Scott, E. (1972). Lactose intolerance in Alaskan Indians and Eskimos. *American Journal of Clinical Nutrition*, 25, 867–868.

The Economist Business Traveller's Guides. (2006). New York: Prentice-Hall.

Eichholzer, M., Tonz, O., & Zimmermann, R. (2006). Folic acid: a public health challenge. *The Lancet*, 367(9519), 1352–1362.

Endo, T., Ozoe, R., Kubota, M., Akiyama, M., & Shimooka, S. (2006). A survey of hypodontia in Japanese orthodontic patients [abstract]. *American Journal of Orthodontics and Dentofacial Orthopedics*, 129(1), 29–35.

Engle, M. (1993, January 4). Japanese New Year's customs demystified. *Star-Bulletin*, (p. A-4).

Epstein, E. (2005, November 17). House OKs funds to preserve WWII internment camps. *The San Francisco Chronicle.* Retrieved June 1, 2006, from Lexis/Nexis Academic Universe database.

Epstein, E. (2006, December 6). Internment-site preservation OK'd sites of WWII prisons for some citizens to serve as remainder of U.S. rights abuses. *San Francisco Chronicle,* Washington Bureau. Retrieved at www.sfgate.com/cgi-bin/article.cgi?file=chronicle/archive/2006/12/06.

Erickson, J. D. (1976). Racial variations in the incidence of congenital malformations. *Annals of Human Genetics,* 39, 315–320.

Evans, G. W., Lepore, S. J., & Allen, K. M. (2000). Cross-cultural differences in tolerance for crowding: fact or fiction? *Journal of Personality and Social Psychology,* 79(2), 204–210.

Fisher, N. (1996). *Cultural and ethnic diversity: a guide for genetic professionals.* Baltimore, Md.: Johns Hopkins University Press.

Flaherty, J. H., Takahashi, R., Teoh, J., Kim, J. I., Habib, S., & Ito, M., et al, (2001). Use of alternative therapies in older outpatients in the United States and Japan: prevalence, reporting patterns, and perceived effectiveness [abstract]. *Journals of Gerontology Series A: Biological Sciences and Medical Science,* 56(10), M650–M655.

Flood, D. M., Weiss, N. S., & Cook, L. S., et al, (2000). Colorectal cancer incidence in Asian migrants to the United States and their descendants. *Cancer Causes and Control,* 11(5), 403–411.

Freeman, A. F., & Shulman, S. T. (2001). Recent developments in Kawasaki disease. *Current Opinion in Infectious Diseases,* 14(3), 357–361.

Fugita, S., Ito, K. L., Abe, J., & Takeuchi, D. T. (1991). Japanese Americans. In Mokuau, N. (Ed.), *Handbook of social services for Asian and Pacific Islanders* (pp. 61–77). New York: Greenwood Press.

Fugita, S. S., & O'Brien, D. J. (1991). *Japanese American Ethnicity: the persistence of community.* Seattle: University of Washington Press.

Fujii, J., Fukushima, S., & Yamamoto, J. (1993). Psychiatric care of Japanese Americans. In Gaw, A. C. (Ed.), *Culture, ethnicity and mental illness* (pp. 305–346). Washington, D.C.: American Psychiatric Press.

Fujimoto, W. Y., Bergstrom, R. W., & Boyko, E. J., et al, (1999). Visceral adiposity and incident coronary heart disease in Japanese-American men. The 10-year follow-up results of the Seattle Japanese-American Community Diabetes Study. *Diabetes Care,* 22(11), 1808–1812.

Fujimoto, W. Y., Bergstrom, R. W., & Boyko, E. J., et al, (2000). Type 2 diabetes and the metabolic syndrome in Japanese Americans. *Diabetes Research & Clinical Practice Supplement,* 5(2), S73–S76.

Galanti, G. A. (1997). *Caring for patients from different cultures: case studies from American hospitals.* (ed. 2), Philadelphia: University of Pennsylvania Press.

Gedalia, A. (2002). Kawasaki disease: an update. *Current Rheumatology Report,* 4(1), 25–29.

Giger, J. N., & Davidhizar, R. E. (1990). Transcultural nursing: a method for advancing nursing care and practices. *International Congress of Nursing Review,* 37 (1), 199–202.

Greendale, G. A., FitsGerald, G., & Huang, M. H., et al, (2002). Soy products may help preserve bone density in Japanese women [abstract]. *American Journal of Epidemiology,* 155, 746–754.

Gudykanst, W. B., & Nishida, T. (1994). *Bridging Japanese/North American differences.* Thousand Oaks, CA: Sage.

Hall, E. T. (1976). *Beyond culture.* New York: Doubleday.

Hamaguchi, E. (1977). Nihonrashiga N. Saihaken. *(Rediscovery of Japaneseness). Nihon Keizai Shaimbun-sha.*

Hashizume, S., & Takano, J. (1983). Nursing care of Japanese American patients. In Orque, M. S., Bloch, B., & Monrroy, L. S. A. (Eds.), *Ethnic nursing care: a multicultural approach* (pp. 219–243). St. Louis: Mosby.

Higa, M. (1974). A comparative study of 3 groups of Japanese mothers' attitudes toward childrearing. In Lebra, W. P. (Ed.), *Youth, socialization, and mental health,* Honolulu: University of Hawaii Press.

Higuchi, S., Parrish, K. M., Dufour, M. C., Towle, L. H., & Harford, T. C. (1994). Relationship between age and drinking patterns and drinking problems among Japanese, Japanese-Americans, and Caucasians. *Alcoholism: Clinical and Experimental Research,* 18(2), 305–310.

Hiratsuka, M., Kishikawa, Y., Takekuma, Y., Matsuura, M., Narahara, K., Inoue, T., et al, (2002). Genotyping of the N-acetyltransferase2 polymorphism in the prediction of adverse drug reactions to isoniazid in Japanese patients [abstract]. *Drug Metabolism and Pharmacokinetics,* 17(4), 357–362.

Ho, M. K. (1976). Social work with Asian Americans. *Social Casework,* 57, 195–201.

Hofstede, G. (1984). *Culture's consequences: International differences in work related values.* Beverly Hills: Sage.

Holman, R. C., Curns, A. T., Belay, E. D., Steiner, C. A., Effler, P. V., Yorita, K. L., et al, (2005). Kawasaki syndrome in Hawaii. *Pediatric Infectious Disease Journal,* 24(5), 429–433.

Hosokawa, G. (2002). *Nisei: the quiet Americans* (revised ed.), Boulder, Colo.: University Press of Colorado.

Houston, J. W., & Houston, J. D. (2002). *Farewell to Manzanar.* Boston: Houghton Mifflin.

Hsu, J., Tseng, W.-S., Ashton, G., McDermott, J. F., & Char, W. (1985). Family interaction patterns among Japanese-American and Caucasian families in Hawaii. *American Journal of Psychiatry*, 142, 577–581.

Huang, B., Rodriguez, B. L., & Burchfiel, C. M., et al, (1996). Acculturation and prevalence of diabetes among Japanese-American men in Hawaii. *American Journal of Epidemiology*, 144(7), 674–681.

Ishihara, A. (1962). Kampo: Japan's traditional medicine. *Japan Quarterly*, 9, 429–437.

Ishii, S. (1987). Nonverbal communication in Japan (Orientation Seminars on Japan, No. 28). Tokyo: Office for the Japanese Studies Center.

Isomura, T., Fine, S., & Lin, T. Y. (1987). Two Japanese families: a cultural perspective. *Canadian Journal of Psychiatry*, 32, 282–286.

Jacobs, A. H., & Walton, R. G. (1976). Incidence of birthmarks in the neonate. *Pediatrics*, 58, 218–222.

Jarvis, J. K., & Miller, G. D. (2002). Overcoming the barrier of lactose intolerance to reduce health disparities. *Journal of the National Medical Association*, 94(2), 55–66.

Johnson, F. A., Marsella, A. J., & Johnson, C. L. (1974). Social and psychological aspects of verbal behavior in Japanese Americans. *American Journal of Psychiatry*, 131, 580–583.

Kakesako, G. K. (1993, March 19). Nisei proved their loyalty on the war front. *The Honolulu Star-Bulletin*, A–1.

Kakuchi, S. (2005, February 25). *Population: young Koreans in Japan shrug off the past. Interpress Service/ Global Information Network.* Retrieved May 24, 2006, from Lexis/Nexis Academic Universe database.

Kalow, W. (1972). Pharmacogenetics of drugs used in anesthesia. *Human Genetics*, 60, 415–427.

Kalow, W. (1986). Conjugation reactions. In Kalow, W., Goedde, H. W., & Agarwal, D. P. (Eds.), *Ethnic differences in reactions to drugs and xenobiotics* New York: Alan R. Liss.

Katada, N. (1991). *Gaman as a preschooler's method of coping during hospitalization.* San Francisco, Calif: Unpublished doctoral dissertation, University of California, San Francisco.

Kataoka-Yahiro, M., Ceria, C., & Caulfield, R. (2004). Grandparent caregiving role in ethnically diverse families. *Journal of Pediatric Nursing*, 19(5), 315–328.

Kiefer, C. W. (1974).*Changing cultures, changing lives*, (pp. 110–129). San Francisco: Jossey-Bass.

Kim, B. S., Yang, P. H., Atkinson, D. R., Wolfe, M. M., & Hong, S. (2001). Cultural value similarities and differences among Asian American ethnic groups. *Cultural Diversity and Ethnic Minority Psychology*, 7, 343–361.

Kim, E. J., O'Neil, J. M., & Owen, S. V. (1996). Asian-American men's acculturation and gender-role conflict. *Psychological Reports*, 79, 95–104.

Kitano, H. H. L. (1969). Japanese-American mental illness. In Plot, S. C., & Edgerton, R. B. (Eds.), *Changing perspectives in mental illness.* New York: Holt, Rinehart & Winston.

Kitano, H. H. L. (1970). Mental illness in four cultures. *Journal of Social Psychology*, 80, 121–134.

Kitano, H. H. L. (1976). *Japanese Americans: the evolution of a subculture.* (ed. 2), Englewood Cliffs, N.J.: Prentice-Hall.

Kitano, H. H. L., & Daniels, R. (2001). *Asian Americans: emerging minorities.* (ed. 3), Englewood Cliffs, N.J.: Prentice-Hall.

Kitano, H. L., Fujino, D., & Takahashi, J. (1998). Interracial marriage: where are the Asian Americans and where are they going? In Lee, L., & Zane, N (Eds.), *Handbook of Asian American psychology* Thousand Oaks, Calif.: Sage.

Klopf, D., Cambra, R., & Ishii, S. (1981). A comparison of communication styles of Japanese and American college students. *Current English Studies*, 53, 22–26.

Klopf, D., & Ishii, S. (1976). A comparison of communication activities of Japanese and American adults. *ELEC Bulletin*, 20, 66–71.

Kobata, F. (1979). The influence of culture on family relations: the Asian American experience. In Ragan, P. K. (Ed.), *Aging parents.* Los Angeles: Ethel Percy Andrus Gerontology Foundation, University of Southern California.

Kobayashi-Winata, H., & Powers, T. (1989). Child rearing and compliance: Japanese and American families in Houston. *Journal of Cross-Cultural Psychology*, 20, 333–356.

Kotani, R. (1982). AJA's and alcohol abuse. *Hawaii Herald*, 3(13), 4.

Kozuki, Y., & Kennedy, M. (2004). Cultural incommensurability in psychodynamic psychotherapy in Western and Japanese traditions. *Journal of Nursing Scholarship*, 36(1), 30–38.

Kudo, Y., Falciglia, G. A., & Couch, S. C. (2000). Evolution of meal patterns and food choices of Japanese-American females born in the United States. *European Journal of Clinical Nutrition*, 54(8), 665–670.

Lauderdale, D. S., Jocobsen, S. J., & Furner, S. E., et al, (1997). Hip fracture incidence among elderly Asian-

American populations. *American Journal of Epidemiology*, 146(6), 502–509.

Lauderdale, D. S., & Rathouz, P. J. (2000). Body mass index in a US national sample of Asian Americans: effects of nativity, years since immigration and socioeconomic status. *International Journal of Obesity and Related Metabolic Disorders*, 24(9), 1188–1194.

Lebenthal, E., Antonowicz, I., & Schwachman, H. (1975). Correlation of lactase activity, lactose tolerance, and milk consumption in different age groups. *American Journal of Clinical Nutrition*, 28, 595–600.

Lebra, T. S. (1976). *Japanese patterns of behavior.* Honolulu: University of Hawaii Press.

Leong, F. T. L. (1986). Counseling and psychotherapy with Asian Americans: review of the literature. *Journal of Counseling Psychology*, 33, 196–206.

Liao, D., Asberry, P. J., & Shofer, J. B., et al, (2002). Improvement of BMI, body composition, and body fat distribution with lifestyle modification in Japanese Americans with impaired glucose tolerance [Abstract]. *Diabetes Care*, 25(9), 1504–1510.

Lin, K. M., & Cheung, F. (1999). Mental health issues for Asian Americans. *Psychiatric Services*, 50(6), 774–780.

Lin, K. M., & Finder, E. (1983). Neuroleptic dosage for Asians. *American Journal of Psychiatry*, 140(4), 490–491.

Lin, K. M., Poland, R., & Nuccio, I., et al, (1989). Longitudinal assessment of haloperidol doses and serous concentrations in Asian and Caucasian schizophrenic patients. *American Journal of Psychiatry*, 146(10), 1307–1311.

Lin, S. S., Clarke, C. A., & Prehn, Q. W., et al, (2002). Survival differences among Asian subpopulations in the United States after prostate, colorectal, breast, and cervical carcinomas. *Cancer*, 94(4), 1175–1182.

Lyman, S. M. (1994). *Color, culture, civilization: race and minority issues in American society.* Urbana, Ill.: University of Illinois.

Madison, J. R., Spies, C., & Schatz, I. J., et al, (2006). Proteinuria and risk for stroke and coronary heart disease during 27 years of follow-up: the Honolulu Heart Program [Abstract]. *Archives of Internal Medicine*, 166(8), 884–889.

Marsella, A. J. (1993). Counseling and psychotherapy with Japanese Americans: cross-cultural considerations. *American Journal of Orthopsychiatry*, 63(2), 200–208.

Marsella, A. J., Johnson, F. A., Johnson, C. L., & Brennan, J. (1998). Ethnic identity in second-(Nisei), third-(Sansei), and fourth-(Yonsei) generation Japanese-Americans in Hawaii. *Asian American and Pacific Islander Journal of Health*, 6(1), 46–52.

Matsumoto, D. (1989). Cultural influences on the perception of emotion. *Journal of Cross-Cultural Psychology*, 20, 92–105.

Matsumoto, M. (1988). *The unspoken way: Haragei: Silence in Japanese business and society.* Tokyo: Kondansha.

Matsumura, S., Bito, S., Liu, H., Kahn, K., Fukuhara, S., & Kagawa-Singer, M., et al, (2002). Acculturation of attitudes toward end-of-life care: a cross-cultural survey of Japanese Americans and Japanese. *Journal of General Internal Medicine*, 17(7), 531–539.

McCormick, W. C., Imai, Y., & Rubenstein, L. Z. (1995). International common denominators in geriatric rehabilitation and long-term care. *Journal of the American Geriatric Society*, 42, 714–715.

McCormick, W. C., Uomoto, J., Young, H., Graves, A. B., Vitaliano, P., & Mortimer, J. A., et al, (1996, July). Attitudes toward use of nursing homes and home care in older Japanese Americans. *Journal of American Geriatrics Society*, 44, 769–777.

McCracken, R. (1971). Lactase deficiency: an example of dietary evolution. *Current Anthropology*, 12(4–5), 479–517.

McDermott, J. F. Jr., Tseng, W. S., & Maretzki, T. W. (1980). *People and cultures of Hawaii: a psychocultural profile.* Honolulu: John A. Burns School of Medicine and the University of Hawaii Press.

McNeill, D. (2006, March 21). The doomsday doctor: Japan's worsening population crisis. *The Japan Times.* Retrieved May 24, 2006, from Lexis/Nexis Academic Universe database.

Mehrabian, A. (1968, June). Communication without words. *Psychology Today*, (p. 53).

Miller, B. A., Kolonel, L. N., & Berstein, L., et al, (Eds.), (1996). *Racial/ethnic patterns of cancer in the United States 1988–1992.* (pub. no. 96–4104). Bethesda, Md.: National Cancer Institute, National Institutes of Health.

Minami, H. (1985). East meets West: some ethical considerations. *International Journal of Nursing Studies*, 4, 311–318.

Minami, H., Yoshii, J., Todoroki, M., Nishikimi, M., Ishimitsu, T., & Fukunaga, T., et al, (2002). Effects of alcohol restriction on ambulatory blood pressure, heart rate, and heart rate variability in Japanese men [abstract]. *American Journal of Hypertension*, 15(2 Pt 1), 125–129.

Ministry of Health, Labour, and Welfare. (2006). Vital Statistics: Abridged Life Tables For Japan 2004, Retrieved May 29, 2006, from http://www.mhlw.go.jp/english/database/db-hw/index.html.

Ministry of Internal Affairs and Communications [MIAC]. (2006a). *Population estimates by age (5 years group) and sex.* Statistic Bureau, Retrieved May 31, 2006, from http://www.stat.go.jp/data/jinsui/tsuki/index.htm.

Ministry of Internal Affairs and Communications. (2006b). *Statistical handbook of Japan. Chapter 2 Population.* Statistics Bureau & Statistical Research and Training Institute. Retrieved May 23, 2006, from http://www.stat.go.jp/English/data/handbook/c02cont.htm#cha2_2.

Modell, J. (1968). The Japanese American family: a perspective for future investigations. *Pacific Historical Review*, 37, 67–81.

Mordkowitz, E. R., & Ginsberg, H. P. (1987). Early academic socialization of successful Asian American college students. *Quarterly Newsletter of the Laboratory of Comparative Human Cognition*, 9, 85–91.

Morris, T. M. (1990). Culturally sensitive family assessment: an evaluation of the family assessment device used with Hawaiian American and Japanese American families. *Family Process*, 29, 105–116.

Nagata, D. (1991). Transgenerational impact of the Japanese American internment: clinical issues in working with children of former internees. *Psychotherapy*, 28, 121–128.

Nagata, D. N., & Takeshita, Y. J. (2002). Psychological reactions to redress: diversity among Japanese Americans interned during World War II. *Cultural Diversity and Ethnic Minority Psychology*, 8(1), 41–59.

Nakawatase, T. V., Yamamoto, J., & Toshiaki, S. (1993). The association between fast-flushing response and alcohol use among Japanese Americans. *Journal of Studies on Alcohol*, 54(1), 48–53.

Nakamura, A. (2005, February 12). Migration expert makes case for helping foreign workers. *The Japan Times.* Retrieved May 24, 2005, from Lexis/Nexis Academic Universe database.

Nakao, A. (2005, July 8). East Bay: Obon season means "people can put on their summer kimono and celebrate." *The San Francisco Chronicle.* Retrieved May 30, 2006, from Lexis/Nexis Academic Universe database.

National Center for Health Statistics. (2005). *Health, United States 2005 with urban and rural chartbook.* Hyattsville, Md.: National Center for Health Statistics.

National Center for Health Statistics. (2006). *Health, United States 2006 with urban and rural chartbook.* Hyattsville, Md.: NCHS.

Nemoto, M., Sasaki, T., Deeb, S. S., Fujimoto, W. Y., & Tajima, N. (2002). Differential effect of PPARgamma2 variants in the development of type 2 diabetes between native Japanese and Japanese Americans [abstract]. *Diabetes Research and Clinical Practice*, 57(2), 131–137.

Newburger, J. W., Takahashi, M., Gerber, M., Gewitz, M. A., Tani, M. H., & Burns, L. Y., et al, (2004). diagnosis, treatment, and long-term management of Kawasaki disease: a statement for health professionals from the Committee on Rheumatic Fever, Endocarditis and Kawasaki Disease, Council on Cardiovascular Disease in the Young, American Heart Association. *Circulation*, 110, 2747–2771.

The new lexicon Webster's dictionary. (1991). New York: Lexicon Publication.

Nomura, A., Stemmerman, G., & Heilbrun, L. (1985). Gastric cancer among the Japanese in Hawaii: a review. *Hawaii Medical Journal*, 44(8), 301–304.

Nomura, A. M., Lee, J., Stemmermann, G. N., Nomura, R. Y., Perez-Perez, G. I., & Blaser, M. J. (2002). *Helicobacter pylori* CagA seropositivity and gastric carcinoma risk in a Japanese American population [abstract]. *The Journal of Infectious Diseases*, 186(8), 1138–1144.

Ohara, S. (2000). We-consciousness and terminal patients: some biomedical reflection on Japanese civil religion. In Becker, S. (Ed.), *The moral status of persons: perspectives on bioethics* (Vol. 96) (pp. 119–127). Amsterdam, Atlanta, Ga.: Rodopi.

Okubo, Y., Suwazono, Y., Kobayashi, E., & Nogawa, K. (2001). Alcohol consumption and blood pressure change: 5-year follow-up study of the association in normotensive workers [abstract]. *Journal of Human Hypertension*, 15(6), 367–372.

Onishi, N. (2005, December 24). Japan's population fell this year, sooner than expected. *The New York Times, Tokyo*, (p. 8). Retrieved May 24, 2006, from Lexis/Nexis Academic Universe database.

Osaka, M. N. (1979). Aging and family among Japanese Americans: the role of ethnic tradition in the adjustment to old age. *Gerontologist*, 19, 448–455.

Overfield, T. (1995). *Biologic variation in health and illness.* Menlo Park, Calif.: Addison-Wesley.

Oyama, N., Sakuma, I., & Kishimoto, N., et al, (2006). Low HDL-cholesterol, hypertension and impaired glucose tolerance as predictors of acute myocardial infarction in northern area of Japan [Abstract]. *Hokkaido Igaku Zasshi*, 81(1), 25–30.

Padilla, A. M., Wagatsuma, Y., & Lindholm, K. J. (1985). Acculturation and personality as predictors of stress in Japanese and Japanese Americans. *Journal of Social Psychology*, 125, 295–305.

Perot, M., & Youdelman, R. T. (2001). *Racial, ethnic, and primary language data collection in the health care system: an assessment of federal policies and practices.* New York: The Commonwealth Fund: 40.

Petersen, W. (1966, January 9). Success story, Japanese American style. *New York Times Magazine.*

Pineda, M. D., White, E., Kristal, A. R., & Taylor, V. (2001). Asian breast cancer survival in the US: a comparison between Asian immigrants, US-born Asian American and Caucasians. *International Epidemiological Association*, 30(5), 976–982.

Reed, D., McGee, D., & Cohen, J., et al, (1982). Acculturation and coronary heart disease among Japanese men in Hawaii. *American Journal of Epidemiology*, 115(6), 894–905.

Reid, T. R. (1993, February 7). Japanese growing taller. *The Sunday Star-Bulletin & Advertiser*, A-32.

Reischauer, E. O. (1977). *The Japanese.* Tokyo: Tuttle Co.

Rice, M. M., Larson, E. B., LaCroix, A. Z., Hutchinson, F., & Drinkwater, B. L. (2001). Diagnosing osteoporosis in Japanese American women. *The American Journal of Medicine*, 110, 241–242.

Rodriguez, B. L., Curb, J. D., & Burchfiel, C. M., et al, (1996). Impaired glucose tolerance, diabetes, and cardiovascular disease risk factor profiles in the elderly. The Honolulu Heart Program. *Diabetes Care*, 19(6), 587–590.

Rodriguez, B. L., D'Agostino, R., & Abbott, R. D., et al, (2002). Risk of hospitalized stroke in men enrolled in the Honolulu Heart Program and the Framingham Study: a comparison of incidence and risk factor effects. *Stroke*, 33(1), 236–246.

Rogers, T., & Izutsu, S. (1980). The Japanese. In McDermott, J. F.Jr., Tseng, W. S., & Maretzki, T. W. (Eds.), *People and cultures of Hawaii: a psychocultural profile* Honolulu: University of Hawaii Press.

Roseblat, R., & Tang, S. W. (1987). Do Oriental psychiatric patients receive different dosages of psychotropic medication when compared with Occidentals? *Canadian Journal of Psychiatry*, 32, 270–274.

Ross, P. D., Horimatsu, H., & Davis, J., et al, (1991). A comparison of hip fracture incidence among native Japanese, Japanese Americans, and American Caucasians. *American Journal of Epidemiology*, 133(8), 801–809.

Sato, H., & Takano, J. (1983). Nursing care of Japanese American patients. In Orque, M. S., Bloch, B., & Monrroy, L. S. A. (Eds.), *Ethnic nursing care: a multicultural approach* (pp. 219–243). St. Louis: Mosby.

Schon, S. P., & Ja, D. A. (2005). Asian families. In McGoldrick, M., Pearce, J. K., & Giordano, J. (Eds.), *Ethnicity and family therapy* New York: Guilford Press.

Simoons, F. (1969). Primary adult lactose intolerance and the milking habit: a problem in biological and cultural interrelations. *American Journal of Digestive Diseases*, 14(12), 819–836.

Spickard, P. R. (1996). *Japanese Americans: The formation and transformations of an ethnic group.* New York: Twayne Publishers.

Storry, R. (1993). Japan—history up to 1952. In *The Far East and Australasia*, (ed. 24) (pp. 372–375). London: Europa Publishers.

Strazar, M., & Fisher, N. (1996). Traditional Japanese culture. In Fisher, N. (Ed.), *Cultural and ethnic diversity: a guide for genetic professionals.* Baltimore, Md.: The Johns Hopkins University Press.

Sue, D. W. (1987). Use and abuse of alcohol by Asian Americans. *Journal of Psychoactive Drugs*, 19, 57–66.

Sue, D. W. (2004). Ethnic identity: the impact of two cultures on the psychological development of Asians in America. In Atkinson, D. R., Morton, G., & Sue, D. W. (Eds.), *Counseling American minorities: a cross cultural perspective* (ed. 6) (pp. 85–96). Boston: McGraw-Hill.

Sue, S., & Okazaki, S. (1990). Asian American educational achievement. *American Psychologist*, 45, 913–920.

Suzuki, S., Kirschling, J., & Inoue, I. (1993). Hospice care in Japan. *American Journal of Hospice and Palliative Care*, 10(4), 35–40.

Syme, S., Marmot, M., & Kagun, A., et al, (1975). Epidemiologic studies of coronary heart disease and stroke in Japanese men living in Japan, Hawaii, and California: an introduction. *American Journal of Epidemiology*, 102(6), 477–480.

Tahara, Y., Moji, K., & Muraki, S., et al, (2003). Comparison of body size and composition between young adult Japanese-American and native Japanese in 1980's. *Annals of Human Biology*, 30(4), 392–401.

Takemura, K. (2007). Institutions and psychological mechanisms behind Japanese collectivism. In Irimoto, T., Takahashi, N., & Yamagishi, T. (Eds.), *Logics and practices of social groups: Psychological and anthropological approached to reciprocity.* Sapporo: Hokkaido University Press (in Japanese), pp 156–170.

Tanaka-Matsumi, M., & Marsella, A. J. (1976). Cross-cultural variations in phenomenological experience of depression, I: word association studies. *Journal of Cross-Cultural Psychology*, 7, 379–396.

Tarn, D. M., Meredith, L. S., Kagawa-Singer, M., Bito, S., Oye, R. K., Liu, H., Kahn, K. L., Fukuhara, S., & Wenger, N. S. (2005). Trust in ones' physician: the role of ethnic match, autonomy, acculturation, and religiosity among Japanese and Japanese Americans. *Annals of Family Medicine*, 3, 339–447.

Tateishi, J. (1999). *And justice for all: an oral history of Japanese American detention camps.* Seattle: University of Washington Press.

Time almanac with information please. (2007). Boston: Information Please, Inc..

Torréns, J. I., Skurnick, J., & Davidow, A. L., et al, (2004). Ethnic differences in insulin sensitivity and beta-cell function in premenopausal or early perimenopausal women without diabetes: the Study of Women's Health Across the Nation (SWAN) [Abstract]. *Diabetes Care*, 27(2), 354–361.

Tracey, T. J., Leong, F. T. L., & Glidden, C. (1986). Help seeking and problem perception among Asian Americans. *Journal of Counseling Psychology*, 33, 331–336.

Tsuchida, T. (1998). A differing perspective on advance directives. In Sass, H. M., Veatch, R. M., & Kimura, R. (Eds.), *Advance directives and surrogate decision making in health care: United States, Germany and Japan.* Baltimore: Johns Hopkins University Press, pp 175–186.

Tweed, R. G., White, K., & Lehman, D. R. (2004). Culture, Stress, and Coping: Internally- and Externally-Targeted Control Strategies of European Canadians, East Asian Canadians, and Japanese Journal of Cross-Cultural Psychology, 35(6), 652–668.

U.S. Department of Commerce, Bureau of the Census. (2000). Population and housing data by race and Hispanic origin, Summary File 1. Washington, D.C.: U.S. Government Printing Office.

U.S. Department of Commerce, Bureau of the Census. (2002). Summary File 3, Population profiles by age, sex, race, and Hispanic origin. Washington, D.C.: U.S. Government Printing Office.

Vessell, E. (1972). Therapy—pharmacogenetics. *The New England Journal of Medicine*, 287(18), 904–909.

Wall, T. L., Peterson, C. M., Peterson, K. P., et al, (1997). Alcohol metabolism in Asian-American men with genetic polymorphisms of aldehyde dehydrogenase. *Annals of Internal Medicine*, 127(5), 376–379.

Watson, O. M. (1980). *Proxemic behavior: a cross-cultural study,* The Hague, the Netherlands: Mouton.

Wenger, A. F. (1991). The role of context in culture-specific care. In Chinn, P. (Ed.), *Anthology on caring.* New York: NLN, pp 95–110.

Wood, K. (2005, October 23). Record of a community destroyed. *The Daily Yomuri.* Retrieved May 31, 2006 from Lexis/Nexis Academic Universe database.

World almanac. (2007). Mahwah, N.J.: World Almanac Books.

Wros, P., Doutrich, D., & Izumi, S. (2004). Ethical concerns: A comparison of values from two cultures. *Nursing and Health Science*, 6, 131–140.

Yamamoto, J. (1982). Japanese Americans. In Gaw, A. (Ed.), *Cross-cultural psychiatry* Littleton, Mass: John Wright–PSG Publishing.

Yamamoto, J., Fung, D., Lo, S., & Reece, S. (1979). Psychopharmacology for Asian Americans and Pacific Islanders. *Psychopharmacology Bulletin*, 15(4), 29–34.

Yano, K., Reed, D., & Kagan, A. (1985). Coronary heart disease, hypertension and stroke among Japanese American men in Hawaii: the Honolulu Heart Program. *Hawaii Medical Journal*, 44(8), 297–325.

Yano, K., Reed, D., & McGee, D. (1984). Ten year incidence of coronary heart disease in the Honolulu Heart Program: relationship to biologic and lifestyle characteristics. *American Journal of Epidemiology*, 119(5), 653–666.

Yeh, C. J., Arora, A. K., & Inose, M., et al, (2003). The cultural adjustment and mental health of Japanese immigrant youth. *Adolescence*, 38(151), 481–501.

Yeh, C. J., & Huang, K. (1996). The collectivistic nature of ethnic identity development among Asian-American college students. *Adolescence*, 31(123), 645–661.

Yoshida, J. (1972). *The two worlds of Jim Yoshida.* New York: William Morrow.

Yoshishige, J. (1993, March 21). Wartime heroics: a nisei history. *The Honolulu Advertiser,* (p. 5). 442nd special section.

Yoo, D. K. (2000). *Growing up Nisei: Race, generation, and culture among Japanese Americans of California, 1924–49.* Urbana, IL: University of Illinois Press.

Young, H. M., McCormick, W. M., & Vitaliano, P. P. (2002 Dec). Evolving values in community-based long-term care services for Japanese Americans. *ANS Advances in Nursing Science*, 25(2), 40–56.

Yukawa, E., Ichimaru, R., & Maki, T., et al, (2003). Interindividual variation of serum haloperidol concentrations in Japanese patients—clinical considerations on steady–state serum level–dose ratios. *Journal of Clinical Pharmacy & Therapeutics*, 28(2), 97–101.

CHAPTER 14 Afghans and Afghan Americans

Juliene G. Lipson, Razia Askaryar Iqbal, and Patricia A. Omidian

Behavioral Objectives

After reading this chapter, the nurse will be able to:

1. Describe differences between the national languages of Afghanistan.
2. Identify topics of conversation that may be considered private by Afghans.
3. Discuss situations in which variations of time are utilized by Afghans.
4. Describe how Afghan beliefs about health and illness and practices affect risk reduction.
5. Describe generational differences that may be observed among Afghans in the United States.
6. List several potential health risks associated with the Afghan refugee experience.

OVERVIEW OF AFGHANISTAN

Afghanistan, a poor, underdeveloped, and land-locked country of approximately 251,825 square miles, is slightly smaller than Texas. It is bordered on the north by Turkmenistan, Uzbekistan, and Tajikistan of the former Soviet Union; on the south by Pakistan; on the east by the extreme northeast of China; and by Iran on the west. Afghanistan is split east and west by the Hindu Kush mountain range that rises in the east to a height of 24,000 feet (7314 m). With the exception of the southwest, most of the country is covered by snow-capped mountains and traversed by deep valleys. It was invaded and colonized for millennia by the Persians, Alexander the Great, the Arabs, Genghis Khan, Tamerlane, and the Moguls of India, all of whom influenced language and religion and created an ethnically diverse population. The largest and most lasting impact on the region that includes the Middle East was the introduction of Islam in the seventh century. There is no census, and no one knows exactly how many people live in the largest cities. Some estimates are the capital, Kabul (about 4 million), Kandahar (459,000), Herat (249,000), and Mazar-I-Sharif (183,000).

Modern Afghanistan emerged in 1921, but the last Afghan king was deposed in 1973. The invasion of USSR troops in 1979, intended to shore up the Communist faction of the government, precipitated one of the largest migrations of people in modern history. Afghanistan's population was reduced from 15.5 million to 8 or 9 million people between 1979 and 1992. More than 1 million Afghans have been killed, and more than 80% of the population has had to move at least once to avoid war or conflict in the last 26 years. The country has been devastated by war and drought and littered with more landmines and unexploded ordinance than there are people in the country. What the war did not destroy, 10 years of the worst drought in modern history devastated. In 2005, the population of Afghanistan was 29,928,987, with an average annual rate of natural increase of 4.77% and a population density of 107 per square mile. Ethnic groups in Afghanistan are Pashtun (42%), Tajik (27%), Uzbek (9%), Hazara (9%), and smaller groups, including Aimaks, Turkmen, and Baloch (Central Intelligence Agency, 2006).

For almost two decades, Afghans were the largest refugee population in the world: at its peak, nearly 6 million people. Of the 4 million refugees in October 2001, 2.3 million have returned to Afghanistan. Although Afghans were coming to the United States for education well into the 1970s, the situation changed dramatically when the United States began processing refugee claims as it fought a proxy war against the USSR on Afghan soil. Between 1980 and 1988, when the USSR withdrew from Afghanistan, between 50,000 and 100,000 Afghan refugees came to the United States. Since 1989, most Afghans have been admitted to the United States under the family reunification classification (immigrants) rather than as refugees.

The first arrivals in the early 1980s were the urban, formerly wealthy, and highly educated elite, and later family reunification brought middle-class relatives who are less educated. The majority are from Kabul and other cities and came through Pakistan and India, and many families spent time in Europe, especially Germany, before coming to the United States. Relatively few people came directly from refugee camps. There is a small group of Afghans from rural areas who had little previous contact with Westerners; they maintain a traditional lifestyle and are illiterate in their own languages.

Although many Afghans in the United States talked about repatriating to Afghanistan, very few did so because of war, food and energy shortages, earthquakes, drought, and famine. Then, despite some peace that followed the takeover of most of the country by the fundamentalist Taliban, repression of women's and human rights further discouraged people from returning. With the demise of the Taliban and a newly elected government, young Afghan Americans in particular are returning to help rebuild the country (Lipson & Omidian, 1996). Those who have returned usually leave their families in the country where they resettled. Very few have returned permanently; most of those hold positions of power and are over 45–50 years of age. Younger Afghans, like those from the San Francisco Bay Area, come for short-term contracts, bringing with them vitally needed expertise and skills, but at a price. Most demand high expatriate salaries and prefer to live with other expatriates. They form a small but very tight community in Kabul because they are not really trusted by Afghans who never left the region, and because they do not share the values or experiences of those who stayed behind. Many find it difficult to live with family members, preferring the international community or their own group of returnees. They return to Western countries for medical care and for a break from the harsh conditions of working in a war-torn country. Afghanistan cannot yet be considered to have post-war stability, another reason that many returnees do not plan to stay.

In Afghanistan, both men's and women's life expectancy is about 43 years. In the United States, both men and women appear to be living at least a decade longer, but the population does not yet reflect national U.S. norms in longevity. Life span is shortened by stressors associated with migrating to a foreign land with no English language skills or expectations for the future. Elderly men tend to suffer from heart disease related to expectations of being breadwinners in the context of lack of jobs and lost status, such as a CEO of a company in Afghanistan now working at a fast-food restaurant. Women tend to suffer from depression, dealt with by constantly visiting physicians to complain of physical symptoms based on psychological difficulties.

LIFE TODAY FOR AFGHANS IN THE UNITED STATES

Afghans are one of the newer U.S. refugee populations, having fled a war that began in 1978 and continued to 2001. Afghans have been mistakenly called Afghanis in the media; in actuality, the unit of money is the afghani. The term *Afghan(s)* is used as a noun, while *Afghan* (not plural) is used as an adjective.

There are no national demographic data on life span, health status, or prevalence of disease among Afghans in the United States. Indeed, it is difficult to know just how many Afghans live in the country. Therefore, this chapter is based on the authors'

knowledge of the Afghan community based on their research. Community leaders indicate that this description is current and generalizable to Afghans in other areas of the country, with minor variations.

In this young population, there are far more younger- than older-generation Afghans, with very few elderly in comparison to the number of children. Because families are large, with an average of four children, the median age is 25 to 35. The children of the many families that arrived in the United States with young children in the late 1970s or early 1980s are now in that age bracket.

According to the U.S. Census Bureau, there are 53,709 persons of Afghan descent residing in the United States (U.S. Department of Commerce, Bureau of the Census, Summary File 3, 2002). The Census Bureau figure significantly underrepresents the number of Afghans living in the United States. One reason is that many Afghans report their ethnicity to census takers rather than their national origin. Estimates range from 60,000 to 100,000. The Afghan Coalition suggests that the largest population, in the San Francisco Bay area, numbers 50,000 to 60,000 people, many of whom are second generation. The Afghan American Association estimated at least 25,000 Afghans in Fremont and 65,000 in the East Bay by counting the number of people who attended simultaneous events commemorating the two holiest Islamic holidays, *Eid al-Fitr* (end of Ramadan fasting) and *Eid al-Adha* (end of the annual pilgrimage to Mecca). The second *Eid* attracted 3000 to 4000 Afghans to each of 12 separate events (Yollin, 2002).

In the San Francisco Bay area, there are eight mosques and many cultural organizations and Afghan-owned businesses. The city of Fremont, in Alameda County, is known as "Little Kabul." Many families live in large apartment complexes that are heavily Afghan, particularly in the Fremont–Union City–Hayward area. Alexandria, Virginia, and the Washington, D.C., area are home to the second largest community, with at least 20,000 people. A third area of concentration is the Los Angeles area, with at least 10,000 Afghans. Other Afghan communities are in Flushing, New York; Atlanta, Georgia; Chicago, Illinois; and the states of Oregon and Texas. Many who lived in Europe for a few years resettled on the East Coast. There are some variations in economics and ethnic clustering in different communities; for example, Afghans in Los Angeles are spread throughout the city and are wealthier overall than Afghans in the San Francisco Bay area, mainly because of a lower cost of living.

The mean salary of Afghans and Afghan Americans is difficult to estimate. The largest group, including the formerly wealthy, has a middle-class income; very few are currently wealthy, and a significant number depend on public assistance. In 1994, community leaders estimated that 90% of San Francisco Bay area Afghan families were supported by Aid to Families with Dependent Children (AFDC). The percentage of people on public assistance in the Bay area has reportedly dropped to about 55% in 2006 because of welfare reform and the young adults who have graduated and moved into the job market. The number on public assistance is lower in other areas of the country.

Occupational issues are most difficult for middle-aged men educated in Afghanistan. Although those from middle-class backgrounds have been more willing to accept entry-level jobs, well-educated professionals and former government officials are rarely able to obtain the kind of work they did in Afghanistan. They lack experience perceived as relevant and "connections," face discrimination because of an accent or being Muslim, and are unfamiliar with job interview expectations and multiple-choice tests. Most physicians, for example, are unable to pass the licensure exam because of finances, English-language problems, or outdated medical training.

In Islam, education is more highly valued than wealth. However, war, poverty, and the recent fundamentalist emphasis on teaching only Islam have ruined the educational system of Afghanistan. In 2000, 43% of men could read and write but only 13% of the women were literate (Central Intelligence Agency, 2006). In the rural areas today, the literacy rate for women is below 2%. It is hard to find women who can write their names, much less read. Afghanistan also experienced a "brain drain" in which many of the best-educated people fled to other countries.

In the 1980s, the refugees who fled from urban areas became one of the most highly educated refugee populations in the United States, with an average education level of 15 years among men and 14 years among women and a literacy rate of about 90%. Later refugees and immigrants had less education. However, there is an extremely wide range of educational levels, from no formal education among some women and many elderly to doctoral and professional preparation, especially among Afghan Americans.

Education is very important to the young generation, illustrated by their high enrollments in San Francisco Bay area universities and community colleges, which have increased markedly over the past 3 to 5 years. During this time, even older men have entered college. However, the children of the first arrivals in the early 1980s, who then ranged in age from 3 to 15 years, have been unable to pursue higher education because they must work full-time to help support their families. A number of young men with high school diplomas or less work in blue-collar jobs, running restaurants or car repair shops, because the older son or sons in the family are responsible for providing family income, even if they desire a college education. Afghan women are by far more college educated; the ratio of women to men earning their bachelor's degrees or equivalent is 3:1. Women are also attending graduate school more than men are. They more often have the luxury of attending college because their income is not an essential source for the family (Lipson & Omidian, 1992, 1997).

COMMUNICATION

Afghanistan has two national languages: Dari, a dialect of Persian (50%), and Pashto (35%). Other languages are Turkmen and Uzbek (11%) and 30 minor languages (primarily Balochi and Pashai) (4%), and there is considerable bilingualism (Central Intelligence Agency, 2006). Both Dari and Pashto are derived from Persian and are part of the Indo-Iranian branch of the Indo-European language family, but they are mutually unintelligible. In the United States, most Afghans speak either Dari or Pashto with regional variations, or another local mother tongue if not Dari or Pashto, and, for many, two or three other languages in addition to English, such as Urdu, Hindi, or German. Many educated Afghans also speak Russian.

Afghans tend to speak in stories rich in context, rather than providing brief answers to specific questions. Generally, people are reluctant to share personal and family issues with people other than family members, including health care professionals, but women may discuss their problems with friends, including non-Afghans. Men do not discuss their personal problems with others.

Afghan women tend to speak loudly. Westerners observing two women engaging in a conversation tend to interpret this as high-volume speech. Afghan women tend to be very affectionate and, in public settings, speak loudly to express their affection. In private settings, the mother's voice symbolizes power and control of the children at home. Men, on the other hand, tend to speak in soft tones in private or public settings, which denotes being in control of the situation in a relaxed and comfortable manner. Showing aggression or speaking loudly means that men are losing control, and it is seen as disrespectful in public.

There may also be ethnic differences. Those who speak Pashto may sound like they are arguing when they are talking, but this is a style of speech that does not reflect emotional content. Dari speakers tend to speak softly and use polite tones and words, even when they feel strongly about a topic or issue. In some contexts, particularly when one wants to convey respect, silence may mean disagreement.

Afghans generally call elderly persons by respectful terms, such as *uncle, aunt,* or *mother*. Most people have several names: their legal name, which is rarely used, and a familiar name by which family and other Afghans will identify the person. Strangers are never given the legal or familiar name of an adult woman but refer to her by a title, such as *Bibi* or *auntie*. Because of the U.S. system of demanding the legal name on documents, this pattern is changing, and health care providers can call a woman by her legal name without causing insult. But Afghans value politeness, and an honorific or title should also be used.

Determinants of touch are family relationships and gender. Among extended family members and close friends, people often touch each other on the shoulder or leg when conversing. They greet with a kiss on each cheek, a hug, or both. However, couples do not show affection in public. Traditional men and women who are not related do not touch each other at all. They do not socialize or even remain in the same room. Unrelated men and women who are from urban backgrounds or who are more acculturated mix socially and may even greet each other with a kiss. Children and young adults raised in the United States use touch much like those in the dominant culture, although they may not do so at home in respect of their parents' values. However, families strongly disapprove of dating and touch in public.

Greetings between people who are not family members or close friends may be a simple nod or a handshake, but a man should wait for a woman to extend her hand first. However, women often greet each other with a kiss on each cheek, alternating three times or more for special friends or family members. Young or older men may accompany a verbal greeting or farewell with placing the right hand over the heart, which is a sign of respect. This is common when men greet women who are not immediate family members. Men will greet other men with hugs and kisses but greet unrelated women with the right hand on the chest, without touch or eye contact.

Gestures in younger Afghan Americans tend to be similar to those in the dominant society, except when they are with their family or in Afghan social gatherings, where they use typical Afghan gestures and body language. In general, youth do not look elders directly in the eyes, but stand turned slightly to the side, with their heads slightly down to convey proper respect. In addition, a young person should not correct an elder, although this is changing in American society and can vary from family to family. When an elderly person or the head of a family enters the room, people show their respect by standing. People kiss the back of an elderly person's hand as a sign of respect and acknowledgment of his or her wisdom, which comes with age (Lipson & Askaryar, 2005).

Sustained eye contact varies by acculturation and generation. More traditional unrelated men and women do not sustain eye contact, nor do they "insult" someone they perceive to be of higher status by making direct eye contact. In general, health providers should avoid winking at or touching a person of the opposite gender. Winking is seen as flirting and should be avoided.

Implications for Nursing Care

An appropriate interpreter may be needed for patients who speak little or no English. A considerable number of Afghans who speak English may not read or write it; thus, it is important to check for English literacy before asking them to read forms or instructions. Ideally, the interpreter is trained, respected in the community, of the same gender as the patient, and around the same age or older. It is important to translate health education and training materials into both national languages, even though most Afghans read Dari. Be careful not to inadvertently be swept into a political faction, which can be based on language usage. People often insist that Pashto translations are unnecessary, but this plays into the politics of the country and sends a message of favoritism to the whole community. Also, it is important to use Dari or Pashto interpreters and written materials rather than using more available Farsi (Iranian Persian) written materials (or mental health providers), despite the similarity of Dari and Farsi. The subtle differences in language usage are great enough to create major misunderstandings in treatment and follow-up. The differences between Dari and Farsi are analogous to those between Spanish and Portuguese.

SPACE

In Afghanistan, extended families live in large houses or compounds, and women socialize as they cook and do household chores together. Afghans in the United States miss daily the proximity of other family members. For example, despite having a four-bedroom house and plenty of space, the four teenage children of parents who have been in the United States for many years often end up coming into their parents' bedroom in the night, sleeping on mats on the floor, because "we like to be together."

As with other cultural characteristics, space varies with relationship, gender, and acculturation. Physical space between close friends and family engaged in conversation is closer than that between those of northern European heritage, often 1 to 1.5 feet. On the other hand, unrelated men and women who are more traditional keep more distance from each other, often socializing in separate rooms or separate areas of one room.

Spatial comfort depends on the activity and relationship of the people involved and on the setting, such as among all Afghans or with others present. Afghans are extremely modest people who are used to thick walls between rooms. In strictly private activities, such as using the toilet and sexual relations, people may fear that other family members may "hear" such activities through the thin walls of the typical U.S. apartment or house; a couple may avoid sexual relations because a daughter's or mother's bedroom is next door.

Implications for Nursing Care

The topics of sexuality, birth control, and vaginal or breast examinations are considered very private and extremely embarrassing for women; older women may have minimal knowledge of how their bodies work. There is no formal education for these women in terms of sexuality, birth control, and the like. Women prefer to be seen by female gynecologists. If only a male is available, the woman's husband will accompany her to appointments and stay in the room during the examination.

The situation is somewhat different among young adults and teens educated in the United States, although some parents forbid their middle school– and high school–aged children to take sex education classes.

Traditional women avoid being touched by male nurses or physicians. For example, one couple had been promised that their baby would be delivered by a female physician, but when the woman arrived at the hospital in advanced labor, only a male physician was available. As they were leaving the hospital, an enterprising nurse suggested that she deliver the baby, although by law, the physician had to be in the room, so the couple stayed. More acculturated men and women Afghan Americans are more willing to be cared for and touched by nurses of the opposite gender, but they may not be entirely comfortable with the situation.

It is uncommon to leave one's children with baby-sitters. Afghans may leave children with other family members who do not work when the presence of children is forbidden or very difficult, but children usually accompany their parents to health appointments and all social activities. They leave children with family members because of language difficulties or lack of transportation. Expect children and provide art materials or other diversions.

Numerous family members and friends gather at the bedside of a patient who is hospitalized and remain until asked to leave. Visiting a sick person is a very important value, and the room will seem crowded. If an Afghan is crying, it is important just to sit beside him or her, without touching or hugging or calling further attention to him or her.

SOCIAL ORGANIZATION

Family System and Roles

Family life is the core of Afghan culture and psychological well-being. People maintain close ties with extended family, and most spend almost all their free time socializing with family and old friends. New friendships are slow to develop because of distrust of those outside the family circle. Lack of social support is a problem for many Afghans in the United States, particularly homebound women and the elderly. In our study, only 7% stated that they had American friends (Lipson, Omidian, & Paul, 1995). Homebound women are isolated and lonely when they speak insufficient English to talk with American neighbors or are culturally restrained from moving outside their family circle. They miss the constant visiting of their life in Afghanistan, which is now limited by distance, transportation problems, and the fast pace of American life. Many elderly, who rarely speak English, experience severe isolation, depression, and numerous physical symptoms, and sometimes they feel they are a burden to their families (Omidian & Lipson, 1992).

Impact of Immigration and Acculturation

Afghan culture in the United States is in transition. Families range from quite traditional to more cosmopolitan, based on their background and personal choice. The intense family focus can cause culture conflict in the United States. What Western psychiatrists call enmeshment is normal family behavior for Afghans, and extended family obligations, especially to parents and older siblings, often supersede other responsibilities, including allegiance to one's spouse, one's job, and certainly one's own needs (Lipson & Omidian, 1997).

Women in the United States experience some role conflict in the context of divided community opinions. Traditional men expect their wives to stay home and cook for the family, take care of the children, clean house, and socialize only with Afghan female friends. More cosmopolitan women enjoy their freedom and the opportunity to be active in the community. However, all Afghan women are expected to maintain modest behavior over their lifetimes; once a woman's reputation is tarnished, she is no longer respected. Gossip is very common and frequent, both positive and negative, which is how community members know about each other and their reputations.

Given the centrality of marriage and children to Afghan women's identity, remaining single is viewed as unnatural. However, because women acculturate more quickly than men do, it may be difficult for Afghan women to find a spouse when many Afghan men perceive women long in the United States as not being properly naive or submissive. While being married by the late teens is common in Afghanistan, most Afghan American women prefer to finish their educations, despite fear of being an "old maid" at the age of 26. Most single women live with parents or siblings, and it is rare for an Afghan woman to live alone or with peers (Lipson & Miller, 1994).

Adults work very hard but also do extensive visiting or entertaining during weekends and sometimes weeknights as well. Women with small children may prefer to remain at home, but they are also very busy with household responsibilities and entertaining relatives and friends. Hospitality, one of the most important Afghan values, requires elaborate food preparation and a very clean house. But many Afghan women work outside the home to provide or contribute to the family income, and essentially they work a double day.

Husbands tend to experience their wives' earnings as a loss of their paternal leadership as breadwinner, a source of stress and often depression. The traditional husband's power and role as head of the family is further damaged when children learn English quickly and become their parents' translators and spokespersons. While women generally like more independence, even educated and cosmopolitan men who have been in the United States for two decades maintain a tribal consciousness that supports women's submission to their husbands. Islam, however, promotes gender equality and mutual respect between husband and wife (Robson, Lipson, Younos, & Mehdi, 2002).

Children are expected to work hard in school and to come home after school to do homework; strict parents do not allow their children to engage in after-school activities. Some children and teens resort to truancy to spend time with their friends when their parents do not allow them to go out with or visit friends at their homes. Boys, however, have much more freedom than girls do. Teenagers tend to rebel against their parents up until high school (Robson, Lipson, Younos, & Mehdi, 2002). Children acculturate quickly to resemble their American peers, whom their parents see as "having no respect" for their parents. Their independence and assertiveness contradict cultural values of family interdependence and strict obedience to elder family members, particularly the father's authority. Younger Afghans with strict families tend to attend colleges and universities that are sufficiently far away from home that they must live in dormitories. They view this as an opportunity for freedom and some space to "breathe." Their parents allow them to live on campus because they so strongly value higher education, but most students must compromise by coming home on the weekends. Men have less trouble convincing their parents to allow them to go to a university out of the area than women do.

Religion

Afghans are staunch Muslims, with the majority following the Sunni branch (84%). Shi'a Muslims comprise 15% and others, 1%. Sunni Afghans are of the Hanafi school, the most liberal of the four schools of thought. Muslims believe in one God (Allah), and Muhammad is believed to be God's final messenger. They pray directly to God privately or in a *jumat* (congregation) where an imam leads the prayers. They must act in accordance with God's commands, as described in the Qur'an (Koran), which includes rules of cleanliness, diet (e.g., avoidance of pork and alcohol), and prayer (facing Kaaba, in Mecca). Observant Muslims plan to visit Mecca (make a *hajj*) at least once in their lives (Younos, 2002).

The majority of Afghans adhere to Islamic principles of hygiene, modest behavior, and moral values, even though most dress like other Americans. However, individuals and families vary in their adherence to traditional rituals. People vary from being very strict (prayer five times a day; *halal* and *haram* food practices; dressing to cover hair, arms, and legs) to more relaxed, such as praying to oneself rather than at specific times. In the past two decades, many Afghans in the United States have strengthened their beliefs and practices because of the availability of Islamic mosques, classes, and libraries. As part of gaining or maintaining an Islamic identity, some children and young adults have become more orthodox than their parents.

Islam expects modest dress and behavior, including female chastity until marriage. Families are concerned that children will pick up immodest behavior from their non-Muslim classmates, as well as from school itself, for example, sex education, being served pork, and teen drinking. However, even when young people appear to be completely American in their speech and activities, most still maintain an Islamic outlook.

Implications for Nursing Care

Assess for how long the family has been in the United States, acculturation level, urban or rural origin, and whether the family is more cosmopolitan or traditional. Ask who makes decisions for the family:

father, mother, or joint decisions? Nurses must recognize that family obligations and traditional hierarchy may interfere with getting to appointments or compliance. Be especially aware of Afghans' strong aversion to "interference" in family affairs, which they see as private. Most people perceive school and social service agency intervention as undermining parental authority, responsibility, and control: "What right do strangers have to intrude in our family and judge our discipline? Our children are our responsibility."

In the context of abuse education in the schools, children may tell teachers about physical discipline, which may result in a report of "child abuse" and removal of children from the home. However, teachers rarely understand Afghan methods of discipline in cultural context, assuming that when a child says, "My mom hits me," it means "beating" rather than a slap on the back or a pinch (Lipson & Omidian, 1997). Some parents are so frightened that their children might be taken away that they are afraid to discipline their children. However, some children use the system to manipulate their parents by threatening to call the police if their parents do not give them the freedom they desire.

TIME

Afghans have different orientations to time, depending on the situation. Past orientation is evident in tradition and family lineage, present orientation is observable in social interactions, and future orientation is observable in hard work and commitment to children's education. Other commitments or values may conflict with being "on time" for appointments. For example, given the central value of hospitality, if a family has guests, they would be extremely reluctant to indicate that someone has another obligation and that it may be time for the guests to leave. Instead, finishing an interpersonal encounter gracefully and naturally is more important than the ticking clock or being on time for an appointment elsewhere. Acculturation influences stricter use of clock time in business, school, or health care. Some Afghans overcompensate by coming very early for an appointment to make sure they will not be late. However,

transportation problems or other family matters that come up may keep someone from coming to an appointment.

Implications for Nursing Care

Awareness of the importance of hospitality and smooth social interactions should help nurses anticipate whether Afghans may miss appointments. A reminder phone call the day before and asking if the person will have any difficulty with transportation (and if an interpreter will be needed) would be appreciated and may help. With regard to health risks, Afghans rarely tend to be future oriented, which has implications for teaching prevention and health risk reduction. It is more the case that they are unfamiliar with risk reduction than that they are not interested, however. They had little previous experience in Afghanistan, where prevention (except for immunizations) and screening were not done.

ENVIRONMENTAL CONTROL

Most Dari words for the concept of health mean "wholeness" or "completeness" (Shorish-Shamley, 1991). Afghans are very concerned about their health, as illustrated by a woman who said, "If you have health the key to the whole city is in your hand, but if you are sick, what are you going to do with riches?" (Lipson & Omidian, 1992, p. 273). Afghans combine internal and external locus of control, as well as natural and supernatural concepts of health and illness beliefs and behavior.

Individual responsibility is evident in the belief that health is maintained through regular exercise, eating fresh food and a balanced diet, staying warm, and getting enough rest. Natural illnesses are believed to be caused by things that exist in nature, such as "germs," dirt, cold, or wind, such as the belief that people are more vulnerable to colds or flu during the change of seasons (Shorish-Shamley, 1991). One cause of illness is not taking proper care of one's body, such as "when we eat lamb and rice for lunch, it is not digestible here because we don't have time to walk and exercise after, so the amount of cholesterol goes up and blood pressure goes up, creating the possibility of heart disease" (Lipson & Omidian, 1992, p. 273).

Illness is also interpreted as the "will of God" and should be "borne with patience as it cleanses one of individual sins, and God will have mercy on a sick person." This view does not mean that a sick person should not seek treatment, however. Illness is also perceived as a result of not adhering to the principles of Islam. For example, an elderly woman who became acutely ill after someone told her that she had inadvertently eaten pork on pizza said, "I was very stupid. It is against Islam to eat pork, it is forbidden to us by our Book (Qur'an). If we eat it, it means we are against our religion" (Lipson & Omidian, 1992, p. 273). Islam strongly emphasizes personal hygiene; for example, "Afghans are obsessive about cleanliness, we keep our bodies, our houses and our children clean." Ablution before prayer includes washing hands and arms, feet, face, nose, and inside the throat. If a person urinates, defecates, passes gas, falls asleep, vomits, or bleeds, he becomes impure and must wash again. After sexual intercourse, the entire body, head to toe, must be washed before the person is fit to pray, and women are prohibited from prayer or fasting during menstruation, until they perform a full purification ritual at 7 days.

Supernatural illnesses are caused by *jinns*, the evil eye, or punishment from God. The Qur'an mentions *jinns*, and some describe them as ghosts or spirits; "some are good and some are bad, but people don't like them." Epilepsy is believed to be caused by a *jinn*. The evil eye, *nazar*, is the belief that someone can cause illness by looking at another person, with a particularly powerful "gaze" emanating from green-eyed, impure, or ill people. Unintentional *nazar* comes from expressing excessive admiration for someone without remembering to say a preventive phrase. Intentional *nazar* is based on envy or anger and is meant to hurt another person or his property (Shorish-Shamley, 1991). *Nazar* illness is distinguished by its sudden onset and prevented by saying, "In the Name of God" or "With the power of God" when giving a compliment. Susceptible people (e.g., children, beautiful young women, brides, rich or fortunate people) are protected by wearing charms or amulets, such as blue stones or beads. *Espand* (wild

rue) is burned in the fireplace for prevention, which is explained as "forcing the evil spirits out; the sounds of the seeds popping are like the sounds of eyes popping."

The choice of treatment depends to some extent on the perception of the cause of illness, although both folk-traditional and Western biomedical treatments are valued and often used at the same time. Biomedical treatment cannot cure a supernatural illness, but natural illness may also be treated by religious means. Prayer in general or verses of the Qur'an may be used for specific illnesses. A healer may select and write a specific verse on a piece of paper and administer it via *ta'wiz* (wrapped in cloth and worn like a necklace), *shuist* (soaked in water and drunk), or *dudi* (burning it with *rue* near the patient so the smoke kills germs and wards off evil spirits) (Shorish-Shamley, 1991). Natural illnesses, if mild, are treated with home remedies and dietary means alone or, if severe, by seeking biomedical care. In most families, an older woman, having been taught by her mother and grandmothers, knows how to prepare herbal remedies. Examples are *zirk* (arnica) dissolved in hot milk for broken bones or internal injuries, *zuf* (ribwort) for colds, and *sirin buya* (anise) for stomach complaints ("Tagamet is made from it"). These plant remedies are available in Afghan, Iranian, and Indian food stores (Lipson & Omidian, 1992). Traditional medical beliefs are also based on Arabic-Persian humoral concepts brought to Central Asia with the spread of Islam (Penkala, 1980). "Hot" and "cold" imbalances cause sickness, and hot or cold qualities describe food, drink, and medicinal herbs; individual human nature; and specific illnesses. Hot illnesses, such as fever and measles, are treated with a diet emphasizing cold foods and medicines; cold illnesses, such as arthritis, malaria, and chickenpox, are treated with hot foods and herbs.

Illness and Wellness Behaviors and Access to Health Care

Barriers to care are lack of health insurance and almost no culturally specific services. Very few hospitals or clinics employ trained interpreters of both genders. There is an enormous need for health education materials in Pashto and Dari, written and on the radio, TV, or videos for illiterate elderly women. Afghans are responsive to and enthusiastic about health education.

Conditions for which people seek health care differ for new immigrants and longer-established Afghans. Newly arrived refugees in the early 1980s had dental caries (41%), dermatologic disorders (39%), intestinal parasites (36%), gastrointestinal disorders (23%), and musculoskeletal pain (joints, back, 12%) (McCaw & DeLay, 1985). Those arriving now also have tuberculosis, nutritional deficiencies, intestinal parasites, chronic hepatitis B virus infection, lack of immunization, and depression. In addition to a complete history and physical examination, tests for tuberculosis, hepatitis B surface antigen, and ova and parasites, as well as a hemoglobin measurement, are advised for most groups (Ackerman, 1997).

Afghans in the United States a decade or more have diabetes, asthma, and motor vehicle injuries (because of a lack of urban driving experience and, until recently, not wearing seat belts). Public health nurses and interpreters have also noted active tuberculosis, diabetes, hypertension, and positive cultures for ova and parasites; one said, "Birth control is a problem and women don't want pap smears and breast exams" (Lipson & Omidian, 1992, p. 273). The women need education about women's health issues and someone to talk to about them.

Mental Health Issues

Refugees experienced multiple losses. Relatives were killed or left behind; they lost their status, language, and vocational competencies, as well as their country, for which they mourn. The primary problems of one Afghan physician's patients, 75% of whom are Afghan, are depression and psychosomatic illness; their major complaints are headaches and musculoskeletal problems, such as joint and back pain. A community mental health psychiatrist described "lots and lots of depression, we establish them on meds and see some improvement, but they get stuck and never become fully functioning." Afghans themselves comment on the prevalence of

"mental problems" in their community: "Afghans are sick because of thinking too much" and "Sadness is the sickness Afghans are faced with" (Lipson & Omidian, 1992, p. 273).

While there seems to be relatively little serious mental disease, such as schizophrenia or other psychotic disorders, many people experience chronic posttraumatic stress disorder (PTSD) related to horrific experiences in Afghanistan and in transit. PTSD is expressed as sleep disorders and nightmares, reexperiencing the traumatic event, numbing or heightened responses to external stimuli, depression, and persecution reactions. Mghir and Raskin (1999) found ethnic differences in young Afghan refugees in the United States. Those with Tajik parents had significantly less evidence of PTSD and depression than those with Pashtun parents. Their socioeconomic and cultural backgrounds were quite different: Tajik parents are wealthier, more likely to speak English at home, and less religious than the Pashtun parents. Pashtun parents and their children spent more time in Afghanistan during the war, and they experienced or saw more traumatic events.

But Afghans also acknowledge current stressors in the United States: "The things they got from Afghanistan—murder, bombs—and the things they got here—children's freedom and not obeying, fear for children's future—all together makes them mentally sick" (Lipson, 1993). Iqbal (2005) conducted a survey of 60 female Afghan refugees between the ages of 25 and 65, who were born in Afghanistan and migrated to the San Francisco Bay area after the Soviet invasion. She explored the relationship between somatization and depression as they relate to acculturation, finding that these Afghan women had high levels of somatization and depression, and that the higher the depression score, the more they tended to somatize their depression.

Although Afghans agree that mental health is a problem in the community, families tend to seek psychiatric care only as a last resort because it is perceived as shaming the family. As one person noted, "We don't believe in psychiatry, although after 22 years of war, more than 50% of us have some mental health problems." Fears include gossip, losing face, and that a therapist may share "personal" information about the family. Many would prefer a medication (a quick cure) to "talk therapy." However, interviews revealed that Afghan women would go to a female psychologist for services if one were available in their community (Iqbal, 2005).

There are almost no available culturally sensitive mental health services, and mainstream counselors tend to treat Afghans like mainstream Americans. For example, an isolated and depressed elderly woman was told to "get a boyfriend," which so insulted her that she cried. Instead, the counselor could have suggested that she pray and increase her reading of the Qur'an (Robson, Lipson, Younos, & Mehdi, 2002). Group approaches with time for socializing are preferable to individual counseling. Other methods of stress reduction, such as physical activity (walking groups), are often effective in reducing depression. For example, an excellent program for the elderly in Fremont was started more than 10 years ago by taking seven isolated and depressed elderly women to the park so that they could socialize with each other. After a few months, these women began to organize the "Tuesdays" themselves. The group grew, and many of the women showed striking improvement in their mental health (Omidian, 1996). Currently, more than 100 attend the Fremont Senior Center weekly, aided by Dari- or Pashto-speaking staff, where they socialize and are provided with health education and other services.

Death Beliefs and Customs

While Afghans grieve expressively and strongly over the death of a loved one, death is seen not as the termination of life but as the beginning of a new and better life, a spiritual existence and a cherished state in which one solidifies one's relationship with God. Muslims believe that they are on earth to be tested; praying five times a day helps them think about God and avoid committing bad deeds. As God's children, they believe that when their time comes to go, they have no choice but to go to the other world where God is calling upon them. The belief in the power of God over all His creation makes "letting go" easier for some families. However, Afghans may oppose stopping life support, viewing it as "playing God," although they may view beginning life support as a gift of medical technology.

After the death, the body is washed in a ritual manner, only by another Muslim. Although the sooner the better, the time of washing may be delayed if family members must travel from a different state or country. The body is washed by a mullah and an immediate family member, who prays during the washing. The body is wrapped in a white cotton shroud and placed in a coffin. If the deceased is a woman, only close female family members are allowed to see her face. Not even her husband is allowed to see it. If the deceased is a man, only close male friends and family are allowed to see his face, with the exception of his wife. Islam does not permit embalming of the dead; in Afghanistan, people are buried directly into the earth to facilitate the transition from "dust to dust." In the United States, the body is not embalmed but placed in a coffin and taken to a mosque, where men (not women) pray over the body (*Jinaza*).

The coffin is then taken to the chapel for burial. Until very recently, only men were allowed to attend the burial, but now women attend as well. A cloth covering with Qur'anic verses written on it is placed on the coffin, but it is removed when the coffin is buried. Then everyone goes to the deceased's home or a local mosque for prayer (*fatya*). Men and women sit separately for the *fatya*.

Close family members gather together to mourn at specified intervals. Following the *fatya*, close family members gather every Thursday to read a chapter of the Qur'an for the first 40 days (*chil*). *Chil* ends on the fortieth day if the deceased had no children. Otherwise, one day is subtracted for each child, determining the length of *chil*. For example, the last gathering for prayer would be the thirty-fourth day if the person had six children.

For the first 40 days after the death, women in the immediate family do not wear makeup and must wear the chador. After 40 days, they can wear light makeup. Immediate family members mourn for a full year, after which they resume their customary lives. Until a year from the day the family member died, they may not attend any social (happy) gatherings such as weddings or birthday parties where there is music and laughter. If the deceased was elderly, the family finds it easier for life to go on than after the death of a young person.

Implications for Nursing Care

It is essential for the culturally competent nurse to be sensitive to values and beliefs that may be held by Afghans and the effects of such beliefs on health care practices and on behavior related to achieving an optimal state of health. For example, the nurse should enable the client to carry out beliefs related to washing before prayer and other religious practices. It is important for the nurse to appreciate that while the client may believe that illness is the "will of Allah"; nonetheless, the client is also likely to value and seek Western medical care.

BIOLOGICAL VARIATIONS

Afghans are a mixture of original tribes and foreigners who invaded the area throughout history, including Greeks, Kushans (Caucasian nomads), Indians from the south, Huns from the north, Arabs, Turks, and Mongols. Indo-European genetics are evident in Pashtuns and Tajiks, whose skin tones and facial features resemble those of other Mediterranean groups, with coloring ranging from blue or green eyes, light brown hair, and fair skin to nearly black eyes, black hair, and brown skin. Mongolian heritage is evident in such Northern groups as Turkmen, Uzbek, and Aimaks, as well as Hazara, in high cheekbones, narrow slanted eyes, and lighter or yellow-toned skin (Ansary, 1991). Because of the variations in skin color, health care professionals may need to assess jaundice and anemia by examining the sclerae and oral mucosa rather than by relying solely on skin assessments.

Cross-cousin marriage used to be common in Afghanistan, resulting in such diseases and birth defects as epilepsy, blindness, several forms of anemia, and hemophilia. Diabetes is common, but the majority of those who have it are not aware of it, despite clear symptoms. Thalassemia is also common. Glucose-6-phosphate dehydrogenase (G-6-PD)

deficiency surveys in Afghan refugees show that this trait was more common among Pashtun and Uzbek refugees (15.8% and 9.1%, respectively) than Pakistani Pashtuns (7.0%) who live in the same area; the prevalence in Tajik and Turkmen refugees was 2.9% and 2.1%, respectively. Hospital studies showed that the type of G-6-PD deficiency in Pashtuns could cause hemolytic crises when they eat fava beans. G-6-PD deficiency affects drug metabolism, such as increasing sensitivity to primaquine, used to prevent malaria (Bouma, Goris, Akhtar, et al., 1995).

The Afghan diet is generally healthy, based mainly on rice seasoned with herbs, vegetables, and small amounts of meat or poultry. People enjoy fresh fruit, raisins, and nuts as snacks, although some serve cake. Unhealthy practices include cooking food with a large amount of oil, sometimes fatty meats, and loss of nutrients in vegetables that are "cooked to death," except for lettuce, cucumbers, and tomatoes in fresh salads. Since tea is always offered to guests and accompanies meals, some people may ingest too much caffeine. A nurse or nutritionist could teach people to cook traditional Afghan food with unsaturated oil and less of it, and to emphasize fresh fruit over cake. Teens and children are becoming addicted to fast food, which upsets their parents and places them at risk.

Implications for Nursing Care

The nurse should be aware that major public health concerns for most Afghans include trauma related to motor vehicle accidents, maternal and child health, and control of communicable diseases. Concerns related to maternal and child health and communicable diseases may be of more concern to newly immigrated Afghans. The nurse should be aware than the gene–environment interaction of coronary heart disease and that conditions such as diabetes and hypertension, which are emerging as a major problem in Afghanistan, may also be more prevalent among Afghan Americans in the United States.

SUMMARY

Afghans and Afghan Americans are culturally unique individuals with their own customs, norms, beliefs, and practices. In the United States, Afghans are a very young population of people as compared with the median age. These young Afghans tend to highly value education. Many Afghans come to the United States speaking either both or one of the two national languages of Afghanistan. Many Afghans believe that optimal health is an individual responsibility, and this belief is illuminated further by their desire to maintain regular exercise habits, eat appropriate foods, stay warm, and get adequate rest to sustain the body. In contrast, many Afghans believe that illness is the "Will of God," and thus illness should be borne with patience as it cleanses sin. Some Afghans believe that treatment may depend on the cause of the illness. In some cases, both folk-traditional and Western biomedical treatment are not only valued but are often used at the same time.

Case Study

Mrs. Hafiza Ahmadi, 45 years old, was taken to the emergency room after she fainted. Blood tests led to a diagnosis of type 2 diabetes. She also has had hypertension for several years but does not take medication because she has no primary health care provider or health insurance. Mrs. Ahmadi, who lives with her husband and young adult son, has three sisters and a brother who live in the area, and they visit each other very frequently. As part of the strong Afghan value placed on hospitality, food is always involved—black tea with accompaniments like raisins, sugared almonds, or cake and fruit between meals or lunch or dinner. The women socialize while preparing the food and cleaning up.

Mrs. Ahmadi tells an American friend about her diagnosis. The friend helps her make contact with the local public health center, and a public health nurse is assigned to her case. The nurse first helps her to reapply for Medicaid, which she was denied when she applied a few years ago because she had trouble with and made errors on the complex application.

Mrs. Ahmadi is 62 inches tall and weighs 160 pounds. She does not drive, so she walks to the market and used to walk 3 miles to her job at the local community college. She is college educated and speaks accented but fairly good English, and she reads English well. However, she has little knowledge of medical terminology and almost no knowledge of how the body works. She is concerned about her health and motivated to learn. She loves sweets and fatty foods, such as cheesecake, butter, and jam on bread. She cooks typical Afghan food with a lot of oil, large portions of rice at lunch and dinner, traditional wheat bread, and fruit. She is aware that her weight is partially causing her hypertension. She has tried to lose weight in the past, but she explains, "I can't help myself, I can't stop eating the food I love."

CARE PLAN

✳ *Nursing Diagnosis: Health maintenance, impaired, related to lack of knowledge about diabetes and hypertension*

Client Outcomes

1. Client asks to learn more about food and diabetes.
2. Client will learn to balance carbohydrate intake to lower blood sugar to safe levels.
3. Client will ask her sisters to support diet.
4. Client will learn to test blood sugar and take oral medication on a schedule.

Nursing Interventions

1. Identify family health beliefs that would support proper diet.
2. Assess Afghan diet for diabetic balance; suggest exchanges.
3. Assess meaning of food and hospitality in the family.
4. Discuss with family group risks of diabetes and dietary changes to manage it. Provide simple information in English or work with a medical interpreter.
5. Teach blood sugar measurement, and how the medication works.

✳ *Nursing Diagnosis: Nutrition, altered, unbalanced: more than body requirements (fat, carbohydrates)*

Client Outcomes	*Nursing Interventions*
1. Client will learn to alter cooking methods to reduce fat and sugar and use substitutes.	1. Engage culturally competent nutritionist to work with client in altering Afghan food preparation.
2. Client will walk 3 miles at least 3 times a week.	2. Provide support and structure for walking program; invite sisters to join.
3. Client will lose 3–4 pounds a month.	3. Measure blood pressure and record weekly blood sugar levels; provide feedback to encourage client and support her progress.

✳ STUDY QUESTIONS

1. Describe the importance of family in Afghan culture and how the family can contribute to an individual's maintenance of health.
2. Discuss gender roles and how they would affect health teaching and individual or group teaching.
3. How can Afghan beliefs about causes of illness and promotion of health be used in teaching someone how to care for herself in chronic disease?

4. What role would present orientation play in prevention and health promotion in an "invisible" disease like hypertension?
5. Describe alternative ways of providing health education materials in English, Dari, and Pashto to aid in teaching about diabetes and hypertension.

NCLEX-RN REVIEW QUESTIONS

1. While the Afghan or Afghan American client might believe that illness is the "will of Allah," it is important for the nurse to remember that:
   A. Afghans are likely to value and seek Western medical care.
   B. Afghans, in general, refuse all but traditional folk treatment.
   C. Afghans are a genetically homogeneous group with numerous genetically linked diseases.
   D. The traditional Afghan diet is very unhealthy, providing poor nutrition.

2. Afghan or Afghan Americans death beliefs and customs center on:
   A. Muslim practices
   B. Christian practices
   C. Buddhist practices
   D. Zoroastrian practices

3. Determinants of the use of touch among Afghans and Afghan Americans are:
   A. Family relationships and gender
   B. Age and social position
   C. Gender and social position
   D. Eye contact and tribe

References

Ackerman, L. (1997). Health problems of refugees. *Journal of the American Board of Family Practice*, 10, 337–348.

Ansary, M. T. (1991). *Afghanistan: fighting for freedom.* Dillon Press: New York.

Bouma, M., Goris, M., & Akhtar, T., et al, (1995). Prevalence and clinical presentation of glucose-6-phosphate dehydrogenase deficiency in Pakistani Pathan and Afghan refugee communities in Pakistan: implications for the use of primaquine in regional malaria control programmes. *Transactions of the Royal Society of Tropical Medicine and Hygiene*, 89, 62–64.

Central Intelligence Agency (CIA). (2006). World Factbook: Afghanistan. Retrieved June 28, 2007, from: https://www.cia.gov/library/publications/the-world-factbook/geos/af.html.

Iqbal, R. (2005). *Somatization underlying depression as related to acculturation among Afghan Women in the San Francisco Bay area.* Unpublished PsyD dissertation, The California School of Professional Psychology, Alliant International University, San Francisco, Calif.

Lipson, J. (1993). Afghan refugees in California: mental health issues. *Issues in Mental Health Nursing*, 14, 411–423.

Lipson, J., & Askaryar, R. (2005). Afghans. In Lipson, J. & Dibble, S. (Eds.), *Culture and clinical care.* San Francisco: UCSF Nursing Press.

Lipson, J., & Miller, S. (1994). Changing roles of Afghan refugee women in the U.S. *Health Care for Women International*, 15, 171–180.

Lipson, J., & Omidian, P. (1992). Afghan refugees: health issues in the United States. *Western Journal of Medicine*, 157, 271–275.

Lipson, J., & Omidian, P. (1996). Health and the transnational connection: Afghan refugees in the United States. *Refugee Issues Papers*, 4, 2–17Council of Refugee Issues, American Anthropological Association.

Lipson, J., & Omidian, P. (1997). Afghan refugee issues in the U.S. social environment. *Western Journal of Nursing Research*, 19, 110–126.

Lipson, J., Omidian, P., & Paul, S. (1995). Afghan health education project: a community survey. *Public Health Nursing*, 12, 143–150.

McCaw, B., & DeLay, P. (1985). Demographics and disease prevention of two new refugee groups in San Francisco: the Ethiopian and Afghan refugees. *Western Journal of Medicine*, 143, 271–275.

Mghir, R., & Raskin, A. (1999). The psychological effects of the war in Afghanistan on young Afghan refugees from different ethnic backgrounds. *International Journal of Social Psychiatry*, 45, 29–36.

Omidian, P. (1996). *Aging and family in an Afghan refugee community.* Garland: New York.

Omidian, P., & Lipson, J. (1992). Elderly Afghan refugees: tradition and transition in Northern California. In DeVoe, P. (Ed.), *Refugee issues papers* (vol. 1, pp. 27–39). Arlington, Va.: American Anthropological Association.

Penkala, D. (1980). "Hot" and "cold" in the traditional medicine of Afghanistan. *Ethnomedicine*, 6, 201–228.

Robson, B., Lipson, J., Younos, F., & Mehdi, M. (2002). The Afghans: their history and culture. Fact sheet. Washington, D.C.: U.S. Center for Applied Linguistics. Retrieved June 15, 2007, from: http://www.cal.org/co/publications/cultures/afghans.html.

Shorish-Shamley, Z. (1991). *The self and other in Afghan cosmology: concepts of health and illness among Afghan refugees.* Unpublished PhD dissertation, University of Wisconsin, Madison.

U.S. Department of Commerce, Bureau of the Census. (2002). Population profiles by age, sex, race, and Hispanic origin, Summary File 3. Washington, D.C: U.S. Government Printing Office.

Yollin, P. (2002, November 5). Wide array of estimates of Bay Area Afghans. Little Kabul gets even littler. Counting Afghans is an inexact science. *San Francisco Chronicle*, p. A–15.

Younos, F. (2002). Gender equity in Islam, published with Afghan community support. Retrieved from: http://www.1stbooks.com.

CHAPTER 15 Russian Americans

Linda S. Smith

Behavioral Objectives

After reading this chapter, the nurse will be able to:

1. Describe how health care practices in Russia may have affected the health of Russian Americans.
2. Identify at least two health problems specific to Russian Americans.
3. Explain how Russian American people use space and gestures as communication mechanisms.
4. List at least two future-oriented values for Russian Americans.
5. Relate the importance of family to Russian Americans.
6. Describe specific characteristics of the Russian language.
7. Formulate and implement a patient plan of care with clients self-reporting as Russian American.

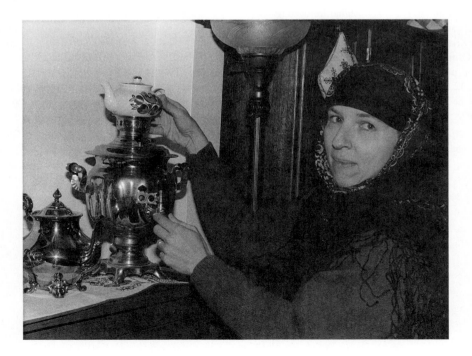

Acknowledgment

This chapter was written with special consultation from four Russian professionals who have now immigrated to the United States. Two of these professionals are Tatiana Victorovna McVay, MD, and Alla Vichinura Powers.

OVERVIEW OF RUSSIA

Russia (Russian Federation) is the largest of the 15 republics once known as the Soviet Union and the largest former republic of the Commonwealth of Independent States (CIS). The CIS was created in December 1991 and currently unifies 12 nations, Russia being the largest. The purpose of the CIS is to provide an economic union among member nations that allows free movement of goods, services, capital, and human resources (CIS, 2006). Before the collapse of the Soviet Union, Russia was known as the Russian Soviet Federative Socialist Republic and the Russian Empire. Russia, occupying much of easternmost Europe and northern Asia, stretches from Norway to the Pacific Ocean and from the Arctic Ocean to the Black sea (Library of Congress, 2005)

Russia occupies 17,075,200 square km and is, therefore, the largest country in the world. This Russian landmass totals roughly 77% of the land once known as the Soviet Union and is almost twice the size of the United States. Of the 142,893,540 people in Russia, 79.8% are Russian, 2% are Ukrainian, 3.8% are Tartar, and 14.4% are other (CIA, 2006). Though the official language is Russian, nearly 100 other languages are spoken (Library of Congress, 2005). It is important to understand that Russian-born nonethnic Russians living inside and outside Russia insist on their separate identities.

Russia's enormous land area is divided by the Urals (a mountain system constituting the traditional boundary between Europe and Asia) into two land localities: European Russia and Siberia. European Russia is smaller in size but includes the greatest number of people, as well as Russia's two largest cities, St. Petersburg (named "Leningrad" until September 1991) and Moscow, Russia's capital.

Though much of Russia is sparsely populated, Russia is the largest country in the world and comprises 89 republics and other subnational jurisdictions, each having its own government. The Russian National Constitution of December 12, 1993, established three government branches: executive, legislative, and judicial, but of the three branches, the executive has the greatest powers (Library of Congress, 2005). Russia's border countries include Azerbaijan, Belarus, China, Estonia, Finland, Georgia, Kazakhstan, North Korea, Latvia, Lithuania, Mongolia, Norway, Poland, and the Ukraine (CIA, 2006). Because of its geographic massiveness, Russia's climate is extremely varied, with all types of weather conditions except tropical. Therefore, Russian land can be plain and grassy, forested, mountainous, frigid, and marshy; despite its size, large portions of Russia lack proper soil and climate for agriculture (CIA, 2006). Russian territory spans 11 time zones, though only 32% of this land has agricultural potential. Oil, natural gas, metals, and timber account for over 80% of Russia's exports (CIA, 2006).

However, despite these natural resources, 18% of Russia's population falls below the poverty line (CIA, 2006) and 40% self-identify as poor (*Russians who*, 2005). Russia has a 7.6% unemployment rate, not including a large underemployed labor force (CIA, 2006). With an 11.7% inflation rate, it now takes 27.11 Russian rubles to equal one U.S. dollar and nearly 34 rubles to equal one euro (Oanda. com, 2006). This compares to nearly 31 rubles per U.S. dollar in 2003 (CIA, 2006)

In the years 1999–2000, the Russian economy improved, mostly because of rising world oil prices. Unfortunately, problems persist. Because Russia depends so heavily on commodity exports, especially fossil fuels and timber, the nation is vulnerable to shifts in world prices (CIA, 2006). Low birthrates, high death rates, and a deteriorating health care system, including an HIV/AIDS epidemic that is one of the worst in the world, have influenced an alarming negative growth rate of −0.37 (CIA, 2006). In just 12 years, the Russian population dropped by 6 million people (World Bank, 2005). Russian industry, accounting for 35% of its gross domestic product (GDP), is too outdated and run-down to sustain any kind of industrial growth (CIA, 2006). Agriculture accounts for 5% of the GDP, with 10.3% of the labor force; service industries make up the remaining 68.3% of the labor force and 60% of Russia's GDP (CIA, 2006). Moreover, widespread corruption, capital flight, and a nationwide brain drain have increased Russia's economic problems. Most Russians are well educated. Approximately one sixth of the world's scientists work in Russia, most Russians have at least a high school education, and there is a 99.6% literacy rate, up from 95% in 1998 (CIA, 2001; CIA, 2006). However, the average Russian enjoys few luxuries.

Moscow is Russia's largest city (nearly 10.1 million people) and also its capital. St. Petersburg, to the north and west of Moscow, has 4.5 million people. Nearly three fourths of Russia's mineral wealth is located in the Siberian regions. Harsh obstacles of climate, distance, and geography thwart exploration and exploitation of these Russian resources (CIA, 2001; CIA, 2006). Though only 8% of Russia is tillable land, some 8 million Russians are farmers. However, farming remains mostly collective, with Russians currently producing only half of the grain, meat, and dairy products needed for the Russian population (CIA, 2006).

June 12, 1991, is the day the Russian Republic declared sovereignty from the Soviet Union (Library of Congress, 2005). After the fall of the Soviet Union on December 21, 1991, Russia and 10 other former Soviet republics joined in the Commonwealth of Independent States. In early 1992, Russia made radical changes that had enormous implications for Russians, including privatization programs and lifting of price freezes, which had stifled free enterprise for decades. Russia became a constitutional federation and a United Nations member, and adopted a constitution in 1993 that includes a multiparty system and scheduled elections. This new constitution gave the president ruling powers independent of the Russian Parliament (CIA, 2006). All citizens 18 years and older may vote. Presidents are elected by popular vote for 4-year terms. On May 7, 2000, Vladimir Putin took office as the Russian president; there was no vice president. The last presidential election was on March 14, 2004, when President Putin was re-elected with a 71.2% majority vote. The next election will take place in 2008 (CIA, 2006).

Life Today in Russia

Today in Russia, life continues to be difficult and frustrating. Anti-Semitism escalates. Railroad stations are crowded with homeless, begging people because of unemployment and underemployment. An estimated 2 million children are homeless in Russia. These children represent the offspring of the unpaid or unemployed. They have been forced into the streets by cruelty, alcoholism, and neglect. They are beggars, glue or gas sniffers, and prostitutes; many have been viciously attacked, are suffering from hypothermia, malnutrition, and depression. The vast majority of these street children have tried to commit suicide at least once (Carpenter, 1997; Harrigan, 2001). Crime has also escalated. After the dissolution of the Soviet Union, few if any controls enforced law and order within the country. What did remain, however, was a tradition of abusing power and innovative officials who had learned how to exploit the system. Thus, crime exploded. Theft and gangs have proliferated, along with weapons and explosives. Murder and crime rates doubled during the early 1990s and were considered some of the highest crime rates worldwide. By the mid-1990s, Russia had 30 murders per 100,000 people. Murders of famous politicians, journalists, and businessmen went unpunished (Kunstel & Albright, 1996; Library of Congress, 2005; Popov, 2004). Russia's police force is plagued by low pay, low prestige, and high levels of corruption. Crimes against women (domestic violence, prostitution, and trafficking) are pervasive and severely underreported (Library of Congress, 2005). Trafficking of girls and young women as foreign brides is pervasive. When performing a Google search using the keywords "Russian girls," 35,400,000 sites were listed; when the words "mail order" were added, 10,200,000 sites appeared.

Russia's economy and infrastructure have recently shown signs of improvement. After more than a decade of steady decline, Russia's gross domestic product (GDP) grew during each of the last seven years, averaging 6.4% annually since 1998 (CIA,

2006). Over the next few years, these increases are expected to continue because of increased investment, private consumption of goods and services, privatization, and oil prices on the world market. The telecommunications industry has expanded, airports and airlines have improved, and road construction and maintenance are increasing, with a decreasing foreign debt. Additionally, governmental control over the economy has been reasseted by the Putin administration (CIA, 2006).

These small gains have not helped improve Russians' health. Health indicators are good social barometers when evaluating the success of any social or economic reform. This is especially true during this transition time for Russians. For Russia, population decline poses a clear threat to national and economic security, the quality of human resources, and the human potential and viability of the nation (Andriouchina, 2002; Koretz, 2003; Marquez, 2005; Starobin, 2003). Russia is in a negative population crisis, with a decline each year of more than 500,000 people. Russian women of child-bearing age have on average 1.1 children (World Bank, 2005), which means there are about 1.5 deaths for each birth in Russia. By the year 2050, Russia's population will have fallen by 28%. Male life expectancy in Russia dropped from 64 to 57 years between 1989 and 1994. Men die far sooner than women because of cardiovascular disease, poisonings, respiratory disorders, traffic and industrial accidents, alcoholism, and suicide (Marquez, 2005). Currently, life expectancy at birth is 59.9 years for men and 73.3 years for women (Library of Congress, 2005). The infant mortality rate is 15.13 per 1000 live births (CIA, 2006). More than 20% of pregnant women in Russia are diagnosed with anemia during labor and delivery. For Russian children ages 1 to 14, the rate of death by accident compares to the death rate for all causes combined in the United States; for Russian children ages 5 to 9, the drowning rate is 10 times higher than in the United States. Sadly, Russian adolescents commit suicide at a rate twice that of the United States (CDC, 2002). Life expectancy in Russia is 66 years, compared with a U.S. life expectancy of 78 years (Marquez, 2005).

Tuberculosis is a major concern, killing more than 100,000 people in the last few years. In that time, more than 2 million Russians have been exposed to tuberculosis. Russian prisons are filled with tuberculosis (TB)-afflicted and HIV-infected inmates. In part because of severe overcrowding, Russia's Ministry of Justice reports that 75% of Russian prisoners have a serious disease, such as HIV positivity or TB and that when released, they spread these infectious diseases to the general population (Burgermeister, 2003). More than half of all new HIV-positive cases in Russia are among injection drug users (IDUs). Since 1990, the number of IDUs has increased 20-fold (Gore-Felton, et al., 2003). Unfortunately, regional hospitals and clinics cannot perform even the most basic TB screenings and diagnostic analyses (Engleman, 2002), and alcohol prevention programs are virtually nonexistent. HIV/AIDS is also a growing but often secret epidemic, with national estimates as many as 2 million HIV-positive cases. In addition to prisoner spread, HIV infection and TB spread rapidly among young, male Russian drug-abusing populations. In 2005, Russia had the most rapid rise in HIV-positive cases outside of Africa (Library of Congress, 2005). On December 8, 2005, thousands of Russian hospital patients learned that they may have been treated with HIV-infected blood. The government's tendency to avoid disclosure of sex-related problems is considered partly to blame (Page, 2005). Medications are terribly expensive and hard to find, with 25% of Russians unable to secure desperately needed medicines (Maximova, 2000; Starobin, 2003). Only a few pharmaceutical firms exist since the August 1998 financial collapse.

According to the World Health Organization (2006), for every 1000 people, Russia has 4.25 physicians, 8.0 nurses, 0.32 dentists, and 0.08 pharmacists. Compare these numbers with those in the United States, which has 2.56 physicians, 9.37 nurses, and 1.63 dentists for every 1000 people. Despite these numbers of health care professionals, the health of Russians has dramatically deteriorated since the fall of communism (Farmer, Sirotkin, Ziganshina, & Greenberg, 2003). Russia's health care system remains mostly public supported and therefore suffers from the problems of inefficiency, incompetence, low salaries, and bribery (Aslund, 2001; Library of Congress, 2005). Hospitals and clinics are poorly managed, equipped, and maintained. Most physicians and nurses are paid dreadfully low salaries; for example, a PhD research scientist can earn only about $50 a month (Larkin, 2000). Health care professionals, teachers, and scientists were the hardest hit during the transition from communism to a free-market economy because the Russian government was unwilling to increased fixed salaries based on inflation. Salaries, therefore, have dropped below poverty levels (Wikipedia, 2006). Russia's per capita spending on health care during 2003 was $325. Compare this with the U.S. expenditure of $2548 (WHO, 2006b). In a study of the fragmented Russian health care system, Danishevski, Balabanova, McKee, and Atkinson (2006) confirm the virtual absence of processes that Russia could use to bring about change. For example, they found that neither regional nor federal governments have been able to improve health and health care. Preventive health care is a low priority, but the Russian Ministry of Health wants to change that by raising the bar for who qualifies for hospital admission, decreasing by one third the number of hospital beds in Russia, and encouraging more MDs to go into general practice (Osborn, 2004). Currently there are 6.76 hospitals and 1071 hospital beds per 100,000 people (WHO, 2004). Nurses are also learning to expand their roles as independent practitioners into community health areas (Ivanov & Paganpegara, 2003; Smith, 2006). This will be essential if the steady increase in alcoholism in Russia is to change course. According to a Russian–American partnered research study by Williams and colleagues (2001), Russian children, when compared to U.S. counterparts, begin drinking earlier, receive fewer prevention messages from their parents, and have fewer prevention programs in schools and communities.

History

Historically, Slavic tribes began migrating into Russia around the fifth century, and the first Russian state was established in the ninth century by Scandinavians. Mongols overran the country until 1480, and Ivan the Terrible became the first tsar in 1547. Peter the Great (1682–1725) tried to westernize Russia, but the pace was slow. Russia had no universities until 1755. In 1917, after Tsar Nicholas II abdicated (and during the October Revolution), Lenin and the Bolsheviks overthrew the government. Between 1918 and 1924, the tsar and his family were murdered, the Bolsheviks declared ideological war on Europe, Joseph Stalin (Josif V. Dzhugashvili) became general secretary, and the Union of Soviet Socialist Republics (USSR) was established.

Recent political change in Russia has been dramatic and historic. The current political situation began on March 11, 1985, when the former USSR KGB chief, Secretary Konstantin Chernenko, died and was replaced by Mikhail Gorbachev.

Between 1985 and 1990, the Gorbachev–Shevardnadze team created a new human rights movement within the USSR. Gorbachev reforms, identified as *perestroika* ("restructuring") and *glasnost* ("openness"), swept the country with promises of democracy and freedom. However, Gorbachev inherited a sad and decaying empire (Anderson, 1992). Gorbachev believed that free enterprise and a carefully controlled form of democracy could be the overhaul needed for communism. To help him with this plan, he heralded a known reformer, Boris Yeltsin.

Yeltsin proved to be forceful, authoritarian, proud, chaotic, and critical of Gorbachev's leadership. Therefore, in a powerful control move, Gorbachev publicly humiliated and fired his former protégé. This embarrassing termination triggered Yeltsin to campaign against the Communist Party and to run as a candidate for a parliamentary seat as the people's deputy from Moscow. Yeltsin achieved enormous popularity among the people, 90% of the vote, and leadership of a growing group of people who opposed communism (Anderson, 1992).

In February 1990, the USSR's Central Committee eliminated a constitutional clause that guaranteed the leading role of the Communist Party. On December 25, 1991, the Russian Federation became an independent republic (Billy, 1993). Yeltsin left the Communist Party in 1990. After confrontations with the Baltic republics, Gorbachev began discussions that would lead toward the creation of a "voluntary" union of the republics.

In May 1991, Soviet citizens were given the right to emigrate. The law titled "On the Procedure for the Exit from the USSR and Entry into the USSR of Citizens of the USSR" came into full effect in January 1993. This law was heralded as one of the most significant steps toward an open Russian society and marked the end of Communist-enforced isolation (Burlatsky, 1991). This law restored the rights of the Russian people to live, work, and travel freely.

In a historic move, the citizens of the Russian Republic elected Yeltsin as president by democratic vote (Kostikov, 1991). However, shortly thereafter, Gorbachev was overpowered in a dramatic conspiracy coup. Since that time, there have been ongoing struggles over rulership of this land as power has passed back and forth between Yeltsin and coup forces. Yeltsin had great power but failed to use this power to make immediate and necessary reforms. Yeltsin's popularity declined dramatically as a result of internal fighting among the 1033-member parliament (also called Congress of People's Deputies).

The Congress (or Duma), Russia's highest legislative body, is dominated by an anti-Yeltsin majority of ex-Communists (Yeltsin rival, 1993). His economic policies received much criticism, and by the spring of 1993, eight attempts on his life had been reported (Eight attempts reported on Yeltsin's life, 1993). However, Yeltsin continued to push for democratic reform (Witt, 1993), including opening classified Soviet archives, allowing Russians the right to own property and businesses, and attempting to stabilize the unit of Russian currency, the ruble. Other reforms included increasing social care for the needy, formalizing a system of granting benefits and privileges (Yeltsin: Main points, 1993), enforcing public disclosure of environmental accidents, dismantling state economic controls, and cutting the military by half, including dramatic nuclear arms cuts, to invest energy in other areas.

In December 1994, Yeltsin drew criticism for sending Russian troops into the southern republic of Chechnya after their drive for independence from Russian control. Fighting continues to be fierce and resistance extremely costly.

Vladimir Putin has been acting president since December 31, 1999, and full president since May 7, 2000 (CIA, 2006). He has inherited the conflict in Chechnya, which continues to draw international and national criticism, especially following the 3-day hostage-taking crisis in 2004 in the North Ossetian town of Beslan, where over 335 persons, mostly children, were killed (Russians rally, 2004). The military draft in Russia includes males ages 18 to 27, and length of required service is two years, though the Ministry of Defense has promised to reduce that to one year by 2008. Because of poor health, violent hazing rituals, poor salaries, poor service conditions, and the public's dissatisfaction with the Chechnyan conflict, the number and quality of military recruits have dramatically dropped (Library of Congress, 2005). Furthermore, a growing percentage of military funding will be targeted for medical, nutritional, and substance abuse programs for the military personnel (Marquez, 2005). In contrast to continued military reductions, Russia's democratic reforms have slowed and in some cases reversed. Today, the greatest danger in Russia is the widespread disregard for democracy and the repression of free speech, such as unbiased radio, television, and newspaper coverage of political issues (Aslund, 2001; Library of Congress).

IMMIGRATION TO THE UNITED STATES

As Russia has undergone rapid changes over the years, life in Russia has been increasingly unbearable to some, and immigration to the United States has dramatically increased. Since the fall of communism, many in Russia have come to think of themselves not as free but rather as abandoned (Starobin, 2003). Thus the likelihood has significantly increased that a nurse in the United States may care for Russian clients and their families and that the nurse herself or himself may be Russian.

The first wave of Russian immigration to the United States occurred after the Revolution (1917) in the 1920s. These immigrants were highly intelligent and generally well educated. The second wave of Russian immigrants occurred after World War II. In this wave, Russian immigrants had a mixture of backgrounds. Russian Jews were and are well educated, with approximately 13.5 years of education. Most entered the United States as refugees because of emerging and ever-increasing anti-Semitism. For many Russian Jews, the Jewish communities in which they settle provide tremendous social and economic support. For most Russian immigrants to the United States, their sphere of family and friends rests primarily with other Russian Americans; this is partly due to U.S. immigration laws, unchanged since 1952, that offer the right to U.S. immigration based on family preference. Therefore, the majority of new Russian Americans are related in some way to earlier Russian immigrants.

For the last 20 years of the Soviet empire, the United States encouraged the USSR to allow free immigration, particularly for the 2 million Soviet Jews residing in that country. A wave of Soviet Jews immigrated to the United States in 1973 as a direct result of a law passed by Congress to facilitate Jewish immigration. Because of this law, more than 66,480 Soviet Jews immigrated to the United States between 1975 and 1980 (Schiff, 1979). As of the 1990 census (U.S. Bureau of the Census, 1998), of the 194,784 Russian-born American residents, 128,249 entered the United States prior to 1980 and 66,535 entered between 1980 and 1990.

From 1971 to 1991, approximately 181,000 Russian Jews entered the United States. In 1991, of the number of Russians entering the United States, almost two thirds were Jewish (In the red, 1992). Historically, Soviet Jews were the most oppressed ethnic group in the USSR (Azarian, Boland, & Skripchenko, 1996). Additionally, policies of the former USSR encouraged, even mandated, the immigration of the family as a unit (Larkin, 2000). Therefore, when younger family members wished to leave Russia, older parents also had to leave. More than half the immigrants to Chicago (62%) stated that leaving Russia was not their decision (Brod & Heurtin-Roberts, 1992; Kohn, Flaherty, &

Levav, 1989). There are only between 400,000 and 550,000 Jews living in Russia. Importantly, the official religion in Russia, Russian Orthodox, has a unique relationship with the Russian government (Library of Congress, 2005). Thus, the Russian Orthodox church has resumed its place at the heart of Russian culture (Jarvik, 2006) and has powerfully dictated policies relative to religious freedom. Violence and hate crimes against Jews, Muslims, and other religious and ethnic minorities have dramatically increased (Library of Congress, 2005), with little or no interference from police or government officials.

For the most part, Russians who immigrate to the United States are well educated (most having college degrees) and courageous people who are voracious readers and passionately devoted to the arts and sciences (Mehler, Scott, Pines, et al., 2001; Trickett & Birman, 2005). Despite years of hardship, Russian immigrants are proud, forward-thinking people. Russian immigrants come to a specific location because they have relatives or other contacts in these locations, which means that pocket populations of Russian Americans have emerged in various regions in the United States.

Recent immigrants did not endure the long delays and confusion that earlier immigrants endured. Some recent immigrants were processed and arrived in the United States within a year or less. In some cases, resentment has surfaced among earlier immigrants, who often endured 10 or more years of frustrated waiting and turmoil.

In 1991, 57,000 people born in the former Soviet Union were granted permanent resident (immigrant) status. With this statistic in mind, the Soviet Union, in its final year as a nation, provided more U.S. immigrants than any other nation of the world. These numbers reflect a dramatic change in Soviet policy. Before 1989, fewer than 3000 Soviet citizens per year were allowed to emigrate. However, in 1988, restrictions on emigration eased. The U.S. Department of Justice's Immigration and Naturalization Service reported 11,000 Soviet immigrants in 1989 and more than 25,000 in 1990. Starting in 1992, Russian immigration was reported separately. However, demographic data based on reported city of birth were compiled for Soviet Union immigrants, and whenever possible the republic of birth origin was identified. From these data, the following Russian immigration statistics were listed and reported. In 1989, most Russian immigrants settled in California. In 1991, most Russian immigrants settled in one of five states: New York (34.2%), California (25.3%), Massachusetts (5.4%), Illinois (4.9%), and Pennsylvania (4.4%). In 1990, Russian immigrants settled in urban settings, primarily in Boston, Chicago, New York, and Philadelphia. In 1991, Portland, Oregon, and Sacramento, Los Angeles, and San Francisco received immigrants (U.S. Department of Justice, 1992). Between 1996 and 2000, the U.S. identified 15,411 legal permanent residents from Russia per year. This jumped to 20,313 in 2000 and 20,771 in 2001. A drop was then noted, with 13,935 in 2003 and 17,410 in 2005. In 2005, 18,083 Russians were considered to have entered the U.S. as legal permanent residents. Of these, 2786 settled in the New York area, 828 in Los Angeles, 678 in Chicago, 680 in Seattle, and 750 in Sacramento (U.S. Department of Homeland Security, 2005a, 2005b).

Immigration also includes a seldom-reported yet growing number of Russian children adopted by U.S. citizens. Since 1992, Russia, with its limited resources to care for orphaned children, has become a major source of foreign children adopted by U.S. citizens, with a total of 3816 children adopted by American adults in 1997 and 2454 in 1996. This number continues to grow. Over 4651 immigrant orphans from Russia were adopted by U.S. citizens in 2005. These children were equally divided between boys and girls; 20% were under one year of age at the time of adoption, 51% were between one and four years, and 28.6% were five years and older (U.S. Department of Homeland Security, 2005c). Importantly, these children are Russian-speaking and usually have special educational and health needs, such as fetal alcohol syndrome (Azarian, Boland, & Skripchenko, 1996; Russia may tighten, 1997). With a resurgence in Russian nationalism, the Russian people and government are becoming more protective of their children; 56% opined that they oppose adoption of Russian children by foreigners (*Russians who*, 2005). An estimated 2,652,214 persons of Russian descent are currently residing in the United States (U.S. Department of Commerce, Bureau of the Census, Summary File 3, 2002).

Life Today for Russians in the United States

Russian Americans report new freedoms in the United States. For example, Russian American Jews and Pentecostal Christians are often able to fully practice their faith for the first time upon arriving in the United States, and Russian parents commend the skills their children learn in schools. They report no longer feeling like persecuted members of minority groups. Russian Americans especially appreciate skills of thinking, analysis, and discussion (generally unheard of in their country). Russian women are familiar with working outside the home in well-paying professions. Russian women make up 47% of the working population. They are also used to doing all or most of the household chores (Sandul, 2002; Weir, 2001). As refugees, Russian American Jews are entitled to resettlement services, training programs, financial help, and permanent resident status in the United States. (A *refugee* comes to the United States because of declared political problems, such as anti-Semitism, and because he or she seeks political safety; an *immigrant* is identified as someone who simply wishes to live in another country.) However, more than half of the newly arriving Russian Jews are over 50 years of age and therefore may have difficulty in adapting to a new culture.

Though the U.S. is currently experiencing an energy crisis, the current low unemployment rates may help improve the transition for new Russian American immigrants, especially those employed in high-tech organizations. Additionally, Russian immigrant communities often provide supportive services, such as career guidance, networking, training programs, classes in English as a second language (Hill, 1992; Mehler et al., 2001), and health care. Russian Americans have high levels of social participation and interactions within Russian communities.

Americans should understand that in Russia, medical treatment, though limited, is free.

Education, including postsecondary university and professional studies, is also often free or low cost, though teachers are poorly paid and less qualified than before 1991. Therefore, many Russian immigrants, including women, have had some form of technical training or advanced education. Nevertheless, Russian immigrants have difficulty in understanding the concepts of insurance, private pay, malpractice, health maintenance organizations (HMOs), and diagnostic related groups. Concepts such as "credit" may be entirely new.

The large and growing Russian American population is, when compared with other immigrant groups, better educated and enjoys higher levels of discretionary income. Russian Americans are also more likely to own their own homes and have health insurance (84.5% have some kind of insurance coverage and of these, 84.6% receive their health insurance as part of employment). Though the median age of Russian Americans is about 42 years, the age composition of the Russian-born U.S. population is skewed toward elders, with 8.6% under age 24, 47.6% between ages 25 and 54 years, and 44.1% over age 55. Clearly, this group of well-educated people is keenly interested in pharmaceuticals and health care (Ethnic population, 2003; U.S. Department of Commerce, Bureau of the Census, 2000).

COMMUNICATION

Dialect, Style, and Volume

The official language of Russia is Russian. This language has a 33-character Cyrillic alphabet named after the ninth-century apostle to the Slavs, St. Cyril. St. Cyril created the alphabet so that the Bible could be translated for liturgy use in the Slavic countries (Moore, 1988). In the tenth century, the Cyrillic alphabet was adopted by Russians, simultaneously with Christianity. The old Cyrillic alphabet was renovated twice, once by Peter the Great and again in 1918. Russian is the most important of all the Slavic languages and belongs to the eastern branch of the Slavic linguistic family. Approximately one sixth of the world's population speaks Russian.

For most Russians, English is the most popular of all the Western languages. This newfound popularity of English on the part of the Russian people is related to media broadcasts, movies, rock video television programs, and Western business opportunities. In addition, professional literature (including health and medicine) is often in English, and medical students are frequently required to read English-language medical journals. In the year 2005, there were 23.7 million Internet users and 1,306,427 Internet hosts, as well as 7306 television stations (CIA, 2006). Therefore, information will be harder to suppress, and English will become even more widely used.

Russian is sometimes referred to as a "house green" language because articles (such as *the*) and verbs (such as *is*) are often unnecessary. The Russian language is a flexible, beautifully rich language. Paralanguage qualities, such as tone, inflection, speed, and verbal pauses, contribute to the variety and meaning of Russian words and sounds. Russians freely use paralanguage and other nonverbal indicators to denote the value being placed on what is said. The spirit of the Russian people, their warmth and love, comes through clearly in this dialect (Binyon, 1983). Just as in the United States, the Russian language carries geographic variances.

Some Russian American people may have studied English in Russia. However, the English they learned is British English, which often is significantly different in sound, spelling, and pronunciation from American English, making language comprehension difficult. Additionally, American geographical accents can cause problems.

Although many well-educated Russians studied English at some point in their education, English proficiency is not always easy, especially for older Russian American immigrants. In the United States, Russian speakers rank fifteenth of total speakers of various languages. Of the 2,652,214 total Russian American population, 484,092 do not speak English at home (U.S. Department of Commerce, Bureau of the Census, 2000). Importantly, younger immigrants have made the adjustment to English with less difficulty. For younger Russian immigrants, the first priority on arrival in the United States is to learn conversational English, the second priority is to enroll children in school, and the third priority is to find employment. When Birman and Trickett (2001) surveyed Jewish families (adolescents and their parents) from the former Soviet Union, they found that American acculturation occurred in a linear pattern over time, with the American culture increasing and Russian culture decreasing. As expected, acculturation gaps between children and parents occurred regarding language.

Using interpreters is important because of potential language barriers. Family, especially younger family members, may be embarrassed and anxious during the crisis of an illness or problem. In a study of elderly Russian immigrants in the Boston area, Tran and his associates (2000) found that more than 50% of the sample reported a poor ability to speak English, even though 85% had college or advanced degrees from Russian schools. These researchers discovered that elderly Russian Americans with English competence enjoy better mental and physical health. Duncan and Simmons (1996) found that in half of the households, no one could read English. Interpreters translate more than words. They must also convey nonverbal and subtle meanings. Therefore, attention must be paid to the issues of confidentiality (Azarian et al., 1996; Kravitz, Helms, Azari, Antonius, & Melnikow, 2000), eliminating family members, especially children, from the interpretation process whenever possible. An additional confidentiality consideration is familiarity. Often interpreters and patients know each other, having both lived and worked in the same isolated Russian American community.

Elderly Jewish immigrants may speak Yiddish. For these people, the practice of speaking Yiddish was greatly discouraged by Russian (and Soviet) authorities as being an "antistate" activity. Younger Jewish immigrants seldom speak Yiddish (Azarian et al., 1996; Gennis, 1989).

Fortunately, many medical, chemical, and scientific terms are cognates, and although the written appearance of the word is different between Russian and English, the sound is similar. A few medical cognates are *organ(ism)*, *appetite*, *function*, *pulse*, *doctor*, *hospital*, *physical*, *diagnosis*, *normal*, and *problem*.

The volume of speech used by Russian Americans is not significantly different from that used by some Irish American people. In Russia, because loud demands were often necessary to receive medical care, some Russians became loud when attempting to be understood or get attention. Thus even normal conversation may seem loud and boisterous.

Touch

Russians often use touch freely with intimate and close friends. It is not unusual to see Russian women embracing and kissing other women, as well as Russian men embracing and kissing other men. Friends who have been separated often greet each other, in public or in private, in this fashion. The technique of kissing each cheek three times seems to be a cultural trait adopted from the Middle East. The gentle kiss of a man on a woman's hand is a gesture of respect and admiration. Also, a handshake of agreement from a Russian is often more binding than a signed document.

Russian people are commonly perceived as kind, caring, and generous. When trust has been established, they express these feelings willingly and publicly. They are by nature and experience, however, cautious. Some Russians evaluate situations and people with great care. Emotions are also freely expressed. Russians have a quick appreciation for jokes and satire, often venting their feelings in this form of expression. It has been said that Russian people cry and laugh easily (R. Feldman, personal communication, April 28, 1998; Smith, 1991).

Context

Russian people who learned English in Russian schools may have learned from a non-native speaker. Therefore, the sound of English will be different. Native Russians who are eager to practice conversational English with a native English speaker often approach tourists traveling in Russia. However, for most new Russian immigrants, conversational English is likely to be unrecognizable.

Russian people have learned through years of Communist rule to look and act neutrally. With strangers and in crowded places, eye contact is avoided, affect is flat, posture is not erect, and eyes are diverted. Upon arriving in the United States, Russian Americans often express great wonder at the freedom with which Americans make nonverbal connections with strangers. However, Americans tend to be cooler and more distant with close friends and family than Russians are. For Russians, it is common to visit friends on a whim, bringing food and gifts without notice, whereas in the United States this practice is uncommon (Gottlieb, 1990).

Kinesics

Until trust and comfort have been established, Russian Americans will use few gestures. They do, however, feel free to maintain eye contact, and they do allow and expect nurses to use touch and gestures freely during the implementation of nursing procedures. Older Russian Americans who are immigrants are more entrenched in social amenities, often preferring to express themselves verbally. "Please" and "thank you" are integral to their speech, and they use these words at every possible opportunity. Nodding one's head is a gesture of approval; outstretching one's hand is a gesture of salute. When compliments are given, they are sincere. Flowers are presented during important meetings as a gesture of tribute. The person seated first in a room is the one with the most authority or prestige.

Implications for Nursing Care

Russian Americans expect the nurse to be warm and caring, to "feel" for them, and to help them cope with physical and emotional problems. The most often expressed expectation of the nurse by the Russian American is that the nurse be friendly. This expectation is demonstrated by an "inviting," open posture; a smile; and a low and calm voice. Touch, when appropriate, is considered a sign of friendliness and caring (Brod & Heurtin-Roberts, 1992). Russian Americans do not appreciate a light, "chatty" approach to health care; they believe appearance and demeanor must always remain professional. Russian Americans want to be certain that the nurse understands them. They can easily become very shy, especially recent immigrants. Because their English may be tenuous, Russian Americans may hesitate to ask for clarification.

When doing histories or intake screenings on Russian Americans with English literacy, nurses need to understand that if they are speaking and thinking in English, they will remember best those health events that have occurred during their English-speaking period. Conversely, Russian Americans speaking in Russian will remember best those events occurring during their Russian-speaking period (Marian & Neisser, 2000). Even if a Russian American is fluent in English, communicating in English during times of pain, stress, and anxiety will be difficult. Knowledge of this difficulty is especially important when working with elder Russian Americans.

Russian Americans, therefore, expect the nurse to speak slowly and clearly and to choose simple words when needed. Russian Americans also tend to be poor listeners, perhaps because of language barriers, and may be unable to represent themselves accurately (Barnathan, 1991). Russians are generally ignorant of many health issues; thus, they tend to assume the nurse and physician will tell them everything they need to know about their health problem. However, gestures and demonstrations, to clarify and promote understanding, are expected and appreciated. "Look at my eyes," explained one Russian American. "My eyes will tell you that I do not understand because I will have a stupid expression!"

In most instances, Russian Americans will comply with medical directives and teachings if they believe that the nurse is trustworthy, sincere, and competent. Nurses will not be believed or trusted by Russian Americans if they are perceived to be masklike, robotic, or phony in their caring behaviors. Nurses should address Russian American clients by "Mr." or "Mrs.," followed by the family name. However, use of the first name, followed by the patronymic (their father's first name plus a feminine or masculine ending, depending on the person's sex) may be an acceptable alternative. Well-educated and professional Russian American women often retain their maiden names. Using this formal method of address will convey the nurse's respect. To address a Russian by his or her first name only is improper and presents a grave social error. Russians also object strongly to terms of endearment, such as "dear,: "hon," "sweetie," and "hi, guy," when used by health care workers (Smith, 1996). As explained by Russian American R. Feldman (personal communication, April 28, 1998), "I want you to believe me when I tell you I have a problem. Here the nurses are perfect. We will respect them and listen to them. They know their job, and they know what they are supposed to do."

Russian Americans tend to speak freely regarding physical problems. Once language is no longer a concern, the nurse will find that clients respond warmly. However, Russian Americans may be uncomfortable using gestures when speaking to the nurse. The nurse must be aware that although younger Russian immigrants adapt well to English, older Russian immigrants may not. Often, elderly Russian immigrants choose to associate only with Russian-speaking friends and relatives, which presents a difficult problem if an interpreter is unavailable. To add to this difficulty, Russian Americans may allow only Russian to be spoken at home. Because many Russian Americans are multilingual (Yiddish, German, French, Polish, and so on), it is an advantage if the nurse understands another language familiar to the client. (However, only 14% of Russian Jews consider Yiddish their mother tongue.) One way to convey respect and an understanding of the culture is to provide avenues for client teaching through Russian literature. Health literature written in Russian may prove to be a better client teaching aid than audiotapes or video films. Additionally, cognate words and interpreters should be used whenever possible. Kravitz et al. (2000) found that Russian Americans occupied an additional 5.6 minutes of physician time for each visit. These authors believed this time was spent because of the extra demands for interpreting health information. Therefore, nurse managers will need to adjust workload requirements for nurses working with Russian American clients.

The challenge is for nurses to expand their own culture to care effectively for members of the Russian American ethnic group. These skills can strengthen the nurse as a person and as a health care professional.

SPACE

The Russian culture exists on two very different levels. To strangers and new acquaintances, a Russian will remain aloof, preferring to speak and work in the social or public zone. However, once friendship and familiarity have been established, Russian people are comfortable within a personal zone. The intimate zone is reserved for spouse or children, except for health care workers performing within a professional capacity. When hospitalized, Russians are extremely compliant and are generally able to tolerate the loss of privacy.

Individuals are perceived according to the boundaries they maintain, which include the degree of permeability and flexibility. Permeability is defined as the degree to which a boundary is open or closed; for the most part, permeability varies from closed to open. When an individual has closed boundaries, very little exchange occurs between this person's internal and external environments, and the person may be perceived as being quiet, withdrawn, and set in his or her ways. On the other hand, if boundaries are open, much exchange occurs between the person's internal and external environments, and this individual may be perceived as being talkative, social, and one who enjoys taking risks. Russian Americans may be very superstitious. Death or other potentially negative events should not be spoken of in the abstract. Joking, teasing, or play-acting is not appropriate in a serious or potentially serious situation.

Flexibility is defined as the ability of a person to move along a permeability continuum. A person who is sometimes closed and sometimes open and who thereby uses the entire permeability continuum is considered flexible. On the other hand, a person who always gravitates toward the closed end of the continuum, which is indicative of a low degree of flexibility, is described as a rigid, closed person. A person who is always open and never closed is described as an open individual. People who are perceived as rigid and closed may be quiet and withdrawn and seldom if ever share intimate secrets, dreams, or thoughts, even with best friends or a spouse (Scott, 1988).

Some Russian persons are perceived as rigid and closed because they remain aloof and distant. However, the word *friend* is not a casual term to Russians. Friendship is taken very seriously by Russian Americans. Close Russian friends may embrace, but mere acquaintances will probably not even shake hands. Russians may prefer to greet and meet acquaintances on a verbal level only.

Implications for Nursing Care

The nurse who cares for Russian American clients will generally find that health-assessment procedures done in the intimate zone are accepted without argument or problem, provided that adequate information and justification have been given before the procedure and permission from the client has been professionally requested and provided. The nurse should be aware that, for the most part, Russians prefer to remain at a social distance rather than an intimate distance with caregivers. If personal distance must be invaded to provide therapeutic assistance, the nurse should provide a careful explanation before the intervention to alleviate the stress and anxiety created by the violation of space. As with all aspects of care, it is important for the nurse to modify approaches based on an evaluation of the individual client and family.

SOCIAL ORGANIZATION

Family

Russian-American people are very family-oriented, and family relations and roles have a significant influence on them. In both Russia and the United States, extended family members often live together, relying on each other for financial and emotional support, child care, and completion of household tasks.

For the Russian American immigrant, who may have left loved ones to come to America, family members in the United States become even more significant. Therefore, Russian Americans are a very close-knit group. Within a few years after immigrating to the United States, Russian children tend to become rapidly assimilated into the American culture, leave home, and may even leave the

geographic area. Remaining family members are often elderly and lack job or language skills. Frequently, they isolate themselves from American contacts (Smith, 1996).

One Russian American explained that her children were also her best friends. Because she had so few other contacts, her son had become enormously important to her. In Russia, even in one- or two-room apartments, parents often live with married children and grandchildren, which may be one reason why Russian couples choose to have just one child. Also related to family size in Russia is the very large number of abortions performed each year. Though abortion rates are falling, Russian women are almost twice as likely to have an abortion as a live birth (National Center for Health Statistics, Health, United States, 2002). One reason for their reliance on abortion as nearly the only birth control method was lack of access to birth control devices and pharmaceuticals, and to birth control education. A history of multiple abortions may severely impact the health status of Russian American women.

Within the Russian family structure, the father tends to have the greatest influence. Children, especially male children, look up to the father and absorb his values and beliefs. Additionally, the husband of the household makes decisions on behalf of the family, though he does consult with his wife, especially when the wife is well educated. Women primarily care for children. Arguing and dish throwing may occur during family disagreements.

Education, family, and cultural activities are values that begin when children are infants. During social gatherings, children are often seen dancing with their parents. Fathers often walk arm in arm with a child through an art museum in an effort to instill an appreciation of history and culture. Children as young as 5 years of age learn to read classic literature and attend the ballet, opera, and concerts. Girls and boys are encouraged to achieve good grades in school and go on to college. For this reason, it has been especially difficult to understand recent trends in high school dropout rates among Russian American teens. In one Oregon-based study,

14% to 19% of Russian-speaking high school students quit school each year (Whites had a 5.7% dropout rate). Study authors reported that Russian students dropped out to earn money and do not feel challenged by classroom study (Russian kids, 2001). Similarly, Birman, Trickett, and Vinokurov (2002) found that acculturation to American culture predicted better grades and perceived support from the youth's American peers, and both American acculturation and Russian acculturation predicted less loneliness and better parental support. Comfort with the English language played a role in this American acculturation process. Trickett and Birman (2005) noted that greater American acculturation among Russian American teens predicted better grades and school belonging and fewer disciplinary infractions. Conversely, Jeltova, Fish, and Revenson (2005) found that recent young immigrants from the former Soviet Union had higher levels of risky sexual behavior (risks for unplanned pregnancy, HIV infection) with higher levels of American culture acculturation.

Most Russians are life-hardened people and come to the United States with few possessions, but they come full of the joy of life, which contributes to their success (Gromov, 2004–2005; Smith, 1991). Another factor contributing to success is that they have made immigration to the United States a family project. Russian Americans complain of feeling stifled and desperate in Russia. A "group" identity has been reinforced by the Russian problems they were forced to endure. Russians proudly express their unresolved questions of the meaning of personal existence and the reasons for their suffering. Theirs is a priority of spiritual values over material ones—the most cherished of all gifts are gifts of the spirit. The Russian cultural identity and love of wisdom and learning have been preserved and reborn (Gromov, 2004–2005). Therefore, a strong bond develops in Russian American communities because of similar backgrounds, culture, language, lifestyles, educational levels, and geographical core. Despite the ethnic bond found in many Russian American communities, Russian Jews have historically felt isolated from dominant Russian life and culture, and this heritage has helped to maintain a strong ethnic identity. Russian Americans rely on person-to-person networks and referrals.

The life of the elderly Russian immigrant can be difficult. In Russia, elders found important roles by helping support their children with child care and household duties, and, in return, Russian adult children cared for their parents. Once here in the United States, parents and children may withdraw from each other. Elders may represent the "old" country, the culture that no longer applies, and parents may lose their authority and family status (Azarian et al., 1996; Smith, 1996; Tran, Khatusky, Aroian, Balsam, & Conway, 2000). This is especially difficult when elders believe that children should accept what they are told without question. If Russian American children become the means for contact and communication because of their English competence, they will sense a reversal of power and authority over their parents. For the elderly, fears may increase because of concerns over the acculturation of their children and grandchildren (Tran et al., 2000). Because of language barriers and age, they may be unwilling and unable to restart their careers.

One Russian American explained, "In Russia, we gathered together many, many people at my house. We could talk endlessly about politics. Russians love to come together with friends and neighbors, forming a very close connection with each person we live and work with. But in the United States, everyone is very busy. They drive in separate cars, have separate houses, and separate neighborhoods. Americans watch television at home rather than go out to the theater or see friends. Here in America I am less social and my friends are few."

Individualism

Russian Americans are hardworking and have very little tolerance for people who do not have the wish to work and stay active. They are self-reliant and independent. Russian Americans who become ill will use home care, hospitalization, or both as much as possible rather than become a burden to their families. They have a strong desire to stay in their own homes and will remain independent until the last possible moment. Caring for aging and elderly parents is considered the duty and responsibility of all children. To place one's parent into a "home" is socially not allowed.

This strong individualism would appear to contradict the former Russian social structure, in which individual achievements were seen in terms of their value to the group. Strong individualism has been a common Russian American response to the forced Soviet collectivism endured in Russia. Being anti-Communists, Russian Americans tend to vote Republican (Gold, 1991). However, being a product of a society in which the individual was not valued, Russian Americans may resist committing anything to writing, fear taking responsibility for their actions (Barnathan, 1991), and find themselves underprepared for a way of life that depends on initiative, creativity, critical thinking, and responsibility (Alaniz, 2001; Brod & Heurtin-Roberts, 1992). One Russian American nurse explained, "Teamwork was the biggest change in terms of the work system. Here, I'm part of a team, but I still have independence. In the Russian system, you have the doctor ... making all the decisions but here I can decide the proper care until the point when I need to call the doctor" (Alaniz, 2001, p. 20).

Problems occur when the nurse or physician expects the Russian American to make independent decisions regarding self-care and self-help, especially when those decisions exclude concepts of holism. Many expect health care professionals to tell them what to do. Furthermore, care regimens will most likely be successful if the nurse includes client and family and presents health care goals as family goals (Azarian et al., 1996). One elderly Russian American explained, "You ask me to tell you all about my health problems. I shouldn't have to tell you—you are supposed to know what they are and then give me medicine to fix them."

Position of Women in the Family and in Society

Russian American women are not liberated at home. Although both husband and wife have full-time employment outside the home, most Russian men prefer to have their wives do the cooking, shopping, housework, and childrearing. Without timesaving conveniences such as microwave ovens, bread machines, washers, dryers, and vacuum cleaners, Russian women spend hundreds of hours a month on household responsibilities.

In Russia, although jobs for women are considered equal, salary and authority are not (Sandul, 2002). Women make up 47% of the working-age population in Russia. In post-Soviet Russia, the gender gap for salaries is growing. The average female worker makes only about 66% of what her male counterpart makes. Women are given positions where they perform secretarial and administrative duties but not positions needing important decisions (Sandul, 2002). The good news is that Russian women are very well educated. The percentage of employed women with at least some university education rose from 19% in 1992 to 27.8% in 2000, and 64% of all women attended higher education while only 50% of Russian men can boast that same level of education. Still, in Russia, women have fewer professional development opportunities than men (Sandul, 2002).

Unfortunately, with the fall of Communism, the percentage of women in government has decreased dramatically (as a result of the change in government-forced quotas). Besides unequal wages for Russian women, sex discrimination permeates Russian society. Hence, most Russian women need to learn assertiveness, positive self-esteem, and a new vision of their important societal role. It is interesting to note that the Russian language has no phrase for sexual harassment (Ross & Searing, 1992; Smith, 1996).

There has been a rapid increase in prostitution among young women in Russia. A current search on Google using "Russian girls" as keywords yielded 35,400,000 listed sites and when "mail order" was added, 10,200,000 sites were displayed. Many escort agencies and personal massage services for men opened within the first 6 months of 1992. With the relaxing of puritanical Communist mores, beautiful, obedient women have become status symbols for Russian men, and the Moscow newspapers are full of advertisements for these kinds of services. Russian women are also exploited via numerous Web sites that promote Russian brides and escorts. Tens of thousands of women from Russia are trafficked yearly all over the world, most especially to the United States. They are attractive, well educated, and desperate to leave a desperate country. Profit margins are high, and without passports or money, these women are easily victimized (Pope, 1997).

Spirituality and Religious Beliefs

Religion in Russia is mainly Eastern Orthodoxy. Until the eighteenth and nineteenth centuries in Russia, literacy was traditionally associated with the Russian Orthodox Church. Historically, the church was highly regarded by the people, mostly uneducated peasants, as a source of guidance, power, and salvation. This undoubtedly contributed to the manner in which the people bowed to authority (Billy, 1993).

Currently, about 20% of Russians are practicing Russian Orthodox and 10% to 15% are practicing Muslims. As a result of over 70 years of Soviet rule, Russia has a large number of nonpracticing believers as well as nonbelievers (CIA, 2006). One Russian American explained, "We were not raised with God; we made fun of the religious" (R. Feldman, personal communication, April 28, 1998).

In Russia, traditionally, Russian Jews could not own property or land, which may explain why many became merchants. As a result of this role, other Russian ethnic groups developed resentment and anti-Semitic feelings. With the relaxation of censorship and a new emphasis on Russian nationalism, there has been a resurgence of anti-Semitism.

Russian Jews immigrated to the United States and other countries in a greater percentage than non-Jewish Russian people. The greater the Jewish oppression and anti-Semitism in Russia, the greater was the rate of immigration. The immigration has led to further discrimination. New freedoms of speech and expression have brought out old, otherwise buried, prejudices. In this newfound climate, Russian Jews feel persecuted and often fear for their children.

Perestroika and *glasnost* changes, along with the dramatic fall of Communism in Russia, witnessed a resurgence of religious freedoms. Christianity has had a remarkable revival. The Russian Orthodox Church requires followers to observe fast days as well as a "no-meat" rule on Wednesdays and Fridays. During Lent, all animal products, including butter and other dairy products, are forbidden. Fasting also occurs during Advent. It is believed that God is served in a more powerful way during periods of fasting. However, even if fasting is strictly observed, special allowances are made for illness and pregnancy. Fear, sin, and punishment have been major themes for the Russian Orthodox Church.

After more than 70 years of war against religion, most Russians hope that the Orthodox Church will be able to positively influence the people's family, moral, and social values and consequently decrease the rate of divorce. As the Russian Orthodox Church attempts to reclaim state-confiscated churches and land, more and more Russians are returning to their once-hidden faith. Before *perestroika* and *glasnost*, religious expressions were prohibited in Russia. However, some churches did remain open. As a result, some people believed that Russian Orthodox Church leaders were obliged to report to the Secret Service and that confessions were not confidential. In addition, the training of Russian Orthodox priests was poor because of the general absence of good academic education programs. Today in Russia the church holds the power of hope for the many people who attend services. This hope is brief, strong, and desperate because of the hardship of Russian life, especially for the elderly.

Implications for Nursing Care

In all human societies, actions that are done for survival, such as eating, elimination, sex, and health practices, though physical, take on cultural and social regulations. Cultural functions and norms dictate behavior patterns in a profound way. It is essential for nurses to understand the role culture plays to provide safe, compassionate, and effective nursing care.

Despite persecution and hardships, Russian Americans maintain a significant degree of individualism. Russian American parents teach their children an appreciation for Russian land and country. One Russian immigrant explained, "Whether good or bad, it is still mine. I still love my homeland." Another Russian American said it this way: "I miss everything—my home, my language, my friends. Here, I am another personality. I am not me. I cannot say what I want because I don't know the right words. This makes me tired and frustrated. I want so much to visit Russia, my country." It is important for the nurse to understand that strong feelings of national pride are only experienced by some Russian immigrants.

Because Russian Americans have strong family ties and values, the nurse must remember to involve the entire family (especially important for teens), including extended family members, in the planning and intervention of care. Because the father and grandfather are perceived as having a paramount role and function in the Russian family, the astute nurse will solicit the opinions and advice of this patriarch before presenting a treatment and intervention plan to the rest of the family. In this instance, if the father's opinions and advice are solicited before the presentation to the rest of the family, the father may be of particular assistance in getting the family's cooperation and support. Because the entire Russian family becomes the client, time, respect, and information must be presented to the entire family.

Some Russian Americans hold particular beliefs in regard to religion, death, and dying. Therefore, it is important for the nurse to respect these beliefs and practices and incorporate them into a therapeutic plan of care that will assist the client in returning to a high level of wellness. Because of a belief that the human body is sacred, Russian Americans will be reluctant to donate organs. More important, the nurse needs to keep imminent death topics away from the terminally ill. Tell the head of the family first. "We choose to give mercy to the person; that person must not know that he or she will soon die. We don't need time to prepare a will because we have so few possessions to write wills about," replied one Russian woman.

Russian Americans, especially elders, tend to feel displaced and isolated. Nurses need to be extremely thorough in gathering data in the psychosocial and physical assessment. The nurse must also remember to expect visitors to Russian American clients. Russian Americans are accustomed to long discussions with friends, which they find socially and spiritually rewarding. Therefore, unless visitors become potentially harmful toward client outcomes, they should generally be permitted and supported.

TIME

Some Russian Americans hold a perspective of time that is past, present, and future oriented. For these people, there is a future within the present and a present within the past. On the other hand, some Russian Americans, particularly the well educated, hold only a future orientation. One example of this cultural attitude is seen in immigration.

Although the study of history and heritage is important to Russian Americans, most look to the future more than to the past, a characteristic related to socialism and Marxism. "Not now," such ideology preaches, "the future!" "Work hard now and have patience; suffer now so that the future will be better." Because living conditions in Russia for most immigrants were desperate, now they feel hope.

Another important example of future orientation is seen in the Russian people's almost universal belief in education for themselves and their children. Education begins early and is reinforced in the home. For Russian Americans who espouse a belief in future orientation, education is viewed as an awakening or a light. Lack of education is viewed as a void or darkness. Self-learning and life-long learning are valued and practiced. On immigration to the United States, Russian children are encouraged to attend school immediately, even before they have any knowledge of English. In fact, Russian children learn English very easily. It is obvious that present efforts are vehicles for future achievements.

Implications for Nursing Care

For the Russian American, the United States offers opportunities for goal establishment and attainment impossible in Russia. For some Russian immigrants who hold a time orientation that is a combination of past, present, and future beliefs, it is important for the nurse to remember that such an individual may be reluctant to seek preventive therapeutic interventions. The nurse must design and implement teaching strategies that will assist the client in developing an understanding about the implications of past and present behavior on future wellness and quality of life.

On the other hand, Russian immigrants who hold a future orientation value preventive therapeutic techniques that have long-range future benefits on wellness and wellness behavior. Because these individuals have a future orientation, the nurse will find it easier to encourage preventive screening techniques than with past-oriented individuals. In fact, the client may even request information on preventive techniques and their benefits. However, routine health mammograms and cholesterol checks were not practiced by Russian Americans in the Duncan and Simmons study (1996).

To a Russian American, punctuality is important, and arriving late for an appointment is considered rude. Therefore, the nurse must remember to keep appointments and be punctual because this will help build rapport and trust with the Russian American client. One Russian explained that to have been late for work under the former Soviet regime meant death; tardiness was considered sabotage of social goals.

ENVIRONMENTAL CONTROL

Locus of Control and Effect on Wellness and Illness Behaviors

The Russian culture instills in its members a belief that man has little control over nature. This external control is especially apparent in health care activities. Spiritually, however, Russian Americans with Russian Orthodox beliefs may have difficulty with current self-help practices. These beliefs center on ideas of Christ's teachings. It is believed that Christ will give as much help as is deserved in relation to the strength of the beliefs, which means that an ill person who is not recovering may somehow not have had enough faith. Illness in this sense is perceived as punishment. Russian Americans who

espouse these beliefs have an external locus of control.

In contrast, some Russian Americans believe that one can control both internal and external forces in the environment, thereby creating opportunities for high levels of wellness. This perception is regarded as an internal locus of control. When Russian Americans have an internal locus-of-control orientation, they are likely to have a unique self-care approach to wellness, illness, and hospitalization.

Russian Methods of Health Treatment

In Russia, *feldshers* deliver a great deal of primary health care. After 3 years of medical school, the feldsher is trained in basic preventive medicine, with a special focus on mothers and preschool children, in suturing, and in emergency care techniques. Some consider feldshers to be similarly placed in Russia as physician's assistants are placed in the U.S. When Russians are ill, they are expected to stay in bed and call the clinic. The physician or feldsher often makes a house call that same day, determines the severity of the problem, and makes a recommendation. Russians expect to be hospitalized.

Although the Russian health care system may lag behind that of the United States, preventive health care is identified as important. Russian people believe that physical screening is the answer to good health care and is widely accepted among Russian immigrants. Female Russian Americans are quite familiar with frequent and routine pelvic and Pap screenings, gastric acid tests, sedimentation rates, and prothrombin times. In contrast, however, they are unfamiliar or unaccepting of mammograms, routine breast examinations, and cholesterol screenings and state that the cholesterol findings are inconclusive and of little or no value.

Other Russian health care alternatives sometimes used are charm men and barbershops. In the past, barbershops and other clinics were equipped to do a procedure called "cupping," which was used primarily for the treatment of respiratory tract disorders. In this procedure, cups with the approximate appearance of a large shot glass are heated, placed up and down the back, and left in place for about 10 minutes. Believed to extract evil humors from the body, the cups leave ecchymosis-like marks that may last for days. Cupping is a technique currently taught to Russian nursing students and is still practiced in some Russian American communities. In addition to cupping, Russian Americans often turn to alternative systems of care: Russian holistic healers, Russian physicians unable to practice in the United States, Russian medications (Azarian et al., 1996), and Russian-based herbal remedies.

One concern Russian Americans have is that the U.S. medicine system lacks a powerful emphasis on prevention. One Russian American responded:

Too many pills. Pills for everything without a clear reason. In Russia, physicians make house calls. If I have a fever, I will stay home, and the doctor will come. This is why United States doctors consider Russians as crying too much and complaining too much. We are used to less intensive medicine. Here, I need to call for an appointment, and it's 1 month away. In Russia we have more alternative medical therapies—the whole cleansing of the body of toxins, massages, acupressure, and acupuncture. In our hospitals, we have prescribed massages. Here, the doctors don't even consider alternative medicine or any Oriental medical practice.

Folk Medicine

Russian immigrants, especially the elderly, may still practice some homeopathic or folk medicine. For example, one client had an amber necklace from Riga and refused to allow treatment for a thyroid condition. The client stated, "Those pills make me sick. My necklace will cure everything with my thyroid except cancer." However, when laboratory work indicated her condition was worsening, she accepted medication (Ruby, 1989). Besides being worn as jewelry, amber is ground into a powder, added to hot water, and used as a kind of medicinal potion.

Other home remedies include herbs, which are prepared as drinks or enemas, and charcoal in water, which is ingested for the treatment of stomach acidity. Hot steam baths are considered healthful for pneumonia and upper respiratory tract infections. Mineral water and plasters are also used. Because of their belief in the healing qualities of mineral water, emerging Russian health care providers are using products that are rich in these properties.

Russian Americans strongly believe in the usefulness of massage. This philosophy seems to stem from a kind of chiropractic idealism related to the spine and back (Avakyan, 1990). In addition, orthopedic shoes for foot or leg pain are commonly used.

Some Russian Americans use dry heat for the treatment of back pain. Others use a raw dough of dark rye flour and honey that is placed on the spinal column. Another back remedy is a loosely knit or compacted pad made of rough, coarse wool or animal hair, which is placed directly on the bare skin in the lower back region.

Headaches are often treated with a strong ointment placed behind the ears and temples and along the back of the neck. For the treatment of rhinitis, Russian Americans may extract raw onion juice and place several drops in each naris with a medicine dropper. A cold may be treated by immersion of both legs in hot water containing strong salts. Sore throats are said to be relieved by a salt and baking soda gargle. Leech therapy is still widely taught and practiced in Russia. Leeches are particularly useful because of the anesthetic, vasodilatation, and anticoagulant properties of leech saliva (Smith, 2000). Leeches are successfully used to treat angina, migraine headaches, and poor circulation to digits or limbs.

Health is seen as the greatest of all gifts and goals. Russians will define health as a mental, physical, and spiritual harmony, the greatest of which is spiritual. One religious requirement is that male Russian Jews are circumcised. Illness, in contrast, is defined as disharmony among body systems. Body systems are blended and functioning as God created them to be, with each part doing its job in perfect interrelatedness. When the mind is troubled, the body will respond negatively. Holistic medicine is a way of life for Russians, through the use of cosmic energy work. Spirituality carries a very important place in Russian medicine. Russians believe a terminally ill person should never be told the prognosis. They believe such disclosure would increase anxiety, decrease hope, and hasten death. This may be changing. The first hospice in Russia opened in Moscow in 1997. During the first two weeks of operation, an honest, sensitive approach overcame communication difficulties related to cultural norms of prognosis disclosure and palliative care (Becker, 1999).

Practices at the Time of Death

Russian families with members who have recently died often keep vigil over the coffin for hours. The family members must wear black. The deceased person is washed, dressed, and placed in the coffin before the wake and funeral. Mourners pool their money to make sure men are dressed in suits and women have fine dresses. There are no funeral homes in Russia, so families must bear the weight of every aspect of the funeral. A black wreath may be placed on the door of the deceased person's home. At the funeral, a priest (if the family is Catholic or Russian Orthodox) places holy oil on the forehead while making the sign of the cross. A paper band is placed on the forehead with this prayer: "Oh God, Father, be merciful to thy servant (name) and accept into thy fold (name)." Each member of the grieving family places a few symbolic grains of soil onto the coffin. Mourners carry carnations, often placing them on the body prior to burial. Russian Orthodox beliefs dictate that friends and family pray for the deceased from the ninth to the fortieth day after death because until the ninth postmortem day, the soul remains with the body. On the ninth day, it begins its journey either to heaven or hell, depending on the consideration given to all the sins committed (Lally, 2000). Immediately after the burial, friends and family return to the host home and enjoy food and liquor in honor of the deceased. One traditional dish is rice with raisins.

Implications for Nursing Care

The nurse should be aware that Russian American clients find the way in which health professionals relate somewhat different from that to which they are accustomed. Traditionally, American physicians and nurses have been taught to have a nondirective, listening approach to client interactions. This approach is unsatisfactory for Russian immigrants, who seem to need almost immediate information and answers. Subjective symptoms may be difficult to assess because of lack of information presented by the client and the tendency to somatize emotional problems. Psychological disorders were rarely appropriately attended to by the Russian health care system.

Russian Americans are nearly 100% compliant with follow-up medical appointments, if they fully understand and believe in the health care instructions. Generally, Russian Americans are respectful and admire their physicians and nurses. They ask appropriate questions and accept what they are told. Russian Americans do not, however, often use walk-in or emergency services. Usually, Russian Americans will call the physician and wait until he or she is available, a practice that is based on their medical experiences in Russia. Furthermore, Russian Americans are not used to medical gatekeepers. American health care professionals have expressed their belief that Russian Americans, especially elders, use and abuse health care services (Aroian, Khatutsky, Tran, & Balsam, 2001; Kravitz et al., 2000). These attitudes result from cultural incompetence and culturally incongruent care. To know Russian American clients is to admire, respect, and validate their courage, intelligence, and unique cultural backgrounds and experiences.

Russian Americans tend to comply with most medical directives, doing whatever is needed to get well and stay independent. However, some Russian Americans may stop taking medications with any sign of a side effect, even if the side effect is unrelated. This is particularly noted with psychotropic drugs. The nurse may also notice a kind of cancer phobia among elderly Russian immigrants, who seem to have an "if it isn't broken, don't fix it" philosophy in relation to screenings for stool guaiac tests, sigmoidoscopies, and mammograms. Diagnostic tests are often refused, resulting in lack of early detection (Ruby, 1989; Vadlamani, Maher, Shaete, et al., 2001). Russian families may further complicate care by forbidding health care professionals from disclosing a cancer diagnosis to loved ones. However, the concept of "do not resuscitate" or hospice care can be a significant problem for Russian family members who are unable to understand not doing everything possible for a loved one.

Unless directly harmful, nurses need to remain open to alternative therapies and medications. It is important that nurses ask for information regarding alternative health care practices that may be practiced. Many traditional Russian medications are available and frequently purchased through the Internet and used. Several large pharmaceutical firms in New York cater to Russian clients in Russian. Russian Americans use the Internet. As evidence, new sites (for example, http://www.rulist.com) have surfaced that list Yellow Pages directories for *family, children, health/wellness,* and many other important topics to Russian Americans. The sites can be accessed in English or Russian. Additionally, Russian Americans can locate Russian-speaking dentists and physicians by using the search tool available at http://www.russiandoctor.com (state/city, specialty) in Russian or English. The *Health Magazine* journal, written in Russian and available online, reports to have a strong commitment to increasing the medical awareness of the Russian-speaking population in the U.S. The Russian American Medical Association (members include physicians, nurses, dentists, and students) also has a Web site with news and articles (http://www.russiandoctors.org/).

BIOLOGICAL VARIATIONS

Body Size

Obesity is especially common among elderly Russian women. This problem is attributed to the lack of fresh fruits and vegetables in Russia. Many culturally preferred foods are high in saturated fats and salt. Many Russian people retain their traditional dietary preferences and, as a result, overuse of saturated fats and salt and underuse of healthy fats, often continues after immigration to the United States. The incidence of overweight adults between ages 25 and 64 years in Russia is about 50% for men and 42% to 60% for women (Marquez, 2005), depending on the region. Duncan and Simmons (1996) found that 65% of their study population was obese. Mehler and associates (2001) also

found an overweight study population. Stature and skin color among Russian Americans are quite similar to those of other White American clients seen by the health care provider because most Russians are White. Even the Russians of Tarta descent have a Europeoid appearance, with any Mongoloid elements being mostly diluted (Hurwitz, 2005).

Enzymatic Variations

Russian Americans do not have problems with hypervitaminosis or hypovitaminosis, and, biochemically, laboratory parameters are the same (Gennis, 1989). Russian Americans do not have diabetes at greater rates than other Americans, nor do Russians have diabetes at greater rates than the rest of the world's population. The one exception is that the cholesterol levels of Russian Americans are generally well above normal (Mehler et al., 2001; Marquez, 2005).

Susceptibility to Disease

Hypertension. Blood pressure screening is routine in Russia. Russian Americans are keenly aware of the causes and effects of hypertension and will identify themselves as either hypertensive or borderline hypertensive. Russian Americans are often very hypertensive, theorized by Mehler and his colleagues (2001) to be due to hyperlipidemia (60% of Russian adults are considered to have high cholesterol levels), obesity, and a diet high in salt and animal fats. Deaths from noncommunicable diseases in Russia account for 70% of all deaths. Russia's cardiovascular disease deaths were 994 per 100,000 population, one of the highest rates in the world—nearly 52% of all deaths, compared to 38% of U.S. deaths). For Russian Americans, especially those recently arrived from Russia, these mortality rates due to cardiovascular disease continue (Mehler et al., 2001; Marquez, 2005).

Tuberculosis. Tuberculosis (TB) exposure has also been noted more often among Russian Americans than in the general populace. TB is rapidly spreading across Russia (including the wealthier and more stable middle and upper classes) because of a debilitated health system, a significant HIV/AIDS infection rate, political instability, prophylaxis resistance, infected prison populations spilling into communities (Russian TB, 1999; USAID, 2005), and an indifference to end it by the medical establishment (TB epidemic, 1998). Two areas of real concern are cases of multidrug- resistant TB cases, at 8.3% of new cases, and the prisoners who have TB rates over 40 times greater than the general public (USAID, 2005).

Cancer. In Russia, respiratory cancers account for 2.4% of all deaths; cancers of the stomach, colon, and rectum account for 3.5% of total deaths (Marquez, 2005). Pomerleau, Gilmore, McKee, Rose, and Haerpher (2004) noted that smoking is a major public health issue in the former Soviet Union, particularly affecting socially vulnerable men and young women living in urbanized areas and with implications for cancer development. Gilmore, Pomerleau, McKee, Rose, Haerpher, Rotman, and Tumanov (2004) reported that the increase in smoking rates among women appears to be related to tobacco company advertising.

After studying the differences in somatic mutation, based on an analysis of peripheral blood lymphocytes, Jones, Thomas, Tucker, et al. (1995) found that because of chronic exposure to environmental toxins, including smoking, DDT-like pesticides, and the Chernobyl nuclear power plant accident, the mutation frequency in Russians was higher; in addition, Russians have a higher risk of health consequences because of accumulated genetic damage. The population of adult Russians accumulated genetic damage at a 250% higher rate than that of Americans. The research work of Vadlamani and colleagues (2001) seems to concur with these findings. These researchers found a high rate of colorectal neoplasms, much higher than control groups or U.S. national averages, for their Russian American study subjects. They recommend greater care and vigilance, with more aggressive cancer screening, for this population group.

Dental Needs

Most Russian Americans tend to value dental care because traditionally they have had access to dental care and often have bridges and removable plates.

Russians in Virginia identified dental health as a major priority, with more than 75% self-identifying as having dental problems (Duncan & Simmons, 1996). There are only 32 dentists for every 100,000 people in Russia (WHO, 2006a).

Eye Care Needs

Because eye care and eye surgery traditionally received a great deal of Russian money and attention, most Russians have had access to eye care.

Nutritional Preferences and Deficiencies

The Russian immigrant who has come from a rural district will prefer to eat cabbage, buckwheat, millet, barley, and bread, along with sour milk and salted pork (if the person is non-Jewish). Russian bread is a kind of heavy rye bread that can weigh as much as 12 pounds per loaf. Salted meats are usually kept in a barrel and stored all winter in a kind of fruit cellar. Meat, as a delicacy, may be severely rationed. Thus, most Russians respect food and handle it with great care. Not a single morsel of food, especially meat, is wasted.

Psychological Characteristics

Illness and Wellness Behaviors. Many Russian American people believe that American medicine is the best in the world. Russian Americans, accustomed to home visits by health care workers in Russia, would like to have U.S. physicians and nurses provide home care when possible. In emergency departments, some Russian Americans may become frustrated by the voluminous paperwork required to establish financial competence, including Medicaid and Medicare sources. Mehler and colleagues (2001) reported that though 71% of their Denver-based sample ($n = 204$) had Medicaid insurance, 14% were medically indigent. Moreover, older Russian American people may consider the medical system a natural place for seeking help. For these immigrants, the clinic and its staff are viewed in a social context. Russian Americans, familiar with making loud demands to receive care in Russia, may appear pushy, manipulative, abrasive, and excessive.

Having endured a lifetime of poor medical care, poor nutrition, and continued frustration, elderly Russian Americans also have a higher number of somatic complaints than other groups the nurse may encounter (Gutkovich, Rosenthal, Galynker, et al., 1999; Tran et al., 2000). These complaints may be caused partially by the cultural stigma of psychiatric illness and treatment by "just talking." Russian Americans do not trust psychiatrists, psychologists, or other counseling services. Thus they may magnify aches and pains disproportionately to their primary care providers rather than describe an emotional problem (Brod & Heurtin-Roberts, 1992; Tran et al., 1999). Azarian, Boland, and Skripchenko (1996) and Tran, Khatusky, Aroian, Balsam, and Conway (2000) also noted expression of psychosocial problems, such as depression, through somatic complaints.

Russian clients have commonly related complaints, such as pain, paresthesia, vertigo, anorexia, hysteria, fatigue, and gastrointestinal distress, to a disease. Unfortunately, these diseases were sometimes present but have not been adequately treated.

Russian Americans tend to perceive health care professionals as high-status people. Feelings of poor self-concept are lifted when attention is received; for example, "I must have some worth if a high-status person pays attention to me." Russian Americans may thus seek health care as a social exercise to increase feelings of worth.

Russian Americans generally have many important health-promoting behaviors. For example, Russian Americans usually do not smoke, drink alcohol excessively (Mehler et al., 2001), or engage in violent crime. Having been accustomed to media portrayals of average people doing extraordinary deeds, Russian Americans long for high-quality newspapers and television programs that provide enthusiasm and inspiration for them. Russian Americans are familiar with hard work and difficulties, but most enjoy American freedoms and believe in the future. Azarian and colleagues (1996) described a common saying among Russian immigrants: "Every US newcomer should bring with him two stones. During the first two years, he will hit his head with one stone saying, 'Why did I come to this country?' The second one he will use afterwards saying, 'Why did I come here so late?'" (p. 324). Gottlieb (1990) wrote of an interview with a Russian American who proclaimed, "This is land of achievable dreams. If you want something and you are willing to work hard for it, you can get it. . . . I have my pride, and I am going somewhere."

Mental Health. In Russia, citizens with mental disorders could expect years of prison-like hospitalization under the influence of potent mind-numbing drugs. Psychiatric wards contained many clients who had refused military service (Langone, 1989; Pope, 1996). Russian citizens who tried to evangelize others, organize labor unions, or speak out against Communist dogma were perceived as state enemies, labeled as insane, and hospitalized in prison-like psychiatric facilities. This practice was scorned by the rest of the world's psychiatric community, who found the diagnosis of "sluggish schizophrenia" used in Russia to describe these persons very objectionable. Hospitalization occurred despite Soviet law, which stated that citizens could be forcibly hospitalized only if they displayed signs of deep depression, were suicidal, or threatened the lives of others.

There are indications that such psychiatric practices changed after the mid-1980s. In 1987 the May 1 issue of *Psychiatric News* carried a report of a change in policy in the USSR regarding psychiatric treatment and treatment of the homeless (APA representatives, 1987). Apparently, Soviet psychiatrists were trying to improve their tarnished image by releasing political prisoners and placing psychiatry under the governance of the Ministry of Health rather than the Ministry of Internal Affairs (police) (Langone, 1989). Traditional Russian psychiatric therapies included hydrotherapy, physiotherapy, insulin therapy, inhalation therapy, work therapy, and drug therapy (Hess, 1971). Further evidence of this shift has been the exchange of training and information with Russian psychiatric nurses (Bloor et al., 2004). Though Russian psychiatric institutions are underfunded, goals to improve services and move into more holistic care for the mentally ill have been established.

In the United States, the most common mental health problem diagnosed in Russian Americans is depression. Working in a primary care setting, Gutkovich and colleagues (1999) found 82% of their sample reporting psychological distress, and of these 82%, 53% were clinically depressed. Importantly, these researchers excluded all persons with known mental or terminal disorders.

Though relocating to a new nation and unfamiliar culture is enormously stressful for any immigrant group, this problem is identified primarily in elderly Russian immigrants who traveled with their children to the United States. They are unfamiliar with the language and customs, have left home and family, and often can get only minimum-wage jobs because of their age. Even after a mental diagnosis is given, they may remain reluctant to adhere to antidepressant drugs because of a fear of such medications in general and a reluctance to experience any side effects. Because of decreased emotional, physical, and financial resources and the realities of illnesses that may accompany aging, including impaired mobility, diabetes, and heart disease, older Russian American immigrants are at great risk for depression. Many Russian immigrants experienced a lifetime of stress, including two world wars, political turmoil and fear, religious persecution, poor health care, financial problems, and nutritional deficits. Often dependent on family or themselves for the first time in their lives, older Russian Americans may feel noncontributive, depressed, helpless, isolated, and demoralized (Azarian et al., 1996; Brod & Heurtin-Roberts, 1992; Gutkovich et al., 1999; Smith, 1996; Tran et al., 2000).

Alcoholism. In Russia, alcoholism is a major and growing national health problem. Alcoholism, since the Soviet Union breakup, is worsening because of the chronic stress of unstable prices, inflation, unsafe living and working conditions, and social upheavals. Unfortunately, two groups hit hardest by increased alcoholism are women and teenagers. Approximately 70% of men, 47% of women, and 30% of teens are considered drinkers; the morbidity and mortality due to alcohol consumption are greater in poor rural areas (Marquez, 2005).

Since the collapse of the Soviet Union, alcoholism has taken a severe toll on the nation's productivity and health. Alcohol addiction contributes to traffic fatalities, domestic violence, and industrial accidents (Marquez, 2005). One *Seattle Times* news article (Study: Russian men, 2000) indicated that two thirds of Russian men die drunk: "Everyone is drunk: murderers and their victims, drowning victims, suicides, drivers and pedestrians killed in traffic accidents, victims of heart attacks and ulcers" (p. A21).

Although alcoholism is an enormous problem in Russia, it has not emerged as a significant mental health problem among Russian American immigrants. A plausible explanation is that Russian immigrants want to survive in the United States, and Russian alcoholics stay in Russia; Russian alcoholics have lost hope and vision (Williams, 1992). Another reason for the low rate of alcoholism is the religious sanctions on alcohol consumption among Jewish and Christian Pentecostal groups. In addition, Russian Americans do not generally use illegal drugs, which might lead to promiscuous sexual behavior. Perhaps the lack of these self-abuse problems is attributable to attitudes and values, an internal locus of control, high levels of education, future orientation, and the cohesiveness of this skewed Russian population. Unfortunately, because Russian Jews did not drink in the homeland, they were often ridiculed and further ostracized by Russian society.

Radiation Accidents and Toxic Pollution

Environmental pollution in the Commonwealth of Independent States is a growing concern for its European and Asian neighbors. It has also been a major health problem for Russians as a result of polluted air and contaminated soil, food, and water. Unfortunately, Communism and an indiscriminate industrialization policy left Russia and the other former Soviet republics too poor and disorganized to fix the massive pollution problems. Much of Russia's air pollution has been caused by industrial waste, and motor vehicle emissions are becoming an increasing problem. With few to no regulations, lead, carbon monoxide, and nitrogen oxide are entering the environment. As more and more vehicles are on Russian roads, this problem will worsen. More than 50,000 square miles of land were radioactively contaminated after the 1986 Chernobyl disaster (Prokhorov, 1990; Stanglin & Pope, 1992). Russian nuclear reactors have been called old, huge time bombs. The Chernobyl disaster, according to the U.S. Department of Energy, will cause an additional 6000 deaths in the European community over the next 50 years (Hofheinz, 1992). Within the last decade, the disastrous results of Soviet industrialization policies have been realized, and awareness regarding the need for environmental protections have yielded important policy changes. This is due to international pressure, especially from the European Union, as well as the hope of the Russian people to reduce or eliminate existing problems (EIA, 2004).

Implications for Nursing Care

American nurses quickly recognize that Russian Americans are very friendly, generous, interesting, likable, intelligent, and well educated. The nurse should be aware, however, that Russian immigrants might be very skeptical of psychiatric services because psychiatric treatment often appears similar to persecution. Education about psychiatric symptoms and the modalities of treatment available in the United States are an essential part of a psychosocial intervention strategy. The client and the family should believe that they are participants and decision makers in treatment selections and strategies.

The nurse who cares for Russian Americans must be aware of possible nutritional implications for nursing care. Because very recent immigrants may be unable to tolerate American foods, the nurse would be wise to introduce new foods slowly. Religious dietary restrictions may also be a concern. Additionally, nutritional deficits such as anemia and goiter must be identified and immediately treated with dietary and medical supplements.

Although alcoholism is not a reported problem among Russian Americans, residual effects of alcoholism, whether physiological or psychological, must be looked for in individuals and families.

In addition, the nurse must assist Russian American clients in identifying culturally sanctioned coping strategies that will reduce anxiety and tension, depression, and low self-worth, thereby reducing the potential for mental health disorders.

Large numbers of Russian Americans are hypertensive. The nurse should use motivational strategies to devise teaching techniques that emphasize the benefits of dietary restraints, weight control, and adequate exercise. In addition, the Russian American client who is hospitalized for hypertension needs to appreciate the importance of medication adherence and timely reporting of all unusual and untoward signs and symptoms.

Although undocumented in current literature, Russian Americans may be suffering physically and psychologically from the ill effects of water, air, and land pollution. The nurse should be keenly alert to these possible effects and assess clients accordingly.

For Russian Americans, U.S. nurses and primary care physicians represent the frontline liaison to a whole array of social and medical benefits. Russian immigrants tend to expect the health care professional to provide social and financial as well as medical services for them. If medical benefits are financially available, as in many Russian Jewish immigrant groups, this may not be a severe problem. However, many Russian Americans arrive without the ability to access appropriate health care services. If they are underpaid or unemployed, Russian immigrants may not have any insurance coverage. The nurse must also understand that Russian Americans are a very proud and noble people, perhaps too proud to go on public assistance. One response offered by the Russian immigrant may be, "If I am sick, I'll have to go back to Russia to get care." Therefore, as a resource liaison, the nurse should identify and facilitate access to all possible health and assistance programs, keeping vigilance over possible exploitation.

SUMMARY

As nurses transcend their own cultural mindset, they learn to celebrate and use cultural uniqueness as an indicator for nursing interventions. Among experiences that are assisting nurses in gaining transcultural perspectives are transcultural educational experiences, such as those offered by the United States–Russian Nurse Exchange Consortium Organization. Since 1993 this group has sponsored more than 24 exchanges of health care professionals between the United States and Russia.

In addition to gaining an understanding of persons in other cultures, the nurse must gain the knowledge to provide culturally appropriate care to immigrant clients. Complexity, variety, and cultural diversity contribute to the nurse's challenge, responsibility, and enjoyment while caring for Russian Americans.

Case Study

Victor and Vera have immigrated to Milwaukee, Wisconsin, from St. Petersburg, the second largest city in Russia. They are Jewish and believe that the strong anti-Semitism they felt in Russia had become unbearable. Their only alternative, they decided, was to leave the country and join relatives in Milwaukee. Mt. Sinai Samaritan Medical Center offered 1 year of free health care to them when they arrived. Now, 3 years later, Victor and Vera continue to seek services at this large teaching hospital and clinic. Victor and Vera are both 58 years old, and Vera speaks very little English. Victor has found a new peer group at the brewery, his place of employment. However, Vera has been unable to find work and prefers to stay near family and friends. Milwaukee Jewish Family Services has been minimally successful in involving Vera in social activities. Vera reads and sits in her chair most of the day. Recently, she has become more withdrawn, with an overwhelming feeling of sadness and loneliness for her native land. She regrets immigrating and has focused her bitter feelings inward.

A painful venous occlusion brings Vera to the health clinic, where the nurse examines her lower extremities and finds swelling, tenderness, edema, and a positive Homan's sign on Vera's left leg. A health history is difficult because of the language barrier, but with the help of Victor and a professional health care interpreter, the nurse learns about Vera's sedentary lifestyle, high-fat and high-cholesterol diet, and recent episodes of sadness. Victor is supportive but impatient for his wife to "get back on her feet again." Vera says very little.

On laboratory examination, Vera's plasma low-density lipoprotein cholesterol level is 240 mg/dL. Left ventricular hypertrophy is noted on the electrocardiogram. Vera is obese and has a blood pressure of 180/116 mm Hg. Slight hemorrhages of the retinas are also noted.

Vera is presented with two medical diagnoses: symptomatic hypertension and clinical depression. The nurse realizes that Vera's dietary instructions need to be presented with great care and attention given to cultural habits and beliefs. The nurse shows Vera an extensive list of "good" foods (written in Russian) and asks her to identify her favorites. With Vera's help and the help of the culturally competent dietitian, the nurse works out a weekly menu. The nurse must also teach Vera specific techniques for controlling her hypertension. Vera is instructed to take her own weight and blood pressure every morning, record them on a graph, and bring the graphs with her for her every-other-week clinic visits. It is explained to Vera that she will need to diligently follow medication, dietary, and exercise regimens to decrease her risk of further disability. Vera is especially motivated to help herself because of her fear of losing her eyesight and thus being unable to read (her favorite pastime). Walking is encouraged after Vera's leg becomes asymptomatic.

After all instructions are repeated carefully and slowly several times (Russian and English), Vera is escorted into a private office. The nurse, who has known Vera for 3 years, asks her about her sadness and isolating behaviors. Vera adamantly rejects the nurse's suggestion that she see a psychiatric consultant.

The nurse understands that a few important psychosocial questions could include: Who do (did) you turn to for help and hope? How is that different (the same) now that you are in the United States? What part in your life does religion play? What was life like in Russia? How is your life different now? What is the most significant difference? What do you miss (not miss) the most about Russia? What were the decisions that brought you to the United States? Help us understand what it's like to leave everything you have ever known—language, culture, friends, family—to come to the United States. I know a great deal about medicine and being a nurse, but I do not know all that you know about getting healthy. From your perspective, what important information do I need to best help you help yourself?

CARE PLAN

✳ *Nursing Diagnosis: Imbalanced nutrition: more than body requirements (animal fat, salt), related to excessive intake in relation to metabolic need.*

Client Outcomes

1. Client will decrease her weight by 4 pounds per month.
2. Client will walk 2 miles per day (after leg has healed).
3. Client will learn to swim and will swim twice weekly at the Jewish Activity Center.

Nursing Interventions

1. Teach client about importance of exercise.
2. Teach client about menu planning in relation to avoidance of high-salt, high-fat foods.
3. Encourage and support compliance with medications, exercise, diet, and follow-up care.

✳ *Nursing Diagnosis: Individual coping, ineffective, related to chronic feelings of loneliness and isolation*

Client Outcomes

1. Client will attend social activities at Jewish Family Services twice a week.
2. Client will enroll in English at the Milwaukee Area Technical College (MATC).

Nursing Interventions

1. Introduce client to Jewish Family Services and involve Victor and other family members in relation to therapeutic adherence.
2. Arrange for client to visit the library of Russian books and journals located at Jewish Family Services.
3. Help client make initial contacts for classes in English as a second language held at MATC. (MATC is a short two-block walk from the clinic and hospital.)
4. Arrange transportation for client for all activities and clinic visits.

✳ *Nursing Diagnosis: Social isolation: related to inadequate personal resources.*

Client Outcome

1. Client will network with other Soviet immigrants.

Nursing Interventions

1. Encourage and support social networking; with Vera's permission, set up appointments with Russian-based self-help and social groups.
2. Respect and honor client's cultural preferences.
3. Provide Russian reading materials for client.
4. Introduce client to other Russian immigrants outside her family and follow up with kindness, caring, and honest concern.
5. Explore employment or volunteer opportunities with Vera, connecting her with available services at the Jewish Family Services Center.

✳ STUDY QUESTIONS

1. Why is it important that Vera's own list of foods be used when the nurse is creating a weekly menu?
2. How will the nurse keep Vera motivated toward self-help and self-care?
3. What role will Vera's family play in her recovery?
4. During client teaching, how much space should be between the nurse and Vera?
5. How may the nurse use Vera's spiritual values and beliefs to the best advantage?
6. What role does language play in this nurse–client relationship?
7. In addition to what is listed in the care plan, how else might the nurse increase Vera's self-esteem and decision-making potential?
8. When talking with Vera, what should the nurse be careful not to do?
9. How may Vera's attitudes toward self-learning and life-long learning enhance nursing care strategies?
10. Why did Vera adamantly refuse psychiatric consultation? What should the nurse do now?

NCLEX-RN REVIEW QUESTIONS

1. When communicating with Russian American clients, it is important for the nurse to address the client by:
   A. Mr. or Mrs. followed by last name.
   B. First name only
   C. Terms of endearment
   D. Using a friendly outgoing manner

2. When caring for a Russian American client the nurse should be aware that, for the most part, Russians prefer:
   A. To remain at an intimate distance rather than a social distance with caregivers
   B. To remain at a social distance rather than an intimate distance with caregivers
   C. That health assessment procedures be done in the intimate zone
   D. That boundaries are open between internal and external environments

3. When assessing Russian American clients, the nurse should use a direct approach to client interaction because the Russian client:
   A. Is used to home care by nurses and physicians
   B. Values the American medical system
   C. Believes in being direct
   D. Has a tendency for somatization of emotional problems

References

Alaniz, J. (2001, September 3). Crossing cultures: Russian nurses navigate the unfamiliar US health care system, finding career advantages and obstacles. *Nursing and Allied Healthweek*, 6(18), 20–21.

Anderson, J. (1992, Novermber 1). Two men clashed and a nation rose. *Parade Magazine*, p. 10.

Andriouchina, E. (2002, July 11–14). *Health of the population of Russia under the transition*. Paper presented at the meeting of the First International Conference on Economics and Human Biology in Tubingen.

APA representatives meet with Soviets to discuss abuse of psychiatry in USSR. (1987, May 1). *Psychiatric News*, p. 37.

Aroian, K. J., Khatutsky, G., Tran, T. V., & Balsam, A. L. (2001). Health and social service utilization among elderly immigrants from the former Soviet Union. *Journal of Nursing Scholarship*, 33(3), 265–271.

Aslund, A. (2001, July–August). Think again: Russia. *Foreign Policy: The Magazine of Global Politics, Economics, and Ideas*. Retrieved June 9, 2002, from http://www.foreignpolicy.com/issue_julyaug_2001/tajulyaug.html.

Avakyan, G. N. (1990). Pressure and massage therapy to relieve fatigue. *Advancing Clinical Care*, 5(5), 12–11.

Azarian, A., Boland, R. J., & Skripchenko, V. (1996). Providing health care for the Russian-speaking patient. *Medicine and Health*, 79(9), 323–327.

Barnathan, J. (1991, November 4). The Russians aren't coming. They're here. *Business Week*, p. 100.

Becker, R. (1999). Adult/elderly care nursing. Teaching communication with the dying across cultural boundaries. *British Journal of Nursing*, 8(14), 938–942.

Billy, C. (1993). *Fodor's Russia and the Baltic countries.* New York: Random House.

Binyon, M. (1983). *Life in Russia.* New York: Berkley.

Birman, D., Trickett, E. J., & Vinokurov, A. (2002). Acculturation and adaptation of Soviet Jewish refugee adolescents: predictors of adjustment across life domains. *American Journal of Community Psychology*, 30(5), 585–607.

Bloor, R., McHugh, A., Pearson, D., & Wain, I. (2004). A training course for psychiatric nurses in Russia. *Nursing Standard*, 18(39), 39–41.

Briman, D., & Trickett, E. J. (2001). Cultural transitions in first-generation immigrants: acculturation of Soviet Jewish refugee adolescents and parents. *Journal of Cross-Cultural Psychology*, 32(4), 456–477.

Brod, M., & Heurtin-Roberts, S. (1992). Older Russian émigrés and medical care. *Western Journal of Medicine*, 157(3), 333–336.

Burgermeister, J. (2003). Three quarters of Russia's prisoners have serious diseases. *British Medical Journal*, 327(7423), 1066.

Burlatsky, F. (1991). Coming and going in the USSR. *Soviet Life*, 7(418), 14, 45.

Carpenter, D. (1997, April 21). Victims of change, homeless children pose new troubles for reformed Russia. *The Greenville News*, p. 4A.

Centers for Disease Control and Prevention (CDC). (2002, March 27). *NCHS: 1999 fact sheet.* Retrieved July 12, 2002, from http://www.cdc.gov/nchs/releases/99facts/russian.htm.

Central Intelligence Agency (CIA). (2001). *The world factbook: Russia.* Retrieved July 5, 2002, from http://www.cia.gov/cia/publications/factbook/geos/rs.html.

Central Intelligence Agency (CIA). (2006, June 13). *The world factbook: Russia.* Retrieved June 24, 2006, from https://www.cia.gov/cia/publications/factbook/geos/rs.html.

Commonwealth of Independent States (CIS). (2006). *Database statistics of the CIS.* Interstate Statistical Committee of the Commonwealth of Independent States. Retrieved June 24, 2006, from https://www.cis-stat.com/eng/cis.htm.

Danishevski, K., Balabanova, D., McKee, M., & Atkinson, S. (2006). The fragmentary federation: experiences with the decentralized health system in Russia. *Health Policy and Planning*, 21(3), 183–194.

Duncan, L., & Simmons, M. (1996). Health practices among Russian and Ukrainian immigrants. *Journal of Community Health Nursing*, 13(2), 129–137.

Energy Information Administration (EIA). (2004, May). *Russia: Environmental issues.* Energy Information Administration official energy statistics from the US government. Retrieved June 25, 2006, from https://www.eia.doe.gov/emeu/cabs/russenv.html.

Eight attempts reported on Yeltsin's life. (1993, February 20). *The Journal Times*, p. 4A.

Engleman, E. (2002, March 22). *Experts warn Russia's fight against TB is far from over* (Associated Press). Retrieved June 9, 2002, from http://www.cdi.org/russia/johnson/6153-7.cfm.

Ethnic population (2003, July 30). Russian-American Advertising, Brooklyn, N.J.: *Media and Information Services,* Brooklyn N.Y. Retrieved June 25, 2006, from www.inforeklama.com/contacts.htm.

Farmer, R. G., Sirotkin, A. Y., Ziganshina, L. E., & Greenberg, H. M. (2003). The Russian health care system today: can American-Russian CME programs help? *Cleveland Clinic Journal of Medicine*, 70(11), 937–938, 941–942, 944.

Feldman, R. (1998, April 28). Personal communication.

Gennis, M. (1989, September). Personal communication with assistant professor of medicine and program director of Internal Medicine, Sinai Samaritan Medical Center/University of Wisconsin.

Gilmore, A., Pomerleau, J., McKee, M., Rose, R., Haerpfer, C., Rotman, D., & Tumanov, S. (2004, December). Prevalence of smoking in 8 countries of the former Soviet Union: results from the living conditions, lifestyles, and health study. *American Journal of Public Health*, 12(2), 2177–2187.

Gold, S. (1991, November–December). Russian Jews in California. *Society*, pp. 76–80.

Gore-Felton, C., Somlai, A. M., Benotsch, E. G., Kelly, J. A., Ostrovski, D., & Kozlov, A. (2003). The influence of gender on factors associated with HIV transmission risk among young Russian injection drug users. *American Journal of Drug and Alcohol Abuse*, 29(4), 881–894.

Gottlieb, A. (1990, March). Coming to America. *McCalls*, 117, 70–79.

Gromov, M. N. (2004–2005). The eternal values of Russian culture: on the interpretation of our fatherland's philosophy. *Russian Studies in Philosophy*, 43(3), 90–100.

Gutkovich, Z., Rosenthal, R. N., & Galynker, I., et al, (1999). Depression and demoralization among Russian-Jewish immigrants in primary care. *Psychosomatics*, 40(2), 117–125.

Harrigan, S. (2001, July 2). "Child by child," group aids homeless street kids. Retrieved June 25, 2006, from www.familycare.org/network/e01_cnn_art2.htm/.

Hess, G. (1971). Impressions of mental health service delivery systems in Finland, Poland, Soviet Russia, and Czechoslovakia. *International Journal of Nursing Studies*, 8(4), 223–235.

Hill, R. (1992, March 3). Recession sours Soviet immigrants' first taste of capitalism. *The Washington Post*, pp. C1, C4.

Hofheinz, P. (1992, July 27). The new Soviet threat: pollution. *Fortune*, pp. 110–114.

Hurwitz, P. (2005, November–December). Readers letters: Scratching Tartas. *Russian Life*, 48(6), 5.

In the red. (1992, March 23). *New Yorker*, p. 25.

Ivanov, L. L., & Paganpegara, G. (2005, November–December). Public health nursing education in Russia. *Journal of Nursing Education*, 42(7), 292–295.

Jarvik, L. (2006). Cultural challenges to democratization in Russia. *Orbis*, 50(1), 167–186.

Jeltova, I., Fish, M. C., & Revenson, T. A. (2005). Risky sexual behaviors in immigrant adolescent girls from the former Soviet Union: role of natal and host culture. *Journal of School Psychology*, 43(1), 3–22.

Jones, I., Thomas, C., Tucker, B., et al, (1995). Impact of age and environment on somatic mutation at the hprt gene of T lymphocytes in humans. *Mutation Research*, 338(1–6), 129–139.

Kohn, R., Flaherty, J. A., & Levav, I. (1989). Somatic symptoms among older Soviet immigrants: an exploratory study. *International Journal of Social Psychiatry*, 35(4), 350–360.

Koretz, G. (2003, October 13). Russia's huge health hurdle: as its economy booms, life spans are still falling [Electronic version]. *Business Week*, 3853.

Kostikov, V. (1991). Boris Yeltsin's political victory. *Soviet Life*, 7(418), 2–5.

Kravitz, R. L., Helms, L. J., Azari, R., Antonius, D., & Melnikow, J. (2000). Comparing the use of physician time and health care resources among patients speaking English, Spanish, and Russian. *Medical Care*, 38(7), 728–738.

Kunstel, M., & Albright, J. (1996, November 17). Russian mobsters growing bolder. *The Atlanta Journal-Constitution*, p. C2.

Lally, K. (2000, January 10). Death offers no relief for woes of Russians. *Baltimore Sun*, p. 1A.

Langone, J. (1989). A profession under stress. *Time*, 133 (15), 94–95.

Larkin, M. (2000). Russian biomedical science survives against all odds. *Lancet*, 355(9200), 294.

Library of Congress. (2005, August). *Country profile: Russia*. Library of Congress–Federal Research Division. Retrieved June 24, 2006, from http://lcweb2.loc.gov/frd/cs/profiles/Russia.pdf.

Marian, V., & Neisser, U. (2000). Language-dependent recall of autobiographical memories. *Journal of Experimental Psychology: General*, 129(3), 361–368.

Marquez, P. V. (2005). *Dying too young: addressing premature mortality and ill health due to non-communicable diseases and injuries in the Russian Federation*. Europe and Central Asia Human Development Department: The World Bank. Retrieved June 24, 2006, from http://siteresources.worldbank.org/INTECA/Resources/DTY-Final.pdf.

Maximova, T. M. (2000, July 10). *Socio-economic conditions and health in Russia*. Semashko Research Institute, Russian Academy of Medical Sciences, Moscow, Russia. Retrieved July 12, 2002, from http://members.tripod.com/~tokourov/socio1.htm.

Mehler, P. S., Scott, J. Y., Pines, I., et al, (2001). Russian immigrant cardiovascular risk assessment. *Journal of Health Care for the Poor and Underserved*, 12(2), 224–235.

Moore, R. (Ed.), *Fodor's 89 Soviet Union*. New York: Fodor's Travel Publications.

National Center for Health Statistics, *Health, United States (2002) with urban and rural chartbook*. Hyattsville, Md.: National Center for Health Statistics.

OANDA.com (2006, June 25). FXConverter-164 currency converter USDollar—Russian Ruble. Retrieved June 25, 2006, from http://www.oanda.com/convert/classic.

Osborn, A. (2004). Half of Russia's doctors face sack in healthcare reforms. *British Medical Journal*, 328 (7448), 1092.

Page, J. (2005, December 9). Patients panic over HIV exposure [Electronic version]. *The (United Kingdom) Times*.

Pomerleau, J., Gillmore, A., McKee, M., Rose, R., & Haerpfer, C. (2004, December). Determinants of smoking in eight countries of the former Soviet Union: results from the living conditions, lifestyles, and health study. *Addiction*, 99(12), 1577–1585.

Pope, V. (1996). Mad Russians. *U.S. News & World Report*, 121(24), 38–43.

Pope, V. (1997). Trafficking in women. *U.S. News & World Report, 122*(13), 38–44.

Popov, V. (2004, November). The state in the New Russia (1992–2004): from collapse to gradual revival? *PONARS Policy Memo 342.* Retrieved June 24, 2006, from www.nes.ru/~vpopov/documents/state-collapse-PONARS.pdf.

Prokhorov, D. (1990). The geography of disease. *Business in the USSR,* 730–31.

Ross, J., & Searing, S. E. (1992). Women's studies take on Russian flavor. *Wingspread: The Journal, 14*(2), 8–91.

Ruby, M. (1989). Sinai Samaritan to double free care for Soviets. *Jewish Chronicle,* p. 8.

Russia may tighten controls on adoptions by foreigners. (1997, November 29). *The Journal Times* (Racine, Wisc., AP), 7A.

Russian kids top dropout list. (2001, January 2). (Associated Press). *Herald and News,* Klamath Falls, Oregon, p. A3.

Russian TB in the US? Not yet, but may be soon. (1999). *TB Monitor, 6*(5), 56.

Russians rally against terror after bloodbath. (2004, September 7). Associated Press, Retrieved September 7, 2004, from http://msnbc.msn.com/id/5881958/print/1/displaymode/1098/.

Russians who. (2005, September/October). *Russian Life, 48*(5), 10.

Sandul, I. (2002, March 22–28). Trying to break through the glass ceiling. *The Russia Journal.* Retrieved June 9, 2002, from http://www.cdi.org/russia/johnson/6152-15.cfm.

Schiff, A. (1979). Language, culture and Jewish acculturation of Soviet Jewish émigrés. *Journal of Jewish Communal Service,* 44–57.

Scott, A. (1988). Human interaction and personal boundaries. *Journal of Psychosocial Nursing, 26*(8), 23–27.

Smith, H. (1991). *The new Russians.* New York: Random House.

Smith, L. S. (1996). New Russian immigrants: health problems, practices, and values. *Journal of Cultural Diversity, 3*(3), 68–73.

Smith, L. S. (2000). Leeches: primitive performers. *Nursing 2000, 30*(6), 9.

Smith, L. S. (2006). Nursing in Russia: an overview of healthcare, nursing education, and practice. In P.S. Cowen & S. Moorhead (Eds.), *Current issues in nursing* (7th ed.), (pp. 828–842). St. Louis, Mo.: Mosby.

Stanglin, D., & Pope, V. (1992). The wreck of Russia. *U.S. News & World Report, 113*(22), 40–49.

Starobin, P. (2003, August 4). The enigma of Russia [Electron version]. *Business Week,* 3844.

Study: Russian kids sicker than during USSR days. (1998, March 13). *The Journal Times* (Racine, Wisc., AP), p. 10A.

Study: Russian men die drunk. (2000, May 21). *The Seattle Times,* p. A21.

TB epidemic in Europe (1998, March 25). *The Journal Times* (Racine, Wisc., AP), p. 6A.

Tran, T. V., Khatutsky, G., Aroian, K., Balsam, A., & Conway, K. (2000). Living arrangements, depression, and health status among elderly Russian-speaking immigrants. *Journal of Gerontological Social Work, 33*(2), 63–77.

Trickett, E. J., & Birman, D. (2005). Acculturation, school context, and school outcomes: adaptation of refugee adolescents from the former Soviet Union. *Psychology in the Schools, 42*(1), 27–38. U.S. Department of Commerce, Bureau of the Census. (1998, February 18, Internet release date). Selected characteristics for persons of Russian Ancestry: 1990. Retrieved July 13, 2002, from http://www.census.gov/population/socdemo/ancestry/Russian.txt.

U.S. Department of Commerce, Bureau of the Census (2002). Population profiles by age, sex, race, and Hispanic origin, Summary File 3. Washington, D.C.: U.S. Government Printing Office.

U.S. Department of Justice (USDOJ), Immigration and Naturalization Service. (1992, April). *Immigration from the former Soviet Union, 1989–1991* (Bulletin no. 10). Washington, D.C.: U.S. Government Printing Office.

U.S. Department of Commerce, Bureau of the Census (2000). Census 2000 demographic profile highlights: Selected population group: Russian, Summary File 4 (pp. 148–151). Retrieved June 25, 2006, from http://factfinder.census.gov/sevlet/SAFFIteratedFacts?_event.

USAID. (2005, February 16). Russia. *USAID Health: Infectious Diseases, Tuberculosis, Countries,* Russia. Retrieved June 25, 2006, from www.usaid.gov/our_work/global_health/id/tuberculosis/countries.

U.S. Department of Homeland Security. (2005a). *Yearbook of immigration statistics: 2005.* Supplemental Table 2. Legal permanent resident flow by leading core-based statistical areas (CBSAs) of residence and region and country of birth: fiscal year 2005. Retrieved

June 25, 2006, from www.uscis.gov/graphics/shared/statistcs/yearbook.

U.S. Department of Homeland Security. (2005b). *Yearbook of immigration statistics: 2005*, Table 3, Legal permanent resident flow by region and country by birth: fiscal years 1995–2005. Retrieved June 25, 2006, from http://www.uscis.gov/graphics/shared/statistcs/yearbook.

U.S. Department of Homeland Security. (2005c). *Yearbook of immigration statistics: 2005*, Table 12. Immigrant orphans adopted by US citizens by gender, age, and region and country of birth: fiscal year 2005. Retrieved June 25, 2006, from http://www.uscis.gov/graphics/shared/statistcs/yearbook.

Vadlamani, A., Maher, J. F., Shaete, M., et al, (2001). Colorectal cancer in Russian-speaking Jewish emigres: community-based screening. *American Journal of Gastroenterology*, 96(9), 2755–2760.

Weir, F. (2001, March 8). Women's day in Russia: showers of flowers. *The Christian Science Monitor*. Retrieved January 23, 2005, from http://www.csmonitor.com/2001/0308/p7s1.html.

World Health Organization. (2006a). *Health workers: a global profile*. The World Health Report 2006, Chapter 1—Working together for health (annex table 4), pp. 197–199.

World Health Organization. (2006b). *World health statistics 2006: health systems*. WHO Statistical Information System: WHOSIS. Retrieved June 26, 2006, from www.who.int/whosis/whostat2006/en/index.html.

World Health Organization. (2005, January 14). *Country profile*. Retrieved January 16, 2006, from http://hfadb.who.dk/hfa/hfaoverw2.

Wikipedia. (2006, May). *Economy of Russia*, Wikipedia Foundation, Inc. Retrieved June 24, 2006, from http://en.wikipedia.org/wiki/economy_of_Russia.

Williams, C. L., Grechanaia, T., Romanova, O., Komro, K. A., Perry, C. L., & Farbakhsh, K. (2001). Public health practice: Russian-American partners for prevention. *The European Journal of Public Health*, 11(3), 314–321.

Williams, J. (Reporter) (1992, June 26). *Russian doctors visit Milwaukee* (WITI Television).

Witt, H. (1993, March 24). Inside the Russian court. *Chicago Tribune*, pp. 1, 13.

Yeltsin rival backs down. (1993, March 26). *The Journal Times*, p. 3A.

Yeltsin: Main points. (1993, March 21). *The Journal Times*, p. 11A.

CHAPTER 16 Chinese Americans

Yu Xu and Karen Chang

Behavioral Objectives

After reading this chapter, the nurse will be able to:

1. Describe Chinese philosophy, beliefs, and values.
2. Explain the ways that Chinese Americans communicate.
3. Describe the influences of the family system on Chinese Americans.
4. Explain the time concept of Chinese Americans.
5. Describe the illness behaviors of Chinese Americans.
6. Identify the biological variations of Chinese Americans.
7. Articulate the implications of providing effective nursing care for Chinese Americans.

OVERVIEW OF CHINA

China (The People's Republic of China), literally "Central Kingdom," occupies the eastern portion of Asia and is slightly larger in area than the United States (*Time Almanac with Information Please*, 2007). In fact, China occupies roughly 3,705,386 square miles (9,596,960 square kilometers) (Central Intelligence Agency, 2006; *Time Almanac with Information Please*, 2007). The coastline of China is roughly a semicircle. The greater part of China is mountainous; it is only in the lower portions of the Yellow and Yangtze rivers that there are any extensive low plains. The principal mountain ranges include the Tien Shan ("Celestial Mountains") in the northwest part of the country; the Kunlun chain, which runs south of the Takla Makan and Gobi deserts; the Tanggula mountain range, which connects the Kunlun chain with Tibet (modified from *Time Almanac with Information Please*, 2007); and the Da Xing, a mountain range in northeast China. Mount Everest on the border with Nepal is the world's tallest peak. The major plains in China include the Northeast Plain, the Inner Mongolia Plain, the Central Plain, the lower Yangtze Plain, and the Pearl River Delta Plain.

In 2005, the total population of China was 1,306,313,812, including Taiwan, which is part of Republic of China (National Bureau of Statistics of China, 2006; *Time Almanac with Information Please*, 2007). Compared with the 1990 census, the average annual growth was 12.79 million, or an average rate of natural increase of 0.96% (National Bureau of Statistics of China, 2006; *Time Almanac with Information Please*, 2007). The birth rate in China is 13.1 per 1000, compared with 16.3 per 1000 for the United States (*Time Almanac with Information Please*, 2007). In 2006, the infant mortality rate in China was 24.2 per 1000, compared with 9.8 per 1000 for the United States (*Time Almanac with Information Please*, 2007; National Center for Health Statistics, Health United States, 2006). The population of China makes it one of the densest countries in the world (353 people per square mile).

The capital city of China is Beijing ("northern capital"; previous spelling, *Peking*), which has an estimated population of 10,848,000. The largest city in China is Shanghai ("on-sea"), which has an estimated population of 12,887,000. Other large cities include Tianjin (5,350,000 metro area), Guangzhou (3,935,193), Wuhan (4,040,113), and Xi'an (2,954,872) (*Time Almanac with Information Please*, 2007; *World Almanac*, 2007).

The principal agriculture products of China include rice, wheat, potatoes, grains, tea, and cotton. In 1998, the makeup of the labor force by occupation sector was as follows: agriculture, 50%; industry, 24%; and services, 26% (Central Intelligence Agency, 2006; *Time Almanac with Information Please*, 2007; *World Almanac*, 2007). Major exports are machinery and equipment, textiles and clothing, footwear, toys and sporting goods, and mineral fuels (Central Intelligence Agency, 2006; *Time Almanac with Information Please*, 2007; *World Almanac*, 2007).

The president of China is Hu Jinato (2003–) and the premier is Wen Jiabao (2003–). The ruling governmental authority in China is the Communist Party. The National People's Congress is the chief legislative organ. Within the governmental hierarchy, the State Council has the executive authority. It is the Congress, however, that elects the premier and the deputy premiers. In China, the ministries are under the auspices of the State Council, which is headed by the premier.

According to incomplete statistics, today China has 100 million religious believers. Among them, there are 14 million Christians (10 million Protestants, 4 million Catholics) and 18 million Muslims. In addition, there are 13,000 Buddhist and 1500 Taoist temples (Lin, 2000).

OVERVIEW OF CHINESE AMERICANS

The majority of Chinese Americans are immigrants from Taiwan, Hong Kong, and mainland China. Today, the 2,734,841 Chinese Americans constitute the largest group of Asian Americans (*Time Almanac with Information Please*, 2007; U.S. Department of Commerce, Bureau of the Census, 2002). This new figure represents a 47.5% growth rate from 1990 to 2000. This figure compares with 104.1%

from 1980 to 1990. Chinese Americans residing in the United States represent 0.7% of the total U.S. population (*Time Almanac with Information Please*, 2007; U.S. Department of Commerce, Bureau of the Census, Summary File 3, 2002). Of the number of Chinese Americans residing in this country, 52.4% live in the West, 27.0% live in the Northeast, 12.4% live in the South, and 8.1% live in the Midwest (*Time Almanac with Information Please*, 2007; U.S. Department of Commerce, Bureau of the Census, Summary File 3, 2002). The states with the largest populations of Chinese Americans are California (704,850), New York (284,144), and Hawaii (68,804). A total of 66% of Chinese Americans live in five states: California, New York, Hawaii, Illinois, and Texas (*Time Almanac with Information Please*, 2007; U.S. Department of Commerce, Bureau of the Census, Summary File 3, 2002).

Of the Chinese Americans residing in the United States before 1975, 18.5% were foreign born; of the number residing in the United States between 1975 and 1979, 11.4% were foreign born; and between 1980 and 1990, 39.4% were foreign born. Immigration has definitely contributed to the growth in the Chinese American population over the past two decades. It is interesting to note, however, that the percentage of Chinese Americans who are foreign born differs considerably across time periods. The median age of Chinese Americans residing in the United States is 32.1 years, compared with 33 years for the general U.S. population. In addition, only 7.5% of all Asian Americans are 65 years of age or older, compared with 13% of the general U.S. population (*Time Almanac with Information Please*, 2007; U.S. Department of Commerce, Bureau of the Census, Summary File 3, 2002).

Chinese Americans are noted for maintaining high educational standards. For example, in 1990, 77.2% of Chinese American males and 70.2% of Chinese American females 25 years of age or older held a high school diploma; in 2000, 46.7% of Chinese American males and 35.0% of Chinese American females held a bachelor's degree (*Time Almanac with Information Please*, 2007; U.S. Department of Commerce, Bureau of the Census, Summary File 3, 2002).

Of the number of Chinese Americans in the United States, 65.9% participate in the workforce. Chinese Americans have lower labor force participation rates than Filipinos (75.4%) and Asian Indians (72.3%). Although the per capita income for most Japanese Americans is $19,375, Chinese Americans have a per capita income of only $14,876. The poverty rate for Chinese Americans is 14.0%, compared with 13.0% for the general U. S. population (*Time Almanac with Information Please*, 2007; U.S. Department of Commerce, Bureau of the Census, Summary File 3, 2002).

There is a bimodal distribution with regard to socioeconomic status and educational attainment in the U.S. Asian and Pacific Islander population, including Chinese Americans (U.S. Census Bureau, 2000). As a subgroup, the socioeconomic status and educational attainment of Chinese Americans are comparable to those of Japanese and Korean Americans and Asian Indians but higher than those of other subgroups, such as Filipinos, Vietnamese, Laotians, Cambodians, and Thais. In other words, there is a significant segment of Chinese Americans who are college-educated professionals. At the same time, there are a large number of barely literate individuals working in low-paying occupations (Wong, 2006).

The contrasting socioeconomic characteristics of the Chinese immigrants in different historical periods determined, to a large extent, their educational attainment and their occupations. Before 1965, most Chinese immigrants had little or no education, and many were alone because their families were not allowed to immigrate with them. They were forced to immigrate for political, social, or economic reasons. The majority of them came from Guangdong Province and took up occupations such as mining, railroad construction, and farming, or engaged in small family businesses, such as restaurants, laundries, and groceries. After 1965, when immigration laws eased in the United States, the better-educated professionals and specialists began to immigrate. Now families were allowed to immigrate together. These immigrants came from Taiwan, mainland China, and Hong Kong. As a result, a wide cultural and linguistic diversity exists among Chinese Americans.

Chinese culture is dominated by Confucianism, which encourages individuals to pursue filial piety, righteousness, decorum, and wisdom. A harmonious relationship with nature and other people is stressed, and a person is expected to accommodate rather than confront. If individual interests conflict with community interests, a person is expected to submit to the interest of the group. Public debating of conflicting views is perceived as socially unacceptable. A person is expected to be sensitive to what other people perceive and think and to be gracious toward others so as not to make them "lose face." Self-expression and individualism are discouraged, whereas showing filial piety to parents and loyalty to family, friends, and government is highly praised. Modesty, self-control, self-reliance, self-restraint, and face-saving are frequently taught to Chinese people. When they fail to follow these cultural practices, many Chinese may feel shame or guilt. Consequently, the Chinese appear to be quiet, polite, pleasant, and unassertive and often suppress personal feelings such as frustration, disagreement, anger, or pain.

Reciprocation, or treating others as one would wish to be treated, is often used in interpersonal relationships. Interpersonal interactions have a hierarchical structure, so that older or higher-status people have authority over younger or lower-status people. A person's status is always referred to during interactions. For example, brothers address each other as "older brother" and "younger brother" in addition to the first name. Educational achievement and professional success are highly valued because pride and honor are brought to the family and the community as a result. Therefore, Chinese parents not only willingly support their children who pursue education but also frequently sacrifice, at almost any cost, to ensure a good education for their children.

The sharp contrasts between the Chinese and American cultures often cause a high level of stress among Chinese Americans during the acculturation process. Some may hold onto traditional Chinese culture, observe holidays according to the lunar calendar, and maintain Chinese customs; some may reject all their traditional heritage; and some may assimilate both the Chinese culture and the American culture. Poorly adjusted individuals may not be able to perform tasks productively, may have low self-esteem, and may exhibit some lawless behaviors. Second- and third-generation Chinese Americans, who are already well assimilated into Western culture, may not be influenced much by traditional Chinese culture. However, they may experience the identity problem of being culturally and linguistically American, even though others perceive them as Chinese (Wong, 2006).

COMMUNICATION

Dialect

A wide cultural and linguistic diversity exists among Chinese Americans. Linguistic diversity may cause communication problems among Chinese people. Although the official Chinese language is Mandarin (Pǔtonghùa), there are many dialects spoken that are not understood by other groups of Chinese. However, all the dialects have the same written characters and grammatical structures, which have been relatively stable for 3000 years despite having undergone great changes. This stability in the language permits all literate Chinese to be able to communicate in writing. Each Chinese character (or logogram) consists of only one syllable. Each character has its own meaning, but if one character is combined with one or more characters, the combination produces words or phrases with different concepts. There are four tones in Mandarin (as well as a neutral tone), and changes of tone produce complete changes in the meaning of a syllable or a word. For instance, ma may mean "mother" with the flat tone, "numbness" with the rising tone, "horse" with the curving tone, and "scold" or "curse" in the falling tone. Undoubtedly, the complexity arising from toning is one of the toughest challenges for any non-Chinese trying to master the spoken language. On the other hand, the Chinese language generally does not use copulas and plurals (though both exist) and has no tenses.

Style, Volume, and Touch

The Chinese value silence and avoid disagreeing or criticizing, especially in public. Disagreements are not verbalized so that harmonious relationships will be maintained, at least outwardly. To raise one's voice to make a point, a common behavior for some Americans, is viewed by many Chinese as being associated with anger and a sign of loss of self-control. To avoid confrontation and subsequent "loss of face," a direct "no" is rarely used. On the other hand, the word *yes* with or without nodding may merely mean "I heard you" and may not indicate agreement or consent. In some circumstances, "yes" can even mean "no" or "perhaps." Hesitancy, ambiguity, subtlety, and implicity are dominant features in Chinese speech. Understanding nonverbal cues and contextual meanings is also necessary to communicate effectively with some Chinese Americans.

Touching and touching different parts of the body have different meanings that are largely defined culturally. Chinese people do not ordinarily touch each other during conversation. Touching someone's head indicates a serious breach of etiquette, particularly when the involved person is elderly or of higher social status. Touching during an argument indicates shameful loss of self-control. In the same respect, putting one's feet on a desk, table, or chair is regarded as impolite and disrespectful. On the other hand, public displays of affection toward a person of the same sex are quite permissible in the Chinese culture. Unlike the American culture, however, public displays between the opposite sexes are considered socially unacceptable (Burkett, 1995). The Chinese are often viewed as polite but reserved, shy, cold, unassertive, or uninterested (Fisher, 1996; Chen & Yang, 1986; Watson, 1970).

Context

Communication among the Chinese is high-context, in contrast to communication among mainstream Americans. A high-context communication is one in which most of the information is either in the physical context or internalized in the persons involved, whereas very little is in the coded, explicit, transmitted message. A low-context communication is just the opposite; that is, the mass of the information is vested in the explicit code (Hall, 1981; Hall, 1989).

The Chinese people tend to perceive, value, and rely on nonverbal and contextual cues during communication and do not communicate explicitly. For example, facial expressions, tensions, movements, pace of speech, and location of interactions are perceived during interactions to formulate specific meanings. They expect others to figure out the underlying meanings of communicated words (Gudykunst, 2001). Again, it cannot be overemphasized that understanding nonverbal cues and contextual meaning is necessary for effective communication with the Chinese people.

Kinesics

In the past, Chinese people greeted others by bowing. It is more commonplace now to greet people with "Have you had your breakfast (lunch, dinner)?" The greeting person is not really interested in the question literally. Instead, it is merely a culturally determined format of greeting other people. Nodding the head may indicate "yes," whereas shaking the head may indicate "no." To answer a question such as "Haven't you had anything to eat?" is problematic for many Chinese Americans. They may be confused about whether to answer affirmatively or negatively: "Yes, I haven't had anything," or "No, I would like something."

Many Chinese Americans experience feelings of shame and embarrassment when they cannot communicate well. Some apologize frequently and repeatedly for their linguistic inadequacies because they think they are inconveniencing others. Although, most Chinese Americans will often refrain from expressing their emotions openly, some may narrow their eyes to express anger and disgust (Chin, 2005). In general, Chinese Americans tend to have less eye contact than other Americans have because, in the Chinese culture, excessive eye contact may indicate impoliteness and rudeness (Watson, 1970), it and may also be perceived as threatening (Chin, 2005).

Chinese Americans, like other immigrants, experience a great amount of stress when they are in health care facilities. The language barrier and their different cultural background often cause confusion, depression, frustration, helplessness, and powerlessness. However, they tend not to discuss their concerns or express their emotional problems with health care professionals (Cheung et al., 2005). Some Chinese Americans believe that emotional problems are personal issues and are often embarrassed to ask questions when no health care workers speak their language. These emotional experiences are often not orally expressed but may be indicated by nonverbal cues. Frequently, observing nonverbal behaviors and encouraging clients to verbalize will help identify these psychological problems.

Implications for Nursing Care

It is important for the nurse to remember that there are diverse Chinese dialects that are not comprehensible to other Chinese groups. If the client needs a translator in the health care setting, the nurse must first find out which dialect the client speaks and then find a translator who can speak that dialect.

Because the Chinese language is quite different from English, the nurse must remember that when Chinese Americans communicate in English they often experience a high level of stress. The nurse may observe and validate its associated symptoms and help the client control and lower the stress level. Because Chinese Americans tend to be "good patients"—quiet and polite, with few requests—and tend to suppress feelings such as anxiety, fear, depression, or pain, it is important for the nurse to recognize nonverbal cues and their cultural meanings to develop culturally appropriate nursing care plans. The nurse can never assume that a Chinese patient has no unmet need if he or she does not request anything.

Some Chinese Americans hesitate to ask questions when they do not understand; therefore, after rapport has been established, the nurse should elicit and encourage Chinese Americans to verbalize their feelings and ask questions. Because of culturally determined communication patterns, the nurse would do best to validate the patient's understanding by asking questions or having the patient do a return demonstration, instead of relying solely on patient's verbal and nonverbal responses. In addition, the nurse should avoid using negative questions to elicit responses because negative questions are comprehended differently in the Chinese language.

In addition, because some Chinese Americans do not ordinarily touch another person during conversation, it is important for the nurse to explain the necessity of touching for therapeutic purposes. Showing respect, demonstrating empathy, and being nonjudgmental can help establish rapport with Chinese American patients. The nurse can communicate better with Chinese Americans by understanding their cultural norms, values, and practices and unique communication styles. Therapeutic communication techniques can also be used to promote conversations to help Chinese American patients express thoughts and feelings and to ensure mutual understanding, especially when the nurse believes that the patient is experiencing anxiety, fear, depression, or pain.

SPACE

In studying human spatial relationships, Hall (1981) divided humans into two groups: contact and noncontact. People from a contact group interact with each other by facing each other more directly, being closer, touching more, making more eye contact, and speaking more loudly than members of a noncontact group. People from a contact group may perceive people from a noncontact group as being shy, uninterested, cold, and impolite. Conversely, people from a noncontact group may view people from a contact group as being pushy, aggressive, obnoxious, and impolite (Hall, 1981). Both Chinese Americans and most middle-class mainstream Americans are categorized as noncontact individuals. However, from the Asian person's point of view, Americans face each other more, touch more, and have more visual contact than Asians do. Chinese people feel more comfortable in a side-by-side or right-angle arrangement and may feel uncomfortable when placed in a face-to-face situation. Americans prefer to sit face to face or at right angles to each other. In the Asian culture, the person of higher status has the prerogative of sitting as proximally as desired; thus the burden of correct behavior is on the person of lesser status (Samovar & Porter, 2003; Watson, 1970).

Implications for Nursing Care

Because Chinese Americans are categorized as non-contact, it is important for the nurse to remember that some Chinese Americans may be erroneously perceived as being extremely shy or withdrawn. It is equally important for the nurse to remember that some Chinese Americans may view tasks that are associated with closeness, increased eye contact, and touch as being impolite or offensive. The nurse can reduce these misunderstandings by providing explanations when performing these tasks. Because some Chinese Americans feel uncomfortable with face-to-face arrangements, the nurse may seek the client's input in terms of comfortable seating arrangements and remain alert and sensitive to the patient's comfort level of personal space.

SOCIAL ORGANIZATION

Effect of Immigration on Social Organization

Many early Chinese immigrants came to this country as contract laborers or with money that was borrowed from various Chinese American organizations. These organizations assumed a supervisory role for these early immigrants once they arrived in the United States. The Chinese immigrants were similar to immigrants from other ethnic and cultural groups in that most of them were unfamiliar with the language and the culture of the United States. Therefore, many of the early Chinese immigrants worked as laborers in gangs. Although many of these individuals were physically smaller than those in other ethnic or cultural groups in the United States, they were hard workers. Historically, Chinese Americans helped build the United States by constructing railroads and working at other equally taxing jobs. Early Chinese immigrants worked cheaply and saved money by living frugally. These virtues made many of the early Chinese immigrants employable, but they were feared and hated as competitors by American workers (Wong, 2006; Lyman, 1974).

By 1851 there were 25,000 Chinese Americans living in California alone (Sung, 1967). By 1870 the number of Chinese immigrants in the United States had increased to 63,000. In 1880 approximately 6000 Chinese persons entered the United States. Nearly twice as many entered the United States in 1881, and nearly five times as many entered in 1882 (Sung, 1967). However, in 1882 an exclusionary immigration law reduced the inflow of Chinese immigrants to less than 1000 until the year 1890. Because of this law, the initial Chinese immigration was almost exclusively male. The immigration of Chinese men to the United States was believed to be a tentative rather than a permanent move, and during the 1880s the number of Chinese persons leaving the United States was greater than the number entering.

In addition to the Chinese Exclusion Act of 1882, other laws that severely curtailed not only immigration but also the possibility of a Chinese person's becoming a naturalized citizen were enacted in the United States. Furthermore, some of these laws were specific enough to require citizenship as a prerequisite for entering many occupations and for owning land (Sowell, 1981). From 1854 to 1874, there were laws that prevented Chinese people from testifying in court against White men (Lyman, 1974). Some historians believe that such laws in effect made it possible to declare "open season" on Chinese Americans because many of these individuals had no legal recourse when robbed, vandalized, or assaulted. The almost total exclusion of Chinese immigration from 1882 to 1890 had devastating long-range effects on Chinese Americans that are still evident. Because the early Chinese immigrants were almost exclusively male, there was little hope for a normal social or family life. Many of these early male immigrants had wives and children in China, whom they would not see for many years, if at all. Because of the severe restrictions on economic opportunities, it was impossible to earn enough money to book passage to China.

Over the years, the few Chinese women who had managed to immigrate to the United States were able to produce a small number of first-generation children. When these children grew up, there was a slight ease in the serious shortage of women that remained characteristic of Chinese Americans from the early immigration period until World War II.

In addition, an unknown number of Chinese women were smuggled into the United States for the specific purpose of prostitution (Lyman, 1974). As recently as the 1960s, many illegal aliens from China entered the United States to pursue a better life. As a result, many Chinese residents deliberately avoided census takers.

Despite the fact that economic opportunities for early Chinese immigrants were highly restricted, many Chinatown communities took care of their own indigents. This fact may explain why even during such disasters as the San Francisco earthquake in 1906 and the Great Depression of the 1930s, many Chinese Americans did not seek or receive federal aid.

In 1943, the Chinese Exclusion Act of 1882 was repealed, and that repeal did help ease the imbalance of the male-to-female ratio and permitted a more normal family life to develop among a very family-oriented people. After the repeal of the Chinese Exclusion Act of 1882, the bulk of the new Chinese immigrants were female (Sung, 1967). The labor shortages of World War II opened many new job opportunities that were not previously available to Chinese Americans. Thus many Chinese Americans abandoned traditional Chinatown occupations to move into these new jobs (Sowell, 1981).

In 1940 only 3% of Chinese Americans in California had jobs that were considered "professional," compared with 8% of the White population. By 1950 the percentage of Chinese Americans in professional fields had doubled to 6%. Over the next decade the percentage of Chinese Americans working in professional fields tripled and for the first time passed the percentage of Whites working in professional fields. By 1970 it was reported that Chinese Americans in general had a higher income or higher occupational status than most other Americans. In 1970 at least one fourth of all employed Chinese Americans were working in scientific or professional fields (Sowell, 1981).

Family

The Chinese family can be classified into five categories: old immigrant families, professional immigrant families, American-born Chinese families, new working-class immigrant families, and biracial/bicultural Chinese families (Wong, 2006). The socioeconomic, educational, or acculturation status of these families vary. The old immigrant families may own small grocery stores or restaurants, speak limited English, and hold on to traditional Chinese values. The parents of professional immigrant families mostly came to the U.S. as international students and have professional jobs after graduation. They may sponsor their parents for immigration to the U.S. and form an extended family. The American-born Chinese families may have children ranging from first-generation to fifth-generation. The children of these families may be well acculturated, receive college degrees, and have high occupational status and income. However, the children of the working-class immigrant families may not acculturate well. Both parents may be employed in the labor-intensive market (such as tourist shops, restaurants, and garment sweatshops) with enclave economy. Because of their work schedule, they have little time with their children. The biracial Chinese families happen mostly among the U.S.-born population. The children of these families may identify themselves as Chinese and another race.

Chinese, like other Asian Americans, have a culture of collectivism. This culture of collectivism emphasizes loyalty to family and devotion to tradition and de-emphasizes individual feelings (Gudykunst, 2001). The Chinese are willing to submit individual interests to those of the family to maintain a strong and cohesive bond. In return, the family is expected to take care of its members, both immediate and extended. Doing so brings honor to the family; not doing so brings shame (Kim, 2003).

The Chinese family generally has a hierarchical structure. The older children have authority over the younger children, and the younger children must show deference to authority figures, usually the elderly male in the household (Chin, 2005). Boys may be more valued than girls. Husbands may have more authority over their wives. Wives may be expected to be obedient to parents and parents-in-law (Cheung et al., 2005). Failure to do so causes shame for the family. The authority figure has more influence on decision making. In most cases, decisions are made on the basis of consensus rather than majority rule. The individual learns to submit to prevailing opinion rather than disagree (Gudykunst, Stewart, & Toomey, 1985). However, the values of the Chinese American family are eroding in the acculturation process. Many youngsters do not show respect to the elderly, and many elderly cannot count on their children or relatives for needed help. Consequently, many older Chinese Americans suffer from mental illnesses, and may commit suicide (Surgeon General's Supplemental Report, 1999).

Marital Status

Because of the early Chinese Exclusion Act in the United States, there was a disproportionately large number of Chinese men compared with Chinese women. Many of the early unmarried Chinese men who came to the United States had virtually no opportunity to marry; thus in 1890 only 26.1% of the total number of Chinese American men were married. The percentage of married Chinese American women from 1890 to 1950 ranged from 57.4% to 69.1%. During this time there appeared to be a lower percentage of single Chinese women who immigrated, which was partially accounted for by the Chinese tradition of females marrying at a younger age. Chinese Americans divorce less frequently than their American counterparts (Sung, 1967).

Today, Chinese Americans remain family-oriented. Married couples may experience conflicts, but will avoid divorce or separation, which may be viewed as a shame. According to the 2000 census, 62% of Chinese Americans are married, 28.7% have never married, 1% are separated, 4.4% are widowed, and 3.8% are divorced (U.S. Department of Commerce, Bureau of the Census, Summary File 3, 2002; Reeves & Bennet, 2004).

Religion

There are four primary religions in China: Buddhism, Taoism, Islam, and Christianity (Catholicism and Protestantism). Of these four primary religions, Buddhism has the largest number of professed followers while Taoism has the smallest number. Among Chinese and Chinese Americans, Christianity is regarded as a newcomer; nevertheless, its effects are pronounced. Christianity is viewed as being partially responsible for the introduction of Western culture into China as well as to Chinese Americans. Today the number of Chinese Roman Catholics is increasing rapidly, particularly among foreign-born Chinese Americans (Fisher, 1996; Sowell, 1981).

Implications for Nursing Care

It is important for the nurse to remember that Chinese Americans are a family-oriented people who normally put family commitments before personal interests. In addition, the Chinese American family has traditionally had a hierarchical structure. By assessing the client's kinship relationship and identifying the authoritative family member, the nurse can effectively use the influential family members to achieve the therapeutic goals. Chinese Americans believe that they have a major responsibility in taking care of family members and relatives. Therefore, family members may view hospitalization or health care needs of a family member as a personal concern. The nurse needs to understand this sense of responsibility and be sensitive to the family's needs. Opinions and ideas of the family members should be incorporated into the plan of care. Also, it is important to provide health care education to all family members, not just the client, when procedures are to be done. However, parents of the ill child may not want the siblings to know about the illness to avoid unnecessary worry. The nurse should assess the family situation to avoid disclosing information to inappropriate family members (Cheung et al., 2005). A rule of thumb with regard to caring for Chinese Americans is to involve the family to the highest possible extent. Otherwise, the family may take away the health professional's access to the patient. The notion that an individual has rights independent of his or her family is alien to many Chinese and Chinese Americans. In addition, Chinese American women may be very uncomfortable and uneasy when examined by male health professionals. Therefore, a female nurse should be present and assist in the examination.

Chinese Americans vary widely in educational background and socioeconomic status, have varied cultural and religious values and practices, and have different levels of acculturation. For example, some Chinese Americans speak English very poorly, whereas others can communicate in English without any problem. Some have medical insurance, whereas others do not. Some use herbal medicine, whereas others do not. Language deficiency is one of the primary barriers to health care access and utilization for Chinese Americans (Smedley, Stith, & Nelson, 2003). If the client has a language barrier, a translator is needed and can usually be found in the local Chinese community. Visual displays, flip charts, or exhibits can be used to facilitate the client's understanding. The nurse can also use patient education materials written in Chinese from the following Web sites: http://www.imunize.org/catg.d/noneng.htm#Chinese, http://spiral.tufts.edu/chinese_simp/index.html.

TIME

The Chinese have a different perception and experience regarding time; it is not past, present, or future oriented. Some Chinese Americans perceive time as a dynamic wheel with circular movements and the present as a reflection of the eternal. This metaphoric wheel continually turns in an unforeseeable direction, and individuals are expected to adjust to the present, which surrounds the rotating wheel, and seek a harmonious relationship with their surroundings (Kim, 2003).

Hall (1981) has described the time concept of Asians as polychronic and that of Westerners as monochronic. An individual with a polychronic time orientation adheres less rigidly to time as a distinct and linear entity, focuses on the completion of the present, and often implements more than one activity simultaneously. On the other hand, an individual with a monochronic orientation to time emphasizes schedules, promptness, standardization of activities, and synchronization with clocks.

When making decisions regarding current and future events, some Chinese people may be affected by traditions and customs. Before making decisions, they may seek symbols, correlations, and intuitive understanding, as well as consider significance, consequences, future situations, and present factors. They do not make decisions according to an individual's own benefit (Gudykunst, Stewart, & Toomey, 1985).

Implications for Nursing Care

Because Chinese Americans are perceived as being polychronic, it is important for the nurse to remember that some Chinese Americans may not adhere to fixed schedules. Polychronic individuals may arrive late for appointments; may insist on completing a task before moving on to a new one, even though the new task may be time sensitive and more urgent; and may implement more than one task at a time. It is important for the nurse to recognize that when some Chinese Americans make important decisions related to current events, they may appear hesitant and request time for deliberation because of the need to consider as many variables as possible, including consultation with family members.

ENVIRONMENTAL CONTROL

Many Chinese Americans, especially first-generation Chinese Americans, may not believe that they have control over nature because they subscribe to a belief in fatalism and may view people as adjusting to the physical world, not controlling or changing the environment (McBride, Morioka-Douglas, & Yeo, 1996). In traditional Chinese philosophy, a harmonious relationship with nature is stressed. Ancient Chinese philosophers believed that *qi* (or *chi*) was the vital life energy flowing around the universe and differentiated *qi* into two forces, *yin* and *yang*. While *yin* and *yang* are opposites; they exist only by virtue of each other. *Yin* and *yang* regulate the universe, including the body and food. *Yang* represents the positive, active, or "male" force, and *yin* represents the negative, inactive, or "female" force. Consequently, body organs are categorized into *yin* and *yang* groups. For example, the liver, heart, spleen, lungs, and kidneys are *yin*, whereas the gallbladder, stomach, large intestine, small intestine, bladder, and lymphatic system are *yang*. The *yin* forces store the strength of life while the *yang* forces protect the body from outside invasions. Some Chinese Americans believe that an imbalance between *yin* and *yang* will result in illness while a balance between the two maintains and enhances health.

Likewise, food is divided into *yin* ("cold") and *yang* ("hot") groups and is considered to be either the cause or the treatment of illnesses. A person with leukemia may believe that too many "cold" foods have been consumed. Diseases with excessive *yin* forces, such as cancer, postpartum psychosis, menstruation, or lactation, are treated with foods with *yang* qualities, such as beef, chicken, eggs, fried foods, spicy foods, hot foods, vinegar, and wine. Diseases or conditions with excessive *yang* forces, such as infection, fever, hypertension, sore throat, or toothache, require foods with *yin* properties, such as bean curd, honey, carrot, turnip, green vegetable, fruit, cold foods, and duck (Ludman & Newman, 1984). In addition, Chinese Americans often use tea, honey, prunes, or vegetables such as bok choy to treat constipation; they use chrysanthemum, crystal (preserved ginger), ginseng, or other herbal decoctions to treat indigestion (Hess, 1986).

Feng shui (translated literally to mean "wind [and] water"), which some Chinese Americans subscribe to, is the art of spatial arrangement of physical structures to achieve proper harmony and balance with nature (Fisher, 1996). Positive *feng shui* wards off evil spirits and promotes good health and prosperity. Shapes of objects, buildings, and so on take on significance for some Chinese Americans and can be correlated with good or bad luck. For example, a triangular building is considered to lead to bad luck and would not usually be used by Chinese Americans for house construction. Likewise, it is believed that doors should not open to direct traffic because this would allow evil spirits ready access into the home. Similarly, it is believed that the best location for a building is directly facing water while its rear is backed by mountains. Such

an arrangement encourages prosperity while offering protection.

Some Chinese Americans hold beliefs related to colors and numbers that may take on significance to health and health care. For example, the number 4 (*sì*), because it is pronounced the same as the word for "death" in Mandarin, is considered bad luck; whereas the number 8 (*ba*), which sounds like the word for "prosperity" in Cantonese, is considered good luck. On the other hand, the color white is considered bad luck because it is a color of mourning, whereas the color red is considered good luck and is associated with happiness and celebration. Thus a person born on 8/8/88 would be considered to be extremely fortunate or lucky, whereas a person born on 4/4/44 would be considered to be extremely unlucky. It is conceivable that a Chinese American subscribing to these beliefs might have considerable difficulty going for diagnostic testing in a triangular building that was located at 444 Fourth Street, where all the personnel wear white laboratory coats (Fisher, 1996).

Illness and Wellness Behaviors

Cultural differences, language barriers, and financial status play a major role in the utilization of health services by Chinese Americans. Jang, Lee, and Woo (1998) found that income, language ability, and citizenship status are associated with health care access and utilization in Chinese Americans.

Many Chinese Americans underutilize health services because of their socioeconomic status, associated high cost, and perceived cultural insensitiveness of the health care system. Although unemployment rates for the Chinese Americans are lower than for the general U.S. population, underemployment among Chinese Americans is much higher, underemployment is evidenced by a shorter work week, a mismatch between education and employment, and longer working hours for the same pay. In addition, at least 14% of Chinese Americans live at or below the poverty level. Many elderly Chinese Americans live alone with a fixed income, and this may be a direct result of early discriminatory immigration laws. Chinese immigrant families may have no health insurance because they may not believe in insuring health, or may be unable to afford it (Fisher, 1996). In fact, Takeuchi, Chung, and Shen (1998) noted that factors such as marital status, length of residence in the United States, education, employment, and average household income were associated with health insurance coverage among Chinese Americans. In addition, Jang, Lee, and Woo (1998) noted that income, language ability, and citizenship are all associated with health care access and utilization among Chinese Americans. Chinese Americans may fear medical institutions due to language barriers and unfamiliarity with the U.S. health care system. As a result, some Chinese Americans may not access or comply with medical treatments. Cultural beliefs and practices may also underscore such underutilization.

Many diagnostic tests, such as amniocentesis, glucose tolerance testing, ultrasonography, or drawing blood, are often perceived as being dangerous and unnecessary (Minkler, 1983). For instance, the invasive procedure of drawing blood on a daily basis not only is perceived as unnecessary but also is tolerated poorly by Chinese Americans because blood is believed to be part of the irreplaceable vital energy of the body and the belief in the intactness of the body (wholism). There was a report that a department store in Beijing had to resort to a lottery to determine whose turn it was to give blood "voluntarily," even with a bonus equivalent to a 2-month salary and 15 days of vacation (Fang, 1998). In addition, many Chinese Americans have a tendency to self-medicate with over-the-counter drugs, herbal remedies, tranquilizers, and antibiotics (Zhan & Chen, 2004). In this regard, some Chinese Americans may save part of a prescribed medicine and take it at their own discretion at a later time (Campbell & Chang, 1973).

Many Chinese Americans use Western and Chinese health providers simultaneously (Chen, 1995; Zhan & Chen, 2004), often failing to inform either. The failure to inform either Chinese or Western health providers (often intentional) when using both Chinese medicines and Western medicines at the same time can lead to increased safety risks and even tragedies (Zhan & Chen, 2004). Because some herbal and Western medicines have similar effects, using both can create problems. For example, ginseng is a tonic stimulant and an antihypertensive medicine. A client may overmedicate by taking antihypertensive drugs and ginseng at the same time.

Typically, Chinese Americans seek opinion and treatment of minor or chronic illnesses first within the informal health care system (that is, family, relatives, and friends) and try to manage on their own. If unsuccessful, then they tend to consult with and seek treatment from Chinese medical providers. Western physicians tend to be the last option. However, Western physicians may be the first choice if the conditions are acute or serious (Liu, 1986). The delay for treatment is especially common among Chinese American psychiatric clients because of the sociocultural stigma associated with mental illnesses (Zhan, 2004). This practice also accounts for the observed phenomenon that admitted Chinese patients tend to be sicker and more symptomatic (Louie, 1999; Xu, Sun, Zhang, & Xu, 2001).

The preparation and administration of Chinese medicine are unique. Chinese herbal medicines are boiled in a specified amount of water over low heat until the desired concentration is reached. The medicines are then taken as a single dose. If the client does not feel better after the initial dose, the client may need to return to the herbalist. Because of this tradition, some Chinese Americans are unfamiliar with the Western practice of continuing to take medications such as antibiotics over the entire prescribed duration even when feeling better (Zhan & Chen, 2004). In addition, the Western practice of taking multiple drugs in tablet or capsule form at various times and over several days or weeks is inconvenient and can be confusing.

Traditionally, Chinese Americans as a group are health-conscious and believe in preventive health practices, frequently incorporating health promotion activities such as walking into their daily lives. Confucianism mandates that one should treat one's own physical well-being as an expression and duty of filial piety (Hui, 1999). For this reason, many Chinese Americans are reluctant to take medications unless absolutely necessary because they believe every medication has side effects. Some Chinese people respond to pain stoically because they fear addiction to analgesics and because of the cultural value on self-control and the belief that suffering is inherent in life (Hui, 1999).

Death and Dying Issues and Practices

Like birth, death is an important life event. However, it is a cultural taboo for Chinese Americans to talk about death and related issues for fear of bringing bad luck or even jinxing their lives (Yick & Gupta, 2002; Zheng, 1999). Euphemisms are used when death or dying has to be dealt with (Yick & Gupta, 2002). Therefore, it is unlikely that Chinese Americans will have a living will and power of attorney at hospital admission, especially for first-generation Chinese immigrants. Where some Chinese Americans are concerned, talk or even mention of death is to be avoided during daily conversation. Although life is mortal, Chinese Americans believe in "natural and peaceful death" (*shou zhong zheng qin*). It is essential for the health care professional to remember that for some Chinese American, dying at home surrounded by family members is more desirable than dying at a health care facility. It is also important to remember that euthanasia and suicide in general are inconsistent with Chinese bioethics. In addition, according to traditional Chinese teaching, life is given by one's parents, and, moreover, it is the extension of one's family's life (Zheng, 1999); therefore, one has no right to take it away. This belief may serve as a protective factor against suicide at the cultural level.

For Chinese Americans, the rituals surrounding death can be very elaborate, with the primary purpose to help the dead live a comfortable and rich afterlife. Upon death, the body is washed and clean clothes are put on. Among Chinese Americans, burial in the ground is preferred, signifying that the body returns to where it came from (that is, nature). Food offerings and burning of fake paper money at burial time, as well as annual visitations in the spring at the Qing Ming Festival, are commonly practiced so that the dead will not be hungry and poor in the afterlife (Zheng, 1999). Many of these rituals are symbolic, with no practical reasons for the dead, but they serve the important purpose of comforting and relieving the burden of the living. Organ donation is inconsistent with the Chinese belief in wholism, which mandates that the body must remain intact, even after death (Yick & Gupta, 2002)

FOLKLORE AND FOLK PRACTICES

Maintaining the balance of *yin* and *yang* is the fundamental principle of Chinese medicine (Chen, 2001). Chinese medical practice includes acupuncture, herbal medicines, moxibustion, massage, coining, cupping, and so forth. Acupuncture involves the insertion of fine sterile metal needles through specific body points to treat or cure illnesses such as pain, stroke, or asthma. Herbal medicines are also categorized according to the properties of *yin* or *yang* and their therapeutic functions and are prescribed on the basis of the *yin–yang* nature of the particular illness. Moxibustion involves heat treatment of illnesses such as mumps or convulsions. When moxibustion is used as a treatment, the ignited moxa plants are placed near specific areas of the body. After moxibustion, tiny craters about 1 centimeter in diameter can be observed on the skin. Massage is used to stimulate the circulation, to increase the flexibility of the joints, and to improve the body's resistance to illnesses. Massage is a useful technique to relieve tension and stress. Coining involves applying a special oil to a symptomatic area and rubbing the area with the edge of a coin in a firm, downward motion. This treatment is used to treat cold, heatstroke, headache, and indigestion. Linear multiple bruises may be observed on the skin as a result of this process. Cupping is used to treat headaches, arthritis, and abdominal pain. A vacuum is created inside a glass jar by burning a special material. Then the inverted jar is placed immediately on the selected area and kept there over the designated duration until it is removed. Circular, ecchymotic marks 2 inches in diameter can be observed on the skin after this treatment (Andrews & Boyle, 2003; Spector, 2004).

Implications for Nursing Care

Because Chinese Americans often believe that they do not have control over nature and maintain a fatalistic outlook on life, they may be hesitant about seeking health care treatment. In addition, because some Chinese Americans subscribe to the theory of *yin* and *yang*, which attempts to restore balance to the body, such individuals are more likely to engage in self-treatment. Therefore, the nurse must be able to distinguish between practices that could be harmful, neutral, or beneficial to the client's particular medical problem. For example, some Chinese Americans from Southeast Asia or urban areas in China may practice native healing processes in which they may tie a string around the wrist, burn incense, or make food offerings to the spirits. As long as these practices are not harmful, the nurse should respect and allow them to continue. In addition, the nurse who observes that a Chinese American client is taking herbal medicine concurrently with prescribed Western medications should inform the attending physician and caution the client about the possibility of overmedicating and the possible side effects of drug interactions. For those Chinese Americans who subscribe to the theory of *yin* and *yang* and believe that food has *yin* and *yang* qualities, the nurse should assist the clients to select the appropriate foods accordingly. Finally, the nurse should encourage the family of a Chinese American client to bring familiar and more tasteful foods from home if (a) the client wishes and (b) there is no contraindication. For dying Chinese American patients, home hospice is more culturally congruent because the dying are often surrounded by family members in a familiar and intimate environment. The nurse should allow and make adaptation to the request for death rituals if safety and health risks are nonissues or can be minimized. Being empathetic, sensitive, and supportive is the key to meeting the family needs at this critical and trying time.

BIOLOGICAL VARIATIONS

Physical variations among races have been the subject of study for physical anthropologists. People are the product of both genetic factors and environmental influences. For example, it has been hypothesized that the epicanthic fold that gives the Chinese a slant-eyed look may have evolved as a protection against blinding blizzards of snow or sand (Bleibtreu & Downs, 1971). Others have theorized that Chinese people may have a thickened corneum, creating the yellowish skin color (Molnar, 2006). Most Chinese people have thick, straight hair. Chinese men tend to have less facial hair compared with Whites.

Body Size and Structure

Chinese Americans tend to be shorter at all ages, with long trunks and short legs, and complete their growth earlier (Molnar, 2006). On the standard growth charts, the mean height and weight of Chinese American children fall in the 10th percentile, whereas the mean height and weight of mainstream American children fall in the 50th percentile (Andrews & Boyle, 2003). The children of Chinese immigrants are generally taller than native Chinese children, perhaps because of better nutrition in a large part, but their sitting and standing height ratios do not change. On the average, Asians have longer trunks and shorter limbs than Whites. Asians have smaller chest volumes than Whites. The average forced expiratory volume for Chinese Americans is 2.53 liters, compared with 3.22 liters for White Americans; average forced vital capacity is 3.27 liters for Chinese Americans, compared with 4.30 liters for White Americans (Overfield, 1995).

Skin Color

The "yellow" color of the Chinese skin is believed to be caused by a smaller amount of melanin in the skin than in the skin of Black people (Race and ability, 1967). Others have theorized that Chinese people may have a thickened corneum, creating the yellowish skin color (Molnar, 2006). The majority of Chinese infants have mongolian spots (irregular areas of deep blue pigmentation observed primarily in the sacral and gluteal regions and occasionally in other areas of the body). Neonatal jaundice is seen in 50% of Chinese infants. The bilirubin level peaks on the fifth and sixth days of life, compared with the second and third days for other races. Bilirubin levels higher than 12 mg/dL occur in 25% to 40% of Chinese infants. Breastfeeding elevates the bilirubin level. The physician may suggest that the mother stop breastfeeding until the baby's bilirubin levels return to normal (Andrews & Boyle, 2003; Overfield, 1995).

Enzymatic and Genetic Variations

A majority of Chinese Americans have a lactase deficiency and are unable to tolerate fresh milk. Lactase splits milk sugar (lactose) into simple glucose and galactose. Lactase deficiency may cause a person who drinks fresh milk to have flatus, abdominal cramps, diarrhea, or vomiting. However, the person can often eat cheese to relieve or avoid the effects of this deficiency because bacteria do the work of lactase. This enzyme may also be induced by long-term consumption of fresh milk.

Chinese people have relatively higher incidences of thalassemia and G-6-PD deficiency (Molnar, 2006). Thalassemia is a type of hemoglobin abnormality characterized by a high rate of red blood cell destruction, necessitating frequent blood transfusions. The G-6-PD deficiency is another red blood cell defect, causing fragility of the red blood cells. Persons with G-6-PD deficiency are prone to anemia when exposed to certain drugs, such as analgesics (aspirin, phenacetin), sulfonamides and sulfones, antimalarials (primaquine, quinacrine), antibacterials (nitrofurantoin, chloramphenicol, para-aminosalicylic acid), vitamin K, probenecid, and quinidine (Molnar, 2006; Overfield, 1995).

Another genetic difference is that Chinese people usually experience noticeable facial flushing and vasomotor symptoms after drinking alcohol. This may explain the low alcoholism rate among the Chinese (Overfield, 1995)(see Chapter 7).

Susceptibility to Disease

There is a lack of national health statistics on Chinese Americans, primarily because existing census and health databases contain only aggregate data on Asian Americans and/or Pacific Islanders (Ghosh, 2003). In other words, the data on Chinese Americans have been dispersed in the lump sum data. Although Census 2000 created "Asians" as a stand-alone category, there will be continuing methodological and statistical challenges to separate data (often impossible) to study Chinese Americans, one among about 30 ethnic subgroups of Asian Americans in the United States. Moreover, the compatibility of the current and future data categories with the existing ones will remain an issue.

Infectious Diseases. Immigrants from Indochina and mainland China share many increased health risks, such as tuberculosis (TB), intestinal parasites, malaria, malnutrition, anemia, and hepatitis. Most Southeast Asians received vaccinations (bacille Calmette-Guérin [BCG]) against tuberculosis in their childhood (Overfield, 1995). However, the exposure to BCG vaccinations tends to produce false-positive results on the Mantoux test. This situation makes it harder to differentiate an authentic TB case from a false-positive one (Overfield, 1995).

Cancer. The burden of cancer for Asian Americans and Pacific Islanders (AAPIs), including Chinese Americans, is "unusual," "unequal," and "unnecessary" (Chen, 2000). The burden of cancer is unusual in that cancer is and has been the leading cause of death for AAPI females since 1980, when these statistics were first collected. No other racial-ethnic-gender group has experienced this. Cancer is also the leading cause of death for AAPIs age 25 to 64; by comparison, cancer does not become the leading cause of death for Whites until they reach the 45- to 64-year age bracket (Chen, 2000).

The burden of cancer for AAPIs is unequal. Cancer death rates for AAPIs have increased at higher rates than for any other racial or ethnic group. Between 1980 and 1996, the number of cancer deaths for AAPI females increased 323.6%, compared with 132.6% for White females. In addition, the number of cancer deaths for AAPI males increased 276.8%, compared with 123.1% for White males (Chen, 2000). The incidence of liver cancer in Chinese, Filipino, Japanese, Korean, and Vietnamese populations is 1.7 to 11.3 times higher than rates among White Americans (Miller, Kolonel, Bernstein, et al., 1996).

The burden of cancer for AAPIs is also unnecessary in many respects. Smoking is the single most important preventable cause of death. AAPI men smoke at rates higher than most other racial and ethnic groups (U.S. Department of Health and Human Services, 1998). Studies (Chen, Unger, Cruz, & Johnson, 1999; Chen, Unger, & Johnson, 1999) demonstrated that smoking patterns of Asian American youth, including Chinese youth, are different from those of their White peers in California. Although Asian American youth have lower smoking rates and later age of smoking onset, high levels of acculturation are associated with higher smoking prevalence rates and earlier age of smoking onset. Tu, Walsh, Tseng, and Thompson (2000) explored the social and cultural functions of smoking among 34 Chinese American men in Seattle, Washington. Forty percent of the study subjects identified family as a significant reason to quit smoking. In a more recent study on smoking among Chinese Americans in Chicago's Chinatown, Yu, Abdulrahim, Chen, and Kim (2002) found that the smoking rate for Chinese men was 34%, significantly higher than for the U.S. general population. Low education, use of a non-Western physician or clinic for health care, and no knowledge of early cancer warning signs and symptoms were significantly associated with smoking. Lam, Ho, Hedley, Mak, and Peto (2001) noted that the proportion of male deaths between 35 and 65 years of age attributable to tobacco will jump from 13% in 1998 to about 33% over the next few decades in mainland China, which has 20% of the world's population and consumes 30% of the world's tobacco. In China, many studies have confirmed that physician advice is the most effective intervention to stop smoking. Li and Rosenblood (1996) examined physicians' smoking behavior and their antismoking counseling practices in the city of Wuhan, China. The study found that 50.9% of male and 4.8% of female physicians were current smokers and that physicians' own smoking status and age were among the significant factors influencing antismoking counseling. In a related study, Li, Fish, and Zhou (1999) reported that the smoking rates for the two groups increased to 61.3% and 12.2%, respectively, from 1987 to 1996. The sharp increase in smoking prevalence among female physicians was alarming and disturbing, while the antismoking counseling of both groups declined. What impact these data will have on Chinese Americans and smoking behaviors is still largely unknown.

East and Southeast Asian women, including Chinese American women, have the lowest rates of breast cancer screening (Carey Jackson, Taylor, Chitnarong, et al., 2000; Juon, Choi, & Kim, 2000; Tu, Yasui, Kuniyuki, et al., 2000). General findings from those studies reveal that because of cultural, educational, institutional, and logistical barriers, East and Southeast Asian women as a group tend to underuse existing cancer screening and early detection programs, thus putting them at increased risks for cancer. The identified contributing factors include, among others, language barriers, lack of knowledge of biomedicine, unfamiliarity with the U.S. health care system, distrust in Western physicians, poverty, and lack of health insurance.

Recognizing the disproportionate cancer risks, the National Cancer Institute launched two multisite studies to increase the awareness, training, and research on cancer control in Asian Americans (Chen, 2000). The two major studies have evolved into two major networks (one based first at Ohio State University in Columbus, Ohio, and now headquartered at University of California at Davis, and the other one based at Temple University in Philadelphia) that intend to build and provide the infrastructure to study cancer control in Asian Americans (Chen, 2000).

Chinese people are also known to be at higher risk for cancers of the nasopharynx, esophagus, stomach, liver, and cervix. The intake of fermented and moldy foods and of the nitrosamines contained in corn, bran, millet, and pickled vegetables is believed to be a possible contributing factor for esophageal and liver cancers. In addition, salted fish has been linked with stomach cancer in East and Southeast Asians, including Chinese. Recent studies have revealed a downward trend for these cancers among Chinese Americans. On the other hand, cancers that were of low risk in the past (such as cancers of the colon, rectum, lung, and female breast and leukemia) are gradually increasing among Chinese Americans (King & Locke, 1988; Overfield, 1995). One significant study (Ziegler, Hoover, Pike, et al., 1993) confirmed that increased acculturation is linked with increased risks for breast cancer in Asian American women. Acculturation is also increasing eating disorders in Chinese college students in the United States (Davis & Katzman, 1999), along with fat-related dietary behavior (Liou & Contento, 2001).

Mortality and Leading Causes of Death

In 2004, mortality data revealed the four leading causes of death for Chinese Americans to be identical to those for White Americans: heart disease, cerebral vascular disease, cancer, and chronic respiratory disorders (National Center for Health Statistics, Health United States, 2006). However, the proportional mortalities are different. Chinese Americans have a lower mortality from heart disease (32%) than White Americans (39%) and a higher mortality from cancer (27%) than White Americans (21%). The fifth leading cause of death for Chinese Americans is pneumonia and influenza. Suicide ranks ninth as a cause of death for Chinese Americans compared with eleventh for White Americans. Chinese women have a higher suicide rate than White women (National Center for Health Statistics, Health, United States, 2006). The specific causes of the higher suicide rate warrant further investigation.

Psychological Characteristics

There is a deeply entrenched sociocultural stigma associated with mental illnesses among Chinese and Chinese Americans (Zhan, 2004). For instance, mental hospitals in China recently were renamed "brain hospitals" to translate literarily. Many Chinese Americans believe that psychiatric illnesses indicate an inability to exert control of one's behavior, bringing shame to the individual client as well as the family. Therefore, the family will often attempt to manage the sick family member on their own for as long as possible. As a result, hospitalized Chinese psychiatric clients tend to appear more symptomatic (Chen, 1995). Research cited by Chen (1995) identified five phases regarding family help-seeking behaviors with mental ill family members for Chinese individuals residing in Vancouver, Canada, that included: (1) exclusive intrafamilial coping; (2) inclusion of certain trusted outsiders in the intrafamilial attempt at coping; (3) consultation with outside helping agencies, physicians, and finally a psychiatrist while keeping the patient at home; (4) the labeling of mental illness and a subsequent series of hospitalizations; and (5) scapegoating and rejection.

Chinese Americans, like other immigrants, experience multiple psychosocial stresses while adapting to the new culture and environment, including cultural conflicts, language difficulties, poverty, and discrimination. Many Chinese Americans experience depression and loneliness (Casado & Leung, 2001), but few seek help until associated psychosomatic symptoms are more severe (Chen, 1995). Chinese Americans tend to seek help from other physicians rather than psychiatrists or related mental health professionals for psychosomatic complaints. Somatization is the most common form of symptom manifestation, frequently caused by mental issues such as experienced shame with no pathological etiology (Chen, 1995). Studies are needed to differentiate whether the low admission rate of

Asian Americans, including Chinese Americans, to psychiatric units across the country should be attributed to the "protective factors" offered by the Asian family and social network, or to the social pressure to confine the mentally ill to closely guarded family circles, or to both.

Recent research has confirmed different reactions to the same prescribed pharmacological agents among different racial and ethnic groups due to drug polymorphisms during metabolism. After reviewing research and clinical evidence, Kudzma (1999, 2001) reported that Asian Americans, including Chinese Americans, respond differently to some psychotropic and antihypertensive agents. Specifically, Asian American patients need lower doses of haloperidol (Haldol), diazepam (Valium), and propranolol (Inderal) to achieve the same therapeutic effect, even after body weight and stature (that is, surface area) have been taken into consideration. Recent empirical research has also revealed that Asian Americans require lower dosages than Whites for psychotropic medications, such as lithium, antidepressants, and neuroleptics. The plasma levels of desipramine (Norpramin) are higher and peak earlier for Asian Americans than for Whites. Asian Americans experience extrapyramidal effects at lower neuroleptic doses than Whites. The plasma levels of diazepam of the same oral dose are higher in Asian Americans than in Whites. Asian Americans are reported to tolerate the sedating effects of diphenhydramine (Benadryl) better. The causes for such differences are considered to be both genetic and environmental and need to be further investigated to ensure patient safety. Another plausible explanation is that the standard dosage is based on clinical trials in which Asian Americans and other ethnic minorities were either underrepresented or not represented at all. The National Institutes of Health, the primary health research agency in this country, has taken steps to correct the problem (National Institutes of Health, 1994, 2001). One major action implemented was mandating that all studies include minority subjects, unless strong explanations were offered, to ensure that the research findings can be generalized to the entire population.

Implications for Nursing Care

It is important for the nurse to know that growth and development norms for Chinese Americans are different from White American standards. A standard growth chart for healthy Chinese children and adolescents is available (Wong & Hockenberry-Eaton, 2001). However, the nurse should not rely on the growth chart alone. A comprehensive assessment of general health status is necessary to identify malnutrition, anemia, or growth retardation (Gallo, Edwards, & Vessey, 1980).

The nurse should reassure the Chinese American mother that it is normal for her newborn to exhibit more jaundice than other American babies do. Otherwise, the mother may feel guilty and believe that the jaundice is caused by something she ate. The observed mongolian spots in Chinese American infants should not be interpreted as lesions.

When working with a Chinese American family that has a family member with a physical or mental problem, the astute nurse will make use of general or mental health facilities easier by providing information regarding available services, encouraging the family to seek help early, and arranging for follow-up care. Rather than waiting until the symptoms are advanced, the nurse should assist the family in getting appropriate care for their family member as soon as possible.

The following case report illustrates the profound effect of the Chinese culture on a client with a medical problem and psychotic symptoms. An 83-year-old Chinese woman exhibited psychotic symptoms at home for 15 months until the family could not handle the situation any longer and admitted her to a hospital. The family members felt guilty and ashamed because they could not take care of their mother. After admission, a health history revealed that the client had had a gastrectomy about 13 years earlier, and her blood level of vitamin B_{12} was 91 mg/dL (normal is 180 to 900 mg/dL). She was treated with vitamin B_{12}, and the psychotic symptoms disappeared. If the family had brought the patient to the hospital earlier, perhaps they could have avoided 15 months of agony (Binder, 1983).

Client and family teaching are important in providing care for the Chinese American client and family. Lack of knowledge related to illnesses and treatments is a common problem and causes fear and anxiety. The nurse can assess the family's understanding of illnesses and treatments and provide education accordingly. If the client takes herbal medicines, which are not currently regulated by the government, the nurse should provide education to increase the client and family's awareness of the possible synergistic and antagonistic effects of Western and herbal medicines taken together.

Because Asians are known to require lower dosages of psychotropic medications, the nurse should provide education about these medications and keep a watchful eye on their possible side effects. The nurse needs to remain alert to possible adverse effects from one-size-fits-all prescriptions. The nurse should also emphasize the importance of taking medicines as prescribed and discourage the practice of taking medicines only when symptoms are present. In addition, the nurse should keep in mind that Chinese Americans have a relatively high incidence of G-6-PD deficiency; therefore, it is essential to urge the client to seek help early when any side effects of medications are experienced.

The need for teaching about medication is illustrated by the following example. A Chinese American man took captopril (Capoten) at home as prescribed for 1 week and developed severe thirst and hyponatremia, leading to irreversible neurological damage (Al-Mufti & Arieff, 1985). He was polydipsic and drank about 7 liters daily. If he had been taught the side effects of captopril and encouraged to seek help when he experienced this side effect, his death could possibly have been avoided.

Although many Chinese women breastfeed their babies, recently many Chinese American women who have been adapting to Western culture have changed to bottle-feeding. The nurse should provide information regarding the benefits of breast-feeding and encourage mothers to breastfeed for at least 6 weeks (Minkler, 1983). If the mother has to stop breastfeeding because of jaundice, the nurse can teach the mother to express milk to continue breastfeeding when the baby is ready to be breastfed again.

Dietary education is also very important in providing care for the Chinese American client and family (Kolonel, 1988). Some Chinese Americans believe in the theory of *yin* and *yang* and eat foods accordingly when they are sick. For example, postpartum and after surgery, some Chinese Americans will not drink or eat anything with *yin* qualities, such as cold drinks, vegetables, salad, or cold meat; they will eat only chicken, beef, or fried foods. The nurse should help the client select foods and encourage the family to bring the desired foods from home.

Chinese foods usually are cooked with soy sauce and monosodium glutamate (MSG). The nurse must remember that many preserved foods are also high in salt content. Therefore, the nurse should advise patients who require a salt-restricted diet to reduce their sodium intake gradually by reducing the use of soy sauce, MSG, and preserved foods and discourage high intake of fermented and moldy foods, which are thought to contribute to the high incidence of esophageal and liver cancer. The nurse should also encourage clients to reduce their intake of foods that have no nutritional value. Because many Chinese Americans may be unable to tolerate fresh milk because of a lactase deficiency, the nurse should encourage the use of tofu (bean curd) and other protein- and calcium-rich foods to provide the needed nutrients.

SUMMARY

Chinese Americans are one of the fastest-growing ethnic groups in the United States. As Chinese immigrants continue to increase, the nurse will encounter more Chinese Americans in health care facilities. Because of the complex cultural values and beliefs, diverse degrees of acculturation, and various educational levels among Chinese Americans, the nurse needs to work with individuals to assess their unique values, communication styles, social organization, time concepts, illness behaviors, and biological variations to provide effective and individualized care. For example, the health beliefs, attitudes, and health-seeking behaviors of the second or third generation of Chinese Americans are different in important ways from those of their parents and grandparents (Willgerodt, Miller, & McElmurry, 2002; Yick & Gupta, 2002), although some of the core values remain unchanged. As a general rule for caring for Chinese Americans, the nurse should involve the family, convey respect for the client, encourage pride in the Chinese culture, reduce feelings of shame, and facilitate adaptation to the Western culture.

Case Study

A 40-year-old Chinese American woman is admitted to a local hospital with the diagnosis of uremia. Her blood urea nitrogen (BUN) level is 168 mg/dL (normal is 8 to 18 mg/dL). She has a history of hypertension and was previously given a prescription for hydrochlorothiazide (HCTZ), which she stopped taking because of increasing dizziness, dry mouth, and weakness. She is single, lives alone, has no immediate family nearby, has a temporary job, and has no medical insurance. Her physician prescribes peritoneal dialysis and HCTZ. The following are noted by the nurse on assessment: blood pressure, 180/100 mm Hg; respirations, 20 per minute; pulse, 110 per minute; height, 5 feet, 1 inch; weight, 100 pounds; dry skin with multiple scratching marks; no urine output; and complaints of blurred vision, itchiness, weakness, and insomnia. Her gait is slightly unsteady. She talks with a soft and low voice and speaks English slowly but not fluently. She sometimes asks questions that have already been discussed. Although she smiles frequently during conversation, she appears tense and restless. The nurse notices some hand tremors, a shaky voice, and twisting fingers. Although she has limited information about peritoneal dialysis, the woman changes the subject as the nurse explains the procedure.

CARE PLAN

✳ Nursing Diagnosis: Pain related to pruritus

Client Outcome

1. Client will verbalize discomfort to others when it exists and will relate relief with therapeutic measures.

Nursing Interventions

1. Explain pruritus will be decreased when client's BUN level is down.
2. Keep client's room cool and avoid excessive warmth from clothes or blankets because warmth will increase itchiness.
3. Apply cool lotions to dry and itchy areas.
4. Apply cool, wet soaks to reduce itchiness if client desires.
5. Ask client's doctor if any medicines can be used to decrease itchiness.
6. Encourage client to engage in diversional activities.
7. Advise client to keep her fingernails short to avoid injury to her skin when she scratches.

✳ *Nursing Diagnosis: Anxiety related to peritoneal dialysis*

Client Outcome

1. Client will verbalize her understanding of peritoneal dialysis and will experience less anxiety after teaching.

Nursing Interventions

1. Assess client's understanding of peritoneal dialysis.
2. Present information to client related to peritoneal dialysis by using pamphlets and drawings.
3. Explain rationale for peritoneal dialysis.
4. Describe feelings the client may have during dialysis
5. Contact dialysis nurses to obtain some audiovisual aids to help client understand.

✳ *Nursing Diagnosis: Noncompliance related to side effects of HCTZ*

Client Outcome

1. Client will describe the experience that caused her to stop taking HCTZ, describe appropriate treatment of side effects, and demonstrate appropriate alternatives to the previous plan.

Nursing Interventions

1. Assess any other contributing factors for stopping HCTZ (such as cost, refer to social worker to seek any financial help).
2. Identify current effects and side effects of HCTZ on client.
3. Teach effects and side effects of HCTZ.
4. Assist client in reducing discomfort (such as dizziness—change positions slowly; dry mouth—ice chips, hard candy; weakness—get plenty of sleep and ask for help for what she is limited in doing).
5. Explain client's dizziness; weakness could be improved when her BUN level is down.
6. Ask client to verbalize what she understands.

✳ *Nursing Diagnosis: Communication, impaired verbal, related to foreign-language barrier*

Client Outcome

1. Client will be able to communicate basic needs and relate feelings of acceptance

Nursing Interventions

1. Talk slowly and clearly to client.
2. Write down important information.
3. Use gestures, actions, pictures, and drawings to facilitate client's understanding.
4. Encourage client to teach others some Chinese words.
5. Seek a translator to discuss important matters.

✳ STUDY QUESTIONS

1. List at least three contributing factors for hypertension among Chinese Americans.
2. Delineate at least two things that the nurse can do to facilitate the communication process between the nurse and the Chinese American client.
3. Identify at least two factors about lack of family structure and its significance to the Chinese culture that may contribute to the difficulties of hospitalization for the Chinese American client.
4. Describe factors regarding the time concept that may hinder health care services for a Chinese American client.
5. Describe health and illness practices that may augment problems associated with the treatment of hypertension for Chinese American clients.

NCLEX-RN REVIEW QUESTIONS

1. Mr. Chan, an 81-year-old Chinese American man, has been admitted to the hospital for abdominal pain. His oldest son answers questions for him and expresses his needs. Mr. Chan's wife, who does speak English although not fluently, defers to the son when asked to participate in discussion. This is an example of:
   A. The cultural value of male-female hierarchy
   B. The cultural value of giving authority for decision making to the young
   C. An attempt by the son to gain control of the situation
   D. The need for family members to participate in care-giving decisions

2. A Chinese American who is experiencing a symptom such as diarrhea (which is felt to be "yin") is likely to try to treat it with:
   A. High doses of medicines thought to be "cold"
   B. No treatment at all, since diarrhea is an expected part of life
   C. Foods that are "hot" or "yang"
   D. Readings and Eastern medicine meditations

3. People from Chinese American cultures, although valuing family, are generally more often inclined toward individualistic behavior.
   A. True
   B. False

References

Al-Mufti, H. I., & Arieff, A. I. (1985). Captopril-induced hyponatremia with irreversible neurologic damage. *American Journal of Medicine*, 79, 769–770.

Andrews, M., & Boyle, J. (2003). *Transcultural concepts in nursing care* (ed. 4). Philadelphia: Lippincott Williams & Wilkins.

Binder, R. L. (1983). Cultural factors complicating the treatment of psychosis caused by B_{12} deficiency. *Hospital and Community Psychiatry*, 34(1), 67–69.

Bleibtreu, H. K., & Downs, J. F. (1971). *Human variations: readings in physical anthropology* (revised ed.). Beverly Hills, Calif.: Glencoe Press.

Burkett, H. (1995). Being culturally correct. *Health Traveler*, 2(4), 4–46.

Campbell, T., & Chang, B. (1973). Health care of the Chinese in America. *Nursing Outlook*, 21(4), 245–249.

Carey Jackson, J., Taylor, V. M., & Chitnarong, K., et al. (2000). Development of a cervical cancer control intervention program for Cambodian American women. *Journal of Community Health*, 25(5), 359–375.

Casado, B. L., & Leung, P. L. (2001). Migratory grief and depression among elderly Chinese American immigrants. In Choi, N. G. (Ed.), *Social work practice with the Asian American elderly* (pp. 5–26). New York: The Haworth Social Work Practice Press.

Central Intelligence Agency. (2006). *The World Factbook*, Retrieved July 17, 2002, from https://www.odci.gov/cia/publications/factbook/geos/ch.html.

Chen, D. (1995). Cultural and psychological influences on mental health issues for Chinese Americans. In Adler, L. L. & Mukherji, B. R. (Eds.), *Spirit versus scalpel: traditional healing and modern psychotherapy* (pp. 186–196). Westport, Conn.: Bergin & Garvey.

Chen, C. L., & Yang, D. C. V. (1986). The self-image of Chinese-American adolescents: a cross-cultural comparison. *International Journal of Social Psychiatry*, 32(4), 19–26.

Chen, M. S. Jr. (2000). Launching of the Asian American Network for Cancer Awareness Research and Training (AANCART). *Asian American and Pacific Islander Journal of Health*, 8(1), 1–3.

Chen, Y. C. (2001). Chinese values, health and nursing. *Journal of Advanced Nursing*, 36(2), 270–273.

Chen, X., Unger, J. B., Cruz, T. B., & Johnson, C. A. (1999). Smoking patterns of Asian-American youth in California and their relationship with acculturation. *Journal of Adolescent Health*, 24(5), 321–328.

Chen, X., Unger, J. B., & Johnson, C. A. (1999). Is acculturation a risk factor for early smoking initiation among Chinese American minors? A comparative perspective. *Tobacco Control*, 8, 402–410.

Cheung, R., Nelson, W., & Advincula, L., et al. (2005). Understanding the culture of Chinese children and families. *The Journal of School Nursing*, 21(1), 3–9.

Chin, P. (2005). Chinese. In Lipson, J. G., & Dibble, S. L. (Eds.), *Culture & clinical care* (pp. 98–108). San Francisco: USCF Nursing Press.

Davis, C., & Katzman, M. A. (1999). Perfection as acculturation: psychological correlates of eating problems in Chinese male and female students living in the United States. *International Journal of Eating Disorders*, 25, 65–70.

Fang, B. (1998, November 9). Why it's really hard to draw blood in China. *U.S. News & World Report*, 44.

Fisher, N. L. (1996). *Culture and ethnic diversity: a guide for genetic professionals*. Baltimore: Johns Hopkins University Press.

Gallo, A. M., Edwards, J., & Vessey, J. (1980). Indochina moves to main street: little refugees with big needs (part 4). *RN*, 43, 45–48.

Ghosh, C. (2003). Healthy People 2010 and Asian Americans/Pacific Islanders: defining a baseline of information. *American Journal of Public Health*, 93(12), 2093–2098.

Gudykunst, W. B. (2001). *Asian American ethnicity and communication*. Thousand Oaks, Calif.: Sage Publications.

Gudykunst, W. B., Stewart, L. P., & Toomey, S. T. (1985). *Communication, culture, and organizational process*. Newbury Park, Calif.: Sage.

Hall, E. T. (1981). A system for the notation of proxemic behavior. *American Anthropologist*, 65, 1003–1026.

Hall, E. T. (1989). *Beyond culture*. New York: Anchor Books.

Hess, P. (1986). Chinese and Hispanic elders and OTC drugs. *Geriatric Nursing*, 7(6), 314–318.

Hui, E. (1999). A Confucian ethic of medical futility. In Fan, R. (Ed.), *Confucian bioethics* (pp. 127–163). Boston: Kluwer Academic Publishers.

Jang, M., Lee, E., & Woo, K. (1998). Income, language, and citizenship status: factors affecting the health care access and utilization of Chinese Americans. *Health and Social Work*, 23(2), 136–145.

Juon, H. S., Choi, Y., & Kim, M. T. (2000). Cancer screening behaviors among Korean American women. *Cancer Detection and Prevention*, 24(6), 589–601.

Kim, Y. Y. (2003). Intercultural personhood: an integration of Eastern and Western perspectives. In Samovar, L. A., & Porter, R. E. (Eds.), *Intercultural communication: a reader* (ed. 10). Belmont, Calif.: Wadsworth/Thomson Learning.

King, H., & Locke, F. B. (1988). The national mortality survey of China: implications for cancer control and prevention. *Cancer Detection and Prevention*, 13(3–4), 157–166.

Kolonel, L. N. (1988). Variability in diet and its relation to risk in ethnic and migrant groups. *Basic Life Science*, 43, 129–135.

Kudzma, E. C. (1999). Culturally competent drug administration. *American Journal of Nursing*, 99(8), 46–51.

Kudzma, E. C. (2001). Cultural competence: cardiovascular medications. *Progress in Cardiovascular Nursing*, 16(4), 152–160, 169.

Lam, T. H., Ho, S. Y., Hedley, A. J., Mak, K. H., & Peto, R. (2001). Mortality and smoking in Hong Kong: case-control study of all adult deaths in 1998. *British Medical Journal*, 323, 1–6.

Li, H. Z., Fish, D., & Zhou, X. C. (1999). Increase in cigarette smoking and decline of anti-smoking counseling among Chinese physicians: 1987–1996. *Health Promotion International*, 14(2), 123–131.

Li, H. Z., & Rosenblood, L. (1996). Chinese physicians' cigarette smoking habits and their anti-smoking counseling practices. *Health Promotion International*, 11(2), 89–94.

Lin, L. Q. (2000). *China: facts and figures 2000*. Beijing: New Star Publishers.

Liou, D., & Contento, I. R. (2001). Usefulness of psychosocial theory variables in explaining fat-related dietary behavior in Chinese Americans: association with degree of acculturation. *Journal of Nutrition Education*, 33(6), 322–331.

Liu, W. T. (1986). Health services for Asian elderly. *Research on Aging*, 8(1), 156–175.

Louie, K. B. (1999). Status of mental heath needs of Asian elderly. In Wykle, M. L., & Ford, A. B. (Eds.), *Serving minority elders in the 21st century* (pp. 147–159). New York: Springer.

Ludman, E. K., & Newman, J. M. (1984). The health-related food practices of three Chinese groups. *Journal of Nutrition Education*, 16, 4.

Lyman, S. (1974). *Chinese Americans*. New York: Random House.

McBride, M., Morioka-Douglas, N., & Yeo, G. (1996). *Aging and health: Asian and Pacific Islander American elders* (ed. 2) ethnographic reviews working paper series 3. Palo Alto, Calif.: Stanford Geriatric Education Center.

Miller, B. A., Kolonel, L. N., & Bernstein, L., et al. (Eds.). (1996). *Racial/ethnic patterns of cancer in the United States 1988–1992*. Retrieved July 25, 2002, from http://seer.cancer.gov/publications/ethnicity/index.html.

Minkler, D. H. (1983). The role of community-based satellite clinics in the perinatal care of non-English speaking immigrants. *Western Journal of Medicine*, 139 (6), 905–909.

Molnar, S. (2006). *Human variation: races, types, and ethnic groups*. (ed. 6). Upper Saddle River, N.J.: Pearson Prentice Hall.

National Bureau of Statistics of China. (2001, March 28). *Communiqué on major figures of the 2000 population census (no. 1)*. Retrieved July 17, 2006, from http://www.stats.gov.cn/english/newrelease/statisticalreports/200204 230084.htm.

National Center for Health Statistics. (1998). *Health, United States, 1998, with socioeconomic status and chartbook*. Hyattsville, Md.: National Center for Health Statistics.

National Center for Health Statistics (2006). *Health, United States, 2005 with urban and rural chartbook*. Hyattsville, Md.: National Center for Health Statistics.

National Institutes of Health (1994, March 18). NIH guidelines on the inclusion of women and minorities as subjects in clinical research. *NIH Guide*. Bethesda, Md.: National Institutes of Health.

National Institutes of Health. Office of Extramural Research. (2001). *Monitoring adherence to the NIH policy on the including of women and minorities as subjects in clinical research*. Retrieved July 25, 2002, from http://www4.od.nih.gov/orwh/salmonrpt.pdf.

Overfield, T. (1995). *Biological variations in health and illness*. Reading, Mass.: Addison-Wesley.

Race and ability. (1967, September 29) *Time*, pp. 46–47.

Reeves, T. J., & Bennett, C. E. (2004). *We the People: Asians in the United States*. Retrieved June 2, 2006, from http://www.census.gov/prod/2004pubs/censr-17.pdf.

Samovar, L. A., & Porter, R. E. (2003). *Intercultural communication: a reader*. (ed. 10). Belmont, Calif.: Wadsworth/Thomson Learning.

Smedley, B. D., Stith, A. Y., & Nelson, A. R. (2003). *Unequal treatment: confronting racial and ethnic disparities in health care*. Washington, D.C.: National Academy Press.

Sowell, T. (1981). *Ethnic America*. New York: Basic Books.

Spector, R. E. (2004). *Cultural diversity in health and illness* (ed. 6). Upper Saddle River, N.J.: Pearson Prentice Hall.

Sung, B. (1967). *Mountain of gold: a story of Chinese in America*. New York: McMillan.

Surgeon General's report. (1999). Mental health: Culture, race, and ethnicity. A Supplement to Mental Health: A Report of the Surgeon General. Washington, D.C.: U.S. Government Printing Office.

Takeuchi, D. T., Chung, R. C. Y., & Shen, H. K. (1998). Health insurance coverage among Chinese Americans in Los Angeles County. *American Journal of Public Health*, 88(3), 451–453.

Time Almanac with Information Please. (2007). Boston: Information Please Inc.

Tu, S. P., Walsh, M., Tseng, B., & Thompson, B. (2000). Tobacco use by Chinese-American men: an exploratory study of the factors associated with cigarette use and smoking cessation. *Asian American and Pacific Islander Journal of Health*, 8(1), 46–57.

Tu, S. P., Yasui, Y., & Kuniyuki, A., et al. (2000). Breast cancer screening among Cambodian American women. *Cancer Detection and Prevention*, 24(6), 549–563.

U.S. Census Bureau. (2000). The Asian and Pacific Islander population in the United States. Retrieved July 24, 2002, from http://www.census.gov/prod/2000pubs/p20–529.pdf.

U.S. Department of Commerce, Bureau of the Census. (2002). Population profiles by age, sex, race, and Hispanic origin, Summary File 3. Washington, D.C.: U.S. Government Printing Office.

U.S. Department of Health and Human Services. (1998). *Tobacco use among U.S. racial/ethnic minority groups—African Americans, American Indians and Alaska Natives, Asian Americans and Pacific Islanders, and Hispanics: a report of the surgeon general*. Atlanta: U.S. Department of Health and Human Services, Centers for Disease Control and Prevention, National Center for Chronic Disease Prevention and Health Promotion, Office on Smoking and Health.

Watson, O. M. (1970). *Proxemic behavior: a cross-cultural study*. The Hague, the Netherlands: Mouton.

Willgerodt, M. A., Miller, A. M., & McElmurry, B. J. (2002). Becoming bicultural: Chinese American women and their development. *Health Care for Women International*, 23, 467–480.

Wong, B. P. (2006). *The Chinese in Silicon Valley: Globalization, social networks, and ethnic identity*. Lanham, Md: Rowman & Littlefield.

Wong, D., & Hockenberry-Eaton, M. (2001). *Wong's essentials of pediatric nursing*. (ed. 6). St. Louis: Mosby.

World almanac. (2007). Mahwah, N.J.: World Almanac Books.

Xu, Y., Sun, J., Zhang, J., & Xu, Z. (2001). Health-seeking behaviors of Southeast Asian immigrants and barriers to health care: implications for the home health nurse. *Home Health Care Management and Practice*, 14(1), 22–30.

Yick, A. G., & Gupta, R. (2002). Chinese cultural dimensions of death, dying, and bereavement: Focus group findings. *Journal of Cultural Diversity,* 9(2), 32–42.

Yu, E. S. H., Abdulrahim, S., Chen, E. H., & Kim, K. K. (2002). Smoking among Chinese Americans: behavior, knowledge, and beliefs. *American Journal of Public Health,* 92(6), 1007–1012.

Zhan, L. (2004). Caring for family members with Alzheimer's disease: perspectives from Chinese caregivers. *Journal of Gerontological Nursing,* 30(8), 19–29.

Zhan, L., & Chen, J. (2004). Medication practices among Chinese American older adults: a study of cultural influences. *Journal of Gerontological Nursing,* 30(4), 24–33.

Zheng, X. J. (1999). *Good death: the Chinese philosophy on death.* Kunming, Yunnan: Yunnan People's Press (in Chinese).

Ziegler, R. C., Hoover, R. R., & Pike, M. C., et al. (1993). Migration patterns and breast cancer risk in Asian-American women. *Journal of National Cancer Institute,* 86, 1819–1827.

CHAPTER 17 Filipino Americans

Anna R. Vance

Behavioral Objectives

After reading this chapter, the nurse will be able to:

1. Describe the problems encountered regarding communication when giving culturally appropriate nursing care to Filipino American clients.
2. Explain the Filipino American orientation to time and space and the relevance to culturally appropriate nursing care.
3. Describe how health care beliefs, values, behaviors, medical and folk practices, and attitudes affect health-seeking behaviors of Filipino American clients.
4. Identify how beliefs of Filipino Americans affect the internal locus of control and subsequently the environmental control variable.
5. Describe biological variations that may be found in the Filipino American client.

OVERVIEW OF THE PHILIPPINES

The Philippine Islands constitute an independent nation located in the Pacific Ocean approximately 450 miles off the southeastern coast of China. Taiwan is the nearest neighbor, approximately 65 miles to the north; Indonesia is 150 miles to the south.

More than 7000 islands compose the Philippine Archipelago; however, the largest islands, Luzon (40,420 square miles) and Mindanao (36,537 square miles), account for 94% of the country's total land area. All the remaining islands are less than 6000 square miles in area. Most of the Philippine Islands are hilly and mountainous, with very little level land. The principal island, Luzon, has several mountains that run from the north to the south of the island. The range, known as the Sierra Madre, runs parallel with the northeastern coast combined with the central Cordillera to form the spine of the Philippines. The highest mountain is Mount Apo (6690 feet) on Mindanao. The islands are of volcanic origin (*Time Almanac with Information Please,* 2007).

The Philippine Islands enjoy warm, even temperatures throughout the year. The average monthly temperature in the Philippines ranges from 76° F to 84° F. Cooler temperatures are found at higher altitudes; however, temperatures below 60° F are a rare occurrence. Typhoons usually strike the Philippines at least once a year. The average rainfall for most of the islands is at least 60 inches of rain per year, with some areas receiving up to 125 inches of rain.

The population of the Philippines in 2006 was estimated at 89,468,677, with a birth rate of 24.89 live births per 1000 persons and an infant mortality rate of 22.81 per 1000, down from 35.2 per 1000 in 1997. The population density is 759 per square mile, with the Philippines ranking the thirteenth most populous country (*Time Almanac with Information Please,* 2007; *World Almanac,* 2007). Of the population, 35% is under age 15 and 4.1% is 65 or older. The life expectancy is 67.32 years for males and 73.24 years for females. Most of the people in the Philippines are of Malaysian (that is, Austronesian) descent, with the two major ethnic groups being Christian Malay (91.5%) and Muslim Malay

(4%) (*World Almanac,* 2007). However, people of Chinese, American, and Spanish origin are also native to the Philippines. The population is unevenly distributed, with Luzon, Cebu, Negros, Bohol, Leyte, and Panay being the most heavily populated islands. Education on the islands is free and compulsory for ages 7 to 12, resulting in a literacy rate of 96% (*World Almanac,* 2007).

The economy of the Philippines is based on agriculture. One of the principal crops is rice, which occupies about half the farmed land in the Philippines. Corn and coconuts are also very important crops. Other crops of some significance include root crops, fruits, nuts, sugarcane, abaca, tobacco, ramie, kapok, and rubber. Although agriculture is the principal industry, the yields per crop per acre are among the lowest in Asia (Ennis & Inaba, 1977). Causes of low productivity of agriculture in the Philippines include poor farm management, inadequate use of fertilizers, poor seeds, and lack of incentive on the part of the farmers because many are tenant farmers (Ennis & Inaba, 1977). The lack of agricultural productivity has resulted in a variety of dietary deficiencies among the people, including insufficient iron and vitamins (Cheong, Kuizon, & Tajaon, 1991; Solon, Solon, Mehansho, et al., 1996). The living environment also results in the prevalence of *Ascaris lumbricoides* worm populations in Filipino children in both urban and rural areas (Monzon, 1991). Fishing is also a major industry in the Philippines, with the number of persons engaged in fishing being second only to those in agriculture, and it provides one of the primary dietary mainstays, second only to rice. Major industries include textiles, pharmaceuticals, chemicals, food processing, and electronics assembly. Natural resources include forests, crude oil, and metallic and nonmetallic minerals. Approximately 36% of the labor force is agricultural. The rest of the work force is divided between industry (16%) and services (48%) (*World Almanac,* 2007). The gross domestic product (2004) is $430.6 billion, which is $5000 per capita, up from $2530 in 1997 (*World Almanac,* 2007). The unemployment rate was 11.7% in 2006 (*Time Almanac with Information Please,* 2007; *World Almanac,* 2007).

More than 40% of the country is covered by forest. Resources found in the forest include Philippine mahogany and pine. Minerals mined in the Philippines include gold, copper ore, and chromite. The country continues to lack adequate supplies of mineral fuels, though coal is mined on the islands of Cebu and Mindanao.

The ancestors of the Malay people probably migrated from Southeast Asia and were undoubtedly hunters, fishers, and unsettled cultivators (*World Almanac*, 2007). Magellan first visited the archipelago in 1521. Twenty-one years later, the islands were named in honor of King Philip II of Spain, and Spain retained possession of the islands for 350 years. Following the Spanish-American War, in 1898, Spain ceded the islands to the United States for $20 million. However, the Filipinos declared their independence and initiated guerrilla warfare against the troops from the United States until peace was established in 1902 and a civilian governor-general from the United States assumed control. Throughout the early 1900s, a Philippine legislature was established and steps set in motion to establish a commonwealth (*Time Almanac with Information Please*, 2006). When Japan attacked the Philippines in 1941 and occupied the islands in World War II, enormous destruction occurred (McKay, Hill, & Buckler, 2007). During the war, the United States extended economic aid to the Philippines as compensation for the large military bases established on the island, and following the war, the Philippines were granted independence. The Republic of the Philippines was established in 1946. From 1946 to 1965, the Philippines pursued an American-style, two-party government. However, in 1965 President Ferdinand Marcos subverted the constitution and ruled as a lifetime dictator. Marcos abolished martial law in 1981 but retained most of his own power. From 1981 to 1986 there was a growing resistance to Marcos's rule. In 1986 Corazón Aquino, whose politically involved husband had been assassinated, possibly by Marcos's supporters, won a spectacular electoral victory over Marcos and forced him to flee the country (McKay, Hill, & Buckler, 2007). In the year that followed, the Aquino government survived coup attempts by

Marcos supporters. Negotiations on renewal of leases for U.S. military bases threatened to sour relations between the two countries. However, when volcanic eruptions from Mount Pinatubo severely damaged Clark Air Base in July 1991, the United States simply abandoned the base. In 1992 General Fidel Ramos, who had the support of outgoing President Corazón Aquino, won the presidency, and the opposition gained control of Congress. In 1992 the U.S. Navy officially ended a long U.S. military presence and turned over Subic Bay Naval Base to the Philippines. A cease-fire agreement was signed between the government and Muslim separatist guerrillas in 1994, but the rebels did not abide by the accord. A new treaty providing for the development of an autonomous Muslim region on Mindanao was signed in 1996. This treaty formally ended the 24-year rebellion, which had claimed more than 120,000 lives. Joseph Estrada won the presidential election in 1998 but was impeached in 2000 for bribery. In 2000, the government repeatedly clashed with the Moro Islamic Liberation Front, which abducted several groups of hostages, including tourists, while demanding money for their release (*Time Almanac with Information Please*, 2007). In the spring of 2001, Vice President Gloria Macapagal-Arroyo became president (*World Almanac*, 2007). After battles with an Islamic guerrilla group and assistance from the U.S., the insurgents were suppressed and President Arroyo won reelection in 2004. Tropical storms and flooding in 2004 displaced 880,000 and left 1060 dead and 560 missing (*World Almanac*, 2007).

IMMIGRATION TO THE UNITED STATES

Three different waves of Filipino immigrants have come to the United States: the first-wave, or pioneer, group; the second-wave group; and the third-wave, or new immigrant, group (Orque, 1983). Although "Philipino American" is the correct spelling, because there is no F in the Philipino alphabet, "Filipino American" is the accepted English spelling (Cantos & Rivera, 1996). The feminine form, "Filipina," is acceptable usage, though not appearing often. Today, Filipinos are the second largest Asian American subpopulation in the

United States, and represent 4.4% of all foreign-born U.S. residents.

First-Wave Immigrants

The first-wave, or pioneer, group is diverse, particularly because of the different times of arrival of its members in the United States and their reasons for immigrating. The first-wave Filipino immigrants were originally drafted to work on trade ships that were traveling from China to the United States (Bartlett, 1977). From 1565 to 1815, hundreds of Filipinos escaped from the trading ships and went first to Mexico and finally to Louisiana and other regions throughout the United States. In 1907, with the passage of the gentleman's agreement that restricted Japanese immigration, Filipinos were recruited to work in Hawaii on sugar plantations (Daniels & Kitano, 1970; Lasker, 1969). Many of the first-wave Filipino immigrants worked on California farms or in Alaskan canneries, and still others worked as cooks or domestic helpers. From 1907 to 1930, Filipinos provided inexpensive and unskilled labor, such as housekeepers, janitors, farmhands, and cooks. Most of the first-wave immigrants were men who came from the Ilocos region, though some did come from the Bisayan and Manila areas of the Philippines (Hart, 1981; Melendy, 1977). In 1934 the United States passed what was known as the Tydings-McDuffie Act, which held Filipino immigration to an annual quota of no more than 50 persons. This act established a Philippine commonwealth and changed the legal status of Filipinos from "nationals" to "aliens" in the United States. When Filipinos were labeled "nationals," they had the rights of citizenship except the rights to vote, own property, or marry. However, with the new alien status, the technical rights of limited citizenship were abolished (Parreno, 1977).

Second-Wave Immigrants

The second wave of immigration began after the Philippine Islands won independence from the United States in 1946, when the annual quota was raised to 100 persons. Many Filipinos who served in the U.S. Armed Forces immigrated to the United States with their families after World War II. Lott (1976) noted that during this period many of the Filipino men were physically separated from their immediate kin and denied full participation in the larger American society. Therefore, many of the second-wave group, particularly the men, relied on communal arrangements as their social group.

Third-Wave Immigrants

The new immigration group, or the third wave of immigrants, is composed of those Filipinos who have immigrated to the United States since 1965 as a result of the liberalization of the immigration quota. In 1974, Urban Associates reported that in the 10-year period from 1960 to 1970, the Filipino population residing in the United States doubled, from 343,000 to 774,652. From 1965 to 2000, the population of Filipino Americans almost doubled again, to number 1,850,314 (U.S. Department of Commerce, Bureau of the Census, Summary File 3, 2002). In 2005, a total of 2,364,815 Filipinos called the United States home. Today, Filipinos represent approximately 0.7% of the total U.S. population. This number represents a 30.3% increase in the Filipino population since the 1990 census (Infoplease.com, 2006; U.S. Department of Commerce, Bureau of the Census, Summary File 3, 2002). Currently, Filipino Americans are the largest Asian group in California, where more than half of the Filipinos in the United States reside. By geographical location, 52.4% of Filipino Americans reside in the West, 27.0% reside in the Northeast, 8.1% in the Midwest, and 12.4% in the South (U.S. Department of Commerce, Bureau of the Census, Summary File 3, 2002). In 2000, Filipino Americans again constituted the second largest group of Asians in the United States, outnumbered in terms of population only by Chinese Americans (U.S. Department of Commerce, Bureau of the Census, Summary File 3, 2002).

Of the number of Filipino Americans residing in this country before 1975, 21.7% were foreign born. Of the number residing in this country between 1975 and 1979, 11.1% were foreign born; between 1980 and 1990, 31.6% were foreign born; and between 1990 and 2000, 35.7% were foreign-born

(U.S. Department of Commerce, Bureau of the Census, Summary File 3, 2002). The median age of Filipino American people residing in the United States is 31.3 years, compared with 32.7 for other Asian Americans and 33 years for the general U.S. population. In addition, only 6% of all Asian Americans are 65 years of age or older, compared with 13% of the general U.S. population (U.S. Department of Commerce, Bureau of the Census, Summary File 3, 2002).

Among Filipino Americans, third-wave immigrants appear to be better educated than members of the first and second waves; however, some of these people still experienced discrimination. In general, Filipino Americans are noted for high educational standards, with parents placing high value on education (Champeau, 1998). In 2000, 84.2% of Filipino American males and 81.4% of Filipino American females 25 years of age or older held a high school diploma, and 36.2% of males and 41.6% of females held a bachelor's degree (U.S. Department of Commerce, Bureau of the Census, Summary File 3, 2002).

The median earnings in 2000 for Filipino Americans ranges from slightly lower to slightly higher than that for the general U.S. population, depending on whether it is the aggregate income or individual by gender income being analyzed. The median earnings in the aggregate for Filipino Americans over 16 years of age were $25,284. It was $27,090 for Filipino men and $23,339 for Filipino American women as compared with $23,755 for the general U.S. population and $29,458 for men in the general U.S. population and $18,957 for women in the general U.S. population (Infoplease.com, 2006). Likewise, the per capita income when compared to their White counterparts is also slightly lower at $19,259 versus $24,819 (APIAHF, 2005). It is interesting to note that the opposite is true for the poverty rate among Filipino Americans, which is slightly lower than that among their White counterpart (7% versus 8%) (APIAHF, 2005).

Takaki (1998) reports in *Strangers from a Different Shore* that for many Filipinos, though they toil in America, they still experience an "unfinished dream," with a society unwilling to embrace its own diversity. On the other hand, many Filipino Americans are being recognized across the United States for excellence, including achievement in academia (Champeau, 1999), in theater (De Leon, 1999), in higher education (De La Cruz, 1999), in medicine (Bofill, 1999), in politics (Pilapil, 1999), and in poetry (Gloria, 1999). Unlike other Asian Americans, recent Filipino immigrants tend not to stand out as much; they speak English fluently, are highly educated, have economic well-being, and are Christians (Agbayani-Siewert, 2004). The label of "Invisible Minority" also extends to the relative lack of political power and representation of, by, and for Filipino Americans. Congress has established two months in celebration of Filipino American culture in the United States. "Asian Pacific American Heritage Month" is celebrated in May. Upon Filipinos' becoming the largest Asian American group, "Filipino American History Month" was established for October, commemorating the first landing of Filipinos on October 18, 1587, in Morro Bay, California.

Since the 1960s, there has been an exodus of nurses from the Philippines to the United States (Cantore, 2001). Nurses educated in the Philippines have been attracted to the United States because of job opportunities, which have become especially attractive in the present nursing shortage. While most nurses coming from the Philippines have a BSN, and graduate education offers additional opportunities to advance, many continue to work in staff positions, often with a second job, in order to maintain a steady financial support for family members still living in the Philippines (Cantore, 2001). Filipino nurses have had to make many adjustments to deliver nursing care in the United States, including learning new technologies and the American work ethic and value system. Cantore (2001) noted that cultural attributes common in the Philippines that may be retained by the Filipino nurse working in the United States can be negative but may also be positive—for example, showing deference to elders and persons who outrank them, thus appearing timid, and working very hard and not complaining. While Filipino American nurses have their own unique ethnic identity and rich cultural heritage, Filipino nurses are often lumped into the general category of "Asian nurses." Because they are not given a separate ethnic grouping in statistics collected by the Health Resources and Services Administration's National Sample Survey of Registered Nurses, Cantore (2001) notes that Filipino nurses are, for the most part, a "hidden minority." Berg, Rodriguez, Kading, and De Guzman (2004) noted that a significant number of nurses who have emigrated from the Philippines and have enjoyed full-time employment and high job satisfaction are now at retirement age, which will negatively affect the RN population in the United States.

COMMUNICATION

Dialect and Language

One of the greatest difficulties that faced Filipinos during the 1960s was the task of forming a more integrated national community. This task was made even more difficult because of sociological diversity and because more than 93 dialects were spoken in the Philippines at the time (Voegelin & Voegelin, 1997). The boundary between "language" and "dialect" in the Philippines is blurred. The most common languages are Ilocano, Cebuano, Bicolano, Pampango, and Chabacano (Cantos & Rivera, 1996). Although 86% of Filipinos speak one of eight major languages as their mother tongue, the fact remains that many diverse languages and dialects are spoken across the country. Filipinos have long recognized the problem with dialect and language, and in 1930 the government adopted a policy to develop a national language based on Tagalog. In addition to Tagalog, English and Spanish were also adopted as official languages of the Philippines. However, adoption of a national language by the people was slow, and by 1960 only 44.5% of Filipinos spoke Tagalog, 39.5% spoke English, and 2% spoke Spanish (Corpuz, 1965). At that time more than 93 Filipino languages were being spoken in the country (Melendy, 1977). Today most Filipinos speak the national language, Tagalog (also known as Filipino), but use English for business, legal transactions, and school instruction beyond the third grade. A hybrid of Tagalog and English (Taglish) is used commonly in business and social interactions as well as in health interactions (Pacquiao, 2003).

In the United States, Filipino immigrants have been willing to undergo discomfort and cultural alienation with the hope that their children might improve the economic status of the people through education. However, one tragic flaw in this scheme is the language barrier encountered by the children in the public school systems in the United States (Melendy, 1977). Even today, the public schools are not able to cope with the problem of bilingual education in languages other than Spanish and English. In 2005, 61% of Filipino Americans spoke a language other than English at home. Even today, Filipino Americans continue to have the fourth largest percentage (21%) of linguistically isolated people among all of the Asian groups residing in the U.S. Some 20% of Filipino Americans live in linguistically isolated households (APIAHF, 2005). A great number of Filipinos speak Tagalog, Visayan, Taglish and Ilokano at home. Tagalog is the sixth most spoken language in the United States (APIAHF, 2005).

Style

Shimamoto (1977) noted that the elderly Filipino man is generally concrete in thinking and pragmatic in problem solving. Shimamoto also noted that when a Filipino man acknowledges emotions in a verbal manner, this may be interpreted as a sign of unmanliness or weakness. Cultural values emphasize group harmony and smooth interpersonal relationships; decision making may be shared among family members according to a patient's needs. A clinician could develop a family decision tree or algorithm. Decisions may be referred to family members living outside the United States, or birth order may be used to designate decisions (McBride & Parreno, 2006; Tompar-Tiu & Sustento-Seneriches, 1995).

Tone

Filipino Americans tend to use tone of voice to emote or to romanticize the language (Cantos & Rivera, 1996). An individual may get loud in the presence of a group of family members or may become agitated or emotional when nervous or frightened. Typically, however, Filipinos are soft spoken and will say nothing rather than disagree.

Context

Filipino Americans are "laid-back, easy-going, serene people" (Santiago, 2001). Thus, there is a tendency for Filipinos to avoid direct expression of disagreement. This protects them from losing face or respect. For example, it was noted in a Midwestern psychiatric hospital that a Filipino male physician, who was a family practitioner, would not disagree directly with a female psychiatrist. In areas of disagreement, the physician would communicate information to the psychiatrist by telling the nursing staff to relay the message (Davidhizar, 1997). In this scenario, the difficulties were encountered because Filipinos are a polite people who do not like to disagree, particularly with people in authority, and because some Filipino men experience discomfort with women as authority figures.

Some Filipino people experience difficulties when discussing topics that are considered personal, including sex, tuberculosis, and socioeconomic status. The issues of sex and sex education are considered so sensitive that Filipino parents generally do not openly or deliberately discuss them with their children (Guthrie & Jacobs, 1976). Because tuberculosis is a dreaded and feared disease among Filipino people (in the Philippines the morbidity and mortality for this disease remain high as a result of unsanitary living conditions), some Filipino people may also avoid discussion about tuberculosis (Hooper, 1958; Orque, 1983; Wooley, 1972).

Some Filipinos have an expressed need for modesty, privacy, and confidentiality. Therefore, it is often difficult for the nurse to begin interventions immediately without a period of small talk on topics considered safe conversation, such as the weather, the condition of family members, or sports events. It is also important for the nurse to remember that Filipino American clients may be hesitant to express feelings and emotions in a group setting. Filipinos are sensitive to the concept of shame or saving face. It may be only out of strong respect

for the health care professional that they will disclose personal information that is needed to plan adequately for health care (Orque, 1983).

Kinesics

Nonverbal language is important for Filipino persons. For example, direct eye contact in the Filipino culture between an older man and a younger woman may be indicative of either seduction or anger. Little eye contact is likely to be used with superiors and authority figures. Another situation in which a nurse may encounter nonverbal communication on the part of a Filipino American client is in a group setting. Because some Filipino people fear losing face in public situations, the Filipino American client may be very hesitant to express personal feelings in a group setting and may resort to remaining silent. It is important to assess the meaning of silence and to determine if it means approval or not.

Filipinos tend to be very polite and therefore tend to behave agreeably even to the extent of personal inconvenience (Cantos & Rivera, 1996). The term for this form of agreement is *pakikisama*, which means "getting along with others at all costs." Some Filipino nurses have difficulty giving commands to staff but rather prefer to request politely that they do an assignment. Another trait for which some Filipinos are known is *amor propio*, which is actually a Spanish term adapted to the Filipino language, meaning "self-esteem." Therefore, when a Filipino's *amor propio* is wounded, there is a tendency to preserve personal dignity by silence or aloofness to demonstrate self-pride. Filipinos will tend to agree even when they mistrust the physician or nurse because they do not want to risk hurting the other person's feelings. Therefore, for some Filipinos a hesitant "yes" could be indicative of a positive "no" because they wish to avoid a direct, blunt "no." In the Filipino language, there are hierarchical terms for "yes" and "no." The term used depends on whether one is speaking to a person of lower, equal, or superior status. When uncertain as to the status of the person with whom they are conversing, some Filipino Americans will use a silent nod to avoid giving possible offense. Also, a Filipino American client will commonly address a physician or nurse as "Doctor" or "Mrs."; however, if the name is unknown, this same individual may only nod (DeGracia, 1979).

Touching is not uncommon, though handshakes are not commonly practiced by Filipino Americans. Elderly people are shown respect by being kissed on the hand, forehead, or cheeks (Wilson & Billones, 1994).

Implications for Nursing Care

It is important for the nurse to remember that a large majority of first-wave Filipino immigrants came to this country with little or no education and may have extreme difficulty comprehending English, especially English spoken in medical jargon (Vance & Davidhizar, 1999). Therefore, the nurse should use interpretive aids such as pictures and interpreters. It is also important for the nurse to remember that if an interpreter is used, the interpreter should speak the same language and same dialect as the client. The nurse should be aware that many Filipinos use a nonverbal response, such as a smile or a raised eyebrow, as an acknowledgment to what has been said, rather than giving a verbal response (Espíritu, 1995). It is important for the nurse to watch the Filipino client when speaking rather than waiting for a verbal response.

Regardless of immigration-wave status, the Filipino American client may view the nurse as an authority figure and therefore relate to the nurse with formality and modesty. Because gender and age differences also have particular significance in the Filipino culture, it would be wise for the nurse to consider both gender and age when communicating with the client. For example, because an elderly person is highly revered in the Filipino culture, it would be inappropriate as well as disrespectful for the nurse to address the elderly Filipino American client by a first name. The nurse might try using such Tagalog designations as *opo* or *oho*, which are used to show respect and honor to the person being addressed (Orque, 1983). The Tagalog designation *po* should be inserted when an elderly Filipino American is addressed because it conveys respect and is similar to designations in the English

language such as "madam" or "sir" (Guthrie & Jacobs, 1976).

It is important for the nurse to remember that direct eye contact for Filipinos has various connotations. A young female nurse who is assigned to an elderly Filipino American male client may encounter difficulties when communicating with this client, who may remain aloof and reserved and avoid eye contact altogether (Bush & Babich, 1986).

Because Filipino men, regardless of age, have great difficulty acknowledging emotions verbally, Shimamoto (1977) recommended that the nurse assume an authority-figure role during the development of the nurse–client relationship. Because of the Filipino trait of deference toward authority figures, Filipino American men, regardless of age, are likely to respect the nurse's position and to listen and adhere to the nurse's suggestions because of the position. It is important for the nurse to appear knowledgeable and competent when communicating with a Filipino American client and to avoid talking down to the client. It is also important for the nurse to remember that because some Filipino men experience discomfort with women as authority figures, difficulties may arise even in nurse–physician relationships. For example, when a female nurse is communicating with a Filipino American male doctor, the nurse should use sensitivity in offering suggestions or criticism. Some Filipino Americans encounter difficulties in group settings, particularly in situations where both men and women are present. Therefore, one-on-one encounters may be best, so that the client or professional with whom the nurse is talking feels free to express true feelings and emotions (Orque, 1983).

Because Filipino American clients tend to be modest, it is important to offer female clients not only a gown but also a robe. Male clients should be offered pants as well as a gown (Cantos & Rivera, 1996).

Because Filipinos have arrived in the United States in different groups and have adapted to the culture at different levels, it is important for the nurse to recognize that different acculturation patterns will be present and to assess for level of acculturation. Dela Cruz, Padilla, and Agustin (2000) have adapted for use with Filipino Americans an acculturation tool first developed for Hispanics. The 12-item instrument, ASASFA (Acculturation Scale for Filipino Americans), has been validated with experts and psychometric testing and is available in two versions, English and Tagalog. Use of the ASASFA can provide a measure for comparing the acculturation patterns of individuals and lead to broader cross-cultural knowledge and understanding.

SPACE

Some Filipino Americans tend to collapse their space inward and limit the amount of personal space available. This is caused in part by the Filipinos' strong feeling for family (Cantore, 2001). On immigration to the United States, the personal space of Filipino Americans also collapsed inward because some of the people lived in urban ghettos, "little Manilas," that were vastly overpopulated (Burma, 1974).

Implications for Nursing Care

Filipino Americans are perceived as a family-oriented cultural group. Therefore, it is not uncommon for a Filipino client to have the entire family, which includes nuclear and extended family members, hovering at the bedside. Even an adult who is unmarried with no relatives in the vicinity is likely to have a number of Filipino American visitors because they are sensitive to the loneliness that illness can provoke. The astute nurse will use family members to the advantage of the client. Rather than viewing their presence as an overcrowding of space in the hospital for both the health care professionals and the client, the nurse should capitalize on these customs and traditions by involving family members in educational training programs that will assist the client in returning to an optimal level of functioning. In addition, it is important to solicit family and client input to develop shared goals.

It is also important for the nurse to remember that Filipino Americans are familiar with a limited personal space because it is always shared with other family members. Therefore, the space provided in a hospital setting may appear to be overextended, thus leading the client to collapse personal space inward even more so. While hospitalized, Filipino Americans may be reluctant to venture out of the personal space that is allocated or leave their room for any reason (DeGracia, 1979).

In response to illness, Filipino elders may often follow a pathway to seeking professional health care that begins with self-monitoring of symptoms to ascertain possible cause, severity, threat to one's functional capacity, and economic and/or emotional inconvenience to the family. The extended trajectory from symptom onset to medical treatment may also be affected by sociopolitical and historical experiences of injustice, by racial or gender discrimination felt by the elders themselves, or by attitudes passed on to them by family members who had difficult experiences (Yeo, Hikoyeda, McBride, et al., 1998).

SOCIAL ORGANIZATION
Family

Most of the first-wave immigrants who came to the United States were not allowed to immigrate with their wives. This immigration pattern was responsible for a disproportionate ratio of males to females. The male-to-female ratio in 1930 for Filipinos residing in the United States was 14 to 1, compared with 1.1 to 1 for the rest of the population (Melendy, 1977). Lott (1976) noted that because Filipino men were separated from their families, they tended to rely on communal arrangements with other Filipino immigrants, who often came from the same island in the Philippines. Most of the first-wave immigrants had little or no education and, because of discriminatory practices that existed throughout the United States, did not receive more education or a better job.

After World War II, when the immigration policies became more relaxed in the United States, more Filipino women began to enter the country, and a more normal family pattern followed. Despite the fact that more women were able to immigrate during the second and third waves, it has been noted that the age of Filipino American husbands continues to exceed that of their wives. Because of their disproportionate ages, many young Filipino American women have been widowed early, thus leading to the establishment of the Filipino matriarchal system. In 1974, 69% of Filipino American families were matriarchal with young children, and at least 23% of all Filipino American families were extended (Urban Associates, 1974). Wagner (1973) noted that the ratio of extended families to nuclear families was at least twice that of the rest of the U.S. population. Today, however, married couples represent approximately 83.6% of all Filipino American households, whereas female-headed households (matriarchal) make up only 11.8% of Filipino American families (U.S. Department of Commerce, Bureau of the Census, Summary File 3, 2002).

In 1974, 38% of all Filipino American families had five or more members (Urban Associates, 1974). Today, this number is decreasing somewhat, and the average Filipino American family has 4.0 persons, compared with the national average of 3.2 (U.S. Department of Commerce, Bureau of the Census, Summary File 3, 2002). Pollard (1995) studied ethnic groups in relation to twinning rates in California. Numbers of Filipino twins were similar to those of Chinese and Japanese but higher than those of Koreans, Thai, and Vietnamese, an indication that twinning rates are modified by both migration and interethnic mixing.

Although the number of matrifocal families has decreased, the matriarchal system remains an integral part of Filipino cultural values. The matriarchal system may be the reason that the family has taken on paramount importance for Filipino Americans. This is evidenced even during times of illness. When a member of a Filipino American family becomes ill, family members often keep a bedside vigil and participate in client care. Burr and Mutchler (1993) noted that Filipino-born women who are less acculturated are more likely than women from some other ethnic groups to move in with others who are more acculturated.

Family Systems and the Relationship to Culture

The Filipino culture is a blend of various heritages, though there are some basic traits that most Filipino people manifest. Individualization is a key to understanding the Filipino culture and an individual of Filipino descent. As a result of the Chinese influence on family solidarity, Filipinos on the Philippine islands tend to socialize with people from the same region. This same clannishness is evident in the United States among the many organizations in the Filipino communities. Persons in the younger generations may have values that are in direct opposition to the traditional values held by older persons. In the Philippine Islands today, many youths resemble their Western counterparts, particularly in areas of social values, dress, and music (DeGracia, 1979). Although these same similarities exist among adolescents in the mainstream United States and Filipino American adolescents, many Filipino American youths still observe such traditional values as respect for elders, love of family, and preservation of self-esteem.

In the Filipino culture there is a strong feeling for family, which is a result of the Chinese influence. Today, these strong feelings for family continue and may be manifested by old-fashioned patterns imposed by the family patriarch or the equally authoritarian matriarch. Lee (2004) noted Filipino American men traditionally have positions of power, dominance, and privilege and are concerned about challenges to their family leadership and to "losing face." The Filipino child is taught always to give deference to an elder and never to question the decision of an elder. In return for such obedience, the Filipino child receives solicitous protection from elders. In the absence of both parents, the eldest Filipino child becomes the ruling authority and must be obeyed. Kataoka-Yahiro, Ceria, and Yoder (2004) conducted qualitative research with Filipino American grandparents and noted that rather than viewing grandparenting as a burden it is viewed as an integral part of the role and part of the "give and take" of family responsibility.

Parent–adolescent communication about sex has been found to be sometimes limited, resulting in limited sex education (Chung, Borneo, Kilpatrick, Lopez, Travis, Lui, Khandwala, & Schuster, 2005). On the other hand, a study by Lantican and Corona (1992) noted that social support for pregnant women was extensive and included a network size of 5.74. For the most part, in the Filipinos studied, immediate family members provided the support. Filipinos also reported that sisters were most likely to be the first to receive information about the pregnancy, with husbands listed third. This was in contrast to the Mexican Americans studied, who reported discussing the pregnancy first with their husbands

Religion

Filipinos are predominantly Roman Catholic, which has been attributed to the influence of the Spanish missionaries in the Philippines as early as 1520. In 2006, chief religions included Roman Catholic, 81%, and Muslim, 5% (*World Almanac*, 2007). The remaining religious groups include Evangelical, Aglipayan, Iglesia ni Kristo, other Christian, and other (Central Intelligence Agency, 2006).

Birth Rituals

Filipino mothers are encouraged to eat well and to get plenty of sleep at night. In the last few months of pregnancy, they are discouraged from staying in a dependent position, such as sitting or sleeping during the day, for fear of water retention. Sexual intercourse during the last 2 months of pregnancy is considered taboo. Eating prunes, sweet foods, or squid is also considered taboo for a pregnant woman (Kittler & Sucher, 2001; White, Linhart, & Medley, 1996). It is believed that such foods will, respectively, make the baby wrinkled, lead to a large baby and difficult delivery, and tangle the baby's cord inside the mother. If a physician is not available, a midwife may be called on to assist in the delivery. Fathers are usually not present but rather are with male friends for support while their wives deliver. A pregnant Filipino woman may walk around the room to promote dilatation. Most Filipino women will moan or grunt during labor. Others may become loud and almost hysterical (Weber, 1996). A symbolic unlocking ritual may be performed during labor. Traditionally, showers and bathing were prohibited for 10 days postpartum (Spector, 2004).

Traditionally, it was an expectation of all Filipino mothers to breastfeed. This tradition is changing.

In a study by Adair and Popkin (1996), Filipino women who ceased breastfeeding early or did not breastfeed were studied. It was found that a low birth weight reduced the likelihood of breastfeeding. This is significant because there are already high risks related to low birth weight and proved benefits of breastfeeding. Thus, these researchers noted that nurses should give special emphasis to promoting breastfeeding. For example, a working mother may have the baby fed formula while she is at work or may have breast milk left for the baby.

Traditionally male circumcision was not done at birth. Today it is more common for a male baby to be circumcised before discharge from the hospital.

Rituals Related to Death and Dying

If a client has a diagnosis of terminal disease, the client should not be told before the family is consulted. The family will usually want to disclose the prognosis to the client and in some cases will prefer to protect the client from knowing the diagnosis (Geissler, 1998). The health care professional should generally continue to communicate with the head of the family outside of the patient's presence regarding the health status. If the family is Catholic, the family will usually want the Catholic chaplain to give the "sacrament of the sick," in which religious objects such as a rosary are used. A Filipino client given a terminal diagnosis will probably prefer to die at home with dignity. A decision to not resuscitate is usually very difficult and will be determined by the entire family. Death is given very high regard by Filipino Americans. Death is a spiritual event, and the client and family may ask for religious medallions, rosary beads, and other objects of spiritual significance to be near the client. The family may pray at the bedside of a dying family member. If a client dies in a hospital room, the family members will usually want to say goodbye before having the body taken out of the room and may want to wash the body. Muslims will want Muslim rites performed (Geissler, 1998). McAdam, Stotts, Padilla, and Puntillo (2005) investigated attitudes of critically ill Filipino American patients and their families toward advance directives and noted that the overall attitude was positive. However, the completion rate and knowledge of advance directives were low, which suggested to the researchers that participants may have wished to avoid disagreement. Terminally ill Filipino American patients usually prefer to die at home, and Becker (2002) notes that in a study of 78 Filipino Americans contemplating death, many expressed a desire to die in their homelands. Becker notes that the preoccupation of respondents with where to die apparently reflects the desire to reconcile issues of continuity, as well as cultural meanings surrounding memory, ritual, and family.

Funerals in the Philippines can be simple or elaborate, with a band accompaniment, several priests officiating, and a large group of mourners. Rituals generally include a wake, novenas, and establishing a burial site acceptable to all the members of the family. A first-year anniversary of the death event in which the family unites draws closure to the mourning. For the traditional Filipino, women related to the deceased may wear white during this period, and weddings and other celebrations may be delayed as a show of respect. Most Filipinos believe in life after death and believe that caring for the spiritual needs of the dying is necessary for peaceful transition of the soul to the afterlife (Pacquiao, 2003).

Implications for Nursing Care

In the Philippine Islands, the family unit is the basic unit of social organization. Several generations of Filipinos are linked by descent and marriage. For some Filipinos, family relationships are so important that many of the kinfolk live under the same roof or as close to each other as possible. Furthermore, membership in a family union is perceived by some Filipinos as being more important than membership in a trade union (Caringer, 1977). Therefore, many nursing implications are based on family structure and organization. Because Filipino American clients are very family oriented, the nurse must remember that these clients may always have their families hovering about them. The sick Filipino child may feel lost without the mother constantly at the bedside, and when grandparents are ill, the entire family may keep vigil at the bedside

out of respect for the elderly. Whenever it is possible, the nurse should arrange for family members to stay at the client's bedside during a hospital stay. Family members will want to bring food from home that is soothing for the body, such as rice soup, and in most cases clients will expect that this will occur.

It is important for the nurse to remember that the family structure of first-wave and second-wave immigrants may be significantly different from that of third-wave immigrants in that more matriarchal family structures may be found in the earlier generations. Thus the varying family structures may present the need for unique and varying approaches to health care needs. Another implication for nursing care is associated with the fact that some first-wave and second-wave immigrants have a limited education compared with third-wave immigrants, who were better educated when they came to this country. When a Filipino American client from the first-wave or second-wave group is hospitalized, it is important that the nurse not only involve families but also recognize the need to modify educational approaches to the family's and client's level of understanding.

It is helpful for the nurse to be aware that throughout the United States and particularly in California, Filipino American centers are being established (Manila, 1999). Filipino student organizations are available at some universities (Suzara, 1999), and the location of Filipino organizations, including the Web site of the Philippine Nurses Association (http://pna-ph.org), are available online.

TIME

Filipino Americans appear to have both a past- and a present-time orientation. According to Kluckhohn and Strodtbeck (1973), human nature has a postulated range of variations, including evil, good and evil, and good. People react to these value orientations by virtue of a time frame of reference. For example, past-time oriented people view human nature as being basically evil, and so control and discipline of the self are continuously required if any real good is to be achieved. On the other hand, present-time oriented people view human nature as a mixture of good and evil, and so although control and effort are needed, lapses in control and effort can be understood and need not always be severely condemned. For some Filipino Americans there is a prevailing attitude that one should unquestionably accept what life and death bring because, regardless of human effort, supernatural forces are mitigating and control the world. It is this attitude that influences some Filipino Americans' time orientation.

Because Filipino Americans are both past- and present-time oriented, they distinguish between social and business time. They tend not to become too aggravated when social functions do not start on time, and so they operate on "Filipino time." This trait results in part from their past-time orientation, which values human relationships and human nature over current events. However, Filipino Americans do equate success in business in Western society with a prompt observation of business time, which is perceived as being both present- and future-time oriented (Orque, 1983). Nevertheless, for some Filipino Americans there is a prevailing attitude that time and providence will solve all (Corpuz, 1965).

Implications for Nursing Care

Because Filipino Americans are both past- and present-time oriented, it is important for the nurse to remember that often a Filipino-American client may ignore health-related issues, preferring to leave these things in the hands of God (*bahala na*). Some Filipino Americans may use the term *talaga*, which means "destined" or "inevitable." When some Filipino Americans are ill, past-time orientation becomes obvious because of a tendency to attribute conditions to the will of God and to cope with illness by praying and hoping that whatever God's will is, it is best for the individual.

Because of their past-time orientation, there is a tendency among some Filipino Americans toward noncompliance regarding medical regimens. In addition, these same individuals may not adhere to appointments or scheduled deadlines for health-related matters. Filipino immigrants are considered at risk for hypertension, coronary heart disease, and diabetes at midlife and at old age, along with other metabolic conditions.

ENVIRONMENTAL CONTROL

As indicated, Filipino Americans are perceived as being both past- and present-time oriented and have a tendency to believe that events, particularly illnesses, are related to supernatural forces. As a result of this belief, some Filipino Americans have a value orientation that is perceived as fatalistic. Thus some Filipino Americans have an external locus of control that is evidenced by a belief in supernatural forces and by the treatment methods of illness.

Physical and mental health and illness are viewed holistically as an equilibrium model. Explanatory models may include mystical, personalistic, or naturalistic causes. The basic logic of health and illness consists of prevention and curing; it is a system oriented to moderation. Parallel to this holistic belief system is the understanding of modern medicine, with its own basic logic and principles, that treats certain types of diseases. Filipino elders use a dual system of health care: avoiding inappropriate behavior that leads to imbalance and restoring balance (Pacquiao, 2003).

Folk Medicine

Filipinos and Filipino Americans support at least two, often competing, medical systems. A Filipino individual who becomes ill might consult both a folk healer and a Western-trained physician. Filipino Americans are like other ethnic groups in that they continue to practice folk medicine simply because it works (McKenzie & Chrisman, 1977). In some situations, folk remedies may be the only treatments available for Filipino Americans, whereas in other situations some Filipino Americans will combine folk remedies with the therapy prescribed by Western health professionals. It is important for the nurse to remember that folk beliefs are an important part of some Filipino Americans' lives and therefore may significantly influence health practices. In a study of ethnic reactions to chronic illness in African-Americans, Latinos, and Filipino Americans, Becker, Beyene,

Newson, and Rodgers (1998) noted that while the illness patterns were similar, responses to and management of the illnesses varied between the groups and was related to self-care practices and knowledge about the illness.

Folk medicine has enjoyed a long history; in fact, folk medicine is believed to be older than contemporary scientific medicine. Some anthropologists believe that folk beliefs have persisted through the generations because they are so closely interwoven with other aspects of culture. Moreover, the therapeutic value of many of the health practices has been verified scientifically (McKenzie & Chrisman, 1977). The Filipino folk medicine system is based primarily on the Malaysian culture but may also be based on the Bisayan culture. The Filipino culture has been influenced by Indian, Chinese, Arabian, Spanish, Mexican, and American belief systems. It is believed that many of the elements of the health practices found in the Philippines may actually have been borrowed from these cultures.

In the Filipino culture, certain illnesses may be assigned to natural causes, such as overeating, poor diet, or excessive drinking. These illnesses would normally be treated with home remedies, including herbal preparations, decoctions, massage, sleep, and exercise.

Illnesses are believed to be caused by supernatural agents. Some Filipino people associate disease with the total life situation, with the result that disease can have both natural and supernatural causes. Some Filipinos believe that there are invisible spirits that replicate the life of the individual and possess supernatural powers that are generally denied to most humans (Hart, 1966; McNall, 1989).

Individuals who subscribe to supernatural causes of disease may feel protected from harmful supernatural influences by such things as talismans, amulets, prayer, and seeking advice from a folk healer. Sickness and death are believed by some Filipinos to be the result of actions of angry ancestral spirits or witches, evil eyes, or the lethal bite or power of a supernatural animal. In such cases, if the client does not recover or if the illness worsens, the client will generally seek the advice of various folk medicine specialists. The client may also seek the advice

of a conventional medical practitioner if resources are available. In the Philippine Islands, it is not uncommon for a physician to incorporate certain aspects of the folk medicine belief system, such as the theory of hot and cold, when implementing the treatment plan (Hart, Rajadhon, & Coughlin, 1965).

Filipino culture has a variety of folk medicine healers, including shamans and curers. A shaman is a priest or priestess who practices folk remedies. A curer diagnoses illness by palpating the pulse. Many Filipino curers believe that the pulse is the best place to detect an illness because the pulse is an outlet, or a substation, of the heart. They believe that, if the pulse lies, the heart lies (Lieban, 1967). An ill person's pulse may be either "hot" or "cold," depending on the type of illness. Some Filipinos believe that a healthy person has a balance regarding hot and cold air elements in the body; however, if the body becomes too hot or subsequently too cold, the circulation of the blood will be increased or decreased and the person will experience a loss of appetite and fatigue that will ultimately lower the body's natural defenses against the illness. It is believed by some Filipinos that both metaphysical and real hot and cold temperatures will cause an illness if absorbed by the body in excessive amounts.

Many Filipino individuals also believe in the theory of the four humors. The body humors include phlegm or mucus, air or vapors, bile, and blood. Filipinos who subscribe to this theory accept one overriding theme that involves health in relationship to air or wind (*mal aire*). For these Filipinos, there are two ways in which one can become ill. One way is related to air and includes exposure to a normal draft or breeze that results in an illness such as a cold. The other way is by absorbing excessive amounts of hot or cold air, which ultimately will cause an imbalance of these principles in the body. A Filipino mother may wrap the navel of her baby with a cloth to prevent air from entering the body through the navel cord. Some Filipinos use coconut oil to soak or rub the skin in order to prevent wind from entering the pores. Some Filipinos believe that air circulates in the veins and, if hot air is absorbed through the pores, the blood will carry it to the brain, resulting in mental illness (Hart, 1981). Another *mal aire* illness includes the means by which the spirits penetrate the body by magically propelling thorns, pebbles, bones, and other foreign objects into the body.

Illness and Wellness Behaviors

Three concepts underlie Filipino health beliefs and practices: flushing, heating, and protection. Flushing is believed to keep the body free from debris, heating is believed to maintain a balanced internal temperature, and protection is believed to guard the body from outside influences. Flushing is based on the premise that the body is a container that can collect impurities. Heating involves the belief that hot and cold qualities must be in balance in the body. Protection involves safeguarding the natural boundaries of the body from supernatural as well as natural forces. Among Filipinos who subscribe to the theory of flushing, there is a complex system of beliefs based on the theory that flushing is a complex system of stimulating perspiration, vomiting, flatulence, or menstrual bleeding for the sole purpose of removing evil forces from the body. A common home remedy used to promote flushing is vinegar. Vinegar may be used to flush the body to cure an ailment such as a fever or a chest cold. In such cases the vinegar is mixed with water, salt, or hot pepper. Drinking this mixture will stimulate perspiration and subsequently remove all the evil or bad things from the body. It must be remembered that such practices are not all that unorthodox when compared with the Western medical system (McKenzie & Chrisman, 1977).

Because Filipinos are deeply religious and a God-fearing people, they believe that many diseases and illnesses are the will of God. When a Filipino client is given a poor prognosis, the client may continue to hope for a cure, despite the severity of the problem. This attitude may help to explain why some Filipino clients are uncomplaining and frequently suffer in silence.

Implications for Nursing Care

It is important for the nurse to remember that Filipino folk-related health practices may be beneficial, neutral, or harmful. Folk practices that are beneficial or neutral should be incorporated into the plan of care. However, the nurse should develop educational training programs that will help the client and family identify and eliminate folk practices that are harmful.

Some Filipino Americans have an external locus of control that is based on the belief that illness is caused by external forces, which may be either natural or supernatural. Therefore, it is important for the nurse to remember that the client's noncompliance with medical regimens may be based on a fatalism-oriented system. It is important for the nurse to ascertain whether the client's noncompliance is based on fatalistic beliefs or a lack of understanding.

The nurse should be aware that many Filipino Americans relate health to food. For example, eating healthful food such as vegetables, meat, chicken, and fruits are related to maintaining health. Eating pigeon soup is related to protecting health or preventing illness. Eating chicken soup is related to restoring health. In addition, some Filipino Americans believe actions taken relate to health. For example, praying relates to maintaining health. Soaking one's feet in salted water after working in the fields and avoiding too much sun or rain protect health and prevent illness. Herbal medicines and special home remedies, such as pounding ginger with coconut oil and massaging painful joints, are cures that will restore health. Another home remedy is toasting uncooked rice until brown, adding water, and drinking the resulting mix for stomachache. Wounds may be treated by boiling guava leaves and drinking the fluid (Spector, 2004).

BIOLOGICAL VARIATIONS

Body Size and Structure

In the United States, prematurity is defined as a birth weight of less than 2500 g (5 pounds, 8 ounces). When controls for income, maternal age, parity, and smoking were done, Filipino Americans tended to have a lower mean birth weight than their White counterparts (Morton, 1977). Morton suggested that the birth-weight requirement for maturity should be lowered for some ethnic groups, including Filipino Americans, and recommended that prematurity be redefined as less than 2200 g (4 pounds, 14 ounces) for Filipino Americans and Blacks.

Filipinos are short and tend to have very small frames. Some Filipinos have short limbs in comparison with the trunk size. At 3 years of age, the mean standing height is 85.7 cm (33.7 inches) for Filipino boys and 84.8 cm (33.4 inches) for Filipino girls. Thus Filipino children are considerably shorter than White children, for whom the mean standing height is 95 cm (37.4 inches) for boys and 93.9 cm (37 inches) for girls (Meredith, 1978). However, the average height and weight of Filipinos are quite similar to those of Thais and Vietnamese persons. Filipinos tend to lag behind Japanese persons in both height and weight. The height of Japanese boys and girls from birth to 1 year of age exceeds the height of Filipinos (Matawaran et al., 1966). It is believed, however, that Filipinos overcome this difference by 21 years of age and that their growth increments are quite similar to those of Japanese persons.

In a classic 1958 study, José and Salcedo observed that Filipino American women tended to be leaner and slimmer than their White counterparts. Anchacosa-Angala and Márquez-Sumabat (1964) noted that body weight for Filipino Americans increased significantly when an increase in skinfold thickness occurred. Based on data, they concluded that skinfold thickness could be used as an index of leanness and fatness for Filipino Americans.

Kusumoto, Suzuki, Kumakura, and Ashizawa (1996) compared foot morphology between Filipino and Japanese women and found that Filipino women showed pronounced deformity of the great toe laterally, "like a hallux valgus," without any complaints (p. 373). A pathological deformity of the hallux valgus appears to be related to the Filipino genetic structure.

Skin Color

Mongolian spots are commonly found at birth on Filipino infants. Normal pigmentation among Filipinos ranges from brown to peach brown, and it is extremely difficult to detect conditions such as cyanosis in darker-pigmented skin. In addition, some darker-skinned Filipinos may also have heavy deposits of subconjunctival fat, which contains high levels of carotene in sufficient quantities to mimic conditions similar to jaundice. If the nurse is to distinguish between carotenemia and jaundice, it is necessary for the nurse to inspect the posterior portions of the hard palate of the client in an extremely good light or in bright daylight (Roach, 1977).

Other Visible Physical Characteristics

Filipinos are classified as members of the Mongoloid race because of very common racial characteristics, including brown skin color, almond-shaped inner eye folds, and extremely sparse body hair, particularly in men, on whom chest hair is often absent. Hair on the head is typically coarse and also either straight or wavy (Garn, 1971). In addition, male pattern baldness appears to be a rarity among Filipino Americans (Garn, 1971).

Chung and Kau (1985) noted that the tendency for cleft lip or cleft palate was higher for Japanese, Chinese, and Filipinos than for Whites and Hawaiians. These researchers also noted that the high-risk groups had smaller dimensions than Whites and Hawaiians in regard to cranial-base measurement, facial height, palatal length, and mandibular length, which might be contributing factors to the higher incidence of cleft lip and cleft palate.

Enzymatic and Genetic Variations

Motulsky, Stransky, and Fraser (1964) found a high prevalence of glucose-6-phosphate dehydrogenase (G-6-PD) deficiency among Filipinos. It would appear that G-6-PD deficiency affects Filipinos as severely and as quantitatively as it affects persons in the Mediterranean group. In addition, alpha-thalassemia, a form of which is known as hemoglobin H disease, is prevalent in Filipinos, Chinese, Thais, and Greeks (Wallerstein, 1976).

Susceptibility to Disease

Cardiovascular Disease. Gerber (1980) noted that White mortalities for coronary artery disease are higher than those for either Japanese Americans or Filipino Americans. Gerber's study also suggested that mortalities for coronary artery disease are higher in urban areas than in rural areas and that differences in mortality noted among races are probably not attributable to genetic factors but rather to environmental ones. This conclusion was based on the fact that when Japanese Americans or Filipino Americans moved from rural to urban areas, their mortality for coronary artery disease rose, which was believed to be directly related to changes in lifestyle, diet, and work patterns. Ryan, Shaw, Pliam, et al. (2000) investigated 527 Filipino American patients and 3176 Caucasian patients from a center treating coronary artery disease in California. The researchers concluded that Filipino Americans have a higher prevalence of hypertension and diabetes and a lower prevalence of smoking and obesity than Caucasians. Ethnicity was an independent predictor of higher mortality after catheterization intervention and increased need for late reintervention. This data suggested that Filipino American patients need to be followed closely after percutaneous intervention or cardiac surgery procedures. Brown, James, and Nordloh (1998) evaluated Filipino American and Caucasian female health care workers, relating ethnicity to blood pressure variation. They concluded that cultural background and emotional state influence the extent of blood pressure variation in daily life.

Among Filipino Americans, heart disease is the leading cause of death for Filipino Americans, with stroke the third leading cause of death (Hoyert & Kung, 1997). In addition, relatively higher rates of hypertension have been reported, with a prevalence rate of 79% as compared with 61% for their White counterparts (Ryan, Shaw, Pliam, et al., 2000).

Hypertension. Stavig, Igra, and Leonard (1988) found that the prevalence of controlled and uncontrolled hypertension in the United States is lower for persons of Asian descent, except for Filipinos. In fact, the California Department of Health Services hypertension study found that Filipino Americans have one of the highest prevalences of hypertension, second only to that of Blacks (Requiro, 1981). The analysis of the data from the

study by Stavig, Igra, and Leonard (1988) indicated that Asians and Pacific Islanders with hypertension are less likely to be aware of the condition, to seek treatment or take medication for the condition, or to control the condition through diet. In addition, these ethnic groups recorded lower frequencies of hospital stays for the condition, fewer days of bed disability, and fewer days of not feeling well as a result of hypertension than all other ethnic groups. The study concluded that because of their high levels of poverty and lack of education and the relationship of these factors to health-seeking behavior for hypertension, additional study is needed to improve health care for Filipino Americans.

Klatsky and Armstrong (1991) reported a study in which 4211 Filipino men and women were compared with Japanese, Chinese, and other Asians for incidence of hypertension. This study noted that the Filipino men and women had the highest rate of hypertension of any of the groups.

Young, Lichton, Hamilton, et al. (1987) noted a high positive relationship between sodium intake and the prevalence of hypertensive disease. This study examined the relationship between ethnicity and blood pressure in young adults of six ethnic groups residing in Hawaii. The findings suggested that body weights and heights of Whites and Hawaiians tended to exceed those of Chinese, Filipinos, Japanese, and Koreans. The study noted that both systolic and diastolic pressures were significantly higher in men than in women across all races. The study also found no significant differences between sexes or across races regarding urinary excretion of sodium and potassium.

Stavig, Igra, Leonard, et al. (1986) conducted a study to determine the death rates in California for hypertension-related diseases for the periods 1969 to 1971 and 1979 to 1981. The data indicated that during both periods, age-standardized rates for composite hypertension-related mortality were highest for Blacks, followed by Whites, and lowest for Asians and Pacific Islanders. Filipinos, who were noted to have high prevalence rates of hypertension, tended to have a lower rate of hypertension-related mortality. Findings from this study suggest that the possible reasons for the decline in hypertension-related mortality may include population awareness, level of treatment, control of hypertension, knowledge of cardiovascular risk factors, improved medical technology, and modification of behavior. A study by Klatsky and Armstrong (1991) also found that Filipino men and women had the highest prevalence of hypertension when Chinese, Japanese, other Asians, and Filipinos were studied.

Diabetes Mellitus. There is an increased incidence of diabetes mellitus among Filipino Americans (Araneta & Barrett-Connor, 2005). Sloan (1963) concluded that diabetes mellitus occurs three times more often among Filipino Americans than it does among White Americans. Cuasay, Lee, Orlander, Steffen-Batey, and Hanis (2001) studied 831 Filipino Americans and noted an overall prevalence for type 2 diabetes of 16.1%, supporting earlier studies that Filipinos are at higher risk than the U.S. non-Hispanic White population.

Cancer. Kolonel (1985) conducted a study comparing the cancer incidence rates for Filipinos in Hawaii. Filipino women in Hawaii had the highest incidence of thyroid cancer among all ethnic groups in Hawaii. In addition, the data indicated a lack of increase in female breast cancer rates among Filipinos in Hawaii and a lower than expected increase in colon cancer rates. In contrast to this study, Goodman, Yoshizawa, and Kolonel (1988) noted that the incidence rates for thyroid cancer remained relatively stable from 1960 to 1984. However, this study also concluded that when Filipinos in Hawaii were compared with other ethnic groups in Hawaii, Filipinos were found to have the highest reported incidence rates for thyroid cancer. The conclusion of this study was that environmental influences may be responsible for the unusually high rate of thyroid cancer among Filipinos in Hawaii.

Young, Ries, and Pollach (1984) found that the rates of gallbladder and urinary bladder cancer for women exceeded those for men among the Filipino population. The primary site of cancer associated with the highest survival rate for both Filipino men and women was found to be the thyroid gland. The 5-year relative survival rate for cancer of the thyroid gland was 91%, whereas the survival rate

for other primary sites of cancer, including the esophagus and the pancreas, were found to be uniformly low. Rosenblatt, Weiss, and Schwartz (1996) compared the incidence of primary liver cancer among ethnic groups and found Filipino males born in the United States to be 6.5 per 100,000 compared with Whites at 3.4 per 100,000 and Filipino women 0 per 100,000 compared with 1.1 for Whites. The incidence of liver cancer was lower for Filipinos born in the United States than for those born in the Philippines.

Gallbladder Disease. Yamase and McNamara (1977) examined the hospital admission rates for gallbladder disease in Chinese, Japanese, Koreans, Filipinos, Hawaiians, Portuguese, Puerto Ricans, and Whites. This study found that although differences in admission rates among races were statistically significant they were not clinically significant.

Amyotrophic Lateral Sclerosis. Studies have indicated that the prevalence for amyotrophic lateral sclerosis among Filipino Hawaiians exceeds that found among Whites and Japanese Hawaiians (Matsumoto, Worth, Kurland, & Okazaki, 1972). However, the findings from other studies suggest that the excess in regard to amyotrophic lateral sclerosis found among Filipinos in Hawaii is more or less a function of population and age distribution, rather than a true racial or ethnic difference (Kurtzke, 1982).

Palatal Mucosal Changes. The habit of reverse smoking is practiced in various parts of the world, including the Philippines (Ortiz, Pierce, & Wilson, 1996). A study of reverse smokers compared with conventional smokers in Cabanatuan City in the Philippines found that 96.7% of reverse smokers exhibited palatal mucosal changes, including leukoplakia, mucosal thickening, fissuring, pigmentation, nodularity, erythema, and ulceration, compared with only 26.7% of conventional smokers (Mercado-Ortiz, Wilson, & Jiang, 1996). This study provides a basis for classification of the palatal mucosal changes among reverse smokers and has implications for nurses in terms of health care teaching with Filipino women.

Patterns of smoking differ from one cultural group to the next, with the Filipino rate at 24%, higher than the 19% rate of non-Hispanic whites, the 20% rate of Hispanics, and the 14% rate of Chinese Americans and lower than that of American Indians/Alaska Natives (29%) and Pacific Islanders (32%). In a study by Chen and Unger (1999), 20,482 subjects between 12 and 17 years of age were randomly sampled in California. The investigators concluded that Filipino Americans showed the highest risk of smoking initiation, Japanese and Korean were in between, and Chinese Americans were at the lowest risk.

AIDS. Research by Woo, Rutherford, Payne, et al. (1988) in San Francisco indicates that the number of AIDS cases has disproportionately increased among Asians and Pacific Islanders (177%), compared with increases among Blacks, Whites, Hispanics, Native Americans, and Alaska Natives (54%). The incidence of AIDS among Filipinos was reported to be 92 per 100,000. Longitudinal studies are being done with children born to HIV-1 antibody–positive Filipino women (Manaloto, Caringal, Santiago, et al., 1996). Maxwell, Bastani, and Warda (2000) interviewed 211 Filipino American adolescents and young adults in Los Angeles to assess AIDS-related knowledge and behaviors. More than half reported condom use at last intercourse. Statistically significant correlates with condom use were higher self-efficacy and the practice of carrying condoms.

Hepatitis B. Chronic carrier rates of hepatitis B virus infection and tuberculosis range from 5% to 15% in Chinese, Koreans, Filipinos, and Southeast Asians, compared with the 0.2% rate found in the total U.S. population (Franks, Berg, Kane, et al., 1989).

Glaucoma. Aghaian, Choe, Lin, and Stamper (2004) investigated central corneal thickness of various ethnic groups. Chinese, Hispanics, and Filipinos were all found to have similar central corneal thickness; in comparison, central corneal thickness in African Americans was thinner. Other parameters also differed between these ethnic groups.

Nutritional Preferences

Some Filipino Americans reflect their culture through their preparation and consumption of specific foods. Because some Filipino Americans subscribe to a theory of hot and cold, foods with these properties are incorporated into their dietary regimen. For example, it is customary to include both "hot" and "cold" foods in cooking, such as mixing beans, which are considered hot foods, with green vegetables, which are considered cold foods, regardless of how they are prepared (Orque, 1983). In addition, Filipino Americans who practice imitative magic may incorporate the concept of magic into the preparation and consumption of foods. For example, a pregnant Filipino woman may believe that eating dark foods such as prunes will produce a dark-complected baby (Affonso, 1978; Pimentel, 1968).

For some Filipino Americans, religious or family customs also dictate the foods that are prepared and consumed. For example, Filipino Catholics may abstain from eating meat during Lent, particularly on Ash Wednesday and Good Friday. Zaide (1961) concluded that Filipino beliefs and customs are so entrenched in the culture that some Filipinos may even refrain from eating meat during the burial of a relative.

The traditional foods for Filipinos include rice, fish, and vegetables. For Filipino Americans, typical dishes include *adobo, pancit*, and *lupia. Adobo* is a method of preparation that includes cooking certain meats, such as pork, chicken, or beef, that have been marinated in vinegar, garlic, and other typical Filipino condiments. The meat is simmered slowly until it becomes tender and brown (Day, 1974). *Pancit* is pasta made of rice or wheat noodles that is cooked with chicken, ham, shrimp, or pork in a soy- and garlic-flavored sauce. *Lupia* is similar to the Chinese egg roll and is either deep-fried or prepared fresh with selected vegetables (Day, 1974). Although Filipino Americans have changed their diets to reflect customs traditionally found in the United States, they also tend to retain ethnic food habits (Lewis & Glasby, 1975). Althaus (1999) notes that dietary patterns are related to degree of acculturation; in particular, the immigrants in the "first wave" tend to eat a more traditional diet, while "second and third wavers" are much different, eating primarily American fare with "just a sprinkling" of Filipino foods.

Psychological Characteristics

Flaskerud (1984) conducted a study to determine whether there was a difference in perspective placed on problematic behaviors exhibited by six minority groups: African Americans, Native Americans, Chinese Americans, Mexican Americans, Filipino Americans, and Appalachians. The findings of the study indicated that there are differences in perceptions of problematic behavior and its management between mental health professionals and minority groups. Flaskerud also concluded that although these differences are related to different levels of education and expertise, they are also likely to be related to cultural influences on conceptual explanations of problematic behavior and appropriate management. Cultural groups that were considered dominant viewed problematic behavior as mental illness and recommended psychiatric treatment, whereas cultural groups that were considered ethnic minority groups (including Filipino Americans, Chinese Americans, Mexican Americans, African Americans, Native Americans, and Appalachians) viewed the behavior from a broader perspective that encompassed spiritual, moral, social, economic, vocational, recreational, personal, physical, and psychological assessments. Bjorck, Cuthbertson, Thurman, and Lee (2001) examined appraisal, coping, and distress among Korean American, Filipino American, and White American Protestants. Filipino Americans reported more problem-solving strategies than White Americans, and both Asian American groups reported using more strategies of accepting responsibility, religious coping, distancing, and escape avoidance than the White Americans.

Psychological defenses vary by culture and thus result in a different configuration of depression (Rosenbaum, 1989). Marsella (1997), who studied depression in various cultural settings, reported that depression occurred infrequently in Filipinos.

A culture-bound syndrome, *amok*, was first reported among persons from Malaysia. A similar behavior pattern has been found in the Philippines, Polynesia, Laos, New Guinea, and Puerto Rico and among the Navajo (Bonder, Martin, & Miracle, 2002). This is classified as a dissociative episode, characterized by a period of brooding, followed by an outburst of violent, aggressive, or homicidal behavior directed at people and objects (American Psychiatric Association, 2000). Instances of *amok* may occur during a brief psychotic episode or at the onset of an exacerbation of a chronic psychotic process.

Alcohol Use. A study by Danko, Johnson, Nagoshi, et al. (1988) found that although Filipinos and Hawaiians who drink have substantial alcohol usage, a large proportion of Filipino Americans are abstainers. Lubben, Chi, and Kitano (1988) found that approximately 50% of the women in a population sample of 298 Filipinos were abstainers, whereas approximately 80% of the men in the sample were drinkers, an indication that heavy drinking is almost exclusively a male activity among Filipinos. The study concluded that the only significant variable found among Filipino men and women in regard to drinking was regular participation in religious services.

Implications for Nursing Care

Because Filipino Americans tend to have darker-pigmented skin than White Americans, the nurse must be able to distinguish between the norm and carotenemia, jaundice, or cyanosis. When the nurse is inspecting the skin of a Filipino American, it is important to inspect the buccal mucosa for petechiae. When looking for evidence of carotenemia, the nurse can substantiate this finding if a yellow tint is absent in the palate when the sclerae are yellow (Roach, 1977). If the nurse is unable to determine the presence of carotenemia, the client's stool may be observed to determine if it is light or clay-colored, and the urine may be examined to determine if it is a dark golden color.

Because some Filipino Americans have a prevalence for enzymatic conditions, such as G-6-PD deficiency, lactose intolerance, or thalassemia, it is important for the nurse to encourage the client to eat meals that are high in protein and to replace whole milk with high-calcium substitutes such as buttermilk, yogurt, and sharp cheese or to add lactic aids to foods or other dairy products.

Filipino Americans are essentially very gentle and mild and have passive temperaments. It is believed that the reason for the passive temperament is the desire of Filipinos to maintain a harmonious balance between people and nature. These people generally are neither assertive nor aggressive and may often appear guarded or reticent. The nurse may often misunderstand this need for passivity and misconstrue and mislabel this behavior as an inferiority complex. Very often Filipino Americans are erroneously labeled as passive-aggressive and as having a personality disorder with anger as the underlying cause. When angry, Filipino Americans do have a temperament that is passive-aggressive, and this anger often produces anxiety, which is usually handled through covert and passive means. Behavioral manifestations of passive-aggressive behavior are evidenced through procrastination, stubbornness, intense craving for acceptance, and varying demands for attention (DeGracia, 1979).

The nurse should be cognizant that some Filipino foods are high in purine, such as *dinuguan* (from *dugu*, "blood"), which is a food prepared from the small intestines, liver, heart, kidney, and blood of pork. Because *dinuguan* is extremely high in purine, a client who is following a purine-restricted diet should be instructed to modify the diet with leaner meats than pork organs. Because Filipinos, particularly men, have been reported to be hypertensive, the nurse should instruct these clients to modify traditional high-sodium Filipino diets. Foods that are considered high in sodium include traditional Filipino condiments such as soy sauce. For the client following a diet moderately restricted in sodium, the nurse may suggest brands of soy sauce that have a lower or reduced sodium content. The client who is following a diet totally restricted in sodium can be taught to prepare certain dishes, such as *adobo*, by marinating the meat overnight in a mixture of lemon juice, onions, garlic, sugar, and crushed peppercorns (Orque, 1983).

The nurse should also be aware that intercultural differences in expression of depression may be the result of differences in social structure and worldview. The concept of self is culture specific and must be considered in transcultural care of depressed people (Rosenbaum, 1989).

SUMMARY

The literature dealing with Filipino Americans has sometimes been confusing because Filipinos have been lumped together in the literature with Asians, Spanish-speaking people, and "other" categories (Orque, 1983); therefore, the nurse must carefully apply data from the literature to Filipino American clients who receive care. In addition, the nurse should be careful to notice the dates on research studies of Filipino Americans because many studies in the literature are old and may not reflect current needs. It is important for the nurse to assess the Filipino American client carefully and to keep in mind what is known about the client's cultural background so that culturally appropriate care can be provided.

Case Study

Mr. Rom Recio, a 46-year-old Filipino American, is admitted to the hospital with a diagnosis of hypertension. Mr. Recio has lived in an urban area in Los Angeles, after coming from the Philippines 2 years earlier. This is Mr. Recio's third admission to the hospital because his hypertension is uncontrolled. Mr. Recio has repeatedly refused to comply and take the Aldomet (methyldopa) the physician prescribed for him during the initial diagnostic hospitalization. The nurse notes on examination that Mr. Recio's blood pressure is 140/104 mm Hg, his pulse is 88, his respirations are 16, and his temperature is 98.6° F.

Although Mr. Recio speaks English, occasionally he has difficulty understanding what is being communicated in English terminology. Mr. Recio has a wife and three children, ages 10, 12, and 15. Mr. Recio's wife speaks very little English; however, all the children are proficient in English. When Mr. Recio is examined by the nurse, he states that he believes the problem with his blood has occurred because of disfavor with God.

CARE PLAN

✳ Nursing Diagnosis: Ineffective health maintenance, related to ineffective coping

Client Outcomes

1. Client and family will verbalize desire to learn more about condition and preventive techniques to reduce symptoms.
2. Client and family will verbalize a willingness to comply with prescribed medical regimen.
3. Client will verbalize an understanding of the need to comply with routine schedule for antihypertensive drugs.

Nursing Interventions

1. Identify with client and family sociocultural factors that influence health-seeking behavior
2. Determine with client and family knowledge of hypertension and severity of illness.
3. Determine with client and family knowledge and level of adaptation to news about condition of hypertension.
4. Identify with client and family necessity for adherence to prescribed time limits for taking antihypertensive drugs.

✳ Nursing Diagnosis: Communication, impaired verbal, related to cultural difference (ineffective health, recent immigration, and the use of English as a second language)

Client Outcomes

1. Client and family will be able to communicate basic needs to health personnel.

Nursing Interventions

1. Use visual aids that will aid client in undersanding the condition.
2. Use gestures or actions that communicate various tasks and procedures to be done.
3. Write down messages to provide visual stimulation about procedures to be accomplished.
4. Encourage client and family to express their needs to health personnel.

✳ Nursing Diagnosis: Interrupted family processes related to shift in health status of family member

Client Outcomes

1. Family will participate in care of the ill family member.
2. Family will assist nurse in assisting client in returning to a high level of wellness.

Nursing Interventions

1. Determine family's understanding of client's condition.
2. Determine support systems available to family.
3. Determine with family a supportive network with friends available.
4. Involve family in care and scheduling of client-centered activities (such as taking Aldomet on time).

✳ STUDY QUESTIONS

1. What factors related to culture are most likely to influence the noncompliance exhibited by Mr. Recio?
2. Explain how the Filipino-American orientation to time may influence Mr. Recio's health-seeking behavior and his adherence to specific schedules.
3. Describe the locus-of-control variable that some Filipino Americans have that may influence health-seeking behavior.
4. Describe at least three other nursing interventions that can be implemented to facilitate communication between Mr. Recio, his family, and the health care team.
5. Describe the structure of some Filipino American families and the relationship the family may have on health-seeking behavior.

NCLEX-RN REVIEW QUESTIONS

1. Filipinos tend to have a higher incidence of which of the following?
   A. G-6-PD and alpha-thalassemia
   B. Metabolic syndrome and Tay-Sachs disease
   C. G-6-PD and Mediterranean spotted fever
   D. Mediterranean spotted fever and Rocky Mountain spotted fever

2. The official language of the Philippines is:
   A. English
   B. Patois
   C. Tagalog
   D. Spanish

3. The universal language spoken in the Philippines is:
   A. Patois
   B. Spanish
   C. English
   D. Arabic

References

Adair, L. S., & Popkin, B. M. (1996, January). Low birth weight reduces the likelihood of breast-feeding among Filipino infants. *Journal of Nutrition*, 126(1), 103–112.

Affonso, D. (1978). The Filipino American. In Clark, D. (Ed.), *Culture, childbearing, health professionals* (pp. 128–153). Philadelphia: F.A. Davis.

Agbayani-Siewert, P. (2004, January). Assumptions of Asian American similarity: the case of Filipino and Chinese American students. *Social Work*, 49(1), 39–51.

Aghaian, E., Choe, J., Lin, S., & Stamper, R. (2004, December). Central corneal thickness of Caucasians, Chinese, Hispanics, Filipinos, African Americans, and Japanese in the glaucoma clinic. *Ophthalmology*, 111 (12), 2211–2219.

Althaus, C. (1999, July). Food: multi-cultural mix shifts diet patterns. *Food Service Director*, 12(7), 50.

American Psychiatric Association. (2000). *Diagnostic and statistical manual of mental disorders.* (ed. 4, revised). Washington, D.C.: American Psychiatric Association.

Anchacosa-Angala, S., & Márquez-Sumabat, L. (1964). Skinfold thickness as indication of leanness-fatness in some female college students. *Philippine Journal of Nutrition*, 17, 176–197.

APIAHF (2006, revised August 2006). *Asian and Pacific Islander American Health Forum, Health Brief, Filipinos in the United States.* San Francisco: Asian and Pacific Islander American Health Forum.

Araneta, M., & Barrett-Connor, E. (2005, August). Ethnic differences in visceral adipose tissue and type 2 diabetes: Filipino, African-American, and white women. *Obesity Research*, 13(8), 1458–1465.

Bartlett, L. (1977, June). The Filipino "Cajuns." *Dixie*, p. 9.

Becker, G. (2002, March). Dying away from home: quandaries of migration for elders in two ethnic groups. *Journals of Gerontology. Series B, Psychological Sciences and Social Sciences*, 57(2), S79–S95.

Becker, G., Beyene, Y., Newson, E., & Rodgers, D. (1998, March). Knowledge and care of chronic illness in three ethnic minority groups. *Family Medicine*, 173–178.

Berg, J. A., Rodriguez, D., Kading, V., & De Guzman, C. (2004). Demographic survey of Filipino American nurses. *Nurs Adm Q*, 28(3), 199–206.

Bjorck, J., Cuthbertson, W., Thurman, J., & Lee, Y. (2001, August). Ethnicity, coping, and distress among Korean Americans, Filipino Americans, and Caucasian Americans. *Journal of Social Psychology*, 141(4), 421–442.

Bofill, M. (1999, Summer). Dr. Rano S. Bofill, the music man. *Heritage*, 13(2), 33.

Bonder, B., Martin, L., & Miracle, A. (2002). *Culture in clinical care.* Thorofare, N.J.: Slack.

Brown, D., James, G., & Nordloh, L. (1998, July). Comparison of factors affecting daily variation of blood pressure in Filipino-American and Caucasian nurses in Hawaii. *American Journal of Physical Anthropology*, 106(3), 373–383.

Burma, J. (1974). *Spanish-speaking groups in the United States.* Detroit: Blaine Ethridge Books.

Burr, J., & Mutchler, J. (1993). Nativity, acculturation, and economic status: explanations of Asian American living arrangements in later life. *Journal of Gerontology*, 48(2), 55–63.

Bush, M., & Babich, K. (1986). Cultural variation. In Longo, D., & Williams, R. (Eds.), *Clinical practice in psychosocial nursing: assessment and intervention* (ed. 2). Norwalk, Conn.: Appleton-Century-Crofts.

Cantore, J. (2001, Spring). Giving voice to the "invisible minority." *Minority Nurse*, 26–30.

Cantos, A., & Rivera, E. (1996). Filipinos. In Lipson, J., Dibble, S., & Minarik, P. (Eds.), *Culture and nursing care.* San Francisco: UCSF Nursing Press.

Caringer, B. (1977). Caring for the institutionalized Filipino. *Journal of Gerontological Nursing*, 3(7), 33–37.

Central Intelligence Agency. *The World Factbook.* (2006). Philippines. Retrieved June 14, 2007, from https://www.cia.gov/cia/publications/factbook/geos/rp.html.

Champeau, A. (1998, Fall). Indiana's bountiful crop of Filipino American graduates. *Heritage*, 12(3), 19.

Champeau, A. (1999, Fall). Gallery of Filipino American graduates in Indiana. *Heritage*, 13(3), 32.

Chen, X., & Unger, J. (1999, June). Hazards of smoking initiation among Asian American and non-Asian adolescents in California: a survival model analysis, *Preventive Medicine*, 589–599.

Cheong, R., Kuizon, M., & Tajaon, R. (1991, December). Menstrual blood loss and iron nutrition in Filipino women. *Southeast Asian Journal of Tropical Medicine in Public Health*, 22(12), 595–604.

Chung, C. S., & Kau, M. C. (1985). Racial differences in cephalometric measurements and incidence of cleft lip with or without cleft palate. *Journal of Craniofacial Genetic Development and Biology*, 5(4), 341–349.

Chung, P., Borneo, H., Kilpatrick, S., Lopez, D., Travis, R., Lui, C., Khandwala, S., & Schuster, M. (2005, January–February). Parent-adolescent communication about sex in Filipino American families: a demonstration of community based participatory research. *Ambulatory Pediatrics*, 5(10), 50–55.

Corpuz, O. (1965). *The Philippines.* Englewood Cliffs, N.J.: Prentice Hall.

Cuasay, L., Lee, E., Orlander, P., Steffen-Batey, L., & Hanis, C. (2001, December 24). *Diabetes Care*, 2054–2058.

Daniels, R., & Kitano, H. (1970). *American racism: exploration of the nature of prejudice.* Englewood Cliffs, N.J.: Prentice Hall.

Danko, G. P., Johnson, R. C., & Nagoshi, C. T., et al. (1988). Judgments of "normal" and "problem" alcohol use as related to reported alcohol consumption. *Alcoholism*, 12(6), 760–768.

D'Avanzo, E., & Geissler, E. (2003). *Pocket guide: cultural assessment* (ed. 3). St. Louis: Mosby.

Davidhizar, R. (1997, November). Personal communication about her experience as a nursing director in a psychiatric hospital.

Day, B. (1974, August). Philippine fare. *Gourmet*, p. 25.

DeGracia, R. T. (1979, August). Cultural influences on Filipino patients. *American Journal of Nursing*, 1412–1414.

De La Cruz, E. (1999, Fall). De La Cruz honored as 1999 outstanding teacher. *Heritage*, 13(3), 8.

Dela Cruz, F., Padilla, G., & Agustin, E. (2000, July). Adapting a measure of acculturation for cross-cultural research. *Journal of Transcultural Nursing*, 11(3), 191–198.

De Leon, R. (1999, Fall). Conversations with actor Fran de Leon. *Heritage*, 13(3), 9.

Ennis, T., & Inaba, M. (1977). *Philippines. The volume library,* Nashville, Tenn.: Southwestern Company.

Espíritu, Y. L. (1995). *Filipino American lives.* Philadelphia: Temple University Press.

Flaskerud, J. (1984). A comparison of perceptions of problematic behavior by six minority groups and mental health professionals. *Nursing Research*, 33(4), 190–197.

Franks, A., Berg, C., & Kane, M., et al. (1989). Hepatitis B virus infection among children born in the United States to Southeast Asian refugees. *New England Journal of Medicine*, 321, 1301–1305.

Garn, S. (1971). *Human races* (ed. 3). Springfield, Ill.: Thomas.

Geissler, E. (1998). *Pocket guide: cultural assessment.* St. Louis: Mosby.

Gerber, L. M. (1980). The influence of environmental factors on mortality from coronary heart disease among Filipinos in Hawaii. *Human Biology*, 52(2), 269–278.

Gloria, E. (1999, Fall). Gloria honored with poetry awards. *Heritage*, 13(3), 41.

Goodman, M. T., Yoshizawa, C. N., & Kolonel, L. N. (1988). Descriptive epidemiology of thyroid cancer in Hawaii. *Cancer*, 61(6), 1272–1281.

Guthrie, G., & Jacobs, P. (1976). *Childrearing and personality development in the Philippines.* University Park, Pa.: Pennsylvania State University Press.

Hart, D. V. (1966). The Filipino villager and his spirits. *Solidarity*, 1, 66.

Hart, D. V. (1981). Bisayan Filipino and Malayan folk medicine. In Henderson, D. V., & Primeaux, M. (Eds.), *Transcultural health care.* Reading, Mass.: Addison-Wesley.

Hart, D. V., Rajadhon, P. A., & Coughlin, R. J. (1965). *Southeast Asian birth customs: three studies in human reproduction.* New Haven, Conn.: Human Relations Area Files.

Hooper, H. (1958). A Filipino in California copes with anxiety. In Seward, G. (Ed.), *Clinical studies in cultural conflict.* New York: Ronald Press.

Hoyert, D. L., & Kung, H. C. (1997). Asian or Pacific Islander mortality, 1992. *Monthly Vital Statistic Report*, 46 (1 suppl), 1–63.

Infoplease.com. Retrieved December 11, 2006, from www.infoplease.com.

Kataoka-Yahiro, M., Ceria, C., & Yoder, M. (2004, Fall). Grandparent caregiving role in Filipino American families. *Journal of Cultural Diversity*, 11(3), 110–117.

Kittler, P., & Sucher, K. (2001). *Food and culture in America* (ed. 3). Belmont, Calif.: Wadsworth/Thomson Learning.

Klatsky, A. L., & Armstrong, M. A. (1991). Cardiovascular risk factors among Asian Americans living in northern California. *American Journal of Public Health*, 81(11), 1423–1428.

Kluckhohn, F., & Strodtbeck, F. (1973). *Variations in value orientations*. Westport, Conn.: Freeport Press.

Kolonel, L. N. (1985, December). Cancer incidence among Filipinos in Hawaii and the Philippines. *National Cancer Institute Monogram*, 69, 93–98.

Kurtzke, J. F. (1982). Epidemiology of amyotrophic lateral sclerosis. *Advances in Neurology*, 36, 281–302.

Kusumoto, A., Suzuki, T., Kumakura, C., & Ashizawa, K. (1996, September–October). A comparative study of foot morphology between Filipino and Japanese women, with reference to the significance of a deformity like hallux valgus as a normal variation. *Annals of Human Biology*, 23(5), 373–385.

Lantican, L. S., & Corona, D. F. (1992, October–December). Comparison of the social support networks of Filipino and Mexican-American primigravidas. *Health Care of Women International*, 13(4), 329–338.

Lasker, B. (1969). *Filipino immigration*. New York: Arno Press.

Lee, R. (2004, September). Filipino men's familial roles and domestic violence: implications and strategies for community-based intervention. *Health and social care in the community*, 12(5), 422–429.

Lewis, J., & Glasby, M. (1975). Food habits and nutrient intakes of Filipino women in Los Angeles. *Journal of American Dietetic Association*, 67, 122–125.

Lieban, R. W. (1967). *Cebuano sorcery: malign magic in the Philippines*. Berkeley: University of California Press.

Lott, J. (1976). Migration of a mentality: the Filipino community. *Social Casework*, 57, 165–172.

Lubben, J. E., Chi, I., & Kitano, H. H. (1988). Exploring Filipino American drinking behavior. *Journal of Studies of Alcohol*, 49(1), 26–29.

Manaloto, C., Caringal, L., Santiago, E., et al. (1996, May–June). Longitudinal studies of children born to HIV-1 antibody positive Filipino commercial sex workers (CSW): diagnostic dilemmas. *International Journal of the Study of AIDS*, 7(3), 212–220.

Manila, E. (1999, Fall). The Filipino American center. *Heritage*, 13(3), 7.

Marsella, A. (1997). Depressive experience and disorder across cultures. In Triandis, H., & Draguns, J. (Eds.) *Handbook of cross-cultural psychology* (ed. 2). Boston: Allyn & Bacon.

Matawaran, A., et al. (1966). Preliminary report on the average heights and weights of some Filipinos. *Philippine Journal of Nutrition*, 19, 318–332.

Matsumoto, N., Worth, R. M., Kurland, L. T., & Okazaki, H. (1972). Epidemiology study of amyotrophic lateral sclerosis in Hawaii: identification of high incidence among Filipino men. *Neurology*, 22, 934–940.

Maxwell, A., Bastani, R., & Warda, U. (2000, Winter). Knowledge and attitudes toward condom use—do they predict behavior among Filipino Americans? *Ethnicity and Disease*, 19(1), 113–124.

McAdam, J., Stotts, N., Padilla, G., & Puntillo, K. (2005, January). Attitudes of critically ill Filipino patients and their families toward advance directives. *American Journal of Critical Care*, 14(1), 17–25.

McBride, M., & Parreno, H. (2006). Filipino American families and caregiving. In Yeo, G., & Gallagher-Thompson, D. (Eds.), *Ethnicity and the dementias* (ed. 2). New York: Rutledge.

McKay, J., Hill, B., & Buckler, J. (2007). *A history of world societies* (ed. 7). Boston: Houghton Mifflin.

McKenzie, J., & Chrisman, N. (1977). Healing herbs, gods, and magics. *Nursing Outlook*, 25, 326–328.

Melendy, H. (1977). *Asians in America: Filipinos, Koreans, and East Indians*. Boston: Twayne.

McNall, C. (1989). Healing we cannot explain. *American Journal of Nursing*, 89(9), 1162–1164.

Mercado-Ortiz, G., Wilson, D., & Jiang, D. (1996, October). Reverse smoking and palatal mucosal changes in Filipino women. Epidemiological features. *Australian Dental Journal*, 41(10), 300–303.

Meredith, H. (1978). Research between 1960 and 1970 on the standing heights of young children in different parts of the world. In Reese, H., & Lipsitt, L. (Eds.), Advances in child development and behavior (pp. 1-59). New York: Academic Press.

Monzon, R. B. (1991, December). Replacement patterns of *Ascaris lumbricoides* populations in Filipino children. *Southeast Asian Journal of Tropical Medicine in Public Health*, 22(4), 605–610.

Morton, N. E. (1977). Genetic aspects of prematurity. In Reed, D. M., & Stanley, F. J. (Eds.), *The epidemiology of prematurity.* Baltimore: Urban & Schwartzenberg.

Motulsky, A. G., Stransky, E., & Fraser, G. R. (1964). Glucose-6-phosphate dehydrogenase (G6PD) deficiency, thalassaemia, and abnormal haemoglobins in the Philippines. *Journal of Medical Genetics,* 1, 102–106.

Orque, M. (1983). Nursing care of Filipino American patients. In Orque, M., Bloch, M. S., & Monrroy, B. (Eds.), *Ethnic nursing care: a multicultural approach.* St. Louis: Mosby.

Ortiz, G., Pierce, A., & Wilson, D. (1996, September). Palatal changes associated with reverse smoking in Filipino women. *Oral Disease,* 2(9), 232–237.

Pacquiao, D. (2003). People of Filipino heritage. In Purnell, L., & Paulanka, B. (Eds.), *Transcultural health care* (ed. 2). Philadelphia: F.A. Davis.

Parreno, H. (1977). How Filipinos deal with stress. *Washington State Journal of Nursing,* 49, 3–6.

Pilapil, V. (1999, Summer). The truth about the first Pinoy in the US Congress. *Heritage,* 13(2), 34.

Pimentel, L. (1968). *The perception of illness among the immigrant Filipinos in Sacramento Valley.* Master's thesis, Sacramento State College, Sacramento, California.

Pollard, R. (1995, December). Ethnic comparison of twinning rates in California. *Human Biology,* 67(6), 921–931.

Requiro, R. (1981). Filipino hypertension rate leads Asian-Pacific group. *Philippine News,* 20, 12.

Roach, L. (1977). Color changes in dark skin. *Nursing '77,* 7, 48–51.

Rosenbaum, J. (1989). Depression: viewed from a transcultural nursing theoretical perspective. *Journal of Advanced Nursing,* 14, 7–12.

Rosenblatt, K. A., Weiss, N. S., & Schwartz, S. M. (1996, May). Liver cancer in Asian migrants to the United States and their descendants. *Cancer Causes Control,* 7(3), 345–350.

Ryan, C., Shaw, R., & Pliam, M., et al. (2000, March). Coronary heart disease in Filipino and Filipino-American patients: prevalence of risk factors and outcomes of treatment. *Journal of Invasive Cardiology,* 12(3), 134–139.

Santiago, M. (2001). Personal conversation with Jean Ann Contore in Giving voice to the "invisible minority." *Minority Nurse* (2001, Spring), 27.

Shimamoto, Y. (1977). Health care to the elderly Filipino in Hawaii: its cultural aspects. In Leininger, M., & Carbol, K. (Eds.), *Transcultural nursing care of the elderly, proceedings from the second National Transcultural Nursing Conference.* Salt Lake City: University of Utah College of Nursing.

Sloan, N. (1963). Ethnic distribution of diabetes mellitus in Hawaii. *Journal of the American Medical Association,* 183, 419–424.

Solon, F., Solon, M., & Mehansho, H., et al. (1996, November). Evaluation of the effect of vitamin A-fortified margarine on the vitamin A status of preschool Filipino children. *Europe Journal of Clinical Nutrition,* 50(11), 720–723.

Spector, R. (2004). *Cultural diversity in health and illness* (ed. 6). Upper Saddle River, N.J.: Pearson Prentice Hall.

Spector, R. (2004). *Culture care: Guide to heritage assessment and health tradition* (ed. 3). Upper Saddle River, N.J.: Pearson Prentice Hall.

Stavig, G. R., Igra, A., & Leonard, A. R. (1988). Hypertension and related health issues among Asians and Pacific Islanders in California. *Public Health Reports,* 103(1), 28–37.

Stavig, G. R., Igra, A., & Leonard, A. R., et al. (1986). Hypertension-related mortality in California. *Public Health Reports,* 101(1), 39–49.

Suzara, A. (1999, Fall). Suzara named director of student cultural center. *Heritage,* 13(3), 5.

Takaki, R. (1998). *Strangers from a different shore* (revised ed.). Boston: Little, Brown & Co.

Time almanac with information please. (2007). Boston: Information Please, Inc.

Tompar-Tiu, A., & Sustento-Seneriches, J. (1995). *Depression and other mental health issues: the Filipino American experience.* San Francisco: Jossey-Bass.

Urban Associates, Inc. (1974). *A study of selected socioeconomic characteristics of ethnic minorities based on the 1970 census* (HEW publication no. 5). Arlington, Va.: U.S. Department of Health, Education, and Welfare.

U.S. Department of Commerce, Bureau of the Census. (2002). Population profiles by age, sex, race, and Hispanic origin, Summary File 3. Washington, D.C.: U.S. Government Printing Office.

Vance, A., & Davidhizar, R. (1999, December). Developing cultural sensitivity: when your client is Filipino American. *Journal of Practical Nursing,* 16–20.

Voegelin, C. F., & Voegelin, F. M. (1997). *Classification and index of the world's languages.* New York: Elsevier.

Wagner, N. (1973). Filipinos: a minority within a minority. In Stanley, S., & Wagner, N. (Eds.), *Asian-Americans: psychological perspectives.* Palo Alto, Calif.: Science & Behavior Books.

Wallerstein, R. (1976). Blood. In Krupp, M., & Chatton, M. (Eds.), *Current medical diagnosis and treatment.* Stamford, Conn.: Appleton & Lange.

Weber, S. E. (1996). Cultural aspects of pain in childbearing women. *Journal of Obstetric, Gynecologic and Neonatal Nursing,* 25(1), 67–72.

White, J., Linhart, J., & Medley, L. (1996, September). Culture, diet, and the maternity. *Advance for Nurse Practitioners,* 26–28.

Wilson, S., & Billones, H. (1994). The Filipino elder: implications for nursing practice. *Journal of Gerontological Nursing,* 20(8), 31–36.

Woo, J. M., Rutherford, G. W., & Payne, S. F., et al. (1988). The epidemiology of AIDS in Asian and Pacific Islander populations in San Francisco. *AIDS,* 2(6), 473–475.

Wooley, P. (1972). *Syncrisis: the dynamics of health—an analytic series on the interactions of health and socioeconomic development: Vol. 4. The Philippines.* Washington, D.C.: U.S. Department of Health, Education, and Welfare.

World almanac (2007). New York: World Almanac Books.

Yamase, H., & McNamara, J. (1977). Geographic differences in the incidence of gallbladder disease: influence of environment and ethnic background. *American Journal of Surgery,* 123, 667–670.

Yeo, G., Hikoyeda, N., McBride, M., et al. (1998). *Cohort analysis as a tool in ethnogeriatrics: historical profiles of elders from eight ethnic populations in the United States* (ed. 2) SGEC working papers series 12. Stanford, Calif.: Stanford Geriatric Education Center.

Young, F., Lichton, I. J., & Hamilton, R. M., et al. (1987). Body weight, blood pressure, and electrolyte excretion of young adults from six ethnic groups in Hawaii. *American Journal of Clinical Nutrition,* 45(1), 126–130.

Young, J. L., Ries, L. G., & Pollach, E. S. (1984). Cancer patient survival among ethnic groups in the United States. *Journal of National Cancer Institute,* 73(2), 341–352.

Zaide, G. (1961). *Philippine history: developing our nation.* Manila: Bookman.

CHAPTER 18 Vietnamese Americans

Ruth Yoder Stauffer*

Behavioral Objectives

After reading this chapter, the nurse will be able to:

1. Identify communication barriers a Vietnamese American may encounter when using the U.S. health care system.
2. Identify beliefs about space that may influence how Vietnamese people feel about care given to females.
3. Describe the organization of the Vietnamese family.
4. Articulate ways the nurse might modify instructions to a Vietnamese American client based on differences in time perception.

5. Discuss briefly the basic *yin* and *yang* theory of Chinese medicine and how it is expressed in the cause and treatment of disease.
6. Articulate at least three explanations for the causes of illness that influence traditional Vietnamese thinking.
7. Discuss implications for care of the small body size of many Vietnamese Americans.

*Former Mennonite Central Committee relief worker in Vietnam; more recently worked with the Mennonite church in the Vietnamese communities in Honolulu, Hawaii, and the Washington, D.C., area.

OVERVIEW OF VIETNAM

Vietnam is situated on the eastern coast of the Indochina peninsula, bordered on the north by China, with the Gulf of Thailand surrounding the Mekong Delta on the south. On the west, Vietnam is bordered by Cambodia (Kampuchea) and Laos and, on the east, by the South China Sea. The country is slightly smaller than Japan, with 127,000 square miles. Vietnam, along with Laos and Cambodia, is often referred to as Indochina or Southeast Asia. These three countries are strikingly dissimilar, with different languages, unrelated social roots, long histories of unique development, and varying sources of strife.

The northern part of Vietnam is mountainous, with deep valleys and the industrial Red River Delta. The central ribbon is a long, narrow corridor with a mountain range, coastal plain, and miles of beautiful white sand beaches. The southern part of Vietnam is mostly the flat Mekong Delta, the agricultural area where most of the rice for the country and for export is grown. Vietnam is considered a tropical country, though the north has four distinct seasons and the south has two seasons: rainy and dry.

The population of Vietnam is 84,402,966 (2006 estimate) (Central Intelligence Agency, 2007; *World Almanac*, 2007), which includes "lowland people" (often urban and more educated), rural village people (with varying degrees of sophistication and education), and mountain people (made up of at least 30 different groups or tribes with a culture all their own). Ethnic groups include Kinh (Viet), 86.2%; Tay, 1.9%; Thai, 1.7%; Muong, 1.5%; Khome, 1.4%; Hoa, 1.1%; Nun, 1.1%; Hmong, 1%; and others, 4.1% (1999 census) (Central Intelligence Agency, 2007). The mountain people number approximately 1 million (*World Almanac*, 2007). The life expectancy is 70.6 (2005 estimate), with an infant mortality rate of 25.9. The literacy rate is 90.3% (*Time Almanac with Information Please*, 2006; *World Almanac*, 2007).

Vietnam has a recorded history of more than 2000 years, with legends that cover an additional 2000 years. Earliest records are of dynasty rule and domination by the Chinese (111 B.C. to 938 A.D.). There were 900 years of independence until the French came in 1858. Throughout the French domination (until 1954), the Vietnamese continued to work toward independence.

The country was divided into the Communist north and the non-Communist south by the Geneva Accords in 1954, when it became clear that the "nationalist" movement in the north had been monopolized by leaders leaning toward Communist ideology. The struggle between the Soviet-assisted North Vietnam and the United States–assisted South Vietnam ended in 1975, when Vietnam was reunited under the victorious Socialist Republic of Vietnam. More than 30 years of war had physically, economically, and socially devastated the country. There were a great deal of turmoil and isolation during the next 15 years, as the Communists attempted to rebuild the country under a new philosophy. Floods and drought added to the crises and poverty. Thousands of people left the country for hope in the outside world, especially France, the United States, Canada, and Australia. By the late 1980s, however, the need and opportunity for economic exchange helped ease restrictions, and there was a pronounced influx of economic interests and business with countries around the world. By 1993, the country had a trade surplus and was the world's third largest exporter of rice (Hiebert, 1993). The years-long trade embargoes from the United States were lifted in 1994, and in 1995 the United States extended Vietnam full diplomatic recognition. The 25% unemployment rate of 1995 has decreased to an estimated 2.4% in 2005, and the Vietnamese have become less anxious to leave the country (Central Intelligence Agency, 2007). The 2004 estimate of the gross domestic product was $232.2 billion, with a per capita income of $2800 (Central Intelligence Agency, 2007). Some 19.5% of the people live below the poverty line (2004 estimate). Today, 56.8% of the labor force is agricultural, 37% is industrial, and 6.2% is services. By 2002, "going back" to visit Vietnam was a common occurrence in most United States Vietnamese communities. Dollars carried in by friends still provide welcome help for improving the quality of life for many Vietnamese. Today, tourism provides many jobs for the people of Vietnam (personal conversation with Luke Martin, August 12, 2002). The U.S. has become Vietnam's top export market with an annual trade totalling over $6 billion (*Time Almanac with Information Please*, 2006)

IMMIGRATION TO THE UNITED STATES

In 2000, 1,223,736 or 0.37% of the population of the United States identified Vietnam as their country of origin. The Vietnamese population ranked as the fourth largest Asian American group, preceded only by Mexicans, Filipinos, Chinese, and Asian Indians (Infoplease.com, 2006; U.S. Department of Commerce, Bureau of the Census, Summary File 3, 2002). Vietnamese make up approximately 11.0% of the total Asian American population.

Of the Asian Americans residing in the United States, 20.7% reside in the Northeast, 11.7% in the Midwest, 18.8% in the South, and 48.8% in the West (U.S. Department of Commerce, Bureau of the Census, The Asian Population: Census Brief, 2000). The highest concentrations of Vietnamese Americans are in California, Virginia, Texas, and Florida. Approximately 80.9% of Vietnamese persons in the United States today were born in a foreign country (U.S. Department of Commerce, Bureau of the Census, The Asian Population: Census Brief, 2000). Between 1980 and 1990, 69.7% of all Vietnamese residing in the United States were immigrants, compared with 27.1% between 1975 and 1979. The number of Vietnamese immigrants slowed somewhat between 1990 and 2000. In fact, while the Vietnamese population grew by 134.8% from 1980 to 1990, the growth rate slowed considerably to 35.1% from 1990 to 2000 (U.S. Department of Commerce, Bureau of the Census, The Asian Population: Census Brief, 2000). The median age for Vietnamese Americans is 25.9 years, compared with 33.1 years for the rest of the U.S. population (Central Intelligence Agency, 2007; U.S. Department of Commerce, Bureau of the Census, The Asian Population: Census Brief, 2000). Approximately 48% of Vietnamese Americans are females, compared with 51% for the total nation (U.S. Department of Commerce, Bureau of the Census, The Asian Population: Census Brief, 2000).

First-Wave Immigrants

The first group of refugees, who began arriving in 1975, included lowlanders, professionals, ranking South Vietnamese military personnel, and those with close U.S. connections. This group also included those who had the means to get out of the country and those who stood to lose the most under the new regime. A high percentage of these immigrants were educated in Vietnam or abroad, and some spoke English. Many were young and single, or married with small children. The children moved into the school systems and could soon speak English more fluently than their parents, and in some cases more fluently than they could speak Vietnamese.

Some of these immigrants had been exposed to European cultures or to the American culture for years and had economic or vocational assets. They generally did not go through a long, stressful period of economic and psychological deprivation affecting their health. Of the 145,000 Vietnamese persons who came to the United States in 1975, 14% lived in single-family households, 42% were under 18 years of age, and 11.6% were over 44 years of age. Approximately 90% were employed 1 year after arrival (Coelho & Stein, 1980).

Second-Wave Immigrants

A higher percentage of the second-wave refugees (1979 to 1980) were Chinese-Vietnamese extended family groups who left Vietnam under duress and pressure from the government. These immigrants were educated and part of the business community in or near Saigon and had as much social status as was permitted under the existing regime. For many persons in the second wave of refugees, however, Vietnamese was a second language, and fewer spoke English than in the earlier group. These immigrants also included elderly persons and other extended family members who often had health needs.

Third-Wave Immigrants

Most of the Vietnamese refugees during the 1980s were "boat people," who in many cases had lived through not only economic struggles but also political and social change while at home. In addition, the boat people had survived life-threatening situations for days at sea. Persons in the third wave often spent months or even years in refugee camps along the way, and these earlier experiences caused turmoil that needed to be dealt with once they arrived and got settled in the United States. Third-wave immigrants were even more diversified than those in the two former groups. Many were in poorer physical condition than those arriving earlier, and generally the adjustment was more difficult and more complex. Although many refugee education programs and school systems had organized programs to absorb the newly arrived children and adults in the first and second waves, these programs were not as effective with persons in the third wave. Life in camps did not encourage rigorous study habits or academic excellence, and many children in the third wave were not able to read or write well in either Vietnamese or English. For the boat people, education to assist in adjustment to the new environment needed to be much more comprehensive.

By 1986, nations surrounding Vietnam, Cambodia, and Laos had tightened laws for illegal travelers to their shores, and the traffic of boat people slowed down. At the same time, the government of Vietnam gave new economic life to the country by allowing the people some private marketing and land use. In 1989 the government agreed to voluntary repatriation of Vietnamese who had left the country, and during the next 3 years, with the United Nations' help, more than 32,000 boat people returned from camps, especially from where they had been held in Hong Kong (Balfour, 1993). Foreign-born Vietnamese usually represent one of the three waves of immigration. In addition, it is helpful to know if the individual is first, second, or third generation in the United States, since these factors will influence adherence to cultural behaviors that are practiced (Bonder, Martin, & Miracle, 2002).

COMMUNICATION

Language

In the United States, Vietnamese is the language of most of the 1,223,736 people who call or have called Vietnam their home. In 2000, 65.0% of all Vietnamese 5 years of age or older could not speak English well (Infoplease.com, 2006; U.S. Department of Commerce, Bureau of the Census, The Asian Population: Census Brief, 2000).

Vietnamese is not mutually intelligible with any other Asian language. It is monosyllabic and disyllabic and polytonal (five to six tones), and so a syllable when spoken with different tones has an entirely different meaning. The language is flowing and musical, and for the most part, pronunciation is consistent and the grammar simple.

Until the 1960s, French was the language of educated Vietnamese people, along with Vietnamese; therefore, much of the scientific and technical vocabulary was borrowed from French or, more recently, English. After 1975 in Vietnam, English was more common as the choice for a second language in high schools and colleges. Three distinct dialects of Vietnamese separate the northern, central, and southern regions of Vietnam. Dialects identify the speaker's origins and are understood by others regardless of region.

For many years before the Vietnam War, Vietnam had a large Chinese minority who had their own schools with classes conducted in Chinese. In the Chinese suburb of Saigon called Cholon, many older Chinese persons spoke only Chinese, and the children learned Vietnamese as a second language. This explains why many persons in the large Chinese–Vietnamese refugee group can speak both Chinese and Vietnamese or only Chinese. In contrast to this, the ethnic mountain people, or *Montagnards*, have their own tribal languages (usually of Austronesian type and, in the north, Miao-Yao type) and often do not understand Vietnamese.

Style

Respect is very evident in communication and is a cornerstone of Vietnamese society (Huynh, 1987). The proliferation of titles in the Vietnamese language is evidence of the cultural focus on respect. For example, when describing family relationships, English users have titles reserved for family members that include *mother, father, sister, brother, uncle, aunt, cousin, grandmother,* and *grandfather.* However, the language and style of the Vietnamese not only encompass family descriptors such as *uncle* but also designate which side of the family a family member represents (mother's or father's) and further indicate whether that relative is the eldest brother or sister. Grandparent titles also reflect paternal or maternal side. When a sister or brother is being described, the term used indicates if the sister or brother is younger (*em*) or older (*chi* or *anh*).

Context

The word *yes* is used in English to express agreement and does not reflect an attitude of respect or disrespect. For Vietnamese people, *ya* indicates respect and not necessarily agreement. Therefore, a troubling verbal communication between health workers and Vietnamese American clients is the polite *Ya, ya, Thua bà, ya, ya,* response, which Americans interpret as "Yes, yes, I understand, and I'll do it." For the Vietnamese, the "yes" of *ya* is simply being respectful, indicating "I'm listening, and I respect what you're saying" (even though the request may not be within the realm of possibility). Nurses often reflect later, "But he said, 'Yes, yes,' and agreed to. . . ." Noncompliance by Vietnamese Americans can often be traced to this misinterpretation of *ya.*

Vietnamese people often use personal pronouns to describe various roles held. For example, the speaker may refer to self as *con* (referring to a child) when addressing parents and as *em* to the nurse or to any superior. However, the same individual may refer to himself or herself as *thây* ("teacher") when addressing students. It is common for Vietnamese persons to use only the title of a person, -such as "Uncle" or "Teacher," except with family and close friends. Especially when there is considerable distance between the speaker and the listener, the title alone is most correct. This custom is practiced even in the United States. For example, people often say "Madam Chair" or "Mr. President," indicating that the title is more important than the name.

A distinct feature of the Vietnamese culture and consequently the language is moderation and caution (Huynh, 1987). Vietnamese people are taught from childhood to think before speaking. High value is placed on modesty of action and speech. A Vietnamese proverb suggests that "bragging reflects an empty soul." There is also concern that a slip of the tongue may bring discord and be disruptive to harmony and respect. Ethnic Vietnamese lowlanders, as well as those from the mountain tribes, place high value on showing respect: communication should always be in a formal, polite manner (Rairdan & Higgs, 1992). Table 18-1 highlights some differences between Asian and American communication styles.

Touch

Traditionally, the high value of emotional self-control and the general esteem for correct behavior have limited touch as a form of communication. Physical behavior, including backslapping, is not considered proper by the well bred. The young people have been less formal, and in Vietnam in the 1970s it was not uncommon to see groups of Vietnamese boys jostling each other in the street or girls walking arm in arm on the sidewalk. Today in the United States, many Vietnamese youths are taking cues from their American counterparts. For some Vietnamese people, the head is considered the "seat," and touching it, even in the process of giving care, may cause some vital force to escape (Hoang & Erickson, 1982).

Kinesics

In the Vietnamese culture, respect is also conveyed by nonverbal communication. By the time standing

Table 18-1	Communication Style and Expression of Emotion	
Asian	**American**
Nonverbal	Verbal
Subtle, indirect	Open, direct
Serene, stoic, suppress negative emotions	Expressive, spontaneous
Indirect expression of affection by fulfilling obligations, needs	Direct verbal and physical expression of affection

From Nilchaikovit, K., Hill, J., & Holland, J. (1993). The effects of culture on illness behavior and medical care. *General Hospital Psychiatry,* 15, 41–50.

is possible, the child is taught to cross the arms over the chest, lower the head, and bend the upper torso slightly forward when greeting an elder or a guest coming into the house. Nonverbal methods to communicate respect continue to be used throughout life. Deference to others shows a Confucian and Buddhist influence in that how something is done is often more important than what is done. Posture and manner of walking can be used to indicate self-concept (Sideleau, 1992). Respect is also shown by avoiding eye contact when talking with someone who does not have equal standing in education, social standing, age, or gender. A student avoids eye contact with a teacher, an employee with the boss, a younger member of the family with the elders, and so on. Direct eye contact in these settings generally means a challenge or an expression of deep passion. Bowing the head slightly when entering the presence of an elderly person conveys respect. Using both hands to give something to, or receive something from an adult, especially an elder, or person of higher status, shows respect. The head may be considered sacred, and care should be taken in touching and patting. Feet are the lowliest body parts and should be kept on the floor.

A silent form of communication may also be used that relies heavily on implied understanding between people of the culture. Because of cultural norms, sometimes implicit concerns are not allowed to be discussed verbally. For example, it may be very unusual or could be considered improper for a son or daughter to discuss issues of death and dying with parents, yet concern by either of them may be expressed by nonverbal cues, such as bowing of the head or direct eye contact. When dealing with Western health care professionals, these understandings are not overtly stated. Unless the health care professional knows the culture well enough to address the unspoken, this valuable information is lost and often leads to misunderstanding of family–patient dynamics or lack of agreement with the plan of care (McLaughlin & Braun, 1998).

In contrast to the usual palm-up position used by persons in the dominant culture in the United States, Vietnamese persons beckon for someone to come by turning the palm downward and waving the fingers. The upturned palm is used to call a dog or other animal, or as an insult. It is never proper to snap one's fingers or wave violently to gain someone's attention.

Except in private circumstances, open expression of emotions is considered in bad taste. Emotions interfere with self-control and can be considered weaknesses. Romantic overtures and demonstrative joyous expressions are reserved for home or other private settings. One exception to the usual restraint is the expected behavior of a widow at the grave for the burial of her husband, when she may wail or attempt to throw herself into the grave.

Implications for Nursing Care

Because respect and harmony are highly valued in relationships, there is a great desire in the Vietnamese culture not to disappoint, upset, embarrass, or cause another person to lose face. The desire to maintain harmony takes precedence over what the actual truth of a situation may be. When a Vietnamese American client is confronted with a difficult or delicate question, particularly if the answer is negative, such as "Did you take your medication?" the client may choose not to give a direct answer in favor of the higher good of keeping peace with the nurse. In the Western culture, this avoidance might be considered an attempt to avoid the truth; however, in the Vietnamese culture the answer would be considered the correct way to handle a delicate situation.

The nurse should recognize that negative emotions or expressions of disagreement are usually conveyed by silence or a reluctant smile. For the Vietnamese a smile may express joy, but more often it is used to convey many other messages, such as stoicism in the face of difficulty or an apology for a minor social offense. A smile may be a proper response to a scolding to show sincere acknowledgment for the wrongdoing, as well as to convey that there are no ill feelings. A smile is also a way to respond when it is improper to say "thank you" or "I'm sorry" because of age or status. A smile is often present, regardless of the situation. Even if angry, feeling neglected, or in need, the Vietnamese

American client will rarely express this to the health care professional but rather will speak quietly and smile. Instead of asking questions that allow an answer, such as "Are you having pain?" or "Do you want something for pain?" the nurse should acknowledge the likelihood of pain and state, "Please let me get you something for pain."

The nurse may experience difficulty with gathering information from Vietnamese American clients. Vietnamese American clients tend to be discreet and passive, quietly understanding problems and rarely expressing feelings. Usually there is even more difficulty obtaining information in the area of emotional problems or sexual difficulties because these topics are considered private and to be avoided in public (Nilchaikovit, Hill, & Holland, 1993). In short-term relationships, it is crucial to have a same-sex Vietnamese interpreter; for the long term, the health professional should work toward a trusting relationship. For the Vietnamese client, a caring, accepting attitude helps bridge the gap to true understanding.

Because most Vietnamese American clients entering the health care system in the United States do not speak medical English, an interpreter or bicultural medical translator can assist in accurate communication. It is important that the translator be culturally aware and conscientious to bridge the gap between the culture of the client and members of the health care team. Accurate translation can be assisted if the interpreter is Vietnamese because of the built-in cultural awareness. However, the Vietnamese interpreter may be hesitant to translate certain complaints that are unacceptable to Western practitioners, such as symptoms the client states are "caused by the wind," a common problem. Other important factors are the effect of differences in social class between interpreter and client, the possible effect of a male interpreter with a female client, and the need for a female interpreter or companion when a physical examination is done on a female client. When an interpreter is unavailable, it is important for the nurse to choose vocabulary carefully, to keep instructions simple and brief, and to avoid medical jargon (Tran, 1980) (Box 18-1).

The nurse should be aware that English phonetic practices applied to Vietnamese names often result in pronunciations that are unintelligible to the Vietnamese. Nguyên Thị Hồng, who has been responding to approximately /Wee-un /Tee-hung/ for 23 years, can hardly be expected to appear at the clinic desk when she hears /Hung Thigh Nugooen/ summoned. (In Vietnam, the family name—for example, Nguyên—is spoken first and always appears first on listings. In the United States the family name is always spoken last, though it appears first on listings.) In a clinic where clients must be called, it may be useful to have the clients take numbers because numbers are more readily understood. It is important for the nurse to appreciate that pronunciation may also cause difficulties with questions regarding addresses and phone numbers. It may be easier for the client to write answers to such questions. Such a client should be encouraged to carry instructions in written form.

A question about age may also be difficult for the Vietnamese American client. A Vietnamese mother may be able to indicate the year a child was born but may not be able to state the child's exact age. In Vietnam individual birthdays are not usually celebrated; rather, everyone becomes a year older at the beginning of each new year (Tết). Thus a newborn who arrives during the week before New Year would be considered 1 year old following the first (Tết) celebration. Another reason for confusion about age, especially for persons who immigrated as teenagers, is that new birth certificates may show an age adjustment of 2 or 3 years earlier. This adjustment may have been done in Vietnam to avoid the draft or in the United States to facilitate entrance into high school. (After 18 years of age, the student was not usually accepted into high school regardless of educational level attained in Vietnam.) The slight build of many Vietnamese persons facilitates this age adjustment. Elderly Vietnamese persons without birth certificates usually know the year of their birth and are officially assigned, on arrival in the United States, a birthday of January 1. Finally, the nurse should be cognizant of the fact that for many Vietnamese

---

Box 18-1

USING AN INTERPRETER

Unless there are large numbers of a specific cultural group, most hospitals or medical centers cannot afford professional interpreters. But with careful selection and guidance, good interpreters can be home grown.

1. Find a good bilingual person in the Vietnamese community who lives near enough to be called upon to help, either in person or on the phone, when needed. Often Vietnamese can suggest suitable candidates. Except in real emergencies, avoid using the family's 10-year-old daughter, friends, or "the cleaning lady."
2. Get to know the interpreter beforehand and practice saying the Vietnamese name correctly. Usually a title should be used.
3. Be sure the interpreter understands the idea of confidentiality, "a commitment of all members on the health team."
4. Impress on the interpreter that you consider him or her a bridge between the two groups of people involved, the family and the health team, and in a special way an important member of both teams.
5. If the terminology for the anticipated causes, symptoms, suspected diagnosis, and other matters is not routine or familiar, review it briefly with the interpreter so these can be looked up or clarified before the interview.

DURING THE INTERVIEW

1. The interpreter's seat should be about half way between you and the patient group. This helps communicate that the interpreter is a bridge, not a member of only the health team or of only the family.
2. Greet the family, and then introduce the interpreter by name to the patient. If the patient is elderly, show respect by introducing the interpreter to the patient, but then also include the accompanying family, who likely will be doing much of the communicating.
3. Always look and talk directly to the patient family group, not at or to the interpreter. Remember, the interpreter is the bridge, not the original messenger. (An exception is when you and the interpreter need to clarify something with each other.)
4. To make it easier:
   - Use short, direct sentences.
   - Plan questions carefully. Do not use double negatives. Focus on one item for yes–no questions.
   - Avoid technical jargon, idioms, and metaphors.
   - Avoid humor or jokes, which are often difficult to translate.
   - Be aware that questions related to the reproductive system or sexual behavior are sensitive areas.
5. Be prepared to hear new names for familiar symptoms without showing surprise or scorn. One way of handling unfamiliar diagnoses can be to ask, "Can you tell me what I need to know about [the specific diagnosis mentioned]?" (McPhee, 2002, p. 499).
6. At the end of the interview, thank the family and specifically thank the interpreter.

The interpreter is not only bilingual but also bicultural. With sensitivity and respect in working together, the professional will be fortunate to come to depend on him or her not only to translate words but also to translate culture, raising the caution flag when the culture is being inadvertently violated in some way. Often the interpreter can come up with a good solution to the situation if the professional can be depended on for respect and understanding.

AFTER THE INTERVIEW

1. Document the interpreter's name on the medical record.
2. Discuss any part of the interview that was problematic, and attempt to learn the cause and find possible options for the solutions.
3. Validate any information or important decisions the professional understood had been made, including the plan of action.
4. Thank the interpreter and check that the institutional plan for reimbursement is clear.

Americans the numerous questions asked by health professionals in the United States raise doubt about the competency of the health professionals. The nurse should attempt to communicate both acceptance of varying cultural practices and genuine concern in order to bridge the gap between the cultures and to increase the client's trust in the caregivers.

SPACE

Intimate Zone

Beliefs about space are rooted deep in Vietnamese culture. For traditional Vietnamese persons, intimate-zone activities are confined to private settings. Holding hands in public, especially with members of the opposite sex, is considered in poor taste, and hugging or emotionally touching in public, even by close friends or family members, is embarrassing to the traditional Vietnamese.

Beliefs about space also influence how Vietnamese people feel about care given to females. Until the early 1900s, traditional practitioners were not to touch the bodies of their female clients except to take their pulse. Figurines were used for the female client to indicate where she was having problems. Today, many Vietnamese persons still emphasize virginity at the time of marriage, especially for the woman, and have strong feelings about unmarried young women having pelvic examinations.

Personal, Social, and Public Zones

Vietnamese individuals are likely to feel more comfortable with more distance during personal and social relationships than that required by persons in the dominant culture. Social exchanges generally do not involve physical contact other than handshaking, which may be practiced between men.

Living Space

In Vietnam, extended families live comfortably in relatively small areas. The moderate or warm climate allows many family activities to be carried on outside. Often the kitchen is separate from the rest of the house, and the two or three main rooms double as living rooms and bedrooms, with the mosquito nets neatly tied back during the day. Even in spacious homes, family members often prefer to spend much of their time in proximity to each other. In rural Vietnam, homes are typically arranged in communities and villages with several homes near each other.

Although many Vietnamese persons were used to living in close proximity, refugee camps brought a new kind of cramped and confined closeness. As refugees, many Vietnamese persons lived for several months or years with 8 to 10 persons occupying a one-room space, sometimes enclosed only by a blanket curtain. Special adjustment was required by most refugees when they received housing in the United States because many well-intentioned sponsors made an effort to provide single-home dwellings for the refugees because "they've been so crowded so long." Unfortunately, this space lacked the familiar sounds, smells, and people and soon brought feelings of loneliness. Today, many Vietnamese Americans have homes with room for parents and additional family members and desire to have relatives and friends in close proximity.

Implications for Nursing Care

When caring for Vietnamese American clients, the nurse should be cognizant of the effect space may have on client care. For example, the nurse should be aware that if a pelvic examination is to be conducted, it is important for a female translator to explain carefully why it is necessary and what will be done and to remain with the client during the examination.

The nurse should also be aware that a back rub from a stranger could cause feelings of uneasiness. The nurse should use discretion in including a back rub as a routine part of nursing care.

SOCIAL ORGANIZATION

Family

In Vietnam, the family is the basic institution of society and provides lifelong protection and guidance for the individual members. The roles and structure are well defined, with extensive terminology designating kinship relationships. The lineage is patriarchal, with the father considered the head of the household. The mother often handles much of the household responsibilities and management.

The immediate family includes the parents, unmarried children, daughters, sometimes the husband's parents, and sons with their wives and children. In addition, the extended family includes other close relatives (usually with the same family name and ancestors) who live in the same community (Box 18-2). The oldest son has the heavy responsibility of carrying on the family name, of taking over for the parents when they become elderly, of seeing to their care, and of following through with the religious and ancestral observances. The oldest daughter takes responsibility for the care of the household in the absence of the mother.

Box 18-2

NAMES

Many Vietnamese family names originated during the various dynasties that ruled in Indochina during the past 3000 years. There were about 100 family names for more than 56 million people, and of those 100 names, "only a score" are in common usage today (Huynh, 1987). *Nguyên* (near pronunciation is /Nwee-un/) is the family name for more than 25% of the Vietnamese family units in the United States and Canada. With so many persons having the same family name, it has limited usefulness in identification; therefore, given names are used.

Names in Vietnam are always written family name first, middle name (or names) second, and given name last, for example, "Nguyên Thị Hồng" or "Trần Văn Hai." The same names may be used for males and females, and the middle name can be a clue as to gender. "Văn" used as a middle name usually indicates male gender ("Trần Văn Hai") compared with "Thị." (pronounced /Tee/), which is used for females (Nguyên Thị Hồng). Sometimes several middle names are used, and therefore there is no gender indicator.

After marriage, a woman keeps her maiden name and does not combine it with her husband's name. Informally she may be called by her given name or her husband's given name ("Mrs. Hai"), but formally she uses her full maiden name preceded by "*Bà*," which can be used as a respectful "Mrs." Children take their father's family name. Customs are changing in the United States, but to avoid confusion, many Vietnamese American wives are adopting their husband's family name. Either name may be used, depending on the setting, and children have interesting choices when asked for "mother's name."

Given names usually have special meanings, often describing the baby or expressing the hopes of the parents for the baby. Names can be chosen from virtues or from nature or music; for example, "Hồng" means "rose" and "Xuân" means "spring." At home or in the village, people may be called by their number in the sibling ranking, rather than by their given names, which explains the nicknames of Nam ("fifth") or "Bảy" ("seventh").

Today, many babies born in the United States are given both an American name and a Vietnamese name. This is not a new practice for the Vietnamese. During the past half-century, for example, the Chinese Vietnamese were commanded by law to change their Chinese given names to Vietnamese names. These persons may also have taken a Christian name when they converted to Christianity. In this resettlement period, almost every Vietnamese child who has an English first name can also give a Vietnamese name if asked.

Except for close friends and coworkers, Vietnamese custom dictates that a person's name is used with a title, never alone. An example of this in English would be "Mr. Bill," "Mrs. Mary," "Director James," or "Uncle John." Titles are important and therefore should be selected carefully by the speaker to convey appropriate respect as well as sometimes to place emotional distance between the speaker and the listener.

The family has been the chief source of cohesion and continuity for the Vietnamese for hundreds of years. In comparison with Chinese and other Southeast Asian groups, the Vietnamese family is seen "as the backbone of tradition and heritage" (Davis, 2000, p. 137), the center around which ancient traditions, customs, and ways of life continue (Fong & Mokuau, 1994).

The crux of family loyalty is "filial piety," which commands children to obey and honor their parents. According to Huynh (1987), the worst insult a Vietnamese can receive is to be accused of failure to fulfill the obligation of filial piety. Along with the three major historical religions of Vietnam, "Honor your father and mother" is also commanded in the Christian faith (Exodus 20:12).

Parents consider it important to train their children, and this responsibility is usually shared by members of the extended family living in the household. Obedience and honor are shown in several ways: obedient behavior and attitudes, using the detailed kinship terminology for each person, and contributing to the family name through outstanding achievements. Personal interests and destiny are seldom considered outside the framework of the immediate and extended family. Behavior or misbehavior (juvenile delinquency, academic failure, mental disorders, and so on) reflects on the entire family and has great significance beyond the person involved. It has often served to curb antisocial behavior, especially among the young.

If personal feelings or ambitions do not contribute to the good of the family or cause disharmony, the individual is expected to bend toward the family and give up personal wishes. In a study utilizing open interviews to understand Vietnamese culture, Laura, a 26-year-old, reflected on how parents or other older members of the family direct children in making life decisions: "Actually my older brother he really wanted to become a doctor. But my uncle said, 'You can't do that. You know that, you have to bring them (rest of the family) here, so you have to study something that take a short time. Engineering, something like that.' And my brother, he listened to my uncle" (Davis, 2000, p. 142).

As Vietnamese point out, Vietnamese family traditions began to change decades before immigration to the United States. With the years of war, the prescribed gender roles and decision making had to be taken on by the females of the family. Large extended families were less common or more scattered, or family homes were located in inaccessible territory. The intergenerational households in the United States create stress in the family, with young family members becoming acculturated into the American way of life, while parents and grandparents retain more traditional values (Tran, 1989).

The Vietnamese concept of family and extended family that has existed across generations as a "super organic unit" is profoundly different from the individualism of the nuclear family in the United States in the beginning of the twenty-first century. And this disparity continues to strongly affect the stress levels of Vietnamese communities in the many pressures toward acculturation. Every culture has particular characteristics that help a member of the culture meet everyday life situations. When a cornerstone of the cultural structure is attacked, the cost of the resulting anxiety cannot be overestimated.

Socialized Role of Children

Children are socialized to their roles in the family at an early age. Children are to obey and respect all elders, address them by correct titles, and correctly cross their arms over the chest and bow slightly from the hips when introduced or coming into the presence of elders.

There is increasing concern noted in the literature with the practice in the West of equating the Asian concept of "training" with the Western idea of "authoritarian" and "control" type of child rearing. Chao (1994) noted that these terms may have entirely different implications for Asians because they are from different cultural systems, an American-European cultural tradition Asians do not necessarily share. The Asian concept of "training" describes the responsibility of parents to be highly involved, caring, and concerned. The mother as the central caretaker has major responsibility for promoting the success of the child, having the child physically near her, even through the night. Chao notes that Asian immigrant children do well in our schools, often not true for our own "authoritarian-type"–parented offspring.

Rudy and Grusec (2001) examine "authoritarian" Asian parenting and the transmission of values. Again, control seemed to be less the determinant; rather the warmth, involvement, and kindness perceived by the child make the difference. Also, the importance of whether the culture is an individualistic or collectivistic culture and the dilemma of the immigrant parents (and African American parents) raising children as minorities in a culture seen as a high risk environment for the child personally, and for the group. "Best values" may be best values for the whole group rather than simply the individual.

Although not mentioning Vietnamese specifically, in the article, "Understanding Context and Culture in the Parenting Approaches of Immigrant South Asian Mothers," the *Social Work* authors, caution social workers against counseling these parents to accept Western culture, but rather establish support groups where parents support each other while finding their way as they "train" their children to survive in their new culture—and also survive in their old one (Maiter and George, 2003).

Vietnamese children in the United States who are in school and learning English at a faster rate than their seniors at home are often placed in the role of translator. This situation, continued over a period of time, gives the child a sense of power in the family hierarchy that is difficult for both the child and the family.

Education

Before 1954, Hanoi was the educational center for Vietnam and contained most of the medical and dental schools. After the Geneva Accords, South Vietnam had its own educational centers in Saigon, Hue, and Can Tho, but the demand far exceeded the supply. The high demand and limited seats in the high schools and universities caused many students to delay their education, go abroad, or, for the men, be drafted.

Today in the United States, education continues to be highly valued in the Vietnamese community. While the census has not yet broken out Vietnamese, they, like their other Asian American counterparts, continue to excel in educational attainment. These data illuminate some interesting trends. For example, Asian Americans are more likely than their White counterparts to have less than a high school education (15% versus 5%), more likely to hold a bachelor's degree than their White counterparts (42% versus 28%), and slightly less likely to have a high school diploma than their White counterparts (85% versus 88%). In 2000, among Asian American men 25 years of age and older, 13% had less than a high school diploma, 20% were high school graduates, 21% had some college education, and 46% held a bachelor's degree or higher. Similarly, among Asian American women 25 years of age and older, 17% had less than a high school diploma, 25% were college graduates, 19% had some college, and 39% held a bachelor's degree or higher (U.S. Department of Commerce, Bureau of the Census, The Asian Population: Census Brief, 2000). Nonetheless, these statistics are remarkable, considering that either these students or their families have come to this country within the past 25 years.

Religion

Vietnam has a history of religious tolerance except for the period immediately before the French takeover, when Christians were suspected of being spies. More recently, the official government position is religious tolerance, with much of the governance being left to the local officials.

Three major religions from China have combined to strongly influence Vietnamese thought and practice and become an ingrained part of the culture during the past centuries: Buddhism, Confucianism, and Taoism. Buddhism is considered less an organized orthodoxy than a state of mind, using the Four Noble Truths taught by Buddha: (1) life is suffering, (2) suffering is caused by desire, (3) suffering can be eliminated by eliminating desire, and (4) to eliminate desire, one must follow the eightfold path.

Confucianism is a code of ethics and emphasizes hierarchy of society, worship of ancestors, and respect for age, customs, teacher, and family. Taoism from Tao, or "The Way," originated in the sixth century B.C. and is a creative principle that governs the physical universe. When things are allowed to take their natural course, they move toward harmony and perfection. Therefore, individuals should attempt to blend into the natural world rather than try to conquer it (U.S. Department of Commerce, Bureau of the Census, The Asian Population: Census Brief, 2000).

Two minor religious sects, Cao Dai and Hoa Hao (harmony) began in Vietnam during the past century, with a present combined following of about 3 million followers. Another belief system, Animism, continues to have a strong influence among the mountain tribal groups. It includes practices to deal with demons, evil spirits, angry gods, and elements of the natural world.

The first Catholic missionary arrived in Vietnam in 1513, and Jesuits arrived in the early 1600s. The Protestants came in the early 1900s. Today Christians number over 2 million. Buddhists (along with many Vietnamese who consider themselves Buddhists because of their practices relating to their ancestors) claim approximately two thirds of the country's 79 million people. Many Vietnamese have turned to both Eastern and Western religions following the 1975 change of government.

Values

Respect and harmony are the two most important values in the Vietnamese culture and are based on the three major religious belief systems that have dominated the country. The strength of filial piety in the culture expresses the first value in many ways and throughout the life cycle.

Preserving harmony affects the lifestyle of a culture, from the highest government echelons to the most remote villages, from handling information to dealing with world conflicts. Specifically, it can affect health care decision making. Families may be less willing to share bad news with the group. Family members tend to be more likely to accept decisions made by the family, feeling the decisions were made for the overall good. Clients may be more willing to endure hardship or pain quietly to avoid causing problems or inconvenience for the family. When the belief values common to the Oriental or Eastern system found in Vietnam and those of the Occidental or Western system found in the United States are compared (Table 18-2), the nature and extent of the tasks of acculturation faced by the Vietnamese who must mesh two systems are apparent.

The API (Asian and Pacific Islanders) as a Group

Although many surveys handle the API as a single group, it is imperative to keep in mind that the 1990 U.S. census identified 30 Asian and 21 Pacific Islands groups in the API. The label includes more than 30 distinct ethnocentric entities, each with its own languages and customs. With this diversity, unless the specific ethnicity of the individual is known, generalizations must be avoided.

The "model minority" is a good example of the extreme unevenness within the API designation. According to the 1980 census, there were many API immigrants above the $50,000/year income, but even greater numbers had income at or below the poverty level. In education, the API group could boast the highest percentage of women age 23 years and older who had completed college in 1980, but 7.5% had fewer than 5 years of elementary school.

The disparity has been referred to as the "bipolar nature" of the API status, in which the successes of some API groups mask the severe problems of other API groups (Braun & Browne, 1998). For example, McPhee (2002) notes that Asian immigrants as a whole are healthier than their U.S. counterparts; however, the pattern is not uniform, and data used to estimate the whole API population are deceptive. To ensure accurate research data, it is important to ascertain the specific ethnic identity of the test group and not to mix populations (Fong & Mokuau, 1994).

Implications for Nursing Care

Because of the high priority placed on respect, harmony, filial piety, and material sharing found in most Vietnamese family systems, both immediate and extended family serve a significant role in providing emotional, physical, and economic support for the Vietnamese patient. A restriction to two visitors per patient in a hospital is incomprehensible to many Vietnamese, who may be used to large family gatherings in the home during illness. The feeling of support from the family outweighs any

---

Table 18-2 Comparison of Eastern and Western Value Systems

Eastern System	Western System
Harmony with nature	Mastery of nature (skyscraper)
Tradition	Change, innovation
Hierarchy	Mobility, upward or downward movement
Age	Youth
Extended family (few family names)	Nuclear family, small, individualistic
Convergent thinking	Divergent thinking
Cyclical concept of time	Specific point, schedules, clocks
Group orientation and reward	Self-concept and self-actualization
Rote learning	Discovery learning
Conformity	Competition

From Cao, A.Q. (1986). Linguistic and cultural issues in refugees. In The next decade: the 1986 conference on refugee health care issues and management. 1986 Refugee Health Care Conference Proceedings (pp. 70–75). Miami, Fla.: University of Miami; Nguyen, D. (1988a, September). Culture shock: a study of Vietnamese culture and the concept of health and disease. *Journal of the Association of Vietnamese Medical Professionals in Canada*, 98, 26–30.

extra burden from the presence of additional family members and friends.

The culturally competent nurse will include family members in planning care and assisting with care whenever possible. If the client cannot speak English, the family will usually be appreciative if the nurse asks someone to stay with the client to serve as translator.

In most cases, communication about plan of care, legal documents needed, or preference of treatment options should be handled with a person designated by the family. Depending on the English proficiency within the family, the person speaking with the staff may be an interpreter. When an interpreter is used, adequate time should be given for the family to clearly understand treatment options. The value of respect and harmony can cause reluctance to tell family members of the client the true diagnosis or prognosis, especially if they are elderly. For example, a family may ask that the client not be told of a terminal diagnosis.

In addition to the potential to upset harmony in the group, it is sometimes believed that the diagnosis will hasten the death and cause the patient to give up prematurely. For many Buddhists, karma determines when death comes. This orientation makes the signing of informed consent and advance directives at best puzzling and, at worst, totally irrelevant. The nurse should appreciate that an elderly patient may delay signing papers until a designated family member arrives. Understanding the values of each individual client and family is essential to providing culturally competent care.

TIME

The Vietnamese culture dates back thousands of years, and this antiquity is reflected in time orientation. Emphasis is placed on ancestors and their wishes, memories, and graves. Most Vietnamese people have been oriented to think of time in terms of cycles, events, or occurrences (Hoang & Erickson, 1982). Since many Vietnamese individuals, even those who are not Buddhist, have some belief in reincarnation, time is less of a fixed point (here and gone) and more of a recurring reality. In other words, there was yesterday, there is today, and

there will be tomorrow ... which will in fact be today, followed by tomorrow ... and so on. This belief results in a less stressful and less time-conscious pace than that commonly experienced in the West. Being late or early is not considered a problem.

As refugees, Vietnamese people practiced a present- and future-time orientation as they struggled to survive and focused on food, housing, employment, transportation, child care, and education. Today, Vietnamese Americans have goals and save for the future, and for many the motivation to live wisely may not only be to please the ancestors (past) but may also be connected with "the good life" (present) or the anticipation of heaven or reincarnation (future).

Implications for Nursing Care

The nurse should be aware that the concept of illness prevention requires both a future- and a present-time orientation. Illness prevention is a difficult concept if a person lacks a scientific understanding of disease processes. The nurse should also be aware that Vietnamese American clients may believe that luck and fate play a significant role in suffering and that illness may easily be considered a result of spiritual failure or punishment. Agreeing to vaccinations for children, having a Pap smear or a mammogram, or even just the act of seeking medical care is influenced by many factors, including time orientation.

Noncompliance with keeping appointments is often a result of factors other than time orientation. Some noncompliance can be traced to not understanding oral or appointment card communications or not being able to read the instructions. The nurse needs to review carefully the appointment card and any instructions given to be certain the client understands what is written. When a client is given a phone number to call for an appointment or for assistance, it is important to determine for sure that the client has a telephone available, knows how to use it, and has the correct clinic telephone number. Arriving at a clinic appointment on time can be a complex assignment for a Vietnamese American client, considering the usual work schedule of Vietnamese households, transportation by bus or subway, child care for those left at home, and the translation and challenges along the way.

Time orientation also contributes to the frustration of the nurse attempting to obtain a chronological sequence of the history of an illness. Especially rural Vietnamese may use life events such as births, marriages, or deaths rather than a specific date on the calendar to mark points of time. Sometimes the nurse can clarify historic events by referring to one of these events: "Did you start having these stomach pains before your husband died or since then?"

ENVIRONMENTAL CONTROL

Concepts of Illness

The medical system in Vietnam is a complex one, providing various options for health care from which the Vietnamese person may choose. Many traditional Vietnamese individuals tend to combine Chinese medicine with scientific techniques brought in from the West (Tran, 1972, 1980, 1989). For most, the choice is usually deliberate and purposeful but rarely rigid or restricted in any single direction. "The baseline is often a set of time-honored beliefs, customs, and usages that are faithfully followed by some, fiercely contested by others, but more or less consciously incorporated by the majority. . . ." (Tran, 1989).

Tran (1980, 1989) divided the explanations of cause of illness into three types: naturalistic (folk medicine), supernaturalistic (animistic beliefs), and metaphysical (the theory of hot and cold). None of these theories excludes the others, and a client may explain illness by aspects of all three. A fourth explanation of germs as a cause of illness is gaining an increased following as Vietnamese interact with persons in Western cultures.

Natural Causes. The naturalistic explanation for illness encourages a search for a natural or obvious cause of the symptoms, such as bad food or contaminated water or an obvious cause-and-effect relationship. To counteract the effects of these natural elements, an informal body of knowledge

has been collected about indigenous medicinal herbs, therapeutic diets, and simple medical and hygienic measures. The information is usually transmitted orally and often treated with secrecy, remaining inside the clan or extended family. Vietnamese folk medicine may fall into the category of either *thuốc nam* ("southern medicine") or *thuốc bắc* ("northern medicine"), which more closely resembles Chinese medicine (Box 18-3).

Supernatural Causes. The supernaturalistic explanation for disease lays the blame on supernatural powers, such as gods, demons, or spirits. The illness is considered a punishment for a fault, for a violation of religious or ethical codes, or for an act of omission causing displeasure to a deity. In the supernaturalistic theory, disease may be caused by black magic or the evil incantation of an enemy who has bought the services of a sorcerer (Westermeyer & Winthrop, 1979).

The supernatural explanation for illness is the more likely choice of the mountain tribespeople or peasants from the rural areas. The Hmong (meaning "free"), for example, believe the individual's spirit is the guardian of the person's well-being. If the spirit is happy, the person is happy and well. A severe shock or scare may cause the individual's spirit to leave, and the individual will become ill. The shaman then must come and call the spirit to return. Copper or silver bracelets, necklaces, or anklets lock the soul to oneself so that it cannot leave.

Metaphysical Causes. A metaphysical explanation for illness may be found in areas of Vietnam heavily influenced by the Chinese (Box 18-4). The metaphysical explanation is built on the theory that nature and the body operate within a delicate balance between two opposite elements: the *Am* and *Duong* (Vietnamese) or the *yin* and the *yang* (Chinese), such as female and male, dark and light, or hard and soft. In medicine the opposites are expressed as "hot" and "cold," and health is the result of a balance between hot and cold elements, which results in harmonious functioning of the viscera and harmony with the environment. An excess or shortage in either direction causes discomfort and illness.

Box 18-3

COMMON FOLK PRACTICES

---

1. *Cạo gió* ("rub-wind": skin rubbing with a coin) is a folk practice used for diseases caused by wind entering the body, such as a common cold or flu-like symptoms. A layer of balm or ointment is spread on the skin over the affected area—often the chest, upper back, or shoulders. A coin (preferably the size of a nickel or quarter) is pressed on the skin and drawn in one direction, and the coin is moved a short distance on the skin without breaking the skin. This is repeated several times, and if dark blood appears under the skin, the treatment is considered to be working. Often these ecchymotic stripes are continued in symmetrical rows down the back or chest. The purpose is to create areas where the offending wind or air may escape from the body. It is usually not a painful procedure for children or adults, and most report feeling improved by the procedure (Lan, 1988; Rosenblat & Hong, 1989).

2. *Bắtgió* ("catch-wind": skin pinching) is a folk practice used for a headache. Fingers and thumbs are pressed on both temples in an attempt to move the blood across the forehead toward a spot between the eyes. After this has been repeated several times, the area on the forehead between the eyes is pinched between the thumb and forefinger and twisted slightly. If petechiae or ecchymoses appear, the treatment is considered successful. Skin pinching is also used on the neck for sore throat.

3. *Xông* is a folk practice in which Vicks VapoRub or a similar agent or herb is stirred into scalding water. Depending on the reason for the treatment, the patient may simply inhale the vapor or may be treated under a blanket as in a steam tent.

4. Inhalation of aromatic oils or liniments, such as menthol, eucalyptus, or mint-based aromatic oils, is used as a folk practice for symptoms such as motion sickness, indigestion, or cold or wind illness. The oils and liniments may be carried in vials in a pocket or purse for ready access and may be smelled when necessary; rubbed on the temple, under the nose, or on the abdomen; or taken internally in small amounts.

5. Balm and medicated plasters are a folk practice involving direct application to the skin. Many common balms, such as Red Tiger Balm, *Cù-Là-Mác-Su*, or *Nhị Thiên Đu'ò'ng* oil, are available in Asian shops, with certain balms obtainable only from an Asian pharmacy. *Salonpas* is a Japanese preparation (Hisamitsu Pharmaceutical Co., Tosu Sagu, Japan) with widespread availability and use. Many of the ointments have a mild "deep heat" quality on application and are used for bone and muscle problems as well as a variety of other ills.

6. Herbal decoctions, soups, and condiments are used as a folk practice for a variety of symptoms and to maintain health (Spector, 2004). The more complex, involving a variety of ingredients and combinations, are prepared by a pharmacist, whereas the simpler ones are prepared at home. The recipes may be generations old and have a mystical or secret quality about them. Many medicines are prepared to be given as soups. A treatment that may have a familiar ring is the use of garlic for hypertension. There is increasing interest and experimental evaluation of Eastern herbs in Western pharmaceutical firms.

7. *Giác ho'i* ("cup-vapor": cup suction) is a folk practice in which small, heated, cuplike forms applied to the skin cause a suction on the skin as the cups cool. The suction is used to remove unwanted wind or other elements from the body and is a favorite remedy for joint and muscle pains.

8. String tying is a folk practice to control spirits. This practice is more common among the mountain people. Although the string, which stays on the arm, on the leg, or around the neck for long periods, may become dirty, it is relatively harmless and is a source of security for the wearer and significant others. Usually it can be left on without difficulty for anyone except health care workers, who may not understand the possible significance of this practice.

All illnesses, foods, medications, and herbs are classified along a continuum according to their "hot" and "cold" qualities. Hot medications and food are used to balance the need in cold diseases and vice versa. Fever, ulcers, and infections are usually hot, though some febrile illnesses are cold. Severity, cause, and duration can influence where diseases are placed. Hot usually includes strong, rough, spicy, and oily foods. Beef, eggs, cheese, and chocolates are usually hot; chicken, fish, honey, and fresh vegetables are cold. Some fruits are hot; tropical fruits are cold. The source and how food is prepared can be significant. Almost all Western medicines are considered hot and Oriental herbs, cold. Water is usually cold but is not always advised for treatment.

Different countries and locales develop their own version of the Chinese system, and there is considerable variation in application. Knowledgeable practitioners seem reluctant to construct "lists" of

---

Box 18-4

CHINESE MEDICINE

Any attempt at probing into the nature of Asian health practices must begin with a search into the age-old philosophy from which they—and indeed all Eastern concepts of health and illness, cure, and death—evolved (Branch & Paxton, 1976).

Chinese medicine is a 5000-year-old system of medicine in which an 81-volume classic on the philosophy of life became the primary medical textbook. Body, mind, and soul are integrated and never separated. Man is seen in relationship to the environment. The system encompasses all of the following (in order of their importance as preventive concepts): philosophy, meditation, nutrition, martial arts, herbology, acumassage, acupressure, moxibustion, acupuncture, and spiritual healing (Branch & Paxton, 1976; Huard & Wong, 1968).

Part of the theoretical and philosophical basis for Chinese medicine comes from the Taoist concept that nature maintains a balance in all things and that as part of the universe, man interacts with this balance. The balance is measured in terms of energy and is articulated by the principle of *yin* and *yang* (negative–positive, dark–light, cold–hot, feminine–masculine, and so on).

An important difference between Chinese and Western medicine is the emphasis on prevention rather than disease and crisis intervention. This difference can be illustrated by the Chinese story of the "old days," when people would go to their physician to have their energy balanced. The physician, knowing the client well, would prescribe the specific approach to life, type of meditation, exercise, diet, and occasional herbs to keep the client healthy. For this service the doctor would be paid regularly. If the client became ill, however, the client stopped paying, and the treatment was free of charge. This may not be as true for Chinese medicine today, but it does underline a major difference in approach from Western medicine.

Disease theory and "germs" is another area where the basic approach separates the two systems. Western medicine has spent the past 200 years identifying disease-causing organisms under the microscope and finding ways of destroying them, in many cases with dramatic success. The goal of the treatment is to destroy the microorganisms causing the illness.

In Chinese medicine, when illness results in an imbalance caused by faulty diet or strong emotional feelings, body harmony can be restored through self-restraint and the use of a corrective diet, often aided by herbs. Action is taken not to kill organisms but to restore a balanced state, countering the effects of unwise lifestyles or food. When the *yin–yang* balance is disturbed, the body is more likely to become ill. Use of massage, steam baths, and the application of Tiger Oil are methods to protect health and prevent illness (Spector, 2004).

---

hot and cold specifics, possibly because of the complexities involved in correct use. Lay people, on the other hand, often seem quite certain of what should be used and when, probably because of what their family has practiced for generations. These ideas are strongly integrated into the thought systems of many Vietnamese and can cause major stress and conflict for the client and family in the Western setting.

Germs. There is widespread understanding that disease can come from contaminants (germs) in the environment. The basic sciences were studied in the upper levels in the schools, and through decades of French occupation and more recently the American influence, even the most rural Vietnamese have become acquainted with the healing power of antibiotics in eye ointments, oral medications, and injections.

Death Beliefs and Practices

Many of the beliefs and practices about death are so woven into the fabric of Vietnamese life that it is difficult to separate them into either religious or cultural concepts (Table 18-3). An important aspect of filial piety and family loyalty is an obligation that extends beyond death; observing the anniversary day of the death, gathering at the family home and altar, and cleaning the ancestral tombs. For Buddhists, typically there are special observances, usually with elaborate rites at 100 days, and one and two years after the death.

Remembrance of deceased elders is culminated during Memory Day, a day set aside annually in homage of the person on the anniversary of the day on which the family member died. Memory Day is more important in most families in Vietnam

Table 18-3	The Meaning of Life, Illness, and Death	

Asian	American
Life	
Life = suffering	Life = happiness, health, opportunity
One's life is determined by various factors out of one's control	One has control over one's own life
Your life is not yours	Your life is your own
Death and illness	
Part of normal life cycle	Disruption of normal life cycle
Bad luck, result of former deeds, and so forth	Personal failure
Something to be accepted and dealt with calmly	Something to be beaten
Response to illness	
Ideal response: serenity, stoicism	Seeking control, fighting (beating) illness, heroic self-healing
Possible problems	
Helplessness	The burden of having to be positive
Denial	Sense of personal failure
Depression	Anger, depression, difficulty letting go
Sick role	
Permission for regression and dependency	Little permission for regression and dependency
Cooperation	Participation
Conflicts over unmet expectations and dependency needs	Conflicts over losing independence and control

From Nilchaikovit, K., Hill, J., & Holland, J. (1993). The effects of culture on illness behavior and medical care. *General Hospital Psychiatry, 15*, 41–50.

than birthdays. In the United States, a 48-year-old mother of two had a large portrait of her late father-in-law displayed in her living room. She said, "I do in Vietnam the same as I do here. Memory Day. Like my husband ... the day his father died is June 30, that day my kids, never mind about where they are, they have to come home to celebrate that day, the Memory Day for your grandfather dead. ... The only one I do the same thing in Vietnam" (Davis, 2000, p. 143). Although most of the ancestors are buried in Vietnam and the custom of gathering in the family home, around the family altar and ancestral graves, is not possible, nevertheless, for many Vietnamese in the United States, Memory Day continues to be observed.

White or black is the color of mourning, and at the time of death and for a period following, black clothing may be worn by family members (Dinh, Kemp, & Rasbridge, 2000). Traditionally in Vietnam and somewhat in the United States, for a specified period of time some family members wear a black armband or a small piece of black cloth pinned on the shirt or blouse.

Burial in Vietnam is preferred, although cremation is also practiced. Especially for older people, cremation is chosen so the ashes can be taken back to Vietnam and buried near the family, a very important promise to fulfill. For some, only through the proper observance of age-old traditions is the soul of the loved one set free, thus traditions after death are the ultimate familial duty and sign of respect.

Implications for Nursing Care

Vietnamese American clients who are oriented to Eastern beliefs and practices regarding illness may explain their illness by entities totally unfamiliar to Western practitioners. The nurse should not be surprised by complaints of being hit by the wind, bad karma problems, "the evil eye," or problems with the spirits (Box 18-5).

If the disease is understood to be a problem of hot and cold balance, the nurse should attempt to learn which the patient understands to be lacking and what corrective plan has been utilized. If fever or diarrhea, which are both "cold" diseases, is the problem, then the Eastern system of treatment would restrict fluids. On the other hand, Western-style treatment would consider fluids to be very important. A brief explanation should be given. For example, if the patient is losing fluids from the body through perspiring, through diarrhea, to restore the balance, it must be replaced. Promptly giving medication to lower the temperature and stop the diarrhea will also help. Since verbal disagreement with the caregiver would be rare, and if the situation involves an elderly person or a baby,

---

Box 18-5

COMMON MISUNDERSTANDINGS ABOUT ILLNESS AND DIAGNOSTIC OR TREATMENT PROCEDURES

1. Drawing blood for diagnostic purposes may cause a crisis for a Vietnamese American patient. The patient may complain, though often not to the health care worker, of feeling weak and tired for varying periods after the procedure. Such symptoms may last for months. A Vietnamese American client may feel that any body tissue or fluid removed cannot be replaced, and that once it is removed, the body will continue to suffer the loss, not only in this life but also in the next life.

2. Donating blood may be a major decision for Vietnamese. In one rural hospital in Vietnam, Western staff members made an effort not only to teach the Vietnamese staff the "facts" about donating blood but also to have the Vietnamese staff assist as the Western staff donated blood and, after a short recovery time, rejoined the medical team. Vietnamese staff members were invited to have their blood typed and to place their names on a possible donor list for emergency situations. Some did donate blood when the need arose (though, because Vietnamese often weigh less than 100 pounds, only one half or three fourths of a unit was drawn).

3. Donation of body parts, such as the donation of an eye after death, is an act that is often viewed with much skepticism by many Vietnamese individuals, who have been heavily influenced by Buddhist beliefs that a body part cannot be replaced once it is removed and that the body may suffer in the next life. Even those who have been Christians for several generations may be very serious about care given to the body after death and are unlikely to feel comfortable with such practices.

4. Hospitalization and surgery were often considered a last resort in Vietnam. Unless insurance considerations are important, outpatient care for the refugee is likely to cause much less anxiety and should be offered as an option when possible.

5. Clergy visitation is usually associated with "last rites" by the Vietnamese, especially those who have been influenced by the Catholic religion. A visit by the clergy may be considered an indication that the situation is grave, and the common practice of chaplains visiting clients in hospitals in the United States can be quite upsetting for Vietnamese American clients. It is important to provide the client with a careful explanation of a visit by the hospital clergy.

6. Giving flowers to the sick is a practice that may surprise and upset a Vietnamese American client who has not been given an explanation of this practice. In Vietnam, flowers are usually reserved for the rites of the dead.

7. American medicines are considered by Vietnamese to be much more concentrated than Eastern medicines. American medicine is likely to be given in tablet form, rather than in tea or soups. Also, Americans are often much larger than the average Vietnamese; therefore, medication needs to be carefully titrated so that it will not harm the Vietnamese American client. It is important for the professional to let the client know that small stature has been considered when the dosage was calculated, which can be done by either weighing the client or by orally discussing this when the prescription is written. It is not an uncommon practice for some Vietnamese American clients to take only half of their prescribed dosage.

8. The germ theory can be very confusing to some of the mountain tribes people who may have had less exposure to Western ideas. Clients with animistic beliefs have a supernatural or spirit-world disease-cause orientation. In an effort to move the client's understanding into the scientific, or natural, world, germs are presented as the cause of disease because they are a component of the real Western world. For all practical purposes, however, germs also cannot be seen and are far less real to the refugee with animistic beliefs than the spirits and demons that the client knows can cause trouble.

---

it may be wise to keep the family in the care area for a period to demonstrate and see that fluids are given. Fluids may need to be given intravenously.

Serious problems may result during longer-term illness when food is restricted to correct an imbalance. Fresh fruits and vegetables (considered cold) are often banned in the case of pregnancy. Pork or chicken, but not beef, is added to the diet slowly. Maternity clients who eat a very salty diet with almost no fruits or vegetables may acquire a nutritional deficiency. Since the theory of hot and cold has been used by many people for generations with some success, it is important to understand that these beliefs will not be discarded immediately just because Western health care providers do not approve. The nurse should try to work with the family in combining approaches to facilitate a high level of wellness.

Probably the most serious problem in the use of Eastern remedies as the first line of treatment is the delay in getting help. Fatalism, denial, acceptance of illness as part of one's destiny, or identification of the cause as non-Western may all be reasons for delay in seeking medical care. Usually Vietnamese have had no or very little preventive care experience and tend to go for help when they have symptoms. When the symptoms disappear, often medications are stopped until the next episode.

The nurse who does physical assessments of Vietnamese American patients should be aware that ecchymotic areas may be the result of "coin rubbing" on the skin to rid the body of harmful substances. After 25 years of blaming Vietnamese parents or caregivers for child abuse and the like, Western practitioners are at last being told to accept the practice as a nurturant and not a harmful folk practice (Yeatman & Dang, 1980).

The Vietnamese use of herbal medicines in soups and teas is not surprising since herbal medicine has official government sanction through the Institute of Popular and Traditional Medicine and is taught in the medical school curriculum in Vietnam. Imported medications are expensive and less familiar.

Although the benefits of folk medicine are likely to outweigh the risks, the nurse relating to Vietnamese American clients should be aware of possible risks:

1. Toxicity may result from the use of remedies containing heavy metals (lead, mercury, arsenic). On several occasions, high blood lead levels among Vietnamese and Hmong children were tentatively blamed on folk medicine; however, a well-controlled study of all under-7, newly arrived refugee children in Massachusetts in a 4-year period indicated that 27% of the Vietnamese group had elevated blood lead levels. Country of origin was the chief predictor, and the cause is not certain (Geltman, Brown, & Cochran, 2001).

2. Inadequate labeling of Chinese medicines may result in excessive use of chemicals, such as phenylbutazone or aminopyrine, neither of which is listed as an ingredient. Agranulocytosis cases are blamed on this.

3. Human error. Many herbs and plants such as mushrooms and seeds found in the United States are new to Southeast Asians. Some have been mistaken, resulting in poisonings.

As Vietnamese American clients experience success with Western medicine and develop positive relationships with health care providers and the system, and as children move through the school systems, new understandings will emerge for both the Eastern clients and the Western health care givers.

It is interesting to note that while for many Vietnamese Western medicine is foreign, the growth of the Vietnam drug market has been considered the most promising in the world. Some 400 drug companies now operate in the country. Drug advertising from manufacturers to prescribers, dispensers, and consumers is intensive and not always accurate or within ethical guidelines. David Finer, a Swedish medical reporter, has published documentaries warning both the Vietnamese and the world that lack of regulation can have critical effects. However, despite the efforts of the World Health Organization (WHO) and Sida to develop the national drug policy in 1996, the drug market in Vietnam is "effectively unregulated" (Finer, 1999, p. 21).

BIOLOGICAL VARIATIONS

Body Size and Structure

Vietnamese people generally have small frames and build, with average body weights between 80 and 130 pounds. An overweight Vietnamese person is uncommon, except among the Vietnamese-Chinese population (Williams & Westermeyer, 1986).

Blood Type

Approximately 30% of the Vietnamese have type B blood group. Type B blood group is present in only 8% of White people. Fortunately, the availability of type O (including O+) red blood cells from the "universal donor" group, and good transportation systems have helped keep the ratio (more than 30% of Vietnamese Americans) from becoming a concern in the areas of high Vietnamese concentration throughout the United States (American Red Cross, 2006).

Skin Color

The skin coloring is usually light to medium with yellow tones. Newborns are usually fair skinned.

In the United States there appears to be a higher-than-average incidence of newborn icterus among Vietnamese Americans, as compared with the rest of the general population.

Other Visible Physical Characteristics

Noses may be small and "classically Oriental" or larger with a less defined bridge. The eyelids usually have an epicanthic fold and a slight droop over the cartilage plate. Both variations are common to Asians.

Teeth are usually proportionately large, with a high incidence of mandibular torus (lump on the inner side of the mandible near the second molar). Some dentists who have treated Vietnamese clients estimate that at least 40% of Vietnamese Americans have these tori, compared with 7% of the White U.S. population (Nguyen, 1988b).

Enzymatic and Genetic Variations

Although some Vietnamese people enjoy milk, cheese, and ice cream, an unknown percentage, possibly as high as 50%, have some congenital lactase deficiency. For most Vietnamese people, the intolerance is not a total one, and many Vietnamese persons can digest some milk in small amounts without incidence. For some Vietnamese individuals, a glass of milk can simply be an inexpensive solution for constipation. Vietnamese babies show a lesser degree of the deficiency by their ability to accept the usual formula preparations without difficulty.

Alcohol is broken down in the body by two enzymes: one converts the alcohol to acetaldehyde, which the other enzyme then breaks down to acetate. Several genes code for the second enzyme, ALDH, and a variant of one of these produces an inactive enzyme, which then allows the buildup of acetaldehyde in the body. Depending on the combination of genes inherited, the accumulated acetaldehyde causes the "flushing" reaction—various amounts of facial flushing, nausea, headache, dizziness, or rapid heart beat (Makimoto, 1998).

This unpleasantness may discourage people from drinking, even casually, and was thought to possibly lower the likelihood of alcoholism among Vietnamese. However, studies over the years suggest that drinking norms and the availability of alcoholic beverages probably have at least as great an impact on alcohol consumption in Asian populations as do genetic factors (Makimoto, 1998).

Medical Problems Among Vietnamese Refugees

Twenty-five years ago Hoang and Erickson (1982) reported on a survey identifying the major medical problems of 594 Vietnamese refugees (see following list). The present health care literature indicates numbers 1, 5, 7, and 9 have all but disappeared. Numbers 2, 3, and 6 are present but not in dangerous percentages. However, numbers 4, 8, and 10 continue and are of even more concern than they were in the original survey.

1. Skin: superficial fungal infections and scabies, 10% to 15%.
2. Teeth: moderate to severe dental problems, 90%.
3. Endocrine system: thyroid diseases, especially goiters, 10% in the group of 400 and 6% in the group of 194.
4. Cardiovascular system: mitral valve prolapse, 1.7%; hypertension, 7% of adults over 30 years of age; rheumatic heart disease, 1%.
5. Renal system: microscopic hematuria may be present with no specific cause.
6. Blood: anemia, 16%.
7. Parasites: ascariasis, hookworm infestation, giardiasis, trichuriasis (most common), and amebiasis.
8. Hepatitis B surface antigen (HBsAg): 13%.
9. Malaria: 2.5% of the sample of 194 persons had a history of malaria, and 1% of this number developed an acute episode.
10. Psyche: 5% in the sample of 194 persons had "significant" psychiatric problems.

Hypertension. Hoang and Erickson (1982) found that only 7% of the Vietnamese adult immigrants over age 30 had hypertension. However, risk factors were brought from Vietnam. The universal use of fish sauce daily in food preparation and seasoning produces a built-in high-sodium diet, and smoking among the men was common, especially in the military. In Vietnam, a diet normally low in red meats and fat and higher in fruits and green leafy vegetables, as well as the physical exercise of walking, biking, and working, made obesity and hypertension uncommon problems for the average villager, except for the Chinese or Chinese-Vietnamese.

However, newly arrived refugees faced stressors with communication and language problems; a diet high in red meats and fats and lower in fish, fruits, and vegetables; and, often, work that requires less physical exercise. In a classic and culturally sensitive work, Duong, Bohannon and Ross (2001) interacted with 201 Vietnamese in two Gulf Coast communities. For this study, one of the meeting places was the only Vietnamese market in a 50-mile radius on a weekend shopping day. Findings from this study suggested that 88 (43%) had a blood pressure over 139 mm Hg systolic, over 89 mm Hg diastolic, or both. Of the 88 participants, 24 of them had blood pressures in excess of 179/100, and 13 were referred for a blood pressure of 180/110 or higher. One was sent for immediate attention for a blood pressure over 210/120. More than 75% of the sample had never been hospitalized or had surgery, 52% paid for their own medical care, and 59% did not see a medical provider regularly. About half were middle-aged, and 47% worked full-time. Risk factors identified include a "profound" need for health education related to cardiovascular disease, smoking, and alcohol use, as well as increased understanding of the need and ways to control diet, weight gain, and stress in their new setting and way of life. The research team begins the final discussion of the report by stating "hypertension is likely to be a significant health risk in Vietnamese people and screening should be a part of all interaction between Vietnamese-Americans and care providers" (Duong, Bohannon, & Ross, 2001, p.10).

Hepatitis B. Hepatitis B is the leading cause of liver cancer worldwide. Each year in the United States, 5000 people die of cirrhosis of the liver that is related to hepatitis B, and another 1500 succumb because of hepatitis B itself, and another 1500 die of hepatitis B–related cancer of the liver (Wiecha, 1999). Hepatitis B virus (HBV) is endemic in South Asian populations, including the Vietnamese. Studies of Vietnamese adults in the U.S. verify rates from 7% to 14% (McPhee et al., 2003; Hoang & Erickson, 1982). The high rate of chronic infection is almost certainly linked with the high rates of liver and intrahepatic bile duct cancers among Vietnamese American males (41.8 per 100,000 compared with 3 per 100,000 for U.S. White males). About two thirds of these cancers are hepatocellular carcinomas associated with hepatitis B and C virus infection (McPhee, 2002).

Hepatitis B can be transmitted horizontally through contact with blood products, through sexual contact, and through casual contact in the household. It can also be transmitted vertically in the newborn child. A neonatal infection often persists in a carrier state with significant risk of cirrhosis and hepatocellular carcinoma in early childhood. It is estimated that 25% of those chronically infected as infants or young children and 5% of adolescents and adults who become chronically infected die prematurely from chronic liver disease (McPhee et al., 2003). Infection during adolescence or adulthood presents a lower risk to the individual, but can become a serious public health problem.

In the United States, HBV is already a national public health priority. A study near Boston assessed knowledge of the definition and risk factors of hepatitis B among 2816 middle- and high-school students in five ethnic groups, including 226 Vietnamese adolescents. The Vietnamese students (who had been tested for hepatitis B at three times the percentages in other groups) responded with the most correct definition (35.3% versus 22.6%). However, sexual contact with an infected person was correctly identified as a risk for infection by 880 (31.3%) of all the respondents, compared with 13.7% of the Vietnamese, the group with the highest seroprevalence of hepatitis B (Wiecha, 1999).

In transcultural studies, when there are unusual correlations, it is imperative to check for contributing factors. For example, when a disease is sexually transmitted and the traditional culture does not discuss sex openly or value sexual permissiveness, Vietnamese sons and daughters would be expected to simply avoid the subject—and the problem, taking their cues from their family, at lease for the present. The result is that surveys report seemingly low concern and low-risk behaviors, despite incidence statistics relative to the cultural group.

To respond to the needs of this high-risk population, it is imperative that the facts of the disease be known and that cultural constraints alone not be counted on to provide the critical protection needed in the future. Noninfected persons can be protected against HBV and the sequelae by having three doses of HepV vaccine. The Centers for Disease Control and Prevention (CDC) recommends universal vaccination of all children ages 0 to 18 years. As of 2003, 42 states require protection to enter middle school (McPhee et al., 2003). Progress is being made, and data from the 1996 National Immunization Survey report that 88% of Asian/Pacific Islander (not specifically Vietnamese, but including Vietnamese) children age 19 to 35 months had received three doses of the HepB vaccine (McPhee et al., 2003). But beyond these covered groups are many unknowing and unprotected persons.

Dr. Stephen McPhee and his group, working with Suc Khoe La Vang (Health Is Gold), the Vietnamese Community Health Promotion Project of the University of California, San Francisco, Department of Medicine designed and led a 3-year experiment on several ways to change this. The goal was to improve Vietnamese American parents' awareness and knowledge about HBV, and the need for their children to get the available free vaccinations. They also organized a media education campaign in the large Houston, Texas, community (over 58,000) and a community mobilization strategy in Dallas (41,000), with 38,000 from the Washington, D.C., area serving as a control group. Success was measured by the proportion of parents responding correctly to various knowledge questions, and the vaccinations recommended. In Houston, a 2-year blitz involved print and electronic media, billboards, calendars, and a 26-page, 4-color booklet completed entirely in the Vietnamese language to showcase a campaign titled "Immunize Against Hepatitis B to Protect Future

Generations," and more. For Dallas, a local Vietnamese American community-based group contracted to plan and execute the Community Mobilization Strategy. The 19-member coalition consisted of medical, public health, and education professionals; business leaders; editors; seniors; and homemakers, who worked together over a 3-year period to get the word out and the vaccinations "caught up." The pre- and post-campaign contacts with the parents in both locations were encouraging and confirmed the good potential of these culturally appropriate efforts. According to McPhee et al. (2003), "In every community where Vietnamese Americans have settled in large numbers, they have established vibrant Vietnamese-language print, radio and television media. These media have flourished because [they] ... are avid consumers of news, community information and advertising."

Economic considerations are also important for public policy and an economic analysis of the preceding study by a group working with the CDC demonstrates in detail the advantages of hepatitis B prevention (Zhou et al., 2000). Longitudinal studies are needed to tell the story about how preventive medicine can affect the Vietnamese.

Tuberculosis Risk. Although the bacille Calmette-Guérin (BCG) vaccine was widely used in Vietnam during the 1960s and was given to babies shortly after birth in hospitals across the country, the living conditions and general upheaval during the next 25 years affected the long-term effectiveness of any preventive effort. Between 1968 and 1974, the movement of people from the less secure countryside to the cities, with the accompanying overcrowding and poor nutritional status, simply exacerbated an already precarious situation.

BCG vaccination often produces a positive skin test, and there is no reliable way to distinguish a skin test reaction to BCG from that caused by tuberculosis (TB). Furthermore, people with latent infection have no symptoms of the illness and cannot spread TB to others. In their work with refugees from Vietnam, Hoang and Erickson (1982) recommended the use of isoniazid prophylactically for 1 year for all refugees under 35 years of age with positive skin tests, and that children with negative skin readings on arrival in the United States be checked in 3 to 6 months to single out false-negative readings. This practice continues in various forms in much of the country today.

According to a CDC report in 1994, there were more than 24,000 cases of active tuberculosis in the United States. Of that number, approximately one third of the cases were in foreign-born persons; of these more than 7000 cases, 869 or 11.4% were from Vietnamese (CDC, 1995). The 1994 tuberculosis incidence in Vietnam was approximately 150 cases per 100,000 as compared with 9.4 cases in the United States (Carey, Oxtoby, Nguyen, et al, 1997; Mac, Doordan, & Carr, 1999). According to a CDC report in 2005, there were 14,093 cases of active tuberculosis in the United States, and of these, 7656 (54.3%) were foreign born, with Vietnam as the third highest contributor with 576 of these cases (CDC, 2005).

Effective medications are available, but improper and sporadic use of the medicines often contributes to the emergence of multidrug-resistant (MDR) strains, an increasing problem worldwide (Lindsay, Narayan, & Rea, 1998). In the United States there was an MDR increase to 128 cases for 2004, 10 of them from Vietnam (CDC, 2005). For the first time in 50 years, six new TB drugs will soon be tested by humans. The hope is that the new medications will reduce the length of therapy time by 30% to 70%, making completion of the treatment more likely and, if effective, give more options in the treatment of persons with MDR bacilli.

Directly observed therapy (DOT) is a plan in which health care workers observe or assist tuberculosis patients as they take their medications. The plan can be clinic or field-based in the home, school, workplace, park, or any other convenient location. The average cost of a 6-month tuberculosis DOT program is approximately $1000 more than a non-DOT program, which compares favorably with the cost of treating multidrug-resistant tuberculosis, with an average cost of over $200,000 (Mac, Doordan, & Carr, 1999).

During the early 1990s, the number of tuberculosis cases steadily rose in Santa Clara County, California, to 18.2 cases per 100,000 population in 1996. The county health department made the DOT plan an option for the Vietnamese and did a study among 30 of the patients (5 in the DOT program and 25 on the usual regimens) to check effectiveness. Results of the comparisons between the two groups showed that among the DOT group, all completed therapy, there were no relapses, and the sputum conversion rate was 2 to 7 weeks. On the other hand, among the non-DOT group, only 21 patients completed the course, 2 patients relapsed, and sputum conversion rates ranged from 4 to 16 weeks. These data suggest that DOT programs can effectively control tuberculosis (Mac, Doordan, & Carr, 1999).

Cancer. Records from the Cancer Hospital in Ho Chi Minh City (Saigon) from 1976 to 1981 showed that cervical cancer accounted for 53.3% of all cancers diagnosed among their female patients (Phipps, Cohen, Sorn, & Braitman, 1999). During the years following that finding in Saigon, thousands of women left Vietnam and settled in the United States, surrounded by people speaking a different language, in a culture very different in many ways, with differing ways of accessing a strange medical system and help. These factors, coupled with the stresses of resettlement, would surely affect the cancer statistics that accompanied them to their new home.

As compared with breast cancer, cervical cancer is a disease of the "developing world," with 80% of over 470,000 cases worldwide as reported by the WHO. Until the 1970s, 75% to 80% of cervical cancer in the United States was in the invasive stage at the time of diagnosis. Today with Pap smears and vaginal exams, 78% of cervical cancers are instead diagnosed in the *in situ* stage, reducing the mortality of cervical cancer by approximately 40% (Phipps, Cohen, Sorn, & Braitman, 1999). Stage of disease at time of diagnosis appears to be a major predictor of survival. Present mortality rates in Vietnam are twice those in the U.S., and it is hoped that recent Vietnamese arrivals will have chances of lowering the risks the longer they are in the United States (Ho et al., 2005).

In the 1980s, breast cancer was reported as the leading cancer among Vietnamese females in the United States. But by 1996, the National Cancer Institute released its findings on cancer incidence and mortality in 11 U.S. racial and ethnic groups, and cervical cancer (43 per 100,000) was the most commonly diagnosed cancer among Vietnamese women, even though breast cancer was the most common for the other 10 groups. The rate was more than 2.5 times the rate for any of the other groups and nearly 5 times higher than that of American White women (Schulmeister & Lifsey, 1999).

Because of the urgency of early diagnosis of cervical cancer, there is frequent documentation of efforts (Ho et al., 2005) to "get the word out" to Vietnamese communities regarding the importance of screening programs. This is also true in other countries, such as Canada and Australia (Taylor et al., 2003), where screening use is also 10% to 12% lower than use by the local non-Vietnamese populations, but survey results present similar findings. As was true of White women in the U.S. 30 years ago, high percentages of Vietnamese females over 65 have never had a Pap test or a vaginal exam as a preventive measure. This was true for 10 of the 11 eldest women in one study of 96 women (Schulmeister & Lifsey, 1999), and may explain why this age group contained 25% of the patients with cervical cancer but 40% of the deaths—too many with advanced invasive cancer at diagnosis. Some common reasons given by women for not having the tests were feeling their risk was low because of no family history of cancer (29%) and not being sick (24%). Other common barriers were having no female doctor, the cost (lack of insurance), fear of the embarrassing procedures, and time.

Knowledge, attitudes, and beliefs about cancer are important in determining behavior, but as is also true for the dominant culture population, these do not explain all behavior. The natural reticence of Vietnamese to openly discuss sexual problems, disease, or activity, especially with a new doctor and in a different language, makes a Pap smear, vaginal examination, or a mammogram a troubling request indeed. To complicate the request, the patient is expected to do this when feeling healthy.

Worldwide cervical cancer is second only to breast cancer as the most common female malignancy, in both incidence and mortality. Breast cancer claims over one million cases a year worldwide. In fact, 55% of these cases occur in "more developed" countries. It is interesting to note that the age-adjusted mortality rate for cervical cancer is much the same throughout the world (Ho et al., 2005). The incidence of breast cancer in Vietnam as reported is 3% lower than that in the U.S., with a mortality rate of 6% (Ho et al., 2005; http://www.cdc.gov). These findings may suggest that Vietnamese women are at a lower risk of both developing and dying of breast cancer (in Vietnam) than are women in the U.S.

In a survey study done to determine predictors in a breast and cervical screening program in a large Vietnamese community near Houston, Texas, one surprise result was that the Vietnamese women were far more worried about breast cancer (52%) than they were about cervical cancer (2%). Though unexplainable, the information was helpful in planning approaches to breast self-examination (BSE) and medical self-examination (MSE) and mammography screening. Further findings from this study assisted in the creation of lists of beliefs about the barriers and benefits as reported by the 209 participants in the study. The findings indicate the most significant predictors of the use of the Pap test, BSE, MSE, and mammography were being married, high education level, lack of barriers, a family history of cancer, older age, and increased concern about cancer (Ho et al., 2005). In "Differences in Breast Cancer, Stage, Treatment, and Survival by Race and Ethnicity," the authors observed that across races and ethnicities, the differences in the treatment received are likely to be "solely the result of socioeconomic and cultural factors." For health care providers this means that targeting women with low socioeconomic status, and improving their treatment programs may be the means not only toward early detection, but also improved survival rates in these populations (Li, Malone, & Daling, 2003).

It is imperative for the nurse to be understanding of the cultural beliefs that Vietnamese women face in order to decrease their risk for cervical cancer during the period of resettlement (Labun, 2000, 2001). By building positive relationships with clients and appreciating a common humanity, health teaching can be effective. Behaviors that can address this high risk include the following:

- Determine the adequacy of the patient's understanding of cancer, risk factors, and hope of treatment. Use translation if at all needed and possible; brochures may be available (McPhee, 2002).
- Encourage and prepare the Vietnamese client by explaining the procedures, draping well, granting that there may be some discomfort, practicing relaxation breathing, and always staying with the client throughout the procedure. Assist after the procedure as needed.
- Give an estimate about how soon and in what way the client will be told of the results.
- Discuss strategies for reminders of upcoming routine exams in the future.
- Keep alert for opportunities to share the information with all Vietnamese females as situations arise, remembering that older Vietnamese (who do not speak English) are at especially high risk for having advanced cervical cancer at the time of diagnosis.

Perhaps the most significant information about lung cancer and the Vietnamese is the findings from one study done in 1995. The study was conducted with face-to-face interviews with men and women 18 years of age and older in Hanoi and a rural community in North Vietnam and in Ho Chi Minh City and a rural community in South Vietnam. Approximately 500 interviews were done at each site for a total of 2001 participants. Findings from this study suggested that smoking prevalence was 72.8% among the men and 4.3% among the women. Males had smoked a mean of 15 years beginning at a median age of 19. Vietnam had the highest reported male smoking prevalence in the world (Jenkins et al., 1997). For the men, smoking seemed an integral part of the serious business, social, and cultural landscape, from top government negotiations on down to family functions. In fact, the offering of cigarettes was found to be a common courtesy. Foreign cigarettes especially were often given as gifts to one's boss, or those in high places. Smoking rates for the younger women are among the lowest in the world because smoking is considered unfeminine and unattractive socially and culturally and thus is a taboo, especially for older women.

Smoking is a habit among the Vietnamese, and as such is not easily given up because it also serves social or cultural purpose (hospitality, maleness). Jochelson reports from Australia that the Vietnamese and Lebanese immigrant communities have the highest and next-to-highest smoking prevalences in Australia, respectively (Jochelson, Hua, & Rissel, 2003). The level of knowledge and type of attitudes and behaviors of the Vietnamese and Arabic communities were very similar to the research previously done in the English-speaking community. The major difference was the fact that the English-speaking group did not associate the problem of environmental tobacco smoke with the problem of sociability and hospitality and asked, "How can we ask our friends not to smoke in our homes?" (Jochelson, Hua, & Rissel, 2003).

In "Cancer Risk Factors of Vietnamese Americans in Rural South Alabama," Xu et al. (2005) surveyed 284 Vietnamese, most of whom lived in a semi-isolated fishing village, had spent most of their lives in Vietnam, and had had fewer education and acculturation experiences in the U.S. than Vietnamese Americans who participated in urban health surveys. A total of 73.8% of the current smokers began smoking in their teens, and 41.5% of the sample currently live with a family member who smokes. The statement was made that a "culture of smoking" is believed to be the primary culprit for the high smoking rate. For many of the men smoking was a way of life to "initiate rapport, strengthen bonding, and maintain relationships" (Xu et al., 2005, p. 237).

It is an understatement to suggest that the challenge to reduce smoking calls for the best efforts of health care providers. All the multidisciplinary team members must collaborate to bring changes in social, political, and economic arenas to discourage smoking (such as banning smoking in public places, cigarette taxes, restraining the tobacco industry's aggressive foreign marketing). Nurses know that smoking is the single most preventable cause of premature death, increasing the risk of lung cancer, emphysema, heart disease, stroke, and other diseases. Nurses also understand the powerful cultural components that help determine habits. The implications for nursing care are to use health status promoters to discourage "the culture of smoking," and help patients—and friends—to find more healthful ways to take care of themselves (Levy et al., 2006; Morrow and Barraclough, 2003, p. 376).

HIV/AIDS. A study used a random sample of 319 students attending four community colleges in Orange County, California, to determine HIV/AIDS knowledge and past and present sexual behavior. The Vietnamese appeared to have low knowledge of the disease, little concern about AIDS, reluctance to be tested, and the lowest incidence of high-risk behavior. Most of the survey sample had been born in Vietnam, had lived in the United States for 5 to 10 years, and probably were still taking cues from family rather than from non-Vietnamese peers. The main concern of the research team was what will happen if and when that allegiance changes and they join the dominant culture in their sexual practices (Shapiro, Radecki, Charchian, & Josephson, 1999).

Nutritional Preferences

The common food staple in Vietnam is rice, eaten from a large bowl with chopsticks two or three times a day. One way a client may describe a medical problem to the doctor is to hold a hand up in the form of a bowl and say, "Now I eat only one bowl of rice instead of three the way I used to do." During the French occupation, bread was introduced and widely consumed in the form of small tasty French rolls, available fresh daily on the street corners everywhere. Today many Vietnamese in the United States replace some of their rice with fresh white bread.

In Vietnam, brown unpolished grains were considered the food of the mountain people and

were almost never eaten by the more sophisticated lowlanders. In the United States, except for those Vietnamese Americans who take nutrition facts seriously, polished rice and white bread continue to be favorites among the Vietnamese people.

Rice and many other cooked dishes are seasoned with the unique condiment *nuoc mam*, a "fish sauce" made by marinating small fish in salt in kegs for a month or more. Depending on use, some sugar, fresh lime juice, garlic, chili peppers, and water are added. Fish sauce is a serious, continuing, major source of salt in the Vietnamese diet.

Fish is usually readily available, and meats served are cut into bite-size pieces and served with rice and vegetables. Chicken and duck eggs are often available. Tofu is served in many vegetable dishes, but dry bean dishes are uncommon.

In Vietnam, green leafy vines or plants are gathered from gardens or the countryside and brought to the local markets in truckloads each morning. Although they are not served in large quantities, the regular presence of these greens, raw or lightly stir-fried and served with rice, contributes to a diet unusually high in vegetable nutrients.

In 1988 the U.S. Department of Agriculture described the traditional Vietnamese diet as "low in fat and sugar, high in complex carbohydrates and moderate in fiber," comparing very favorably with the best U.S. dietary guidelines (Burtis, Davis, & Martin, 1988). About 59% of the more than a million Southeast Asians who had immigrated to the United States since 1975 were Vietnamese, and 25% of those were children. What effect has acculturation had on this diet, which, except for the present emphasis on calcium consumption, was flawed only by its lack of dairy products?

In 2001 a survey team used a simple questionnaire ("How many servings of fruits, vegetables, and dairy foods do you eat each day?") for 2618 adolescents in two middle schools and two high schools near Boston. Vietnamese, White, African-American, and Hispanic students were involved. There were 226 Vietnamese, 64 of whom had either been born in the United States or had lived here more than 10 years, and 162 had been here 10 years or less.

Compared with the Whites, the Vietnamese were much more likely to eat five servings of fruits and vegetables (35.5% and 15.3%, respectively), but more than 44% less likely to take in three or more dairy servings. Younger Vietnamese students were more likely to eat the five servings of fruits and vegetables than the older students (Wiecha, Fink, Wiecha, & Herbert, 2001).

When other aspects of the diet such as fat and sugar intake are considered, indications are that Southeast Asians tend to adopt a less healthy diet in the United States. This study indicates that at least preference for fruits and vegetables seems to persist during the acculturation period. This practice is quite protective against disease and should definitely be encouraged.

Milk and dairy foods have not traditionally been staples of Vietnamese rural or urban diets. Some canned evaporated milk may be used in cooking, or sweetened condensed milk used to prepare *sinto* ("vitamin"), a delicious drink made by blending a small amount of the milk with ice and fresh chopped fruit, sold along the sidewalks in towns and cities. Too often the sweetened milk was placed in a baby bottle and warm water added to make formula, especially during travel. But milk and ice cream were not common or valued tastes or consistencies to the Vietnamese palates.

While a low calcium intake has always been a feature of traditional Asian diets, the effects of it may have been offset by an active lifestyle. Osteoporosis, apparently associated with low calcium intake, is a major public health concern in the United States at present, with the highest risk group being Asian women—and Vietnamese women presenting as the fastest-growing group numerically.

In Louisiana, five focus group discussions were held with 34 Vietnamese mothers, ages 25 to 47, with incomes up to $30,000 a year, to learn what they knew about calcium intake and what barriers there may be to increasing it (Reed, Meeks, Nguyen, Cross, & Garrison, 1998). For these study participants, a perceived negative taste of dairy products was the most common problem with including these foods in the regular diet. Only two mothers stated that milk was a desirable dietary component,

and only one felt that drinking milk would improve her diet. Unfamiliarity with milk foods, cost, time, and, to a lesser degree, problems with lactose intolerance were also given as reasons.

The study participants were not aware of how serious the lack of calcium could be for their future and were open to trying high-calcium recipes using both American and Vietnamese foods, adding milk to Vietnamese pancakes, and using milk in drinks and puddings (Reed, Meeks, Nguyen, Cross, & Garrison, 1998). Their children with school cafeteria experience may find these tastes familiar.

Thirty years into their "new life in a new country," many Vietnamese are joining their American friends struggling to control weight gain as they watch their blood pressure, and/or glucose or cholesterol readings rise to dangerously high levels. Understandably those without insurance (often 50% or more) do not see a doctor regularly and one study identified as a risk factor a profound need for increased understanding of the need and ways to control diet and weight gain in their new setting and way of life (Duong, Bohannon, & Ross, 2001). Among those Vietnamese Americans with average adult weights of 80 to 130 pounds, it is suggested that they are more oriented to attaining or maintaining weight, rather than concern with grams of fat. Their children, however, are having many opportunities to become sensitized to the problems of weight as their peers are targeted in schools and community preventive programs today.

Dioxin

More than 40 years ago in Operation Ranch Hand (1962–1971) during the Vietnam conflict, some 19 million gallons of Agent Orange were sprayed as a defoliant over selected areas of Vietnam and Laos to remove cover on Viet Cong supply routes and troop movements from the north. The herbicide, named from the color-coded drums it was shipped in, contained minute amounts (3 parts per million, but 1000 times more powerful than domestic weed killers) of TCDD or dioxin, a persistent organic pollutant with a half-life of 8.7 years. In the time since, dioxin has become linked to health problems such as immune system suppression, birth defects, and soft tissue sarcomas (Satchell, 1999).

The Air Force Health Study (Pavuk et al., 2005) is a 20-year longitudinal study (1982–2003) detailing the health, mortality, and reproductive outcomes in the U.S. Air Force veterans of Operation Ranch Hand, the unit responsible for 85% of all Agent Orange sprayed in Vietnam. Included in the study was a comparison Air Force group of veterans matched for age, race, and military occupation who flew or serviced aircraft in Southeast Asia (SEA), but did not handle or spray the herbicides as did the Ranch Hand Veterans. Previous studies after 5 and 15 years showed no increases in Ranch Hand morbidity or mortality. But more recent comparisons with the U.S. general White male population to December 1999 showed increases in prostrate cancer and melanoma in Ranch Hand veterans. However, the comparison Air Force veterans also reported an increase in prostrate cancer. The final results reported in a 2005 article were that "TCDD and years of SEA service interacted with all sites cancer, but the risk was greatest in those with the highest TCDD levels and the longest time served in Southeast Asia" (Pavuk et al., 2005).

Dioxin enters the body primarily through food, possibly animal fat. The U.S. miliary base at Bien Hoa, about 20 miles north of Saigon, was the location of the Ranch Hand Spraying operations, the Agent Orange storage facility, and in 1971, a substantial leak of more than 5000 gallons of Agent Orange (Dalton, 2001). In the early 1970s, some dioxin levels of human breast milk in areas of the spraying were recorded at over 300 times the usual accepted range of 5 ppt, which correlated with the extremely high levels found in certain local fish, a main source of food for the mothers.

Now more than 30 years later, in 5 years of following the dioxin content in blood samples of 43 Vietnamese residents of Bien Hoa, approximately 95% proved to be above the 5 ppt level (Schecter et al., 2003, August). This study was done to determine if food is the current route of intake in the dioxin "hot spots" in Vietnam today. The highest levels were in free-ranging duck fat (over 20 ppt)

and certain fish. Researchers caution that significant studies of Agent Orange alone do not explain all the dioxin-like toxicity measured in the Vietnamese people or their food (Schecter et al., 2002).

In January 2001 the National Toxicology Program added TCDD to the Report on Carcinogens as a known human carcinogen (Booker, 2001). All 2.6 million U.S. military personnel who served in Vietnam are eligible to apply for benefits for themselves and their children if either suffer from any of 10 proven or suspected dioxin-related conditions (Satchell, 1999).

Epidemiologists, toxicologists, and environmental scientists gathered for four days of meetings in Hanoi in March 2001, after which Vietnam and the United States formally established a joint research program. Although the passing of time has been helpful, the several significant handicaps inherent in the situation predict it will take wisdom and commitment to follow through on the plans: for the U.S, concern about exposing the damage, and for the Vietnamese, protecting their fishing and food export industries (Cyranoski, 2002).

It is hoped that the results of these efforts will not only add to the worldwide state of the science regarding the health effects of dioxin, but also be helpful for the Vietnamese in Vietnam. Although the long-term picture is not yet clear, it is important that the nurse understand the dioxin event and its possible significance in the "history of the present illness" of Vietnamese clients currently and for some years to come.

Psychological Characteristics

Mental Health. Vietnamese believe the nervous system to be the source of all mental and physical activities. Therefore, when there is a disturbance in mental or physical activity, the nervous system is considered central to the malfunction. Neuroses are called "weakness of the nerves," a term used to describe many kinds of anxiety, depression, weariness, mental deterioration, or retardation. Psychoses are known as "turmoil of the nerves," more accurately reflecting the client's behavior or feelings (Tran, 1989). The two possible sources of mental disease are the organic model, which considers damaged nerves or brain, and the inorganic model, which may attribute bizarre behavior to various causes, such as disobedience, sin, or demons (more common in tribal groups).

The term *psychiatrist* or *mental doctor* has no direct Vietnamese translation. *Nerve doctor* is slightly better, but the best comprehension comes with an explanation of "a specialist who treats crazy people" (Tran, 1989). The following are some Vietnamese words that may be helpful to health care givers to identify what could be causing symptoms:

- *Lu lan:* confusion related to retardation
- *Lang tri* and *dang tri:* slipping away of memory, loss of memory caused by the absence of the mind
- *mat tri nho:* the mind is already lost
- *lmat tri giac:* if the mind is lost quickly (as in multiinfarct dementia)
- *binh tam than:* indicates mental illness or high anxiety
- *dien:* usual lay term for "crazy" (Braun & Browne, 1998, p. 268)

In Vietnam, often there was some optimism regarding most illness affecting the nerves, with the possibility of using folk remedies, a nerve tonic to restore strength to weak nerves, or a calming medicine to quiet inner turmoil. In the United States, some feel medication is the logical answer, although there is some concern over oversedation or dependency.

Probably the most important single factor in accessing mental health care for Vietnamese Americans is the cultural pattern of keeping family psychiatric problems within the family and solving them there if at all possible. The value of "face saving" in the tradition continues, and discussing or expressing emotions, especially with a stranger, is avoided unless absolutely necessary. Working with traditional doctors and healers when possible can be an effective treatment plan when this kind of cooperation is available and the illness is not of a psychotic nature (Bernier, 1999). Otherwise, persons with mental health problems may not enter the health care system until their problems have become critical. Evaluation of severity and decisions on treatment of refugee psychiatric problems by Western professionals are extremely difficult.

Emotional and Behavioral Manifestations of Distress in Refugees. The Vietnamese are used to dealing with the problems of life, within the family as a unit. However, in the refugee/immigrant situation, the family is often incomplete, with few or no elderly to give balance and stability because many of the ancestors are far away in a very different setting. On the one hand is the anticipated freedom for the middle-aged and younger in the group to make independent decisions, but on the other hand is the unexpected uncertainty and loneliness of that independence. Anxiety and depression are not uncommon in Vietnamese immigrant communities, sometimes handicapping their best efforts to embrace their new home.

It is easy to assume acculturation challenges lessen as time in the new setting passes. And with concentrated effort, this is usually true for the language. Bernier (1999) observed that among the Vietnamese Americans with repeated failures and frustrations over time, the psychological stresses of change may accumulate. Families go through acculturation together but each member reacts individually. With the growing family with children in school, learning the language in "fast forward," and interacting daily with new ideas is a challenge. In addition, for some Vietnamese American families, children moving into the teenage years rarely decrease the stress in American families as the teens "acculturate" into the current peer culture. This is especially true for the "strong" Vietnamese family with "two-culture" children. Among the understandably concerned elder members in the home, the value conflicts can become even more focused as the children grow older and move toward the values of the host culture. With much change, and without help, the family ties can deteriorate and the family conflicts unfortunately may lead to disruptive family crises (Nguyen, 1988b).

By the early 2000s, longitudinal studies were attempting to examine the complex phenomenon of depression in Vietnamese communities. Especially for the middle-aged and elders, the societal cornerstone values of self-control, harmony, and respect continued largely intact (if not more appreciated and cherished) against the 30-year backdrop of war, boats, refugee camps, and settling into a very different culture, all with a relatively small family or community support group.

Earlier research has shown mixed results for the role of social support in psychological distress. As expected, persons with a strong support network do better in a crisis than those with a weak support system. However, the immigration experience, by definition, involves disruption of the immigrant's social support systems, and successful acculturation is accomplished when new reference points and networks are integrated into or alongside the old. This may explain why other studies find that immigrants with strong ties only to their ethnic group tend to have more psychological distress than those with additional nonethnic social supports. Strong and meaningful emotional commitments to personal relationships and networks provide good mental health, but that does not mean that change will be easy or painless, especially if it involves major life adjustments.

In 2003, Gellis reported a study on the relationship of social support and depression and the effect of "kin" and "nonkin" support groups, as experienced by a sample of 79 Vietnamese immigrant men and women receiving mental health services in a psychiatric hospital. These study participants had immigrated between the ages of 26 and 35 and had lived in the U.S. an average of 14 years. Most were diagnosed with major depressive disorder and had an average hospital stay of almost 2 months. Their kin group averaged five people to whom they could turn for advice and discussion of personal problems, and with whom they had disagreements. The nonkin group averaged four people who were friends, coworkers, or mental health service providers.

A common problem during the acculturation years for families is the different rates and patterns of change, which easily become sources of conflict causing strained relation within the entire family. The strong Vietnamese family will likely continue to try to support its own, sometimes increasing the psychological stress for everyone. Depending on the severity of the problems and the management options, medical services may be required.

With this history and a diagnosis of major depressive disorder, the client may be unable to translate the efforts of a family support group (kin) into evidence of their efforts to help in recovery. In this event, perhaps the nonkin support team can be perceived to be more helpful. Gellis (2003) calls for caregivers who can assess therapeutic support networks, social workers who understand cultural family dynamics, and appropriate follow-up services.

General Patterns of Coping and Adaptation. A general pattern of coping and adaptation is experienced by many persons in their cultural adjustment to immigration (Cook & Timberlake, 1984).

Stage I. For the first few months, there is a positive attitude with high expectations; energy is focused toward language, employment, and meeting basic needs. The excitement of a new physical environment and "things" helps suppress the pain of the multiple losses.

Stage II. The period of "psychological arrival" occurs 6 to 18 months after immigration, when the person becomes more aware of losses and "the past" becomes idealized. This agrees with Hoang and Erickson (1982), who noted that psychiatric problems may become more obvious 6 to 12 months after immigration. Survivor's guilt (Why did I survive and my child did not?) must be faced. Posttraumatic stress disorder (PTSD) is common, and the normal tensions of close family life are magnified. Interpersonal conflict is common. Other symptoms may be feelings of hopelessness, acute distress and grief, fatigue, and mood instability. The period may be transitory or long-lasting, mild or severe, and it seems to occur regardless of how much help or support has been given. It is usually a very frustrating time for sponsors and "helping persons," who feel inadequate to help. During this period somatization is common. Somatization is not new among Southeast Asian refugees. In a culture where overt expression of anxiety, disappointment, or anger is considered failure, a high value is placed on suppressing negative feelings; then, expressing mental distress through various physical ailments is a preferred and acceptable option. It is less worrisome to see a physician for a physical problem (Eyton & Neuwirth, 1984).

Stage III. After roughly 18 to 24 months, the person is able to reformulate the grief and get involved with the tasks at hand. There is less idealizing of the past, and helping those left behind becomes important. Adaptation moves ahead at a more rapid rate as former ways of coping are given up for more effective ones. A new self-identity emerges.

A Vietnamese nurse on a Canadian university nursing faculty, Tan Truong Donnelly (2002), examined the Western approach to coping with stress as a personality style or trait, especially as it informs health care professionals in their understanding and counseling of clients. She makes the case that "coping theories should emphasize the contextual nature of stress and that coping should be viewed as a dynamic process that varies under different social, cultural, political, economic, and historical conditions." The author refers specifically to the needs of the recent Vietnamese immigrants entering Canada. Using the dominant view of coping as a personality trait leads to unfairly categorizing and understanding these clients whose culture, perception of power structures, history, ethnicity, and personal place in their group influences their response to "stress." Traditional Vietnamese women are taught and expected to be the caretakers of their children, spouses, and elderly members of their extended family. They accept these responsibilities and hardships as a part of life, to be handled in the best way possible. These methods of coping are supported by their community and the high regard given to "good mothers" and "good daughters." This "passive coping" is considered successful in the context of the collectivist society. But it becomes an important source of stress when judged by an individualistic western society, which applauds self-assertiveness and grieves the "unsuccessful coping" they observe. Coping happens contextually, and how the challenge is met depends on many factors in the situation. The factors vary at any given time and influence the "coping response."

Cook and Timberlake (1984) list denial as the defense mechanism most often used by Vietnamese refugees. The authors believe that denial is congruent with the values of the culture: submission to the common good (and to fate), harmony, and self-sacrifice. Denial is needed to lessen the profound effect of losses and to allow the refugees to go on with the task of survival. When denial fails, facing the hard realities without the needed support systems may encourage withdrawal or the turn to alcohol, drugs, or medication abuse (Cook & Timberlake, 1984).

Alcohol and Drug Abuse. Few well-controlled longitudinal studies are available on substance abuse among the Vietnamese. But evidence suggests that pockets of trouble are beginning to emerge in the communities, and these appear to be directly related to a host of psychosocial stressors (O'Hare & Tran, 1998). Some of the Vietnamese have come to the United States following a refugee and immigration experience that was among the more traumatic in recent memory (see discussion of PTSD), resulting in significant stress in many areas. This may well place them and their children at increased risk for alcohol and substance abuse (Makimoto, 1998).

Depression seriously slows the ability of the sufferer to successfully meet the daily challenges without being overwhelmed and discouraged. One Vietnamese immigrant study reported that 14% of the study group had trouble with other drugs "some of the time," a much higher percentage (40%) reported using alcohol as a means of "coping with sorrow," and almost 12% reported using drugs for the same purpose (O'Hare & Tran, 1998).

Women rarely drank in Vietnam, and the effect of men drinking a bottle of "33" (*Ba Muoi Ba*) beer at the village café with friends in the evening seems to have little in common with "drinking" in the United States. Here, wine and liquor are readily available, and drinking is more acceptable in the dominant culture. Drinks were served at weddings in Vietnam, but guests rarely became drunk, a not uncommon occurrence at Vietnamese weddings in the United States at the present time. The effects of the increased drinking on the persons, their families, and community can be expected to become more apparent in the coming years as acculturation continues.

In working with Vietnamese clients in abuse problems, it is wise to remember the cultural importance of "face saving" and of not openly disagreeing or confronting another. Also helpful will be sensitivity to the guilt and shame to the family, especially for the older Vietnamese clients.

Insight-oriented therapies or pressuring clients to admit "alcoholism" or "addiction," for example, may seem so rude and unprofessional, especially to older clients, and be such a foreign approach to handling a problem that it may only call into question the competence of the caregiver. Cognitive-behavioral therapies (CBT) appear to have more promise for effective intervention (O'Hare & Tran, 1998).

CBT for persons with addiction problems typically include some combination of the following: (1) self-monitoring thoughts, feelings, and events likely to "trigger" the impulse to abuse; (2) teaching more effective social skills to deal with situations in which the client is pressured to use drugs; and (3) teaching stress management skills to lower anxiety and deal with somatic complaints (O'Hare & Tran, 1998). These skills can also be helpful with depression and anxiety, which often co-occur with substance abuse.

Cognitive-behavioral therapies may feel more comfortable to Vietnamese clients because they are easily adapted to family- and community-based approaches. They feel less personally intrusive, often complement Asian values, and use stress management techniques that clients may find familiar. More work is being done using CBT, which may provide insight into other helpful approaches. For valid statistics on drug abuse in Vietnamese, more studies using Vietnamese are needed, rather than Southeast Asian, Asian-American, or API.

Posttraumatic Stress Disorder (PTSD). The exact relationship between premigration and postmigration experiences and adaptation challenges continues to be debated. Nicholson (1997) noted that current stressors best predicted mental health outcomes. However, experienced events better predicted posttraumatic stress disorder than did either anxiety or depression.

The exact causes of the increased number of mental health disorders in the Vietnamese resettlement communities are often evasive and are difficult to isolate, identify, or even test; possibilities include language, the high value of communicating only positive feelings, the somatization option, or the cultural practice of handling psychiatric problems within the family if at all possible.

The stresses of immigration have been found to be particularly difficult for women. Fox, Cowell, and Johnson (1995) identified the chief role of the Southeast Asian women as meeting the needs of husband, children, and extended family. They had the responsibility of home and children while husbands were in the army for years and then in re-education camps. They were with their children; were abused as "boat people"; and lost family members through sickness, exposure, drowning, and killing. Men were also traumatized for years, and it is not clear how much these premigration experiences have continued to produce great emotional stress and handicap years into the resettlement period (Fox, Cowell, & Johnson, 1995).

Although first described in war veterans, PTSD is now being recognized by health professionals in other settings, and the definition is broadening to include more than "exposure to actual or threatened death or injury." Not only did Vietnamese immigrants have war and violence in their history, they also had the added difficulty of upheaval inherent in the refugee immigration experience, which affected every area of life for the individual, family, and "village." In "Contextual Analysis of Coping: Implications for Immigrants' Mental Health Care," a Vietnamese nurse named Tan Truong Donnelly uses Vietnamese immigrant experiences to make the case that "coping theories should emphasize the contextual nature of stress and coping, and that coping should be viewed as a dynamic process that varies under different social, cultural, political, economic, and historical conditions."

One way of categorizing symptoms of PTSD can be to consider three groupings: intrusion—nightmares, flashbacks, memories with intense emotional and physical distress; avoidance—avoiding people, activities, thoughts connected with the trauma, becoming numb to all emotions, positive or negative; and arousal—being constantly on guard, resulting in problems concentrating, insomnia, emotional outbursts, and instability (Harvard Women's Health Watch, 2005).

Many of these symptoms are normal experiences after trauma, but if after a month the symptoms are getting worse or interfering with ability to function, the diagnosis may be an acute stress disorder. After three months, chronic PTSD can be considered and sometimes requires treatment over an extended period of time. As of 1990, 15 years after the Vietnam Conflict ended, over 9% of Vietnam veterans still suffered from PTSD, and 15 years beyond that, in 2005, many continued to be compensated for PTSD-like symptoms (McNally, 2006). PTSD can occur with other stressors, such as an unexpected death or mental illness, making diagnosis and recovery more difficult. Also, treatment for substance abuse will likely be unsuccessful in the presence of underlying PTSD (Harvard Women's Health Watch, 2005).

Exposure therapy, a cognitive behavioral therapy approach, is a type of psychotherapy that is a good fit culturally for Vietnamese adults and elders. Often, anti-anxiety and anti-depressant medications are part of the regimen. The selective serotonin reuptake inhibitors Paxil and Zoloft have been approved by the Food and Drug Administration for the treatment of PTSD.

The Indochinese Psychiatry Clinic near Boston served many Vietnamese who came as refugees under the 1989 Released Reeducation Center Detainees Resettlement Program. These refugees were former South Vietnamese political prisoners who had worked for the United States and came with their spouses and unmarried children. All of them had experienced suffering. Men averaged 7 to 8 years of brainwashing and hard labor in the camps, while the women and children were at home, were unable to get jobs or buy food, and were ostracized in their villages in many areas. Both men and women were diagnosed with PTSD, and half also experienced a major depressive disorder (Allden, 1998).

Although the Boston setting is not a typical Vietnamese resettlement community, most Vietnamese communities have some common history with this group in their premigration experiences. PTSD and the accompanying or resulting anxiety and depression are becoming more recognized in the communities, and efforts are being made to work with those who are suffering. Without help, adjustment and adaptation to a new culture are slow and extremely taxing, learning a new language is very difficult, and people understandably become emotionally and physically isolated and increasingly discouraged.

Drug Interactions and Metabolism

Caffeine, a component of many drugs as well as coffee, tea, and colas, appears to be metabolized and excreted faster by Whites than by Asians (Grant, 1983). Alcohol is also metabolized differently (see discussion of enzymatic and genetic variations).

Many Chinese herbs and medicines are given as soups or teas. Most Vietnamese believe that Western medicines in tablets, capsules, or injections are "too strong" or "hot" and upset their internal balance, and unfortunately there is poor understanding of the possible serious effects of underdosage, sudden withdrawal, or, for antibiotics, short-term usage. Immediate results are anticipated, and often the medication is discontinued when the patient feels better or there is no improvement, behavior similar to that in many of their American counterparts.

Many Vietnamese believe that they have a different physical constitution from Americans so that Western drug dosages may not be appropriate for them. It is true that many Vietnamese weigh less than Americans, and, especially in the case of sedative or psychiatric medications, many of their experiences have been very troubling and encouraged the practice of "halving the dosage" (experience of the author). Current research into ethnopharmacology indicates that, indeed, Vietnamese do have a pharmacodynamic difference in therapeutic response to psychotropics. In one study the Asian clients' mean required dose for haloperidol was significantly lower than the average for optimal therapeutic response, and extrapyramidal symptoms emerged (Lin, Poland, Nuccio, et al., 1989). This study and others suggest that Asian clients also generally respond to substantially lower doses of neuroleptics (Murphy, 1969; Rosenblat, & Tang, 1987). It is a wise and kind practitioner who makes an obvious effort to take these factors (weight, ethnicity, increased sensitivity) into account when prescribing medication for Vietnamese clients by checking the weight and asking about previous experience with medications. Vietnamese want to please those trying to help them—and also want to be healthy.

Implications for Nursing Care

The small body size of many Vietnamese American clients has an important implication in terms of nursing treatment. Some nurses have delayed giving pain medication to a Vietnamese American client in pain "since the client is so tiny" (Tien-Hyatt, 1989). Because Vietnamese American clients may be stoic, it is important for the nurse to evaluate carefully the need for pain medication and to provide sufficient medication without delay (Lin & Finder, 1983; Tien, 1984; Tien-Hyatt, 1989). Offering medication for pain rather than asking if it's needed may result in a more accurate response.

Smither and Rodríguez-Giegling (1979) have noted that within the first 5 years after leaving Vietnam, personality and coping are the more important determinants of which acculturation patterns develop. Other significant factors are level of income and social class (Smither & Rodríguez-Giegling, 1979). Allden (1998), however, in her work with persons who had undergone very traumatic premigration experiences in Vietnam and Cambodia, has been treating a number of clients with PTSD diagnoses and sees these premigration stresses as continuing to slow down adaptation for years into the resettlement period. It will take time and more studies to resolve the differences in these and other similar findings.

In the difficult everyday situations that require translations in psychiatric evaluation and counseling, the use of bilingual paraprofessionals is gaining increasing attention (Leung, 1988). Professionals and clients readily recognize that the person communicating between them is indeed a key person in determining the outcome of this effort. When the inherent potential of the "translator" is recognized, persons should be selected and trained in techniques of information gathering, importance of not screening the reporting, confidentiality, and so on (McPhee, 2002). When this interpreter is welcomed as a colleague on the team, the client also comes to see this person not only as a member of "my" team, the only possibility of communicating the problem, but also as a respected member of "their" team who is trying to help. Trained or untrained, the paraprofessional often becomes the first source of help Vietnamese American clients turn to because they are hesitant to contact the professional with personal or family matters.

The nurse should also recognize that for many Vietnamese American clients, food is medicine. Many Vietnamese Americans are able to practice their food beliefs without difficulty. However, if a client develops a health problem and encounters Western medical practitioners, the need to adopt Western food practices may be considered necessary for survival, such as the need for fluids, the restriction of salt, the need for specific medications (such as cardiac medications), and the need for specific nutrients in the diet. Helping the client to understand why dietary restrictions have been recommended is essential. A client may be willing to limit the amount of *nuoc mam* in the diet when health care professionals carefully explain the reason for this request. For many Vietnamese Americans, eating habits are changing. Children are learning to eat hamburgers, french fries, pizza, spaghetti, and tacos in school lunch programs. Vietnamese Americans are pragmatists, and teaching about dietary practices in relation to Western medicine can result in changed behavior (Reed, Meeks, Nguyen, Cross, & Garrison, 1998).

Another important health care issue for the nurse who provides care for Vietnamese American clients is utilization of health care resources. Tran (1980) suggested that utilization of health care services is related to the identification of a problem and the availability of an appropriate service. A study by Strand and Jones (1983) found that health services utilization is not directly correlated with education and English-language skills but is related to a variety of factors. For example, working two jobs makes it difficult to make time for a clinic appointment. The person who speaks English best and those persons who should accompany the client to the health facility are usually at work or at school. A car or a babysitter may be unavailable. Choosing health care may be difficult. The options for health care are fewer than they were in Vietnam, and even wealthy Vietnamese persons may have problems finding health care providers who understand the Vietnamese language. Phan (1996) reports how taking the clinic to the community and working with individual families in their own environment helped eliminate many of the utilization problems.

The importance of the nurse in teaching, modeling, and encouraging health promotion and illness prevention practices among the children cannot be overemphasized. As Nguyen (1988b) observes, "Children can learn to make positive health behaviors an integral part of their lives." Understandably for parents, ideas of illness and treatment are deeply ingrained. Vietnamese American children are immersed in new ideas and change, understand the new language, and will make important health decisions that will influence their lives, the lives of their children, and the lives of their parents.

The majority of health care problems do not occur or at least are not reported by Vietnamese refugees during the initial settlement period. This may result from the fact that immediately before or after arrival the refugees are routinely screened and treated for existing problems. After the excitement of arriving and getting settled, however, previously untreated health problems often become evident, and eventually the patient finds the way into the health system.

Another deterrent for a few Vietnamese Americans in the utilization of health services is integration into ethnic subcommunities. For a small group of persons, especially the elderly, who have found learning English and the process of adaptation too difficult, surrounding themselves with familiar lifestyles, language, friends, and family has made loneliness less of a problem. In these subcommunities, traditional beliefs and superstitions survive more comfortably than in the "outside world." Health care givers should keep in mind that these sometimes are the persons being admitted to the hospital for emergency care by a very concerned family. It is crucial and helpful that the nurse has some cultural awareness and sensitivity.

SUMMARY

The initial arrival of large groups of Vietnamese to the United States began 30 years ago. It is important for the nurse to recognize that the present Vietnamese American clients are a diverse group, moving through differing stages of acculturation to life in a new setting and a different health care system. The Vietnamese are survivors, and how rapidly this is happening depends on many factors in their past as well as many experiences in their day-to-day life here: length of time, group support, language proficiency, place in the family and community, economic stability, general mental health, and the quality of the contacts with the host culture. Encouraging the children toward healthy lifestyles and illness prevention is a key to the future.

The customs, values, health beliefs, and practices the Vietnamese American clients have brought with them are an important consideration for the Western health care provider. The nurse who develops an appreciation of these will promote more effective health care delivery, and will encourage use of, and comfort in the new health care system.

Age, sex, and individual idiosyncrasies also contribute to variations in response to the American health care system. The customs, values, and health beliefs and practices of Vietnamese American clients are an important consideration for the Western health care professional (Tripp-Reimer & Thieman, 1981). Most adult Vietnamese Americans have retained some folk medicine beliefs that affect not only explanations for causes of symptoms but also the type of treatment that will be selected. The nurse who develops a knowledge and understanding of these beliefs will promote more effective health care delivery and will ease the adjustment and comfort in the new health care system.

Case Study

Mr. Yen Van Nguyen is a 26-year-old man who has recently arrived in the United States from Vietnam with his wife and 2-year-old son, Tran. Yen arrives at a local emergency room one evening carrying his son, Tran, and gesturing that his son needs medical attention because he has been running a low-grade fever, sneezing, and coughing for the past 2 days. Yen speaks very poor English and appears to be somewhat excited.

The emergency room nurse takes Tran back to an examination room, where she can get him undressed and into a gown for examination by the physician. While undressing Tran, the nurse notices bruising over the sternum and along the spine and immediately summons the physician. On examination, the physician notices that the bruised areas do not appear tender but nevertheless suspects child abuse. The child's father, Yen, is escorted back to the child's room by a hospital security officer, where he is questioned by the physician. Yen speaks very poor English, and communication is difficult. The harder the physician tries to communicate with Yen, the more frustrated both the physician and Yen become.

A young Vietnamese woman who works in housekeeping is requested to report to the emergency department to help with the communication problem between the emergency room staff and Yen. After a short discussion with Yen, the young Vietnamese woman explains the custom of *cạo gió* ("rub-wind"), or "coin rubbing," to the emergency room staff. On further examination, the physician can find no other evidence of child abuse. The emergency staff realize that the bruising is from the coin rubbing and not from child abuse, as initially suspected. The child is given an injection of an antibiotic and discharged.

CARE PLAN

✳ *Nursing Diagnosis: Communication, impaired verbal, related to foreign-language barrier*

Client Outcome

1. Parent will be able to communicate more effectively about customs and beliefs used in treating illnesses, and nurse will better understand these customs.

Nursing Interventions

1. Determine parent's understanding and ability to communicate in English.
2. Talk slowly, enunciating words.
3. Face parent and speak in a slow, clear voice.
4. Use gestures to convey meanings, but do not use excessive "touching."
5. Attempt to locate a translator for assistance.
6. Provide parent adequate space to communicate without "crowding."
7. Keep language simple.

✳ *Nursing Diagnosis: Fear related to Americans' misunderstanding of Vietnamese culture with a potential for prosecution for child abuse*

Client Outcome

1. Parent will experience reduced fear with awareness of nurse's understanding of Vietnamese cultural folk medicine.

Nursing Interventions

1. Allow parent to explain Vietnamese traditional folk medicine.
2. Provide parent with a quiet area to help reduce fears.
3. Attempt to communicate in a nonthreatening manner.
4. Recruit others familiar with Vietnamese culture to help parent explain.
5. Remove persons perceived as threatening to parent.

(Continued)

✳ *Nursing Diagnosis: Knowledge deficit related to modern medical practices secondary to cultural differences*

Client Outcome

1. Parent will demonstrate an understanding of the importance of modern medical treatment in conjunction with traditional folk medicine.

Nursing Interventions

1. Explain to parent the importance of modern medical care in conjunction with cultural folk medicine.
2. Determine parent's perception of medical model of treatment.
3. Keep language simple; avoid long medical terms.
4. Explain importance of compliance with medical treatment ordered.
5. Keep instructions simple and brief.
6. Arrange for an interpreter to help explain importance of seeking medical attention for illness or injury.

✳ *Nursing Diagnosis: Parental role conflict related to child's present illness and need to seek "foreign" medical attention*

Client Outcome

1. Parent will demonstrate an understanding of the importance of seeking qualified medical attention for the betterment of the child's well-being.

Nursing Interventions

1. Educate parent on importance of seeking medical attention to treat illnesses.
2. Provide parent the opportunity to describe how similar situations were handled.
3. Assess past medical practices and folklore that the parent normally uses in similar situations.
4. Allow parent time to ask questions related to child's health care.
5. Provide information in a clear, concise, easy-to-understand manner.

✳ *Nursing Diagnosis: Noncompliance (risk for) related to misunderstanding of the prescribed treatment secondary to the belief that medications in the Western world are much stronger than those found in the Far East*

Client Outcome

1. Parent will demonstrate an understanding of prescribed treatment and importance of following prescribed medical regimen.

Nursing Interventions

1. Assess parent's fear of prescribed treatment.
2. Promote health teaching to educate parent on the effects, desired outcome, and side effects of prescribed medicine.
3. Warn parent that some medications may make the client sleepy and that this is an expected occurrence.
4. Teach parent about importance of adhering to prescribed medical treatment.
5. Reassure parent that prescribed medication is appropriate and safe for client.
6. Review medication, dosage, and proper administration technique to help parent feel more comfortable with the treatment.

✳ *Nursing Diagnosis: Coping, ineffective family: compromised, related to illness of a family member and the necessity to seek culturally unfamiliar medical treatment*

Client Outcome

1. Family members will be better able to cope with illness-related problems after obtaining information on prescribed medical treatment.

Nursing Interventions

1. Reassure parent of appropriateness of prescribed medical treatment.
2. Provide parent the opportunity to express fears and concerns.
3. Encourage parent to verbalize familiar treatments that family sought in Vietnam, including customs and folk medicine.

4. Direct parent to areas of potential help (such as churches, Vietnamese communities, social workers).
5. Instruct parent how to perform prescribed treatment to increase feelings of being needed.

✳ *Nursing Diagnosis: Role performance, altered (risk for), related to undue stress of an ill family member in an unfamiliar culture*

Client Outcome

1. Parent will discuss feelings of altered role performance and identify areas of undue stress.

Nursing Interventions

1. Encourage parent to talk openly about actual or potential areas of stress.
2. Provide quiet area for parent to gather thoughts.
3. Help parent to understand what resources are available in the community (such as self-help groups).
4. Reassure client.
5. Avoid negative criticism.
6. Encourage parent to openly discuss concerns about the health of child and about the care that child will receive.

✳ STUDY QUESTIONS

1. List several ways that the nurse and the emergency room staff might better communicate with the Vietnamese American client.
2. Should the client be told that his folk medicine treatment is foolish and that he should abandon it? Why or why not?
3. How could the nurse effectively teach the client about the benefits of seeking conventional medical treatment in the United States?
4. When asked questions, Yen answers, "Yes." Does this always indicate that he necessarily means "yes"?

5. List some strategies and techniques to help the nurse communicate more effectively with the Vietnamese American family.
6. Describe the misconceptions that Vietnamese Americans have concerning Western medical practices and medications.
7. In American society, hospitalization and visitation by clergy is a common, almost expected, act by some. How do the Vietnamese view hospitalization and clergy visitation?
8. Describe the importance of folk medicine and folk healers to Vietnamese Americans.

NCLEX-RN REVIEW QUESTIONS

1. A nurse in a doctor's office explains to a Vietnamese female client the medication regimen for the prescription the client has been given. The client nods her head and smiles as the explanation is given. However, in 2 weeks she returns. Her condition has deteriorated, and the nurse discovers that she has not taken any medication. Initially, the nurse should:
   A. Find out if she understood the instructions as they were provided in English.
   B. Firmly explain that she needs this medication to improve.
   C. Call in the client's husband and explain the schedule again.

   D. Provide her with printed directions in Vietnamese on how to take the medication.

2. Mrs. Nguyen, a Vietnamese client, is to undergo cancer surgery. She seemed frightened. The best way for the nurse to initiate a therapeutic relationship is to:
   A. Give Mrs. Nguyen a hug and pray with her.
   B. Ask Mrs. Nguyen how she is feeling.
   C. Tell Mrs. Nguyen that the outcome of the surgery should be favorable.
   D. Tell Mrs. Nguyen the nurse will call the hospital chaplain.

3. A Vietnamese resident in a nursing home does not want to follow the nursing care plan regarding diet. The best course of action for the nursing staff would be to:
   A. Insist the resident accept the diet as ordered.
   B. Document the stubbornness of this resident.
   C. Avoid making an issue of his noncompliance.
   D. Consider the possibility of cultural differences.

References

Allden, K. (1998, April). The Indochinese Psychiatry Clinic: trauma and refugee mental health treatment in the 1990s. *Journal of Ambulatory Care Management*, 21(2), 30–38.

Balfour, F. (1993). Return of the boat people. *World Press Review*, 40(7), 10–12.

Bernier, D. (1999). The Indochinese refugees: a perspective from various stress theories. *Journal of Multicultural Social Work*, 2(1), 15–30.

Bonder, B., Martin, L., & Miracle, A. (2002). *Culture in clinical care*. Thorofare, N.J.: Slack.

Booker, S. (2001, March). Dioxin in Vietnam: fighting a legacy of war. *Environmental Health Perspectives*, 109(3), A116, 2P, IBW.

Braun, K., & Browne, C. (1998). Perceptions of dementia, caregiving, and help seeking among Asians and Pacific Islander Americans. *National Association of Social Workers*, 23(4), 262–274.

Burtis, G., Davis, J., & Martin, S. (1988). *Applied nutrition and diet therapy*. Philadelphia: W.B. Saunders.

Cao, A. Q. (1986). Linguistic and cultural issues in refugees. In the next decade: the 1986 conference on refugee health care issues and management. *1986 Refugee Health Care Conference Proceedings* (pp. 70–75). Miami, Fla.: University of Miami.

Carey, J., Oxtoby, M., & Nguyen, L., et al, (1997, January). Tuberculosis beliefs among recent Vietnamese refugees in New York state. *Public Health Reports*, 112(1), 66–72.

Centers for Disease Control and Prevention, Division of Tuberculosis Elimination. (1995). *Reported tuberculosis in the United States, 1994*. Atlanta: Centers for Disease Control and Prevention.

Centers for Disease Control and Prevention, *Trends in Tuberculosis—United States*. (2005), Atlanta: Centers for Disease Control and Prevention.

Central Intelligence Agency. *The World Factbook* (2007). Vietnam. Retrieved from https://www.cia.gov/cia/publications/factbook/geos/vm.html. Date retrieved: October 7, 2006.

Chao, R (1994). Beyond parental control and authoritarian parenting style: understanding Chinese parenting through the cultural notion of training. *Child Development*, 65, 1111–1119.

Coelho, G., & Stein, J. (1980). Change, vulnerability, and coping: stresses of uprooting and overcrowding. In Coelho, G., & Ahmed, P. (Eds.), *Uprooting and development*. New York: Plenum Press.

Cook, K., & Timberlake, E. (1984). Working with Vietnamese refugees. *Social Work*, 29(2), 108–113.

Cyranoski, D. (2002, March). U.S. and Vietnam join forces to count cost of Agent Orange. *Nature*, 416(21), 252.

Dalton, R. (2001, October). Bilateral Vietnam study plans to assess war fallout of dioxin. *Nature*, 413 (6855), 442.

Davis, R. (2000, May). The convergence of health and family in the Vietnamese culture. *Journal of Family Nursing*, 6(2), 136–156.

Dinh, A., Kemp, C., & Rasbridge, L. (2000, July). Culture and the end of life: Vietnamese health beliefs and practices related to the end of life. *Journal of Hospice and Palliative Nursing*, 2(3), 111–117.

Donnelly, T. (2002). Contextual analysis of coping: implication for immigrants' mental health care. *Issues in Mental Health Nursing*, 23, 715–732.

Duong, D., Bohannon, A., & Ross, M. (2001, Spring). A descriptive study of hypertension in Vietnamese Americans. *Journal of Community Health Nursing*, 18(1), 1–11.

Eyton, J., & Neuwirth, G. (1984). Cross-cultural validity: ethnocentrism in health studies with special reference to the Vietnamese. *Social Science and Medicine*, 18 (5), 447–453.

Finer, D. (1999). Pressing priorities. *Consumer drug information in the Vietnamese marketplace* Stockholm: IHCAR, Karolinska Institute.

Fong, R., & Mokuau, N. (1994, May). Not simply "Asian Americans": periodical literature review on Asians and Pacific Islanders. *Social Work*, 39(3), 298–305.

Fox, P. G., Cowell, J. M., & Johnson, M. M. (1995). Effects of family disruption on Southeast Asian refugee women. *International Nursing Review*, 42(1), 27–30.

Gellis, Z. (2003, April). Kin and nonkin social supports in a community sample of Vietnamese immigrants. *Social Work*, 48(2), 248–258.

Geltman, P., Brown, M., & Cochran, J. (2001, July). Lead poisoning among refugee children resettled in Massachusetts, 1995–1999. *Pediatrics*, 108(1), 158–162.

Grant, D. M. (1983). Variability in caffeine metabolism. *Clinical Pharmacology Therapy*, 33, 591–602.

Hiebert, M. (1993). Miles to go. *Far Eastern Economic Review*, 156(30), 24–26.

Ho, V., Amal, J., Atkinson, E., Bassen-Enquist, K., Tortolero-Luna, G., & Follen, M. (2005). *Predictors of breast and cervical screening in Vietnamese women in Harris County*. Houston, Texas.

Hoang, G., & Erickson, R. (1982). Guidelines for providing medical care for Southeast Asian refugees. *Journal of the American Medical Association*, 248(6), 710–714.

Huynh, T. D. (1987). *Introduction to Vietnamese culture*. San Diego, Calif: Multifunctional Resource Center, San Diego State University.

Infoplease.com. Retrieved December 11, 2006, from www.infoplease.com.

Jenkins, C., Pham, D., Do, N., Hoang, K., Truong, H., Bales, S., Stewart, S., & McPhee, S. J. (1997, June). Tobacco use in Vietnam prevalence, predictors, and the role of transnational tobacco companies. *Journal of the American Medical Association*, 277(21), 1726–1731.

Jochelson, T., Hua, M., & Rissel, C. (2003). Knowledge, attitudes and behaviors of caregivers regarding children's exposure to environmental tobacco smoke among Arabic and Vietnamese-speaking communities in Sydney, Australia. *Ethnicity and Health*, 8(4), 339–351.

Labun, E. (2000, Summer). Discovering our common humanity: developing partnerships in a Vietnamese community. *Journal of Christian Nursing*, 17(3), 8–11, 39.

Labun, E. (2001, September). Cultural discovery in nursing practice with Vietnamese clients. *Journal of Advanced Nursing*, 35(6), 874–881.

Lan, L. V. (1988, September). Folk medicine among the Southeast Asian refugees in the U.S.A.: risks, benefits, and uncertainties. *Journal of the Association of Vietnamese Medical Professionals in Canada*, 98, 31–36.

Leung, L. (1988). Training bilingual paraprofessionals for counseling services. *Hawaii Journal of Counseling and Development*, 4(1), 16–22.

Levy, D. T., Bales, S., Lan, N. T., & Nikolayex, L. (2006). The role of public policies in reducing smoking and deaths caused by smoking in Vietnam: results from the Vietnam tobacco policy simulation model. *Social Science and Medicine*, 62, 1819–1830.

Li, C., Malone, K., & Daling, J. (2003, January). Differences in breast cancer stage, treatment, and survival by race and ethnicity. *Archives of Internal Medicine*, 163, 49–56.

Lin, K. M., & Finder, E. (1983). Neuroleptic dosage for Asians. *American Journal of Psychiatry*, 140, 490–491.

Lin, K. M., Poland, R., & Nuccio, I., et al, (1989). Longitudinal assessment of haloperidol doses and serous concentrations in Asian and Caucasian schizophrenic patients. *American Journal of Psychiatry*, 146(10), 1307–1311.

Lindsay, J., Narayan, M., & Rea, K. (1998, October). Nursing across cultures: the Vietnamese client. *Home Healthcare Nurse*, 16(10), 693–700.

Mac, J., Doordan, A., & Carr, C. (1999, December). Evaluation of the effectiveness of a directly observed therapy program with Vietnamese tuberculosis patients. *Public Health Nursing*, 16(6), 426–431.

Maiter, S., & George, U. (2003, Winter). Understanding context and culture in the parenting approaches of immigrant South Asian mothers, *Affilia*, 18(4), 411–428.

Makimoto, K. (1998). Spotlight on special populations. Drinking patterns and drinking problems among Asian-Americans and Pacific Islanders. *Alcohol Health and Research World*, 22(4), 270–275.

McLaughlin, L., & Braun, K. (1998, May). Asian and Pacific Islander cultural values: considerations for health care decision making. *Health and Social Work*, 24(2), 116–126.

McNally, R. J. (2006, March). Psychiatric casualties of war. *Science*, 313, 923–924.

McPhee, S. (2002, January). Caring for a 70-year-old Vietnamese woman. *Journal of the American Medical Association*, 287(4), 495–505.

McPhee, S. J., Nguyen, T., Euler, G., Mock, J., Wong, C., Tram, L., Nguyen, W., Nguyen, S., Ha, M., Do, S., & Buu, C. (2003, June). Successful promotion of hepatitis B vaccinations among Vietnamese-American children ages 3–18: results of a controlled trial. *Pediatrics*, 111(6), 1278–1288.

Morrow, M., & Barraclough, S. (2003). Tobacco control and gender in South-East Asia. Part II: Singapore and Vietnam. *Health Promotion International*, 18(4), 373–380.

Murphy, H. B. (1969). Ethnic variations in drug responses. *Transcultural Psychiatric Research Review*, 6, 6–23.

Nguyen, D. (1988a, September). Culture shock: a study of Vietnamese culture and the concept of health and disease. *Journal of the Association of Vietnamese Medical Professionals in Canada*, 98, 26–30.

Nguyen, D. (1988b). Personal communication.

Nicholson, B. (1997). The influence of pre-emigration and postemigration stressors on mental health: a study of SEA refugees. *Social Work Research*, 21(1), 12–15.

Nilchaikovit, K., Hill, J., & Holland, J. (1993). The effects of culture on illness behavior and medical care. *General Hospital Psychiatry*, 15, 41–50.

Not getting over it: post-traumatic stress disorder. *Harvard Women's Health Watch*, March 2005, pp. 4–6.

O'Hare, T., & Tran, T. (1998). Substance abuse among Southeast Asians in the U.S.: implications for practice and research. *Social Work in Health*, 26(3), 69–80.

Pavuk, M., Michalak, J., Schecter, A., Ketchum, N., Akhtar, F., & Fox, K. (2005, April). Did TCDD exposure or service in Southeast Asia increase the risk of cancer in Air Force Vietnam Veterans who did not spray Agent Orange? *Journal of Occupational Environmental Medicine*, 47(4), 335–342.

Phan, T. (1996). Ethnic and cultural specificities of domestic violence: a research and clinical discourse with references to the Vietnamese emigrant community. *International Journal of Psychiatric Nursing Research*, 2(2), 187–197.

Phipps, E., Cohen, M., Sorn, S., & Braitman, L. (1999, March–April). A pilot study of cancer knowledge and screening behaviors of Vietnamese and Cambodian women. *Health Care for Women International*, 20(2), 195–207.

Rairdan, B., & Higgs, Z. R. (1992). When your patient is a Hmong refugee. *American Journal of Nursing*, 92(3), 52–55.

Reed, D. B., Meeks, P. M., Nguyen, L., Cross, E.W, & Garrison, M. E. (1998, May–June). Assessment of nutrition education needs related to increasing dietary calcium intake in low-income Vietnamese mothers using focus group discussions. *Journal of Nutrition Education*, 30(3), 155–163.

Rosenblat, H., & Hong, P. (1989). Coin rubbing misdiagnosed as child abuse. *Canadian Medical Association Journal*, 140(4), 417.

Rosenblat, H., & Tang, S. W. (1987). Do Asian patients receive different dosages of psychotropic medication when compared to Occidentals? *Canadian Journal of Psychiatry*, 32, 270–274.

Rudy, D., & Grusec, J. (2001, March). Correlates of authoritarian parenting in individualist and collectivist cultures and implications for understanding the transmission of values. *Journal of Cross-Cultural Psychology*, 32(2), 202–212.

Satchell, M. (1999, April 26). Questions in a village: did Agent Orange cause Vietnamese birth defects? *U.S. News and World Report*, 126(16), 62.

Schecter, A., Hoang, Q., Pavuk, M, Papke, O., Malish, R., & Constable, J. (2003, August). Food as a source of dioxin exposure in the residents of Bien Hoa City, Vietnam. *Journal of Environmental Medicine*, 45(8), 781–788.

Schecter, A., Pavuk, M., Constable, J. D., Le, C. D., & Papke, O. (2002, March). A follow-up: high level of dioxin contamination in Vietnamese from Agent Orange, three decades after the end of spraying [letter]. *Journal of Occupational and Environmental Medicine*, 44(3), 218–220.

Schulmeister, L., & Lifsey, D. S. (1999, June). Cervical cancer screening knowledge, behaviors, and beliefs of Vietnamese women. *Oncology Nursing Forum*, 26(5), 879–887.

Shapiro, J., Radecki, S., Charchian, A., & Josephson, V. (1999, February). Sexual behavior and AIDS-related knowledge among community college students in Orange County, California. *Journal of Community Health*, 24(1), 29–43.

Sideleau, B. (1992). Space and time. In Haber, J., Leach McMahon, A., Price-Hoskins, P., & Sidleau, B. (Eds.), *Comprehensive psychiatric nursing* (ed. 4) (pp. 193–209). St. Louis: Mosby.

Smither, R., & Rodríguez-Giegling, R. (1979, December). Marginality, modernity, and anxiety in Indochinese refugees. *Journal of Cross-Cultural Psychiatry*, 10, 469–478.

Spector, R. (2004). *Cultural diversity in health and illness* (ed. 6). Upper Saddle River, N.J.: Pearson Prentice Hall.

Strand, P., & Jones, W. (1983). Health service utilization by Indochinese refugees. *Medical Care*, 21(11), 1089–1098.

Taylor, R., Morrel, S., Mamoon, H., Macansh, S., Ross, J., & Wain, G. (2003). Cervical cancer screening in a

Vietnamese nominal cohort. *Ethnicity & Health*, 8(3), 251–261.

Tien, J. L. (1984). Do Asians need less medication? Issues in clinical assessment and psychopharmacology. *Journal of Psychosocial Nursing and Mental Health Services,*, 22, 19–22.

Tien-Hyatt, J. (1989, May). Keying in on the unique care needs of Asian clients. *Nursing and Health Care*, 11, 269–271.

Time almanac with information please. (2006). Boston: Information Please, Inc.

Tran, T. M. (1972). The family and the management of mental health problems in Vietnam. In Lebra, W. P. (Ed.), *Transcultural research in mental health.* Honolulu: University of Hawaii Press.

Tran, T. M. (1980). *Indochinese patients.* Falls Church, Va.: Action for Southeast Asians.

Tran, T. M. (1989, October). Personal communication.

Tripp-Reimer, T., & Thieman, K. (1981). Traditional health beliefs/practices of Vietnamese refugees. *Journal of Iowa Medical Society*, 71(12), 533–535.

U.S. Department of Commerce, Bureau of the Census. (2000). *The Asian population 2000: census 2000 brief.* Washington, D.C.: Government Printing Office.

U.S. Department of Commerce, Bureau of the Census. (2002). Population profiles by age, sex, race, and Hispanic origin, Summary File 3, 2002. Washington, D.C.: U.S. Government Printing Office.

Westermeyer, J., & Winthrop, R. (1979). Folk criteria for the diagnosis of mental illness in rural Laos. *American Journal of Psychiatry*, 136, 136–161.

Wiecha, J. (1999, November). Differences in knowledge of hepatitis B among Vietnamese, African-American, Hispanic and White adolescents in Worcester, Massachusetts. *Pediatrics*, 104(5 part 2), 1212–1216.

Wiecha, J. M., Fink, A. K., Wiecha, J., & Herbert, J. (2001, February). Differences in dietary patterns of Vietnamese, White, African-American, and Hispanic adolescents in Worcester, Mass. *Journal of the American Dietetic Association*, 101(2), 248–251.

Williams, C., & Westermeyer, J. (1986). *Refugee mental health in resettlement countries.* New York: Hemisphere.

World almanac. (2006). New York: World Almanac Books.

Xu, Y., Ross, C., Ryan, R., & Wang, B. (2005). Cancer risk factors of Vietnamese-Americans in rural south Alabama. *Journal of Nursing Scholarship,*, 37(3), 237–244.

Yeatman, G. W., & Dang, V. V. (1980). Cạo gió (coin rubbing). Vietnamese attitudes toward health care. *Journal of the American Medical Association*, 244(24), 2748–2749.

Zhou, F., Euler, G., McPhee, S. J., Nguyen, T., Tram, L., Wong, C., & Mock, J. (2000, June). Economic analysis of promotion of hepatitis B vaccinations among Vietnamese-American children and adolescents in Houston and Dallas. *Pediatrics*, 111(6), 1289–1296.

CHAPTER 19 East Indian Hindu Americans

Scott Wilson Miller and Kira Ann Lass

Behavioral Objectives

After reading this chapter, the nurse will be able to:

1. Identify two important East Indian Hindu cultural values that influence the behavior of East Indian Hindus living in the United States and Canada.
2. Describe concepts of health and illness influencing East Indian Hindus in relation to illness and health-seeking behaviors.
3. Outline the characteristics of the three waves of immigrants who have come to the United States and Canada from India.
4. Describe the effect culture has had on symptoms of mental illness experienced by the East Indian Hindu in India and after immigration.
5. Understand the unique beliefs about touch held by East Indian Hindus and explain how these beliefs may influence attitudes and reactions of East Indian Hindu Americans to caregivers.
6. Describe the beliefs and values held by East Indian Hindus concerning the family.
7. Explain the past-, present-, and future-time orientation held by East Indian Hindus.
8. Describe the Ayurvedic system and the way this system explains illness.

OVERVIEW OF INDIA AND HINDUISM

The Republic of India is a subcontinent that is a vast, wedge-shaped triangular peninsula jutting from the south mainland of Asia into the Indian Ocean. India includes an area of about 1,269,338 square miles and stretches about 2000 miles from north to south. It has three major land regions: the Himalayas and associated mountain ranges to the north, the Indus-Ganges-Brahmaputra Plain in the north central, and the Deccan Plateau in the south. The country contains a large part of the great Indo-Gangetic plain, extending from the Bay of Bengal on the east to the Afghan frontier and the Arabian Sea on the west. This plain is the richest and most densely populated part of the subcontinent.

The climate of India varies according to region. The Himalayas shield the Indian subcontinent from the main body of the Eurasian landmass, resulting in a unique climate. High-pressure winds moving down the Gangetic Plain into the Bay of Bengal result in winters that are generally dry on most of the continent. The Ganges Valley is noted for summer monsoons and rain, though rainfall may vary considerably. In the Ganges-Brahmaputra delta and surrounding areas, rainfall may exceed 80 inches per year, whereas in the northeastern portions of the Deccan region and along the southeastern coast, the total rainfall ranges from 40 to 80 inches per year. In the areas around the western half of the Deccan region, the annual rainfall is 20 to 40 inches per year. In the southern half of the country, temperatures are tropical and vary little from month to month. In northern India, however, the annual range is considerable, and in January the average temperature in the north may be 30° F lower than in the south (Simons, 1976).

About 70% of India's working population is engaged in agriculture. Living in small villages, working farms that average 2 acres per family, and using age-old cultivation techniques based on human or animal power, the average Indian farmer lacks efficiency and is seldom able to provide more than the bare subsistence for the family. Rice wheat, peanuts, corn, and millet are traditional crops. Cash crops include sugarcane, tea, tobacco, jute, and cotton (United Nations, 2006). Cultivation potential is further handicapped by lack of water, allowing only 50% of the land to be cultivated. About 49% of the land is suitable for crop production, and only 3% of that contains permanent crops (McKay, Hill, & Buckler, 2007; Simons, 1976; Information Please Almanac, 2002; Central Intelligence Agency, 2006). The Indian constitution prohibits the slaughter of cattle. India has one of the largest livestock populations in the world, yet most of the animals are undernourished and diseased.

While the majority of the country is involved in agricultural activities, the urban areas of India are indeed heavily industrialized. The textile industry is an important area. Other industry includes iron and steel as well as machine tools, transportation equipment, and chemicals (United Nations, 2006).

India is a federal republic with a parliamentary system of government. The head of state is a president who is elected for a 5-year term by members of the national and state legislatures. Effective executive power is exercised by a prime minister who is normally the leader of the majority political party. Prime ministers have included Jawaharlal Nehru (1984–1989); Chandra Shekhar (1989–1991), and P.V. Narasimha Rao (1991–1996). In 1991, Prime Minister Shekhar resigned. Two months after Shekhar's resignation (May 22, 1991), former Prime Minister Rajiv Gandhi was assassinated (*World Almanac*, 2007). In November 1991, an election was held and P. V. Narasimha Rao was chosen to form a new government. In May 1996, the ruling Congress Party lost the parliamentary elections. At that time, Atal Bihari Vajpayee of the Hindu nationalist Bharatiya Janata Party became prime minister for 13 days. After this short regime, Deve Gowda of the United Front Coalition became prime minister. However, Prime Minister Gowda lost a confidence vote in April 1997. At that time Foreign Minister Gujral was sworn in as Prime Minister. In 1998, Atal Bihari Vajpayee once again became Prime Minister. On July 25, 1997, Kocheril Raman Narayanan was elected president. In 2002, A.P.J. Abdul Kalam was elected president, a position he currently still holds. In 2004, the Indian National Congress Party led by

Sonia Gandhi prevailed in the parliamentary elections, thus prompting Prime Minister Atal Bihari Vajpayee to resign. Because of a variety of reasons, the Congress Party ultimately chose to elect former finance minister Manmohan Singh as the new Prime Minister in 2004 (*Information Please Almanac*, 2007; Central Intelligence Agency, 2006).

Despite a large land mass, India is overpopulated. The most densely populated state is West Bengal, with 767 people/274 km^2. The most densely populated union territory is Delhi, with 6352 people/274 km^2. The most densely populated district is Calcutta, with 23,783 people/274 km^2 (Census of India, 2006).

Most of the population, crowded into the Ganges River Valley and the eastern and western coastal regions, is of diverse racial genotypes. The people of India speak approximately 200 different languages, including 1652 dialects. Some of the languages spoken include Hindi (40%), Bengali (8%), Telugu (8%), Marathi (8%), and Tamil (6%) (Census of India, 2006).

In 1989, the Indian subcontinent numbered more than 685 million people (United Nations, 2006). In 1997 the (estimated) population of India numbered 967,612,804, an increase of 1.59%; and by 2001 the estimated population was 1,207,015,247, with a natural increase of 1.55% (*Information Please Almanac*, 2007). India and China are the only two countries in the world that have a population of over one billion (Census India, 2002). In 2003 the population numbered 1,068,512,000 and in 2004 the population increased to 1,095,351,995 (United Nations, 2006; Central Intelligence Agency, 2006).

Based upon 1997 statistics, the birth rate in India was 25.53 births per 1000 persons; in 2002 the birth rate had decreased to 23.8 per 1000 persons. In 2006 the birth rate was 22.01 births per 1000. Infant mortality for 1997 was 69.2 per 1000, with a slight decrease in 2002 to 61.5 per 1000. In 2006, the infant mortality was 54.63 deaths per 1000. The death rate was 8.18 deaths per 1000. The Hindu population is increasing at the rate of 1.8%, or almost 13 million people each year. The median age of the population is currently 24.9 years. Life expectancy for the general population is 64.71 years (*Information Please Almanac*, 2007).

In the slums of Calcutta, Mumbai (formerly Bombay), and other large cities, thousands die yearly from malnutrition and disease. Some of these diseases include bacterial diarrhea, hepatitis, typhoid fever, dengue fever, and malaria. The prevalence of HIV in adults is 0.9%, and it is estimated that 5.1 million people live with HIV or AIDS (*Information Please Almanac*, 2007). Under the pressure of population increases, the economic, political, and social aspects of life are strained (Warshaw, 1988).

Today the situation in the region is further complicated by the forces of religion and nationalism. The people of the subcontinent are deeply divided by the Hindu and Muslim faiths. Their loyalties are divided between the nation-states of India, Pakistan, and Bangladesh, which share the subcontinent. Indian society is composed of many separate fragments coexisting through mutual tolerance and general agreement on the states and functions of various groups. The regions vary considerably in their historic traditions, cultural patterns, and complement of castes. Within each region, contrasts in customs and traditions parallel class and caste differences. Cutting across linguistic and class divisions are the "communities," which are large aggregates of people defined by some common denominator, such as religion, ethnic affiliation, or area of origin (Melendy, 1977). Some Indians believe that there is no need for people in these diverse groups to conform to a single set of practices and beliefs. The underlying unity of the country is derived from the larger arena of cultural traditions shared by most groups and from the dominance of certain national elites.

Hinduism is the title given for convenience to the religion of most of the population of the Indian subcontinent (Warshaw, 1988). Consequently, approximately 82% to 85% of the population is classified as Hindu (Central Intelligence Agency, 2002). Other religions include Islam (13%); Christianity (2%), and Sikhism (2%) (Central Intelligence Agency, 2006).

Hinduism is a culture as much as it is a religion, and the balance of culture and religion forms the social structure of the Hindu society. Social and religious mores are so predominant that if an Orthodox Hindu were to abandon Hindu belief for another religion, this individual, like the Orthodox Jew, would become an outcast from the people.

Hindus agree on a philosophy rather than doctrine. Although Hindus built magnificent temples, they developed no church. The priesthood is hereditary and can be achieved only through reincarnation. Of the few beliefs shared by all Hindus, respect for a priest is among the foremost. Hinduism evolved over the last 4000 years and has no single founder or creed; rather, it consists of a vast variety of beliefs and spiritually based health practices and customs. Formal organization is minimal and a religious hierarchy is nonexistent.

A common belief shared by most Hindus is veneration of life, especially regarding the cow, which is believed to embody fertility. Although rivers, trees, and other forms of life are also regarded as sacred, the cow is considered the holiest life form.

Early Hindus were united in other philosophical respects. The transmigration of the soul represented one essential element of faith. In the backward or forward movement of the soul, there existed an underlying moral responsibility (*dharma*, which may be translated as law, religion, virtue, morality, or custom). It was *dharma* that obliged each member of society to maintain the role that was assigned at birth. On the individual level, *dharma* required the pursuit of *nirva* in ways that were defined by the priests (Warshaw, 1988).

The doctrine of reincarnation, of which transmigration is an integral part, provided a vital link between the religion of Brahmanism and the social order in which it was practiced. The religion claimed a divine mandate to separate people by castes, otherwise known as the vara (color) system. At the same time, it suggested to members of the toiling lower castes that they might become reincarnated at a higher level in another life. To attain advancement in the other life, the individual must fulfill moral obligations in the present one. Thus the doctrine of reincarnation was an incentive for members of the lower caste to be dutiful. The ultimate bliss of final union with Brahma, though

dim and distant, was a realizable goal. Although this union might be achieved through correct actions, the nature of action was limited by each caste (Warshaw, 1988).

The relationship between the people's beliefs concerning the causes of illness and attempts to seek relief from its effects is learned from local folk practitioners. Illness and its treatment are perceived as biological as well as social phenomena (Kakar, 1977).

Many health professionals do not recognize that the health beliefs and practices of Hindus evolved over the centuries and that every cultural trait has direct relevance to the environment. Although beliefs concerning the causes of prevalent disease may appear illogical, they are difficult to dismiss or substitute with Western medical practices. Adequate knowledge about these beliefs can assist nurses in the formulation of nursing diagnosis and nursing interventions and guard against undue conflicts with the practice of folk medicine.

IMMIGRATION TO THE UNITED STATES AND CANADA
First-Wave Immigrants

The arrival of East Indians from the Indian subcontinent during the first two decades of the twentieth century caused considerable uproar along the Pacific Coast of Canada and the United States (Melendy, 1977). Although East Indians immigrated to these countries in very small numbers, their immigration coincided with increasing American hostility toward the Japanese. Before the nineteenth century, very few Hindu Indians migrated oversees from the Indian subcontinent because most Hindu Indians believed that crossing the "black waters" was dangerous to the Hindu soul. By 1900 the U.S. Bureau of the Census reported that 2050 East Indian residents had immigrated to the United States. Many of the immigrants in this group were non-Indians who were born in India, some were Indian students, and some were Indian businessmen (Melendy, 1977).

In 1901, East Indian students began arriving in the United States to enroll in various colleges and universities throughout the East Coast area. Many of these students enrolled in such prestigious institutions as Cornell University. It was not until 1904 or 1905 that East Indian students began to immigrate to the western portion of the United States to enroll in such universities as the University of California and the California Polytechnic Institute. Students were not the only immigrants who were included in this first major wave of Hindu Indians. During this period, U.S. ports of entry began to register major increases in East Indian immigrants; from 1904 to 1906, 674 East Indians immigrated, compared with only 9 in 1900. The majority of the East Indian immigrants were unskilled agriculturalists and small entrepreneurs from the arid lands of the Punjab, the United provinces, Bengal, and Gujarat (Melendy, 1977).

From the onset of the first wave of East Indian immigrants, these people were classified as Hindus (or Hindoos) regardless of their home, culture, or religion. The U.S. Immigration Commission in 1911 mandated that any native of India was to be considered a Hindu for immigration purposes (Divine, 1972; U.S. Immigration Commission, 1911). In 1917 Congress passed, over President Wilson's veto, an immigration restriction act for East Indians. This new law required a literacy test and also encompassed a barred zone for immigration. All Asians who resided in India, Southeast Asia, the Indonesian islands, new Guinea, or regions of Arabia, Afghanistan, or Siberia were excluded by the new immigration law (Melendy, 1977).

Second-Wave Immigrants

In 1909 Canada closed its doors to East Indian immigrants; however, immigration of East Indians to the United States continued for another 5 years. The Immigration Exclusion Act of 1917, which excluded most persons of East Indian descent, including Hindu Indians, severely curtailed the number of Hindus in the United States. The number of East Indian immigrants residing in the United States began to decline sharply in 1910. In that year, the U.S. Commission reported that there were some 5000 East Indians residing in the United States, but in 1930 this number was disputed by the U.S. Bureau of the Census, which reported that there were only 2544 East Indians residing in the United States, most in California. In 1946, President Harry Truman signed into law a bill that allowed East Indian immigration on a quota basis and allowed naturalization of East Indians. This law is credited with beginning the second wave of immigration of East Indian Hindus to the United States.

These new immigrants, who arrived after World War II and before 1965, were mostly professional Hindu people and their families. These immigrants came mostly from large cities of Mumbai (formerly called Bombay) and Calcutta (Ramakrishna & Weiss, 1992).

Third-Wave Immigrants

In 1965, an immigration law marking the beginning of a third wave of immigrants to the United States was enacted. The Immigration Act raised quotas for Asians to the same level as Europeans, facilitating entry to the Unites States (Koshy, 2001). Although the first-wave immigrants were primarily agriculturists with some students and the second-wave immigrants were primarily businessmen and their families, the third-wave immigrants were entirely different. These new generations of immigrants were very young, with 3 out of 5 under 30 years of age and 1 out of 7 less than 10 years of age. In 1974 approximately 12,777 East Indians resided in the United States; by 2000 this number significantly increased to 1,678,765 (U.S. Department of Commerce, Bureau of the Census, 2002).

These immigrants were predominantly male, coming to the U.S. for graduate education in the science and business fields. Eventually, in the 1980s, women who wanted an education started arriving. Among Asian males, 89.4% have at least a high school education compared with 79% of females; 65.7% of males and 48.7% of females have at least a bachelor's degree (U.S. Department of Commerce, Bureau of the Census, 2002). Additionally, these new immigrants may not be coming directly from India. Many have emigrated from other countries in Asia and Europe before coming to the United States (Korom, 2001; Singh & Unnithan, 1999).

In 1998, there were 570,000 people of East Indian descent residing in the United States (*Information Please Almanac*, 2007), with 107,954 living in the South, 85,245 in the Midwest, 159,641 in the Northeast, and 97,566 in the West (U.S. Department of Commerce, Bureau of the Census, 2002, 2006). The median age of East Indian Hindus in 1990 was 30.1 years and has stayed the same during the 2000 census. The number of married-couple East Indian Hindu Americans represented 91% of that population, compared with 83% for the rest of the general U.S. population. In 1990, the per capita income of East Indian Hindu Americans was 17,777 compared with 14,143 for the rest of the general U.S. population. Data from the 2000 census show that the per capita income of Asian Indians is 27,514 and the median family income is 70,708 (U.S. Department of Commerce, Bureau of the Census, 2006).

COMMUNICATION

Origins of Hindustani Dialect

Language is a means of communication, and it disseminates new ideas. It is the storehouse of tradition and literature that provides a people with a sense of pride, self-confidence, and emotional unity. The national elite groups of a culture emphasize the value of a common language as a unifying force and the necessity for the development of language and literature. The study of linguistic heritage not only is an end in itself but also serves to establish the conditions for nationhood (Pye, 1976).

Hindustani (the name given by Europeans to an Indo-Aryan dialect), as a result of political causes, has become the great *lingua franca* of modern India. The name is not used by natives of India, except as an imitation of the English nomenclature. Hindustani is by origin a Hindi dialect of western India. Hindustani has been called a mongrel pidgin form of speech composed of contributions from the various languages spoken in a Delhi bazaar. This theory has not been disproved because of the discovery that the language is the actual living dialect of western India, which has existed for centuries in its present form (Singh, 1966).

Hindustani is the natural language of the people of Delhi. Because the origin of Hindustani began with the people in the Delhi bazaar, it became known as "bazaar language." From the inception of Hindustani, this language became the *lingua franca* of the mongrel camp and was transported everywhere in India by the lieutenants of the empire. Several recognized forms of the dialect exists, such as Dakhini, Urdu, Rekhta, and Hindi. Dakhini, or "southern," is the form in current use in southern India and the first to be employed in the literature. It contains many archaic expressions now extinct in the standard dialect. Urdu, "the language of the camp," is the name usually employed for the Hindustani by natives and is now the standard form of speech used by Muslims. All the early Hindustani literature was written as poetry, and this literary form of speech was named Rekhta, or "scattered," from the way in which words borrowed from Persia were scattered through it. Hindustani is the dialect used in poetry, with Urdu being the dialect of prose and conversation (Singh, 1966).

There are approximately 18 languages spoken in India, Hindi being the most prevalent (40.2%). Bengali is spoken by 8.3% of the population, Telugu by 7.9%, Marathi by 7.5%, Tamil by 6.32%, Urdu by 5.2%, Gujarati by 4.8%, Kannada by 3.9%, Malayalam by 3.6%, Oriya by 3.4%, Punjabi by 2.8%, Assamese by 1.6%, Sindhi by 0.3%, Nepali by 0.3%, Konkani by 0.2%, Manipuri by 0.2%, Kasmiri by 0.01%, and Sanskrit by 0.01%. All but Nepali, Konkami, and Manipuri are considered official languages (Census India, 2002; Central Intelligence Agency, 2002).

Hindi is the official language of India. English is considered to be an associate official language, with some states declaring it as their official language. The use of English in India is in a fairly fluid state because of the political ideology of each state. The languages taught in the education system are variable, as is the timeframe in which the various languages are introduced. In general, the languages would be the regional dialect pertinent to the school system, Hindi because it is the national official language, and English as a means to improve social mobility and compete in the workforce (Bayer & Gupta, 2006).

Style

The term "Hindi" is ambiguous and therefore the source of much controversy because it is not easily defined. It is considered a regional dialect with a variety of common structural and interchangeable content elements. Its usage depends on both the regional affiliation and the social background of the speaker. Hindi is a highly open language closely related to other Indo-Aryan languages; therefore the degree of stylization is determined by the degree of language-orientation consciousness in the speaker's mind (Corlett & Moore, 1980). Hindi encompasses three areas of stylization: high, medium, and low. An individual may shift between high and low stylization according to situational requirements, as in formal discourse, during conversations with equals, and in giving instruction to subordinates.

Volume and Kinetics

East Indians are generally noted for their soft-spoken manner, almost considered mumbling by some. Frequently, head movements and hand gestures accentuate conversations, adding vitality to the speaker's content. Men maintain direct eye contact with each other when conversing, but women usually draw their eyes downward when addressing their husband, father, or grandfather. This gesture demonstrates a sign of respect.

Touch

Displays of public affection are prohibited and viewed as disrespectful in the eyes of the gods. Married East Indian couples may show signs of affection in the privacy of their own home but not in view of children or elders. Affectionate touching among friends, relatives, and acquaintances is not a socially acceptable Hindu practice.

Implications for Nursing Care

The use of Hindi among East Indian Hindus is the one culturally unifying trait these people possessed after immigration to the United States or Canada. Reluctantly, East Indian Hindus have recognized the need for adoption of English as a communicative norm in the Western culture. Still, most elderly family members are unwilling to abandon the native language, which is regarded as meaningful to their cultural identity, and find it difficult to learn and communicate in English. On the other hand, younger family members, especially children, easily adapt to the Western culture and are more inclined to incorporate English into their language skills. Whenever possible, translators should be utilized by the nurse and other health care personnel when administering care to persons in the East Indian Hindu American population.

When obtaining a health history from an East Indian Hindu American client or family, both Hindi- and English-speaking family members should be involved. Because of uncertainty with the English language, the client may feel frustrated and not communicate conditions thoroughly. When a Hindi-speaking client becomes frustrated, the client may first attempt to translate needs by using Hindi; therefore it may be necessary to translate Hindi responses into English. This process preserves the client's cultural identity while promoting client confidence.

When interacting with recently immigrated traditional Hindu patients, it is important for the nurse to remember that it is considered taboo for a man other than the woman's husband to extend his hand toward her in greeting. In introducing oneself to a female Hindu client, the greeting is first addressed to the husband or eldest female companion.

It is also considered taboo for a man other than a woman's husband to initiate or maintain direct eye contact with a woman. This may be perceived by the husband as a seductive gesture. The wife, as a show of respect and out of fear of reprisal, may divert her eyes downward during conversation.

SPACE

In countries that are vastly overpopulated, such as India, the time lag between a decline in death rate and the acceptance and practice of rational control of fertility presents a serious strain on the economy of the country. India is making positive efforts to reduce the birth rate and thus reduce the phenomenon of overcrowding that currently exists (Moore, 1963). The automobile has been poorly adapted in

India because the cities are so physically crowded, and the Indian society has buildings with elaborate architectural designs (Hall, 1990). Most Hindu Americans are surprised to find that internal ornaments such as ceiling fixtures do not fit into American houses because the ceilings are too low, the rooms are too small, and privacy from the outside is viewed as inadequate (Hall, 1990).

Implications for Nursing Care

East Indian Hindus are a family-oriented people who do not view family as intrusive in personal space parameters. When an East Indian Hindu Americans becomes ill and is hospitalized, the entire family may gather at the bedside. It is important for the nurse to remember that the client may feel that the space in the hospital is overextended and that the family's presence is essential to collapse the space inward. In this case it is important for the nurse to involve family members in the plan of care and to ascertain which family members will provide personal care. This may eliminate the feelings of overcrowding on the part of the nurse and other health care professionals.

SOCIAL ORGANIZATION

Family

In a traditional East Indian Hindu household, married sons live with the family under the parental roof and are subject to parental authority. Frequently the joint family includes approximately 25 individuals and may include up to 200 people. The average joint family is composed of 6 or 7 family members, and the family may comprise several generations. It is of note that the average household size of the East Indian family residing in the U.S. is 3.0 (U.S. Department of Commerce, Bureau of the Census, 2006).

The patriarch controls the finances of the group, giving the sons allowances from their earnings. With globalization and the impact of the growing middle class, men are still considered the primary provider for the family. Thus, the primary role of men in these households is to provide financial income to support the family (Larson, Verma, &

Dworkin, 2001). The matriarch is the autocrat of the home, and her daughters-in-law are subject to her rule. Although this system provides the members of the family with security and sustenance, it has been suggested that it encourages dependence and lack of initiative among many family members (Reddy, 1986). In the past, East Indian Hindu girls have wept at the prospect of marriage, not because of objections to little-known bridegrooms but in fear of their future mothers-in-law (Reddy, 1986). The joint family is a powerful social unit, whose pressures on the individual are greater than most Westerners can imagine. It has also been suggested that the East Indian family demands much sacrifice and devotion and consequently fosters timidity and lassitude in its members (Reddy, 1986).

The hierarchy of the joint family places the father or eldest brother at the highest level. However, the family relies heavily on a democratic system of governance, and decisions of prime importance are determined by a vote in which heads of family may be overruled. Although the head of the family (the patriarch) is the undisputed overseer of other male members of the household, the matriarch is responsible for the family's female members and is instrumental in determining other domestic concerns. Modern East Indian women continue to be the dominant force in home life activities even if they enter the workforce and also provide income for the family (Larson, Verma, & Dworkin, 2001). Recent efforts to promote family planning to reduce the burden of the mushrooming population for the most part has resulted in action by women. Indian men appear to reject sterilization for both psychological and religious reasons, fearing it will destroy their male power or will interfere with God's will (McKay, Hill, & Buckler, 2007; Nossiter, 1970).

The East Indian Hindu father is perceived as being distant from his children, who prefer to bond closely with their mother (Kurian & Ghosh, 1983). The eldest son is destined to continue the family name and perform the holy death rites that will ensure peace for his father's soul. It is this expectation that places the eldest son in the position of being one of the closest family members to the patriarch. Throughout his life the eldest son, even when fully mature, rises when his father enters a room or is near him and greets his father with the *pranām*, the sign of deference in which one touches the feet of a highly respected figure. East Indian Hindus tend to be respectful of authority figures but are more distant with male superiors than with their female counterparts. These people cherish courtesy, which is reflected in the traditional greeting, wherein the head is bowed, the hands are clasped, as if in prayer, and the Hindu word *namaste* ("I bow to thee") is uttered softly.

It is the family, above all other institutions, that is responsible for the implantation of social mores and values in the Hindu culture. Ancient traditions that are suggestive of the existence of external rituals are strictly practiced, and it is the adherence to these ancient traditions that determines whether young East Indians become conservative or rebellious (Warshaw, 1988).

Marriage

In India, marriages of Hindu Indians have always been arranged by parents or other intermediaries. Because marriage was regarded as a union of families rather than of individuals, the marriage traditionally took place when the husband and wife were only children. In 1955 in India, it became illegal to arrange for the marriage of girls under 15 and boys under 18 years of age. This law has been amended in subsequent years to reflect the current legal age for marriage to be 18 years of age for girls and 21 years of age for boys (UNICEF, 2006). However, this law is not easily enforced, and almost 20% of girls are married before they reach 18 years of age. Poverty is a major risk factor in the practice of child marriages. The National Family Health Survey from 1988 to 1999 found that up to 65% of girls were already married by the time they reached 18 years of age. Marriage at a young age brings about difficult challenges, such as financial responsibility, early and frequent pregnancies, and poor health (UNICEF, 2006).

The long-standing practice of courtship rituals, which is primarily a Western phenomenon, is beginning to gain wide acceptance as traditional arranged marriages are being displaced. Now only the educated elite are able to personally arrange marriages, and these marriages account for less than 10% of the total marriages in India (Warshaw, 1988).

The nuclear family, at 38.74%, is the predominant household classification type in India. Couples with married children and relatives residing in the home, termed *extended* and *supplemented* nuclear families, are also common. Males are overwhelmingly (91.2%) considered the head of household (Census India, 2002).

East Indians have long considered marriage a financial and social arrangement designed to strengthen the position of the whole family, and traditionally one of the most important factors determining the choice of a bride has been the size of the dowry, that is, the property a woman brings to her husband at marriage (Warshaw, 1988). In India marriage proposals traditionally have been elicited through a third party who may or may not be a member of the immediate or extended family. In contrast to this, today in the United States, East Indian Hindus frequently place a classified advertisement in their search for a suitable candidate for a prospective bride or groom (Warshaw, 1988).

According to Singh and Unnithan (1999), "the divorce rate is one of the lowest in the world" (p. 642). Because of societal pressures, the majority of married couples stay together even when there is dissatisfaction with their partner. Women are especially vulnerable to miserable, imbalanced, constricting, and even violent relationships. Fernandez (1997) states that "it is not just the husband but also members of his family, especially the mother in law, who abuses directly as an oppressor or indirectly as an instigator" (p. 445). In Indian society oppression of women was considered the norm, and continued use of this oppression in a different social setting, such as in the United States, is thought to be "one way of recapturing a familiar primordial order in an alien setting" (Singh and Unnithan, 1999, p. 653). Thereby, acceptance of violence against women can be traced back to cultural beliefs.

Position of Women in the Family and in Society

In the past, East Indian women ranked far below men in social status. Marriage became obligatory because the unmarried woman was believed to have no place in heaven. Traditionally the belief has been held by East Indian Hindus that the role of a woman is faithfulness and servility to her husband. Because women were deprived of inheritance, a male descendent was essential (Reddy, 1986).

Traditionally the wife had few legal rights and could not publicly contradict or challenge her husband. Mentioning her husband's name in public was also not permitted. This taboo proved particularly confusing when she was required to identify herself for legal purposes (Warshaw, 1988). Among the upper class in the Hindu communities of the Northern regions of India and in some areas of Southern India, many wives practice *purdah*, the anglicized form of Hindi *parda*, meaning "veil." This tradition decrees that in public a wife hides her face behind a veil to ensure that she will be seen only by her husband. This custom is intended to protect her husband's rights over her (Warshaw, 1988).

Mahātma Gandhi was one of the first champions for women's political and social rights in India. In addition, the Women's Indian Association (1917) and the All-India Women's Conference (1927) were organized to unite women in their quest for status attainment through education, social reform, and politics. The association and conference included political picketing and voluntary social work. Although the Indian women's organizations provided tremendous support for the independence movement, it has been reported that they were unable to promote the essential issues related to women's emancipation. It has even been alleged that these organizations were means of maintaining and gaining status to move into higher echelons of power and that only upper- and middle-class women benefited from them (Reddy, 1986). Cumulatively, change in the status of women in post-independence Indian society has been moderate and not far reaching in its influence; for example,

the issues of marriage (particularly regarding the remarriage of widows), divorce, and property inheritance serve to illustrate the inequities still occurring in India where women are concerned (Mukherjee, 1983; Sinha, 1977).

In concurrence with modern feminist movements throughout the world, a "sisterhood of women" hoping to establish "a global female community" is flourishing in the Indian province of the Madras presidency (Raman, 2001, p. 131). The goals of these women include improving literacy, abolishing caste traditions, and the option to delay marriage.

Caste Systems in India

For centuries East Indians have divided themselves by caste, by language, and by religion (Spear, 1972). The Hindu population was divided into four *váras* (colors), which became castes (Box 19-1). These segregated castes were the *Brahmin*, or priestly caste; the *Kshatriya*, or warrior caste; the *Vaiśyas*, or trading and farming caste; and the *Aasādra*, or artisan caste. Approximately 60% of the population held membership in one of these four castes. Outside the caste system, another group of people were referred to as "untouchables." Gandhi renamed the untouchables the *Harijans* or "children of God." These people were the handlers of slaughtered animals, garbage, and the dead. Although the members of the highest caste, the Brahmins, were regarded as pure, Harijans were thought of as polluted and defiled (Spear, 1972). See Box 19-1 for a description of each caste's or noncaste's role in Hindu society.

An individual became a member of a caste at birth, and it was believed that only death could release an individual. Individuals were expected not to marry outside of caste. The exception to this rule was when a man took a bride from a lower caste. Work, acquisition of property, and education could not enable an individual from a lower caste to move to a higher caste.

Historically in India, an intricate system of subcastes known as *jātis*, interlaced with the four main varas. The members of a *jāti* ("caste, lineage") were

---

Box 19-1

CASTE SYSTEM IN INDIA

1. *Brahmins.* The *Brahmins* ("possessing sacred knowledge") were the priests and occupied a position of prestige and influence. These priests performed scholarly pursuits. The distinguishing color of the *Brahmins* was white.
2. *Kshatriyas.* The *Kshatriyas* were the warriors who in ancient times had been the head of society and later were ranked second to the priests. The color of their dress was red to symbolize their work of providing military and political leadership. Warfare was considered a duty of the *Kshatriyas*, and any hesitancy to fight, even against one's own kin, was considered a violation of the *dharma,* or "law," of the caste.
3. *Vaisyas.* The *Vaisyas* ("community men settled on soil"), who made up the largest caste, were involved in commerce. The ritual color of this caste was yellow. The members of this caste had the more mundane tasks of raising cattle, tilling the soil, shopkeeping, and lending money. Although the *Vaisyas* lacked the social, ritualistic, and political privileges associated with *Brahmins* and the *Kshatriyas*, they ultimately gained great power and wealth as a mercantile order.
4. *Śūdras.* The function of the *Śūdras* was to perform menial tasks for the higher groups. Most members of this caste were poor tenant farmers and artisans. The most the *Śūdras* could hope for was that they would be reborn in a higher caste. The ritual color of this lower caste was black.
5. *Untouchables.* *Untouchables* were not allowed to live within the boundaries of a community or to have access to the village water well. They had to perform those duties that were considered unclean, such as tanning leather, cremating the dead, and executing criminals.

From Spear, P. (1972). India: a modern history. Ann Arbor, University of Michigan Press.

---

closely united by family, village, and region. A *jāti* had more prestige and gained greater rewards for services than other people had. Often the members of a *jāti* would claim to have descended from a common ancestor, whether they had or not, to proclaim kinship with one another. These people shared customs, traditions, and usually a dialect. Based on an occupation or a set of related occupations, the *jāti* did not encourage members to seek social relationships outside of the group. Tailors, sweepers, or moneylenders (some of the occupations included in the *jātis*) did business with one another but maintained a social distance (Spear, 1972).

The caste system was officially abolished by the Indian constitution in 1950 (Warshaw, 1988). Today, in most large cities, educated workers and professionals of many castes intermingle. Caste taboos on eating and drinking with others tend to be ignored. Schools, public transportation, facilities, restaurants, and apartment houses have been almost entirely desegregated. Caste lines in major cities are so blurred that a person of the merchant caste may be an officer in the army, whereas a person of the military caste may be a prosperous business executive. However, although commercial practices are forcing East Indians to abandon old castes, family life continues to use them.

Religion

The Hindu religion may be the oldest religion in the world (Eshleman, 1992). In India, Hindu (83%) is the most prevalent religion. Other religions practiced are Islam (12%), Christianity (2.3%), Sikhism (1.9%), Buddhism (0.8%), and Jainism (0.4%) (Census India, 2002).

There are at least 910,000 practicing Hindus in the United States, including those of East Indian descent, and there are over 400 Hindu temples (*Information Please Almanac*, 2007; *World Almanac*, 2007; Yang & Edbaugh, 2001). Hinduism, especially as learned and practiced in the United States, is a religion of disciplined acts, *karma yoga* ("the path of deeds") (Miller, 1995). Key teachings of Hinduism emphasize the importance of *satya* ("truthfulness, reality"), self-control, and respect for others. Many practicing Hindus engage in meditation, *prāṇāyama* ("breathing exercises"), singing *bhajans* ("sacred hymns"), yoga, and daily prayer.

The Hindu religion is polytheistic in the sense that there are numerous gods and goddesses, but there is an overriding sense of a supreme spirit. The origin of Hinduism is based on the Vedas, the sacred written scriptures. In Hinduism, the belief is that Brahma is the principle and source of the universe and the center from which all things proceed and to which all things return. Reincarnation is a central belief in Hinduism. Life is determined by the law of karma, which states that rebirth is dependent on moral behavior in a previous stage of existence. In Hinduism, life on earth is transient and a burden. The goal of existence is liberation from the cycle of rebirth and redeath and entrance into *nirvāṇa* (literally, "outblowing"), a state of extinction of passion.

Religion continues to play a part in assimilation into a new culture and of preserving one's native culture and identity. As East Indians assimilate into the American culture, their religious customs may have changed. Hindu religious leaders in the United States and India are returning to classic texts and turning away from certain modern adaptations in an effort to unify the practitioners of the religion. Also, the World Hindu Council is in the process of completing a code of conduct manuscript based on Hindu beliefs and traditions. This return to the classics is a way of combining different views, beliefs, and attitudes to one common goal. Hindus are protective of their religion, especially so in the United States, where pressures come from the mainstream Christian culture. The challenge of preserving ethnic identity in light of cultural assimilation may have made many East Indians present a "model minority image of themselves and their culture" (Kurien, 1999; Yang & Edbaugh, 2001).

Hinduism is a common part of life for most Hindu Indians. Religious shrines are prevalent within many Hindu households and are located in various parts of the home, based on family preference. Each family has a set of specific gods and goddesses to whom they pray, and by popular account the Hindu pantheon numbers some 33 million gods. The shrines contain statues and pictures of the chosen gods, candles, incense, and offering of milk, flowers, and fruits. Times for prayer and meditation are reserved for the early morning (after bathing) and early evening, as time permits.

The common Hindu custom of fasting is observed on specific days of the week, depending on which god the individual worships. This practice is predominant among the women of the family, and children are not allowed to participate. Based on the family's degree of compliance to orthodox Hindu laws, fasting rituals may vary from abstinence to consuming only one meal a day. This practice may span over a 1-month time period or merely an observance of a holy day. Pittsburgh is a major center of Hindu cultural and religious strength. The first major Hindu temple in the United States, the Śri Venkateswars Temple in Penn Hills (a suburb of Pittsburgh), is an internationally known pilgrimage site for Hindus. Other major temples have been established in Washington D.C., Chicago, Austin, Berkeley, Los Angeles, and Boston. Temples serve as the centers of community, promoting the retention of Hindu values and instruction in the scriptures and key teaching, such as *ahiṁsā* ("nonviolence"), vegetarianism, and self-control. The temples often sponsor cultural events, language classes, and secular activities (Miller, 1995). There is a World Hindu Council of America, a subset of the international organization, which seeks to promote the Hindu religion in the United States by offering information via a wide variety of formats (World Hindu Council of America, 2006).

Effect of Immigration to the United States on Social Organization

The restricted immigration policies that were in place before 1965 in the United States created fear for many East Indian Hindu Americans because it appeared that the culture was losing its significance. Before 1965 there were so few East Indian Hindus residing in the United States that the few who did reside there chose to remain culturally isolated. Those Hindu Indians who did choose to assimilate believed that there was no free access to the White community and therefore chose to assimilate the Mexican American culture, particularly because there were so few East Indian Hindu women residing in the United States before 1865. Some sociologists concluded that the assimilation between East Indians and Mexicans occurred as a result of their similarities in physical characteristics. In addition, some sociologists believe that East Indian Hindus may have lost their ethnicity entirely in the Mexican subculture, but others regard the fact of intermarriage between East Indian Hindu Americans and Mexican Americans as evidence of mutual acceptance (Melendy, 1977). In a classic study of 50 East Indian Hindu men, 26 had wives in the United States, 22 of whom were Mexican. Consequently, the children from these Mexican-East Indian marriages were raised predominantly in the Mexican culture (Dadabhay, 1954).

As a new wave of East Indian Hindu immigrants began to assert themselves in the 1960s, the sagging Hindu culture and traditions were revived and prospered. This was attributable in part to the fact that after 1965, more East Indian Hindu wives and families began to arrive in the United States, which facilitated a revival of the traditional culture. On arrival, these wives continued to wear saris, the traditional dress, whereas only 10% of the men continued to wear traditional garb because many of the men felt the need to conform to the business community in the United States (Wenzel, 1965). Most of the newer immigrants were more adaptable and moved more easily into the American way of life, whereas the older generation remained apart from the mainstream society. Although the older groups of East Indian Hindus, who continued to live in rural areas, managed to adjust to economic demands, the social acculturation of this group remained significantly behind that of the newer generation of immigrants (Melendy, 1977). Some East Indian Hindu wives in the United States continued to practice bindī ("forehead dots," also called *tilak*) as a sign of the husband's well-being and prosperity.

Urbanization, industrialization, and education are major interacting forces disrupting the framework of the joint family system traditionally found in the East Indian culture and consequently are affecting the East Indians family value system in the United States.

The concepts of ethnic identity and acculturation are important to note. Ethnic identity is at the level of the individual and that particular person's feeling of belonging and the amount of involvement they have to a particular ethnic group. Acculturation is the process by which the individual changes, adapts, or interacts with the new culture that they are in contact with. In general, Asian Indian families have maintained their cultural identity and value such as the importance of family, traditional gender roles, and group dynamics (Farver, Narang, & Bhadha, 2002).

Education is so highly valued among East Indian Hindu culture that approximately 80.1% of East Hindu Americans 25 years of age or older have a high school education, compared with 66% for the rest of the general U.S. population. Of the U.S. population 25 years of age or older, East Indian Hindus have the highest percentage of college graduates, with approximately 68% of Hindu men and 36% of Hindu women obtaining a college education as compared with approximately 20% of men and 13% of women for the general U.S. population (U.S. Department of Commerce, Bureau of the Census, 2006). Indian college students in the United States have expressed a desire to improve communication between their parents and with other family members, along with improved emotional and financial independence. Conversations are typically one-sided, especially on the sensitive subjects of dating, marriage, and sexuality. Change has been slow because of societal, cultural, and financial limitations (Medora, Larson, & Dave, 2000).

Since the third-wave immigration period (1965), East Indian Hindus have integrated into the U.S. labor force, with approximately 51% of all East Indian Hindus working. The per capita income for East Indian Hindu Americans is $27,514 versus $21,587 for the general population. The median family income for East Indian Hindu Americans in 1999 was $70,708, compared with $50,046 for the general population (U.S. Department of Commerce, Bureau of the Census, 2006)

Politically, the adult East Indian Hindu community in the United States tends to favor a low profile, with fewer members serving in public office. Relationships between East Indian immigrants and U.S. society vary based on the community where they reside. According to Miller (1995), "discrimination against East Indian groups can be severe, ranging from 'dot buster' violence in New Jersey (perpetrated by white racist 'skinheads') to subtle forms of job discrimination that are difficult to document statistically."

An increasing number of young East Indian Hindu Americans are relocating to large urban centers in New York, New Jersey, Pittsburgh, Texas, and California (Helweg & Helweg, 1990) and are living in apartments. As a result the joint family system has been rendered impractical. In school and at work, more East Indian Hindu Americans have learned to depend on ability rather than the caste system formerly found in India. The development of individualism among family members has resulted in uncertainty about the need for elaborate rituals of the past. Some of the values learned from the family are therefore extinct, especially as more young people detach themselves from the traditions that previously controlled them.

Recent East Indian immigrants to the United States, coming predominantly from western India, continue to bring their religious and cultural beliefs with them. Some of these beliefs as stated by Singh and Unnithan (1999) include the following: "religion, caste, and regional affiliations are important criteria for mate selection, the families of both partners play crucial roles in mate selection and choice, patriarchy is the norm, and the status of women is predominantly secondary and dependent" (p. 642). As East Indian communities flourish in the United States, the communities have strived to maintain their cultural and ethnic identity.

Implications for Nursing Care

It is important for nurses to appreciate that the traditional East Indian Hindu family is the basic unit wherein values, manners, and morals are learned as part of its social structure. The pursuit of individualism, which is so predominant in Western culture, is not the accepted norm. The nurse should appreciate that the father is highly regarded as the head of the family and is the primary spokesman concerning important family matters, including the health care of the individual members. It is unusual for the East Indian Hindu American to seek medical care outside the confines of the family because of the fear that the family will be subjected to public scrutiny by strangers.

The nurse who cares for traditional, newly immigrated East Indian Hindu American clients should expect that the wife will usually sit passively by her husband, expecting all questions and inquiries to be directed toward him. He in turn may consult with his wife regarding the health status of other family members. The nurse who ignores the husband and seeks information directly from the wife may precipitate, on the part of the husband, feelings of mutual humiliation and disrespect in the eyes of his family. The major objective in developing an effective nurse–client relationship is to develop trust by gaining the husband's confidence so that the husband no longer views the nurse as an intruder but, instead, as a health care advocate.

TIME

The sense of time is an important concept for East Indian Hindus, who are past, present, and future oriented. East Indian Hindus are perceived as past oriented because of the traditions and rituals that are inherent to the culture. On the other hand, they are perceived as present oriented because of the view that they are "beings-in-becoming" (Kluckhohn & Strodtbeck, 1973). Finally, they are perceived as future oriented because life in the present is lived with an emphasis of the hereafter.

At the highest intellectual level, Hindus seek the one reality, whether this is conceived impersonally or theistically. Once they succeed in reaching this reality, they may continue to live in the world but without emotional attachment to it. They will have passed beyond sorrow and joy, pain and pleasure, and good and evil (Warshaw, 1988). In other words, the present is transcended by concern for the future and future reward.

Hindus, through cremation of their dead, hope to release the individual's spirit for union with an all-pervading one. The act is suggestive of the existence of a timeless presence in which all Hindus may share. The doctrine of rebirth—that every living being, animal or heavenly, will again be reborn and for all eternity—is a popular Hindu belief. The precise form of each rebirth is determined by the balancing of the being's deeds, good and evil, in previous existences. Escape from the cycle of birth constitutes salvation, a state of perfect, blissful consciousness that may be gained by acquiring perfect knowledge and performing one's duty flawlessly. Most Hindus aim only to improve their condition in the next existence.

Implications for Nursing Care

Because East Indian Hindu Americans are perceived as being past, present, and future oriented, it is important for the nurse to remember that the client may place little or no value on some present things, such as being on time for appointments, but may place considerable importance on other present-oriented concepts, such as the spiritual atonement of the self. At the same time, the same client may place equal importance on past-oriented things, such as traditions and rituals, and on future-oriented concepts, such as the preparation of the soul for the life hereafter.

ENVIRONMENTAL CONTROL

According to Kluckhohn and Strodtbeck (1973), it is essential for a people to answer the question of whether humans are innately good or bad. In regard to this question, there exists a range of variabilities, including evil, good and evil, and good. Hindus believe that the goodness in the soul of man is recaptured by virtue of the process of reincarnation. In addition, they believe in the man-to-nature orientation, as proposed by Kluckhohn and Strodtbeck, that man is not only subjected to nature but also has the need to live in harmony with nature. Being a past-, present-, and future-oriented cultural group that subscribes to a multiple man-to-nature orientation, some Hindus believe that because man is a mixture of good and evil, there is a need for constant control and discipline of the self if any real goodness is to be achieved.

Hindus are viewed as having both an internal and an external locus of control, meaning that some Hindu people believe that although external forces control destiny, internal forces, such as feeling states or misuse of the body, can also control destiny. For example, Hindu Americans who subscribe to both an internal and an external locus of control believe that internal conditions are influenced by psychological factors such as anger, jealousy, envy, fright, and shame. This belief is supported by the premise that when an individual is unable to control internal conditions that are self-perpetuated, a possibility exists for a susceptibility to disease (Henderson & Primeaux, 1981). The external locus of control is evident in that illness is an external event or misfortune, the cause of which may be related to the fault of a family member or the wrath of a disease goddess against the entire family. It is not uncommon for Hindus to believe that the malevolent spirits of dead ancestors, sins committed in a previous life, or jealous living relatives are responsible for one's ill health. Such phenomena as "soul loss," "breach of taboo," and "wrath of a goddess" are viewed as symbolic expressions of internal conflict. Hindus believe that people make themselves vulnerable to such calamities through conscious or unconscious transgressions against the ghosts and spirits. Agents empowered by evildoers to precipitate illness are numerous and varied; thus, to avert the vile intentions of these demons, Hindus wear charms, make offerings to the saints and their ancestors, and avoid visiting areas in the village where spirits are believed to reside.

Perception of Illness

According to classical East Indian theory, the human body consists of five natural elements: earth (bones and muscles), water (phlegm or *kapha*), fire (gall or *pittá*), wind (*vāyú*), and space (in hollow organs) (Andrews & Boyle, 2003). Water, fire, and wind are the three elements that interact in harmony to produce wellness. Illness results from an excess or deficiency of one of these elements, which are also referred to as the *tridosha* or the "three troubles." *Prāṇá* deals not only with respiration but also with a pneumatic element circulating in channels, distributing the "humors" and body fluids (bile, blood, and phlegm) throughout the body. In addition to giving attention to the five natural elements, East Indian theory also identifies bone, flesh, marrow, fat, chyle, blood, and sperm as seven essential constituents of the body. Although the nomenclature of bones is extensive, the viscera are given less attention in East Indian theory.

A great deal of attention traditionally was devoted to the source of disease and to the hygienic prescription. The intention of medical treatment addressed not only the disease symptoms but also the diagnosis of causes. For example, the treatment of fever consisted of giving antithermic drugs in addition to prescribing medication against *pittá* or the causative element involved (Dash, 1974). Hindus believe that praying for health is the lowest form of prayer. Among East Indian Hindus, it is preferable to be stoic rather than pray for recovery (Peck, 1981).

Folk Medicine

Significance of Folk Beliefs in the Hindu Culture. Today, there is a growing sense among psychologists, sociologists, and biologists that illness and its treatment are both biological and sociological phenomena (Kakar, 1977). It is believed there are at least three different types of medical systems practiced at three different cultural levels. On the first level are primitive or preliterate people, who practice a form of primitive medicine based predominantly on a supernatural theory of disease causation. These people are believed to seek treatment through magicoreligious means. On the second level are people who belong to the folk culture level and practice folk medicine, which encompasses a theory of illness that involves both supernatural and physical treatments as well as causations. On the third level are people who subscribe to a modern theory of treatment and disease causation. At this level, people recognize natural rather than supernatural causes of disease. When East Indian medicine is traced back historically, there is a magicoreligious mixture of theology. In early East Indian history, disease causation as attributed to gods and goddesses and was explained on the basis of a cause and effect relationship with these gods

and goddesses or with ghosts and evil spirits. However, Indian folk beliefs have undergone centuries of transition and now include herbal medicines and the ayurvedic system (Kakar, 1977).

The belief that certain diseases have natural or physical origins does not preclude the simultaneous role of a supernatural antecedent. For example, diarrhea in a child is generally attributed to consumption of a combination of incompatible foods. However, the possibility of someone casting an "evil eye" or "evil mouth" on the child is also recognized (Kakar, 1977).

Another system of beliefs is that ayurvedic doctrine, which dictates that disease not only has a germ causation but also occurs because of an imbalance of the essential body elements. *Āyurveda* is a term that is composed of two words: *āyus* and *veda*. The literal translation for the word *Āyurveda* is "science of life." A primary concern for East Indian Hindus is knowledge of favorable or unfavorable conditions that assist in the introduction or resistance of the growth of harmful or nonharmful germs. East Indian Hindus believe that there are three fundamental elements in the body—*dosha*, *dhātu*, and *mála*—which must be in balance if a state of optimal equilibrium is to exist. *Dosha* ("disease") governs the physiochemical and physiological activities of the body; *dhātu* ("layer") forms the basic structure of the body cell; *mála* ("dirt") consists of substances partly utilized in the body and partly excreted in modified form after their physiological function has been completed (Kakar, 1977; Ramakrishna & Weiss, 1992).

Many medications may be prescribed in the ayurvedic system of medicine. For example, drugs for rejuvenation may be prescribed by an ayurvedic physician (Dash, 1974). Another example for ayurvedic medicine is found with the treatment of amebic dysentery, which is caused by the organism *Entamoeba histolytica*. In ayurvedic medicine, the belief is that the organism is not the major etiological factor of the condition. Rather, the major cause is attributed to irregularity of diet; intake of heavy, indigestible foods; and emotional factors, such as worry, anxiety, and anger (Dash, 1974). As a folk remedy for amebic dysentery, the drug *cyávana prâśa* ("disease causer–eating") is used, but this drug is considered more a food than a medicine. Two tablespoons of this medication are taken in a glass of milk, and the client is instructed to avoid salt in excess as well as sour things. Another part of the treatment includes avoidance of anxiety, worry, and sexual indulgence (Dash, 1974; Ramakrishna & Weiss, 1992).

Emphasis on the diet of a client is a unique feature of ayurvedic medicine. The popular belief is that the client does not require any medication if he or she has a wholesome diet. According to this belief system, even if errors and diagnoses are made, most of the ayurvedic herbal medicines will not produce any harmful effect; however, if a diagnosis is correct, these herbal medications will act instantaneously.

Diseases in ayurvedic medicine are considered to be psychosomatic, involving both the body and the mind. This point is always kept in mind when medicines and regimens are prescribed for the client (Dash, 1974; Ramakrishna & Weiss, 1992).

Types of Folk Practitioners. A majority of East Indians obtain their beliefs in relation to the cause, prevention, and elimination of illnesses from their families, their parents-in-law (particularly the mother-in-law), elderly women of the neighborhood, indigenous midwives, other folk practitioners, and government health care workers. Usually the decision to seek medical treatment is influenced by factors such as the client's sex, the economic condition of the family, the family's perception about the cause of the illness, and the family's relationship with the local practitioner (Kakar, 1977).

Therapeutic advice is generally obtained at five different levels: family level, *mohalla* (properly, *mahalla*) level, caste level, village level, and beyond the village level (Kakar, 1977).

1. At the family level, the mother-in-law, regarded as the family practitioner and well versed in the use of home remedies, is the source of treatment for any illness. Her authority is highly regarded and usually unchallenged in the scope of maternal and child care. Acting as diagnostician and therapist, she uses such healing techniques as the purgatives, massages, and various body-stretching devices.

2. At the *mohalla* (*mahalla*, "eunuch in palace or harem") level, there exists 2 or 3 highly respected *syānas* or *syānis* ("wise or holy men"), who are readily available and consulted only for certain illnesses. Intervention by the *syānas* is decided by the mother-in-law, and it is assumed that the importance of not relinquishing the family's secrets and affairs to the community is understood.

3. At the caste level, the intervention by one or two *syānas* is often sought. The practitioners cater to people's needs, especially members of their own caste. They are highly respected members of the caste and recipients of special treatment on socially important occasions.

4. At the village level, the faith healer, the most religious member, is a popular practitioner of choice and is employed for his free services regardless of caste or creed.

5. Beyond the village level, consultation is sought with a variety of folk and indigenous practitioners, ranging from exorcists to spirit mediums. There have been instances where a simple reassurance of the client by the spirit medium, without any actual medication, had resulted in instant relief (Kakar, 1977).

Principles of Hygiene

Personal hygiene is extremely important to East Indian Hindus. As part of the religious duty, a bath is required at least once every day. Some Hindus believe that bathing after a meal is injurious and that a cold bath may prevent a blood disease, whereas a hot bath may cause an alterative effect on blood diseases. East Indian Hindus also believe that if the bath is too hot, injuries to the eyes may occur. Hot water may be added to cold water, but cold water is not to be added to hot water when one is preparing a bath. When the bath is completed, the body is to be carefully rubbed dry with a towel and properly dressed (Jee, 1981).

Perception of Death

Death, according to the Hindu belief, is perceived as a passage from one existence to another. From the scriptures and the inspiration of "seers," the Hindu learns that all creatures are in a process of spiritual evolution extending through limitless cycles of time. A person's lifetime is like a bead on a necklace whose other beads represent past and future lifetimes. Each *atman* ("basic self") strives through successful rebirths to ascend the scale of merit until, after a life of rectitude, self-control, nonviolence, charity, reverence for all living creatures, and devotion to ritual, it wins liberation from worldly existence to achieve union with Brahma (Chakravarty, 1978).

In India, the preparation of the body for cremation involves bathing the remains with a milk and yogurt solution, which symbolically cleanses the soul of the disease. When a married woman dies, she is attired in a traditional white wedding sari, devoid of make-up or jewelry, the wearing of which is considered a bad omen. A man is attired in a plain, off-white, East Indian suit. Religious prayers and chanting are continually offered by friends, family members, and priests before and after death to promote safe passage of the soul. Outward displays of grief are accepted practice within the Hindu faith. Open grieving by family, friends, and acquaintances encompasses wailing, crying, and even fainting. Men are as expressive in their grief as women and do not project a stoic demeanor (Chakravarty, 1978). The eldest son of the deceased carries the body to the funeral pyre, and all other children are prohibited from approaching the funeral site. During the cremation ceremony, a priest chants prayers while the body is cremated. The ashes are then placed in a container and transported by the eldest son to a designated holy ground and scattered.

Implications for Nursing Care

It is important for the nurse to remember when working with Hindu Americans that there may be a belief that self-control of strong feelings is one of the keys to balancing health or a wellness state. In addition, some Hindu Americans believe in a value orientation that encompasses the belief that man is subjected to nature and at the same time is expected to live in harmony with nature. Because

of this belief, it is important for the astute nurse to keep in mind that the client may believe that illness has a twofold causation, which may include ill favor or overindulgence of self.

Because Hindu Americans have very strict beliefs regarding things such as bathing, it is important for the nurse to remember that the Hindu American may refuse to take a bath after breakfast, which may be a common policy in some health care facilities. In addition, because some Hindu Americans believe that it is not permissible to add cold water to hot water, if the water is too hot, the nurse should pour the water out and begin the process again rather than risk offending the Hindu client.

Because some Hindu Americans subscribe to a theory that encompasses the belief that there are three elements in the body that must be in harmony to produce wellness, it is important for the nurse to identify with the client those beliefs that are beneficial, neutral, or harmful. If the client has beliefs that are beneficial, it is important for the nurse to identify these beliefs and practices, and incorporate them into the plan of care. It is equally important for the nurse to identify those beliefs and practices that are considered neutral, having no effect one way or the other on the outcome of treatment, and that therefore do not need to be eliminated from the daily rituals of the client. Finally, it is extremely important for the nurse to identify those practices that could be considered harmful and therefore need to eliminated from the practices and daily rituals of the client.

When a Hindu American client dies, the nurse should not be surprised by the religious rites after death. For example, the priest may tie a thread around the neck or wrist to signify a blessing, and this thread should not be removed. The nurse should expect that after death, a priest will pour water into the mouth of the body and the family will request to wash the body. Because Hindus are particular about who touches the body after death, it is essential that the nurse communicate respect, and provide privacy for the family so that these rites can be carried out (Murray & Huelskoetter, 1991; Potter & Perry, 2001).

BIOLOGICAL VARIATIONS

Variations According to Racial Strain

The modern population of India can be classified into six major racial strains. Two of the six racial groups can be related to a geographical region and the other four groups may be found throughout India. Persons in the upper classes are different in physical type from those in the lower social strata. East Indians can be regarded as a separate racial group occupying an intermediate position between the peoples of Asia on the one hand and those of Europe on the other.

1. Mediterranean strain. These people are characterized by a long head, moderate stature, slight build, and dark skin. The face is narrow, the nose is small and moderately broad, and the hair is wavy or curly. These are the dominant features among the Dravidin-speaking people of southern India.

2. Broad-headed strain. This section of the population varies in stature from short to medium and in skin color from light to dark brown. The head is broad and sometimes high. The nose is prominent, and the hair is straight and usually abundant on the face and body.

3. Nordic strain. A distinguishing characteristic of this people is their long head. They are tall, long-faced with a straight and narrow nose, and light-skinned. This type of strain predominates in the upper caste in northern India.

4. Mongoloid strain. The head on these people varies from long to medium and the skin color varies from light to dark brown. Their stature is medium, and the hair is sparse on the face and body. The face is short, with predominant cheekbones, and the eye sockets are slanted, giving a slit-like appearance to the eye.

5. Negritos. These people represent earlier inhabitants of India. Their stature is less than 5 feet, and frizzy hair is among the chief distinguishing features.

6. Proto-australoids. This strain is predominant with tribal people of central, western, and southern India. A long head; short stature; broad, short face, with strongly marked brow edges and a small, flat nose; and wavy to curly hair are features of the lowest social strata of the population. The skin is dark to black. The strain is so-named because of certain resemblances of people of this type and the Australian aborigines (Guha, 1945), but genetic evidence of such a relationship is exceedingly weak (Cavalli-Sforza, Menozzi, & Piazza, 1994).

Enzymatic and Genetic Variations

Thalassemia, a genetic condition that can result in various degrees of anemia, is believed to have a high incidence in people of the Mediterranean region, the Middle East, and Southeast Asia. It is believed that thalassemia has a range of variability in occurrence of people of Indian descent (Overfield, 1995). In addition, G-6-PD deficiency, which also causes anemia, is believed to have a high occurrence in high-risk malarial areas. What is believed to occur in high-risk malarial areas is that the malarial parasite attacks red blood cells that contain the G-6-PD enzyme. Therefore, cells with a deficiency are less likely to be parasitized, which lowers the parasite load and consequently lowers the G-6-PD deficiency.

Lactose intolerance is another condition that affects persons of East Indian descent. Lactose intolerance is believed to occur among African and Asian populations because of genetic selection that may lead some groups of people to have adequate levels of intestinal lactase and others to have inadequate levels (Bayless, Rothfield, Massa, et al., 1975; Overfield, 1995). It is believed that although lactose intolerance varies by race, at least 80% to 90% of the world's population become lactose intolerant in adult life, except for some Whites (Overfield, 1995).

Susceptibility to Disease

The average life expectancy for the East Indian Hindu is 64.71 years of age, as opposed to 77.85 years of age for of the general U.S. population. Additionally, the infant mortality rate in India is 54.63 deaths per 1000 live births as opposed to 6.43 deaths per 1000 live births in the United States (Central Intelligence Agency, 2006).

It is believed that susceptibility to heat stress is influenced by factors such as age, race, body build, body fat, climatic experience, and possibly gender (Wagner, 1972). According to Frisancho (1981), there is a possibility that certain races have the ability to withstand heat stress better than other races do; however, the racial effect is compounded by climatic exposure. Frisancho (1981) concluded that persons brought up in hot climates, such as that in India, are better able to tolerate heat than those persons raised in cooler regions, such as certain regions of the United States. In general it is believed that Blacks, southwestern American Indians, Asian Indians, East Indians, and Australian aborigines have the ability to withstand heat better than their White counterparts (Frisancho, 1981; Riggs & Sergent, 1964). The belief is that these people have lower sweat rates than Whites but similar body temperatures and therefore may have more efficient sweat production (Dill, Yousef, & Nelson, 1983). It is believed that part of the climatic influence on heat tolerance is directly related to the effect of heat on the development of the body during childhood. Eveleth (1966) concluded that children who grew up in hot climates, such as conditions found in India, have a tendency to be more slender than their counterparts raised in more temperate areas. In addition, these children also have thinner arms and legs.

In the area of stroke, public awareness in India of signs and symptoms, as well as affected organs, is marginal, which is comparable to knowledge in other nations. There has been an identified need to improve public education regarding stroke, as the data suggest that the population is aging putting them at higher risk. Current stroke prevalence in India is variable, from 40 to 270 per 100,000 people, 12% of which occur in people less than 40 years of age. Should the incidence of stroke increase, there needs to be further discussion regarding the availability of resources for caring for the acute and rehabilitative needs of this population (Pandian, Jaison, Deepak, et al., 2005).

Nutritional Preferences and Deficiencies

Most caste Hindus are vegetarians. However, strictness in adherence to the vegetarian diet varies. In most cases, the vegetarian diet consists primarily of grains (wheat, rice, millet, and barley) and legumes (grains, beans, and pulses, the edible seeds of plants having pods). In northern and western India, baked or fried cakes made with wheat are common. *Chapātī*, a popular form of bread, is a round, flat cake made of whole wheat flour and water and baked on a convex iron plate. *Pūrī* is similar to *chapātī*, except for the addition of shortening and being fried in deep fat. *Parāṭhā*, a third form of bread, is cooked on a convex metal pan.

In eastern and southern India, rice is the staple food. It is usually boiled, but it can be combined with *ghee* (*ghi*, clarified butter) and spices to become *pilau* (or pilaf). Corn, barley, and millet are served alone or as supplements to wheat and rice dishes. The primary sources of protein are the grains and pulses, which include *chanā* (chick pea) and *arhar* (pigeon pea), which when split and dried is referred to as *dāl*. Vegetables include most of the green leafy vegetables, especially spinach, mustard, and radish greens, as well as gourds, eggplant, okra, cucumbers, cabbage, turnips, and potatoes.

Most East Indians eat a very light breakfast on rising in the morning, a heavy meal at midday, and a light meal between 7 and 9 P.M. (Ashraf, 2000). Before partaking of the meal, traditional Hindus chant the name of their god of preference, as if offering food to him or her before they eat. East Indian dietary laws dictate that the right hand is used for eating, whereas the left hand is used for personal hygiene and toileting.

Psychological Characteristics

Community tolerance for mental illness is high in India, and in many cases any idiosyncrasies are channeled into occupations or lifestyles in which the behavior can be carried out. For example, a marginally schizophrenic Indian person may wander the country doing odd jobs and living off handouts. Approximately 500 years ago *ambalams* were built throughout India to house travelers. Today, these ancient buildings are used by many persons who wander through India, including the mentally ill, as places to obtain food, beg, get water, and bathe.

For the East Indian Hindu, environment has a significant effect on mental illnesses that may develop (Ali, 1989). For example, because of the strong belief in supernatural forces, when a client becomes psychotic, delusions and hallucinations are often related to possession by a god, demons, or a witch, rather than to the minds being influenced by equipment being placed, or fears that the place is "bugged," which is more often the case in Western societies. An East Indian immigrant who has difficulty with English and with understanding what is occurring in the environment and who becomes psychotic will often manifest a paranoid reaction rather than one of the other psychotic illnesses. The delusions of the new immigrant frequently relate to the supernatural and reflect the culture of India. However, as East Indians have become assimilated into the western culture, the nature of these delusions has changed to more "Western" symptoms.

Because mental illness is consistent with the sociological beliefs of the people, the treatment is also sociologically based and must be appropriate for the beliefs about the cause of the illness, such as exorcism of a spirit, demon, or god. The most effective exorcism is dramatically performed in a room with others in the family or in front of neighbors and friends (Ali, 1989).

Many drugs that are restricted in the United States are legal in India, such as cocaine, opium, and marijuana. Although these drugs are cheap and available, abuse is much less common than in the United States. Drugs that are commonly abused in the United Sates may be used in India for therapeutic purposes. For example, marijuana leaves in water may be used for a baby's cramps, and opium may be used for diarrhea. Although Judeo-Christian beliefs regarding drug use as wrong have been present in India since the British arrived and to some extent have been adopted by the upper-class people, most East Indian Hindus still retain the value that although drugs may not be "good" their use is not "wrong."

Implications for Nursing Care

The most crucial aspect for proper nutrition is to make Hindus aware of the advantage of diet in relation to the survival of children. As East Indian Hindu Americans become assimilated into Western culture, it is important for them to understand the significance of using available foods in a nutritious manner. The nurse must keep in mind that a Hindu person may be reluctant to use Western foods because of sociocultural restrictions. Therefore, because dietary considerations are of utmost importance to some Hindu Americans, the astute nurse will involve the nutritionist or dietitian in the development of a culturally appropriate plan of care. The nurse should also be aware that fasting is an important part of religious practice and that this practice may have consequences for persons on special diets or with diabetes, or with other diseases related to food (Murray & Huelskoetter, 1991).

Nurses and other health care workers must be aware that the joint family is an important characteristic of the East Indian Hindu community. In planning culturally relevant nutritional programs, the nurse must understand the nutritional patterns in relation to other aspects of the culture and to identify those elements that can be changed without disorganization of the whole cultural scheme. The nurse also needs to explore the beliefs and attitudes of not only the people, but also the authorities from whom these beliefs are derived.

It is also important for the nurse to remember that because some East Indian Hindu Americans have a genetic predisposition for G-6-PD deficiency, thalassemia, and lactose intolerance, alternative methods of supplying calcium in the adult diet may be necessary. Another consideration for the nurse is the theory that people from warmer climates have a more efficient heat production system and thus can better tolerate heat. In this case it is important to teach the client that overexposure to heat does have profound effects on the body. In addition, they should also be taught about risk factors for stroke as well as the signs and symptoms of a stroke.

Because of the concept that health results from the body's ability to help itself, the traditional East Indian Hindu American may discount Western medical practices while responding positively to traditional folk healing practices. It is important for the nurse to appreciate that these clients may believe that the treatment they receive for an illness is more likely to be effective if both a pill and a solution are prescribed. A physician who is aware of this belief may prescribe both types of medication because this is what the client believes will effect a cure.

SUMMARY

Nurses who work in a transcultural setting providing health care services to clients of East Indian descent and Hindu affiliation are challenged by the multiplicity of norms, mores, and values, all of which influence and shape the delivery of nursing acre. It is essential that the professional nurse and other health care providers use a holistic approach toward the assessment, planning, intervention, and evaluation of nursing care activities.

Case Study

Vaidya Chuttani is admitted to the hospital with a diagnosis of Cooley's anemia (thalassemia major). Although Vaidya is only 16 years old, she is a student at the local university. Vaidya speaks English, but she is experiencing difficulty communicating her needs to the health care team. Her family, which consists of her mother and father and five brothers and sisters, all reside in Bombay, India. Vaidya has not seen her family or talked with them for the 3 months that she has been enrolled in the American school. She tells the nurse that it is not unusual for some Indian families to allow their children to come to the United States to study at such a young age. In addition, she relates to the nurse that after she receives her degree, she will return to her country to assist her family by working and contributing to the family's monetary resources.

On admission, Vaidya's presenting complaints include (1) cholelithiasis as revealed on radiographic examination, (2) a right leg ulcer about 1 inch in diameter, (3) jaundice, and (4) an enlarged spleen as revealed on radiographic examination. The nurse notes the following on examination: blood pressure, 140/70 mm Hg; pulse, 88; respirations, 20; and temperature, 99.2°F.

CARE PLAN

✳ *Nursing Diagnosis: Communication, impaired verbal, related to cultural differences (recent arrival from India and use of English as a second language)*

Client Outcomes

1. Client will be able to communicate basic needs to health care personnel.
2. Client will relate feelings of acceptance, reduced frustration, and decreased feelings of isolation.

Nursing Interventions

1. Use gestures or actions instead of words to communicate information.
2. Use visual aids that will communicate to client necessary procedures to be done.
3. Write down messages in the hope that client can understand written English better than spoken English.
4. Obtain a translator, if necessary, to communicate important information.

✳ *Nursing Diagnosis: Tissue perfusion, ineffective: peripheral, secondary to Cooley's anemia related to decreased hemoglobin concentration in blood*

Client Outcomes

1. Client will verbalize activities that promote vasodilatation.
2. Client will verbalize factors that inhibit circulation.
3. Client will communicate existence of pain from right leg ulceration to health care professionals.

Nursing Interventions

1. Assess causative and contributing factors of right leg ulceration as related to Cooley's anemia.
2. Promote factors that will improve arterial blood flow and explain factors to client.

3. Encourage client to keep right leg in a dependent position and explain reasons.
4. Encourage client to change position every hour when in bed and discuss rationale.
5. Assess right leg in regards to pain and sensation.

Nursing Diagnosis: Health maintenance, ineffective, related to inability to make thoughtful judgments and lack of information about Cooley's anemia (thalassemia major)

Client Outcomes

1. Client will verbalize a willingness to comply with treatment regimen.

Nursing Interventions

1. Identify sociocultural factors that affect health-seeking behaviors.
2. Determine present knowledge of illness severity and prognosis.
3. Determine client's level and stage of adaptation to present condition (such as disbelief, denial, depression).
4. Using appropriate visual aids, describe necessity for blood transfusions to correct Cooley's anemia.

Nursing Diagnosis: Family processes, interrupted, related to separation from family because of schooling in another country

Client Outcomes

1. Client will verbalize fears and anxiety related to separation from family.
2. Client will identify support systems available within school and community and from external resources that will facilitate return to optimal health.
3. Client will verbalize desire to be involved in health care and scheduling of client-centered activities.

Nursing Interventions

1. Encourage client to express feelings related to being separated from her family.
2. Determine client's understanding of present medical condition.
3. Determine support systems available in school and community from external outside resources that will facilitate return to optimal functioning.
4. Involve client in care and scheduling of client-centered activities (such as wound care for right leg ulceration).

STUDY QUESTIONS

1. List other nursing interventions that can be implemented to facilitate communication between Vaidya and the health care team.
2. Describe the family structure of some East Indian Hindu families and the effect the family organization may have on health-seeking behavior, as well as how this may affect nursing interventions for Vaidya.
3. Describe why Cooley's anemia is perceived as a biological variation for East Indian descent.
4. Identify at least two other biological variations that are common to East Indian descent.
5. Identify how Vaidya's health-seeking behavior may be affected by time and space variables.

NCLEX-RN REVIEW QUESTIONS

1. In bathing an East Indian American client, the nurse should:
   A. Add hot water to cold water
   B. Add cold water to hot water
   C. Provide a bath after breakfast
   D. Have a family member assist with the bath

2. When a Hindu American client dies the nurse should prepare for the family to:
   A. Anoint the body with oils
   B. Cleanse the body
   C. Celebrate the passing of their loved one.
   D. Chant Hindu prayers to the soul

3. In providing morning care to a Hindu client, the nurse takes into consideration the very strict beliefs regarding:
A. Bathing
B. Medication
C. Drinking fluids
D. Body massage

References

Ali, S. (1989, November 1). *Personal communication.* (Dr. S. Ali was former district medical officer in Silon, Madhya Pradesh, India.)

Andrews, M., & Boyle, J. (2003). *Transcultural concepts in nursing care* (4th ed.). Philadelphia: Lippincott Williams & Wilkins.

Ashraf, K. M. (2000). *Life and conditions of the people of Hindustan.* New Delhi: Gyan Pub. House.

Bayer, J. M., & Gupta, A. (2006). Englishes in India. In *Language in India,* Retrieved May 28, 2006, from http://www.languageindia.com.

Bayless, T. M., Rothfield, B., & Massa, C., et al, (1975). Lactose and milk tolerance: clinical implications. *New England Journal of Medicine,* 292, 1156–1159.

Cavalli-Sforza, L. L., Menozzi, P., & Piazza, A. (1994). *The history and geography of human genes.* Princeton, N.J.: Princeton University Press.

Census of India. (2006). Retrieved May 28, 2006, from http://www.censusindia.net.

Census of India. (2002). Retrieved May 2, 2002, from http://www.censusindia.net.

Central Intelligence Agency. *World factbook.* (2006). Retrieved May 28, 2006, from http:// https://www.cia.gov/cia/publications/factbook/geos/in.html.

Central Intelligence Agency. *World Factbook.* (2002). Retrieved May 9, 2002, from http://www.cia.gov/cia/publications/factbook/geos/in.htm.

Chakravarty, A. (1978). *Quest for the universal one: great religions of the world.* Washington, D.C.: National Geographic Book Society.

Choudhry, U. (1997). Traditional practices of women from India: pregnancy, childbirth, and newborn care. *Journal of Obstetric, Gynecologic, and Neonatal Nursing,* 26, 533–539.

Corlett, W., & Moore, J. (1980). *The Hindu sound.* Scarsdale, N.Y.: Bradbury Press.

Dadabhay, Y. (1954). Circuitous assimilation among rural Hindustani in California. *Social Forces,* 33, 141.

Dash, V. B. (1974). *Ayurvedic treatment for common diseases.* Delhi: Delhi Diary.

Dill, E., Yousef, M., & Nelson, J. (1983). Volume and composition of hand sweat of White and Black men and women in desert walks. *American Journal of Physical Anthropology,* 61(1), 67–73.

Divine, R. (1972). *American immigration policy, 1924–1952.* New York: Da Capo Press.

Eshleman, J. (1992, November). Death with dignity: significance of religious beliefs and practices in Hinduism, Buddhism, and Islam. *Today's OR Nurse,* 19–20.

Eveleth, P. (1966). The effects of climate on growth. *Annals of the New York Academy of Sciences,* 134(2), 750–759.

Farver, J. A.M, Narang, S. K., & Bhadha, B. R. (2002). East meets west: ethnic identity, acculturation, and conflict in Asian Indian families. *Journal of Family Psychiatry,* 16(3), 338–350.

Fernandez, M. (1997). Domestic violence by extended family members in India: interplay of gender and generation. *Journal of Interpersonal Violence,* 12, 433–455.

Frisancho, A. (1981). *Human adaptation.* Ann Arbor: University of Michigan Press.

Guha, B. S. (1944). *Racial elements in the population of India.* Milfod: Oxford University Press.

Hall, E. (1990). *The hidden dimension.* New York: Doubleday.

Helweg, A. W., & Helweg, U. M. (1990). *An immigrant success story: East Indians in America.* Philadelphia: University of Pennsylvania Press.

Henderson, G., & Primeaux, M. (1981). *Transcultural health care.* Reading, Mass.: Addison-Wesley.

Information Please Almanac. (2007). Retrieved May 28, 2006, from http://www.informationplease.com. December 22, 2002.

Jee, H. H. (1981). *Aryan medical science: a short history.* Delhi: Maharaja of Gundal.

Kakar, D. (1977). *Folk and modern medicine.* New Delhi: New Asian Publishers.

Kluckhohn, F., & Strodtbeck, F. L. (1973). *Variations in value orientations.* Westport, Conn: Freeport Press.

Korom, F. J. (2001). Live like the banyan tree: images of the Indian American experience. *Journal of American Folklore,* 114(451), 70–73.

Koshy, S. (2001). Morphing race into ethnicity: Asian Americans and critical transformations of whiteness. *Boundary 2,* 28(1), 153–194.

Kurian, G., & Ghosh, R. (1983). Child-rearing in transition in Indian immigration families in Canada. *Journal of Comparative Family Studies,* 83, 132–133.

Kurien, P. (1999). Gendered ethnicity: creating Hindu Indian identity in the United States. *The American Behavioral Scientist,* 42(4), 648–670.

Larson, R., Verma, S., & Dworkin, J. (2001). Men's work and family lives in India: the daily organization of time and emotion. *Journal of Family Psychiatry,* 15(2), 206–224.

McKay, J., Hill, B., & Buckler, J. (2007). *A history of world societies* (ed. 7). Boston: Houghton Mifflin.

Medora, N. P., Larson, J. H., & Dave, P. B. (2000). East-Indian college students' perceptions of family strengths. *Journal of Comparative Family Studies,* 31(4), 407–425.

Melendy, H. (1977). *Asians in America.* Boston: G.K. Hall.

Miller, B. D. (1995, Spring). *Precepts and practices: researching identity formation among Indian Hindu adolescents in the United States: New Directions for Child Development.* San Francisco, Calif.: Jossey-Bass.

Moore, W. (1963). *Man, time and society.* New York: John Wiley & Sons.

Mukherjee, P. (1983). The image of women in Hinduism. *Woman's Studies International Forum,* 6, 375–381.

Murray, B. M., & Huelskoetter, M. M. (1991). *Psychiatric mental health nursing* (ed. 3). San Mateo, CA: Appleton & Lange.

Nossiter, B. (1970). *Soft state: a newspaperman's chronicle of India.* New York: Harper & Row.

Overfield, T. (1995). *Biological variation in health and illness: race, age, and sex differences* (ed. 2). Boca Raton, Fla.: CRC Press.

Pandian, J. D., Jaison, A., Deepak, S. S., Kalra, G., Shamsher, S., Lincoln, D. J., & Abraham, G. (2005). Public awareness of warning symptoms, risk factors, and treatment of stroke in northwest India. *Stroke,* 644–648.

Peck, M. F. (1981). The therapeutic effect of faith. *Nursing Forum,* 22(2), 153.

Potter, P. A., & Perry, A. G. (2001). *Fundamentals of nursing* (ed. 5). St. Louis: Mosby.

Pye, L. (1976). *Politics, personality, and nation building: Burma's search for identity.* Westport, Conn.: Greenwood Press.

Ramakrishna, J., & Weiss, M. (1992, September). Health, illness, and immigration: East Indians in the United States. *Western Journal of Medicine,* 157, 265–270.

Raman, S. A. (2001). Crossing cultural boundaries: Indian matriarchs and sisters in service. *Journal of Third World Science,* 18(2), 131–148.

Reddy, G. (1986). Women's movement: the Indian scene. *The Indian Journal of Social Work,* 46(4), 507–514.

Riggs, S., & Sargent, F. (1964). Physiological regulation in moist heat by young American Negro and White males. *Human Biology,* 36(4), 339–353.

Simons, B. (1976). *The volume library.* Nashville, Tenn.: Southwestern.

Singh, B. (1966). *The dialect of Delhi.* New Delhi: Lakherwal Press.

Singh, R. N., & Unnithan, N. P. (1999). Wife burning: cultural clues for lethal violence against women among Asian Indians in the United States. *Violence against Women,* 5(6), 641–653.

Sinha, D. (1977). Ambiguity of role-models and values among youth. *Indian Journal of Social Work,* 38, 241–247.

Spear, P. (1972). *India: a modern history.* Ann Arbor: University of Michigan Press.

Time almanac with information please. (2007). Boston: Information Please, Inc.

UNICEF. (2006). Retrieved May 28, 2006, from www.unicef.org/india/child_protection.

United Nations. (2006). Retrieved May 28, 2006, from www.un.org/english.

U.S. Department of Commerce. Bureau of the Census. (2006). Retrieved May 28, 2006, from http://factfinder.census.gov.

U.S. Department of Commerce, Bureau of the Census. (2002). *Population profiles by age, sex, race, and Hispanic origin.* Summary File 3, Washington, D.C.: Government Printing Office.

U.S. Immigration Commission. (1911). *Dictionary of races of people.* 63rd Congress, 3rd Session, pp. 52–54, 75–76.

Wagner, J. (1972). Heat intolerance and acclimatization to work in the heat in relation to age. *Journal of Applied Physiology,* 33(5), 616–622.

Warshaw, S. (1988). *India emerges.* Berkeley, Calif.: Diablo Press.

Wenzel, L. (1965). East Indians of Sutter County. *California Living,* 17, 3–15.

World almanac. (2007). New York: World Almanac Books.

World Hindu Council of America. (2006). Retrieved May 28, 2006, from www.vhp-america.org/aboutus.

Yang, F., & Edbaugh, H. R. (2001). Transformations in new immigrant religions and their global implications. *American Sociological Review,* 66(2), 269–288.

CHAPTER 20 Haitian Americans

Robert E. Cosgray

Behavioral Objectives

After reading this chapter, the nurse will be able to:

1. Describe the etiology of the Haitian Creole language.
2. Explain the tradition of spatial behavior often found among Haitian Americans.
3. Understand the Haitian family structure and the relevance to assimilation of Haitian Americans into the Western culture.
4. Describe the relationship of time and social class in Haitian Americans.
5. Identify the beliefs regarding Voodoo commonly found in the Haitian culture and how they pertain to healing.
6. Identify diseases that are prominent in Haitian American people.

The small republic of Haiti in the West Indies has a colorful but tormented history. To provide appropriate care to Haitian American clients, the nurse needs to have knowledge about the social and political turmoil that Haiti has experienced. In addition, the nurse should be aware of the difficulties that have surrounded migration as Haitians have sought sanctuary from their troubled homeland. It is only through an understanding of Haitian culture and health beliefs that the nurse can adequately meet the needs of Haitian American clients. In addition to discussing the land of Haiti, the immigration process, and the influence of the six cultural phenomena on nursing care of Haitian American clients, this chapter explores the struggles that Haitians have experienced in their attempts to assimilate the cultural traits of the dominant culture in North America.

OVERVIEW OF HAITI

Social History

Haiti (République d'Haïti) is situated in the western third of the island of Hispaniola. The other two thirds of the island is occupied by the Dominican Republic. Haiti is in the Caribbean Sea, with Cuba to the northwest, Jamaica to the southwest, and Puerto Rico to the east. Haiti, about the size of Maryland, is two thirds mountainous, and the rest of the country is characterized by great valleys, extensive plateaus, and small plains (*Time Almanac with Information Please*, 2007; *World Almanac*, 2007). Columbus discovered the island of Hispaniola on Christmas Eve in 1492, when his flagship, the Santa María, ran aground and was wrecked at Cap Haitien, a historic town on Haiti's northern coast. As the French took over the island, the native Indians were either exterminated or removed to Mexican gold mines. Black slaves were imported from Africa as the French became owners of flourishing sugarcane plantations. By 1681 there were 2000 slaves in St. Domingue, the French name for Haiti. A little more than 100 years later, there were at least 500,000 African slaves and some estimate as many as 700,000, compared with 40,000 Whites and 28,000 freemen of color—offspring of masters and slaves (Wilentz, 1989). Many slaves were newly imported because many died of overwork, beatings, disease, and undernourishment. The masters were obviously outnumbered, necessitating harsh measures to keep the slaves in line.

Interestingly, the African religions were seen as a source of resisting the French (Thomas, 1997). Although night ceremonies and dances were often forbidden, they continued and fomented the desire for power and freedom. Legend has it that one night the slaves on half a dozen plantations rose up and burned down their masters' homes, killing their masters. This revolt spread throughout the country, continuing for some 13 years. In 1802 Napoleon's troops landed at Cap Haitien, planning to recapture the island from the slaves and use it as a jumping-off place for an invasion of the United States. However, because of yellow fever epidemics, which assisted the Haitians in killing the French soldiers, the Haitians altered the course of world history, and the French admitted defeat. In 1804 Haiti was freed from France and became the second independent nation in the Western Hemisphere and the first independent Black republic in the world. According to Hobsbawn (1996), the failure of Napoleonic France to recapture Haiti was one of the main reasons why France liquidated its entire remaining American empire, which was sold by the Louisiana Purchase to the United States. Thus a consequence of the revolution in Haiti was to make the United States a continental world power.

Unfortunately, independence from France did not end the misery for the poor in Haiti. Although they were no longer slaves, the poor soon found that the oppressive French rulers had been almost immediately replaced by equally oppressive new Black rulers, the mulattos. With the advantage of money inherited from their French fathers, the mulattos became educated and wealthy and continued to monopolize Haiti's resources, with little regard for the social conditions of the poor (Seligman, 1977).

The American occupation, from 1915 to 1934, resulted in reorganization and improvements of the country regarding its road system, telecommunications, health care system, universities, banking system, and so on but did not effect permanent change. This assistance failed to solve the economic and social problems, and when the majority of

Americans left in the 1930s, the country once again regressed.

In addition to the attempt at revitalization by the Americans, François Duvalier, who came to power in 1957 and was to become president for life (Abbott, 1991), can be credited with initiating comprehensive programs to alleviate economic and technological problems. Unfortunately, Duvalier, preoccupied with wealth and power and the programs that were initiated, failed to have long-lasting effects, and the country's money was squandered. In 1963 Duvalier murdered countless enemies and managed to incur the wrath of Haiti's neighbor, the Dominican Republic, by harboring enemies of its new president. Upon his death in 1971, his son Jean Claude succeeded him. A drought in 1975–1977 brought famine, and in 1980 Hurricane Allen destroyed most of the rice, bean, and coffee crops. In 1986, following weeks of political unrest, President Jean Claude Duvalier fled Haiti aboard a U.S. Air Force plane. Democracy was attempted, but the country was soon taken over by a military coup (Masland, 1992). In 1991, the United States joined members of the Organization of American States in a regional embargo aimed at reinstating Haiti's first democratically elected president, Jean-Bertrand Aristide. The economic blockade led to a sharp downturn in an already poor economy. In July 1991, Aristide and the army signed an accord to return the exiled president to power. When the military leaders failed to resign, the United Nations reimposed an embargo. The embargo had a severe effect on the health of the population because it created difficulties in distributing aid and health care in Haiti. Although food and medicine are exempt from United Nations sanctions, an increase in AIDS, tuberculosis, and malnourishment among children occurred (Chelala, 1994). After Aristide's return to Haiti in October 1993, he quickly replaced the police force, downsized the military, and purged the officer corps. In 1996, René Préval, the winner of the second free election in the country's history, was sworn in as president of Haiti, with the UN Security Council remaining in the country to assist in maintaining peace. However, Préval had not even been sworn in

before supporters of Aristide urged his return to office (Rohter, 1996). In fact, Aristide's Lavalas Family party swept parliamentary and local elections, and in 2000 Aristide again became President. Other countries threatened Haiti with sanctions unless democratic procedures were strengthened. Aristide, once a charismatic champion of democracy, grew more authoritarian and seemed incapable of improving the lot of his people. In January 2004, violent protests rocked the country and demanded Aristide resign. In 2004, about 8000 peacekeepers from the United Nations Stabilization Mission (MINUSTAH) entered the chaos-engulfed country and assisted an interim government to take over. Tragically, flooding in May 2004 and Hurricane Jeanne in September 2004 killed more than 3400 (*Time Almanac with Information Please*, 2007; *World Almanac*, 2007). Continued violence and technical delays have prompted repeated postponements, and Haiti missed the constitutionally mandated presidential inauguration date of February 7, 2006 (*Central Intelligence Agency*, 2007). However, on May 14, 2006, Rene Préval was elected president in Port-au-Prince, and it is hoped that stability can be regained (Miami Herald.com; United Haitians Home Page, 2006).

Not only has there been social and political unrest in Haiti but also this has contributed to despoiling the land. In 1996, it was estimated that only 2% of the country is forested and more than half of the land has been destroyed by erosion (United Nations Program Development, 1996). The remaining agricultural land is capable of producing food for only half of the population. Still, Haitian farmers continue to despoil remaining land by removal of roots and stumps for charcoal manufacture to heat their cooking stoves in order to survive. The lack of farming land in the country has resulted in dependence on food from foreign aid (Hiebert, 1997). There are at present efforts in the country by charitable groups to assist the country economically. One example of this is the Mennonite Economic Development Association, which has 20 paid staff who assist Haitians in developing their own small business by giving them small loans for start-up money. This organization has been very effective in helping hardworking Haitians have a chance to be self-supporting (Claude, 1997). The Mennonite Central Committee has also had workers doing projects, including producing seedlings in 20 community-based tree nurseries (Dening, 2001).

Life in Haiti

Today, Haiti is an independent republic with 8,121,622 inhabitants (2006 estimate) (*World Almanac*, 2007). Between 90% and 95% of the population is descendants of West African slaves; 5% of the population are mulatto and White, while 95% are Black. Fifty-three percent live in rural settings, 37% live in urban settings, and 10% are overseas. Haiti is considered to be the poorest nation in the Western hemisphere, with a gross domestic product of $12.1 billion (2004 estimate) and a per capita income of $1700 (Central Intelligence Agency, 2007). However, other estimates of the income for most rural Haitians is probably more realistically set at $1.26 a day (Cowley, 2002), with 80% living below the poverty line. Haiti's real economic growth rate is −3.5%, with an inflation rate of 22% (*Time Almanac with Information Please*, 2007); this has dramatically decreased the purchasing power of the population. In 2000, the local currency drastically declined in value, dropping from 16 to 22 gourdes per U.S. dollar (Dening, 2001) and further plummeting to 41.87 in 2005 (*World Almanac*, 2007).

More than two-thirds of the labor force does not have formal jobs, and there is widespread unemployment and underemployment (2002 estimate) (*Time Almanac with Information Please*, 2007). Some 92% of the population live in small, rural hamlets in small straw shacks without light, water, or windows. In sharp contrast to the destitute living situations is the pride of the Haitians, their value of self-respect, and their strong work ethic. Much time is spent daily in washing clothes, and at the beginning of each day the typical Haitian has clean and often ironed clothing (Hiebert, 1997).

Although the issues and problems confronting the people of Haiti are similar to those of many other countries, they seem to be more numerous and more intensified. The country is drastically overpopulated, with a density of 758 persons per square mile (*Time Almanac with Information Please*, 2007). The annual population growth rate is 2.3%. The life expectancy is 52.9 years overall, 51.6 years for males, and 54.3 years for females. The birth rate is 36.6 per 1000 and the death rate is 12.3 per 1000. Infant mortality is 73.5 per 1000. Haiti has a young population: 42.4% of the population is 0 to 14 years old, and the median age is 18.2 years (Central Intelligence Agency, 2007).

Haiti has numerous unresolved obstacles to public hygiene, including an inadequate water supply for 77% of the rural population and 62% of the urban population. There is inadequate access to sanitation for 64% of the rural population and 59% of the urban population. Some 80% of the population suffers from malnutrition. Health care services are lacking throughout Haiti. A national health service is responsible for the medical care of the population, but only 50% of the population (47% of the rural population) has access to health care. There is one physician for 8800 people and one nurse for 8600 people. This is even more problematic than it appears because most of the physicians are on the government payroll and are disproportionately concentrated in the capital city, Port-au-Prince (United Nations Program Development, 1996).

Health care is also provided by private foundations such as the Mellon Foundation, which sponsors the Hôpital Albert Schweitzer in central Haiti. To make health care more available to the people, small medical teams go out from this hospital into the rural areas to provide village-based health services. In this program, rural farmers, both men and women, are trained in primary health skills and provide direct services to clients. Health service delivered to the natives has resulted in a significant decrease in tetanus, which formerly ranked with tuberculosis and malnutrition as one of the three major health problems (Grant, 1989; Reichman, 1989; Stauffer, 2006; Westphal, 1989). However, although this hospital operates as a charity to the local people, it is not without exposure to the unrest in Haiti. For example, administrators are sometimes threatened that their family members will be harmed if they do not hire certain Haitians who come seeking employment (Venton, 1997). A number of nursing and medical schools in the United States use Haiti for transcultural experiences in a third-world setting (Gregg, 2001). Recently, nurses from the United States and Canada have gone to Haiti to assist with flooding and disaster recovery (Benedict, 2004; Barnard & Sincox, 2004; & Hardcastle, 2004).

IMMIGRATION TO THE UNITED STATES

Most of the immigrating Haitians in the early years were upper-class individuals who came to the United States as resident aliens. These upper-class Haitians were able to obtain permanent residence and citizenship with little difficulty and became assimilated into the dominant culture.

In 1980 an explosion of Haitian immigration took place as a result of a short-lived (April to October 1980) change in the U.S. immigration policy. More than 14,000 Haitian refugees landed on the shores of southern Florida in 1980 (Dempsey & Gesse, 1983), which includes the Mariel boatlift from Cuba. The influx of Cuban refugees required that a special status be created by the U.S. State Department, called "Cuban-Haitian entrant, status pending." Haitian refugees were included in this status to prevent the policy from being discriminatory (Metropolitan Dade County, 1981; Walsh, 1980). The "entrant" status described a temporary status and was used rather than granting the new arrivals political asylum. However, this "entrant" status placed the Haitian immigrants in a bureaucratic limbo that cannot lead to citizenship (Wilk, 1986).

The immigration policies changed in October 1980. A maritime interdiction program was initiated to turn back Haitian refugees at sea. Haitians who arrived in the United States were not classified as entrants but as parolees and were subject to deportation. Haitians were kept in detention along with Cubans while their cases were processed in the courts. Unlike other refugees arriving at the time (such as Indochinese refugees), resettlement was not guided by the federal government. The federal government's refusal to grant asylum deprived the refugees of benefits under the new 1980 Refugee Act. Emergency aid was limited, and most of it had lapsed by 1983 (Holcomb, Parsons, Giger, & Davidhizar, 1996). Lacking either jobs or government assistance, many refugees were compelled to rely on private charity and to invent jobs in a burgeoning "informal" economy in Miami. In 1991 mass migration of Haitians led to 34,000 Haitians being held at the U.S. Naval Base in Guantánamo Bay, Cuba, while their immigration status was determined (Lillibridge, Conrad, Stinson, & Noji, 1994). Numerous health problems, including active tuberculosis and AIDS, were addressed by the uniformed service medical support personnel (Bonnlander, 1996; Granich, Sfeir, & Jacobs, 1994). In 1993 the Supreme Court of the United States ruled that repatriation was legal and that illegal aliens could be returned to Haiti (Holcomb, Parsons, Giger, & Davidhizar, 1996). Despite this ruling, thousands of Haitians still attempt to enter the United States each year by trying to travel from Haiti to the United States by boat. Some have given all their money to private entrepreneurs and boarded barely seaworthy crafts for a chance to escape to a better life in the United States (Portes & Stepick, 1985). Many Haitians do not survive because the conditions at sea are too harsh or the boat is too full to permit safe travel. When weather conditions are too harsh, older Haitians have been thrown into the sea to lighten the load (Veeken, 1993). Still, perilous as the journey may be, many Haitians would rather try for the hope of the opportunities of living in the United States. Of those who do arrive, only a fraction (5%) are allowed to stay under the status of political refugees. The United States has steadfastly clung to a policy that makes it difficult for Haitians to meet the requirements for political refugee status. For example, since the immigration act of 1990, mandatory HIV testing with indefinite detention without treatment in HIV-positive detention camps has discriminatively singled out Haitians from other immigrants (that is, Cubans, Vietnamese, Chinese) and required that persons with HIV be held rather than "paroled" (Annas, 1993). In 1998, the Omnibus Budget Bill made changes in the Haitian Refugee Immigration

Fairness Act, which allowed amnesty for some Haitian immigrants in the United States (Isgro, 1998).

These waves of immigrants have resulted in four classifications or categories of Haitians in the United States: (1) citizens, (2) residents or legal aliens, (3) entrants, and (4) illegal aliens. Illegal aliens have all the pressures and fears of discovery, which could result in sudden deportation. Entrants, on the other hand, suffer from the uncertainty of whether they will be able to remain and from being unable to make permanent plans or feel entirely settled (Wilk, 1986). Because possibly half of the Haitians in the United States are here illegally, few programs exist to provide assistance. Some Haitians are understandably reluctant to discuss their difficulty, and they attempt to maintain a low profile with government agencies that might return them to Haiti. Another effect of an uncertain status in North America is infrequent use of health care services after immigration. The nurse should be aware that the Haitian immigrant probably will not seek medical treatment until the condition is severe or has become chronic (Bryan, 1988). The nurse should also be aware that hope is related to economic factors, and lack of economic assets results in feelings of hopelessness (Holt & Reeves, 2001).

Despite these difficulties and the possibility of deportation, many, primarily poor, Haitians continue to try to enter the United States. Those who do make it to North America are in one of the most at-risk populations now living in the United States. This high risk becomes actualized in several ways; for example, a study by Moskowitz, Kory, Chan, et al. (1983) reported unusual cases of death among Haitians residing in Miami and a high prevalence of opportunistic infections. The nurse should expect, when caring for a Haitian, that the client may never have had immunizations. If a client needs a tetanus immunization, it is unlikely that a tetanus booster is appropriate because the client probably has not received the series.

Adaptation of post-1980 Haitians to the dominant culture in the United States and Canada has been especially problematic because the proportion of refugees having a high school or college education and skills in English has declined. With limited education and money, many Haitians arriving in North America have been restricted to occupations such as migrant agricultural work and service industry jobs in restaurants and hotels (Eshleman & Davidhizar, 1997). Only a few of the more educated Haitians have been able to find work as mechanics and construction workers. Gaining the requirements needed to adjust to the urban, industrialized culture encountered in the United States and Canada is for most Haitians a stressful, overwhelming, and slow process because the people continue to cling to their cultural values and beliefs. Potocky (1996) noted that although many other refugees are faring moderately well in the United States, Nicaraguans and Haitians tend to be faring poorly. Assimilation to U.S. culture for Haitians has been particularly difficult. When they are compared with other groups, Potocky (1996) noted that Haitians on the average had a significantly lower economic status in regard to yearly earnings, percentage employed, and percentage never employed and living in poverty. A substantial proportion of Haitians arriving in the United States are children, who often arrive without their parents and are placed with extended family or in foster care (Office of Refugee Resettlement, 1993). Children who are with families face intergenerational problems. Children often experience a role reversal because they tend to more quickly adopt the language and culture of the United States and then must translate English for their parents. Because most of the asylum cases of Haitians are denied (U.S. Committee for Refugees, 1995), many Haitians in the United States are considered illegal aliens. Children who are denied asylum but remain in the country illegally have suffered from nonhumanitarian treatment even into their adult years. Whereas other immigrants have been welcomed, the lack of welcome experienced by many Haitians has had a negative effect (Fernández-Kelly & Schauffler, 1994). Haitians have not consistently received the same treatment as other asylum-seeking refugees. It was not until May 1995 that the Clinton administration reversed the *de facto* policy that granted virtual blanket asylum to all Cubans (Epstein, Lantigua, & Cavanaugh, 1995).

In 1975 Haitians could be found in 45 of the 50 states (Seligman, 1977). Large settlements of Haitian people are located in the southern and eastern parts of the United States, with 75% to 95% residing in Florida (Boswell, 1982; Wilk, 1986). New York City (especially Brooklyn) and Montreal have large, established Haitian communities that have mushroomed during times of revolution and political unrest in Haiti. For example, in 1960 there were reported to be 2584 Haitians living in New York City (Laguerre, 1984; Rosenwarke, 1972). It was estimated that 34,000 Haitians had arrived in the United States in 1968, and in 1970 it was estimated that 50,000 Haitians were living in New York City alone (McMorrow, 1970). According to the U.S. Census Bureau, in 2000, there were 548,199 people of Haitian descent residing in the United States (U.S. Department of Commerce, Bureau of the Census, Summary File 3, 2002). This census figure may underrepresent the true numbers because of the number of illegal aliens from Haiti. The Bahamas, which lie between Haiti and Florida, have been inundated with an estimated 60,000 Haitians who have failed in their attempt to cross the sea and instead have been shipwrecked on the vast Bahamian chain of some 700 islands (Fineman, 2001). Haitians report paying as much as $5000 for the privilege of the odyssey, only to land undetected on the tourist-dependent islands hoping to raise the fare to go on to Florida (Fineman, 2001).

Some Americans have been supportive of the plight of Haitians in Haiti and of the treatment of Haitians who have come to America (Barnes, 2000). In 2000, Haitian Americans marched in New York to protest policy brutality against Haitians in New York City and demanded the resignation of New York City Mayor Giuliani. Cases of mistaken identity have resulted in violence against Haitian Americans (Barstow, 2000). Others have protested deportation practices in which the Immigration and Naturalization Service has made Haitian immigrants who have received deportation orders choose between leaving their children in the

United States in hopes of giving them the opportunity for a better life or taking the children back to Haiti (Bragg, 2000).

COMMUNICATION

Issues related to communication present a variety of problems for Haitians living in the United States or Canada. In Haiti there are two official languages: Haitian Creole (Kreyòl) and French. French is the official national language and is understood and spoken only by the upper or wealthy class. Although Haitian Creole is the language of the rural or poor population, it is also the primary language and is understood and spoken throughout the country (Weil, 1973). Speaking only Haitian Creole, a hybrid of old French vocabulary and African grammar, is perceived as a sign of poverty and a lack of education. Both Haitian Creole and French are often spoken so fast that one word is slurred into another. Because many Haitian immigrants in the United States continue to combine Haitian Creole and French, a dialect undergoing further creolization has been created, and it creates language barriers for some Haitian immigrants because most people in the dominant U.S. society are unfamiliar with it.

Haitians frequently use hand gestures to complement their speech. Hand gesturing and tone of voice become more pronounced during communication. Primarily, hand gesturing is used as an addition to verbalizations. Touch and direct eye contact are also used in both casual and formal conversation. The Haitians' use of touch in conversation is perceived as friendship and does not violate personal space. Direct eye contact is used to gain the attention and respect of the other person during conversation. The Haitian cultural uses of touch and direct eye contact and the perception of friendship through conversation are much like those used throughout the United States.

Implications for Nursing Care

Language is often an area where problems arise between refugees and health care providers. One reason Haitians have received limited health care in the United States is the failure of many Haitians to speak either of the dominant languages: English or Spanish. Many schools in the United States have extensive bilingual programs for native Spanish speakers but have paid little attention to other non-English speakers. The problem of providing bilingual education for Haitians is complex and begins with a lack of materials for teaching English to Haitian Creole speakers. There are also varying opinions on the best way to teach literacy skills. Some persons believe that Haitians who have immigrated to the United States must be taught literacy in their native language. The view is that if Haitian Creole is used as a teaching tool, it can facilitate acquisition of reading and writing skills in English (Dejean, 1983).

The nurse should promote the Haitian American client's interest in gaining English-language skills to facilitate the client's adjustment to the dominant culture. Although most Haitians are eager to learn English, learning to read and write as an adult is often difficult and time consuming, and support from health care professionals can encourage the Haitian individual to stick with this difficult task. Many Haitians who use French as their primary language have retained it, even though they have made a permanent move to the United States or Canada. Although many in the United States and Canada share the French-speaking Haitian's view that French is the language of the culturally elite, it should be noted that French-speaking Haitians have as much difficulty learning English as any other non-English speakers do.

If the client does not speak English, the nurse should first determine what language the client does speak. If the nurse does not know Haitian Creole or French, an interpreter may be necessary. When possible, a bilingual family member can help convey to the client and nurse information essential to health care. The nurse may find that Haitian Americans with children are more likely to speak correct English because speaking correct English is a status symbol and parents who know English will usually speak correct English in the home. The nurse caring for a Haitian American client should be aware that Haitians value a touch or a smile by the nurse as a sign of friendship. Nonverbal communication

can assist in bridging gaps between the differences in language because it can facilitate an understanding of client needs.

Haitian Americans who have newly arrived from Haiti may be unfamiliar with modern technology, including use of the telephone since Haiti has only 140,000 main lines, many of which may be down for a month after a rain (*Time Almanac with Information Please*, 2007). Access to the Internet is new in Haiti, with only four local servers and limited satellite links. It is estimated that fewer than 5000 Haitians have access to the Internet and that limited numbers have the skills to use a computer (Corbett, 1999).

SPACE

Personal space to the Haitian can be defined as a public zone. Haitians as a cultural group are a sharing population. If they possess something that another person could or might benefit from, it will be shared. Another factor that tends to make the culture a public zone is the closeness of the living arrangements or dwellings. As a result, the Haitians are a public-oriented society. Haitians in the United States, for the most part, usually socialize with other immigrants arriving from their own town in Haiti and maintain primary loyalty to family members, many of whom remain in Haiti. Legal immigrants look forward to spending holidays in Haiti and regard the allowed time each year as a focal point. Illegal aliens are more isolated because they cannot maintain family contact. This represents a great change from the lifestyle led in Haiti, where extended family and the closeness of the community are emphasized.

Implications for Nursing Care

It is important for the nurse caring for a Haitian American client to know that data from studies have indicated that Haitians find touch by caregivers to be supportive, comforting, and reassuring (Dempsey & Gesse, 1983). In a study of 10 women, Dempsey and Gesse noted that there were diverse views on whether these women preferred to be touched during delivery and if the preference was for a man or woman to touch them. In the study two women specified a preference for being touched by a woman, three preferred to be touched by a man, and three did not have a preference. Nine stated that the father should be present. What is implied by this is that Haitian women may be less likely than women from some cultural groups to insist on having female nurses in the delivery room.

Although Haitians and African-Americans share a heritage that extends back to Africa, the two groups do very little social mixing and tend to mistrust each other (Dempsey & Gesse, 1983). It is important for the nurse to understand that just because two clients may be Black does not mean they will share common interests or find each other suitable companions for sharing a hospital room. Some Haitians, like some other people from other social groups, are not free of social prejudice. Appreciation of these cultural socioeconomic issues by the nurse will facilitate assignment of staff to care for Haitian clients as well as room assignments of clients.

Because of the large gap in social classes, it is important for the nurse to consider the economic background of Haitian American clients before placing them in the same area. For example, a poor client and a wealthy client with a Haitian background, though from the same country, may find a room assignment together in a hospital very distasteful.

SOCIAL ORGANIZATION

Social Class

The Haitian masses are essentially divided into two class structures: the wealthy and the poor. Statistically, 85% of the Haitian population is classified as poor, 10% as middle class, and 5% as wealthy (Bell, 1981). Class is demonstrated in many interesting ways. Wearing shoes is a requirement by law in the capital city, but many Haitians, especially in the small towns and villages, go barefoot. This is by no means a matter of choice but a mark of social standing. As an illustration of this, a Haitian physician who was enjoying a little recreation in one of the small towns was told that a client was waiting for him nearby. The physician asked if the client had shoes on. What was implied in this question was that if

the client had shoes on, the physician would be obliged to go immediately. On the other hand, if the client did not, the client would be in for a wait (Jeanty, 1989). Regardless of class, Haitians are a proud and independent people.

Education

Education in Haitian schools differs greatly from that in American schools. Until 1979 French was the only officially recognized language and the language that was required to be used in school. The educational system and schools are strict and authoritarian. Children who are financially able to attend must wear starched uniforms. The Haitian teacher has the right to use corporal punishment on a misbehaving child. Thus the lack of structure and discipline of many American schools meets with disapproval from Haitians. Much of the information given to students in the Haitian schools is memorized; memorization through repetition is the primary source of learning. Haitian children can be heard reciting multiplication tables through rhyme and song throughout the community. Sheer repetition of the same formula, problem after problem written on the blackboard, manages to register the information in the student's mind. Haitian teachers enunciate clearly when communicating with their students (Verdet, 1985).

Rather than attend the public high schools, Haitian Americans prefer to remain out of the mainstream of education and often strive to accelerate the educational process and obtain the credentials they value by seeking a high school equivalency diploma. Haitian Americans view a college education as a form of prestige and status.

Family

The commonality among Haitians in Haiti and Haitians in the United States, whether wealthy or poor, is family. The family structure or system is very different from that of the American system. The practice of common-law marriage is predominant, particularly among the poor. Most legal marriages occur among the wealthy as a result of their economic status. Common-law marriage gives the father of the family much freedom and imposes much of the responsibility of caring for and meeting the needs of the family unit on the mother. The father, perhaps dividing his time between several family units, becomes a powerful but unreliable figure. The concept of a single-parent family, primarily the single mother, is similar to that in the United States but more prevalent in Haiti. The Haitian mother is commonly left to raise the children without the support system of the father.

The term *plaçage* may be defined as the union of a man and woman who desire to live together and who fulfill certain obligations and perform certain ceremonies at the home of the woman's parents, after which a new household is established. These unions are said to endure as long as recognized church marriages and constitute two thirds of all unions in Haiti (Herskovits, 1971; Schaedel, 1962). Haitian women involved in *plaçage* can be classified into four groups according to their relationship with Haitian men:

1. *Femme caille* (common-law): a woman who shares her home with a man in a common-law marriage situation.
2. *Mama petite* ("mother of my children"): a woman who is the mother of some of the man's children but does not share his house. This is similar to some *plaçage* unions with children, but in this situation the husband continues to live with his first wife while maintaining the second relationship.
3. *Femme plaçage* (woman whom a man "goes with" or a friend): a woman who neither lives with nor has had children by a man but who shares his bed intermittently and often maintains a garden, usually furnished by him.
4. *Femme avec* (woman who is lived with): a woman with whom the man cohabits for pleasure and without firm economic ties (Williams, Murthy, & Berggren, 1975).

Affection from both parents is readily given to children, and physical punishment is given as a form of discipline. Haitian mothers rely less on parent–child dialogue and more on physical punishment to effect changes in the child's behavior and to instill proper attitudes and values (Charles, 1979). Although Haitian mothers are extremely affectionate with their children, the children are taught from infancy that there is an unquestioned obedience to adult wishes. Haitian children do not presume to question parents or seek information concerning matters such as sex education because this would be seen as disrespectful of adult authority (Bestman, 1979). Childrearing is shared by siblings as well as by the parents.

The Haitian family is traditionally extended, with each dwelling or residence paralleling a small community. Outside the extended family, godparents play a very important role in the family organization and are generally considered part of the natural family. Rural or poor families tend to be matriarchal and child centered, with parents exercising strong influence and authority over their offspring, even when the children are grown. Haitians view their children as direct reflections of themselves and the family. If children fail to fulfill obligations or meet expectations, they are seen as having failed the family and as having brought disgrace on the parents (Desantis & Thomas, 1987). Because of the parent–child ties, many Haitian couples separate only temporarily when immigrating. The wife usually immigrates with the younger children, and the husband remains in Haiti with the older children until the entire family can obtain authorization to relocate. One-parent families are quite common among this immigrant group in the United States. Immigrants often lack support of extended families in child rearing (Prudent, Johnson, Carroll, & Culpepper, 2005).

DeSantis and Ugarriza (1995) investigated Haitian mothers and their childrearing practices. They identified the need for psychiatric mental health nurses to assist immigrant Haitian families in handling intergenerational conflict because there are significant differences between the culture of origin and the culture encountered in the United States. Conflicts arise for children between what their parents say and what they see in the culture around them. Adolescent Haitians tend to fit the profile of high school leavers in that they are often poor and Black and live in households with high levels of stress. Social support for education is necessary if the adolescents are to remain in school (Rosenthal, 1995).

Traditionally, Haitian parents have a strong voice in their children's selection of a mate and in their choice of a career. Haitians tend to be an extremely status-conscious group and desire marriages or careers that enhance the status of the family. For most Haitian immigrants in the United States, home ties to Haiti remain strong. Even though there may be little opportunity for travel back and forth because of cost and the illegal status of many, ties to the motherland and home remain. Letters, packages, and money are sent regularly. Because many Haitians are illiterate, sending cassettes to relatives in the United States or home to Haiti is a common form of communication (Jeanty, 1989).

Some older Haitian immigrants have been found to depend more on the members of their social support network than other Haitian age groups (Degazon, 1994; Seabrooks, 1992). The older immigrants experienced more changes in life events and loss of network members because of age, in addition to problems associated with migration. The older Haitian immigrants also reported that they encountered hostility and stress because of their African heritage and skin color (Seabrooks, 1992). On the other hand, Robinson (1994) reported that aides in nursing homes caring for Black clients from three cultural groups were generally positive toward the elderly but negative toward the families of the elderly residents who did not take care of the elderly at home. Findings indicated the need for education for aides related to differences among people in different cultural groups.

Implications for Nursing Care

Cultural factors related to social organization have an important influence on health and health care behavior. Fundamental norms, such as the desirability of having many children and the traditional roles of men and women, affect reproductive behavior. Because the legal status of many is either questionable, as for entrants, or undesirable, as for illegal aliens, Haitians frequently use different names, giving one name at one clinic and another

name at another clinic. In addition to causing confusion to health care providers, this practice leads to people "falling through the cracks" because of records not being available. Consequently, there is a loss in continuity of care for some Haitian clients. In addition, because of the repeated intake procedures on the same client, health care services may be delayed (Wilk, 1986).

An astute nurse should keep in mind that because the Haitian family is traditionally extended, the opinions and ideas of the family must be incorporated into a culturally sensitive plan of care. It is also important to remember that because Haitian children are taught from infancy to be unquestionably obedient to adult wishes, it is especially important to provide parents with adequate health education if children are to benefit from improved and knowledgeable health care.

The nurse should also be aware that bisexuality may be an occurrence among Haitian men. Even when this information is important, the client may not readily offer it. The nurse may need to elicit this information by asking if the client has ever had sex with another man, rather than using the labels of homosexuality or bisexuality (Laguerre, 1981; Randall-David, 1989).

Immigrant Haitian mothers have been found to believe that little can be done to avoid childhood illnesses considered medically preventable in the United States (DeSantis & Thomas, 1992). Many Haitian mothers adhere to the beliefs and practices of Haitian folk medicine because they have not been taught or do not believe in preventive health care. This has important implications for the health education of parents and children (DeSantis & Thomas, 1992). DeSantis and Thomas (1992) found that nurses were considered the best persons to do health teaching. Teaching is valuable when it is understandable, is practical, reinforces parenting abilities, and allows time for questions.

TIME

Traditionally, Haitians have not been committed to time or a schedule. It is not considered impolite to arrive late for an appointment. Everyone and anything can wait. Nelson (2002), a Haitian business consultant in Florida, describes how present-time orientation, which might include conducting a personal conversation rather than waiting on a customer, can cause Haitian-owned businesses in the United States to fail. On the other hand, some Haitian Americans have learned to compensate for lack of time orientation by manipulating timing of activities. For example, a wedding invitation will show a starting time of 6 P.M. when the actual starting time is actually 7 or 7:30 (Colin, 2005).

The time orientation of Haitian Americans is related to social class. Poor or lower-class Haitian Americans tend to be relatively past- and present-time oriented because they find it necessary to live from day to day, looking for food and trying to sustain a meager living. Because of their economic and educational status, the future for some of these people remains bleak. If a poor Haitian American has little to no chance of getting ahead, it is unlikely that a future-time orientation will be developed.

On the other hand, wealthy Haitian Americans may perceive time from a totally different perspective. For these people, time orientation may be a combination of both present and future orientations. It would appear that as a result of adequate financial resources, upper-class Haitians and Haitian immigrants do make plans for the future. Because wealth may ensure educational attainment, which may translate into status and prestige, it is likely that a well-educated upper-class Haitian may have a future-time orientation.

Implications for Nursing Care

Because Haitians may have different orientations to time, depending on their social status and class, it is important for the nurse to adequately assess each individual client. It is also important for the nurse to remember that personal ethnocentric attitudes toward time may negatively affect planning care for clients. Persons with a present-time orientation may view future-oriented tasks as irrelevant or unimportant to present situations. Thus a present-time orientation may restrain a Haitian from gaining upward mobility because future-time orientation is required in gaining an education and planning to achieve future goals. It is also

important to remember that when a Haitian immigrant does not keep an appointment or does not arrive for a clinic appointment on time, it may be a result of both a present-time orientation and economic constraints. It is important for the nurse to assess not only the time variable but also other socioeconomic variables, including the availability of transportation to and from clinic appointments. If a Haitian American is to arrive at clinic appointments on time, it is very important for the nurse to emphasize the importance of adhering to the clinic's schedule. The nurse should be aware that Haitian Americans frequently stop a treatment regimen as soon as the symptoms appear to be relieved. It is also very likely that the Haitian American will fail to follow through with a treatment regimen or preventive health care because cultural beliefs do not relate personal actions to health status.

ENVIRONMENTAL CONTROL

Although Haitians and African-Americans share a lineage that extends back to Africans who were seized from their countries and enslaved, some individuals have surmised that these two cultural groups fraternize very little socially and tend to mistrust and be suspicious of each other (Wilentz, 1989). It is believed that Haitians place a high value on personal liberty and are therefore resentful of American prejudice and at times indignant and critical of African-Americans, whom they discern as too submissive and accepting of discrimination (Wilentz, 1989). At the same time, African-American militancy and violent protest seem to be contrary to the Haitian personality and are generally regarded by Haitians with disapproval (Wilentz, 1989).

Traditionally, the upper classes in Haiti have been the lighter-skinned Blacks, whose skin color results from crossbreeding with lighter-skinned people. Light skin traditionally has been regarded as more prestigious than dark skin in Haiti (Leyburn, 1980), with the upper-class, lighter-skinned Haitians dealing with the lower-class, darker-skinned persons in an authoritarian manner. Therefore, because of indoctrination regarding the color of the skin and its perceived relationship to social status or class, some Haitians have developed a social prejudice that causes difficulty in the assimilation process in the United States. As a result of social prejudice formed by such variables as color grading and social status, some Haitians living in the United States or Canada continue to have trouble adjusting to other groups and thereby choose to remain in isolated areas, socializing only with other Haitians and family members.

Some Haitians view illness and disease as natural or unnatural events. Natural events keep balance between nature and humankind and as such are believed to be designed by God. Natural laws are believed to give life predictability (Snow, 1981). Unnatural events are believed to upset the balance of nature and at their worst represent forces of evil and the devil. Unnatural events lack predictability because they exist beyond the parameters of nature and are beyond the control of "mere mortals." This view is in sharp contrast to traditional Western medical beliefs. It is essential that the nurse remember that some Haitians believe illness is a result of witchcraft. People who supposedly possess supernatural power are believed to be able to alter the health status of others (Snow, 1981).

Voodoo Practices

The practice of Voodoo, the primary religion in Haiti, is prevalent throughout the country. Voodoo is a religious cult practice that dates back to the preslavery days in the West African homeland (Miller, 2000). Today, the term *voodoo* is commonly used both as a derogatory term by non-Haitians to describe the illogical and unexplainable and as a catchword of ethnomedical or ethnoreligious beliefs that involve magic and spirit possession (Miller, 2000).

In the 1600s, slavery was rationalized by the Code Noir, instituted by Louis XIV, by mandatory evangelization on arrival to a French colony (Thomas, 1997). Catholicism was implemented by required religious assemblies. Nevertheless, the outlawed African religious practices were loosely incorporated, as the slaves identified their deities with the saints of the Catholic church. European religious and decorative objects were also

incorporated, allowing the slaves to appear nominally Catholic while still preserving the basic structure common to West African religious systems (Mena, 1996). However, when the sovereignty of the country was not recognized by the Catholic church from 1804 to 1858, the Catholic church forbade priests to enter the country, and all ordained priests were ordered to leave. During this time, Voodoo flourished and became the dominant belief practice. In 1860, partly as a result of the spread of Protestant missions on the islands, a concordat was approved in Rome, a bishop was consecrated in Port-au-Prince, and Catholicism was once again the official religion recognized by the state. Nevertheless, the new priests sent by the church faced an ineradicable folk religion and a people who were able to reconcile living with two parallel albeit often contradictory spiritual beliefs systems (Laguerre, 1989; Mena, 1996; Miller, 2000). Today, the majority of Haitians combine some degree of both Voodoo and Christianity (Mena, 1996).

Today many Haitians still believe that man is surrounded or enveloped by a variety of powerful, dominant spirits and that it is essential to invoke spirits. In the Haitian culture, the invoked spirits are called *loas*, *mystères*, or saints. Some Haitians believe that Voodoo spirits manifest and reveal themselves by possessing or "riding" the devoted believer. It is believed that the personality of the *loa* "mount" may change; he or she may be calm and subdued one minute and then suddenly become violent. Such transformations may be caused primarily by nervous instability under the influence of compelling drum rhythms and mass emotion (Logan, 1975). Haitians trust and depend on their Voodoo beliefs and also rely on "readers" or "diviners," who predict the future by reading cards or hands and cure by means of being possessed by the Voodoo spirit. The readers, or diviners, also considered Voodoo priests, are organized into independent cults.

Voodoo priests may be either male (*hungan*) or female (*mambo*) and are categorized into five classes: shaman (Voodoo practitioner), herbalist (*docte fey*, literally "leaf doctor"), midwife (*matronn*, or *fam saj*), bonesetter (*docte zo*), and injectionist (*pikirist*). Healers are often not well defined, and a Haitian may go to a neighbor who has "extra" medicine or a healing practice in hopes of relief. In terms of the number of practitioners and frequency of use, the herbalists constitute the most significant class of healers. Herbalists are the most generalized caregivers, and thus their role characteristics overlap to a certain extent with those of all other healer types (Coreil, 1983). Haitians often use home remedies and herbs for treating illnesses that are suggested by healers or priests. Many Haitians believe that tea made from leaves of the Bible will cure rheumatism. In this case, the Bible serves as protection against black magic, which is believed to cause rheumatism (Nida, 1954).

Magic powers may be used for purposes other than destroying enemies or healing the sick. The Voodoo sorcerers of Haiti claim to be able to change themselves into animals, to pass through locked doors, and to raise the dead and make them slaves (zombies). Almost everyone who is a native Haitian claims to know someone who has been a genuine zombie. One man requested his family to cut his corpse into two pieces to be buried in separate graves for fear that the local sorcerer, who was his enemy, would bring him to life as a wretched slave. Although the Haitian government has no valid evidence of the existence of zombies, it sanctioned the belief by passing a law against the supposed practice (Nida, 1954).

In Haiti, Voodoo is sometimes actualized as fetishes, which are shared by groups of native Haitians. For example, a Haitian might have a small bottle containing some reddish liquid and a small mirror backed by cardboard facing the bottle, and all this wrapped in coarse red cloth with yards of black thread. This object is safeguarded in the most remote part of the house, with its location kept secret from visitors. If the Haitian could be induced to talk about this, he might explain that his father, who was a kind of Voodoo priest, captured his soul when he was very young and put it in the bottle. As long as the bottle is preserved, the person will live, but once the bottle is broken, the soul will depart and the man must die. Not only would this fetish be held by this individual but also identical or similar fetishes might be shared by others in the community (Nida, 1954).

Many Haitian influences regarding Voodoo practices are evident in the mainstream of American society. For example, in some cities and towns in Louisiana, the Haitian influence is extremely prevalent and is perceived or felt by persons from other cultural groups as well. Louisiana is renowned for its Voodoo society, which is a carryover from Haitian slaves who were brought to areas such as New Orleans for various domestic duties. Even today, because of early Haitian influence, Voodoo and mystical thought remain evident regardless of ethnic or cultural background in cities such as New Orleans (Snow, 1981). Traditionally, some Haitians believed that a spell could be cast with the possession of a lock of the individual's hair (Calypso, 1999).

Although health care is a significant problem in urban Haiti, it is even more of a problem in rural Haiti, with pregnant and postpartum women being particularly vulnerable (Wiese, 1976). Many Haitians know nothing about prenatal care and do not routinely seek such care. Some may never have seen or been to a physician in their lives. Healers are related to protection, and physicians are related to sickness. Use of a midwife is culturally permissible and is much more likely among Haitian people than among other cultural groups in the United States. When a nurse is interacting with a pregnant Haitian woman or is providing care for a baby, using the phrase "We will help you have a strong baby" will often elicit cooperation. Staff who are willing to help the mother have a "strong baby" (rather than a "healthy baby") are more likely to be accepted (Jeanty, 1989).

Some pregnant Haitian women who experience an increase in salivation do not believe they should swallow the saliva. Sometimes they carry a "spit" cup with them and are not embarrassed to use it in public (Colin, 2005). Many dietary precautions are followed by the Haitian pregnant women.

Pregnant women are viewed as special and are likely to be treated with more kindness and respect than other women. Chants or sounds of a woman in labor include praying, singing, crying, and moaning in various combinations, which is done to call on their Voodoo protectors (Dempsey & Gesse, 1983).

A study conducted by Scott in 1978 identified the postpartum period as the most crucial and decisive period of childbearing for the Haitian woman. During the postpartum period of 6 to 11 weeks, the Haitian woman follows a cultural regimen of baths, teas, vapor baths (see below), and dressing warmly. This practice is supposed to make the client healthy and clean again after the birth. For the first 3 days, the mother bathes in hot water in which herb leaves have been boiled. She also drinks a decoction made from boiled herb leaves. (Also during the first few days after childbirth, the mother takes "vapor baths." She sits above a pot of steaming water with leaves in it, especially orange tree leaves, and drapes a cloth over her head and shoulders.) For the next 3 consecutive days, the mother takes her second series of baths, which are prepared with leaves in water warmed by the sun. At this point the mother drinks only water warmed by the sun or an infusion made with leaves steeped in water warmed by the sun. The mother takes constant special care to keep her body warm. She stays inside her dwelling for at least 3 days after the birth and keeps the doors and windows closed to keep out the cool air. She wears long sleeves, keeps her head covered, and wears heavy socks and shoes.

After 2 weeks to 1 month, the mother takes another bath. She may take a cold bath or perhaps jump into a cold stream. After this ritual, she may self-induce vomiting to cleanse her inner body. After all of this is completed, she can again resume normal activities and is considered clean (Harris, 1987).

The Miami Health Ecology Project (Scott, 1978) reported beliefs about menstruation among Haitians, a majority of whom believed the function of menstruation was to rid the body of "unclean," "waste," or "unnecessary" blood. Many Haitians also described menstruation in this manner: "It means you are a woman," with "woman" meaning that the individual has sexual feelings or needs and is not sterile. The Haitian girl reportedly learns

about menstruation at a median age of 10 years. For 85% of the sample, this information was obtained from their mothers or in classes at school.

Rituals Related to Death and Dying

Laguerre (1981) has studied patterns of bereavement among Haitian American families. Death arrangements are usually taken care of by a male kinsman of the deceased who has had experience with American bureaucracies. Death appears to mobilize the entire extended family, including matrilateral and patrilateral members. Because Haitians frequently believe that illness and death can be of a supernatural as well as natural origin (Métraux, 1953), death is often accompanied by feelings of guilt and anger. The surviving relatives may believe that the death was a result of failure to relate appropriately to the Voodoo spirit. Recurrent dreams of the deceased person, so much a part of grief work, take on a particular meaning to the Haitian. Haitians commonly evaluate illness in terms of symptoms previously experienced by close kin (Laguerre, 1981), and grief work frequently includes taking on symptoms of the deceased person's last illness (Eisenbruch, 1984).

Colin (2005) notes that health care professionals should tell the family spokesperson when death is imminent so family members can assemble at the bedside. Family members try to meet the spiritual needs of the dying person by religious medallions, pictures of saints, or fetishes/talismans for protection or as good luck for a peaceful death and restful afterlife. A kinsman usually makes the arrangements of telling the family and preburial arrangements, including purchase of a coffin and prayer services before the funeral. Traditional Haitians have seven days of consecutive prayer to assist the passage of the soul to the next world. This is terminated by a mass that begins the official mourning process.

Implications for Nursing Care

The nurse should be aware that the healing systems associated with Voodoo and Haitian ethnomedicine may be seen by some health care professionals as barriers to health care and even as adversely affecting health care (Carrazana, DeToledo, Tatum, et al., 1999). If Haitian Americans do use conventional means of health care, they tend to use emergency rooms or clinics and to seek health care only when they are quite ill (Orque, Bloch, & Monrroy, 1983; Samet, Retondo, Freedberg, et al., 1994). Haitian Americans may also seek relief from their symptoms through a physician and at the same time consult a cultural healer. The client's having both a faith healer and a physician should not be perceived as incongruent (Jeanty, 1989). A client's fear and anxiety that he or she has been "hexed" may be alleviated or reduced if the therapist combines conventional treatment with the assistance of a cultural healer who is believed to be able to remove the hex or spell. Nurses, as primary health care providers, must formulate and use a treatment plan that displays respect and understanding of the client's cultural healing system or systems and must accept that a Haitian American client may use a variety of sources to obtain relief when sick.

It is important for the nurse to understand that for many Haitians, leaves have a special significance. When the client comes into the hospital or the clinic for an examination, leaves may be found in the clothes and on various parts of the body. Leaves are believed to have mystical power, and therefore keeping them close to the body is related to regaining or keeping health (Jeanty, 1989). The nurse should be accepting of this practice and avoid being shocked if leaves are found in the luggage or on the body of a client being treated. The nurse should also appreciate that religious medallions, rosary beads, or figures of a saint to whom the Haitian client is devoted may have special significance and be felt to offer protection; they should be left with the client (Colin, 2005). The nurse should be cautious about forming negative judgments about a client who may have practices with Voodoo origins (Quillen, 1999).

Haitians have grown accustomed to receiving some direction from authority figures in their lives—parents as well as religious and social leaders. The nurse, as an authority figure, will usually find that Haitian Americans respond well to counseling approaches that foster self-help and independence and should consider the need for heightened self-esteem, which is manifested by the pride and willingness to work that is present in most Haitians.

Haitian Americans need to have occupational options expanded for them and need to understand the steps involved in achieving an occupational goal. Because Haitians have not traditionally had the freedom to set goals, the nurse may be of assistance in this process, as well as in problem solving, to achieve the established goals.

A variety of tools have been used to measure Haitians' beliefs about illness and wellness (Neilson, McMillan, & Díaz, 1992). Neilsen (1989) used a semistructured interview for three Black cultures, including Haitian. This work is ongoing (Neilsen, 1989).

BIOLOGICAL VARIATIONS

Body Size and Structure, Skin Color, and Other Visible Physical Characteristics

Haitians and African Americans are similar biologically. As with some other racial groups, the body size and structure of Haitians vary greatly. Haitians have no specific or distinctive size that can be linked genetically. This phenomenon may be a result of crossbreeding with other races throughout history. For this reason, Haitians can be short or tall, light skinned or dark skinned. Haitians are characterized as having shades of brown to black skin as well as brown to black eyes. The hair on the head is often tightly curled, and the body hair is sparsely distributed. The "true" Haitian is tall and exhibits an erect stature. The skull is dolichocephalic in form, being long and relatively narrow. The eyebrow ridges are scant or absent, and the forehead is moderately wide. The form of the orbits is almost square, and their margins are strongly built. The cheeks are wide and, with their supports or zygomatic arches, are bowed laterally in keeping with the powerful jaw musculature. The eyes are set widely apart by the broad and flattened nasal bones. The nose is flat, and the nostrils are widely expanded. The face is large and prominent. The jaws are prognathic and covered by full, fleshy lips, the prominent mucosae of which are reddish black or purple in color (Godsby, 1971).

Some years ago, anthropologists and scientists discovered that two different types of earwax are present among the human race and that the composition of the earwax determines racial origin. Haitian earwax is described as moist and adhesive (Godsby, 1971).

Susceptibility to Disease and Other Health Concerns

Several major areas of health concerns have been identified in the Haitian culture, including intestinal problems, malnutrition, venereal disease, high birth rate, tuberculosis, sickle cell anemia, hypertension, and cancer. AIDS has also become a serious and increasing health issue for Haitians since the 1970s both in Haiti and in the United States.

Intestinal Problems and Malnutrition. Intestinal problems stemming from malnutrition and ranging from stomach ailments to peptic ulcers are common. The peasant Haitian suffers more from these types of ailments than the wealthy or elite Haitian does. Typically, the Haitian diet tends to be very spicy and greasy. Haitians cook almost everything in oil or grease. Even after immigration to the United States, some Haitians continue to prepare foods that are spicy and greasy.

In Haiti the poor Haitian will consume virtually any type of food to sustain human life. Because many Haitians who have immigrated to the United States have remained at or below the poverty level, they will most likely continue to consume any type of food available. Chronic abdominal discomfort is primarily caused by parasites that are common to the Haitian population (Wilk, 1986).

Venereal Disease. Another problem is venereal disease. Haitian men tend to be more susceptible to different kinds of venereal diseases as a result of promiscuity (Jeanty, 1989). Because most marriages are common-law, the man of the family generally lacks commitment to one woman and usually has more than one sexual partner. In addition, the venereal disease is difficult to treat because the medication is usually taken only as long as the symptoms persist. Premature discontinuation of medication results in an incomplete cure. The problem of venereal disease is also extremely difficult to treat

because Haitians do not equate venereal disease with sexual intercourse.

Because there are numerous illegal Haitian immigrants, the prevalence of venereal disease among Haitians in the United States is likely, but the extent is unknown. Testing for syphilis has been required since the Immigration Act of 1990 (Herip, 1993). When Haitians were interdicted at sea and subsequently tested, 5% of Haitians had serological evidence of past or present syphilis (Herip, 1993).

High Birth Rate. The high birth rate has many health and cultural implications for Haitians. One factor contributing to the population explosion is the lack of contraception, which is virtually nonexistent in the conventional manner. This is attributed to a lack of education and technology. An unusually large number of very young Haitian women become pregnant (Jeanty, 1989), and Haitian women also tend to become pregnant at older ages. Pregnancy in women 35 years of age and older in Haiti is fairly common (Wilk, 1986). Williams, Murthy, and Berggren (1975) reported that Haitian women between 35 and 49 years of age have an average of eight pregnancies. Because of this pattern, the nurse must be aware of the high risk among Haitian women in relation to their childbearing habits. Furthermore, family spacing is not an option, and a series of pregnancies within a short time leaves the woman's body unable to fully recover or replenish iron levels.

Tuberculosis. Tuberculosis is another concern to the Haitian population. As a result of the poor economic levels, which lead to poor living conditions and malnutrition, Haiti has one of the world's highest rates of tuberculosis (Wilk, 1986). Another factor is overcrowding, which results in poor sanitation. The majority of the population has no waste facilities. Garbage and human excrement are thrown into the streets or placed in community pits, and the water for drinking is contaminated, resulting in a vast number of diseases, including tuberculosis. Malnutrition complicates the situation. The poor cannot afford the cost of examination or the medication to treat the illness if it is diagnosed. Of the number of Haitians who attempted to immigrate to the United States from

November 1991 to April 1992, 55% tested positive for tuberculosis on a purified protein derivative test. Chest radiographs confirmed pulmonary tuberculosis in approximately 5% of this group (Herip, 1993). Approximately one third of those testing positive had findings suggestive of active infection. In 21% of the cases, culture and sensitivities for tuberculosis isolates were found to be resistant to medication. Because there is a high incidence of tuberculosis among Haitian immigrants, assessment for symptoms of tuberculosis is an important part of health screening when the nurse is caring for Haitian clients.

Sickle Cell Anemia. Sickle cell anemia, or Hb S disease, is a chronic hereditary hemolytic disorder mainly affecting the Black populations of the world and is characterized by the presence of erythrocytes that primarily contain Hb S instead of Hb A. The red blood cell assumes a sickle shape when exposed to lower oxygen levels. Persons who are homozygous for Hb S are estimated to have erythrocytes that contain 80% to 100% abnormal Hb S and only up to 20% normal Hb A. The erythrocytes of persons with sickle cell trait contain approximately 25% to 40% Hb S and 60% to 75% Hb A.

Sickle cell anemia develops as a result of a genetic mutation that is transmitted from parent to child. Laboratory testing is available to determine if the sickle cell trait is present (Sorensen, Luckmann, & Bolander, 1994). It is important for the nurse to have a working knowledge of sickle cell anemia when assessing Haitian American clients and to be able to refer the client to a sickle cell association or support group. It is important to provide the client with information about this illness because most of these clients know little about it (Jeanty, 1989).

Hypertension. Little is known about hypertension among Haitians. A pilot study was conducted with 88 Haitian clients by Preston, Materson, Yoham, and Anapol (1996). This study indicated that hypertension was highly prevalent and unusually severe in terms of blood pressure level, refractoriness to treatment, and target organ consequences.

Malaria. *Plasmodium falciparum* malaria was a major problem among displaced Haitians in temporary camps at the U.S. Naval Base, Guantánamo Bay, Cuba. From December 1991 to March 1992, 235 cases of unmixed falciparum malaria were diagnosed, giving a cumulative attack rate of 160 per 10,000 camp residents. Health professionals in treating Haitian immigrants should plan for malaria, and preventive medicine measures are indicated (Bawden, Slaten, & Malone, 1995).

Cancer. Cancers reported in Haiti include cervical, hepatic, stomach, and intestinal cancer and Kaposi's sarcoma (Mitacek, St. Vallières, & Polednak, 1986). Cervical cancer accounts for 39% of all cancers among Haitian women and may be related to poor feminine hygiene as well as early sexual activity with multiple partners (Sebastian, Leeb, & See, 1978). Failure to have Pap smears, which would allow early detection, may relate to the high incidence of cervical cancer. Fruchter, Wright, Habenstreit, et al. (1985) reported that approximately 50% of Haitian women had never had a Pap smear, compared with 25% of the English-speaking Caribbean immigrants and 10% of U.S.-born Black women studied. In a study by Consedine, Magai, Spiller, Neugut, and Conway (2004), Haitian American women were found to be least knowledgeable about breast cancer and behavior that puts them at risk. Liver, stomach, and intestinal cancers are high among Haitian males. From 1979 to 1984, cancer of the liver (23.4%) and stomach and intestines (20.5%) accounted for 43.9% of all cancers (Mitacek, St. Vallières, & Polednak, 1986). Gastrointestinal cancer is related to the poor nutrition and low vitamin intake. Kaposi's sarcoma is found in some Haitians who are HIV positive. In a study with seven ethnic groups, American Haitian men were noted to report fewer digital rectal examinations and prostate-specific antigen tests than their counterparts. The importance of fear as a psychological determinant to male screening behavior must be considered in designing models to increase male screening frequency (Consedine, Morgenstern, Kudadjie-Gyamfi, Magai, & Neugut, 2006.)

AIDS. Cases of AIDS in Haiti are believed to date back to the late 1970s. Actual incidence is unclear, though Herip (1993) noted that 7% of Haitians interdicted at sea tested positive for HIV.

Unfortunately, Haiti is the country most heavily affected by AIDS in the Caribbean and accounts for more than 50% of all cases in the region. Because of the publicity of AIDS originating in Haiti, Haitians who have immigrated to the United States face constant discrimination. Samet, Retondo, Freedberg, et al. (1994) noted that most Haitian American clients presented for primary care with advanced immune dysfunction. Many had waited a year to initiate medical care after testing positive for HIV. The belief of the prevalence of AIDS in Haitians prompted the U.S. Centers for Disease Control and Prevention in Atlanta to list Haitians as one of the four high-risk groups for AIDS, along with homosexuals, hemophiliacs, and heroin users. Testing of Haitian immigrants for AIDS has been required since the Immigration Act of 1990 (Herip, 1993). Finally in 1991, Haitians were removed from the list. Though Haitians are no longer listed as a high-risk AIDS group, public opinion is slow to change. Tragically, the adult prevalence rate for HIV/AIDS is estimated at 5.6% in Haiti compared to 1% in the United States, with 24,000 deaths annually and 280,000 persons living with HIV/AIDS (2003 estimate) (Central Intelligence Agency, 2006; Key, DeNoon, & Boyles, 1998).

HIV/AIDS among Haitians and Haitian Americans is an illness highly related to cultural beliefs. Fitzgerald, Maxi, Marcelin, Johnson, and Pape (2004) conducted an investigation in Port-au-Prince and found issues related to the belief that HIV can be transmitted by magic, depression during counseling, and female fear of economic ruin and domestic violence related to notifying sexual partners could predict a patient's future adherence to risk reduction counseling and medical referral. However, health disparities can be reduced with culturally sensitive intervention. An integrated prevention and care project in Haiti by Devieux, Malow, Jean-Gilles, Samuels, Deschamps, Ascencio, Jean-Baptiste, and Pape (2004) indicated that since 1993 there was a 50% drop in incidence among pregnant women. Critical to culturally sensitive care is the

reduction of AIDS-related stigma. Preliminary data from research by Castro and Farmer (2005) indicated that with the introduction of quality HIV care, stigma can be reduced and willingness for testing increased.

Haitian American women are particularly vulnerable to health disparities. Santana and Dancy (2000) investigated the long-term effects of AIDS stigmatization in Haitian American women. This study noted effects in five categories: rejection by the dominant society, self-doubt, effect on self-esteem, effect on intimate relationships, and rejection by Haitians within the community. The damaging effect of stigma was found to permeate the lives of the women studied in myriad situations, either daily or on a very frequent basis. In the study by Samet, Retondo, Freedberg, et al. (1994), women presented with significantly higher CD4 cell counts than men did.

Health-illness beliefs are highly significant in intervention strategies. Martin, Rissmiller, and Beal (1995) conducted a qualitative study of health-illness beliefs and practices of Haitian Americans with HIV disease living in Boston. Five themes were identified: (1) incorporation of traditional health–illness beliefs into beliefs about HIV disease, (2) a perceived need to hide HIV disease to avoid rejection, humiliation, and isolation, (3) use of spirituality to help cope with HIV disease, (4) history of limited contact with doctors before diagnosis of HIV disease, and (5) use of traditional healing practices for HIV disease. Malow, Jean-Gilles, Devieux, Rosenberg, and Russell (2004) describe an HIV prevention study among Haitian youths in Florida with Haitian American adolescents. Self-efficacy, behavioral intentions, social factors, and acculturation issues all influence the risk behavior of Haitian American adolescents and can be influenced to reduce health disparity. Ellerbrock et al. (2004) conducted a population-based study in 1986 and 1998–2000 in a rural Florida community and found that HIV prevalence and risk factors can be changed positively with culturally sensitive interventions in the Haitian American communities.

Nutritional Preferences and Deficiencies

There is a critical problem with malnutrition in the agricultural areas of Haiti among the poor (Rodman, 1984). Some estimate that 80% of Haitians suffer from malnutrition (Haitians in America, 1983). For the Haitian peasant, environmental, technological, and economic factors alone account for a substantial amount of poor nutrition.

Haiti's rugged topography combines with a generally limited system of mass transport to accentuate the regional and seasonal nature of many of the crops. The economic status of most Haitians confines their food expenditures to a survival level of foods chosen from among locally produced foodstuffs. In addition, the humeral medical beliefs that classify food into "hot" and "cold" categories further restrict dietary selection (Wiese, 1976). Haitian Americans often combine "cold" foods, natural sedatives and purgatives from herbal medicine, religious treatments, and Western medicine in treating illness (Prudent, Johnson, Carroll, & Culpepper, 2005).

The nurse should be aware of food preferences customary to the Haitian culture (Box 20-1). As a result of the lack of ready availability of food items, Haitians have learned many poor nutritional habits, which have persisted even after immigration to the United States, particularly if similar economic conditions prevail.

Dietary Habits for Childbearing. Childbearing Haitian women are very particular about their dietary habits both before and after delivery. These dietary cultural habits include foods that a woman should and should not eat (Box 20-2). The nurse should assess these foods to ensure that the client maintains adequate nutrition (White, Linhart, & Medley, 1996).

Breastfeeding has traditionally been very common among Haitians because bottle-feeding was considered unnatural (Jeanty, 1989). However, as traditional beliefs are changing among Haitian Americans, breastfeeding is decreasing (Thomas & DeSantis, 1995).

Psychological Characteristics

Psychiatric care is also limited in Haiti. In 1956, Kline (Bordeleau & Kline, 1986) reported the

---

Box 20-1

COMMON CULTURAL FOOD

FRUITS AND NUTS
Rice
Avocados
Cashews
Coconuts
Granadilla flesh
Mangos
Pineapples
Soursop (guanabana) fruit
Star apples (*Chrysophyllum*)
Cassava bread (manioc, tapioca)
Bananas
Limes
Grapefruit
Oranges
Tomatoes
Watermelons

MEAT, VEGETABLES, AND OTHER FOODS
Beef
Beets
Okra
Biscuits (from imported white flour)
Cabbage
Carrots
Imported cheese
Chicken
Milled corn
Eggplant
Fish
Goat meat
Kidney beans
Lima beans
Peas
Pork
Sweet potatoes
Pumpkin
Sugarcane

---

presence of one psychiatrist and one psychiatric hospital in Haiti. In 1989 Gustafson reported that there were fewer than a dozen psychiatrists in Haiti, and all were located in the capital.

The first modern psychiatric hospital was opened in 1959, amid prejudice and resistance, by

---

Box 20-2

CHILDBEARING WOMEN AND FOOD PREFERENCES

FOODS EATEN BY CHILDBEARING WOMEN
Cornmeal porridge with bean sauce
Rice and beans
Plantains
Vegetables
Red fruits

FOODS AVOIDED BY CHILDBEARING WOMEN
Lima beans
Tomatoes
Black mushrooms
White beans
Okra
Lobster
Fish
Eggplant
Black peppers
Milk
Bananas

---

two psychiatrists from Canada and the United States. Because perphenazine (Trilafon) was donated by the three founding pharmaceutical companies and was used abundantly, the psychiatrists were called "Trilafon doctors." Although psychiatric treatment has improved, the frequency of mental illness in Haiti is unknown, and the psychiatric services remain undeveloped. Bordeleau and Kline (1986) have reported that psychiatric symptoms do not appear to be much different from those found in other countries. Projection has been identified as a frequent defense mechanism because paranoid delusions often appear in clients who are psychotic. Delusions are profoundly colored by Voodoo religious beliefs. Aggressivity is seldom directed toward others, with psychomotor hyperactivity being more often noisy than destructive. Affective disorders are more often of the hypomanic or manic type than depressive, and suicide among Haitians is rare. More recently, psychiatric care has advanced with the development of outpatient clients (Azaunce, 1995; Bordeleau & Kline, 1986).

However, in 1986 the Pan-American Health Organization reported no listing of psychiatric diagnoses in Haiti in a study involving the years 1981 to 1984. Rather than psychiatric care, most emotionally disturbed clients sought native healers who treat with amulets, packets of herbs and spices, liquids, baths, powders, rubbing, and massage (Gustafson, 1989). Wilson (1984) noted that disclosure of the belief in Voodoo can result in the diagnosis of psychiatric illness by a Western-trained practitioner.

Possession crisis, which has been diagnosed in some Haitian clients, is not unique to Haitian Voodoo but has also been observed in many African countries and on rare occasions among American Indians. This belief has much similarity with the early Greek Dionysian mysteries, the evil possession of the European Middle Ages, the witch possession in the New England colonies, and the contemporary African-American religious services of certain extreme groups in the South. See Box 20-3 for the conditions that must be present to have a possession crisis (Bordeleau & Kline, 1986).

Implications for Nursing Care

Because stomach ailments are a major problem for Haitians, the astute nurse will carefully assess the Haitian American client for various stomach ailments, including worms, which may be the result of spoiled food. In fact, a nurse may assume that if a Haitian American family has poor nutritional habits and at the same time cannot afford nutritious food, the likelihood that the family members will have worms is increased. Garlic is considered a folk remedy for worms and is boiled and eaten to prevent and treat worms. When a Haitian American client brings in a specimen and hands it to the clinic nurse, it is important for the nurse to understand that this may be a communication about a problem with worms and that the specimen should be analyzed with this in mind. The nurse will be better able to assist the Haitian American client by not trying to convince the client that garlic is inappropriate. The folk remedies should be accepted and combined with Western medicine.

Box 20-3

POSSESSION CRISIS

1. The general population of the local community must believe that a human being can communicate with the deities.
2. The person being "mounted" by the spirit (*loa*) is one of a group involved in a religious ceremony where the drums control the rhythm of the dance and the *hungan* behaves at first as a ritualistic priest.
3. Some spirits "participate" only at a certain time of the year and with a similar type of personality; that is, a gentle *loa* mounts a calm person and a fighting *loa* chooses an aggressive person.
4. The group considers being possessed to be a privilege, not a shameful event.
5. The possession crisis is stereotyped in the sense that someone mounted by a specific *loa* will talk like the *loa*, ask for the needed symbolic ornaments, and generally behave and dance in the way traditions in the region have dictated.

From Bordeleau, J.M., & Kline, N.S. (1986, July). Experience in developing psychiatric services in Haiti. *World Mental Health*, pp. 170–183.

The nurse should appreciate that in addition to diet being important in relation to the health of pregnant women, dietary practices are generally related to health. Eating well and eating fresh foods are related to maintaining health. Drinking tea every day made with *soros*i ("mulberry juice") is believed by many Haitian Americans to increase appetite, protect health, and prevent illness. One can treat fever by mixing castor oil, alcohol, and shallot (*Allium ascalonicum*), heating the mixture, rubbing it together, and rubbing it all over the fevered body (Spector, 1996).

It is important for the nurse to know that many Haitian Americans have very little information about disease or medical problems. Therefore, an illness is more commonly considered a "hex" or the result of an evil curse. The nurse should collect information from the client about the possible cause for the medical problem and should remain nonjudgmental, even when Voodoo is provided as a possible explanation. Health teaching (such as regarding diarrhea or pneu-

monia) is essential to help the Haitian client understand that the illness is not an evil curse imposed by a neighbor but an illness with natural physical causes.

The nurse cannot assume that all Haitian Americans will have the same beliefs. It is useful to ask Haitian American clients how long they have been in the United States, which will provide an indication of how Americanized the client may be. The age of the client is also a consideration when health beliefs are being assessed. Younger people are more likely to have made an effective adjustment to the Western culture, whereas older people often continue to find such things as American food strange and unacceptable.

Haitian American clients are more likely to believe that they are receiving effective treatment when a nurse is seen. In Haiti a nurse is given more authority and status than a physician, and the client will often be more cooperative with directions given by a nurse (Jeanty, 1989). When nursing procedures are being implemented (such as taking the client's blood pressure), the nurse should tell the client orally what is being done and that this is for the client's benefit. Actions by the nurse are related to being helped.

Some Haitian Americans associate wheelchairs with being sick. Therefore, on discharge the client who is allowed to walk out of the hospital will be more likely to feel that care has been effective (Jeanty, 1989).

Great stress has been placed on Haitians as they have attempted to adjust to life in the United States and Canada. Coming from a disadvantaged background and often arriving in the United States with a history of poor health care, Haitians have been hesitant to reach out for health care. For some of these people, a hospital is perceived as a place to go to die, which may contribute to large numbers of visitors when a Haitian is ill (Jeanty, 1989). Health professionals at all levels must communicate a nonjudgmental attitude while trying to encourage the Haitian American client to take advantage of available health services. Not only do Haitian Americans need to be educated regarding health care agencies but also they may need information on health insurance, on how to use health benefits, and on finding a job that has medical benefits. Conway and Buchanan (1985) suggest that what is most helpful to Haitians' adjusting to life in the United States is to focus on the strengths from their cultural heritage, such as attitude, perseverance in the most arduous circumstances, deep religious faith, high self-respect, reliance on the extended family, and the tradition of sharing.

SUMMARY

Haiti is an independent, underdeveloped republic that continues to face many critical issues, such as a poor economy, lack of technology, high mortality, inadequacy in food and water supplies, and lack of adequate health care. With the ever-growing Haitian population immigrating to the United States, the nurse must constantly keep these issues in mind when formulating a treatment plan for a Haitian American client. The holistic approach must take priority when the nurse is assessing, treating, and evaluating the Haitian American client. The Haitian cultural method of health care delivery must be included with conventional methods of treatment, and transcultural issues in nursing must be recognized before high-quality care can be rendered. Cultural behavior is meaningful and should not be ridiculed, judged negatively, or ignored. The nurse must be aware of cultural and behavioral considerations that affect the care of the Haitian immigrant and use this understanding in implementation of the nursing process. High-quality health care that is culturally sensitive to the needs of Haitian refugees is possible when knowledge of their culture and beliefs is used as a basis for intervention.

Case Study

A 33-year-old Haitian man is admitted via the emergency room with symptoms of persistent coughing and spitting up small amounts of blood. Through the nursing assessment and by talking with the client and his family members, the nurse determines that the client has been experiencing a progressive lack of appetite and is visibly underweight. Radiographic examination reveals that the client has an active and communicable case of tuberculosis. Respiratory assessment reveals low Pao_2 and elevated $Paco_2$. When the client and the family are informed that the diagnosis is tuberculosis, there is little reaction. The nurse is informed by the client's family members that the client was initially diagnosed as having a positive Mantoux test in Haiti approximately 2 years previously. At that time the client was given a prescription for isoniazid (INH) by a clinic physician but was noncompliant with his medication regimen.

CARE PLAN

✳ *Nursing Diagnosis: Gas exchange, impaired, as evidenced by low Pao_2 and elevated $Paco_2$*

Client Outcome

1. Client will have no further coughing or viscous secretions.

Nursing Interventions

1. Maintain adequate hydration (increase fluid intake to 2 to 3 quarts per day).
2. Maintain adequate humidity of inspired air.
3. Minimize irritants in inspired air (such as dust, allergens).
4. Provide periods of uninterrupted rest.
5. Administer prescribed medication such as cough suppressant or expectorant as ordered by physician.

✳ *Nursing Diagnosis: Nutrition, imbalanced: less than body requirements, inability to ingest food because of biological factors (tuberculosis) as evidenced by anorexia and weight that is below normal for age, sex, and body stature*

Client Outcome

1. Client will gain weight to be within normal range for body size.

Nursing Interventions

1. Maintain good oral hygiene (make sure client brushes teeth, rinses mouth) before and after ingestion of food.
2. Arrange to have foods with the most protein and calories served at times the client feels most like eating.
3. Use dietitian for meal planning.

✳ *Nursing Diagnosis: Noncompliance related to perceived beliefs of significant others as evidenced by failure of client to take isoniazid*

Client Outcome

1. Client will take prescribed medication as ordered.

Nursing Intervention

1. Allow client an opportunity to make decisions about his own health care; assume an advisory approach when counseling, rather than one that is dictatorial.
2. Consult with an interpreter who speaks both English and Haitian Creole to provide instructions on how to take medication.
3. Consult with an interpreter who speaks both English and Haitian Creole to help client vent his feelings of anxiety and frustration.

✳ *Nursing Diagnosis: Medication noncompliance related to referral process*

Client Outcome

1. Client will keep scheduled follow-up appointments.

Nursing Interventions

1. Whenever possible, allow client to make own appointments.
2. Shorten referral waiting time.
3. Personnel handling referral appointment should inquire about transportation, suggesting help if needed.

✳ *Nursing Diagnosis: Interrupted family processes, related to shift in health status of family members*

Client Outcome

1. Family will achieve functional support for client.

Nursing Interventions

1. Include family members in group education sessions about tuberculosis.
2. Refer family members to support and self-help groups.
3. Obtain Haitian Creole–speaking interpreter to facilitate communication.
4. Facilitate family involvement with social supports.

✳ STUDY QUESTIONS

1. If a Mantoux test is given incorrectly and no wheal appears (because the injection was made too deep), should the nurse repeat the test at another site that is at least 2 inches away from the first injection?

2. What does erythema without induration mean?

3. In tuberculosis, treatment is continued until when?

4. The physician says the client has induration. What does this mean?

5. List the possible side effects of isoniazid (INH).

6. What preventive steps can be taken to avoid the spread of a diagnosed case of tuberculosis?
7. Why is proper nutrition important with a client diagnosed as having tuberculosis?
8. Why is the Haitian population at high risk for being infected by tuberculosis?
9. What is the nurse's role when caring for a client with tuberculosis?
10. Compare the similarities and differences in family structure between the American and Haitian cultures.
11. What are the contributing factors that lead to the high birth rate in Haiti and among Haitian immigrants?
12. Why are Haitian women at risk during pregnancy?
13. Describe the practice of healers and their importance to the Haitian population.
14. Describe the role of the Haitian man as it pertains to family.

NCLEX-RN REVIEW QUESTIONS

1. In planning care for a pregnant Haitian American client, the nurse needs to be alert that the most crucial and decisive cultural compliance associated with childbearing are related to the:
   A. Delivery of the baby
   B. Time of labor
   C. Antepartum period
   D. Postpartum period

2. A Haitian American client comes to the clinic and tells the nurse she has been eating garlic to cure an intestinal problem. The most appropriate action for the nurses is to:
   A. Convince the client that garlic is an inappropriate treatment
   B. Accept folk remedies and combine it with Western medicine
   C. Teach the client to seek medical help earlier
   D. Accept that the intestinal ailment is a curse

3. When assessing the sexuality of Haitian men, it is best for the nurse to ask if the client:
   A. Is bisexual
   B. Is homosexual
   C. Is heterosexual
   D. Has ever had sex with another man

References

Abbott, E. (1991). *Haiti: The Duvaliers and their legacy* (revised ed). New York: Simon & Schuster.

Ambassade d'Haiti. (2000). *Haiti at a glance.* Retrieved July 25, 2002, from http://www.haiti.org/invest. htm#haag.

Annas, G. (1993). Detention of HIV-positive Haitians at Guantánamo. *The New England Journal of Medicine,* 329, 589–592.

Azaunce, M. (1995). Is it schizophrenia or spirit possession? *Journal of Social Distress and the Homeless,* 4 (3), 255–263.

Barnard, R., & Sincox, A. (2004, June–July). A call for help from across the sea. *Michigan Nurse,* 9, 16.

Barnes, J. (2000, April 21). Haitian Americans march to protest brutality by police. *New York Times,* 149 (51364), B3.

Barstow, D. (2000, March 22). Shooting resonates among Haitians. *New York Times,* 149(51335), B6.

Bawden, M. P., Slaten, D. D., & Malone, J. D. (1995, November–December). *Falciparum* malaria in a displaced Haitian population. *Transactions of the Royal Society of Tropical Medicine and Hygiene,* 89(6), 600–603.

Bell, I. (1981). *The Dominican Republic.* Boulder, Colo.: Westview Press.

Benedict, M. (2004, August–October). Vermont nurses venture to Haiti. *Vermont Nurse Connection,* 7(3), 5.

Bestman, E. (1979). *Cultural, linguistic and racial barriers in providing health services to Haitian refugees.* Paper presented at a workshop on improving health services to Haitian refugees, sponsored by the U.S. Health Service Administration, Metro-Dade County, Florida.

Bonnlander, H. (1996, September). Migrant TB treatment in Haiti resulting in U.S. policy change at Guantánamo Bay, Cuba. *Bulletin of the Pan-American Health Organization*, 30(3), 206–211.

Bordeleau, J. M., & Kline, N. S. (1986, July). Experience in developing psychiatric services in Haiti. *World Mental Health* (pp. 170–183).

Boswell, T. (1982). The new Haitian diaspora. *Caribbean Review*, 11(1), 18–21.

Bragg, R. (2000, March 29). Haitian immigrants in U.S. face a wrenching choice. *New York Times*, 149 (51342), A1.

Bryan, S. (1988). *Ethnic disease*, Paper presented at a workshop sponsored by the U.S. Health Service Administration, Metro-Dade County, Florida.

Calypso, A. (1999, November). Tet Grenn. *Essence*, 30(7), 90.

Carrazana, E., DeToledo, J., & Tatum, W., et al. (1999). Epilepsy and religious experiences: Voodoo possession. *Epilepsia*, 40, 239–241.

Castro, A., & Farmer, P. (2005, Jan.) Understanding and addressing AIDS-related stigma: from anthropological theory to clinical practice in Haiti. *American Journal of Public Health*, 95(1), 53–59.

Central Intelligence Agency (2007). *The world factbook*. Haiti. Retrieved June 28, 2007, from https://www.cia.gov/cia/publications/factbook/geos/ha.html.

Charles, C. (1979). *Anthropological consideration of barriers affecting delivery of health services to Haitian refugees in Florida* Paper presented at a workshop on improving health services to Haitian refugees, sponsored by the U.S. Health Service Administration, Metro-Dade County, Florida.

Chelala, C. (1994, August 20–27). Fighting for survival. *British Medical Journal*, 309(6953), 525–526.

Claude, J. (1997, November 7). Presentation on Haiti at the Mennonite Economic Development Conference, Kansas City, Mo.

Colin, J. (2005). Haitians. In Lipson, J., & Dibble, S. (Eds.), *Culture and clinical care*. San Francisco: UCSF Nursing Press.

Conway, F., & Buchanan, S. (1985). Haitians. In Haines, D. (Ed.), *Refugees in the United States* (pp. 95–109). Westport, Conn.: Greenwood Press.

Consedine, N., Magai, C., Spiller, R., Neugut, A., & Conway, F. (2004). Breast cancer knowledge and beliefs in subpopulations of African American and Caribbean women. *American Journal of Health Behavior*, 28(3), 260–271.

Consedine, N., Morgenstern, A., Kudadjie-Gyamfi, E., Magai, C., & Neugut, A. (2006, February). Prostate cancer screening behavior in men from seven ethnic groups; the fear factor. *Cancer Epidemiology Biomarkers Prevention*, 15(2), 228–237.

Corbett, R. (1999, February 1). Cyberspace is striving in Haiti. *Washington Post Foreign Service*. Retrieved July 25, 2002, from http://www.hartford-hwp.com/archives/43a/160.html.

Coreil, J. (1983, July). Parallel structures in professional and folk health care: a model applied to rural Haiti. *Culture, Medicine and Psychiatry*, 70, 131–151.

Cowley, G. (2002, February 4). The biggest bet yet. *Newsweek*, 45–49.

Degazon, C. (1994). Ethnic identification, social support and coping strategies among three groups of ethnic African elders. *Journal of Cultural Diversity*, 1(4), 79–85.

Dejean, Y. (1983). *Revisiting the issues of the native language as a natural medium of instruction*. Master's thesis. New York: Bank Street College of Education.

Dempsey, P. A., & Gesse, T. (1983). The childbearing Haitian refugee: cultural applications to clinical nursing. *Public Health Reports*, 98(3), 261–267.

Dening, E. (2001). Haiti. *Workbook, walking with a hurting world*. Akron, Pa.: Mennonite Central Committee.

DeSantis, L., & Thomas, J. (1987, August). Parental attitudes toward adolescent sexuality: transcultural perspectives. *Nurse Practitioner*, 12, 43–48.

DeSantis, L., & Thomas, J. (1992). Health education and the immigrant Haitian mother: cultural insights for community health nurses. *Public Health Nursing*, 9 (2), 87–96.

DeSantis, L., & Ugarriza, D. (1995, December). Potential for intergenerational conflict in Cuban and Haitian immigrant families. *Archives of Psychiatric Nursing*, 9(6), 354–364.

Devieux, J., Malow, R., Jean-Gilles, M., Samuels, D., Deschamps, M., Ascencio, M., Jean-Baptiste, L., & Pape, J. (2004, November–December). Reducing health disparities through culturally sensitive treatment for HIV+ adults in Haiti. *ABNF Journal*, 25(6), 109–115.

Eisenbruch, M. (1984). Cross-cultural aspects of bereavement: part 2. Ethnic and cultural variations in the development of bereavement practices. *Culture, Medicine and Psychiatry*, 8, 315–347.

Ellerbrock, T., Chamblee, S., Bush, T., Johnson, J., Marsh, B., & Lowell, P, et al. (2004). Human immunodeficiency virus infection in a rural community in the United States. *American Journal of Epidemiology*, 160(6), 582–588.

Epstein, G., Lantigua, J., & Cavanaugh, J. (1995, May 7). U.S. ship taking rafters to Cuba. *Miami Herald*, p. 1A.

Eshleman, J., & Davidhizar, R. (1997, Spring). Life in migrant camps for children: a hazard to health. *Journal of Cultural Diversity*, 4(1), 13–15.

Fernández-Kelly, M., & Schauffler, R. (1994). Divided fates: immigrant children in a restructured U.S. economy. *International Migration Review*, 28, 662–689.

Fineman, M (2001, September 2). Desperate Haitians inundate Bahamas. *The Journal Gazette*, 11A.

Fitzgerald, D., Maxi, A., Marcelin, A., Johnson, W., & Pape, J. (2004, November 18). Notification of positive HIV test results In Haiti: can we better intervene at this critical crossroads in the life of HIV-infected patients in a resource-poor country? *AIDS Patient Care and STDs*, (11), 658–664.

Fruchter, R. G., Wright, C., & Habenstreit, B., et al. (1985). Screening for cervical and breast cancer among Caribbean immigrants. *Journal of Community Health*, 10, 121–135.

Godsby, R. (1971). *A race and races*. New York: Macmillan.

Granich, R., Sfeir, M., & Jacobs, B. (1994, February 3). Detention of HIV-positive Haitians and Cubans. *The New England Journal of Medicine*, 330(5), 372.

Grant, W. (1989, August 6). *The prevalence of antibodies to HTLV-I virus in the Aribonite Valley*. Paper presented at the annual reunion of the Hospital Albert Schweitzer Alumni Association, Burlington, Vermont.

Gregg, V. (2001, Autumn). The world in our classroom. *Emory University, a magazine for alumni and friends*, Atlanta: Nell Hodgson Woordruff School of Nursing.

Gustafson, M. (1989). Western voodoo: providing mental health care to Haitian refugees. *Journal of Psychosocial Nursing*, 27, 22–25.

Haitians in America. (1983, March 2). *National Catholic Reporter*, p. 1.

Hardcastle, M. (2004, May). Reflection. Lessons from Haiti. *Canadian Nurse*, 100(5), 12–13.

Harris, K. (1987). Beliefs and practices among Haitian American women in relation to childbearing. *Journal of Nurse-Midwifery*, 32(3), 149–155.

Herip, D. (1993). Health status of Haitian migrants: U.S. naval base, Guantánamo Bay, Cuba, November 1991–April 1992. *Journal of the American Medical Association*, 269, 1395.

Herskovits, M. J. (1971). *Life in a Haitian valley*. Garden City, N.Y.: Anchor Books.

Hiebert, C. (1997, November 8). Presentation on Haiti at the Mennonite Economic Development Conference in Kansas City, Mori.

Hobsbawn, E. J. (1996). *The age of revolution: 1789–1848*. New York: Vintage Books.

Holcomb, L. O., Parsons, L. C., Giger, J. N., & Davidhizar, R. E. (1996). Haitian Americans: implications for nursing care. *Journal of Community Health Nursing*, 13(4), 249–260.

Holt, J., & Reeves, J. (2001, April). The meaning of hope and generic caring practices to nurture hope in a rural village in the Dominican Republic. *Journal of Transcultural Nursing*, 12(2), 123–131.

Isgro, F. (1998). New law grants amnesty to Haitians. *Migration World Magazine*, 26(5), 41.

Jeanty, M. (1989). Personal communication at Logansport State Hospital, Logansport, Indiana.

Key, S., DeNoon, D., & Boyles, S. (1998, September 21). U.S. film's tying of Haiti to AIDS stirs protests. *AIDS Weekly Plus*, 11.

Laguerre, M. (1981). Haitian Americans. In Harwood, A. (Ed.), *Ethnicity and medical care*. Cambridge, Mass.: Harvard University Press.

Laguerre, M. (1984). *American odyssey: Haitians in New York City*. Ithaca, N.Y.: Cornell University Press.

Laguerre, M. (1989). *Voodoo and politics in Haiti*. New York: St. Martin's.

Leyburn, J. G. (1980). *The Haitian people*. Westport, Conn.: Greenwood Press.

Lillibridge, S., Conrad, K., Stinson, N., & Noji, E. (1994, February). Haitian mass migration: uniformed service medical support, May 1992. *Military Medicine*, 159(2), 149–153.

Logan, M. (1975). Selected references on the hot-cold theory of disease. *Medical Anthropology Newsletter*, 6 (2), 8–11.

Malow, R., Jean-Gilles, M., Devieux, J., Rosenberg, R., & Russell, A. (2004, November–December). Increasing access to preventive health care through cultural adaption of effective HIV prevention interventions: a brief report from the HIV prevention in Haitian youths study. *ABNF Journal*, 15(6), 127–132.

Martin, M., Rissmiller, P., & Beal, J. (1995, November–December). Health-illness beliefs and practices of Haitians with HIV disease living in Boston. *Journal of the Association of Nurses in AIDS Care*, 6(6), 45–53.

Masland, T. (1992, February 24). Haiti: "We could turn our back." *Newsweek*, pp. 30–32.

McMorrow, T. (1970, November 15). Haitians try to adopt U.S. with three strikes on them. *Daily News,* p. B1.

Mena, A. (1996). Cuban Santeria, Haitian voodun, Puerto Rican spiritualism: a multiculturist inquiry into syncretism. *Journal for the Scientific Study of Religion,* 37, 15–27.

Métraux, A. (1953). Médecine et voudou en Haïti. *Acta Tropica,* 10, 28–68.

Metropolitan Dade County. (1981). *Social and economic problems among Cuban and Haitian entrant groups in Dade County, Florida: trends and implications.* Miami, Fla.: Metropolitan Dade County.

MiamiHerald.com. (2006, June 3). *Top Haiti story.* Retrieved June 3, 2006, from http://www.miami.com/mld/miamiherald/news/world/haiti.

Miller, N. (2000, July). Haitian ethnomedical systems and biomedical practitioners: directions for clinicians. *Journal of Transcultural Nursing,* 11(3), 204–211.

Mitacek, E. J., St. Vallières, D., & Polednak, A. P. (1986). Cancer in Haiti 1979–1984: distribution of various forms of cancer according to geographical area and sex. *International Journal of Cancer,* 38, 9–16.

Moskowitz, L., Kory, P., Chan, J., et al. (1983). Unusual causes of deaths in Haitians residing in Miami. *Journal of the American Medical Association,* 250(9), 1187–1191.

Neilsen, B. (1989). Beliefs towards a diagnosis of cancer: a transcultural approach. In Prichard, A. P. (Ed.), *Proceedings of the fifth International Conference on Cancer Nursing* (pp. 129–132). London: Macmillan.

Neilson, B., McMillan, S., & Díaz, E. (1992). Instruments that measure beliefs about cancer from a cultural perspective. *Cancer Nursing* 15(2), 109–115.

Nelson, M. (2002). Haitian-owned businesses: why we often fail. *The United Haitians Home Page.* Retrieved from http://www.business.uhhp.com. Date retrieved: July 25, 2002.

Nida, E. (1954). *Customs and cultures.* New York: Harper & Brothers.

Office of Refugee Resettlement. (1993). Refugee resettlement program: annual report to Congress, FY 1992. Washington, D.C.: U.S. Government Printing Office.

Orque, M. S., Bloch, B., & Monrroy, L. S. A. (1983). *Ethnic nursing care: a multicultural approach.* St. Louis: Mosby.

Portes, A., & Stepick, A. (1985, August). Unwelcome immigrants: the labor market experiences of 1980 (Mariel) Cuban and Haitian refugees in South Florida. *American Sociological Review,* 493–515.

Potocky, M. (1996). Refugee children: how are they faring economically as adults? *Social Work Journal of the National Association of Social Workers,* 41(4), 354–373.

Preston, R. A., Materson, B. J., Yoham, M. A., & Anapol, H. (1996). Hypertension in Haitians. *Journal of Human Hypertension,* 10(11), 743–745.

Prudent, N., Johnson, P., Carroll, J., & Culpepper, L. (2005). Attention-deficit/hyperactivity disorder: presentation and management in the Haitian American child. *Companion Journal of Clinical Psychiatry,* 7(4), 190–197.

Quillen, T. (1999). The voodoo religion [letter]. *Journal of Psychiatric Nursing and Mental Health,* 31(1), 4.

Randall-David, E. (1989). *Strategies for working with culturally diverse communities and clients.* Washington, D.C: U.S. Department of Health and Human Services.

Reichman, L. (1989, August 5). *Treating tuberculosis in developing countries.* Paper presented at the annual reunion of the Hospital Albert Schweitzer Alumni Association, Burlington, Vermont.

Robinson, A. (1994, Winter). Attitudes toward nursing home residents among aides of three cultural groups. *Journal of Cultural Diversity,* 1(1), 16–18.

Rodman, S. (1984). *Haiti: the Black republic* (6th revised ed.). Old Greenwich, Conn.: Devin-Adair.

Rohter, L. (1996, February 9). Preval is Haiti's president, but thoughts focus on Aristide's future. *Professor Corbett Haitian history files.* Retrieved July 24, 2002, from http://haiti.uhhp.com/history/postbabydoc/nytimes_preval_inauguration.htm.

Rosenthal, B. (1995, January). The influence of social support on school completion among Haitians. *Social Work in Education,* 17(1), 30–39.

Rosenwarke, I. (1972). *Population history of New York.* Syracuse, N.Y.: Syracuse University Press.

Samet, J., Retondo, M., & Freedberg, J. G., et al. (1994, October). Factors associated with initiation of primary medical care for HIV-infected persons. *American Journal of Medicine,* 4, 347–353.

Santana, M., & Dancy, B. (2000). The stigma of being named "AIDS carriers" on Haitian-American women. *Health Care for Women International,* 21, 161–171.

Schaedel, R. (1962). *The human resources of Haiti.* Unpublished manuscript.

Scott, C. (1978, November). Health and healing practices among five ethnic groups in Miami, Florida. *Public Health Report,* 55, 524–532.

Seabrooks, P. (1992). *Social supports of older Haitians in Port-au-Prince and Miami: effects on health practices and perceived health status.* Doctor of Nursing Services dissertation, University of California, San Francisco.

Sebastian, J. A., Leeb, B. O., & See, R. (1978). Cancer of the cervix: a sexually transmitted disease. *American Journal of Obstetrics and Gynecology,* 131, 620–623.

Seligman, L. (1977, March). Haitians: a neglected minority. *Personnel and Guidance Journal,* 2, 409–411.

Snow, L. F. (1981). Folk medical beliefs and their implications for the care of patients: a review based on studies among Black Americans. In Henderson, G., & Primeaux, M. (Eds.), *Transcultural health care.* Reading, Mass: Addison-Wesley.

Sorensen, K., Luckmann, J., & Bolander, V. (1994). *Sorenson and Luckmann's basic nursing: a psychophysiologic approach.* Philadelphia: W.B. Saunders.

Spector, R. (1996). *Culture care: guide to heritage assessment and health traditions* (ed. 3.). Upper Saddle River, N.J.: Pearson Prentice Hall.

Stauffer, R. (2006, October). Personal communication with the former Assistant Director of Nursing at Hôpital Albert Schweitzer, Deschapelles, Haiti.

Thomas, H. (1997). *The slave trade: the story of the Atlantic slave trade 1440–1870.* New York: Touchstone.

Thomas, J., & DeSantis, L. (1995, Winter). Feeding and weaning practices in Cuban and Haitian immigrant mothers. *Journal of Transcultural Nursing,* 6(2), 34–42.

Time almanac with information please. (2007). Boston: Information Please, Inc.

United Haitians Home Page. (2006). *Haiti Related Headlines.* Retrieved from http://haiti.uhhp.com. Date retrieved: June 4, 2006.

United Nations Program Development. (1996). Rapport de Coopération au Développement-Haïti. Port-Au-Prince, Haiti.

U.S. Committee for Refugees. (1995). Asylum cases filed with INS, April 1991–Sept. 1995. *Refugee Reports,* 16 (12), 12.

U.S. Department of Commerce, Bureau of the Census, Population profiles by age, sex, race, and Hispanic Origin, Summary File 3. Washington, D.C.: U.S. Government Printing Office.

Veeken, H. (1993). Hope for Haiti. *British Medical Journal,* 307, 312–313.

Venton, D. (1997, November 7). Report on volunteer experiences in Haiti at the Mennonite Economic Development Association Conference in Kansas City, Mori.

Verdet, P. (1985, Winter). Trying times: Haitian youth in an inner city high school. *Social Work in Health Care,* 228–233.

Walsh, B. (1980, May 17). The boat people of South Florida. *America,* pp. 420–421.

Weil, T. E. (1973). *Area handbook for Haiti.* Washington, D.C: U.S. Government Printing Office.

Westphal, R. (1989, August 5). *Transfusion transmitted infectious diseases.* Paper presented at the annual reunion of the Hospital Albert Schweitzer Alumni Association, Burlington, Vermont.

White, J., Linhart, J., & Medley, L. (1996, September). Culture, diet and the maternity. *Advance for Nurse Practitioners,* 26–29.

Wiese, J. (1976). Maternal nutrition and traditional food behavior in Haiti. *Human Organization,* 35(2), 193–200.

Wilentz, A. (1989). *The rainy season.* New York: Simon & Schuster.

Wilk, R. (1986, Winter). The Haitian refugee: concern for health care providers. *Social Work in Health Care,* 11, 61–74.

Williams, S., Murthy, N., & Berggren, G. (1975, November). Conjugal unions among rural Haitian women. *Journal of Marriage and the Family,* 37, 1022–1031.

Wilson, M. (1984). Voodoo believers: some sociological insights. *Journal of Sociology and Social Welfare,* 9, 373–383.

World almanac. (2007). New York: World Almanac Books.

CHAPTER 21 Jewish Americans

Enid A. Schwartz

Behavioral Objectives

After reading this chapter, the nurse will be able to:

1. Identify how the religion of Judaism affects the cultural behaviors of Jewish Americans.
2. Identify some of the differences between health-oriented behaviors demonstrated by various religious groups within Judaism.
3. Identify how the various ethnic backgrounds of Jewish Americans affect their cultural behaviors.
4. Describe attitudes and beliefs affecting health care within and across individuals in various Jewish groups.
5. Identify how the verbal and nonverbal communications of Jewish individuals may affect health care.
6. Identify implications or precautions for providing effective nursing care to Jewish Americans.
7. Recognize those health care practices that are mandated by Jewish law for people who are Jewish.

Explaining what it means to be Jewish is not easy. It is more than just belonging to a religious organization; it is also being a part of a specific people (Glazer, 1989; Popenoe, 2000; Trepp, 1980). It is a shared feeling of "Jewishness." Jewish people are linked together by a common history, common ethical teachings, a common language of prayer (Hebrew), a vast quantity of literature, common folkways, and, above all, a sense of common destiny (Kertzer, 1993). Jewish people share centuries of history as a minority subjected to hostility wherever they go.

The Jewish American culture has many subcultures because of the different areas of the world in which Jews live as well as a diversity of religious observances. Jews came to the United States predominantly from Spain, Portugal, Germany, and Eastern Europe. There are four main religious groups: Orthodox, Conservative, Reform, and Reconstructionist. Within the orthodox group are the Chassidic (or Hasidic) and Lubovitch subgroups, which are the largest subgroups in the United States today.

Despite differences, there are some cultural similarities that are indigenous to this group of people. To understand the culture, one must have knowledge of some of the religious dictates. Through a discussion of the six common variables found within and across cultural groups as they apply to Jewish Americans, this chapter attempts to clarify some behaviors that are commonly found among Jews in order to assist nurses in developing an effective plan of care for the Jewish American client. Attention is also placed on Jewish rituals and the effects of assimilation on their cultural traits.

OVERVIEW OF THE JEWISH PEOPLE IN THE UNITED STATES

The history of American Judaism encompasses three distinct waves of immigration. The first wave of people, who began arriving in the middle 1600s, was relatively small. They were Sephardic Jews from Spain and Portugal, and they had little effect on the development of modern American Judaism (Sachar, 1965). The beginning of the nineteenth century saw a steady German immigration, which swelled after 1836, when Jews sought to escape persecution in Bavaria and other German states (Glazer, 1989). The last tide of immigration began slowly in 1845, when Polish Jews began arriving in the United States, but swelled to tens of thousands in 1881 as a result of a wave of pogroms and a series of new anti-Jewish decrees in Russia. This last wave, consisting of Eastern European Jews and German Jews, has had a profound effect on modern Jewish American culture and religious practices.

To understand Jewish American culture today, it is necessary to consider Europe during the Middle Ages. At that time, most of the internal law in European Jewish communities was strongly controlled by the Talmud (the Rabbinic code). Talmudic law governed not only the religious behavior of Jews but also almost every other aspect of life, such as birth, marriage, and death, as well as the proper foods to eat and the proper clothes to wear. The Jews were kept separate from the general population not only by persecution from others but also by the rigidity of these laws.

In the nineteenth century, not all German Jews were isolated in their communities; some were involved in non-Jewish communities. Many of these Jews were embarrassed by the ancient laws and found them distasteful, especially if they desired the status of full members of the German nation (Glazer, 1989). To maintain their beliefs and yet not appear different from the general culture, German Jews of high social status attempted to start the Reform movement. The freedom experienced in the United States allowed the Reform movement to flourish. The German Jews who immigrated to the United States and wished to become part of the American community were willing to rid themselves of the old traditions and become increasingly "Americanized." They were insistent, however, that the Jews be maintained as a people.

The Eastern European immigrants came predominantly from Russia, Romania, Poland, and Austria. In contrast to many of the German Jewish immigrants who had lived predominantly in non-segregated areas, most of the Eastern European Jews came from all-Jewish villages, known as *shtetls,* where a Jewish culture was created that was almost totally unaffected by the cultures of the people around them. Life was dictated by the religious traditions Eastern European Jews followed and was much the same as it had been during the Middle Ages.

Along with these pious Jews came the radical political and socialist Jews, who believed that the only way to survive was through complete abandonment of religion. A third group who immigrated during this time represented the "middle-of-the-road" Jews, who were both religious and radical (Glazer, 1989).

It is important to understand the differences in religious behavior when caring for Jewish clients. All Jewish beliefs derive from the Torah (the five books of Moses) and the Talmud (the Rabbinic code). From the Torah come 613 commandments. The combination of the Torah and Talmud results in codes of law. Rather than referring to a body of doctrine, Judaism refers to a body of practices (Glazer, 1989).

As mentioned previously, four main religious Jewish groups exist today: Orthodox, Conservative, Reform, and Reconstructionist. The Orthodox Jew maintains a strict code of interpretation of the law, the Conservative Jew maintains a less strict code of interpretation, and the Reform Jew follows a more liberal interpretation of the law. Reconstructionist Judaism is a little difficult to explain. Reconstructionists do not necessarily believe in God as a personified deity, or that God chose the Jewish people. If they follow the laws of Judaism, they do so because of their cultural value. An example of the differences deals with the head coverings worn by men: the Orthodox Jew is obligated to keep his head covered at all times in reverence to God, the Conservative Jew keeps his head covered during times of worship, and the Reform and Reconstructionist Jews are not obligated to keep their heads covered.

The division between Jewish practices started in Germany in the nineteenth century, but it was not until Jews experienced the religious freedom of the United States that the conservative and reform movements thrived. The freedom experienced in the United States allowed the Jewish immigrant to question the narrow confines of orthodoxy and led to a desire to express religious beliefs and traditional practices in a less confining environment. The German Jews had begun to practice Reform Judaism. However, to the Eastern European Jew, Reform Judaism seemed empty (Howe, 1989). A movement known as "Conservatism," which had begun in nineteenth-century Germany, had a small beginning but appealed to the children of many Eastern European immigrants. According to Glazer (1989), Conservatism offered a compromise between the blind religious teachings of the Orthodox Jews and the scholarly endeavors of the Reform movement to break from tradition completely. Today, Reform temples are moving toward more traditional practices but maintain the belief that a person should be able to make choices based on knowledge of customs and their meanings.

In regard to religion, Jewish identity has changed through the generations. In the United States today, the sense of Jewish identity does not lie in the Old World religious observances. Most Jewish Americans do not observe the traditional Jewish Sabbath, nor are they active in their temple or synagogue. According to Sowell (1981), their identity lies not with the historical religious aspects of Judaism but with their ethnic or racial identity.

Changes in immigration laws have decreased the number of Jews entering the United States. However, since the time of the large immigration of Eastern European Jews, Jews from other countries have come to the United States under different circumstances. There are Jews who escaped or lived through the Holocaust, Jews who have emigrated from Communist Russia, Russian Jews who were able to leave after the collapse of the Communist party, and Jews who have arrived from many other countries of the world, including Ethiopia and Israel. Each group has added to the cultural diversity of the Jewish people. All have brought with them the culture of the land from which they emigrated. Because of the close ties that have developed between Jews of all nationalities, cultural traits have begun to blend. For example, descendants of Eastern European Jews talk about eating falafel, a food made from ground chickpeas, which originated in the Middle East.

A fear of many Jewish Americans is the effect of assimilation on their children. Jewish American people do not want to appear different from other Americans because being different has led to thousands of years of persecution. However, many Jewish Americans do not want to lose the common thread that binds them to one another.

Although Jewish Americans make up only about 3% of the U.S. population, they are visible in many areas of U.S. culture. It is estimated that today there are 6,061,000 Jews residing in the United States (*Time Almanac with Information Please*, 2006). Jewish Americans are distinguished members of the arts, academia, the sciences, medicine, law, and the political arena. Education is a large part of the Jewish culture, which has helped Jews in the United States succeed as they never could in other countries.

The desire to succeed, plus intermarriage, has caused some loss of Jewish identity. Some Jews today in the United States do not wish to be identified as Jewish for fear of discrimination in the workplace. Discrimination against Jews does exist in the United States, and many Jews are sensitive to anti-Semitism.

COMMUNICATION

Today the primary language of Jewish Americans is English. In the late 1800s the primary language of the Jews was Yiddish, which is a combination of German, Slavic, Old French, Old Italian, and Hebrew languages (Rosten, 1999). The children of first-generation Jews, born to Eastern European parents, wanted to be accepted by the other children. Although Yiddish may have been spoken in the home, these children spoke English outside the home. Very few second-generation Jewish Americans understand Yiddish. However, almost all Jewish Americans know some Yiddish, and many Jewish conversations are sprinkled with Yiddish words. Some of these words have become a part of American English, such as shtick (or shtück) and tush.

Hebrew, which is the language of Israel, is not spoken by most Jews who do not live there. However, Hebrew is the language of the Torah, and many Jews can read it. An important part of Jewish religious education is the reading, speaking, and writing of Hebrew. *Shalom* is a Hebrew word that is commonly used by Jewish people to mean "peace," "hello," or "good-bye."

The Sephardic Jews have a language of their own, Ladino, which is similar to Old Spanish. It is not commonly spoken in the United States today.

Style

Jews tend to be expressive when communicating, and they tend to be very verbal about how and what they are feeling. Most Jewish people use their hands to express their thoughts; as they talk, their hands emphasize what is being said. They not only punctuate their conversations using hand and arm movements but also use voice inflections. By changing the emphasis on certain words, the Jewish person changes the meaning of the message being conveyed (Rosten, 1999). This change in emphasis is done easily in Yiddish and has been carried over into English. As an example, changing the emphasis on the words "Him you trust?" changes the meaning: "Him you *trust*?" versus "*Him* you trust?" The first questions a person's judgment; the second implies that anyone who would trust the character of such a scoundrel must be an idiot.

Humor is used frequently by Jews, and often the humor is directed at themselves. This self-directed humor has led to comments that Jewish humor comes out of self-hatred. Although Jewish humor may appear to be self-critical and sometimes self-deprecating, it does not stem from a form of Jewish masochism. One of the most popular beliefs is that Jewish humor arose as a way for Jews to cope with the hostility they found around them, sometimes using that hostility against themselves. It appears as if a Jewish person is telling enemies, "You don't have to attack us. We can do that ourselves—and even better" (Novak & Waldoks, 1981).

Jews today are sensitive to humor from "outside" sources. Jokes that are not appreciated when told by non-Jews include "JAP" (Jewish American Princess) jokes and those about "Jewing people down" (referring to Jews being cheap or unmerciful at bartering).

As Jews become more acculturated with each generation, the communication styles change. Jewish people who are third- or fourth-generation Americans are more likely to demonstrate the same communication style as their neighbors rather than that of their parents, grandparents, or great-grandparents. This type of acculturation is part of the history of Jews all over the world (Patai & Wing, 1989).

Touch

The use of touch varies among Jewish people; however, the use or nonuse of touch can be a critical issue with Orthodox Jews and must be carefully considered by the nurse. Because of the Jewish laws regarding personal space and touching others of the opposite sex, it is important to ascertain to which religious group the client belongs. If the client is Orthodox, he or she will be very modest. Over-exposure of or touching the parts of the body associated with sexual activities can cause a great deal of distress. When caring for strict Orthodox Jewish clients of the opposite sex, the nurse should use touch only for hands-on care. To touch the client at any other time could be offensive because of the sexual connotations attached to casual touch. It is also important to note that, according to Jewish law, religious observances are not to be followed if doing so will endanger the person's health.

Implications for Nursing Care

Because older Jewish clients may be very verbal about what and how they are feeling, they may appear to be chronic complainers. Although it is difficult to remain nonjudgmental with a client who is considered a chronic complainer, it is important to remember that letting others know feelings is part of the Jewish culture. It may be difficult to assess pain levels of Jewish clients because they are very emotional when expressing their discomfort, and it may take persistence and patience to pinpoint the problem and its extent. Younger Jewish clients may be more articulate and may also complain less than their parents or grandparents as a result of acculturation.

SPACE

The Orthodox Jew is keenly aware of religious dictates regarding personal space that may or may not be invaded by members of the opposite sex. Many Orthodox Jewish men and women will not shake hands with a member of the opposite sex. This practice stems from the ruling in the Code of Jewish Law that forbids a man to smell the scent of a strange woman, to look upon her hair, or even to gaze upon her little finger (Kolatch, 1985). A very Orthodox Jewish man will not usually touch his wife in public.

Traditionally, Jewish people have also had practices about personal and social space. In times of sickness and during their elderly years, Jewish individuals have an acute desire to have members of their family and other Jews around them. This desire has been illustrated in studies of the elderly that indicate that elderly Jewish people in nursing homes adjust better if they have other Jews around them (Kaplan, 1970).

Implications for Nursing Care

Judaic laws can lead to some misinterpretation by nurses and other health care providers. For example, during childbirth, if a very Orthodox Jewish husband decides to participate in the delivery, his participation will be only verbal. He will not touch his wife during labor. This practice is associated with the laws of separation that dictate that avoidance is necessary during the time a woman has any vaginal bleeding. He will not view the birth because he is not permitted to view his wife's genital area. After the birth, he may lean over his wife (being careful not to touch her), smile, and say, "*Mazel tov*" ("good luck, congratulations") (Bash, 1980; Lutwak, Ney, & White, 1988). Some very Orthodox husbands elect to participate only spiritually. If this is the case, they will sit with their prayerbook and recite from the Book of Psalms. It is important to remember that this practice does not mean the man loves his wife any less than the man who actively participates.

Among the Orthodox Jews there are different groups. The "modern" Orthodox Jew cannot be distinguished by his or her dress, though some traditional Orthodox Jews are often recognizable by their appearance. The men usually have long earlocks and beards and wear a yarmulke (skull cap) or large black hats and long black frock coats. The women are modestly dressed in long-sleeved dresses and have wigs or scarves covering their heads.

With the increase of male nurses, the question arises regarding the assignment of a male nurse to a female Orthodox Jewish client. The Code of Jewish Law (Ganzfried, 1963) states that "a male is not permitted to attend to a woman who is suffering with a belly ache ... but a woman may attend to a male who is so suffering...." This passage may be interpreted to mean that a male nurse should not be assigned to care for a female client. If, however, only male nurses are available, this law would probably be waived because all laws are suspended in the case of severe illness. A law that addresses attendance of a male physician with a female client states that a physician is permitted to let blood and to feel the pulse or any other place of a woman, even if she is married, even the pudenda (external genital organs), as is customary with physicians, because he is merely following his profession (Ganzfried, 1963).

The nurse should be aware that since elderly Jewish clients in non-Jewish hospitals or nursing homes may adjust better with other Jews around them, it may be advantageous to have Jewish clients room together or at least be in proximity. This closeness will allow for increased comfort and offer the Jewish client the chance to interact with someone who "understands" him or her.

SOCIAL ORGANIZATION

The foundation of the Jewish culture is the nuclear family and the greater Jewish community. Controversy exists as to whether the Jewish community or the Jewish family has had the bigger influence on maintaining the Jewish faith and the Jews as a people (Schneider, 1985).

Jewish families tend to be close-knit and child oriented (Schlesinger, 1971). Jewish parents tend to "want better" for their children than they had themselves. It is not unusual to hear parents say

that they have given up something they really wanted for the "sake of the children."

Family life of the Jewish Americans has changed through the years. The earlier Jewish family was male dominated, and the father made the major decisions. The mother's job was to care for the home, the children, and her husband. Today the delineation of duties is more obscure. Usually both parents work, often at jobs of equal financial and professional status.

The Jewish family structure is seen as protective. The Eastern European mother of the past got the reputation of being overbearing and overprotective. In the shtetls of Europe, the mother was the cohesive force in the home. This is still the case today, though younger women are not considered as overbearing or overprotective as their mothers and ancestors were.

In the Jewish family the child is seen as the means of maintaining Jewish existence. Therefore, education of the child in the Jewish faith and traditions is often seen as the most important thing a community, as well as the family, can do. In small Jewish communities, even communities too small for a rabbi, religious education of the children is seen as a priority. The fear of assimilation and annihilation increases the importance to the community of "sticking together" and educating the children.

Among the commandments that Jews are expected to follow are those that dictate the social relationships of family and community. These commandments dictate expected behavior toward parents and people within the community, such as the poor, teachers, rabbis, neighbors, ill people, the dying, and the dead.

Social orientation has helped maintain the Jewish people. When the Eastern European immigrants arrived in the United States, they were an embarrassment for the German Jews. However, commandments that control social behaviors dictated that the German Jews reach out to help the newcomers. This sense of kinship was so strong that Jews felt obliged to help one another, both in the United States and abroad. Today, this dictate is seen in the assistance offered Russian Jews, as well as other smaller groups of Jews from other countries, who immigrate to the United States.

Eastern European Jews brought with them a strong sense of community, which arose from their restricted lives within the shtetls. Furthermore, they were often held responsible for political events that occurred outside the Jewish quarters. Even though each Jew developed his or her own individuality, there was an intense feeling of "groupness," an identification with a common cultural heritage (Kolatch, 1985).

When the immigration laws of the 1920s resulted in decreased numbers of Eastern European Jews entering the United States, increased assimilation began to occur. Several significant events have helped slow the rate of Jewish American assimilation. The event that seems to have had the largest effect was the rise of Nazi anti-Semitism and its American counterparts. The Holocaust caused all Jews to realize that they were indeed brothers (Janowsky, 1964), and the memory of the Holocaust continues to have this effect on Jewish people. Other events that have had an effect on Jewish identification were related to the development of the state of Israel and the struggle of Israel to continue to exist despite a hostile environment. When Israel won the Six-Day War in 1967, the feeling of pride in the Jewish state was almost tangible. There seemed to be a stronger sense of "Jewishness" and an increased willingness to admit to being Jewish. Today, the tension in the Middle East continues to unite Jews.

Today, the Jewish American community is much more mobile than it was in the past. It is not unusual for the children to move away when they leave for college or marry. When a Jewish individual moves, often one of the first things he or she may look for is a Jewish affiliation. A Jew may not join a synagogue until the children are ready for religious school, but often he or she desires the company of other Jews despite the inability to join a synagogue until that time.

Implications for Nursing Care

When a Jewish person becomes ill, family and community resources are mobilized to assist the client.

The Jewish faith contains a commandment to visit the sick. Therefore, friends, relatives, and neighbors will visit an ill Jewish client. If the client is very ill, the visitors will act as client advocates. It is important for the nurse to recognize the cultural implications of these visitors and to expect them to ask about the client.

Because of the protective attitudes of Jewish parents, they will make arrangements to have someone with their child at all times if the child is hospitalized. Jewish parents may appear demanding and aggressive if they believe their child is not getting the care he or she "deserves." Handling the concerns of the parents may take patience on the part of the nurse. The nurse needs to remember that this cultural group highly prizes their children and sees the survival of the Jewish people as a responsibility of the next generation. This view places a large responsibility on the child to get well and on the parents to see that the child does get well.

TIME

The best way to classify Jewish people in relation to time orientation is to say that they are past, present, and future oriented. Jews are aware of their past—all 5000 years of it. They are also concerned about the present and are very involved with current social concerns, both Jewish and non-Jewish. They also look toward the future by insisting that their children be educated, religiously and secularly, and by participating in philanthropic activities to help the future of Israel.

The Jewish concern with the past is very obvious in American society, especially in relation to the Holocaust. Every Jewish person believes that this kind of atrocity should never happen again. By continuing to remind the world of the horrors that happened, not only to Jews but also to people of all faiths and ethnic origins, the Jewish people hope the world will never again let that type of event occur.

During happy occasions, such as a wedding, there is always something to remind Jews of their past. As an example, at the end of the wedding ceremony, the groom breaks a glass. One reason for this custom is to symbolize the destruction of the Jewish temple during the Roman invasion.

Past orientation is also seen following the death of a loved one (such as a parent, sibling, or spouse). On the anniversary of the death each year, a candle is lit and a prayer, the *kaddish* (meaning "holy"), is recited in honor of that person. In addition, the *kaddish* is recited at special times during the year for a loved one. In some congregations the *kaddish* is recited by the whole congregation in memory of those who have recently died or those who have no one to say the prayer for them. In relation to present-time orientation, Jews tend to be very social minded and are often involved in social movements. In many communities, Jewish congregations help run soup kitchens. In a southwestern city a rabbi was involved with the sanctuary movement.

From the Talmud comes the requirement that Jews care for all who are in need whether they are Jewish or non-Jewish. Because the concepts of charity and righteousness are so intertwined, the Hebrew word for "righteousness" (justice), *tzedaka*, has become the Hebrew word for "charity" (Kolatch, 1985). This concept has had an influence on the social system in New York City (Howe, 1989).

Another way that Jewish present-time orientation is apparent is in relation to an afterlife. Although Jews may believe that the spirit continues to live or reside with God after death, they are not concerned about an afterlife. What is considered important is doing good deeds on earth. During an interview regarding the belief in a soul, one woman summed up what has been written by other authors when she stated that it is the memory of one's good deeds that causes one to be immortalized (Schwartz, 1984).

Future-time orientation is apparent in issues concerning the education of children. Establishing schools, supporting schools, and furthering education are top priorities. Throughout the ages, education of the children in the Torah has been regarded as a duty. Originally it was the duty of the parents. Eventually it became the duty of the community (Janowsky, 1964). Today, not only religious but also secular education is seen as important. In most Jewish households the children hear, from the time they are very young, that someday they will go to college. Education is highly prized

as a way of securing the future for the child as well as for the Jewish community as a whole.

Another way that future-time orientation is apparent relates to concerns during illness. Jewish people not only want immediate relief but also worry about what the future implications of their illness will be. They worry about the effect of their illness on the future of their family members, their jobs, and their lives. According to Zborowski (1969), the intensity of their concern is greater than that of other Americans.

Many Jews tend to be punctual when it comes to appointments and become very upset when they arrive on time and have to wait for their appointment to begin. However, some Jewish people also talk about "Jewish standard time," which is at least 10 to 15 minutes later than regular time. Although there are many Jews who are very punctual (especially when it comes to appointments), general Jewish functions, such as weddings or bar mitzvahs, often begin late.

Implications for Nursing Care

Because Jewish people are past, present, and future oriented as well as emotionally expressive, they appear to feel joy, sorrow, illness, and so on with great intensity. They become very anxious when they do not feel well and may appear to be impatient about finding a cure. Jewish people have a tendency to worry about what the illness means in the present as well as the implications it has for the future.

Patience and honesty are necessary qualities for a nurse to display when dealing with Jewish clients. Demonstrating interest and concern will convey the message that the nurse cares about the ill person and may help decrease the amount of anxiety the client is feeling. Until a diagnosis is made, trying to help the anxious Jewish client put events into proper perspective may not work because the client reasons that the nurse cannot know what the future will hold if the physician does not know what is wrong.

It is important to understand that the high degree of outward anxiety the Jewish person may feel is probably more apparent in the older generation of Jews than in the younger generation because assimilation has caused them to exhibit more "acceptable" behavior patterns.

ENVIRONMENTAL CONTROL

Many Jewish people tend to be fatalistic about life. They may believe that they do have some control over their health, but God has the final say. This belief is apparent during Rosh Hashanah and Yom Kippur (the New Year and the Day of Atonement), when Jews pray to be written in the Book of Life for another year.

Health Care Beliefs

Jewish people have a religious requirement to maintain the health of the body as well as the soul. The origin of Jewish health care beliefs dates back to the Torah. Many of the 613 biblical commandments appear to be hygienic in intent. Several chapters in the Book of Leviticus (12 to 14), as well as other books in the Bible, are devoted to the control of disease (Kolatch, 1985). The Talmud continues to stress this concern for health. There are passages that deal with proper exercise, getting enough sleep, eating breakfast, and eating the proper diet.

Physicians are held in high esteem by people in the Jewish culture (Feldman, 1986). In biblical times the priests were physicians. When a Jewish person is ill, it is a duty to go to a physician, and it is the duty of the family to make sure the individual goes. The importance of health care is so great in this culture that Talmudic scholars stated that a person should not settle in a city without a physician (Feldman, 1986).

Jewish people realize that physicians cannot heal without the participation of the client. It is permissible for the Jewish client to question the physician if the client believes the physician is wrong about a diagnosis or treatment (Feldman, 1986; Zborowski, 1969), and the Jewish client may decide not to follow the physician's orders. However, if the client chooses not to listen to the physician or does not agree with the physician, this individual is expected to seek the knowledge of another physician (Feldman, 1986). Seeking the best medical care, even obtaining a second opinion, is a religious dictate.

Health is one of the most frequent topics of conversation among Jewish people. With some Jewish people, especially older ones, health is seen as an exception rather than the rule. The older individual may become preoccupied with the issue of good health because life may be viewed as a temporary lapse between one illness and another (Zborowski, 1969).

The Jewish person believes that prevention of illness is important. Each family member tries to protect and warn the other members of dangers that may cause illnesses, which can make client teaching easier for the nurse. It is important to remember that client teaching in the Jewish family requires the cooperation of all the immediate family members.

There is an increased interest among Jewish adults in alternative or collaborative health care. It is not unusual to hear a group of Jews discussing the issues of fat content in food or the use of herbs to maintain health. In recent years, two healing centers that address prayer and healing have been developed in San Francisco and New York City. Healing services are held periodically in temples throughout the United States.

Illness Behaviors

When a member of a Jewish family is ill, the whole family suffers with the person. Each individual is expected to become a part of the process of helping the ill person feel better.

Complaining about discomforts is expected and accepted, especially in the older generation. Complaining fulfills several important functions: it gives relief through its cathartic function, it is a means of communication, it mobilizes the assistance of the environment, and it reaffirms family solidarity (Zborowski, 1969).

When Jewish clients are admitted to the hospital, they may continue to behave as though they were at home. The Jewish client may attempt to mobilize the attention and sympathy of those in the new environment by using the same methods that worked in the home, so that what the nurse encounters may be a client who complains, cries, moans, and groans. When this behavior does not result in the reactions that would be received from the family, the client may attempt to temper reactions so that feelings of acceptance and being cared for are experienced.

If the client does not verbalize pain, another member of the family will usually do so. The reasoning is that the client may be too ill to tell the physician or nurse and that it is the family member's responsibility to communicate to obtain the attention the family member believes the loved one should have.

Zborowski's (1969) study of first-generation Jewish Americans in pain noted that these clients responded to questions with details that sometimes seemed to relate only marginally to the topic. In the study a simple question released a flow of responses that led to information about pain, illness, anxieties, intrafamily relationships, and so on. Probing was necessary to pinpoint specific information rather than to elicit a fuller answer to a question.

Second-, third-, and fourth-generation Jewish Americans seem to be a little less expressive about their pain. However, they do consider it wrong not to express their feelings. The expressive behavior of Jews seems to indicate that Jewish people believe that one cannot get help unless a complaint is made.

If oral complaining does not result in the type of behavior the client wishes to elicit from those around him or her, crying may be used. Crying, with many first-generation Jewish Americans, is acceptable behavior and is seen as an expression of frustration or pain and often results in the attention desired (Zborowski, 1969).

With increased American acculturation, each succeeding Jewish American generation appears to be less expressive when in pain. The women may cry easily, but the men have adopted the American view that crying is not proper behavior for men. Second-generation Jewish American male clients tend to be less verbal about their pain than their fathers (Zborowski, 1969). For some Jewish people, however, the meaning of pain does not change, just the outward signs. For a Jewish person, pain, discomfort, and change in the state of good health

are seen as a warning that something is wrong and that the professional health care system needs to be utilized.

Jews have been noted to have higher physician utilization rates than other groups, as well as having a heightened concern for maintaining health (Jacobs & Giarelli, 2001). Utilization of the health care system may involve getting the opinions of several physicians. The Jewish client recognizes that the physician is only another human, with the possibility of being incorrect. By getting at least one other opinion, the client can decide if the physician was correct or not. Before choosing the physician to see for a second opinion, the Jewish person will most likely ask a number of people who might have connections in the medical community for recommendations. Not only is a Jewish client likely to get a second or third opinion but also this client may check the medical literature and search the Web for information about their condition and prescribed regimen. Zborowski (1969) has noted that these activities seem to be based on a feeling that the client is the final judge and authority in matters pertaining to his or her health. In this case the physician is seen in the role of consultant and advisor.

Once the Jewish client accepts the physician's opinion, the client will also accept the prescribed treatment. The cultural belief is that to get well, one must cooperate with all therapeutic measures. Although the Jewish client will follow the prescribed regimen, the client expects the medication regimen to be individualized because illness is viewed as being individualized. Jewish patients today take a more active role in health care decisions.

In many cases, the client will want to know all about the prescribed treatment: what is expected of the client, what the side effects are, and, if a drug is being prescribed, the name of the drug. The client is unlikely to be content with, "It's good for you."

The Jewish client tends to observe carefully the effects of the drug or treatment on the system. Since many Jews believe that they are the ultimate judge of their condition, they may change the time they take a drug, increase or decrease the number of drugs taken, or reject the drug completely if they decide it is not helping or is harmful. Many times these decisions are made without consulting the physician. Careful, thorough explanations about the drug, its purpose, side effects, and why it was ordered are essential.

The future-oriented Jewish client may become hesitant to take analgesics because most drugs are viewed as "dope" and Jewish persons often fear addiction. This fear increases the problem for the client in pain who wants to receive pain relief but is afraid of addiction (Zborowski, 1969).

Wellness Behaviors

Jewish American people tend to be more educated than most other American ethnic groups (Sowell, 1981), and the thirst for knowledge is apparent in their wellness behaviors. They tend to be well read on issues of health, and it is not unusual to hear Jews discussing the latest information on maintaining healthy diets, preventing disease, or following health-oriented regimens.

In years past, it was rare to see Jewish children involved in physical activities. Eastern European Jews tended to de-emphasize physical activity in favor of more intellectual activities that kept the children closer to home. This practice may have stemmed from the fears of child abduction that they brought with them from the "old country" (Sowell, 1981). However, this trend seems to be changing. Jewish children are now involved with soccer teams, baseball teams, and other physical activities. Their parents are also more involved in physical exercise. Jogging, tennis, racquetball, and aerobics are some of the activities that are attracting more Jewish participants as the importance of physical exercise is discussed in the media.

Maintaining certain laws is included in the wellness behaviors seen in Orthodox Jewish people. Many of these laws have been incorporated into the everyday habits of most Jewish Americans because they are good hygiene or they have been proved to be medically prudent. The following are examples of these laws taken from the Code of Jewish Law (Ganzfried, 1963):

1. The hands must be washed on awakening from sleep, after elimination of bodily wastes, after hair cutting, after touching a vermin, and after being in proximity to a dead human body.
2. The proper way of washing oneself is to take a bath regularly every week.
3. It is advisable for one to accustom himself to having breakfast in the morning.
4. One is forbidden to eat or drink out of unclean vessels, and the individual should not eat with hands that are not clean.

There is a belief, although there is no empirical evidence to support it, that the custom requiring washing hands before meals has contributed to lower morbidity and mortality rates. Plus, because of better hygiene, infant and child mortality rates have been lower in Jewish than in non-Jewish populations (Jacobs & Giarelli, 2001).

Kosher Diet, Religious Holidays, and Illness

Maintaining a kosher (*kasher*, "fit, proper") diet may pose a problem for some Jewish clients. As mentioned in Chapter 7, kosher meat is usually salted to help drain all the blood. This process presents a problem for a client on a low-salt diet unless the meat is soaked in water to remove as much of the salt as possible.

It is important for the nurse to consider what can be done for the Jewish client following a kosher diet if the hospital does not have a kosher supplier nearby. In this case it is possible to serve any fish that meets the dietary requirements of having fins and scales. It is also possible to serve dairy products as long as they are not contraindicated on the person's diet. These meals should be served on paper plates with plastic utensils because meat and milk products or dishes prepared with milk products should not be mixed.

If, because of medical dietary restrictions and the unavailability of kosher food, maintaining a kosher diet is impossible, the client must decide to waive the dietary restrictions. All commandments are suspended whenever a life is in danger, no matter how remote the likelihood of death (Feldman, 1986). Food is essential to maintain life; therefore, the client would be directed by the rabbi to eat whatever the hospital could provide that would help sustain life.

Yom Kippur (the Day of Atonement) and Passover (based on Hebrew *pesah*, "passing over") are two holidays that require special consideration. On Yom Kippur, Jewish people are required to fast for 24 hours. If this fast is considered physically or medically dangerous, however, the individual is required by law to put aside the law and eat. Passover requires that special foods be served. Passover, which falls in or near the spring of the year, is an eight-day holiday that celebrates the freedom of the Jews from Egypt. During these eight days, certain foods must be "kosher for Passover" (*kasher le-pesah*). In addition, there are other foods that are forbidden, including any foods with leavening (bread, cakes made with baking soda or baking powder) or foods made with even a small amount of a grain product or by-product that is not specifically prepared for Passover. This prohibition includes many drugs and medications, such as those containing starch or grain alcohol. These drugs may be refused by the client unless they cannot be replaced and are urgently needed by the client.

Procreation

The use or nonuse of contraceptives is dictated by Jewish law, which requires one to "be fruitful and multiply." This can cause special problems for the woman who is unable to conceive or the woman who may have physical problems making conception dangerous. There is a lengthy discussion of this issue in the *Mishnah* (a part of the Talmud containing the oral law). The final analysis is that the man is commanded to procreate, but the woman is not, because, it is believed, God would not impose on the "children of Israel" a burden "too difficult for a person to bear" (Gold, 1988). Since childbirth is painful and may be physically dangerous, it would be unfair for the Torah to impose the commandment for procreation on the woman.

When Jewish men were allowed two wives, this commandment was not a problem. Today, because monogamy is the rule in the Jewish community, procreation is seen as the couple's obligation. However, outside of the very Orthodox community, Jewish couples today decide on how many children they want, and most practice some form of birth control. Within the very Orthodox community, the use of birth control is discouraged unless pregnancy or delivery would be dangerous for the woman.

Couples who have a problem with fertility are encouraged to seek medical help. For the very Orthodox Jewish man, however, a problem arises in the collection of semen. Rabbis have declared that masturbation and the use of male contraceptives such as condoms are not permitted because the Talmud outlaws the spilling of seed. For this reason, the woman is usually tested first, and then, if no problem can be detected, the man may be tested. The very Orthodox Jewish husband will have to consult his rabbi before he consents to a sperm count. Since masturbation is considered taboo, it may be emotionally difficult for the man to collect his semen. This is not a problem for most non-Orthodox couples.

It is interesting to note that the role of companionship is given an equal place with procreation in the purpose of a Jewish marriage (Gold, 1988). To add to this idea of companionship, rabbis have also addressed the idea of sexual satisfaction being the right of both men and women within the bonds of marriage (Lutwak, Ney, & White, 1988).

Organ Transplants

According to Jewish law, all body parts should be buried with the body after death (Jakobovits, 1975). However, if an organ transplant would save the life of another human being, it is permissible to donate the organ (Feldman, 1986). Even removal of the heart for transplantation is allowed so long as the dying person has experienced total brainstem death (Feldman, 1986; Kolatch, 1985).

Life-Support Measures

According to Jewish law, nothing may be done to hasten death; a client must be given every chance for life. However, if the use of mechanical systems would delay death rather than prolong life, they should not be used. If mechanical systems have been connected and they are not helping to prolong life but are delaying death, they may be removed (Feldman, 1986).

The Dying Jewish Client

As there are commandments that control living for the Jew, there are also commandments that control dying. These commandments are usually followed strictly only by Orthodox Jews, but some of the behaviors that the nurse may see in other Jews are a result of the cultural knowledge that these commandments have created.

According to Jewish law, a person who is very ill and considered to be dying should not be left alone. One reason for this law is that the spirit is believed to depart from the body at the time of death, and if no one were present, the soul would feel alone and desolate (Sperling, 1968). To satisfy this commandment, family members will often take turns sitting with the critically or terminally ill client. Asking family members to leave may cause family distress.

Jewish law also dictates that a client should be informed that death is near. However, because of two controversial passages in the Torah, some rabbis believe it is important to inform a dying individual about serious illness but not that death is near. Informing a person about a serious illness allows the individual time to put worldly affairs in order, as Isaac and Jacob did when they were told they would die (Heller, 1986). However, to tell a person that death is imminent removes all hope, and some Jewish people fear that this information may hasten death.

Judaism teaches that it is important to lead a good, decent, and helping life on earth. Since good deeds must be done on earth, the law requires a Jew to ask God to forgive those deeds that may have been against God or not in keeping with God's commandments. To fulfill this commandment, the dying person is encouraged to recite the confessional. If the individual is too sick to say the whole confessional, the individual is encouraged to recite the affirmation of faith, the *Shma*. If the dying person cannot repeat any of the confessional, the law says that it is up to the family or friends who are with the person to recite it. The recitation of the confessional is usually seen only with observant Jews.

Once death has been established, the eyes and mouth are closed by the son or nearest relative. In some Orthodox Jewish families, it is customary to remove the body from the bed and place it on a straw mat on the floor, with the person's feet toward the door through which the body will be taken. A candle is placed at the person's head to symbolize the "light," or joy and love the departed brought to others while alive (Trepp, 1980). A sheet is placed over the person's face because it is disrespectful to the dead to permit others to see the ravages of death on the face (Sperling, 1968). The dead body is viewed as being contaminated by Orthodox Jews and is placed on the floor because the bed is viewed as being defiled by contact with the dead body; however, the ground is not considered defiled by contact (Sperling, 1968). It is important to understand that this behavior is rarely seen in most hospitals or nursing homes today.

Autopsy is not allowed by Orthodox Jews unless (1) it is required by governmental regulations, (2) the person had a hereditary disease and autopsy may help safeguard the health of survivors, or (3) another known person is suffering from a similar deadly disease and an autopsy may yield information vital to that person's health (Jakobovits, 1975). If an autopsy is performed, all parts that are removed must be buried with the body. Autopsy does not pose a religious problem for the non-Orthodox Jew.

AIDS

It has been stated that "AIDS will cause psychological and social reactions that may change the character of human social life" (Edelheit, 1989). In the Jewish community, AIDS poses a psychological, social, and religious problem. The problem lies in the traditional belief system of the Jewish people: according to the Torah, homosexuality is an abomination, and premarital sexual activity is not permitted by the traditional rabbinate. This belief system is a potential cause of distress for the Jewish homosexual, or for any Jew who tests HIV positive. They have to live not only with their disease but also with being an outcast of their culture.

Patient education in an Orthodox Jewish environment may be very difficult, and rabbis in all the religious groups are still trying to decide how to handle this situation. Some of them are addressing it and trying to teach about the disease and safe sex. It appears that Orthodox rabbis are handling the issue of "safe sex" by going to the law that states that methods to destroy or block the passage of the seed are not permitted. Rabbi Yonassan Gershom (1998) notes that the issue of safe sex should not be a problem for Orthodox Jews because sex outside of marriage is not permitted. When asked about issues of finger sticks or blood transfusions, Rabbi Gershom responded that each case would be considered on an individual basis. Homosexuality among Reform Jewish rabbis is recognized and accepted. There are Reform synagogues that have predominantly homosexual congregations. In 1997 the Reform Jewish movement agreed to ordain openly homosexual Jewish rabbis.

AIDS and the Jewish client is an area requiring great sensitivity for the nurse. The most important thing that the nurse can do for the Jewish AIDS victim is to be there for support. These victims not only need to deal with a terminal illness and rejection by the general society but also need to deal with possible cultural and religious ostracism.

Circumcision

According to Jewish teaching, God made a covenant with Abraham in which God promised to bless Abraham and make him prosper if Abraham would be loyal to God. This covenant was entered into and sealed by the act of circumcision. Jewish people honor this covenant by having a *brit* (which means "sign of the Covenant," *bĕ rith*) on the eighth day of the baby's life. If the child is ill or was born prematurely, the *brit* is postponed until the infant is in good health. The circumcision is usually done by a *mohel*, who is trained to do circumcisions. This is a time of celebration, and usually the entire family and friends gather at the home of the baby's parents for this important occasion. Since the circumcision is performed in the home, the nurse should review the principles of circumcision care with the mother before discharge.

The postcircumcision care is usually managed by the *mohel*. L'Archevesque and Goldstein-Lohman (1996) note the importance of offering parents information about the different methods of circumcision, types of pain-control measures, and symptoms of possible complications. Parents should be educated about the expected amount of bloody staining and what would be excessive bleeding, as well as signs and symptoms of infection.

Implications for Nursing Care

Caring for Jewish clients may be viewed as difficult by the nurse. Jewish clients tend to be vocal about feelings, anxieties, and pain, but they may not be direct about what is bothering them. This type of verbalization can be difficult for health care providers who expect the client to be compliant, noncomplaining, and direct about needs. Nurses with judgmental attitudes may label the Jewish client as childish, which leads to treating the client as a child or ignoring the client as much as possible. It is important for the nurse to remember that for the Jewish client, this childlike behavior may be part of the culture. The nurse must be patient and let the client know that the nurse cares about needs because this will lead to feelings of trust and may decrease what is seen as demanding behavior.

Demanding behavior is less likely to occur in second-, third-, or fourth-generation Jewish Americans, who are more aware of what is considered acceptable behavior by the general American culture. This awareness does not mean that they feel pain or anxieties any less.

Illness is often viewed by Jews as a family affair. Because the whole family is involved with the ill person's suffering, the whole family wants to know what is happening with or to the client. The family members often do not appear to trust the word of another family member and instead want to get the information directly from the physician or the nurse. To assist the family and decrease the amount of time numerous explanations may take, it may help to have a family conference. However, not all the members may show up at the same time, and the nurse may need to repeat the information. The most important message to convey to the family of a Jewish client is that of caring, not only about the client but also about each family member and the pain they are going through.

Assisting the client who is dying, as well as the family, requires knowledge of Jewish cultural practices and beliefs. The nurse needs to remain sensitive to the need for a confessional if death is imminent and the client is Orthodox. Studies have shown that following cultural practices helps decrease the amount of distress and disorganization felt by loved ones during the death and dying period (Dempsey, 1977; Ross, 1981). Therefore, it is the duty of the nurse to assist families in following customs related to death and dying. When an Orthodox Jew dies, the body must not be touched by a person of the opposite sex. One nurse recounted the story of a young Chassidic boy who died and was washed by the nurses on the floor before the father arrived. The father became so upset that a female had touched his son's body that he told the nurses not to touch him, left the hospital, and returned a few minutes later with some dirt and a bag. He covered the boy's body with the dirt, put him in the bag, and carried him out of the hospital. He did this because the body was considered contaminated. When an Orthodox patient dies, all clothing and dressing material with the patient's blood on it must be left with the patient (Sommer, 1995).

Jewish people are interested in illness prevention and may ask in-depth questions to clarify what is being said. They may ask many questions to weigh information for personal effect, and these questions should not be misconstrued to indicate mistrust of the health care professional.

When caring for a Jewish client, it is helpful for the nurse to know what form of religious practice is adhered to because the Orthodox Jewish client will follow religious practices more strictly than any other group. Unless the nurse works in an area that has a large number of Orthodox Jews, most Jewish clients cared for will be non-Orthodox and may not be affiliated with any group.

BIOLOGICAL VARIATIONS

Some people believe that a Jewish person can be recognized by physical appearance, and the "Semitic appearance" is occasionally related to cultural patterns (Goodman, 1979). However, Jews differ greatly in physical appearance, depending on what part of the world they migrated to when forced out of Israel. Jews are not uniformly the same as far as height, hair and eye color, body structure, or shape of the nose is concerned. European Jews are White, Falashas (Ethiopian Jews) are Black, and Chinese Jews have Asian features. The differences among Jews from different parts of the world are the results of biological adaptation to the area of the world resided in, intermarriage with non-Jews, and converts to Judaism (Goodman, 1979; Mourant, Kopec, & Domaniewsks-Sobczak, 1978).

For determination of the extent of genetic similarity among Jews as opposed to non-Jews, studies of blood phenotypes have been done (Goodman, 1979; Mourant, Kopec, & Domaniewsks-Sobczak, 1978). As opposed to outward appearances, blood characteristics are unaffected by the environment.

Enzymatic and Genetic Variations

Although skin color, body size, and body structure vary, depending on the part of the world resided in, fingerprint patterns indicate a relatedness among Jews from Germany, Turkey, Morocco, and Yemen. The patterns of fingerprint whorls, loops, and arches are similar to those of non-Jews living in the Mediterranean area. This seems to indicate that the Jewish people, though appearing to be diversified genetically, still maintain a remnant of the Mediterranean gene pool.

To classify genetic differences of peoples, polymorphic blood groups, serum and cell proteins, and enzyme variants that have altered catalytic activity, kinetic properties, stability, or electrophoretic mobility are used. Since anthropological structures and simple genetic traits of Jews are difficult to define, Jewish genetic studies have concentrated on the genetic polymorphisms (Rothschild & Chapman, 1981). Data from these studies have concluded that (1) Jewish groups from different parts of the world are very different genetically, (2) Jews of a certain area tend to resemble the surrounding non-Jews more than they resemble Jews from other parts of the world, and (3) European Jews have a residue of non-European genes that resemble Mediterranean genes (Patai & Wing, 1989).

A study by Stevenson, Schanfield, and Sandler (1985) on immunoglobulin allotypes had interesting results. The multivariate analyses indicated that the Jewish populations may be derived from a common gene pool. When the results were plotted, all the Jews, except the Yemenite group, were genetically similar to each other. The European Jewish cluster is the most closely knit in similarity, and the Asian and North African Jewish clusters are closer to Middle Eastern groups than to European non-Jews.

In relation to genetic disorders, the Jewish population is divided into Sephardic Jews, Asian Jews, and Ashkenazi Jews. Since the largest number of Jews in the United States are Ashkenazi Jews (European), the rest of this discussion involves genetic disorders most prevalent in this group.

Of all the genetic disorders that occur most frequently in Eastern European Jews, the one receiving the most publicity is Tay-Sachs disease. This disease is recessively inherited and is characterized by the absence of an enzyme involved in fat metabolism, resulting in the accumulation of fatty substances in the brain and leading to gradual neural and mental degeneration, with death occurring around 3 or 4 years of age. Couples in which both partners are Jews of Eastern European descent should be counseled to have genetic screening done to prevent the possibility of having a child with this deadly disease.

In January 2001, the genetic mutation for another disorder common to Ashkenazi Jews was discovered (Jorde, Carey, Bamshad, & White, 2006; Jaffe-Gill, 2002). This disorder, familial dysautonomia, is a deadly disease affecting children and often causing death before the age of 30. It is characterized by pain; wild fluctuations in blood pressure and body temperature; and impaired chewing, swallowing, and digestion.

Although Gaucher disease is rare, it has a frequency more than 0.03 in Ashkenazi Jews (Jorde, Carey, Bamshad, & White, 2006). The most common allele attributable to Gaucher disease is thought to be produced by an A to G mutation resulting in a single amino acid substitution (Jorde, Carey, Bamshad, & White, 2006). Gaucher disease is characterized by enlarged visceral organs, multi-organ failure, and a debilitating skeletal disease. The DNA tests available today are capable of detecting 97% of the mutations among the five most common Gaucher alleles in the Ashkenazi Jewish population (Jorde, Carey, Bamshad, & White, 2006).

Glucose-6-PD (G-6-PD) deficiency has been linked to severe jaundice that leads to kernicterus or even death in newborns (Kaplan, Renbaum, Levy-Lahad, et al., 1997). Kaplan and associates (1997) conducted a study to determine whether the TA repeat promoter in the gene for uridinediphospho-glucuronate glucuronosyltransferase (EC1.1.1.49; UDPGT1) was associated with benign jaundice noted in adults (Gilbert syndrome) or to determine if this mutation could increase the incidence of neonatal hyperbilirubinemia in G-6-PD deficiency. Findings from this study suggested that neither G-6-PD deficiency nor the variant UDPGTI promoter, by themselves, increased the incidence of hyperbilirubinemia. Findings from this study, however, suggested that UDPGTI promoter, when coupled with G-6-PD deficiency, did ultimately increase the incidence of hyperbilirubinemia (Kaplan, Renbaum, Levy-Lahad, et al., 1997).

Susceptibility to Disease

Susceptibility to disease for Jewish people depends on geographical origin. Some beliefs about Jewish susceptibility have no real scientific basis, such as the belief that Jews are more likely than others to have diabetes mellitus. Some studies have shown that Jews are no more susceptible to this disease than non-Jews from the same area of the world, as had been originally believed (Goodman, 1979).

Cancer. Certain cancers are more frequent in certain groups of Jews than in others. Stomach cancer is more prevalent among Jews from Europe and the United States. Colon and prostate cancer is prevalent in Jews of Eastern European descent. Breast cancer, the most frequent type of cancer for all Jewish female groups except those from Iran (Patai & Wing, 1989), has been found to be more common in Jewish women from Europe and the United States than in those from Asia. Cancer of the ovary is generally higher in Jews from Europe than in those from Asia or Africa. Darwish and associates (2002) conducted a study on subjects residing in the same geographical location. The primary purpose of the study was to evaluate and compare differences in molecular genetics among high-risk (Ashkenazi), intermediate-risk (Sephardic), and low-risk (Palestinian) people for colorectal cancer. Findings from this study suggested that Ashkenazi Jews have the highest rate of colorectal cancer and are generally diagnosed earlier than Sephardic Jews.

Studies indicate that 1% to 2% of American Ashkenazi Jewish women have a high incidence of specific mutations of *BRCA1* and *BRCA2* (Gene mutation, 1995; Jacobs & Giarelli, 2001). These changes have been associated with an increase in ovarian cancer and with a higher risk in breast cancer. A specific alteration (185delAG) appears to be found in Ashkenazi Jews and is considered to be ethnic specific (Key, 1997). While the *BRCA1* and *BRCA2* founder mutations have been clearly delineated among Ashkenazi Jewish women, this knowledge alone has not lead to increased testing among this vulnerable population (Schwartz, Benkendorf, Lerman, et al., 2002). Schwartz, Benkendorf, Lerman, et al. (2002) conducted a study to determine whether a brief educational booklet regarding *BRCA1* and *BRCA2* could influence knowledge and attitudes and generate interest in testing among Ashkenazi women. Findings from this study suggested that, relative to breast cancer education, the genetic testing materials did lead to increased knowledge among these women, increased the perceptions of the risks and the limitations of the testing, and yet decreased the interest of these women in obtaining a *BRCA1/BRCA2* mutation test. Nonetheless, these researchers concluded that educational print material is an innovative way to educate low-risk individuals about *BRCA1/BRCA2* genetic testing (Schwartz, Benkendorf, Lerman, et al., 2002).

Historically, rates of cancer of the cervix have been lower in Jewish women than in non-Jews (Patai & Wing, 1989). However, as Jews become more acculturated and the incidence of multiple sexual partners, as well as partners who are not circumcised, increases, so does the incidence of cervical cancer. Cervical cancer is an area of concern for some Jewish individuals and an area where client teaching is helpful.

Just recently, *HPC1/RNASEL* was identified as a candidate gene for hereditary prostate cancer (Rennert, Bercovich, Hubert, et al., 2002). Rennert and associates (2002) identified a novel founder frameshift mutation *RNASEL*, 47delAAAG, in Ashkenazi Jews. In fact, when these researchers estimated the mutation frequency in this Ashkenazi population, they were able to determine that the frequency among 159 healthy young females was 4% (95% confidence interval [CI]). However, among Ashkenazi Jews, the mutation frequency was significantly higher in subjects with prostate cancer as compared with a control group consisting of elderly males. It was interesting to note that 47delAAAG was not detected in 134 non-Ashkenazi subjects with prostate cancer. Findings from this study also suggest that the 47delAAAG null mutation is associated with prostate cancer in Ashkenazi Jewish men (Rennert, Bercovich, Hubert, et al., 2002).

Heart Disease. Data from a classic 1952 study of serum cholesterol levels in New York indicate a higher frequency of elevated serum cholesterol levels among Jews than among non-Jews. It is believed that elevated serum cholesterol levels may be caused by a single gene (Patai & Wing, 1989). If this is true, Ashkenazi Jews may have a higher frequency of the gene than Asian Jews, who seem to have a relatively low rate of elevated serum cholesterol levels.

It is commonly believed that Ashkenazi Jews are more prone to coronary disease than other Jewish ethnic groups or non-Jews are. In international comparisons of the rate of first-time myocardial infarctions among men, Israel ranks among the highest in the world if all types of infarcts (including clinically unrecognized infarcts) are included (Mourant, Kopec, & Domaniewsks-Sobczak, 1978). Although there is a relatively high incidence of infarcts in Israel, there is a low mortality rate. After numerous studies, the conclusion regarding heart disease in the Jewish population is that further studies need to be done to determine the frequency of the disease among Jews as well as the interplay between heredity and environment (Mourant, Kopec, & Domaniewsks-Sobczak, 1978).

Polycythemia Vera. Evidence indicates that polycythemia vera is more common in Ashkenazi Jews than in other ethnic groups. In addition, there seems to be a higher prevalence of polycythemia vera in Jewish men than in Jewish women (Mourant, Kopec, & Domaniewsks-Sobczak, 1978).

Diabetes Mellitus. Diabetes has been referred to as the "Jewish disease" in Germany. Through ethnic Jewish studies done in Israel, an interesting phenomenon has been noted. A slightly higher percentage of Ashkenazi Jews than Sephardic Jews have diabetes. Also, in Yemenite and Kurdish newcomers to Israel, there are almost no cases of diabetes. However, in Yemenite and Kurdish settlers who have lived in Israel for more than 25 years, the same frequency of diabetes as with Ashkenazi Jews has been identified (Mourant, Kopec, & Domaniewsks-Sobczak, 1978; Patai & Wing, 1989). The results of this study indicate that dietary habits have an influence on the development of diabetes. The main dietary change in the older settlers as compared with the new arrivals has been an increased intake of sugar.

Although the incidence of diabetes in Jewish people has been indicated as being higher than in the general population, there has been no study to confirm this belief. Most of the studies on diabetes among Jews have been done in Israel. For a truer assessment of the prevalence of diabetes in the Jewish community, further studies outside Israel need to be conducted (Mourant, Kopec, & Domaniewsks-Sobczak, 1978).

Crohn's Disease. Studies indicate that Crohn's disease occurs in Jewish males more often than in Jewish females, and in Jews more often than in any other White ethnic group (Mourant, Kopec, & Domaniewsks-Sobczak, 1978). Although the number of young people diagnosed as having this disease has been increasing (Thompson, McFarland, Hirsch, et al., 1989), it is unknown if the increase is a result of a better awareness of the disease and improved diagnostic techniques or if there is an actual increase in the number of cases.

Ulcerative Colitis. Ulcerative colitis is seen more frequently in Ashkenazi Jews than in non-Jews or in any other Jewish ethnic groups. It has many similarities to Crohn's disease and may even be seen with Crohn's disease. The cause of ulcerative colitis is unknown, but familial tendencies have been noted; it occurs 10% to 15% more often in families of clients with ulcerative colitis than in families of control clients without the disease (Mourant, Kopec, & Domaniewsks-Sobczak, 1978).

Myopia. Jews seem to have a higher incidence of myopia than the general population, and it occurs more often in boys than in girls. It is important to understand that myopia is not caused by close bookwork, as was believed many years ago, but by a prevalence of low hypermetropia and factors that allow for a greater or longer development of the length of the eye. Vision screening is an important part of a physical examination for Jewish people, particularly Jewish children.

Nutritional Preferences and Deficiencies

Jewish people tend to eat a lot of dairy products, which becomes a concern in patients with a history of lactose intolerance. Lactose intolerance has been identified among some Jewish ethnic groups, and a study done in Israel identified approximately two thirds of the Jewish population in Israel as being lactase deficient. However, the researchers also noted that most of these clients were not aware of their milk intolerance, leading to the conclusion that the condition was relatively benign and asymptomatic in the Jews studied (Mourant, Kopec, & Domaniewsks-Sobczak, 1978). Any Jewish client with a history of diarrhea, nonspecific lower gastrointestinal symptoms, and abdominal pain should have a good dietary history taken to check for a history of milk intolerance. The nurse needs to determine any family tendency toward lactose intolerance, as well as the relationship between foods and the onset of abdominal symptoms.

It is important for the nurse to remember that not all Jews maintain a kosher diet and that some Jews are stricter about their diet than others. If the nurse is caring for an Orthodox Jewish client who is not eating properly because of the conflict between maintaining a kosher diet and eating institutional food, the nurse should consult with the family about bringing food from home. If the family cannot help with this situation, the client's rabbi may be consulted.

Psychological Characteristics

Jews have been labeled with certain personality traits for over 3000 years. According to the Bible, the Children of Israel, following their exodus from Egypt, were "stiff necked," quarrelsome, disobedient, and rebellious. In Talmudic literature the Jews are described as the "merciful sons of a merciful father." Greek and Roman authors, who were usually anti-Semitic, made derogatory comments on the Jewish character.

It was not until the 1930s that studies began to explore Jewish personality characteristics (Patai & Wing, 1989). All these studies involved Jewish Americans, and most involved college students. The conclusions derived from these studies are as follows (Patai & Wing, 1989):

1. Studies indicate that Jews are superior in intelligence to comparable groups of non-Jews, especially in verbal intelligence. It is questionable whether Jews are genetically more intelligent than non-Jews; the apparent superiority in intelligence may be attributable to the pressures from the Gentile world for Jews to rely on their brains in order to survive.

2. In scholarly, intellectual, literary, and artistic pursuits, Jews seem to be proportionately overrepresented. Whether this phenomenon is proof of special Jewish talent or the result of extraneous circumstances that attracted Jews to concentrate on certain areas is open for debate.

3. As far as character traits are concerned, it is difficult to pinpoint differences between Jews and non-Jews. Character traits seem to be formed more by personal experiences in the immediate environment than by historical conditioning.

As an example, Jewish Americans have been characterized as being aggressive, and this aggressiveness may be attributable to the pressure placed on Jewish children by their parents to "have a better life" than they did.

Anti-Semitism is a concern for Jewish people. Within the Jewish community, mention is often made of Jewish fear in regard to anti-Semitism. Although the relative freedom experienced in the United States has led to a decrease in the practice of many Jewish rituals and possibly to the increased numbers of nonpracticing Jews, there are constant reminders that Jews are different and not always accepted by the general public. Today, in addition to constant reminders of the Holocaust, some Jewish people are also concerned about events in Israel.

Mental Health. The older medical literature indicates that the rate of occurrence of a variety of mental illnesses in Jews is high. In discussing this issue with numerous psychiatrists and leaders in the mental health field, Mourant, Kopec, and Domaniewsks-Sobczak (1978) have concluded that necessary data are lacking to confirm that the old medical literature is correct.

One concern among psychiatrists and mental health workers in Orthodox Jewish sections is the apparent need for but lack of use of mental health facilities. To determine what discourages Orthodox Jews from seeking psychiatric professional help, a study was conducted with 20 Orthodox Jewish mental health outpatients; it revealed that Orthodox Jews attach a stigma to mental health treatment and to Jews who avail themselves of it. This stigma is partly the result of an association of mental health treatment with insanity and partly because of the fear that this knowledge will have a negative effect on matrimonial prospects (Wikler, 1986).

It is important for the nurse to remember that Orthodox Jews do not enter mental health treatment easily. In the case of an Orthodox Jew who may need psychiatric counseling, there may be resistance to overcome before treatment can be started. The prospective client may display a real concern about confidentiality that may be seen as paranoia. This paranoia needs to be understood within the context of the social risk involved.

Orthodox Jews who do seek mental health care usually choose the agency or therapist based on reputation. One agency that opened its office in the Williamsburg section of Brooklyn, New York, in the heart of the Chassidic and Orthodox Jewish sections, was picketed and threatened. Today, however, this center has earned the "grudging" respect of the community (Meer, 1987).

Alcoholism. The literature reports that Jews have had a low incidence of alcoholism in the past (Mourant, Kopec, & Domaniewsks-Sobczak, 1978). This assumption is questionable, and the incidence of cross-addiction, to both alcohol and another substance, may be higher among Jews than among non-Jews (Steinhardt, 1988). Lieberman (1987) has noted that Jews do not acknowledge a problem with alcohol because of their perception of what an alcoholic is. Many Jews view the alcoholic as a skid row bum, not a person who gets drunk and acts silly at a wedding or maybe drinks too much when celebrating a holiday or festival, even if this behavior occurs on a regular basis.

All the behaviors that characterize the alcoholic in general—denial, isolation, ignorance of the disease, and guilt—seem to be intensified in the Jewish alcoholic because of the myth of Jewish sobriety. Orthodox Jews seem to suffer the greatest from these symptoms (Steinhardt, 1988).

Studies done in the United States indicate that drinking disorders tend to increase in Jews as religious affiliation shifts from Orthodox, to Conservative, to Reform, to secular (Mourant, Kopec, & Domaniewsks-Sobczak, 1978). Some sociologists have suggested that alcoholism among Jews may increase as acculturation increases.

Of greatest concern to the Jewish community and to health care workers is the increasing alcohol and drug abuse among Jewish youth. It is important to educate the Jewish community on the facts that alcoholics are not just skid row, homeless people and that the ceremonial and social drinking of the Jewish community can increase the potential for alcoholism if it is not tempered.

Holocaust Survivors. Although the Holocaust has had a profound effect on Jewish feelings regarding "Jewishness" and persecution, the Holocaust survivors have had very little effect on the Jewish culture in the United States as a whole. The reason for this is that a relatively small number of Jewish Americans are Holocaust survivors. Many studies have been done on the effects of the Holocaust on survivors (Kren & Rappoport, 1980; Rose & Garske, 1987). These studies have helped the medical profession, especially the psychiatric medical profession, to determine the effects of war atrocities on survivors.

Since the 1990s, there has been an increase in studies of adults who are child survivors of the Holocaust. The studies indicate that child survivors show an increased level of posttraumatic symptomatology; see the world as more negative, however more controllable and meaningful; and have a high vulnerability to stress (Cohen, Brom, & Dasberg, 2001). Although many of these studies were done in Israel, it is expected that all child Holocaust survivors will have similar symptoms.

Many Jews have a difficult time discussing the effects of the Holocaust and its devastation on Jewish families and communities. Jewish individuals sometimes leave the room when the Holocaust is mentioned or joke to relieve their distress or feelings of anger and bewilderment at how this type of event could occur in modern times in a country that was supposed to be "civilized."

The effects of the Holocaust on the survivors and their children are still being studied. From the literature comes evidence of anger, depression, withdrawal, and anxiety in the survivors (Krystal & Niederland, 1971; Steinitz & Szonyi, 1979). Bearing children was seen as a means for the survivors to replace their loved ones who were lost during "the War," and the children were seen as a source of new hope and meaning. Because of this transference, the children of the survivors were usually overprotected and had unrealistic expectations placed on them (Nadler, Kav-Venaki, & Gleitman, 1985).

Numerous studies have been done on children of Holocaust survivors. The results of these studies indicate that, on the whole, this population is well adjusted, with few significant psychopathological problems (Nadler, Kav-Venaki, & Gleitman, 1985; Rose & Garske, 1987; Steinitz & Szonyi, 1979).

The biggest problems for these children seem to be related to the pressures they feel to protect their parents from any further physical or psychological pain and the desire to fulfill their parents' unrealistic need to have the child compensate for what has been lost. These pressures lead to feelings of guilt when the children attempt to become emancipated from their parents.

Personality characteristics that most studies have discovered in Holocaust survivors are repressed anger, feelings of guilt, depression, fears of abandonment, worries of personal injury, feelings of being different, strong feelings of Jewishness (even if they are nonpracticing Jews), concern for Jewish survival (often more intense than in non–Holocaust survivors), and desires to maintain Jewish traditions that may border on obsession (Nadler, Kav-Venaki, & Gleitman, 1985; Rose & Garske, 1987; Sorscher, 1994; Steinitz & Szonyi, 1979). Daughters of survivors have been found to be more susceptible to Holocaust-related symptoms than sons, and daughters whose parents did not talk about their experience had more problems than those whose parents talked about the experience (Sorscher, 1994).

Some Jewish people believe that it is important that the memory of the Holocaust never die and that no event like this should ever happen again. These same people believe there should never be mass destruction of any people. Perhaps protecting the memory of the Holocaust is one plausible explanation for the vast amount of literature that has been published regarding the Holocaust and its effect on the survivors. Some Jewish people believe that the Holocaust was just one more act of persecution against a people who have endured thousands of years of being victims of ignorance and misunderstanding.

Implications for Nursing Care

The nurse caring for a Jewish American client should get a careful history of the client's eating habits. Many ethnic Jewish foods are high in animal and saturated fats. Since these are known to influence the amount of cholesterol in the body and since high cholesterol is known to be a factor in heart disease, dietary education is important in this cultural group. In addition, many prepared kosher foods are made with eggs as well as palm or coconut oil. Jewish clients who maintain a kosher diet must be cautioned to read labels carefully on all prepared kosher foods.

Because of the use of dairy products by this cultural group, as well as the high incidence of Crohn's disease and ulcerative colitis, a history regarding bowel habits and abdominal problems should be carefully obtained. The nurse needs to remain alert for any symptoms that may indicate lactose intolerance. In addition, the nurse needs to remain alert for signs of drug or alcohol abuse. Since alcohol consumption is considered permissible at religious and secular functions, excessive drinking on a routine basis may not be viewed as a problem by the individual or the family. Cultural beliefs and taboos may make educating the client about the potential for alcohol abuse difficult.

Assisting Orthodox Jewish clients in areas of psychological needs takes patience and understanding on the part of the nurse. Not only may clients have concerns about personal acceptance by peers but also they may worry that knowledge of psychiatric problems in the family will lead to potential problems in finding a suitable mate for themselves or future children. Going to counseling is equated with being "crazy," and being "crazy" is seen as a hereditary problem. Further education on psychiatric and emotional problems is needed to change negative attitudes about treatment.

SUMMARY

It is crucial that the nurse remember that not all Jewish clients are alike. Although some Jewish patients are Orthodox and follow the commandments strictly, other Jewish people, with each successive generation, have become more acculturated to the behavior of the people around them.

Caring for the Jewish American client can be a challenge. Although nursing education traditionally has prepared nurses to view health from a singular professional perspective, health must also be understood from a cultural perspective when care is being provided to clients whose cultural background differs from that of the nurse (Leininger, 1985). Many educational programs are seeking to address this issue by providing transcultural experiences for student nurses. Other health care facilities are offering educational programs to new nurses and to nurses already in practice. One such experience related to the Jewish client is at Baycrest Centre for Geriatric Care in Toronto, Canada (Gorrie, 1989; Gould-Stuart, 1986; Rose, 1981). This program provides a transcultural experience for nurses in orientation and for selected nurses on a continuing care unit of the hospital. During this experience, differences between the Jewish culture and the secular culture are examined. Such educational programs can assist nurses in developing an increased understanding of the universality of various cultural attributes and the importance of culture to all individuals.

Case Study

Esther Rosenbloom was admitted to a nursing home after a fall that resulted in a fractured hip. Esther, age 87, emigrated from Russia with her family in 1920, at 4 years of age. She was brought to the nursing home by her son-in-law, Nat, and her daughter, Bernice. Esther was admitted for physical therapy and is expecting to be discharged to her home after she learns to walk with a walker. Her home is a block away from her daughter and son-in-law's home.

Esther was raised in an Orthodox Jewish home in Brooklyn, New York, but joined the Conservative movement when she married at 24 years of age. Bernice, age 61, informs the nurse that although Esther follows Conservative Jewish thought, she maintains a kosher diet. The nursing home she is admitted to has very few Jewish clients and is unfamiliar with kosher diets. Bernice also mentions that her mother has abdominal difficulties if she ingests too much cheese or milk.

Esther appears worried, is moaning, and is complaining of pain in her hip. Bernice's eyes appear red, as if she has been crying. Bernice is wringing her hands and mentions that her mother has been uncomfortable and that she hopes the nurses at the nursing home will be able to keep Esther comfortable.

When the nurse asks Esther how she is feeling, she states in a whining tone of voice, "My hip hurts, and I want to go home. How are you going to feed me here? What do you know about kosher foods?"

When moving Esther from wheelchair to bed, the nurse notes that Esther does not seem to want to assist, despite the fact that the transfer sheet notes that Esther can move from wheelchair to bed with minimal assistance. When asked why she did not help, Esther replies, "I'm just too tired."

Esther is usually self-sufficient and very busy with her volunteer activities, despite decreased visual acuity, for which she wears glasses. Although Bernice mentions that her mother always worries about her bowels, Esther does not have a history of constipation. She is continent of urine and stool.

CARE PLAN

Nursing Diagnosis: Pain related to fractured hip and anxiety. Supportive data: complains of pain, appears upset and tense, has difficulty transferring from chair to bed

Client Outcome
1. Pain will decrease.

Nursing Interventions
1. Medicate as ordered.
2. Use comfort measures (such as relaxation techniques, diversional activities) to promote relaxation.
3. Assist client to a comfortable position.
4. Spend at least 10 minutes per shift, while client is awake, to allow for expression of feelings.

(Continued)

CARE PLAN — CONT'D

✳ *Nursing Diagnosis: Nutrition, altered, less than body requirements, related to religious and cultural dietary restrictions, plus possible lactose intolerance*

Client Outcome
1. Client will maintain weight within normal limits.

Nursing Interventions
1. Determine client's likes and dislikes in foods that the institution can provide that meet with client's religious restrictions.
2. Request that family bring ethnic foods from home that client would enjoy.
3. Serve foods on paper plates with plastic utensils to avoid serving permissible foods and nonkosher foods on same set of dishes.
4. Offer cheese or milk products in small amounts until tolerance can be determined.
5. If milk products are ingested, assess for abdominal cramps and diarrhea.

✳ *Nursing Diagnosis: Anxiety related to situational crisis*

Client Outcome
1. Client will adjust to new living arrangements with minimal difficulty.

Nursing Interventions
1. Spend time with client to allow verbalization of fears, discomforts.
2. Find activities client is interested in and attempt to have client participate in facility activities.
3. Encourage independence.
4. Include client in decisions related to her care whenever feasible.
5. Allow family to spend as much time as desired with client.
6. Give client clear, concise explanations of anything that is about to occur.
7. Introduce client to other Jewish clients and encourage them to visit with each other.
8. Remain nonjudgmental toward family and client.
9. Contact rabbi and ask him to visit if client wishes.

✳ *Nursing Diagnosis: Anxiety related to maturational crisis*

Client Outcome
1. Client will identify potential and actual sources of anxiety.

Nursing Interventions
1. Encourage client to identify stressful life events experienced within the last year.
2. Spend specific amount of uninterrupted time with client to listen to her concerns.
3. Allow family to spend as much time with client as desired.
4. Involve family in client's care if desired.
5. Assist client in identifying sources of fear or tension.
6. Assist client in identifying activities that help decrease anxiety and encourage the use of these activities.

✳ *Nursing Diagnosis: Mobility, impaired physical, related to discomfort, fractured hip, and possible fear*

Client Outcome
1. Client will be able to transfer easily by self from bed to chair and ambulate with walker with minimal assistance.

Nursing Interventions
1. Provide physical therapy daily.
2. Reinforce what client is learning in physical therapy.
3. Observe client's functional ability daily.
4. Encourage and compliment client liberally.
5. Encourage verbalization of fears and feelings regarding altered state of mobility.

6. Remain nonjudgmental when client is unwilling to perform to her ability.
7. Provide comfort measures, such as medication as ordered and padding of extremities where they may be prone to skin breakdown.
8. Do range-of-motion exercises to increase strength; instruct family in these exercises and encourage them to encourage client.
9. Promote progressive ambulation.
10. Discuss use of distraction and other nonpharmacological pain relief.
11. Explain necessity of moving, even when in pain, to prevent arthritic conditions or contractions and increased stiffness.

Nursing Diagnosis: Injury, risk for, related to impaired mobility, decreased visual acuity, and new environment

Client Outcome
1. Client will sustain no injury.

Nursing Interventions
1. Encourage use of a walker, with assistance.
2. Assist client when she is getting short of breath, getting out of chair, or walking.
3. Be sure floor is dry and furniture and litter are out of the way when client is engaging in activities that may cause falls.
4. Instruct client and family regarding safety practices when client is using walker or transferring.
5. Keep side rails up when client is in bed.
6. Maintain bed in low position.

Nursing Diagnosis: Constipation related to decreased mobility

Client Outcome
1. Client will not develop constipation.

Nursing Interventions
1. Monitor frequency and characteristics of stools; record.
2. Recognize that client may have concerns about bowels because of age and culture.
3. Ask client if she has a specific routine at home, such as a normal time for defecation or use of prune juice (a favorite "remedy" for Eastern European Jews).
4. Encourage fluid intake of 2000 ml per day.

Nursing Diagnosis: Spiritual distress (risk for) related to separation from religious and cultural ties

Client Outcome
1. Client will express feelings of spiritual distress.

Nursing Interventions
1. Listen for cues that client may be having spiritual distress (such as "Why did God do this to me?").
2. Remain nonjudgmental.
3. Acknowledge spiritual concerns and encourage expression of thoughts and feelings.
4. Find ways to help client maintain kosher diet.
5. Encourage client to continue her religious practices during hospitalization and do whatever is necessary to help facilitate this.
6. Ask client if she desires rabbi to visit, and contact synagogue if necessary.
7. Introduce client to and help foster friendships with other Jewish clients.
8. If client can have pass, and family and client desire it, make arrangements for client to attend Friday night or Saturday services.

(Continued)

✳ STUDY QUESTIONS

1. List ways that a kosher diet can be maintained while a client is in the hospital.
2. List religious needs a Jewish client may have while being hospitalized with which nursing staff can assist.
3. Identify three communication barriers that a nurse may encounter when giving care to a Jewish American client.
4. List biological variations a Jewish client may have that will affect care given by a nurse.
5. Explain relationship characteristics that families of Jewish clients usually display toward a hospitalized relative.
6. Explain how Jewish people may react toward the impending death of a relative.

NCLEX-RN REVIEW QUESTIONS

1. When providing care for an Orthodox Jewish client, the nurse should:
   A. Introduce self and shake hands
   B. Use touch as a manner to show caring
   C. Avoid touching the client on the head
   D. Touch the client for "hands on" care only

2. To assist a hospitalized Jewish client following a kosher diet the nurse should:
   A. Serve seafood instead of meat
   B. Suggest the client waive the dietary restriction
   C. Serve meals on paper plates with plastic utensils
   D. Serve different food on a different tray

3. The nurse overheard two nursing assistants talking about a Jewish American client whom they consider to be a chronic complainer. The best way for the nurse to handle the situation is to:
   A. Explain that letting others know feelings is a part of the Jewish culture
   B. Agree with the staff and develop a plan to decrease complaints
   C. Explain that being a perfectionist is a part of the Jewish culture.
   D. Avoid discussing the situation and not assign them to care for their client.

References

Bash, D. M. (1980, September–October). Jewish religious practices related to childbearing. *Journal of Nurse-Midwifery*, 25, 5.

Cohen, M., Brom, D., & Dasberg, H. (2001). Child survivors of the Holocaust: symptoms and coping after fifty years. *Israel Journal of Psychiatry*, 38(1), 3–12.

Darwish, H., Trejo, J., Shapira, I., et al. (2002, September). Fighting colorectal cancer: molecular epidemiology differences between Ashkenazi and Sephardic Hews and Palestinians. *Annals of Oncology*, 13(9), 1497–1501.

Dempsey, D. (1977). *The way we die*. New York: McGraw-Hill.

Edelheit, J. (1989, July–August). The rabbi and the abyss of AIDS. *Tikkun*, 4(4), 67–69.

Feldman, D. M. (1986). *Health and medicine in the Jewish tradition*. New York: Crossroad.

Ganzfried, S. (1963). *Code of Jewish law: a compilation of Jewish laws and customs*. New York: Hebrew Publishing.

Gene mutation in Jewish women. (1995, November). *Harvard Women's Health Watch*, 3(3), 7.

Gershom, Y. (1998).Personal communication, Douglas, Arizona.

Glazer, N. (1989). *American Judaism*. (revised ed. 2.). Chicago: University of Chicago Press.

Gold, M. (1988). *And Hannah wept: infertility, adoption and the Jewish couple*. Philadelphia: Jewish Publication Society.

Goodman, R. (1979). *Genetic disorders among the Jewish people*. Baltimore: Johns Hopkins University Press.

Gorrie, M. (1989). Reaching clients through cross cultural education. *Journal of Gerontological Nursing*, 15(10), 29–31.

Gould-Stuart, J. (1986). Bridging the cultural gap between residents and staff. *Geriatric Nursing*, 7, 319–321.

Heller, Z. (1986). The Jewish view of death: guidelines for dying. In Kubler-Ross, E. (Ed.), *Death: the final stage of growth*. New York: Simon & Schuster.

Howe, I. (1989). *World of our fathers*. New York: Shocken Books.

Jacobs, L. A., & Giarelli, E. (2001, April–June). Jewish culture, health belief systems, and genetic risk for cancer. *Nursing Forum*, 36(2), 5–13.

Jaffe-Gill, E. (2002, June). The next Tay-Sachs? *Moment*, 24.

Jakobovits, I. (1975). *Jewish medical ethics*. New York: Bloch Pub Co.

Janowsky, O. (1964). *The American Jew: a reappraisal*. Philadelphia: Jewish Publication Society.

Jorde, L., Carey, J., Bamshad, M., & White, R. (2006). *Medical genetics*. St Louis: Mosby.

Kaplan, R. (1970, May 26). *An experience with residual populations in Detroit*. Paper presented at the annual meeting of the National Conference of Jewish Communal Service, Boston.

Kaplan, M., Renbaum, P., Levy-Lahad, E., et al. (1997). Gilbert syndrome and glucose-6-phosphate dehydrogenase deficiency: a dose-dependent genetic interaction crucial to neonatal hyperbilirubinemia. *Proceedings of the National Academy of Science of the United States of America*, 94(22), 12128–12132.

Kertzer, M. (1993). *What Is a Jew?* New York: Collier Books.

Key, S. W. (1997, June 2). Three breast cancer gene alterations in Jewish community carry increased cancer. *Cancer Weekly Plus*, pp. 14–17.

Kolatch, A. J. (1985). *The second Jewish book of why*. Middle Village, N.Y.: J. David Publishers.

Kren, G. M., & Rappoport, L. (1980). *The Holocaust and the crisis of human behavior*. New York: Holmes & Meier.

Krystal, H., & Niederland, W. G. (1971). *Psychic traumatization: aftereffects in individuals and communities*. Boston: Little, Brown.

L'Archevesque, C. I., & Goldstein-Lohman, H. (1996). Ritual circumcision: educating parents. *Pediatric Nursing*, 22(3), 228, 230–244.

Leininger, M. (1985). Transcultural nursing: an essential knowledge and practice field for today. *Canadian Nurse*, 80(11), 41–45.

Lieberman, L. (1987). Jewish alcoholics and the disease concept. *Journal of Psychology and Judaism*, 13(3), 165–179.

Lutwak, R., Ney, A. M., & White, J. E. (1988, January). Maternity nursing and Jewish law. *Maternal and Child Health*, 13, 3.

Meer, J. (1987, April). An open door. *Psychology Today*, p. 17.

Mourant, A. E., Kopec, A. C., & Domaniewsks-Sobczak, K. (1978). *The genetics of the Jews*. New York: Clarendon Press.

Nadler, A., Kav-Venaki, S., & Gleitman, B. (1985). Transgenerational effects of the Holocaust: externalization of aggression in second generation of Holocaust survivors. *Journal of Consulting and Clinical Psychology*, 53(3), 365–369.

Novak, W., & Waldoks, M. (1981). *The big book of Jewish humor*. Philadelphia: Harper & Row.

Patai, R., & Wing, J. P. (1989). *The myth of the Jewish race* (revised ed.). Detroit: Wayne University Press.

Popenoe, D. (2000). *Sociology* (ed. 11). Upper Saddle River, N.J.: Prentice Hall.

Rennert, H., Bercovich, D., & Hubert, A., et al. (2002, October). A novel founder mutation in the RNASEL gene, 47delAAAG, is associated with prostate cancer in Ashkenazi Jews. *American Journal of Human Genetics*, 71(4), 981–984.

Rose, A. (1981). The Jewish elderly: behind the myths. In Weinfield, M., Whaffer, W., & Cotler, I. (Eds.). *The Canadian Jewish mosaic* (pp. 199–200). New York: John Wiley & Sons.

Rose, S. L., & Garske, J. (1987). Family environment, adjustment, and coping among children of Holocaust survivors: a comparative investigation. *American Journal of Orthopsychiatrics*, 57(3), 332–342.

Ross, H. M. (1981, October). Societal/cultural views regarding death and dying. *Topics in Clinical Nursing*, 3(3), 1–16.

Rosten, L. (1999). *The joys of Yiddish*. New York: Galahad Books.

Rothschild, H., & Chapman, C. F. (Eds.). *Biocultural aspects of disease*. New York: Academic Press.

Sachar, A. L. (1965). *A history of the Jews* (ed. 5). New York: Knopf.

Schlesinger, B. (1971). *The Jewish family: a survey and annotated bibliography*. Toronto: University of Toronto Press.

Schneider, S. (1985). *The non-Orthodox Jewish perspective of dying and death*. Master's thesis submitted to the University of Arizona, Tucson.

Schwartz, E. (1984). *The non-Orthodox Jewish perspective on dying and death*. Master's thesis, University of Arizona, Tucson.

Schwartz, M., Benkendorf, J., Lerman, C., et al. (2002). Impact of educational print materials on knowledge, attitudes, and interest in BRCA1 and BRCA2 testing among Ashkenazi Jewish women. *Cancer,* 92(4), 932–940.

Sommer, B. (1995). Special consideration for Orthodox Jewish patients in the emergency department. *Journal of Emergency Nursing* 21(6), 569–570.

Sorscher, N. (1994, May). Children of Holocaust survivors may inherit their parents' trauma symptoms. *The Psychology Letter,* 6(5).

Sowell, T. (1981). *Ethnic America.* New York: Basic Books.

Sperling, A. (1968). *Reasons for Jewish customs and traditions.* New York: Bloch.

Steinhardt, D. (1988, February). Alcoholism: the myth of Jewish immunity. *Psychology Today,* p. 10.

Steinitz, L. Y., & Szonyi, D. M. (Eds.). (1979). *Living after the Holocaust: reflections by children of survivors in America.* New York: Bloch.

Stevenson, J. C., Schanfield, M. S., & Sandler, S. G. (1985). Immunoglobulin allotypes in Jewish populations living in Israel and the United States. *American Journal of Physical Anthropology,* 67(3), 195–207.

Thompson, J. M., McFarland, G. K., Hirsch, J. E., et al. (1989). *Mosby's manual of clinical nursing* (ed. 2). St. Louis: Mosby.

Time almanac with information please. (2006). Boston: Information Please, Inc.

Trepp, L. (1980). *The complete book of Jewish observances.* New York: Summit Books.

Wikler, M. (1986, October). Pathways to treatment: how Orthodox Jews enter therapy. *Social Casework: The Journal of Contemporary Social Work,* 113–118.

Zborowski, M. (1969). *People in pain.* San Francisco: Jossey-Bass.

CHAPTER 22 Korean Americans

Jaibum Kim Earp

Behavioral Objectives

After reading this chapter, the nurse will be able to:

1. Describe the communication patterns of Korean Americans and the difficulties encountered when communicating in an English-speaking society.
2. Identify patterns of spatial behavior found among Korean Americans.
3. Relate family and social values commonly held by Korean Americans.
4. Describe the effect of cultural perspectives on time on the behavior of Korean Americans.
5. Relate the significance of Oriental herbal medicine for the health care of Korean Americans in the United States.
6. Describe the biological variations that affect health care for Korean Americans.

OVERVIEW OF KOREA

Korea, known as the "Land of the Morning Calm" (in Japanese, Cho⁻sen) because of its spectacular mornings, is a nation with one of the richest and most original cultures in East Asia (AmeriForce, 2001; Kyong-hee, 1997). A peninsula in the East Sea (Sea of Japan), Korea is bordered by thousands of islands, with China and Russia to the north and neighboring Japan to the east. The peninsula is 125 miles wide at its narrowest point and extends 625 miles from north to south.

Korean history dates back to 2333 B.C., with the founding of the state of Ancient Choson by Tan-Gun (Korean Overseas Information Service, 1993). Korea was united as a kingdom under the Silla Dynasty, 668 A.D. At times Korea was associated with the Chinese empire. A treaty that concluded the Sino-Japanese war of 1895 recognized Korea's complete independence. However, in 1910 Korea was forcibly annexed by Japan. After World War II, Korea was occupied by both the Soviets and the Americans, and the thirty-eighth parallel was designated as the line dividing the Soviet and American areas of occupation. Following the war, efforts to let the Koreans unite the country were blocked by the Soviet military. In 1953, following four years of battle between the north and the south in the Korean War, an armistice was declared. Today the country remains one of the few nations in the world still affected by the Cold War. About 40,000 U.S. troops continue to guard Korea at the thirty-eighth parallel demilitarized zone (DMZ) against another Communist invasion. In 2006, North Korea began a proliferation of its missile testing. While this situation appeared to put the World at large in an extremely vulnerable position, in July 2007, the United Nations verified that North Korea had closed all five of its major nuclear facilities, which was seemingly a milestone in the efforts expended to get the country to give up its nuclear weapons programs (CNN, 2007).

The South Korean landmass is only 38,023 square miles, slightly smaller than Indiana. In contrast, the North Korean land mass is 46,541 square miles, slightly smaller than Pennsylvania. The population of North Korea is 22,912,177. In contrast, the population of South Korea is 48,640,671, which approximates the populations of California and Florida combined (World Almanac, 2006). If South Korea and North Korea were reunited, the country would be about the same size as Iceland or Portugal.

Today, North Korea remains under Communist rule, isolated from the world. The Head of State for North Korea is Kim Jong Il (1994–) and the Prime Minister is Hong Song Nam (1997–). In North Korea, the labor force is 36% agricultural, with many dependent on the scarce farmland (14% arable land) for a basic subsistence. The per capita income is $1700 (World Almanac, 2006).

The president of South Korea is Roh Moo Hyun (2003–) and the Prime Minister is Lee Hae-Chan (2004–). In contrast to North Korea, South Korea has made great strides in developing its potential as one of the Far Eastern powers by blending nationalism, administrative efficiency, and semi-authoritarian rule (Time Almanac with Information Please, 2006). The war left South Korea with virtually no natural resources (Kaltsounis & Shin, 1988). However, South Korea's export successes have been the result of the labor and skills of its people, with 73% of the labor force involved with services, 19% in industry, and 8% in agriculture (World Almanac, 2006). South Korea has made a remarkable economic transformation in the last several decades, with its per capita gross national product (GNP) increasing from $87 in 1962 to $2300 in 1987 (Park, 1988) to $19,200 in 2004 (World Almanac, 2006). Today, South Korea enjoys a hitherto undreamed of standard of living and is the sixth largest trading partner of the United States. The United States is the second largest export recipient of Korean goods, with major exports including electronic products, machinery, and passenger cars (World Almanac, 2006). Sponsorships of the Twenty-Third World Olympics in 1988 and the International Council of Nurses (ICN) Nineteenth Congress in Seoul in 1989 represent a few examples of the economic confidence of the people of South Korea. At an unprecedented summit meeting in Pyongyang in 2000, former South Korean President Kim Dae Jung and North Korean leader Kim Jong II agreed to work at reconciliation and reunification of their two countries. Kim Dae Jung was named winner of the 2000 Nobel Peace Prize for his efforts (*World Almanac*, 2006). Unification of the peninsula is a hope held very close to the hearts of most Korean people (Lee, 1988). However, recent events of 2006, with launch of a nuclear test in North Korea, perhaps makes reconciliation at this time improbable. Nonetheless, South Koreans have not forgotten the United Nation's commitment of the 1950s (Korean Conflict) and continue to partner with the ideals and democratic philosophy of the United States, a staunch economic, political, and military ally. In recent years, there have been unification demonstrations in South Korea by those who did not experience the previous aggression of the North.

Mountains, valleys, and streams dominate the terrain of both North and South Korea. North Korea is almost completely covered by a series of north–south mountain ranges that are separated by narrow valleys. In North Korea, the Yalu River forms a part of the northern border with Manchuria (*Time Almanac with Information Please*, 2002). South Korea is approximately 70% mountainous. In the north and east of South Korea, more than 10% of the land is 3000 feet above sea level. In South Korea, narrow plains and hills between the mountains provide the major land area for agriculture and other economic activities. Approximately 19% of the land is arable and is cultivated for rice, root crops, barley, soybeans, and vegetables (*World Almanac*, 2006).

South Korea has a clear delineation of four seasons, and its climate is characterized by cold winters and hot summers. The average temperature in the coldest winter month is below 28°F and in the warmest month is over 86°F. A humid summer monsoon from the Pacific lasts about 6 weeks in June and July. South Korean weather has been attributed by many as similar to that in Virginia.

The population density in South Korea is 1275 per square mile, with 81% of the people living in cities (*World Almanac*, 2006). The population of Seoul, the capital (the term *Seoul* also means "capital city"), is 9,714,000, and Pusan ("cauldron-mountain") has 3,673,000 inhabitants (*World Almanac*, 2006). In North Korea, the majority of the population is urban (61.1%), with the capital and city of Pyongyang having the largest population, 3,228,000 (*World Almanac*, 2006).

OVERVIEW OF KOREAN AMERICANS

Although Korean immigration to the United States dates back to 1885, when three Korean men claimed to be political refugees, it was not until after the Korean War when sustained immigration started. Early immigrants during this time principally came to Hawaii to work as laborers in the sugar plantations solely for the purpose of making money and with the intention to return home. They had a "sojourner" mentality, never fully participating in American life.

The Immigration Act of 1965, the rapidly rising population level in Korea, and Korea's urbanization and rapid industrialization led to a dramatic increase in Korean immigration to the United States. Additionally, the connection through the political–military alliance with the United States and the stationing of large numbers of U.S. military personnel allowed more female immigrants to the United States. These Koreans were largely well-educated professionals and students who wanted more freedom to live in a truly democratic society and who had no intention of going back (Jo, 1999). This created a "brain drain" phenomenon. However, dramatic improvements in economic and living standards in South Korea and the establishment of a civilian-controlled government in the 1990s caused a drop in immigration rates. Even some people who had immigrated to the United States earlier returned home during this period. It is interesting to note that the emergence of a favorable political, economic, and social climate in South Korea had an immediate effect on Koreans' decisions to immigrate.

LIFE IN THE UNITED STATES TODAY

According to the U.S. Bureau of the Census (2002), 1,228,427 Korean Americans reside in the United States, representing 0.4% of the total U.S. population and 10.3% of the Asian American population. The growth rate for Korean Americans has slowed from 134% between 1980 and 1990 to 35.1% between 1990 and 2002. Koreans are the fifth largest ethnic group among Asian Americans, following the Chinese, Filipinos, Indians, and Vietnamese. Of all Korean Americans residing in the United States, 48% live on the West Coast and 24% live on the East Coast, which is a typical historical settlement pattern for Asian Americans. More than 75% of Korean Americans live in just 10 states: California, New York, New Jersey, Illinois, Washington, Texas, Maryland, Pennsylvania, Hawaii, and Georgia (U.S. Department of Commerce, Bureau of the Census, Summary File 3, 2002).

Of the Korean Americans who resided in the United States between 1975 and 1979, 15.3% were foreign born; between 1980 and 1990, 41.0% were foreign born; and between 1990 and 2000, 60% were foreign born (U.S. Department of Commerce, Bureau of the Census, Summary File 3, 2002). Immigration has obviously contributed immensely to the growth of the Korean American population over the past four decades. However, the percentage of Korean Americans who are foreign born differs considerably across time periods.

The median age of Korean Americans is 29.1 years, compared with 32.7 for other Asian Americans and the national median age of 35.3 years for the general U.S. population. In addition, only 6% of Asian Americans are 65 years of age or older, compared with 13% of the general U.S. population (U.S. Department of Commerce, Bureau of the Census, Summary File 3, 2002).

Korean Americans maintain the highest level of ethnic attachment of any Asian ethnic group. An extremely high percentage of Korean immigrants speak Korean, eat Korean food, and practice Korean customs a majority of the time. Further, a larger population of Korean Americans belong to ethnic associations (75%) than Filipino (50%) or Chinese (19%) do (Asian and Pacific Islander American Health Forum [APIAHF], 2005; Mangiafico, 1988).

There are three major reasons Korean Americans maintain high levels of ethnic attachment. First, Korea is a small, homogeneous country with one language (Min, 2006). Second, most Korean Americans (55%) were affiliated with Korean ethnic churches prior to immigration, and 75% affiliate with Korean churches after settling in the United States, probably for practical and social reasons (Min, 2006). Third, Korean Americans tend to concentrate in small businesses, which strengthens Korean ethnicity. Many Koreans who do not operate small businesses are employed in these enterprises. This ties many Korean Americans together socially and culturally.

Although the ethnic bonds within the Korean American communities provide a high level of nationalistic satisfaction, the same ethnic bonds have hindered Korean American assimilation into the American society. American-born Korean Americans assimilate proportionately according to length of residence and education. Older immigrants cling to Korean food, language, customs, and newspapers, thus slowing assimilation compared with other Asian immigrant groups (Chang, 1999; Hurh & Kim, 1990). Korean Americans who have the opportunity to move through the American educational system, including universities, enhance the rate of assimilation while retaining pride of heritage.

Korean Americans are noted for high educational standards. Of the Korean Americans surveyed by Mangiafico in 1988, 40.9% had completed 4 or more years of university-level studies. In 2000, 89.1% of Korean American males 25 years of age or older and 74.1% of Korean American females 25 years of age or older held a high school diploma. In 2000, 46.9% of Korean American men and 25.9% of Korean American women held a bachelor's degree. Children excel in school, particularly in math and science (APIAHF, 2005; U.S. Department of Commerce, Bureau of the Census, the Asian Population, 2000; Clark, 2000), which can be related to the struggle to achieve economic development after the Korean Conflict and the importance of education, which was emphasized in the home. Each year, over 98% of Korean students move from elementary school into middle school, and about 90% graduate from high school (Kaltsounis & Shin, 1988). Korean children go to school more than 220 days a year for 5 and a half days per week (Clark, 2000). Stress and competition to go to the top-rated schools have created some problems, such as loneliness (Simmons, Klopf, & Park, 1991), depression (Crittenden, Fugita, Bae, Lamug, & Lin, 1992), and suicide.

Many Korean Americans view entering the workforce after college graduation as a serious lifetime commitment. Because of limited job opportunities, some Korean Americans do not look favorably at moving from job to job. In addition, some Korean Americans believe that attendance at the right school plays a major role in landing a prestigious position because many elite companies scout only capable people from the top-rated schools. Korean Americans, like other Asian Americans, are more likely to participate in the U.S. labor force than the U.S. population as a whole. Of the number of Korean Americans in the United States, 76.5% participate in the workforce. In general, Asian American women are reported to have a higher participation rate than all other women in the workforce. In fact, 69% of Asian American women, compared with 57% of all other women in the United States, participate in the labor force (U.S. Department of Commerce, Bureau of the Census, Summary File 3, 2002). The proportion of families with three or more workers in the workforce is 15.3%. Asian Americans and Korean Americans are no exception. They are more likely to work in jobs related to technical, sales, and administrative support (33.3%) and managerial and professional specialties (31.2%). The rest of Asian Americans work in jobs related to service (14.6%); farming, forestry, and fishing (1.1%); precision, production, craft, and repair (7.6%); and operators, fabricators, and laborers (14.9%). In 2000, the median earnings for Asian Americans were $36,051, as compared with $33,955 for their White counterparts. Similarly, Asian Americans fare better than their counterparts regarding median individual income. In 2000, the median income for Asian American women was $31,049, as compared with $27,878 for their White counterparts. Likewise, the median individual income for Asian American men was $40,650, as compared with $39,235 for their White counterparts (U.S. Department of Commerce, Bureau of the Census,

Summary File 3, 2002). Yet, the per capita income for a Korean American woman is only $18,027 as compared to $25,000 for her White counterparts (APIAHF, 2005). Similarly, 14% of Korean Americans live below the federally defined poverty level and another 30% live at 200% of the federal poverty level, compared to 8% and 22%, respectively, for their White counterparts (APIAHF, 2005).

One major issue that prompted Korean adults to immigrate to the United States was consideration for their children's future. However, many elderly Koreans came over without a thorough awareness of their future or a plan (Messaris & Woo, 1991). Many Koreans found difficulty in leaving behind old cultural and social norms and adjusting to new ones (Moon & Pearl, 1991). Many of these individuals faced problems, including financial struggles, poor health, poor care practices, difficulty with social interactions, and mental problems such as *Hwa-byung*, which is a Korean culture–bound syndrome of suppressed anger and depression (Lin, 1983; Pang, 1990). Another major issue involves Korean American men who suffer from loss of control and a sense of not belonging (Hurh & Kim, 1990). Many men followed their spouses who were nurses or physicians (it was easier for females to immigrate because of their professions) without adequate preparation for their own professional future and the "equalization" of the male-female relationship.

COMMUNICATION

Language and Culture

Koreans use their own unique language, Hangeul. Hangeul is spoken by more than 78 million people in 31 different countries, including large groups in the former Soviet Union, Australia, United States, Canada, Brazil, and Japan (Wikipedia, 2007). Although it is a unique language without any near kin, it is considered to have one of the most efficient alphabets in the world and has garnered unanimous praise from language experts for its scientific design and excellence (Korean Cultural Service NY, 2006). The Korean language is entirely different and capable of standing on its own

(14 consonants and 10 vowels). The language and the literature have been greatly influenced by the Chinese (Chang, 1999). More than half of the words now used in Korean are of Chinese origin. With continued emphasis on learning Chinese because of the ruling Neo-Confucian philosophy of the earlier Chosun Dynasty, Chinese characters and Chinese words still occupy more than 50% of the text of Korean newspapers, magazines, and books today. Nonetheless, the Hangeul language was created in 1446 during the Joseon Dynasty to give the Korean people an alphabet that was learnable and usable by all (Korean Cultural Service NY, 2006). The unique simplicity of Hangeul is reinforced by the fact that illiteracy is almost non-existent in Korea. Most Korean children have mastered their language by the time they reach school age (Korean Cultural Service NY, 2006).

The forced annexation of Korea by Japan from 1910 to 1945 prohibited the public use of the Korean language and forced Koreans to learn Japanese (Lee, 1988). Thus, many words used in Korean also have a Japanese origin (many of which are also from Chinese). However, the Korean language has a well-developed and extensive vocabulary, and Hangeul has been at the root of the Korean culture, helping to preserve its national identity and independence. Because of the simplicity and accessibility of the Korean alphabet, Hangeul is easy to learn, which has resulted in 100% literacy in Korea. Scientific design makes it easy to mechanize for computer utilization (Korean Overseas Information Services, 1997). During the occupation many Korean scholars worked to preserve the national language, which was critical in forging a strong national identity (Korean Cultural Service NY, 2006). The Japanese occupation, historical Chinese influence, and other foreign contact have led to the integration of many indigenous words and loan words into the Korean language, mostly technological and scientific terms (Korean Cultural Service NY, 2006).

Dialect and Style

The usual commentary on dialect, style, emotional context, and kinesics does not apply to Hangeul as spoken by Koreans. Breadth of full language use and preciseness of pronunciation are most often the discriminators that identify and delineate higher class (educated) from lower class (less educated) Koreans.

Verbal Communication

When abroad, a Korean being introduced to other Koreans, whether socially or professionally, will listen quite attentively before deciding to interact. This reserved behavior is related to the Korean equation of "reserved familiarity" until the individual has mastered the language and learned to know the individual. During conversation with an unfamiliar person, if there is a match between individuals, the individual is "in" and conversation will ensue. Of the Korean Americans residing in this country, 80.8% speak Korean at home, 65% do not speak English well, and 43.9% are linguistically isolated (U.S. Department of Commerce, Bureau of the Census, 2002).

Use of Eye Contact and Kinesics

In public situations, Koreans are a "noncontact" group. In this sense, some Koreans have some difficulty making eye contact or engaging in physical contact on streets, at markets, on subways, and in the workplace. However, in one-on-one and "acquaintance" situations, Koreans are very similar to Americans in interactions. With a familiar acquaintance, some Korean Americans will engage in eye contact. When conversing with familiar individuals, they will speak in the first person. Some Korean Americans are comfortable in face-to-face situations. However, some Koreans are still offended if, for instance, the sole of a shoe or foot is directed at them. Most Koreans who subscribe to this belief are willing to forgive "lack of knowledge" on the part of some Westerners in this regard. Basic courtesy, when sincerely exhibited by all parties, is a good faith gesture that overcomes traditional Korean mores.

Confucian philosophy forms the basis for behavior and position within the social hierarchy (Van Decar, 1988). Etiquette is very important to Koreans, and it is a mistake to appear too familiar or informal. First names are used only within a family or a circle of close friends. For some Korean Americans, addressing or referring to people by name is considered a lack of proper respect and is believed to invoke evil spirits and lead to ill fortune.

Social Rank and Language

The idea of filial piety (*Hyo*, eternal indebtedness to the parents who gave children life) is so pervasive in Korean culture that the language itself is structured to reflect the junior–senior relationship of the parties in any given conversation (Clark, 2000). Different vocabulary and verb endings are used according to whether the person being addressed is of higher, equal, or lower rank or socioeconomic status than the speaker. Koreans accept filial obligations as part of life; these obligations set the patterns for getting along with other people and make it easier to know how to act in daily situations. Parents have a duty to their own ancestors to be wise, and it is children's duty to obey their parents and to repay them with loyalty and sincere efforts (Clark, 2000).

Relationships outside the family are also modeled by filial piety. People understand how to behave toward others who are above or below them on the social scale (Clark, 2000). Many Korean Americans are very sensitive regarding the feelings of others. In most instances, Korean Americans are generous and agreeable and rarely say no to even an "impossible" request to prevent overt conflict and a breakdown of relationships (Fisher, 1996; Van Decar, 1988).

Implications for Nursing Care

More than 60% of Korean Americans were not able to speak English prior to immigration (Mangiafico, 1988). Many elderly Korean Americans who immigrated late in life may be quite intelligent and trilingual (Korean, Chinese, and Japanese), but they may not be able to communicate in English with health care professionals. Some elderly Korean Americans may have an attitude of "giving up on learning English." It is essential for the nurse to assess the linguistic abilities of the client. When translators are needed and Korean interpreters are not available, sometimes a Japanese or Chinese interpreter may be used to communicate with the client. If the client speaks and understands only Korean, a Japanese or Chinese interpreter might not be helpful. In these instances, the nurse may seek the assistance of a family member who speaks English to serve as a translator. However, children should not be used as translators, because this may create a reversal in the parent–child relationship and cause conflict. When communicating with a Korean American client who has some knowledge of English, it is essential that the nurse speak slowly because this aids understanding. However, it is not necessary to speak loudly. Understanding and applying filial piety are of utmost importance during interaction with Korean Americans, be it polite body posture showing respect to elders or a sincere appearance of attentive listening.

SPACE

Distal spacing—between elderly and young, seniors and juniors, bosses and subordinates—is very subtle but quite distinct within the Korean community. If this spacing is ignored through ignorance or "cockiness," the person is considered a "black sheep" and will not be accepted socially.

Korean Americans, like some other Asian Americans (Chinese Americans, Japanese Americans), have a high tolerance for crowding in public spaces. For Korean Americans who emigrated from Korea, the ability to tolerate crowding probably developed in Korea as a result of the density of the population. In South Korea, it is so crowded that its 49 million people are packed: the density is 1279 per square mile (*World Almanac*, 2006).

Although Korean Americans can tolerate crowding, some avoid physical contact if possible. These individuals are uncomfortable in situations where physical contact is likely to occur. In addition, although some Korean Americans can tolerate higher degrees of crowding, they do not necessarily desire to engage in eye contact with unfamiliar persons.

Implications for Nursing Care

Because Korean Americans are basically a "non-contact" cultural group until a relationship has been established, the nurse should attempt to establish an environment of trust and caring. Korean Americans are often perceived as extremely practical and thus when confronted with sincerity will respond in a manner of "Let's get the job done." When interacting with an elderly Korean who does not speak the language, an interpreter who can convey sincerity should be used. It is essential for the nurse to remember that although some Korean Americans are reported to have a higher tolerance for crowding, physical contact may not be acceptable, despite the closeness to the individual.

SOCIAL ORGANIZATION

Family

The average family size for Korean Americans is 3.6 people. The percentage of Asian American families maintained by a husband and wife is 82%, which is slightly higher than the national average of 79%. Of the number of Korean American families, only 12% are female-headed households, compared with the national average of 17%. During the last 15 years, a watershed percentage of women in the workforce that has both enhanced tradition and extended opportunity to family unit members, especially females, has been maintained (U.S. Department of Commerce, Bureau of the Census, 2000).

Historically, the Korean American family has been the cornerstone of the culture. In most cases, father and sons have enjoyed preeminence as the leaders and undisputed decision makers (Van Decar, 1988). The traditional Korean family has been fixated on the need for a male heir. A male heir is needed to guarantee the family line and lead the family in rituals that pay homage to ancestors, both in the home and at burial sites. The firstborn son inherits the mantle of family leadership and a greater property inheritance. Other sons receive lesser portions. Daughters receive very little, if any, inheritance. However, Pritham and Sammons (1993) investigated women receiving prenatal care in Korea and noted that only 35% felt having a male son was "important."

In Korea, marriages of daughters have been traditionally arranged, and elders have been respected and cared for. Gender biases may be held by some Korean Americans. However, since the Republic of Korea has leaped into the forefront of industrial export and partnership with the Western world, there has been a demand for qualified citizens with bachelor's, master's, and doctoral degrees, regardless of gender. This surge of national output and pride saw the competitive Korean educational system pushing those with potential to the top, regardless of gender. The movement toward equality in rights for women has threatened tradition both domestically and internationally. Although pure tradition is still found in the larger Korean rural society, the profound effect of this change is clearly visible in the matriculation picture at Korean universities. Essentially, modern mobility has strengthened relationships between couples and immediate family and has weakened traditional extended family obligations.

For some Korean American families, problems have arisen when the wife has experienced professional upward mobility and the educationally prepared husband has not been able to find employment. Some Korean American males have not been able to accept this situation and as a result have experienced enormous stress and anxiety. Some Korean American males have discouraged their partners from continuing in competitive job tracks. This reaction appears to be adjusting with time because Koreans not only are rooted in tradition, but also are very pragmatic and realistic.

Koreans as a whole are determined to increase their stock as an international economic partner. Korean Americans are an impressive example of how people can both assimilate and remain true to national heritage and family values. Korean American communities have both become a part of the greater American society and begun to internalize to ensure homogeneity. Almost every major Korean community in the United States (that is, Los Angeles, San Francisco, New York, Baltimore, and Atlanta) and almost every city with a major university have locally organized Korean schools to ensure that the culture, history, language, and tradition are not lost. Korean Americans today strive to balance American opportunity with knowledge and pride of heritage.

In a study on perceptions of elder abuse, elderly Korean American women were substantially less likely to perceive a situation with an elder as abusive than were African-Americans or White Americans (Moon & Williams, 1993). Korean American elderly were more likely to define abuse in a narrow context and were significantly less likely to seek legal help than the other groups.

Religion and Social Values

The social values of modern Korea reflect a blend of both old and new religious viewpoints. Shamanism, Taoism, Buddhism, and Confucianism were practiced in Korea long before Christianity (Clark, 2000; Min, 2006).

Although Buddhism is not the dominant influence in Korean life that it once was, it is still the largest single religion, with 22.9 million (47%) adherents (*World Almanac*, 2006). Buddhism was originally not a religion but rather a doctrine of self-enlightenment, attainment of which would result in a deep understanding of one's own nature and place in the universe. This, in turn, engendered a way of "being-in-the-world" in which suffering would cease to exist and a timeless peace would be enjoyed.

Confucianism, entering Korea four centuries after Buddhism, was not so much a religion as a social ideology, exacting subordination of the son to the father, of the younger to the elder, of the wife to the husband, and of the subject to the throne. It inculcated filial piety, reverence for ancestors, and loyalty to friends, with strong emphasis on decorum, rites, and ceremony. With Japanese rule in 1910, the Confucian system disappeared. However, its basic values and premises lived on and continue to serve as the moral backbone of Korea (Korean Overseas Information Service, 1996).

Christianity in Korea, although more recent, has been accentuated by the presence of 40,000 to 60,000 Westerners for more than 40 years. With the Westerners have come missionaries, astutely armed with modern learning, which isolated and withdrawn Korea badly needed. They had a powerful appeal to Koreans. As a result, approximately 20% of Koreans are church-going Christians. In addition, even more are influenced by the "Christian way." Unlike many Buddhists, Korea's Christians are fervent and devout to a point where they would probably feel quite out of place in a Western congregation (Korean Overseas Information Service, 1996).

Many Koreans honor and practice a blend of traditional and modern religion, as Korea does not have one national religious creed. Although certain conflicts are recognized—that is, Confucianism versus Christianity—Korean Americans are able to harmonize the "best of both worlds." Korean Americans are generally more oriented to the future than to the ancient past and will adopt consistent, provable change, whether religious or political. Today, approximately half of the Korean population is affiliated with Buddhism or Christianity, while essentially the whole population is profoundly influenced by Confucian thought (Korean Overseas Information Service, 1993).

Implications for Nursing Care

Although contemporary changes in traditional family customs have weakened the kinship and family structure, there is no question that Korean Americans are family oriented. Hospitalization of one client becomes an entire family concern. The increasing importance of conjugal family relationships rather than the son–parent relationship has put sons and daughters-in-law at risk of great guilt if the parents become ill. Some Korean Americans may blame the illness of the father or mother on inadequate attention and care on the part of the child.

While Koreans are exposed to many religions, it is important to note that Confucianism became the philosophical basis of family life as well as of government and society. Respect for authority, balanced by affection and a sense of obligation toward one's subordinates, is central to the Korean way of life (Korean Overseas Information Service, 1993). This may affect health care decision making for Korean Americans; for example, if an elder family member believes a medical procedure is necessary, the patient will usually accede. Of course, the reverse may also be true. If culturally appropriate care is to be rendered, it is essential to remember that the family is a primary social unit and family members must be included in the plan of care. In some instances, the client and the family may need counseling services to ensure proper intervention with the family.

TIME

According to Dodd (1998), time is an element of culture that belongs to a unique category in a nonverbal communication system. The organization of time is essential for some cultural groups. In other words, perceptions of time are culturally determined and are not culturally free (Dodd, 1998). Some Korean Americans believe that a person is in this world for only a brief time. For persons subscribing to this belief, life and living are viewed as a harmonious relationship between nature and the human being. Some Korean Americans, like some other Asian Americans, believe that every individual needs to learn to use time wisely. Thus they are likely to believe that time should be used for activities such as performance of service for another person (Dodd, 1998).

Many Korean Americans are future oriented, which is derived from a Confucian belief in reincarnation. In this sense, many individuals who subscribe to this belief are likely to believe that it is essential to finish a task before beginning another one.

By virtue of culture, individuals can be either polychronic or monochronic in the organization of time. Hall (1990) described the time orientation of Asians as polychronic, in contrast to the monochronic orientation of Westerners. Monochronically oriented individuals believe that it is essential to do one thing at a time. Persons who are monochronically oriented believe that accomplishments should be achieved during each task (Dodd, 1998). These individuals have an increased need for closure (finishing a task, ending a relationship). Monochronically oriented individuals generally think in a linear fashion. People who think in a linear fashion tend to internally process information in a sequential, segmented, orderly fashion (Dodd, 1998). For example, these individuals would sequence a meeting in this order: arrival, meeting, conclusion, action. They are likely to cycle through this sequence all day (Dodd, 1998). In contrast, polychronic individuals tend to think about and attempt to do many things at one time (Dodd, 1998). Persons who are polychronic can experience a high degree of information overload because they are trying to process so many things at one time. These individuals may also procrastinate because of information overload (Dodd, 1998). They may also tend to struggle harder to articulate abstractions without visualizations. Dodd (1998) concludes that polychronic individuals are very visually oriented. This orientation appears to be in concert with some research that indicates that these individuals may have either a right-brain or left-brain orientation. Right brain–dominant people tend to think more creatively, visually, and artistically than left brain–dominated individuals do, whereas left brain–dominant people tend to think more mathematically and linearly (Dodd, 1998). Because Korean Americans tend to be polychronically oriented and appear to be visually oriented, they are very likely to be right brain dominant.

For some Korean Americans, having children is an essential life task. Sacrifice to bring up children in the best possible environment is an indescribable quest. For example, parents may be maintaining their living by selling fish at the market, but they may send their children to the best private institution possible.

Many Koreans believe that people are reincarnated. They believe that those who perform good deeds and provide mercy for others in this world will be reborn as another human being, and that those who are bad in this world will be punished and be reborn as some sort of animal. Because of this belief, an intact body is necessary. Organ donation and transplantation are not seen as a virtue but as a threat to reincarnation.

Westerners tend to prioritize and schedule their lives. Compartmentalization of time occurs even in clinical settings such as the hospital. For example, in the hospital, rounds are made, temperatures taken, meals served, medicines dispensed—all on schedule.

Implications for Nursing Care

Time as viewed by Koreans is obviously a concept not held by Westerners in general. Nurses can expect cooperation in matters involving time, but when the client is suffering from anxiety and stress, the nurse must take time to communicate with the client to determine the client's needs.

ENVIRONMENTAL CONTROL

Illness and Wellness Behaviors

Several theories can explain the perceptions of illness by Korean people. One predominant health–illness theory governing Korean people is the equilibrium system, which emphasizes harmony and balance. Health derives from the harmonious relationship among elements of the universe, the human environment, and the supernatural world. Health also derives from the balance of the two major forces: *eum* (cold/dark, Chinese *yin*) and *yang* (hot/bright, Chinese *yang*). Disruption in the harmony of nature and imbalance between the two forces causes illness.

Dominance of *eum* creates problems related to cold, which makes a person depressive, hypoactive, and hypothermic. Examples of diseases from this dominance of *eum* are abdominal cramps, indigestion, and vaginal discharge. In contrast, dominance of *yang* causes a person to be hyperactive, hyperthermic, and irritable. Febrile seizures, stroke, and pimples are some examples of conditions related to *yang* dominance. Treatment for a person with dominant *eum* includes its replacement with *yang* to achieve balance, which includes providing hot food such as onions, peppers, ginger, and scallion roots. Giving cold food such as ice water, myung bean curd, cold noodles, and crab are some of the treatment modalities for those who have dominant *yang* problems (Hwang, 2002; Manderson, 1987).

Elderly Korean Americans consider drawing blood for laboratory work a very unfortunate event and may refuse. This idea stems from the fact that blood is considered life and removing blood from the body is considered as removing *ki* (Chinese *ch'i*), which is the very essence of life energy (Kim, 1992).

Oriental Herbal Medicine

The use of herbal medicines (*Han-yak*, "Chinese medicines") dates back to ancient Chinese practices. However, traditional Korean medicine has developed with its own characteristics (Pang, 1989). There are 396 distinct herbs and spices commercially available that are used either singly or in blended mixtures, such as herbal decoctions (Hwang, 2002).

Today the power and influence of herbal medicine are evident in every city with a large Korean community, where many wholesale and retail herbal medicine shops may be found (Korea Times, 2002; Korean American Journal, 2002). Oriental herbal medicine doctors practice their trade by four common treatment methods: herbal medicine shops, acupuncture, moxibustion, and cupping. They may use one method singly or several in combination to treat clients.

Oriental medicine is based on the visual observation of behavior, physical properties of the body such as build, illness history, verbal responses, and radial pulses. After assessment, symptoms of disease are interpreted, and the treatment plan is devised on the basis of the metaphysical and cosmological philosophy of the concepts of *eum* and *yang* (Hwang, 2002; Pang, 1989, 1990).

If property trained, Oriental medicine doctors have completed at least 6 years of education, with 2 years of premedical school and 4 years of Oriental medical school. To practice in Korea, they also must pass a national licensing examination. Because of the popularity of holistic and alternative forms of health care, not only Asian people are seeking herbal medicinal treatment in the United States but also many Americans are seeking to have their health monitored by the "herbal doctors" (Pang, 1989).

Oriental medicine doctors who have been assimilated into the American culture may incorporate biomedical technologies in making diagnoses.

They may explain and make an analogy of their Oriental treatment in biomedical terms. It is likely that the number of Oriental medical doctors will increase as Korean communities become larger. In Atlanta alone, at least nine Oriental medicine doctors are in official practice (Korean American Journal, 2002).

Pregnancy and Postpartum Practices

Tae-kyo ("prenatal training") is commonly practiced among some Korean American women during pregnancy (Choi, 1986). Using *tae-kyo*, women are supposed to think only about good things in life and to maintain a calm attitude to ensure having a healthy baby. Pregnant Korean American women are taught to eat only the right food in the right form, for example, an apple without nicks or spots (Pritham & Sammons, 1993). Pritham and Sammons (1993) note that in an investigation of Korean women receiving prenatal care at a U.S. military facility, the women reported that they had followed traditional beliefs in *Tae Mong,* a conception dream, and *tae-kyo* rituals for safe childbirth, as well as food taboos, including protein sources. The responses included positive maternal and paternal perceptions of pregnancy.

The nurse should appreciate that the possibility of not having a husband for support during delivery can cause anxiety, particularly when the husband can serve as translator. Limited language ability has been an obstacle for health care for women, which can be enhanced by assistance from a more fluent husband (Park & Peterson, 1991).

During the postpartum period, women were instructed to have 21 days of bed rest with lots of seaweed soup for cleansing the body and providing fluid for adequate lactation (Giger, Davidhizar, & Wieczorek, 1993). However, this practice may be a dysfunctional health care practice because after delivery a woman is in a hypercoagulable state (Giger, Davidhizar, & Wieczorek, 1993).

General Preventive Health Practices

Koreans have many general preventive health patterns. For example, during the hot summers in Korea, individuals tend to sweat more. Too much sweating is considered a loss of energy (*ki*) and negative to good health. Eating dog meat soup just before summer is believed to build stamina and strength by decreasing sweating (Hwang, 2002). Restaurants specializing in dog meat soup are abundant and busy in Korea.

Sex is regarded as a high-energy consumer; therefore, sex drains *ki* from the body. Traditionally, both Korean men and women have been highly considerate of their partner's state of health—if one's health was not at its best or if one was "weak," sex might be abstained from in consideration of the situation.

Influence of Oriental herbal medicine on preventive health is very strong. Many Koreans take Bo Yak (herbal medicine that raises stamina and general health status) regularly at the beginning of spring for the purpose of enjoying health for the rest of the year. It is common for sons to present Bo Yak as their gesture of filial piety to their elderly parents each spring. Frequently, if daughters-in-law do not appear to be as vibrant, energetic, and obedient as they used to be soon after marriage into the family, it is the mother-in-law who suggests that the daughter-in-law take some Bo Yak. These rituals are often practiced in mostly well-to-do families, as Bo Yak is expensive and considered a luxury to many struggling families, although they know and appreciate the power of Bo Yak.

Another preventive health measure many Korean Americans practice is to visit fortune tellers, who may, in turn, forecast a person's health for the year. Visiting various religious shrines brings inner comfort and serenity and therefore is a positive health measure for the supplicant.

In general, Korean Americans have transformed from a culture of family-oriented caregiving and treatment to a culture of outreach to those who need to seek medical attention in which prevention is emphasized. Studies have shown that among Korean Americans, those who are more proficient in English, are higher educated, and have health insurance are more likely to seek out available community health resources (Juon et al., 2004). Culturally appropriate educational programs reaching out to the older, less educated, less English proficient Korean American population should be developed. Nurses involved in community-focused interventions and outreach can play a significant role in acceptance of available services by Korean Americans.

Death and Dying Issues

Many Korean Americans also believe that illness or death is fated and that they have no control over nature (Tien-Hyatt, 1987). Many Korean Americans equate admission to a hospital with a death sentence and may refuse to be admitted. This refusal may occur particularly with elderly Korean Americans, which in turn delays treatment. Among many Korean Americans, a do-not-resuscitate order would be common because prolonging life might be viewed as unacceptable. In stark contrast, discussing a terminal illness with some Korean American might be resisted by both the client and the family. Even today, some Korean Americans view the donation of organs and transplantations as a disturbance in the body. Such subjects much be broached with care by health care professionals (Kwon, 2006).

Many Korean Americans believe that the dying should die at home (Kwon, 2006). This concept is considered to be a "good death" among many Korean Americans (Kwon, 2006). When a Korean or Korean American is dying, it is essential to bring that individual to the warmest part of the bedroom. Next, it is the obligation of the children, which is called *imjong*, to watch at the deathbed of their parents. Oftentimes, a piece of cotton (*sokkweng*) will be placed on the dying person's mouth as this helps to check the last breath of the person (Kwon, 2006). In the past, it was the practice of some Koreans and Korean Americans to take a white shirt of the deceased out into the garden and if possible climb up on the roof and repeat the word "*Bok*" three times. This word meant "to return." The purpose of this past traditional ceremony, which was called *kobok*, literally translated to mean "calling back the spirit of the dead." Today, the *kobok* ceremony is not practiced as much as it once was (Kwon, 2006).

In Korea, the practice of embalming is not observed (Kwon, 2006). Because embalming is required in the United States, and a certified affidavit from five licensed embalmers is required for shipment of the body to any foreign country, this may cause concerns for a Korean American who is attempting to ship the body of a loved one to Korea (Kwon, 2006). Even today, the most important rites in the traditional Korean funeral ritual remains the *sup* (washing of the body) and the *yom* (binding). To observe a traditional Korean ritual with the body of the deceased, the body is washed with a piece of cloth or cotton that has been soaked in warm water. After washing, it is bound in with a long cloth known as a *yom* (Kwon, 2006).

Implications for Nursing Care

Many Korean Americans embrace more than one belief about their health–illness systems. As a result of these multiple beliefs, a variety of health care practices may be encountered by nurses. Persons who believe that sickness is from the action of a supernatural being may delay seeking health care until it is too late. They also may project a guilty conscience about their past behavior and act as though they have given up on recovering from the present illness. Nurses must be very authoritative in carrying out treatment plans for the Koreans who exhibit such attitudes. Healing practices utilized by Korean clients should not be rejected automatically. Careful assessment is essential to provide culturally appropriate care.

It is essential for the nurse to recognize that many Korean Americans who are admitted to acute care or other health care facilities may be using both modern and herbal remedies simultaneously (Pourat, Lubben, Wallace, & Moon, 1999). This creates a problem of allergic and synergistic effects. Several specific cases of herbal-use conflicts have been reported (Lamba, 1993). Some herbal decoctions contain mistletoe, shave grass, horsetail, or sassafras and are certainly unsafe. Mistletoe contains viscotoxin, a mixture of toxic proteins that can produce anemia, hepatic and intestinal hemorrhage, and fatty degeneration of the thymus in experimental animals (Lamba, 1993). Most of these ingredients are crude complex mixtures that are neither uniformly prepared nor assayed for purity. Many contain a variety of unidentified allergens that may cause many potentially adverse effects. Some of the known allergenic materials include pollen (particularly from flower herbs), insect parts, and mold spores. Nurses must monitor the clients closely for potential side effects as well as synergistic effects of medicines in case they are dual users.

Health care practices that are based on the client's cultural beliefs must be honored when possible to ensure client compliance. If a client desires and truly believes in herbal medicine, some sort of collaborative health supervision may be the best solution for the client. Open discussion to enhance rapport and trust is a key ingredient for successful client-oriented care. One of the herbal medicine ingredients that is gaining tremendous popularity in the United States is ginseng (*Panax quinquefolius* and *P. ginseng*). Ginseng is used to raise the stamina and power of thoughts, improve the tone of body organs, and increase longevity. The long-term properties of ginseng have been poorly researched. It is postulated, however, that long-term abuse of ginseng can cause hypertension. Other, less frequently seen side effects of ginseng include nervousness, sleeplessness, skin eruptions, morning diarrhea, and edema (Siegal, 1979). Nonetheless, despite the many hazards that have been alluded to, it should be understood that the majority of herbal products on the U.S. market are safe when properly used (Lamba, 1993).

In assessing the predictive factors of social context and ethnicity on childhood hepatitis B immunization status among Korean American children in an urban area, Kim and Telleen (2001) found that the mother's history of adequate prenatal care was significantly related to immunization status. They found that major perceived barriers in accessing preventive health care were burden of cost, language barrier, and difficulty in remembering the immunization schedule. Preventive health care providers must look beyond the mother's health beliefs and include beliefs and knowledge of the mother's social network.

BIOLOGICAL VARIATIONS

Body Size and Structure

Generally speaking, Korean Americans are shorter than other Americans. A direct correlation exists between age and height among Korean Americans: the older they are, the shorter they are (Molnar, 2006). This correlation exists because in the old days in Korea, meager living and lack of food prevented people from consuming enough nutritious food for growth (Overfield, 1995). Children born since the industrialization of Korea are considerably taller, though they are not so tall as children in the United States. Korean Americans have longer trunks and shorter lower extremities in general (Overfield, 1995). This may be attributable in part to genetic factors but also from cultural habits. Koreans do not wear shoes in the house. They sit on *ondol* ("hypocaust") floors that are generally heated from beneath by coal, called *yun-tan* ("briquettes"). Long years of sitting on the floor in a "Buddha" position prevents vertical blood circulation into the legs, which in turn prevents the legs from stretching and achieving adequate growth. Sitting also contributes to aches and weakening of the legs in many elderly Korean people because of the habitual stretching of thigh muscles above the knees (Overfield, 1995).

Adipose tissue deposition is smaller in Koreans than in Americans, which is largely a result of less fatty-food consumption. Shoulder-to-hip width is about the same in most Koreans (Overfield, 1995). For Korean American women breast-to-hip size is also about equal. Because of their small structure and body size, it is unusual for Korean American women to wear large sizes of clothes.

Some Korean Americans tend to have less body hair than other Americans (Overfield, 1995). In fact, some Korean American women do not have to shave their legs. Usually, hair that does appear on Korean Americans is not shaved because of the Confucian belief that such hair means good luck and that shaving it would be bad luck (Eshleman, 1992).

Skin Color

Koreans have a golden-brown skin tone as a result of a higher melanin composition in their skin

(Molnar, 2006; Overfield, 1995). However, Korean Americans have a wide range of skin tones, mostly attributed to the degree of exposure to the sun. The majority of Korean and Korean American infants have mongolian spots, which are dark pigmentations seen primarily in the posterior iliac crest and buttock areas (Overfield, 1995).

Enzymatic and Genetic Variations

A majority of Korean Americans have lactose intolerance because of a lack of lactase in the body. Thus, the Korean American diet may not necessarily include milk. After consuming dairy products such as milk, cheese, or ice cream, some Korean Americans experience a feeling of bloating, frequent burping, abdominal cramping, diarrhea, and vomiting. Lactose intolerance is a relatively common condition and is found in approximately 90% of Asians (Overfield, 1995).

Bone density among Korean Americans is lower than that in other Americans, creating a higher risk for osteoporosis (Ott, 1991). This low bone density is a result of both hereditary and dietary factors. Some of the risk factors for osteoporosis in Korean American women include a thin, small bone frame and calcium intake of about half that of Western women (NIH OBBD-NFC, 2002). Anemia is common among Koreans because of their predominantly vegetarian diet (Ott, 1991).

Koreans and Korean Americans tend to have a higher prevalence of insulin autoimmune syndrome (Uchigata, Kuwata, Tokunaga, et al., 1992). Insulin autoimmune syndrome is characterized by spontaneous hypoglycemia without evidence of exogenous insulin administration. High serum concentrations of total immunoactive insulin and presence of insulin autoantibodies in high titer are found (Uchigata, Kuwata, Tokunaga, et al., 1992).

Hantavirus disease (HVD), which is characterized by fever, headache, hemorrhagic manifestations, shock, and renal failure, can trace its origin to Korea (Levins, Epstein, Wilson, et al., 1993) and is synonymous with Korean hemorrhagic fever (KHF) with its high mortality. Although found in other parts of the world, this disease in Korea is much more severe. Treatment consists mainly of maintaining careful fluid balance and circulatory support to prevent shock (Levins, Epstein, Wilson, et al., 1993).

Diet

The Korean and Korean American diets are known for high fiber content and spicy seasoning (Kim, Yu, Liu, Kim, & Kohrs, 1993). Two foods that have become synonymous with Korea are *kimchi* and *bulgogi* (Korea.net, 2006). *Kimchi* is a staple dish, eaten with every meal. A typical Korean meal consists of rice, soup, vegetables, meat or fish, and *kimchi*. *Kimchi* is a pungent, fermented dish consisting of salt-seasoned cabbage or turnips with garlic, green onions, ginger, red pepper, and shellfish (Korea.net, 2006). It is very nutritious and rich in vitamins. It is an excellent source of fiber and contains many of the nutrients and naturally occurring chemicals that can help combat certain forms of cancer. The combination of cabbage, garlic, and red chili peppers fermented with the other ingredients creates an ideal health food. To most Koreans, at home or abroad, a meal without *kimchi* is unthinkable (Korea.net, 2006). *Kimchi* is now found, increasingly, on supermarket shelves internationally.

Bulgogi, a marinated meat dish commonly known as Korean barbecue, is extremely popular with Koreans and non-Koreans alike. *Bulgogi* is marinated in soy sauce, sesame, minced garlic, and other seasonings and cooked over a dome-shaped pan, often at the table. The grilled beef is eaten as is or wrapped in lettuce with garlic, green pepper, soybean, or red pepper paste. Chicken, lamb, squid, or octopus can also be cooked in this style, known as *bulgogi* barbecue. *Bulgogi* is tasty, healthy, and versatile (Korea.net, 2006). It can serve as a main course, hors d'oeuvre, or picnic item

Koreans eat a great variety of vegetables and wild herbs, seasoned with various spices and aromatic herbs. Garlic, ginger, soy paste, soy sauce, and red pepper are favorite seasonings, and a liberal use of red pepper is what makes Korean food distinctively hot. Koreans eat only moderate amounts of protein and sugar, and fat intake is lower than in the typical American diet. Obesity is rare among Koreans.

Drug Interactions and Metabolism

Korean Americans, like other Asian Americans, metabolize alcohol by aldehyde dehydrogenase (Kudzma, 1992). This is in stark contrast to White Americans, who metabolize alcohol by the liver enzyme alcohol dehydrogenase. Since Korean Americans tend to metabolize alcohol by aldehyde dehydrogenase, alcohol tends to work faster, causing circulatory and unpleasant effects, such as facial flushing and heart palpitations (Kudzma, 1992). Facial flushing occurs in 45% to 85% of Asian Americans after alcohol consumption (Kudzma, 1992).

Susceptibility to Disease

Because Korean American people have a tendency to consume high amounts of carbohydrates, including vegetables and high-roughage foods, health alterations such as diverticulosis or inflammatory bowel diseases are uncommon. Hypertension is the leading cardiovascular risk factor among elderly Korean Americans (Kim, Juon, Hill, Post, & Kim, 2001). Peptic ulcer disease is also common. These are due to the Korean American's frequent consumption of spicy and salty food. Examples of spicy and salty foods include soybean mash sauce (*dwen jang*), soy sauce (*gan jang*), and hot pepper sauce (*ko choo jang*). Consumption of salty food traces back to earlier days, when refrigeration was unavailable and people were concerned about storing food for long times. Peppers were traditionally used for quick energy because of the backbreaking labor of rice farming.

Cardiovascular Disease. Relatively few studies have been done regarding the cardiovascular risk factors among Asian Americans (Kim, Juon, Hill, Post, & Kim, 2001). Asian Americans are often excluded from clinical trials on various cardiovascular conditions because of the assumption that they do not have cardiovascular risk factors because of their body weight and tendency to follow diets of low animal fat. However, available data suggest more cardiovascular risk factors among Asian Americans than once thought, as a result of Koreans' lifestyle changes after coming to the United States (Lauderdale & Rathouz, 2000).

Klatsky and Armstrong (1991) examined 13,031 Asian people to determine if biological markers for cardiovascular risk factors existed. Findings from this study are suggestive that significant ethnic differences in risk factors exist and that health care professionals must target their public health efforts to reduce obesity, hypercholesterolemia, and hypertension among all Asian Americans. Findings from the study also suggest that smoking cessation among Asian American women is imperative to reduce the potential for cardiovascular conditions (Klatsky & Armstrong, 1991).

Smoking. Smoking by men in Korea is a common thread in their social world and a prime component of Korean men's gender identity (Kim, Son, & Nam, 2005). Compared to their counterparts in Korea, Korean American men show significantly decreased rates of both smoking and drinking. Interestingly, however, acculturated Korean American women are more likely to smoke and drink (Song, et al., 2004). These reports of smoking changes among genders are very likely due in part to the stigmatization of smoking in the workplace (men) and the freedom of Korean American women to smoke by choice without traditional family pressure to abstain.

Body Weight. It is true that Korean Americans do have lower body weight than Americans. But there is a strong association between birthplace and years since immigration, which means that higher levels of body mass index were found in those U.S.-born and those who have been in the United States for a number of years (Lauderdale and Rathouz, 2000). Researchers (Klatsky & Armstrong, 1991; Yano, MacLean, Reed, et al., 1988) asserted that regardless of how low the blood cholesterol was, within 2 years of living in the United States, the blood cholesterol level of Asian Americans will go up to 200 mg/dL unless they continue to follow a diet similar to what they ate in their native land. Younger Korean Americans who have been living in the United States for at least 2 years and who are continuously exposed to diets high in animal fat must be checked for cardiovascular risk factors. Elderly Korean Americans who are set in their ways may be more prone to have salty vegetarian diets and must be monitored closely for cerebrovascular risk factors. When providing health teaching, health care professionals must remember that Korean Americans who were born in the United States may have the same risk factors as the rest of the U.S. population.

Korean Americans who are more acculturated consume more American food and less Korean food. American foods are adapted more at breakfast and Korean foods continue to dominate the dinner meal (Lee, Sobal, & Frongillo, 1999). Compared to their diets in Korea, Korean Americans generally increase their consumption of beef, dairy products, coffee, soda drinks, and bread, while decreasing their intake of fish, rice, and grains. However, the balance between carbohydrates and fat did not indicate dietary problems except for decreased intake of fiber and calcium (Kim, et al., 2000).

There is a definite trend for the more acculturated Korean Americans to consume more western food than the less acculturated Korean Americans. More acculturated Korean Americans tend to dine out more frequently and prepare less traditional Korean food at home (Park, et al., 2003).

HIV/AIDS. Chang and Hill (1996) investigated the HIV-AIDS knowledge, attitudes, and preventive behavior of pregnant Korean women in Seoul, Korea. While the women described high levels of knowledge about HIV and AIDS risk factors, they had less knowledge about transmission of the virus, as well as attitudes of rejection toward unrelated people with HIV-AIDS. They concluded that Korean women are at high risk for heterosexual transmission of HIV despite knowledge of risk factors.

Communicable Disease. The CDC cautions travelers to South Korea concerning malaria. Risk is limited to the demilitarized zone and to rural areas in the provinces along the demilitarized zone (CDC, 2002). Other illnesses that may be carried by insects in the area include dengue, filariasis, Japanese encephalitis, leishmaniasis, and plague (CDC, 2002).

Psychological Characteristics

Influenced by Confucian and Buddhist philosophy, Korean Americans are a very proud and independent people. Generally they do not ask for handouts in either the material or psychological realms. Korean Americans generally view psychological or psychiatric illness as shameful and do not usually reveal such afflictions to the public. In South Korea, mental patients may be locked in their rooms at home or left uncared for during the day when family members have gone to work (Kim, 1998). A number of mentally ill patients live alone when family members are unable to cope with the conflicts at home. In Korea there is a strong conflict between the preference for institutional care and an inability to address the volume of the need.

Hwa-byung (an ailment caused by pent-up resentment) is common among Korean Americans, particularly among elderly Korean females, and is categorized as a Korean culture–bound syndrome (Pang, 1990; Park, Kim, Kang, & Kim, 2001). *Hwa-byung* is believed to be caused by *han*— a bitter feeling, an unsatisfied desire, a discontent caused by life's problems (Kudzma, 1992; Pang, 1990). Since Lee (1977) first studied *Hwa-byung* in 1977, studies related to this illness have increased. However, studies have usually focused on persons in psychiatric departments or clinics. These studies have revealed that *Hwa-byung* prevails in middle-aged, married women of lower socioeconomic status and lower educational background and in up to 11.9% of the population (Chi et al., 1997; Moon, Kim, & Wang, 1988; Park, Min, & Lee, 1997). In a study by Park, Kim, Kang, and Kim (2001) in seven metropolitan areas and six provinces of Korea, 4.9% of women designated themselves as having had *Hwa-byung*. These researchers found rates of *Hwa-byung* were higher among women of low socioeconomic status, those living in rural areas, divorced or separated women, smokers, and drinkers. It is important that health care professionals appreciate the cultural lifeways in the pathogenesis of this illness and respond in a culturally sensitive manner (Park, Kim, Kang, & Kim, 2001).

Kim (1995) notes that depression is higher among Korean Americans than in other ethnic groups and that problems associated with depression, such as family violence, substance abuse, and suicide, have sharply increased among Korean Americans during the immigration and acculturation process. Kim (1995) also suggests that lack of research on the cultural context of health behavior among Korean Americans has obstructed health care professionals from understanding mental health needs and has resulted in lack of culturally appropriate care.

Moon and Williams (1993) studied perceptions of elder abuse and help-seeking patterns among Korean American elderly women and noted that Korean Americans were substantially less likely to perceive a given situation as abusive than the African-American and White women studied. These subjects also differed significantly in intended use of formal and informal sources of help in the case of elder abuse.

Mental Health. Koreans have traditionally viewed mental illness as a family shame and stigma. Rather than actively seeking outside mental health treatment or resources, family members have cared for and protected their relatives suffering from a variety of mental health issues. Korean Americans, however, find themselves in an environment in which mental illness is readily addressed through both individual and group approaches. Culturally relevant psychoeducational intervention has been found to be a useful treatment modality for mentally ill children of Korean Americans (Kim, Shin, Carey, 1999). Family education and community-based treatment programs can encourage Korean Americans to seek treatment for mental health challenges. Today's nurses can further acceptance of mental health treatment by Korean Americans by developing culturally relevant programs to achieve treatment needs (Donelly, 2005).

Implications for Nursing Care

Korean American patients may have food brought in by family members and friends while hospitalized. Some Korean Americans consider American food "too mushy," and many believe it has too many blended tastes. Knowledge of usual Korean diets will allow health care professionals to make informed choices about diet exchanges appropriate to the client's prescribed diet. For example, Korean clients on a bland or full liquid diet will gladly take, instead of orange juice and Jell-O, rice soup and corn decoction, which complements the prescribed diet. Instead of policing of diets and creation of conflicts, mutual understanding can promote client cooperation with satisfactory outcomes.

Health care professionals must also remember that Koreans talk very little during mealtime because of the Confucian belief that the quality of the food should be appreciated in silence by concentrating on eating. Providing a quiet mealtime without interruption is vital and will enhance the client's nutritional intake.

Nursing care givers should be aware that Korean Americans experience various levels of eating behavior changes as a result of cultural assimilation. Korean American dietary behavior will, however, differ by acculturation stage, and interventions should be tailored appropriately.

The nurse who attempts to develop a cultural appreciation of the Korean psyche can bring about more successful client outcomes, enhance family and institutional economics, and improve public attitudes toward our health care system. The nurse's alertness to indicators, some obvious, some subtle, can transcend Asian-Western cultural differences and create opportunities for more desirable physical and psychological results.

If a health-restoration regimen requires Korean American clients to consume milk or any other dairy products, lactose-free milk should be given. Comparable lactose-free food (such as tofu) can be substituted for dairy products.

Korean women tend to avoid sunlight to prevent their faces from becoming darker. They use parasols (*yang-san*) to avoid the sun and often use cosmetics to look lighter than their actual skin color. Most Korean women are sensitive about their skin color, and allowing them in the medical setting to "fix" their faces to their satisfaction will ensure more positive patient attitudes.

Because the development of insulin autoimmune syndrome is associated with a strong genetic predisposition, those Koreans who have insulin autoimmune syndrome should be instructed to carry sugar packs, chewing gum, or gum drops with them at all times.

Calcium intake during childhood has long been related to bone density. Korean American female clients of childbearing age should be encouraged to take calcium supplements to increase bone density. Compliance with their drug regimen must be monitored because Korean Americans have a tendency not to take prescribed medicines if they do not have any obvious symptoms. Iron supplements also should be encouraged to prevent anemia.

For those with psychological or psychiatric problems, the best approach is to establish a relationship of trust with the client. Since Korean Americans are reluctant to reveal their feelings, time should be provided for them to sort through their problems. A consistent and caring approach will eventually cause the clients to open up and allow the health professionals to help them. If this approach is unsuccessful, they should be referred to appropriate psychiatric services. For the elderly, visits by a Korean of the same age group and background will often be the key to cooperation and problem solving. Mental health interventions should be approached with insight, empathy, and patience because of the long-standing negative attitude by Korean people toward mental illness (Kim, 1998).

SUMMARY

Korean Americans, like other Asian Americans, vary in their degree of acculturation. The nurse should recognize this diversity and remember that as much diversity is present as within any cultural group across racial, ethnic, and cultural lines. Some Korean Americans have developed cultural behaviors that are integral to their past and complementary to their present. Therefore, the nurse must develop a respect for the uniqueness of the individual. When the client is Korean American, illness or wellness behaviors should be considered from a cultural perspective so that culturally appropriate and competent care can be rendered.

Case Study

A 9-year-old Korean American boy was admitted to the hospital after an automobile accident. Despite all efforts, he has been in a coma for 2 weeks. Basically, nursing care has been directed toward supportive and comfort measures. Throughout the hospitalization, the mother maintained an obsessive-compulsive (rigid) behavior concerning nursing interventions. For example, if medications were not given on the dot, the mother was angry and hostile to the assigned nurse. She did not allow anyone to touch her son.

Because of the difficulty confronting the staff members, a Korean clinical specialist was called to provide in-service teaching about Koreans in an effort to better understand the client and meet the client's needs. After speaking to the mother a few minutes, the nurse learned that this was the only son in her family. She was driving when the accident occurred, and the boy was not wearing his seat belt. She did not have health insurance. Thus she had tremendous guilt feelings, plus the normal anxiety and fear of having her son in the hospital and possibly losing him. In addition, the mother had the false idea that because her son was under indigent care, medications were not given on time and that this was the main reason so many different staff members were in and out of her son's room.

CARE PLAN

✳ *Nursing Diagnosis: Communication, impaired verbal, related to inability to speak dominant language*

Client Outcome
1. Effective communication between provider and family will be established.

Nursing Interventions
1. Establish rapport with family members.
2. Assess family members' understanding of client's condition.
3. Encourage expression of feelings.
4. Support attempts to improve communication.
5. Assist in correction of faulty perceptions regarding indigent care and medication.
6. Speak slowly and in an unhurried manner.
7. Use translators to facilitate communication.

✳ *Nursing Diagnosis: Coping, ineffective individual, related to situational crisis, guilt, and faulty perceptions*

Client Outcomes
1. Client will verbalize need for more information or clearer understanding relating to the situation.
2. Client will demonstrate understanding of health status and verbalize any concerns.

Nursing Interventions
1. Involve other family members in care of client as much as possible.
2. Clarify misconceptions about number of staff members in and out of room.
3. Expand social networks.
4. Seek to understand client's perspective of situation.
5. Encourage expression of fear of information given.

✳ STUDY QUESTIONS

1. What are the two cultural values, beliefs, and practices unique to Korean Americans that affect health care?
2. Of which biological variations among Korean Americans should the nurse be aware?
3. How does culture affect illness and wellness behaviors exhibited by some Korean American clients?
4. How can the nurse transcend a language barrier when a Korean American client does not speak English?

NCLEX-RN REVIEW QUESTIONS

1. In meeting the dietary needs of Korean American clients who practice the Confucian belief related to the appreciation of food quality, the nurse should:
   A. Provide a quiet mealtime without interruption
   B. Provide a well balanced diet
   C. Permit food brought in by family member
   D. Provide for including rice in various forms

2. The nurse is developing a plan of care to increase bone density for a Korean American client, which should include a diet:
   A. High in Vitamin D
   B. High in Vitamin C
   C. With milk and other dairy products
   D. With lactose-free milk and foods

3. When communicating with a Korean American client, it is important for the nurse to apply filial piety, which includes:
   A. The nurse speaking slowly
   B. The nurse speaking loudly
   C. The nurse using a sincere appearance of attentive listening
   D. The nurse using hand gestures to emphasize the topic

References

AmeriForce Publishing. (2001). PCS-TDY, *Korea 2002: land of morning calm*. Irvine, Calif.: AmeriForce Publishing.

Asian and Pacific Islander American Health Forum (2006, August). Koreans in the United States. Asian and Pacific Islander American Health Forum Health Brief.

Centers for Disease Control and Prevention. (2002, July). Malaria information for travelers to East Asia. Retrieved June 17, 2002, from http://www.cdc.gov/travel/regionalmalaria/easta sia.htm.

Chang, K. (1999). Chinese Americans. In Giger, J., & Davidhizar, R. (Eds.), *Transcultural nursing: assessment and intervention*. St. Louis: Mosby.

Chang, S., & Hill, M. (1996). HIV/AIDS related knowledge, attitudes and preventive behavior of pregnant Korean women. *Image*, 28(4), 321–324.

Chi, S., Kim, J., Whang, W., & Cho, H. (1997). The study of the clinical aspects of Hwa-byung patients. *Journal of Oriental Neuropsychiatry*, 8(2), 63–84.

Choi, E. (1986). Unique aspects of Korean-American mothers. *Journal of Obstetric, Gynecologic, and Neonatal Nursing*, 15(5), 394–400.

Clark, D. N. (2000). *Culture and customs of Korea*. Westport, Conn.: Greenwood Press.

CNN.com. Retrieved August 14, 2007, from http://www.cnn.com/2007/WORLD/asiapcf/07/18/north.korea.inspectors.reut/index.html?iref=newssearch.

Crittenden, K., Fugita, S., Bae, H., Lamug, M., & Lin, K. (1992). A cross-cultural study of self-report depressive symptoms among college students. *Journal of Cross-Cultural Psychology*, 23(2), 163–178.

Dodd, C. (1998). *Dynamics of intercultural communication* (ed. 5). Boston: McGraw-Hill.

Donnelly, P. L. (2005, Summer). Mental health beliefs and help seeking behaviors of Korean American parents of adult children with schizophrenia. *Journal of Multicultural Nursing & Health, Summer*, 43–53.

Eshleman, J. (1992, November). Death with dignity: significance of religious beliefs and practices in Hinduism, Buddhism, and Islam. *Today's OR Nurse*, 19–20.

Fisher, N. E. (1996). *Cultural and ethnic diversity: a guide for genetics professionals*. Baltimore: Johns Hopkins University Press.

Giger, J., Davidhizar, R., & Wieczorek, S. (1993). In Bobak, I., & Jensen, M. (Eds.), *Maternity and gynecological care* (ed. 5) (pp. 43–67). St. Louis: Mosby.

Hall, E. T. (1990). *The silent language*. New York: Anchor Books.

Hurh, W., & Kim, K. (1990). Adaptation and mental health of Korean male immigrants. *International Migration Review*, 24(3), 456–470.

Hwang, I. (2002). *Bang Yak Hap Pyun*. Seoul: Young Lim Publishing.

Jo, M. H. (1999). Korean immigrants and the challenge of adjustment. Westport, Conn.: Greenwood Press.

Kaltsounis, T., & Shin, S. (1988). South Korea: a country on the move. *Social Studies*, 79(4), 137–139.

Kim, K., Yu, E., Chen, E., Cross, N., Kim, J., & Brintnall, R. (2000). Nutritional status of Korean Americans: Implications for cancer risk. *Oncology Nursing Forum*, 27(10), 1573–1583.

Kim, K., Yu, E., Liu, W., Kim, J., & Kohrs, M. (1993, December). Nutritional status of Chinese, Korean, and Japanese American elderly. *Journal of American Dietetic Association*, pp. 1416–1422.

Kim, M. (1995). Cultural influences on depression in Korean Americans. *Journal of Psychosocial Nursing*, 33(2), 13–18.

Kim, M. T., Juon, H. S., Hill, M. N., Post, W., & Kim, K. B. (2001). Cardiovascular disease risk factors in Korean American elderly. *Western Journal of Nursing Research*, 23(3), 269–282.

Kim, S. (1998). Out of darkness. *Reflections*, 3, 7–9.

Kim, S. K. (1992). Korean elderly women in America: every day life, health, and illness. *The Journal of Asian Studies*, June, 402–404.

Kim, W. J., Shin, Y. J., & Carey, M. P. (1999). Comparison of Korean-American adoptees and biological children of their adoptive parents: a pilot study. *Child Psychiatry and Human Development*, 29(3), 221–228.

Kim, Y., & Telleen, S. (2001). Predictors of hepatitis B immunization status in Korean American children, *Journal of Immigrant Health* 3(4), 181–192.

Klatsky, A., & Armstrong, M. (1991). Cardiovascular risk factors among Asian Americans living in Northern California. *American Journal of Public Health*, 81(11), 1423–1428.

Korea Cultural Service, New York, New York. Retrieved July 26, 2007, from www.koreanculture.org/02about_us/KCSaroundworld.htm.

Korea.net. Retrieved on July 27, 2007.

Korean Overseas Information Service. (1993). *The Koreans*. Seoul: Jung Min SaMun Hwa Co.

Korean Overseas Information Service. (1996). *Korea: its history and culture*. Seoul: Jung Min SaMun Hwa Co.

Korean Overseas Information Service. (1997). *Korean cultural heritage*. Seoul: Jung Min SaMun Hwa Co.

Kudzma, E. (1992, December). Drug interactions: all bodies are not created equal. *American Journal of Nursing*, 92, 48–50.

Kwon, SY. (2006, March 22). Grief ministry as homecoming: framing death from a Korean-American perspective. *Pastoral Psychology*, s11089–12005.

Kyong-hee, L. (1997). *Korean culture.* Seoul: The Korean Herald.

Lamba, S. (1993, April 15). Be careful with herbal medicines. *Tallahassee Democrat*, p. D4.

Lauderdale, D.S, & Rathouz, P. J. (2000). Body mass index in a US national sample of Asian Americans: effects of nativity, years since immigration and socioeconomic status. *International Journal of Obesity and Related Metabolic Disorders: Journal of the International Association for the Study of Obesity*, 24(9), 1188–1194.

Lee, J. H. (1988). Features of Korean history. *Social Studies*, 79(4), 147–152.

Lee, S. (1977). A study of the Hwa-byung (anger syndrome). *Journal of Korea General Hospital*, 1(1), 63–69.

Lee, S., Sobal, J., & Frongillo, E. (1999). Acculturation and dietary practices among Korean Americans. *Journal of the American Dietetic Association*, 99(9), 1084–1089.

Levins, R., Epstein, P. R., Wilson, M. E., et al. (1993, November 20). Hantavirus disease emergency. *Lancet*, 342(8802), 1292.

Lin, K. (1983). Hwa-byung: a Korean cultural bound syndrome? *American Journal of Psychiatry*, 140, 105–107.

Manderson, L. (1987). Hot-cold food and medical theories: overview and introduction. *Social Science and Medicine*, 25(4), 329–330.

Mangiafico, L. (1988). *Contemporary American immigrants: patterns of Filipino, Korean, and Chinese settlement in the United States.* New York.: Praeger.

Messaris, P., & Woo, J. S. (1991). Image vs. reality in Korean Americans' responses to mass-mediated depictions of the United States. *Critical Studies in Mass Communication*, 8, 74–90.

Min, P. G. (2006). *Asian Americans: contemporary trends and issues* (ed. 2). Thousand Oaks, Calif.: Pine Forge Press.

Molnar, S. C. (2006). *Human variations: races, types, and ethnic groups* (ed. 6). Upper Saddle River, N.J.: Pearson Prentice Hall.

Moon, A., & Williams, O. (1993). Perceptions of elder abuse and help-seeking patterns among African-American, Caucasian American, and Korean-American elderly women. *Gerontologist*, 33(3), 386–395.

Moon, C., Kim, J., & Wang, W. (1988). The bibliographical study on stress and Hwa. *Journal of Korean Oriental Internal Medicine*, 9(1), 153–159.

Moon, S., & Pearl, J. (1991). Alienation of elderly Korean American immigrants as related to place of residence, age, years of education, time in U.S., living with or without children, living with or without a spouse. *International Journal of Aging and Human Development*, 32(2), 115–124.

National Institutes of Health. Osteoporosis and related bone disease. National Resources Center (NIH-ORBD-NRC). (2002). Washington, D.C.: U.S. Government Printing Office.

News on Korean Americans. *Korean American Journal.* (2002, July 17). Valrico, Florida, p. C3.

Ott, S. M. (1991). Bone density in adolescents. *The New England Journal of Medicine*, 325(23), 1646–1647.

Overfield, T. (1995). *Biologic variation in health and illness: race, age, and sex differences* (ed. 2). New York: CRC.

Pang, K. Y. (1989). The practice of traditional Korean medicine in Washington, D.C. *Social Science and Medicine*, 28(8), 875–884.

Pang, K. Y. (1990). Hwa-byung: the construction of a Korean popular illness among Korean elderly immigrant women in the United States. *Culture, Medicine, and Psychiatry*, 14, 495–512.

Park, J., Min, S., & Lee, M. (1997). A study on the diagnosis of Hwa-byung. *Journal of Korean Neuropsychiatry Association*, 36(3), 496–502.

Park, K., & Peterson, L. (1991). Beliefs, practices, and experiences of Korean women in relation to childbirth. *Health Care for Women International*, 12, 261–269.

Park, S., Paik, H., Skinner, J., Ok, S., & Spindler, A. (2003). Mothers' acculturation and eating behaviors of Korean families in California. *Journal of Nutrition Education and Behavior*, 35(3), 142–147.

Park, Y. (1988). The geography of Korea. *Social Studies*, 79(4), 141–145.

Park, Y., Kim, H., Kang, H., & Kim, J. (2001). A survey of Hwa-byung in middle-age Korean women. *Journal of Transcultural Nursing*, 12(2), 115–122.

Pourat, N., Lubben, J., Wallace, S., & Moon, A. (1999). Predictors of use of traditional Korean healers among elderly Koreans in Los Angeles. *The Gerontologist*, 39(6), 711–719.

Pritham, U., & Sammons, L. (1993). Korean women's attitudes toward pregnancy and prenatal care. *Health Care for Women International*, 14, 145–153.

Siegal, R. K. (1979). Ginseng abuse syndrome: problems with the pancreas. *Journal of the American Medical Association*, 24(15), 614.

Simmons, C., Klopf, D., & Park, M. (1991). Loneliness among Korean and American university students. *Psychological Reports*, 68(3), 754.

Song, Y., Hofstetter, C., Hovell, M., Paik, H., Park, H., Lee, J., & Irvin, V. (2004). Acculturation and health risk behaviors among Californians of Korean descent. *Preventive Medicine*, 39(1), 147–156.

Song, Y., Joung, H., Engelhardt, K., Yoo, S., & Paik, H. (2005). Traditional vs modified dietary patterns and their Influence on adolescents' nutritional profile. *The British Journal of Nutrition*, 93(6), 943–949.

The Korean Times, Florida. (2002). Update on Korean Americans, C2, Altamonte Springs, Florida. July 17.

Tien-Hyatt, T. L. (1987). Keying in on the unique care needs of Asian clients. *Nursing and Health Care*, 8(5), 268–271.

Time almanac with information please. (2002). Boston: Information Please, Inc.

Uchigata, Y., Kuwata, S., & Tokunaga, K., et al. (1992). Strong association of insulin autoimmune syndrome with HLA-DR4. *Lancet*, 339, 393–394.

U.S. Department of Commerce, Bureau of the Census. (2000). *The Asian population 2000.* Census Brief, February 2002. Washington, D.C.: U.S. Government Printing Office.

U.S. Department of Commerce, Bureau of the Census, Summary File 3. (2002). *Population profiles by age, sex, race, and Hispanic Origin.* Washington, D.C.: U.S. Government Printing Office.

Van Decar, P. (1988). Teaching about Korea in secondary school. *Social Studies*, 79(4), 177–193.

Wikipedia. (2007). Retrieved July 27, 2007, from http://en.wikipedia.org/wiki/Main_Page.

World almanac. (2006). New York: World Almanac Books.

Yano, K., MacLean, C., & Reed, D., et al. (1988). A comparison of the 12-year mortality and predictive factors of coronary heart disease among Japanese men in Japan and Hawaii. *American Journal of Epidemiology*, 127, 476–487.

CHAPTER 23 French Canadians of Québec Origin

Mary Reidy

Behavioral Objectives

After reading this chapter, the nurse will be able to:

1. Understand the communication patterns and the dialectal variations of the French Canadian people of Québec.
2. Describe the spatial needs, distance, and intimacy behaviors of the French Canadian people of Québec.
3. Describe the time orientation and effects on treatment regimens of the French Canadian people of Québec.
4. Describe the social organization of family systems among the French-Canadian people of Québec.
5. Identify the illness, wellness, and health-seeking behaviors of the French Canadians of Québec.
6. Identify beliefs, practices, and healers unique to the health value systems of the French Canadians of Québec.
7. Identify susceptibility of the French Canadian people of Québec to specific disease or illness conditions.

OVERVIEW OF QUEBECERS

The people of Québec represent a rich cultural heritage of French settlers, native Canadians, as well as Scottish, Irish, English and other immigrants from around the world. Québec (English /kwuh-bek`/, French/ kay-bek`/, from the Micmac *kepek*, "narrows") is the only society in North America with a preponderance of French speakers (francophones). The early French settlers referred to themselves first as Canadians and later as French Canadians in order to differentiate themselves from British and other immigrants, who also began referring to themselves as Canadians. Today, the descendants of these French colonists call themselves "Québécois" (Quebecer), and the term "French Canadian" has been largely replaced by *Québécois de souche*, designating "old-stock" Quebecer (Québec Government Portal: Society, 2002b). The Quebecers' social identity is the result of their cultural and geographic history, its congruence with personal history, contiguity with other Quebecers, a common language, and the sentiment of the right to exist as an entity (Gohier & Schleifer, 1993). While each French-speaking community across Canada has its own sociocultural history, Quebecers have their own ethnic identify, an essential factor in the planning and providing of culturally appropriate care (Davidhizar & Giger, 2000; Ntetu & Fortin, 1996).

QUÉBEC PROVINCE

Québec, the largest of the 10 Canadian provinces, encompasses about one sixth of the Canadian landmass and is so vast that it could accommodate the United Kingdom five times over. Reaching almost to the Arctic Circle, it takes in the territory north of the Ottawa and St. Lawrence Rivers. To the south of the St. Lawrence, it takes in the lowlands as far as the U.S. border, as well as the Gaspé Peninsula projecting into the Gulf of St. Lawrence. The borders are with Labrador, Newfoundland, and New Brunswick in the east; the American states of Vermont and New York in the south; and Ontario and Hudson Bay in the west. The province's lifeline, the St. Lawrence River, approaching 750 miles in length, together with the St. Lawrence Seaway, forms a direct link between the Atlantic Ocean and the Great Lakes. Because of this geographical location, Quebec possesses three climate zones: humid continental in the central southern areas (warm summers, cold winters), subarctic farther to the north, and arctic in the far northern regions (long, cold winters; short, cool summers) (*World Almanac*, 2006).

According to STATS Canada (2006a), as of January 2006, the estimated population of Canada was 32,422,900, and that of Québec was 7,623,870. The province is home to some 73,000 native people, including 64,000 American Indians from 11 aboriginal nations and 9,000 Inuits (Québec Government Portal: Society, 2002a).

The People and Culture of French Québec

While New France was claimed by Jacques Cartier in 1534, the actual settlement began in 1604. Québec traces its cultural origins to the Catholic colonists who came from Normandy and west central France and to the French explorers and traders who soon penetrated beyond the Great Lakes to the prairies (McGovern, 2002). Conflict between England and France, climaxing in the Seven Years' War (1756–1763), ended with a conquest by England. The colonists of New France formed bonds with the indigenous Huron and developed ties with the arriving Scottish traders, farmers, and merchants. In the years that followed, an agricultural-, family-, and church-oriented culture evolved that had a high degree of homogeneity and rapidly became differentiated from the French culture (Québec Government Portal: Society, 2002b; Rioux, 1974).

With power in the hands of England and extensive British immigration, the urban centers of Montréal and Québec City became predominantly English speaking. While the language of commerce was English and the British controlled business and trade until the mid-nineteenth century, agriculture, law, and medicine proved to be the primary professions of the French in the province. In subsequent years, thousands of British colonists expanded existing settlements and formed new ones. Large scale Scottish mass migration in the eighteenth and nineteenth centuries contributed literate and skilled immigrants to the growing population (Herman, 2001). Further, a poor potato crop in Ireland, causing a widespread famine, prompted another wave of immigrants. A cholera epidemic at the peak of the immigration took numerous lives, resulting in many Irish children arriving as orphans. Although they were assimilated through adoption by French-speaking families, they often kept their own names, explaining names such as McNeill and Ryan among today's French-speaking population. More recent waves of immigration have added a further dimension of sociocultural complexity (Labrie, 1990; Tétu de Labsade, 1990). While immigration came primarily from English-speaking places such as Scotland and Ireland during the eighteenth and nineteenth centuries, a smaller proportion also came from Eastern European countries, such as Poland and Czechoslovakia.

In 2001, with an increase of 15% over 2000, Québec received 37,500 immigrants, including 54% between the ages of 25 and 44 and 56% with university education. Of these, about 60% were entrepreneurs or workers, 23% were joining family members, and 19% were refugees. While most came from French-speaking countries like France, Morocco, Algeria, Congo, and Haiti, 10% were from China, and between 2.5% and 4.5% were from the former Soviet republics, Romania, Sri Lanka, India, Pakistan, the former Yugoslavia, and Libya (Institute de la statistique du Québec, 2002; Wilton, 2002). Only about 15% of these immigrants choose to reside outside the Montréal area. Of the immigrants who entered the country in 1989, during the first 10 years in Québec, a number, particularly among the non–French speaking, returned to Montréal from outlying regions or left the province (Renaud, Gingras, Vachon, et al., 2001). While overt and organized racism or extreme marginalization of Québec's ethnic minorities is rare, certain social and racial barriers on one side, and resistance to total integration on the other, slow the development of a feeling of belonging to a common society (McAndrew & Potvin, 1996).

POLITICAL DEVELOPMENT

After the English conquest, the political system of Canada took on the form of a parliamentary democracy, with the Crown as head of state. In 1867, the British North America Act established Canada as a federal state, with strong central powers. The federal government shares legal, fiscal, and social powers with the provinces. Criminal and international law are under federal jurisdiction in conformity with the British common law tradition. The provinces retain the power to enact civil legislation affecting private property, social welfare, and health. The Québec civil code, recently revised in detail rather than in spirit, is unique as it was inspired by French legal tradition.

"Quiet Revolution"

In the years after World War II, Québec underwent a rapid transition from a rural to an urban technological society. Until the 1960s, Quebecers were oriented to family and to the church. The latter, in Catholic Québec, not only dictated mores and behavior and served as the major social and health resource but also participated actively in political affairs. The so-called Quiet Revolution resulted in social, political, and behavioral transformations as extensive as any produced by violent revolution. Secularization resulted in changes in structure and power rather than in function or values. The state assumed control of schools, health care, and welfare programs. The social classes in Québec evolved to the current three classes: nonspecialized workers, cyclically employed workers, and welfare recipients make up the lower or disadvantaged class; specialized workers, small business owners, and merchants are included in the middle class; and technocrats, writers, artists, and media experts are included in the upper class (Lacroix & Simard, 1984). Starting in the 1950s, the control of political institutions and business enterprises shifted into the hands of French-speaking Quebecers (Bouchard, 1992).

Moreover, the Quiet Revolution stimulated feelings of nationalism and led to legislation to protect language and culture. Also fueled was the movement in favor of the political independence of Québec from Canada, contributing to a charged emotional climate between those "for" and those "against" separatism and augmenting tensions between provincial and federal governments. Separatist sentiments peaked in the referendum on secession in October 1995, which rejected separatism by a narrow margin. While the issue has remained on the political agenda, many Quebecers feel that it is time to make the best of the current constitutional status and to redirect concerns to economic, health, and education priorities (Bauch, 2002).

Economy

The profound change in the politico-economy was associated with more families needing two sources of income to maintain living standards, women with higher education pursuing careers, a decline in the birthrate, and an increase in the number of the elderly (Lacroix & Simard, 1984; Lanthier & Rousseau, 1992). By the year 2000, 71% of men and 56% of women participated in the workforce, and Montréal had become the home to some 100,000 businesses and headquarters for some 50 international organizations (Québec Government Portal: Society, 2002c). While the provincial economy is currently fairly strong, with an unemployment rate of 8.2% (McGovern, 2002), Québec influences and in turn is influenced by the global economy. For example, U.S. tariffs and Russian exports of softwood result in job losses in the Saguenay (Lamey, 2002).

Health Care

Catholic religious orders brought health care and hospitals to New France and were responsible for training many generations of nurses. For example, the Augustines founded the Hôtel Dieu Hospital in Québec City in 1639. Protestant religious groups and Scottish trained physicians provided for the health of the English speaking populace. The latter were influential in the development of scientific medicine and hospital organization in Québec and throughout the rest of Canada. In 1969, the province put into place a medical insurance program, followed in 1970 by the development of a network of social services (Anctil & Bluteau, 1986). Today the health and social services system, based on the

principles of universality, fairness, access, and adaptation of services, is managed by a ministry with 18 regional boards. By law, health care is offered by public access in hospitals, local community health centers, and affiliated community agencies, as well as in centers for residential and extended care, child and youth protection, and rehabilitation (Québec Government Portal: Health, 2002). Currently there is debate on whether it is best to maintain the "core" level of health care provided by Medicare, or whether a greater role should be played by private care providers, which would provide a two-tiered health system (Desrosiers, 2006; Kennedy, 2002). An example of private care providers is the dozen medical imaging clinics thriving in Montréal (Derfel, 2005).

The contemporary vision of nursing care within this system is professional, clinical, and evolving (Ordre des infirmières et infirmiers du Québec [OIIQ], 2001). In 1999, care was provided by more than 66,000 nurses: about 50% prepared in colleges, 40% in universities, and 10% in hospital schools (OIIQ, 1999). Some hospital schools have subsequently closed, and an intense movement is underway to assure the baccalaureate degree as entry into practice. During the last few years, the province has been involved in health care reform and a shift to ambulatory care, with the concurrent problems of high costs and shortages of staff and hospital beds (Sevunts, 2002). Such reforms have increased professionalization in nursing practice and more autonomous roles in patient/family education (Reidy, 2005). Public opinion and the media promote the advancement of nursing education (Editorial, 2002). Additional spaces have been opened in basic and advanced nursing programs and new roles developed for clinical nurse specialists (Allard & Durand, 2006). In order to support nurse practitioner preparation in the universities and employment in the health system, the Ministry of Health has offered substantial bursaries and incentives to employers (OIIQ, 2006).

Education

During the nineteenth and most of the twentieth centuries, free schooling was provided to the eighth grade and high schools and colleges were private, maintained for the most part by Catholic or Protestant religious groups. In 1943, attendance became compulsory in the Canadian school system (Gagnon, 1992). In 1960 and 1961, a series of laws, which provided free universal education through the eleventh grade and compulsory education to 15 years of age, was enacted. By 1998, 80% of the population received a high school diploma, as compared with 60% in 1976 (Audet & Gauthier, 1967; Institute de la Statistique du Québec, 2002). System restructuring led to a network of free postsecondary junior colleges; universities provide 3-year undergraduate programs, as well as graduate and professional education. School boards were originally organized according to religion, with Catholic and Protestant boards operating schools in both French and English. In 1993, the Supreme Court of Canada upheld the constitutionality of a 1988 law that reformed governance of school boards along linguistic rather than religious lines. By 2004 such reorganization had been completed throughout the province. Today, private schools, which may be religious or secular, coexist with the public system. Organizational school reform has centered on devolution of powers based on a philosophy of school-based autonomy, accountability, and parental involvement. Reform has been carried out concurrently with budget constraints and shortages of financial and human resources. Concomitant curriculum reform focuses on competencies rather than teachers' intentions (Foster, Smith, & Donahue, 2000). While such reform is a battlefield upon which ideas, beliefs, and cultures struggle for control of the future, the effects on the educational system of the efforts to transform ethnic rapport and integrate "at risk" groups (such as non–French-speaking immigrants) are yet to be determined (McAndrew & Proulx, 2000).

COMMUNICATION

Language and Culture

The French-Canadian people of Québec are a linguistic minority in North America and, as such, fear the eventual loss of their cultural identity.

Despite their ongoing efforts to preserve the distinct nature of the French-speaking culture, they are bombarded by pervasive American political and cultural influences exerted through various media, including film, radio, television, magazines, and recordings (Lamonde, 1991; Labrie, 1990). The use of the Internet poses a particular dilemma in the reconciliation of international science and business with the protection of linguistic identity (MSNBC, 2000).

A charter (*Charte des Droits et des Lois*), which established French as Québec's official language, was established to protect Québec's language, culture, and identity (McKenzie, 2002). These laws have enabled the French language to prosper, and promote the use of French among newly arrived immigrants and within commercial enterprises and public institutions. Several organizations have been created to monitor and encourage the use of French, for example, the Commission for the Protection of the French Language, which handles complaints concerning the unavailability of health or social services by French-speaking clients, and the Office of the French Language, which is charged with maintaining the quality of the French language and administering French competency tests to individuals entering the health (and other) professions (Gouvernement de Québec, 2002).

French

French is the everyday language of most of the people of Québec and the foundation of their cultural identity. The language brought from the old country was shaped and refined for two centuries from an amalgam of accents and expressions of various regions of France, with the assimilation of American Indian words designating places, lakes, flora, and fauna. In speaking this language, the *r*s can be rolled, and long vowels, *t*s, and *d*s can slide into certain front vowels with a postconsonantal *s* sound (Tétu de Labsade, 1990).

With the migration of rural populations to the cities and the common use of English in the workplace, a popular level of language often referred to as *joual* (literally, "stock of an anchor") was created. This type of speech, reserved for oral communication, incorporates English words into a syntax and grammatical system that is essentially French (Tétu de Labsade, 1990). The resulting speech patterns are, at times, quite remote from the standard French used by intellectuals, writers, and those in the media. *Joual* belongs, for the most part, to the poorly educated and economically underprivileged class (Tétu de Labsade, 1990). Some 83% of the population of Québec are French-speaking descendants of the French (Bailey & Bailey, 1995). English is the language of 12% of the people. Although the English-speaking population has decreased, 30% of the urban population is bilingual, speaking both French and English. Another 35 languages are spoken in the province, including Italian, Greek, Chinese, Native Indian, Inuit, Slavic, Spanish, Chinese, Vietnamese, Persian, and Tamil (STATS Canada, 2002). Immigrants usually learn French as a second language and frequently learn English as a third language. However, the more than 50% non–French-speaking immigrants arriving yearly tax the process of integration into the French-speaking society (McKenzie, 2002).

Communication Behavior

As the French language evolved, so did the behavioral patterns of its speakers. For example, there is a tendency to use the familiar pronoun *tu* ("you") soon after a first meeting or being introduced to someone, a habit frowned on in France (Tétu de Labsade, 1990). Quebecers are warmhearted people who express their thoughts and opinions openly, are expressive, and use their hands for emphasis when speaking. However, they do not use as many nonverbal movements as the Italians, Spaniards, or the continental French. They enjoy the interaction of social gatherings, celebrate important dates, have a quick sense of humor, and enjoy conversation and discourse. They express themselves in the performance, visual, and written arts; cinematography and television production flourish, along with theater, dance, and music; and events such as the yearly jazz festival have become international. Local artists not only are influenced by cultures from all over the world but also are becoming

appreciated internationally (Québec Government Portal: Society, 2002d).

With the older and more rural population, conversation tends to center on subjects having to do with community, farmwork, and day-to-day life. Within the home, discussions take place between women in the kitchen about subjects of mutual concern, such as children. Men may appear to talk less and seem to prefer conversing with other men in the barn, the garage, the club, or the tavern. Little use is made of the living room of the home except on very special occasions. The intelligential and younger, urban, educated people of both sexes discuss politics, art, or world events. When they are married and have young children, they tend to associate with others in similar life situations. Family and friends enjoy meals together, but women often leave for the kitchen as the men retire to the balcony or watch sports on television. Women tend to be well aware of feminist concerns and are increasingly vocal concerning issues of status, needed services, and treatment by various government agencies. Québec women demand respect and heatedly discuss the right to "freedom of choice" versus the "right to life."

Implications for Nursing Care

In Québec, as elsewhere, the nurse must respect the client's choice of language, not only to ensure clear communication but also to meet the requirements of Québec law. The Quebec nurse realizes the centrality of good communication to patient/family care and education (Reidy, 2005). Most nurses and doctors are bilingual, and whether they work in traditionally anglophone (English-speaking) or francophone (French-speaking) health settings, they care for patients and families whose mother tongue may be French, English, or a host of other languages (Derfel, 2002). The ethnic mosaic that exists requires that the nurse be sensitive to the style, mode, and context of the communication patterns, not only of Québécois of different backgrounds and education but also of diverse ethnic groups in different stages of social and linguistic integration into the province (Vissandjée, & Dupéré, 2000).

The nurse must be familiar with the popular Québec expressions used to designate parts of the body (such as *passage* for "vagina") or certain infections (such as *chaude pisse* for "gonorrhea"). Those older or with a rural background might say that a person able to resist illness is as "strong as an ox" or "able as a bear," or when ill that the sufferer has a "weak constitution." If someone faints, the term "all into the apples" may be used. Someone who is unconscious is said to "hit the canvas" (Dulong & Bergeron, 1980). When interacting with the older generation, the nurse should avoid using the familiar *tu* form because such usage is considered to show lack of respect.

SPACE

Conceptualization of Space

The representation of space in Québec's consciousness is process-oriented, related to urban-rural tensions and historical and social-political evolution, as well as to place-based identity (Chapman, 2000). This representation may be seen in three (interrelated rather than sequential) attitudinal themes: (1) spatial possession, depending on the underlying premise that specific groups can own, name, and control space; (2) spatial oppression, or domination or oppression by military force, patriarchy, class system, economy, or capitalism; and (3) spatial mobility, the tension between mobility and stasis, whether physical movement or identified with gender and ethnicity. The frame of reference consists of reterritorializing maps of power, domination, and marginalization.

Interpersonal Space

In public, Quebecers tend to avoid physical contact and maintain a certain physical space. At work they may be in closer contact than in public, but individuals generally attempt to maintain a distance of 18 to 30 inches between themselves and others (Hall, 1990). Among friends and close relations, greater intimacy is permitted. Men may pat each other on the back or shake hands when they meet, but seldom embrace or kiss. Women may embrace or kiss cheeks but seldom walk arm in arm.

Normally, physical contact in public is limited to young lovers, between adults and young children, or between adults at emotional or difficult moments when they require support.

Physical Space

Families generally live in apartments, condominiums, or single-family dwellings in the cities and suburbs, or in single-family dwellings in rural areas. Housing, particularly low-cost and public housing, is in relatively short supply chiefly in the larger cities, and there are homeless among the young, the addicted, and the chronically mentally ill (Desrochers, 2002; Editorial, 2002). Overcrowding is not a problem except in the poorest parts of the inner cities, where the elderly, the poor, and the deinstitutionalized chronically mentally ill live in poorly maintained rooms and apartments. Despite immense territory, some 80% of the population is concentrated in the southern part of the province. Most people reside in the larger cities, the capital, which is Québec City, Montréal, Sherbrooke, Trois Riveres, or Laval.

Implications for Nursing Care

An understanding of cultural geography can help nurses realize that space meanings are subtly constructed through a reworking of the past. Quebecers are jealous and protective of their usually ample physical and personal space. In caring, the nurse avoids overly familiar attitudes, maintains distance when conversing, respects the privacy needs of patients and families, and recognizes the patient's sense of modesty when receiving intimate care.

SOCIAL ORGANIZATION

Family and Church

In early colonial days, families were large and stable, and family members felt a sense of belonging, not only to their land but also to "Holy Mother the Church," accepting its dominance in health care, education, and population management (Fahmy-Eid & Dumont, 1983). During the period preceding the world wars, rural families often had 8 to 14 children, in order to provide additional help with farmwork and out of respect for the teachings of the church. With the advent of the Quiet Revolution of the 1960s, the state assumed responsibility for the family through health and social services. By the late 1970s, changes in social attitudes and legislation permitted divorce, contraception, and abortion (Henripin, Huot, Lapierre-Adamcyk, & Marcil-Gratton, 1981; Lazure, 1990).

Evolution of the Family

In the past, family roles were well defined. The father was head of the family and responsible for its material well-being. The mother had specific household duties and was caregiver and religious educator, and rural mothers also had specific farm duties. These roles remained relatively unchanged until women, in great numbers, began to join the workforce and become the heads of single-parent families. Amid social change, the mother has remained the principal health caregiver in the Québec family and instilled and supervised the practice of healthy habits within the family (Lazure, 1990; Thibaudeau & Reidy, 1985). From colonial times through the 1950s, the mother would depend on her eldest daughter, usually unmarried, who shared and later, if necessary, would assume this caregiver role.

With the transition to the new generation of families, men and women began to reevaluate their familial roles (Valentine, 2001). In 1985, family was defined in Québec as a group of parents and children united by multiple and varied ties, favoring the development of person and society, for mutual support during life (Gouvernement du Québec, 1985). However, family functioning has not evolved without some difficulties. Often the mother has maintained a double burden, still encumbered with her former tasks while assuming the obligations from outside employment. But, despite social change, she has remained the principal health caregiver in the Québec family (Thibaudeau & Reidy, 1985). Nonetheless, the two-parent family remains the ideal, the fathers of young children play a larger role in the care of children and their home environment, and the reconstituted family unit has become an accepted social phenomenon (Lacourse, 1999).

Statistics confirm the evolution of the nuclear family in Québec: by the year 2005 the number of births had dropped to 76,100 from about 98,000 in a 15-year period, and abortions had risen from 1.4 in 1971 per 100 live births to 38.1 in 1999 (Dandurand, 1990; Gouvernement du Québec, 2002; Institut de la Statistique du Québec, 2002, 2006a). The fertility rate had dropped from 1.67 in 1991 to 1.45 children per woman in 1999, as compared with Britain's 1.7 and the United States of America's 2.1 (Globalis, 2005). In 2001, 23.9% of families had one child, 22.5% two, 7% three, and 1.9% had four or more. Some 77% of families with children consisted of married couples, while about 20% were common law. Further, in slightly more than one-third of the marriages, at least one of the partners was previously divorced and 20% of families were headed by a single parent of whom 80% were women, with more than half of these living in poverty (Gouvernement du Québec, 2002; Institut de la Statistique de Québec, 2002, 2006b).

A province-wide study of the health of families with children concluded that the family constitutes an effective setting for the health and welfare of both parents and children, although single-parent and reconstituted families seem more at risk than two-parent families (Létourneau, Bernier, Marchand, & Trudel, 2000). While the regular use of alcohol varied little with type of family, smoking ranges from 28% in two-parent families, to 49% in single-parent families, to 54% in reconstituted families. Elevated psychological distress was reported in 18% of two-parent families but in 32% of the single-parent families and in 29% of the reconstituted families.

New Models of Interdependence

Québec society has evolved in such a way as to dilute traditional networks of support built around family and relatives, the neighborhood, and various religious institutions (Lazure, 1990). However, changing cultural mores and options, emerging lifestyles, or shared problems over the last few years have stimulated the creation of new models of interdependence, individualization, and actualization for women, as well as legalization of gay and lesbian unions and adoptions (Fitterman, 2002; Lacourse, 1999). Regrouping of individuals into new networks of mutual aid or self-help is particularly significant. Community and volunteer organizations that have assumed many social and health functions for a variety of individuals are often inspired by needs no longer met by traditional means or by emerging social and health needs, such as persons living with AIDS (Stewart, Hart, Mann, et al., 2001).

Aging of the Population

Profound demographic changes in the last 25 years have left Québec with a higher percentage of older citizens. The number of persons 65 years of age and over in 2005 totaled 1,045,661 or 13.8% of population, as compared with 650,000 in 1988 (Institut de la Statistique du Québec, 2006c). This general aging of the population (Institut de la Statistique du Québec, 2006d) includes an increase in the number of elderly women (about 606,000) in relation to men (439,000), and an increase in the number of the very old, that is over 80 years (214,995), who often experience chronic illness and serious financial difficulties (Institut de la Statistique du Québec, 2006e). The number of persons 65 years of age and over in 2005 totaled 1,045,661 or 13.8% of population, as compared with 650,000 in 1988 (Institut de la Statistique du Québec, 2006c). This general aging of the population (Institut de la Statistique du Québec, 2006d) includes an increase in the number of elderly women (about 606,000) in relation to men (439,000), and an increase in the number of the very old, that is over 80 years (214,995), who often experience chronic illness and serious financial difficulties (Institut de la Statistique du Québec, 2006e).

Youth

In 2001, in Québec, there were 2,682,400 children, youths and young adults (0–4 years: 375,765; 5–9 years: 457,230: 10–14 years: 458,590; 15–19 years: 462,070; 20–24 years: 487 410; 25–29 years: 44,1335; Institut de la Statistique du Québec, 2006f). While socio-educational problems are present such as street gangs (2006a) child and youth

welfare is a priority for the province. There are provincial programs in pre- and post-partum care, scholastic adaptation for children with learning disabilities, recreation, and job training for youth and young adults. Although the general unemployment rate in Québec is 8.3%, it is 14.4% for youths 15 to 24 years of age (Institut de la Statistique du Québec, 2006g; STATS Canada 2006b). However, in the 2004–2005 period 3974 young adults (aged from 21 to 30 years) moved into the Montréal area, from outside the province, for jobs and professional advancement (Nebenzahl, 2006).

Religion

Even with the British military conquest, the Catholic church remained a social and political force in French Canada, defending faith, language, and culture (Orr, 1992). The church was actively involved in financial, educational, and health affairs. In the 1960s, however, the Quiet Revolution brought about greater separation of church and state. At that time, attendance at church declined greatly, and religious affiliations became more diversified (Orr, 1992). However, despite the decline in Catholicism's influence and practice, more than 6 million Quebecers consider themselves to be Catholic. Many individuals conform to a model whereby one calls oneself "Catholic" and marks certain important life events in life by a church ceremony (baptism, marriage, funeral, and so forth) and also continues to support a school system organized on religious groups (Laperrière, 1992). Today, Québec is noted for a growing interest in spirituality, a search for values, and diversification of beliefs and religious affiliations, including, Protestantism, Judaism, Buddhism, Islam, Sikhism, Hinduism, and Seventh-Day Adventism (Québec Government Portal: Society, 2002c).

Implications for Nursing Care

The integration of extreme diversification of ethnic, cultural, and age groups in Québec presents a challenge for the nurse. By assessing the cultural attitudes of the client and family caregivers toward health, human reproduction, illness, and health care, the nurse takes the first step in assuring clients' enabling and empowerment (Thibaudeau & Reidy, 1985). An investigation of community nurses in Montréal found that family participation was one of the most important facilitators to care, and that patient/family participation in care objectives was one of the most important nursing strategies (Reidy, 2005). Nevertheless, despite Québec's evolving social complexity, the social canvas of the province is still, in many ways, held together by the influence by the older generation, a sense of family, and sharing and mutual aid between generations. In working with single-parent families headed by women with limited financial means, the nurse may work with families whose members suffer from a variety of health and social problems, as well as the intervention of several specialists. With feelings of powerlessness, whatever the family's status, a mother's self-confidence is undermined. The nurse can help the mother understand her situation, participate in the care process, and deal with the health system. With an increase in feelings of confidence as a parent and of self-esteem as an individual, the single mother may learn to function in her role as principal health agent in the family. Further, it is necessary to develop or reinforce family support networks, both for exchange of services and for stimulation of a sense of empowerment, for example, to help maintain neighborhoods free from drugs and prostitution. Within the family itself, efforts can be made to improve functioning in health matters, whether by improving competencies, direct support, information, and advice or by arranging access to resources. The nurse can also become an advocate for these families so that they may obtain the social and health services to which they are entitled (Thibaudeau & Reidy, 1985; Thibaudeau, Reidy, d'Amours, & Frappier, 1984).

An aging population and a diminishing national health budget require that more community services be available to enable elderly people, with functional limits, to remain in their own homes. Day hospitals and centers, staffed by multidisciplinary teams, that offer various social services are increasing in number. Cossette, Lévesque, and Laurin (1995) note that both gender and kinship should be considered with respect to support when assisting French-speaking primary caregivers in providing care for aging and disabled relatives in the home. However, to attain the ultimate goal of health and autonomy of the aged, additional innovative nursing approaches must be created.

TIME

Past and Present

The development and diffusion of time sense (the way we see and live time) is a phenomenon for the people of Québec that is related to the consciousness of time in the context of the value and rhythm of human life of a Catholic and rural society; the preciousness of time and calculation of time within the modernity of the educational system, urban industrialization, and the evolution of a city-based mechanized society; and the importance accorded to time in an era of developing communications (Watelet, 1999). French Quebecers tend to attach primary importance to day-to-day affairs and to living in the present. Pleasure and sorrow are generally accepted as they occur, with an attitude that life goes on from one day to the next (Paquet, 1989). However, climatic and historic conditions have prompted planning to survive long and cold winters and a context of stability that provides structure for these values and attitudes. For older Quebecers, time is intimately associated with religion. They envision the future with the hope of life after death. Anniversaries of the death of family members are often commemorated by a Mass. However, many of the young and urban tend not to follow these traditions because they tend to reject traditional institutions. For women in modern Québec society, time has taken on a new meaning as working women assume a variety of roles (wife, mother, professional person).

Although time is determined by the flow of the successive seasons for rural populations, urban life is characterized by variations in the relationship of time devoted to work, to family, and to leisure (Pronovost, 1989). In 1998, productive time for Quebecers (work and domestic responsibilities) averaged 7.8 hours per day in households without children and 9 hours in those with at least one child

(Laroche & Gauthier, 2002). More than half expressed preference for engaging in free or leisure time activities, about 17% preferred time devoted to family and domestic responsibilities, and about 7% favored work time (Laroche, 2000). Time accorded to leisure activities (media, social, cultural, physical activities, and sports) totaled about 6 hours a week (Québec Government Portal: Society, 2002d). The most popular cultural activities were recreational games, dancing, audiovisual entertainment, plastic arts, and literary activities. Outdoor activities and sports accounted for time spent by people of all ages: more than 40% cycled; about a third camped, fished, or skied; and about 15% golfed, canoed, or rode snowmobiles.

Implications for Nursing Care

The nurse must consider the present-time orientation, often demonstrated by the importance attributed to practical goals, when interacting with families and individuals, as well as in the approach and content of health education. A verbal "contract" between the nurse and patient and family, of prioritized collaborative objectives including a time frame, often proves advantageous in enabling and in supporting self-care within the context of health promotion and therapeutic regimens.

ENVIRONMENTAL CONTROL
Attitudes Toward Health

In intellectual circles in Québec, health is perceived as being in complete possession of one's physical and mental capacities and as a way of improving one's status, professional or otherwise (Paquet, 1989). For financially secure families, health is seen as an ideal state in which illness is absent, while illness is seen as a slow and insidious degradation of health that occurs over time. In lower socioeconomic groups, health is defined as the ability to work, to be self-sufficient, and to satisfy primary needs. The disadvantaged often attach less value to a general state of good health, often seeking resolution of immediate problems without follow-up of long-term goals. Illness is seen as a stroke of bad luck, causing a momentary rupture in one's normal

state of health. Various religious beliefs have encouraged the perception of illness as divine punishment for sins committed by the individual.

Lavasseur (2000) noted that the majority of Quebecers age 15 or older consider themselves to be in a good or excellent state of health. However, those from 45 to 64 evaluated their health more negatively than did the youth; the poorer and less educated rated their health less favorably, and persons employed saw themselves to be in better health than those who were unemployed. Lavasseur (2000) identified factors associated with an unfavorable self-evaluation of health, including problems with weight, limits on activities, consultations with health professionals, and psychological distress.

The practice of medicine has always held a place of prestige and political power in Québec. The older generation had complete confidence in their doctors for the preservation of life and the restoration of health. However, with the advent of consumerism, the people of Québec began to participate more directly in health care decision making, and the ideology of the powerful medical establishment is now being questioned by both ordinary people and other health professionals. In recent years, various "alternative medicine" and spiritual approaches to health have become more popular, apparently in answer to a need for therapies that are global and allow greater personal control (Laforest, 1985; Renaud, Jutras, & Bouchard, 1987). A frequent pattern of behavior is consultation with practitioners of alternative medicine after ordinary medicine has failed to bring about a cure or to avoid chemically derived treatments. Individuals with the "gift" of healing and bonesetters are still quite popular in some rural areas (Desautels, 1984). They have learned through knowledge passed from generation to generation and are often experts in the massage of strained muscles and ligaments or in the setting of certain bones.

Social Environment of Health

Because of the strong interrelationship between an individual's social environment and health, Québec's health and welfare policy is directed to reinforcing family and social networks. In their study of the health and social supports of Quebecers, Julien, Julien, and Lafontaine (2000) concluded that men; persons widowed, separated, or divorced; and persons between the ages of 25 and 64 were more dissatisfied with their level of social interaction and social support. The proportion of persons living alone increased with age. While men were more dissatisfied with living alone, the women in general had better social support. Women between the ages of 45 and 64 were the most likely to miss intimacy. One person in four with a spouse, whether cohabiting or not, reported difficulties in the relationship. Those 25 to 44 years old were more likely than their elders to have experienced the divorce of their parents or to have attributed family problems to alcohol or drug problems of their parents. Even though 65% of the population considered spiritual life to be very important, 64% seldom or never frequented a place of worship (Carkson, Pica, & Lacombe, 2000). Generally, it was those persons who considered themselves to be in a poor state of health, who had at least one health problem, or who were limited in their activities who most valued spiritual life and attendance at religious worship. Those persons who most frequently attended religious services were less likely to report a high level of psychological distress or suicidal ideas.

The work environment in Québec has been found to affect health; that is, 3% of workers reported violence and 18% intimidation, and 8% of women and 2% of men were subjected to unwanted words or gestures of a sexual nature (Arcand, Labrèche, Stock, Messing, & Tissot, 2000). About 30% of them report elevated psychological distress following these incidents. Constraints at work (such as combined low level of work autonomy with a high level of psychological demand) were found to be associated not only with psychological distress but also with perceptions of poorer mental and general health. Certain work conditions (for example, working nights, exposure to solvents or vibrations), as well as certain characteristics of the work environments (such as size of the company, work organization, age of

workers), were found to be associated with a high risk of accidents (Arcand, Labrèche, Stock, Messing, & Tissot, 2000).

Physical Environment

Problems of pollution and waste management constitute a serious challenge to the environment in terms of costs, contamination, and health. A water-purification program, under way in Québec since 1981, involves water-processing plants and greater control of industrial waste (Thibault, 1989). Public awareness programs have been created, including recycling, composting, using natural products, cleaning up lakes and rivers, and disposing of dangerous household wastes. Further, pesticides, which are linked to cancer and diseases affecting children, have been banned from use on private lawns and gardens, as well as on the grounds of schools and other provincially owned green spaces (Dougherty, 2002). However, Québec has the highest number of polluted land sites in Canada, and farm contamination has been recognized as a provincial problem (Canadian Press, 2002).

Illness and Wellness Behavior

Determinants of health and well-being include physical activity and exercise, control of body weight, the practice of behavior proper to women's health, and the practice of safe sex (Chénard, Daveluy, & Émond, 2000). Many Quebecers 15 years or older (70%) undertook physical activity during their free time, and 25% did so at least three times a week. Physical inactivity declined significantly since the early 1980s, going from 82% in 1981 to 62% in 2000 (Institut de la Statistique de Québec, 2006h). However, in Québec, as in the rest of Canada, the number of obese children has tripled since 1981 (Lalonde, 2002). Further, obesity related to health risk has more than doubled in Québec, with 26.5% of the province's adults now overweight compared with just 11.4% in 1985; and obesity-related illnesses cost the Québec health care system more than half a billion dollars annually, or 5% of total direct health care costs in the province (Institut de la Statistique de Québec, 2006i; Physical Activity Monitor, 2004).

In a study by Chénard, Daveluy, and Émond (2000), about 27% of women over age 15 practiced self-examination of breasts, and 50% indicated that they had a medical examination of their breasts, 49% a mammography, and 44% a Pap test within the year. Oral contraceptives were used by about 30% of women age 15 to 17 and 25 to 34 years, by more than 50% of women age 18 to 24, and by about 7% of those over age 35, for a total of 27% of the female population. Further, 36% of women age 45 to 64 years and 18% over 65 used hormone replacement therapy. About 75% of heterosexual respondents reported having only one sexual partner during the previous year. However, 1 in 10 of the sexually active had more than one partner, and 60% of these reported the at-risk behavior of not systematically using a condom. The proportion of homosexual and bisexual people in Québec is estimated at 3% of the population over 15 years of age (Chénard, Daveluy, & Émond, 2000).

Fournier and Piché (2000) noted that health professionals, other than physicians, are assuming increasing importance in the health care system. While health problems, incapacity, and psychological distress prompt consultation with a health professional, the most important factor in seeking health care is perception of one's state of health. Eight percent of persons without health problems, compared with 24% with problems, consulted a health professional. Persons without a health problem were more likely to consult another professional rather than a physician. Most people (85%) found the time between making an appointment and the consultation acceptable. Info-santé (Info-Health), a telephone service in which nurses give information and advice on health and social matters, is available 24 hours a day, 7 days a week (Dunnigan, 2000). Seventy-five percent of the population knew of the availability of telephone service, and 32% of those used it. This service was least known and used by persons whose first language was other than French.

Papillon, Laurier, Barnard, and Baril (2000) reported that in the 2 days prior to their study half of their respondents had consumed at least one prescription or nonprescription medication. The proportion of women who consume medication is greater than that of men, although it should be noted that this utilization includes contraceptives and hormone replacements. Utilization increased with age, and nonprescription utilization increased with revenue and education; groups with greater resources were greater consumers. Trahan, Bégin, and Piché (2000) indicated that 6% of Quebecers had been hospitalized and 4.2% had been treated in day surgery during the previous year. Persons living alone, the chronically ill, aged, and new single-parent mothers were the most likely to receive home care. Family and others close were the principal source of help and care at home, following hospitalization or during long-term care. Families, in partnership with home-care nurses from local community centers, were the principal source of help and care at home, following hospitalization or during long-term illnesses (Reidy, 2005).

Rituals Related to Death and Dying

Functionality, aging, spousal death, and dying are interrelated as the older Quebecer "downsizes" from the family home to a smaller apartment or care environment and to a smaller set of "things." In Québec, such a move, often accompanied by a compulsion to divest themselves of many of their belongings, is called *casser la maison* (literally, "breaking the house"). An ethnographic study, realized in Montréal by Marcoux (2001) and seen as descriptive of life/death across Québec, reveals that to *casser la maison* is not a means of merely separating from one's belongings; more essentially it is a ritualized form of ancestralizing oneself by placing those possessions with kin or other recipients, guaranteeing one's survival in memory. For the aging Quebecer, divestment of belongings becomes a form of investment, part of the social organization of death. Marcoux continues, arguing that *casser la maison* begins with a compulsion toward detachment but evolves into the appropriation of the event in the reconstruction of self: the acceptance of the loss of status through the acceding to the higher status of ancestor (STATS Canada, 2006e).

For earlier generations in Québec, death was formalized and dealt with by adherence to the symbols and ceremonies of the Catholic Church, usually in the context of the family, and by a strong belief in an afterlife. For older Quebecers death remains intimately associated with religion, and the future is envisioned with the hope of life after death. Death and anniversaries of the death of family members are often commemorated by a Mass. However, with increased secularization and urbanization, many younger Quebecers are less likely to continue to follow traditional customs. While funeral Masses remain common, embalming, visitation, and body burials in a cemetery are declining as "baby boomers" choose cremation over burial. While in the 1950s cremation was unacceptable to Québec's Roman Catholics, it is now is requested twice as often as body burials (Johnston, 1996).

Today, the final agony of death and all the emotions it provokes are frequently concealed from public view, as death usually occurs in an institution. Death is often perceived as the ultimate failure, by both family and health professionals, since it cannot be mastered or controlled by technology. However, here in Québec, the attitudes and philosophical outlooks of nurses and doctors, ethical problems of death, and treatment and cessation of treatment are considered central to the care and accompaniment of the terminally ill, as well as being a subject worthy of continued scientific study and philosophical discourse (Volant, 2004).

Implications for Nursing Care

In a multicultural society, health and illness are, in part, determined by the degree of an individual's integration into a society and the social support supplied by the community. Social support has a preventive value if it is associated with networks that are stable, homogeneous, and dense and that provide a variety of links between individuals (Bozzini & Tessier, 1985). Health care planning must be sensitive to such diversity to be effective. A public-centered approach is at the heart of health and social service reform in Québec (Battaglini & Gravel, 2000). It is essential that the nurse work as a part of the interdisciplinary team in effective decision making about health and social services (Trudel, 1995).

Three differentiating factors contribute to health care assessment in a multicultural setting. First, note should be made of the meaning of health and illness in terms of the underlying significance of these concepts in the cultural group. Second, consideration must be given to the socioeconomic level of the individual requiring care. Descriptions of symptoms, compliance with treatment, and reaction to pain will differ according to social level and ethnic origin. Third, the client's gender influences how individuals view their bodies and the adoption of dependent or independent behavior patterns with regard to health (Dorvil, 1985). These factors influence one's representation of illness, the way the client's illness is explained, the assumption of responsibility for personal health through self-care, and participation in the treatment regimen. Because women are ordinarily the principal health agents in the family, nursing interventions should usually be directed toward encouraging their collaboration in fostering healthful living habits.

In the larger cities, polluted air is associated with such problems as asthma, bronchitis, and allergies affecting the skin, eyes, and respiratory tract. Families could be advised to minimize the exposure of infants to automobile fumes during the rush hour and to minimize use of possible allergy-producing substances found in rugs, bedding, and humidifiers in homes with young children, older people, persons suffering from asthma, or individuals with symptoms of acquired immunodeficiency. Prevention of symptoms caused by stagnant air in large buildings or factories also falls within the domain of the nurse concerned with the work environment and the reduction of worker absenteeism.

Since hunting and fishing are popular activities in Québec, it is of concern that certain pollutants may be present in fresh water and soil. Therefore, pregnant women should be advised against consuming freshwater fish or game during pregnancy. Even when women are not pregnant, the federal government recommends that fish from contaminated lakes be consumed no more than once a week to prevent accumulation of polychlorinated biphenyls (PCBs) in body tissues. The nurse's role includes participation in awareness campaigns, in short-term and long-term preventive measures, and in research to determine possible interrelations between such factors as pollution, health, lifestyle, and heredity.

With the aging of the population and the subsequent increase in the incidence of chronic illnesses has come an intensification in the use of various drugs and medicines in the community. It is the nurse's responsibility to help clients maintain their medical regimen and to inform them about the dangers of uncontrolled and irrational use of prescription or nonprescription drugs, of accidental or intentional intoxication, of teratogenic and iatrogenic effects, and of physical and psychological dependency.

BIOLOGICAL VARIATIONS

Genetic Factors

The various social, economic, and cultural practices of a given population influence the eventual formation of a genetic "pool" that determines the biological characteristics of a community and contribute to reducing or increasing the frequency of certain genes in the population (Bouchard & DeBraekeleer, 1991a). Such phenomena as migrations, successive waves of immigration, family inbreeding, and concentration of certain groups in specific areas are of particular consequence. Quebecers of French origin have a specific genotype inherited from the original group of 5000 colonists (Bouchard & DeBraekeleer, 1991b). For example, the genetic abnormalities found in the populations of the Saguenay and Charlevoix regions or Québec represent an important public health problem in these areas. The most striking example is that of muscular dystrophy, a disorder of genetic origin characterized by a progressive increase in muscular debility (Bouchard, 1991). Its worldwide frequency is approximately 1 in 25,000 individuals. In the Saguenay region, the frequency is estimated to be 1 in 514 (DeBraekeleer, 1991). Familial hypercholesterolemia has a worldwide frequency of 1 in 500 in the general population; in the eastern part of

the province, its frequency is estimated to be 1 in 15. Familial hypercholesterolemia has probably been the most carefully studied of the dominant chromosome abnormalities. The principal complication of this disease is coronary thrombosis in the young adult, which is often fatal (Bouchard & DeBraekeleer, 1991b). Cystic fibrosis is the most common fatal hereditary illness among Quebecers. Its frequency of 1 in 895 births in the Saguenay region is higher than that in most other populations. Tay-Sachs disease also seems to occur frequently in Québec. No treatment has been discovered for this condition, which occurs in infants from 2 to 6 months of age (DeBraekeleer, 1991).

Life Expectancy

During the past 30 years, the life expectancy of Quebecers has increased to about 80 years. However, it should be noted that the "disability-free" expectancy, which includes staying mobile and living outside a hospital or nursing home, is just over 70 years. Montréalers have the lowest life expectancy in urban Canada, at 74.8 years for men and 81 for women. Rural and northern Québec residents live shorter lives than the average Canadian; for example, the average life expectancy in Nunavik was only 66.7 years in 2005 (STATS Canada, 2006c). However, the province reported the low infant mortality rate of 4.4 per 1000 births in 2003 (STATS Canada, 2006d).

As in the rest of Canada, the leading causes of death include cancer, heart disease, cerebral vascular disease, chronic pulmonary disease, injuries, pneumonia, diabetes, suicide, and AIDS (STATS Canada, 2002). The most important causes of death in Quebecers are heart disease and cancer, with rates at about 175 per 100,000. Trauma and accidents, with a rate of about 27 per 100,000, and suicide (12 per 100,000) are the major causes of death for persons under 20 years of age (STATS Canada, 2002). Trauma, accidents, and suicide are more common in men than in women. However, while deaths from such accidents have decreased from 585 in 1975 to 112 in 1998, suicides have risen in the same period from 50 to 121 (Institut de la Statistique du Québec, 2002).

Susceptibility to Disease

Approximately two Quebecers out of three report at least one health problem that has imposed limits or required consultation with a health professional. Lavasseur and Goulet (2000) noted that Quebecers reported a range of disease conditions, including arthritis or rheumatism (11.8%), other osteoarthritic disorders (2.3%), hypertension (8.5%), asthma (5%), heart condition (4.6%), thyroid problems (3.7%), high cholesterol (2.8%), diabetes (2.8%), bronchitis or emphysema (2.3%), and kidney problems (1.9%). The rate of report of other health problems includes headache (11.8%), allergies (10.3%), allergic rhinitis (4%), skin allergies (9.1%), respiratory problems (5.4%), digestive problems (5%), mental problems (4.6%), intense nervousness (4.3%), and sleeping problems (2.3%). Other diseases, such as cancer, were reported at less than 1%. Combined categories indicate the importance of allergic manifestations and osteoarthritic conditions, although the rate of arthritis is the lowest in Canada (STATS Canada, 2002). An analysis of health problems by age indicates that allergies, asthma, and other respiratory afflictions are the most important problem for children and adults under age 24 and remain significant throughout the life span. After 24 years of age, Quebecers add headaches, backaches, accidents, intense nervousness and mental problems, and arthritic conditions as significant problems. Between ages 45 and 64, cardiac, cholesterol, and thyroid problems surface, and after age 65 cardiac, digestive, diabetes, and sleep problems assume added importance. Such conditions as diabetes ranged in prevalence from 0.1% of those under age 14 to 11% of those over 65; for the same age groups, cardiac disease ranged from 0.2% to 23.2%. The rate of asthma increased from 3.3% in 1987 to 5% in 1998.

Sexually and Intravenously Transmitted Diseases. Diseases transmitted sexually and through the bloodstream constitute a serious public health problem in Québec. Chlamydiosis is the most frequently reported sexually transmitted diseases, with 8404 cases reported in 2000, a 14% increase from 1999. The greater proportion of reported cases of gonorrhea were found in Montréal among men. In 2000 there were 381 cases, an increase of 29% from 1999. During the past 10 years, the incidence of hepatitis B has declined from 6.5 to 2.4 per 100,000 inhabitants. The incidence of syphilis is low, with about 10 cases, usually among homosexual men, reported yearly (Parent, Alary, Venne, & Dupont, 2001).

Among Canadian provinces, Québec has the second highest number of cases of AIDS. Bisexual and homosexual men under 40 years of age and intravenous drug users account for most cases of AIDS. However, while women infected with HIV constitute a growing group, the number of children infected by vertical transmission is small because of early treatment of infected pregnant women. They are concentrated in the Montréal area, where the women have contracted the disease either from infected male sexual partners or through intravenous drug use. Quebecers have, in general, a positive attitude toward those living with HIV and AIDS. Younger and more educated people and those who know someone who is infected have the most open attitudes (Leaune & Adrien, 1998).

Nutritional Preferences and Habits

From early colonial times, because of the harsh climate, the diet of Quebecers has been rich in starchy foods and fat. A considerable portion of the family budget has been devoted to food. Women have had the predominant role in the choice and preparation of food. Beginning in the 1960s, the practice of eating in restaurants became more frequent, and fast foods, rich in fat and salt and poor in fiber and vitamins, became widely popular. In 1987, Renaud, Jutras, and Bouchard reported that a majority of respondents claimed to have made an effort to balance their diets. However, while consuming less fatty foods, they still report consuming too much sugar and too few milk products, fruits, and vegetables. In 2000, Chénard, Daveluy, and Émond concluded that 85% of Quebecers had a positive perception of their food habits. Nevertheless, 20% reported eating at least four meals prepared outside the home per week, thus losing control of the nutritional quality of food consumed. Furthermore, a poor nutritional state was associated with the perception of a poor state of health, an elevated level of psychological distress, and poor social support. Nearly 1 in 10 Quebecers were unhappy with their nutritional regimen, either because of monotony or insufficient quantity of food available or because of an inability to offer balanced meals to their children. This situation was described in about two of five of the very poor, one of four of the unemployed, and one of five single-parent families. To combat the problem of undernourishment and hunger in disadvantaged children, food and milk programs are subsidized by the province. On the other hand, parental attitudes toward food and dieting are a factor in child and youth eating habits.

Psychological Characteristics and Coping

Tobacco, Alcohol, and Drug Abuse. In 1998, 31% of Quebecers smoked cigarettes daily, with slightly fewer women smoking than men. Of the smokers, 77% came from higher socioeconomic groups. Fewer married persons, 27%, smoked than those in common-law unions, 44%. Some 37% of the population is exposed at home to secondhand smoke, while 26% is exposed in public (Bernier & Brochu, 2000). By the year 2003 it was estimated that $2.8 billion in direct and indirect costs (such as for heath services and absenteeism) was due to tobacco in Québec (Physical Activity Monitor, 2004). However, as of May 2006, not only was smoking banned in public buildings throughout Québec, but it also was prohibited in bars and restaurants (Lamonde, 2006).

In 1998, 80% of persons over age 25 reported consumption of alcohol. Both users and those reporting an elevated consumption were highest in men between the ages of 15 and 44. Daily consumption increased with income (Chevalier & Lemoine, 2000a). Québec rates second in Canada in per capita sales of alcohol. Quebecers buy less hard liquor and more beer. Of all red wine sold in the country, 44% is sold in Québec (Kalbfuss, 2002).

However, in the same year, two thirds of Quebecers affirmed that they had never used drugs or psychoactive substances. Actual use was distinguished by sex, age, and socioeconomic status; it was more common by men, by young people, and, for older users, by higher income and education. The use of marijuana rose from 3.3% in 1985 to 20% in 1998 (Chevalier & Lemoine, 2000b). Illegal drug users have access to substances such as cocaine, crack, hallucinogenics, and, to some extent, heroin. Moisan (1991) reported that in Québec women have a tendency to abuse antidepressants and sleeping pills, while older people abuse psychotropic drugs. The abused drugs are often prescribed.

Mental Health. Chronic mental illness, deinstitutionalization, and drug and alcohol abuse problems have combined with economic factors to contribute to the number of homeless. In the year 1999–2000, about 5300 Quebecers were hospitalized for psychiatric problems. The most common diagnoses included affective and other psychoses, alcoholic psychosis, and schizophrenia (STATS Canada, 2002). In 1998, 4.6% of the population reported mental health problems, and 4.3% reported periods of intense nervousness (Lavasseur & Goulet, 2000). While the majority of people over age 15 described their mental health as excellent (35%), very good (36%), or good (21%), at least 20% reported an elevated level of psychological distress. Distress was strongest in women, youth under 24 years, the unemployed, and persons with low income. Higher psychological stress is related to traumatic events in childhood and youth (Légaré, Préville, Massé, et al., 2000a).

The suicide rate increased from 13 per 100,000 in 1976 to 19 per 100,000 in 1997 (Ministère de la santé et des Services sociaux, 1999). Suicidal ideation is also significant within the population of Québec, affecting 3.9% in 1998 (Légaré, Préville, Massé, et al., 2000b). Of people with suicidal ideation, 69% saw themselves as having an elevated level of psychological distress, and 43% judged their mental health to be bad. Suicidal ideation was found most among the very poor (15%) and poor (7%) and among the unmarried (8%).

Implications for Nursing Care

The particular mortality and morbidity curves occurring in the Québec population, combined with severe budget limitations placed on health services, call for the creation of new approaches in the care of those affected by illness. Target populations include those who suffer from chronic illnesses, osteoarthritic and cardiac conditions, asthma, and diabetes. The evolution of these latter illnesses follows a pattern in which brief hospitalizations occur episodically, followed by long periods of time when the patient and family must learn to function at home within the limits imposed by the condition. As length of allowed hospitalizations become shorter, the nurse must develop educational interventions and home care approaches in order to facilitate the participation of the patient and the family caregiver, as well as enabling self-care and maintaining quality of life.

Health care and counseling in parallel with preventive and health programs, for Quebecers exposed to venereal disease, also fall within the scope of nursing practice. Intervention should be designed to educate the public concerning the dangers of sexually transmitted diseases, especially AIDS, and the part played by intravenous drug use in the transmission of the latter. Moreover, nurses need to maintain open, nonjudgmental attitudes in their interactions with clients suffering from AIDS (Taggart, Reidy, & Grenier, 1992).

A "language of food" indicates not only how society views eating but also how a culture designates foods as normal and healthy. It also includes the personal adaptation that an individual or group makes concerning eating habits. Although socioeconomic and cultural factors influence the way these two concepts function, both must be considered when attempts are made to improve living habits. The perceived social requirement of staying slim, coupled with the burdens of motherhood and outside employment, causes many women to be undernourished or overweight. Given the importance of the relationship between nutrition, the health of newborns and adolescents, and osteoporosis in older women, much remains to be accomplished in the area of proper diets for women and children. The nurse's role includes participating in setting up and maintaining programs designed to reduce malnutrition in schools serving underprivileged children. School nurses are in a good position to assess needs and seek ways to foster healthful living habits among children and to act as a liaison between parents and teachers.

SUMMARY

The ethnic identity of French Canadians of Québec is witnessed in the attitudes and values common to them and in the knowledge they have of what it means to be a *Québécois*. They share a common background of the culture and ways of life of their ancestors, but one must accept that their ethnic identity varies in terms of content and degree relative to disparities such as age, education, and socioeconomic situation (Gohier & Schleifer, 1993). It is essential, however, for the nurse to remember that the people of Québec now live within an evolving multicultural society. To understand the significance of health and social behaviors of *les Québécois* (Quebecers), it is essential that the nurse develop cultural competence and sensitivity to the unique culture of the people of Québec, as well as to the diverse ethnic and racial groups who blend to make up the larger heterogeneous, pluralistic society.

Case Study

Marguerite Tremblay (born McNeill) married in 1929 at 16 years of age. Her husband, Théophile Tremblay, worked at a farm in the Laurentians. They were for the most part self-sufficient, with cows, a few sheep, and a market garden. They traded for certain goods and had a small cash crop. Life was hard, with a day that began before dawn and continued until bedtime.

(Continued)

In 1960, at the death of Théophile, the eldest son, Étienne, took over running the family farm, where he continued to live with his wife, Estelle, and their children. Several years later, the land was expropriated to make room for a highway. The family, now composed of Mrs. Tremblay, Rose (her unmarried daughter), and Étienne and his children, moved to a small farm property in Ste-Rose. Mrs. Tremblay, with the help of Rose, raised Étienne's children after their mother died in childbirth.

Mrs. Tremblay, a good Catholic and farm wife, had 15 children between 1930 and 1956, 8 of whom survived to maturity (see Tremblay Family Tree, Figure 23-1). Two of these children were born dead, two died after premature births, one died of meningitis, one died of polio, and one did not survive a hard winter. One son died in an automobile accident, when drunk, at 18 years of age.

The life situation of the surviving family members demonstrates how the family structure and religious practices have changed within the life span of one family.

Mrs. Tremblay has remained active and involved in the lives of her children and grandchildren. At 80 years of age, she suffered a cerebrovascular accident that left her with a left-sided hemiplegia. She has made only a moderate recovery. She requires help with transfers but can stand with a walker. She requires help with many activities of daily living and spends much of her time in a wheelchair. She speaks slowly but is lucid, if somewhat anxious.

Mrs. Tremblay has been admitted to a long-term care unit because of her physical limitations and her immediate family's inability to care for her at home. She alternates between understanding the need for long-term care and fear that her family no longer needs her. Her family, particularly her eldest son and daughter, with whom she lived, feel guilty and fear that they are not doing their "duty," despite their own health problems and physical limitations.

Rose
Age 63; unmarried; lives with mother; suffers from obesity, diabetes, and osteoporosis; attends church and receives the sacraments regularly.

Étienne
Age 62; widower; farmer and truck driver; father of seven children, five of whom survived to maturity, all of whom have left home; suffers from severe arthritis.

Philippe
Age 59; notary; father of six children, five of whom lived to maturity; smoker; suffers from hypertension and hypercholesterolemia; wife has recovered from breast cancer.

Line
Age 56; married a farmer; worked as a volunteer for the parish church; mother of four children, all of whom survived to maturity.

Victor
Age 55; missionary in Africa; smoker; suffers from certain chronic parasitical infections.

Marie-Madeleine
Age 45; was a nun in a nursing order; after leaving the convent, has worked with adolescents with drug problems; does not practice her religion.

Catherine
Age 43; former teacher; divorced from a doctor; mother of two children; suffers from chronic anxiety and mild abuse of tranquilizers; has become a Christian Scientist.

Denise
Age 34; former commercial artist; unmarried; mother of one child whose father, an actor, died of AIDS; mother and child HIV-positive; activist in AIDS self-help group; very interested in spiritual renewal but refuses her mother's pleas to return to the church.

Figure 23-1 The Tremblay Family Tree.

CARE PLAN

✳ *Nursing Diagnosis: Anxiety, related to change in health status and role function.*

Client Outcomes

1. Client will identify the factors in the situation that provoke anxiety (such as strange room, room shared with other resident).
2. Client will identify those activities, feasible in the new situation, that have helped her relax in the past.
3. Client will begin to accept the limits imposed by stroke and to control the anxiety provoked by life in a long-term setting.

Nursing Interventions

1. Take the time, daily, to talk personally with client in an informal setting such as the lounge or kitchen.
2. When talking about client's stroke, as much as possible use the language and words she uses. Verify client's comprehension of new or technical language.
3. Use the techniques of reminiscence therapy to remind client of past strategies for dealing with anxiety.
4. Identify those strategies appropriate to new environment that have previously helped control anxiety.

✳ *Nursing Diagnosis: Powerlessness, related to the health care environment*

Client Outcomes

1. Client will express her feelings of powerlessness.
2. Client will identify factors she can learn to control in the current situation.
3. Client will succeed in learning to control these factors.
4. Client will learn to use her interpersonal skills to exercise some control over her social environment.

Nursing Interventions

1. Encourage client to express her feelings and health goals.
2. Help client arrange her room and equipment, such as telephone, radio, and call bell, so that she is comfortable in using them.
3. Arrange with client's family to have a telephone with memory for frequently called numbers and a remote control for television (both with "user-friendly" boards).
4. Develop with the client daily routine that incorporates, as much as possible, strategies that give client control in current situation.
5. Develop with the client a prosthetic and secure environment where she compensates for her physical limits and maintains some control of her physical environment.
6. Encourage client to participate in social and recreational activities such as group singing and bingo.
7. Encourage client's interest and sense of responsibility in building the morale of other residents whom she seems to like.

✳ *Nursing Diagnosis: Role performance, ineffective related to health alterations*

Client Outcome

1. Client will maintain and strengthen those aspects of her former social and familiar roles that are possible within the current situation.

Nursing Interventions

1. Encourage the client to express her feelings and wishes concerning the roles she would like to play and the activities she would like to do.
2. Help client's daughter aid the client in exploring the sustainable aspects of her former roles and in developing new roles within the family.
3. Client will identify a role, within the long-term unit, that takes into consideration her limits but makes use of her abilities and the prosthetic environment.
4. Help the client understand and play her role in maintaining effective interrelationships between the generations of her family.
5. Develop a "caring" relationship with the client and explore with her the relationships she can develop and the roles she can play in interacting with other staff members, volunteers, other staff members, and other residents.

✳ *Nursing Diagnosis: Self-esteem (situational) low, functional impairment (right-sided hemiplegia) related to dependence on health care team within long-term care unit.*

Client Outcomes

1. Client will express opinions and her preferences to both staff and family.
2. Client will participate in the various aspects of her care process (such as decision making, physical care, assessment).
3. Client will experience and express, through her body language, an increase in self-esteem.

Nursing Interventions

1. Address the client by her name, Madame Tremblay, never by "Mama" ("Maman") or other diminutives.
2. Respect the client's privacy and her physical space and go slowly in manifesting a physical display of affection. Permit client to set the parameters of her social space.
3. Listen to the client, encourage her to use "I" in her conversation, respect her opinion, encourage her to make decisions, and respect these decisions.
4. Encourage the family to help client maintain her personal appearance by providing clothes that fit and are attractive, personal grooming equipment, and the like.
5. Compliment her on any improvements in appearance.
6. Work with occupational and physical therapy personnel to develop appropriate but practical and worthwhile projects (such as weaving, food preparation).

✳ *Nursing Diagnosis: Disturbed sensory perception (kinesthetic), related to sensory reception, transmission, and integration*

Client Outcomes

1. Client will begin to compensate for inability to identify position of body parts by developing other senses (sight, sensations of unaffected members, and so on).
2. Client will learn to master prosthetic aids to compensate for diminished motor coordination.
3. Client will understand the importance of practicing preventive and safety measures (such as skin care and proper shoes).

Nursing Interventions

1. Validate with the client that she understands the effect of the "stroke" on her ability to function and that she realizes that certain false perceptions can occur because of this condition.
2. Work with the client so that she learns to use her "good" hand routinely and to use visual inspection to verify the position and location of her affected limbs.
3. Develop with the client compensatory routines such as turning her head to improve her visual field or repositioning items in her physical environment.
4. Show the client how to inspect her skin for pressure points, and help her develop a routine for turning and relieving these pressure points.

✳ *Nursing Diagnosis: Compromised family coping related to disabling progression that exhausts supportive capacity of significant persons*

Client Outcomes

1. Family will develop appropriate involvement of all family members in the client's current situation (such as involvement that encourages both affiliation and autonomy).
2. Family will mutually accept new roles of the client and the principal caregiver in the family.

Nursing Interventions

1. Clarify with the daughter, in terms of her limits and abilities, her new role as principal health caregiver in the family, emphasizing the essential nature of this new role.
2. Clarify with family members (especially the eldest son) the importance of visits, family celebrations, development of relationships with grandchildren, and keeping client informed of family events.
3. Include the daughter in the planning of the client's care.
4. Encourage family members to develop joint family projects such as a family photo album.

(Adapted from Ackley & Ludwig, 2002)

✹ STUDY QUESTIONS

1. How is public access to health care authorized in Canada and what group of citizens are included under the authorization?
2. Describe how the work environment in Québec affects the health care of workers in Québec.
3. Describe the most commonly occurring genetic conditions found among French Canadians in Québec.
4. Describe the life expectancy by gender of French Canadians in Québec.
5. Describe the commonly occurring conditions to which French Canadians living in Québec are most susceptible.

NCLEX-RN REVIEW QUESTIONS

1. In promoting self-care for a client from Québec, the nurse needs to be sure to:
   A. Include a spiritual plan of care
   B. Include touch in the plan of care
   C. Include the family in health teaching
   D. Include a time frame with collaborative objectives

2. In providing nursing care in Québec, the nurse realizes that the space meanings are implemented by:
   A. Standing close when communicating with a client
   B. Standing close when discussing familiar attitudes
   C. Maintaining distance when conversing with a client
   D. Shaking hands with the client before providing care

3. A nurse in Québec is doing dietary teaching for a pregnant woman. Because of environmental factors, the nurse should advise the client to:
   A. Consume fish no more than once a week
   B. Avoid consuming fresh-water fish
   C. Consume a vegetarian diet from a variety of sources.
   D. Avoid eating beef that is imported from England

References

Ackley, B. J., & Ludwig, G. (2002). *Nursing diagnosis handbook.* (ed. 5). St. Louis: Mosby.

Allard, M., & Durand, S. (2006). L'infirmiere practicienne specialisee: un nouveur role. [Clinical nurse specialist: a new role]. *Perspective Infirmiere,* 3(5), 10–15.

Anctil, H., & Bluteau, M. A. (1986). *La santé et l'assistance publique au Québec, 1886–1986* [Québec health and social welfare, 1886–1986]. Québec: Ministère de la Santé et des Services sociaux, Direction des Communications.

Arcand, R., Labrèche, F., Stock, S., Messing, K., & Tissot, F. (2000). Travail et santé [Work and health]. *Enquête sociale et de santé* [Health and social inquiry] (pp. 525–570). Québec: Institut de la Statistique du Québec.

Audet, L. P., & Gauthier, A. (1967). *Le système scolaire du Québec: organisation et fonctionnement* [Québec educational system: structure and function]. Montréal: Librairie Beauchemin Limitée.

Bailey, E., & Bailey, R. (1995). *Discover Canada.* Oxford: Berlitz Publishing Company.

Battaglini, A., & Gravel, S. (2000). Diversité culturelle et planification de la santé. [Cultural diversity and health planning]. In *Dans culture, santé et ethnicité-vers une santé publique pluraliste* [Culture, health and ethnicity—toward a pluralist public health]. Montréal: Régie Régionale de Montréal-Centre et des Service Sociaux. Direction de la Santé Publique.

Bauch, H. (2002, July 6). Flagging fervour. (Montreal) The Gazette, p. B1.

Bernier, S., & Brochu, D. (2000). Usage du tabac [Use of tobacco]. In *Enquête sociale et de santé* [Health and social inquiry] (pp. 99–115). Québec: Institut de la Statistique du Québec.

Bouchard, G. (1991). Pour une approche historique et sociale du génome québécois [Historical and social approach to the Québec genome]. In Bouchard, G., & DeBraekeleer, M. (Eds.). *Histoire d'un génome: population et génétique dans l'est du Québec* [History of a genome: population and genetics in eastern Québec] (pp. 3–18). Québec: Les Presses de l'Université de Québec.

Bouchard, G. (1992). Sur les perspectives de la culture québécoise comme francophonie nord-américaine [On the perspectives of Québec culture as a French-speaking community in North America]. In Lanthier, P., & Rousseau, G. (Eds.), *La culture inventée, stratégies culturelles aux XIXe et XXe siècles* [Cultural tendencies and cultural strategies of the nineteenth and twentieth centuries] (pp. 319–328). Québec: Institut Québécois de Recherche sur la Culture.

Bouchard, G., & DeBraekeleer, M.(Eds.). (1991a). *Histoire d'un génome: population et génétique dans l'est du Québec* [History of a genome: population and genetics in eastern Québec]. Québec: Les Presses de l'Université du Québec.

Bouchard, G., & DeBraekeleer, M. (1991b). Mouvements migratoires, effets fondateurs et homogénéisation génétique [Migratory shifts, founders effects and genetic homogenization]. In Bouchard, G., & DeBraekeleer, M. (Eds.), *Histoire d'un génome: population et génétique dans l'est du Québec* [History of a genome: population and genetics in eastern Québec] (pp. 281–321). Québec: Les Presses de l'Université du Québec.

Bozzini, L., & Tessier, R. (1985). Support social et santé [Social support and health]. In Dufresne, J., Dumont, F., & Martin, Y. (Eds.), *Traité d'anthropologie médicale* [Medical anthropology treatise] (pp. 905–939). Québec: Les Presses de l'Université du Québec.

Canadian Press. (2002, July 13). Quebec tops the list of polluted land, p. A12.

Carkson, M., Pica, L., & Lacombe, H. (2000). Spiritualité, religion et santé: une analyse exploratoire. [Spirituality, religion and health: an exploratory analysis]. In *Enquête sociale et de santé* [Health and social inquiry] (pp. 603–623). Québec: Institut de la Statistique du Québec.

Chapman, R. (2000). *Siting the Québec novel.* New York: P. Lang.

Chénard, L., Daveluy, C., & Émond, A. (2000).Conclusion général. [General conclusions]. In *Enquête sociale et de santé* [Health and social inquiry] (pp. 628–643). Québec: Institut de la Statistique du Québec.

Chevalier, S., & Lemoine, O. (2000a). Consommation d'alcool [Consumption of alcohol]. *Enquête sociale et de santé* (pp. 117–133). Québec: Institut de la Statistique du Québec.

Chevalier, S., & Lemoine, O. (2000b). Consommation de drogues et autres substances psychoactives [Consumption of drugs and other psychoactive substances]. In *Enquête sociale et de santé* [Health and social inquiry] (pp. 135–147). Québec: Institut de la Statistique du Québec.

Cossette, S., Lévesque, L., & Laurin, L. (1995). Informal and formal support for caregivers of a demented relative: do gender and kinship make a difference? *Research in Nursing and Health,* 18(5), 437–451.

Dandurand, R.B. (1990). Peut-on encore définir la famille? [Can we still define the family?]. In Dumont, F. (Ed.), *La société québécoise après 30 ans de changements* [Québec society after 30 years of change] (pp. 49–66). Québec: Institut Québécois de Recherche sur la Culture.

Davidhizar, R. & Giger, J. (2000). Cultural competency matters. *International Journal of Health Care Quality Assurance,* 13(6/7), viii–xi.

DeBraekeleer, M. (1991). Les gènes délétères [Deleterious genes]. In Bouchard, G., & DeBraekeleer, M. (Eds.), *Histoire d'un génome: population et génétique dans l'est du Québec* [History of a genome: population and genetics in eastern Québec] (pp. 343–363). Québec: Les Presses de l'Université de Québec.

Derfel, A. (2002, July 1). Health care system is bearing up well. (Montréal.) *The Gazette,* pp. A1, A7.

Derfel, A. (2005). Medical-imaging clinics thrive. (Montréal). *The Gazette.* A1 & A7.

Desautels,Y. (1984). *Les coutumes de nos ancêtres* [Customs of our ancestors]. Montréal: Édition Paulines.

Desrochers, P. (2002, June 29). Shattering shelter myths. (Montréal). *The Gazette,* p. B7.

Desrosiers, G. (2006). Health care: are we moving close to a two-tiered system. *Perspective Imfirmiere,* 3(5), 8–9.

Dorvil, H. (1985). Types de sociétés et representations [Types of societies and representations]. In Dufresne, J., Dumont, F., & Martin, Y. (Eds.), *Traité d'anthropologie médicale* [Medical anthropology treatise]. Québec: Presses de l'Université du Québec.

Dougherty, K. (2002, July 4). Keep off the grass: Québec bans pesticides linked to diseases (Montréal). *The Gazette,* pp. A1, A2.

Dulong, G., & Bergeron, G. (1980). Le parler populaire du Québec et de ses régions voisines [Popular language of Québec and its neighboring regions]. *La documentation québécoise,* 8, 3124–3655.

Dunnigan, L. (2000). Recours au service téléphonique Infosanté CLSC. [Recourse to Info-health telephone service] In *Enquête sociale et de santé* [Health and social inquiry] (pp. 429–443). Québec: Institut de la Statistique de Québec.

Editorial. (2002, June 29). Tackle housing crisis head on. (Montréal) *The Gazette*, p. B6.

Fahmy-Eid, N., & Dumont, M. (1983). *Maîtresses de maison, maîtresses d'écoles: femmes, familles et education dans l'histoire du Québec* [Housewives, school mistresses: women, families, and education in Québec history]. Montréal: Boréal Express.

Fitterman, L. (2002, June 17). Married . . . with controversy. (Montréal) *The Montréal Gazette.*

Foster, W., Smith, W., & Donahue, H. (2000). Systemic education reform in Québec: How far have we come? Where are we headed? *Journal of Educational Administration and Foundations,* 14(2), 12–37.

Fournier, M.-A., & Piché, J. (2000). Recours aux services des professionnels de la santé et des services sociaux [Recourse to the services of health and welfare professionals]. In *Enquête sociale et de santé* [Health and social inquiry] (pp. 388–407). Québec: Institut de la Statistique du Québec.

Gagnon, S. (1992). L'École élémentaire québécoise au XIXe siècle [Québec elementary school in the nineteenth century]. In Lanthier, P., & Rousseau, G. (Eds.), *La culture inventée, stratégies culturelles aux XIXe et XXe siècles* [Cultural tendencies and cultural strategies of the nineteenth and twentieth centuries] (pp. 135–153). Québec: Institut Québécois de Recherche sur la Culture.

Globalis. (2005). Retrieved June 28, 2007, from http://globalis.gvu.unu.edu/indicator_detail.cfm?IndicatorID=138& Country=GB.

Gohier, C., & Schleifer, M. (1993). *La question de l'identité: Qui suis-je? Qui est l'autre?* [The question of identity: Who am I? Who are the others?]. Montreal: Les Éditions Logiques.

Gouvernement du Québec. (1985). *Livre vert: pour les familles Québécoises* [Green book: for Québec families]. Québec: Ministre du Conseil exécutif, Secrétariat à la politique familiale.

Gouvernement de Québec. (2002, avril). La situation démographique au Québec: bilan 2002 [The demographic situation in Québec: Outline 2002]. Québec: Ministre du Conseil exécutif, Secrétariat à la politique familiale.

Hall, E.T. (1990). *The hidden dimension*. New York: Anchor Books.

Henripin, J., Huot, P.M., Lapierre-Adamcyk, E., & Marcil-Gratton, N. (1981). *Les enfants qu'on n'a plus au Québec* [Children that we no longer have in Québec]. Montréal: Les Presses de l'Université de Montréal.

Herman, A. (2001). *How the Scots invented the modern world*. New York: Crown Publishers.

Institut de la Statistique du Québec. (2002). Retrieved June 28, 2007, from http://www.stat.gouv.qc.ca.

Institut de la Statistique de Québec (2006b). Retrieved June 28, 2007, from http://www.stat.gouv.qc.ca/donstat/societe/famls_mengs_nic_vie/menage_famile/men_fam_enf/families/tableau_14.htm.

Institut de la Statistique de Québec (2006b). Retrieved June 28, 2007, from http://www.stat.gouv.qc.ca/donstat/societe/famls_mengs_nic_vie/menage_famile/men_am_enf/families/tableau_18.htm.

Institut de la Statistique de Québec (2006c). Retrieved June 28, 2007, from http://www.stat.gouv.qc.ca/donstat/societe/econm_finnc/ conjn_econm/TSC/pdf/chap1.pdf.

Institut de la Statistique de Québec (2006d). Retrieved June 28, 2007, from http://www.statcan.ca/101/cst01/demo31c. htm.

Institut de la Statistique de Québec (2006e). Retrieved June 28, 2007, from http://www.stat.gouv.qc.ca/donstat/societe/famls_ mengs_nic_vie/menage_famile/men_fam_en f/families/tableau_18.htm.

Institut de la Statistique de Québec (2006f). Retrieved June 28, 2007, from http://www.stat.gouv.qc.ca/regions/lequebec/population_ que/popjeune20_an.htm.

Institut de la Statistique de Québec (2006g). Retrieved June 28, 2007, from http://www.stat.gouv.qc.ca/regions/lequebec/population_ que/popjeune20_an.htm.

Institut de la Statistique de Québec (2006h). Retrieved June 28, 2007, from http://www.cflri.ca/cflri/pa/surveys/2000survey/2000_qc.html.

Institut de la Statistique de Québec (2006i). Retrieved June 28, 2007, from http://www.gpiatlantic.org/releases/pr_quebec.shtml.

Johnston, D. (1996, September 3). Aging boomers put a spin on funeral industry. (Montréal). *The Gazette,* A1.

Julien, M., Julien, D., & Lafontaine, P. (2000). Environnement de soutien [Support environment]. In *Enquête sociale et de santé* [Health and social inquiry] (pp. 499–522). Québec: Institut de la Statistique du Québec.

Kalbfuss, K. (2002, July 13). Québec drinkers in the red. (Montréal). *The Gazette,* pp. 1, 12.

Kennedy, M. (2002, June 15). Public backs health-care changes. (Montréal) *The Gazette,* p. A14.

Labrie, N. (1990). La question linguistique et les communautés culturelles au Québec [Québec linguistic issue and cultural communities]. In Guilbert, L. (Ed.), *Identité ethnique et interculturalité: état de la recherche en ethnologie et en socio-linguistique* [Ethnic identity and interculturalism: state of research in ethnology and in sociolinguistics] (pp. 33–46). Sainte-Foy: CELAT (Centre d'Études sur la Langue, les Arts, et les Traditions populaires des Francophones en Amérique du Nord), Université de Laval.

Lacourse, M.-T. (1999). Famille et société (ed. 2). [Family and society]. Montreal: Chenelière.

Lacroix, B., & Simard, J. (1984). Religion populaire, religion de clercs [Popular religion and clergymen]. In Collection: *Culture Populaire*, No. 2. Québec: Institut Québécois de Recherche sur la Culture.

Laforest, L. (1985). Pratiques médicales et évolution sociale [Medical practices and social evolution]. In Dufresne, J., Dumont, F., & Martin, Y. (Eds.), *Traité d'anthropologie médicale* [Medical anthropology treatise] (pp. 267–280). Québec: Les Presses de l'Université du Québec.

Lalonde, M. (2002, June 18). Parental role seen in the "cycle of obesity." (Montréal). *The Gazette*, p. A4.

Lamey, M. (2002, June 29). Softwood casualties mounting. (Montréal). *The Gazette*, pp. A1, A7.

Lamonde, Y. (1991). *Territoires de la culture québécoise* [Québec cultural territoires]. Québec: Les Presses de l'Université de Laval.

Lamonde, M. (2006, May 27). No smoking... says who? (Montréal). *The Gazette*, 83.

Lanthier, P., & Rousseau, G. (Eds.). (1992). *La culture inventée, stratégies culturelles aux XIXe et XXe siècles* [Cultural tendencies and cultural strategies of the nineteenth and twentieth centuries]. Québec: Institut québécois de Recherche sur la Culture.

Laperrière, G. (1992). La place du catholicisme [The place of Catholicism]. Dossier: Catholicisme et société distincte [Catholicism and distinct society]. *Présence, 2* (5), 21–23.

Laroche, D. (2000). Indicateurs pour des activités quotidienne [Indicators of daily activities]. *Donnée sociodémographique en bref, 4*(6), 5–6 [Sociodemographic data in brief].

Laroche, D., & Gauthier, H. (2002). Quelque résultats sur l'emploi du temps [Some results about the use of time]. *Donnée sociodémographique en bref, 6*(2), 1 [Sociodemographic data in brief].

Lavasseur, M. (2000). Perception de l'état de santé [Perception of health status]. In *Enquête sociale et de santé* [Health and social inquiry] (pp. 259–269). Québec: Institut de la Statistique du Québec.

Lavasseur, M., & Goulet, L. (2000). Problèmes de santé [Health problems]. In *Enquête sociale et de santé* [Health and social inquiry] (pp. 273–293). Québec: Institut de la Statistique du Québec.

Lazure, J. (1990). Mouvance des générations. Condition féminine et masculine [Generational sphere of influence. Female and male status]. In Dumont, F. (Ed.), *La Société québécoise après 30 ans de changements* [Québec society after 30 years of change] (pp. 27–40). Québec: Institut québécois de Recherche sur la Culture.

Leaune, V., & Adrien, A. (1998). *Les Québécois face au sida: Attitudes envers les personnes vivant avec le VIH et gestions des risques* [Québecers in regards to aids: attitudes toward persons living with HIV and the management of risks]. Montréal: Direction de la santé publique, Régie régional de la santé et de services sociaux de Montréal-Centre.

Légaré, G., Préville, M., Massé, R., et al. (2000a). Santé Mentale [Mental health]. In *Enquête sociale et de santé* [Health and social inquiry] (pp. 333–352). Québec: Institut de la Statistique du Québec.

Légaré, G., Préville, M., Massé, R., et al. (2000b). Idées suicidaires et parasuicides [ideas of suicide]. In *Enquête sociale et de santé* [Health and social inquiry] (pp. 354–364). Québec: Institut de la Statistique du Québec.

Létourneau, E., Bernier, B., Marchand, P., & Trudel, G. (2000). Familles et santé [Families and health]. In *Enquête sociale et de santé* [Health and social inquiry] (pp. 271–293). Québec: Institut de la Statistique du Québec.

Marcoux, J. S. (2001). The 'casier maison' ritual. *Journal of Material Culture, 6*(2), 213–235.

McAndrew, M., & Potvin, M. (1996). *Racisme au Québec: éléments d'un diagnostique* [Racism in Québec elements of a diagnosis]. Québec: Ministère des Affaires internationales de l'immigration et des Communications du Québec.

McAndrew, M., & Proulx, J.-P. (2000). Éducation et ethnicité au Québec: un portrait ensemble [Education and ethnicity in Québec: a common portrait]. In McAndrew, M., & Gagnon, F. (Eds.), Relations ethniques et éducation dans les sociétés divisées (pp. 86–110). Paris: l'Harmattan.

McGovern, S. (2002, July 6). 66,000 jobs, jobs, jobs. (Montréal) *The Gazette*, pp. A1, A2.

McKenzie, R. (2002, June 29). Vivre l'immigration français [Long live French immigration]. (Montréal). *The Gazette*, pp. B1, B4.

Ministère de la santé et des Services sociaux. (1999). *Stratégie québécoise face au suicide* [Québec strategies for combating suicide]. Québec: Les Publications du Québec.

Moisan, C. (1991). *Portrait de la consommation d'alcool et de drogues au Québec: principales données de l'Enquête nationale sur l'alcool et les autres drogues* [Portrait of alcohol and drug consumption in Québec: principal data of the national survey on alcohol and other drugs]. Collection: Données statistiques et Indicateurs. Québec: Ministère de la Santé et des Services sociaux.

MSNBC. (2000, July 9). Web-threat to French in Québec: "le combat" over the web. Retrieved from http://www.msnbc.com/news/defalt.asp.

Nebenzahl, D. (2006, May 27). Thrilled to be back. (Montréal). *The Gazette*. G1.

Ntetu, A., & Fortin, J. (1996). Reconsidering nursing interventions among Native people. *Canadian Nurse*, 9(3), 42–46.

Ordre des infirmières et infirmiers du Québec. (1999). Statistiques relatives aux infirmières et infirmiers inscrit au tableau au 31 mars 1999 [Statistics concerning registered nurses] [March 31, 1999]. Retrieved June 28, 2007, from http://www.oiiq.org/ptf/stat99.pdf.

Ordre des infirmières et infirmiers du Québec. (2001). *La vision contemporaine de l'exercice infirmier au Québec* [Contemporary practice of nursing in Québec]. Montréal: Ordre des infirmières et infirmiers du Québec.

Ordre des infirmières et infirmiers du Québec. (2006). L'infirmiere practiciencce specialisee en soin de premiere ligne: le point sur les travaur [The nurse practitioner in primary care: where we are]. *Le Journal*, 3(5), 4.

Orr, R. (1992). Notre héritage Catholique [Our Catholic heritage]. Translated by Serge Gagnon. Dossier: Catholicisme et société distincte [Catholicism and distinct society]. *Présence*, 1(5), 11–13.

Ottawa Citizen. (2002, June 20). Best to keep "core" level of health care. (Montréal). *The Gazette*, p. A13.

Papillon, M.-J., Laurier, C., Barnard, L., & Baril, J. (2000). Consommation de médicaments [Consumption of medications]. In *Enquête sociale et de santé* [Health and social inquiry] (pp. 245–267). Québec: Institut de la Statistique du Québec.

Paquet, G. (1989). *Santé et inégalité sociales: un problème de distance culturelle* [Health and social inequality: cultural gap]. Québec: Institut Québécois de Recherche sur la Culture.

Parent, R., Alary, M., Venne, S., & Dupont, M. (2001). *Analyse des cas d'infection génitale (déclarés au Québec par année civil 1996–2000)* [Analyses of cases of genital infection (declared in Québec by civil years 1996–2000)]. Québec: Santé et Services sociaux Québec.

Physical Activity Monitor. (2004). Retrieved from http://www.cflri.ca/cfiri/resources/pub.php#2004pam.

Pronovost, G. (1989). Les transformations des rapports entre le temps de travail et le temps libre [Transformation in work time and leisure time]. In Pronovost, G., & Mercure, D. (Eds.), *Temps et sociétés* [Time and societies] (pp. 37–61). Québec: Institut québécois de Recherche sur la Culture.

Québec Government Portal: Health. (2002). Retrieved from http://www.gouv.qc/Vision/Sante/Sante_en.html.

Québec Government Portal: Society. (2002a). Retrieved from http://www.gouv.qc/Vision/Societe/ProtraitDemographique_en.html.

Québec Government Portal: Society (2002b). Retrieved from http://www.gouv.qc/Vision/Societe/ProtraitHistorique_en.html.

Québec Government Portal: Society. (2002c). Retrieved from http://www.gouv.qc/Vision/Societe/ProtraitsDistinctives_en.html.

Québec Government Portal: Society. (2002d). Retrieved from http://www.gouv.qc/Vision/Societe/Protraitcultural_en.html.

Reidy, M. (2005). *The educational role of the nurse in the context of the shift to ambulatory ca*re. Ph.D. Dissertation. Universite de Québec a Montréal.

Renaud, J., Gingras, L., Vachon, S., et al. (2001). *Ils sont maintenant d'ici! Les dix premières années au Québec des immigrants admis en 1989* [They are from here now! The ten first years in Québec of immigrants admitted in 1989]. Collection Études, recherches et statistiques. Québec: Les Publications du Québec.

Renaud, M., Jutras, S., & Bouchard, P. (1987). *Les solutions qu'apportent les Québécois à leurs problèmes sociaux et sanitaires* [Solutions brought forth by Québecers concerning social and health problems]. In *Commission d'Enquête sur les Services de santé et les Services sociaux* [Inquiry Commission on Health and Social Services]. Québec: Les Publications du Québec.

Rioux, M. (1974). *Les Québécois* [The Québecers]. Paris: Seuil.

Sevunts, L. (2002, June 17). General's ER patients "packed like sardines." (Montréal). *The Gazette*, p. A3.

STATS Canada. (2002). Retrieved June 28, 2007, from http://www.statcan.ca.

STATS Canada. (2006a). Retrieved June 28, 2007, from http://www.statcan.ca./Daily/English/060328/do60328e.htm.

STATS Canada. (2006b). Retrieved June 28, 2007, from http://www.statcan.ca./English/Subjects/Labour/LFS/lfs-en.htm.

STATS Canada. (2006c). Retrieved June 28, 2007, from http://www.statcan.ca./Daily/English/050201/d050201a.htm.

STATS Canada. (2006d). Retrieved June 28, 2007, from http://www.statcan.ca/101/cst01/health21a.htm?sdi=death%20rate%20quebedDaily/English/.ca./English/Subjects/Labour/LFS/lfs-en.htm.

STATS Canada. (2006e). Retrieved June 28, 2007, from http://www40.statcan.ca/101/health50a.htm?sdi=asthma.

Stewart, M.J., Hart, G., Mann, K., et al. (2001). Telephone support group: intervention for persons with haemophilia and HIV/AIDS and family caregivers. *International Journal of Nursing Studies*, 38(2), 209–225.

Taggart, M.E., Reidy, M., & Grenier, D. (1992). Attitudes d'infirmières francophones face au sida [French-speaking nurses' attitudes toward AIDS]. *Infirmière canadienne/Canadian Nurse*, 88(1), 48–52.

Tétu de Labsade, F. (1990). *Le Québec: un pays, une culture* [Québec: a country, a culture]. Montréal: Boréal.

Thibaudeau, M.F., & Reidy, M. (1985). A nursing care model for the disadvantaged family. In Stewart, M. (Ed.), *Community health nursing in Canada* (pp. 269–286). Toronto: Gage.

Thibaudeau, M.F., Reidy, M., d'Amours, F., & Frappier, G. (1984). *La santé de la famille défavorisée: évaluation de l'application d'un modèle de soins infirmiers auprès de familles défavorisées qui utilisent les services du CLSC* [Health of the disadvantaged family: assessment of the application of a nursing care model in disadvantaged families using community health clinics]. Montréal: Faculté des Sciences infirmières, Université de Montréal.

Thibault, M.T. (1989). Environnement [Environment]. In Asselin, R. (Ed.), *Le Québec statistique 1989* [1989 Québec statistics] (ed. 59) (pp. 261–291). Québec: Les Publications du Québec.

Trahan, L., Bégin, P., & Piché, J. (2000). Recours à l'hospitalisation, à la chirurgie d'un jour et au services posthospitaliers [Recourse to hospitalization, day surgery and post-hospital services]. In *Enquête sociale et de santé* [Health and social inquiry] (pp. 409–428). Québec: Institut de la Statistique de Québec.

Trudel, A. (1995). Nurses as members of administrative boards. *Canadian Nurse*, 91(5), 37–40.

Valentine, H. (2001, November). The increasingly assertive ladies of Québec. *Le Québécois Libre*. 92, Nov. Retrieved June 28, 2007, from http://www.quebecoislibre.org/011110-8.htm.

Vissandjée, B., & Dupéré, S. (2000). La communication interculturelle en contexte clinique: une question de artenariat [Intercultural communication in a clinical context: a question of partnership]. In *Revue canadienne de recherche en sciences infirmières* [Canadian Review of Nursing Research], 32(1), 99–113.

Volant, E. (2004). L'accompagnement des mourants: auz limites du sens -une ethique du seuil [The companionship of the dying: at the end of life—an ethic of the threshold]. *Frontieres*, 17(1), 83–86.

Watelet, H. (1999). Temps et culture [Time and culture]. In *Quatre essais sur temps et culture* [Four essays on time and culture] (pp. 5–8). Montréal: Centre interuniversitaire d'études québécois & Institut d'études canadiennes.

Wilton, K. (2002, March 26). Québec immigration leaps. (Montréal). *The Gazette*, p. A4.

World almanac. (2006). New York: World Almanac Books.

CHAPTER 24 Puerto Rican Americans

Sara Torres

Behavioral Objectives

After reading this chapter the nurse will be able to:

1. Describe methods a nurse can use to enhance communication with a Puerto Rican.
2. Explain the importance of personal space to some Puerto Rican women.
3. Describe the importance of family relationships for Puerto Ricans.
4. Discuss the effect of time orientation on health promotion activities.
5. Identify the role of folk and spiritual healers for some Puerto Ricans.
6. Discuss biological variations that may be found in Puerto Ricans.

OVERVIEW OF PUERTO RICO

The commonwealth of Puerto Rico is located in the Caribbean Sea about 1000 miles east-southeast of Miami. Puerto Rico is to the east of Haiti and the Dominican Republic (La Hispaniola) and to the west of the Virgin Islands. With a land area of 3425 square miles, Puerto Rico is approximately three times the size of Rhode Island (McGovern, 2002). Its territory includes the islands of Culebra, Vieques, Descecheo, and Mona. Puerto Rico has a high central mountain range, dry and fertile northern coastal plains, low eastern mountains, and the El Yunque rain forest (CultureGrams, 2002).

In the fifteenth century, some 50,000 indigenous Taino Indians inhabited the territory and called the island Boriken or Borinquen, which means "the great land of the valiant and noble Lord" or "land of the great lords" (Welcome to Puerto Rico: History, 2006). This word is still used to designate the people and island of Puerto Rico. When Christopher Columbus arrived in 1493 and claimed the island for Spain, the Taino Indians lived in small villages, organized in clans and led by a chief. The Taino lived off the tropical crops, including pineapples, cassava, and sweet potatoes, supplemented by seafood. Spanish colonizers who arrived in 1508 were welcomed by the Taino, who offered them gold nuggets they picked out of the river. The seaside port, which later was named San Juan and today is the capital, quickly became Spain's most important military outpost in the Caribbean. The Spaniards constructed a wall around San Juan. A massive fort on the harbor, San Felipe del Morro Castel, protected the city with garrisoned troops. The Spaniards also established gold-mining operations, which lasted until 1570, when the gold stores were depleted.

Under the rule of Juan Ponce de Leon, the governor appointed by the Spanish crown, the first *repartimiento* of Puerto Rico was established to distribute fixed numbers of Indians to officials and colonists for wage-free and forced labor. When several priests protested the treatment of the Indians, the Spanish crown instituted the *encomienda*, which required

Indians to be paid for the labor and taught the Christian religion. However, the Indians continued to be treated as slaves, men who resisted were killed, and much of the male population was annihilated. Only a few Indians escaped into the remote mountains. Many of the remaining women were taken by the Spanish settlers for mates, and their offspring become known as *jibaros*. With industrialization and migration to the cities, few *jibaros* remain today (Welcome to Puerto Rico: People, 2006). African slaves were brought to the island as sugarcane was introduced, with slavery continuing until 1873 (CultureGrams, 2002). The slaves imported from Africa came from Sudan, Congo, Senegal, Guinea, Sierra Leone, the Ivory Coast, and the Gold Coast, adding further diversity to the island's racial mix. Furthermore, some French families from both Louisiana and Haiti, farmers from Scotland and Ireland escaping depressed economies, Italians, Germans, and even Lebanese people moved to Puerto Rico and contributed to the cultural and racial mix that makes the Puerto Rican culture unlike any other. This historic intermingling has resulted in an island where racial problems are minimal (Welcome to Puerto Rico: Puerto Rican Culture, 2006).

Over the centuries, the Spaniards fought off attempts by the French, Dutch, and British to capture control of the island. Nevertheless, after the Spanish–American War, the Treaty of Paris ceded Puerto Rico to the United States in 1898, thus adding American influence to the culture. In 1917 Puerto Ricans were given U.S. citizenship. In 1952 the people voted in favor of commonwealth status. As a commonwealth, Puerto Rico is a self-governing part of the United States. Puerto Rico's executive power resides in the governor and a bicameral legislature made up of a Chamber of Representatives of 53 members and a Senate of 27 members, who have control over the internal affairs of Puerto Rico. Puerto Rico is divided into 78 municipalities, each of which has an elected mayor and municipal assembly (Welcome to Puerto Rico: Government, 2006). Puerto Rico has one resident commissioner with a voice but no vote in the Congress of the

United States. As U.S. citizens, Puerto Ricans are subject to military service and most federal laws, and they have free movement in and out of the United States. However, as residents of the commonwealth, they pay no federal income tax on locally generated earnings, nor can electoral votes be cast by Puerto Rico in the U.S. presidential elections. Today, Puerto Ricans are divided over whether to request the United States for statehood or to remain a commonwealth (CultureGrams, 2002). A view of the Internet version of the *Puerto Rico Herald* (http://www.puertorico-herald.org) indicates numerous articles related to the political future of Puerto Rico, including an article in volume 6, number 34, "What should the U.S. Congress do about Puerto Rico's political status?"

Puerto Rico is a strategic location for the U.S. military in the Caribbean. This setting gives the U.S. military access to North, Central, and South America, and Puerto Rico is a center for U.S. military training, surveillance, and weapons testing (Welcome to Puerto Rico: Government, 2006). Since the closure of U.S. bases in Panama in 1999, Puerto Rico has provided the home for military forces in Latin America and for the U.S. Army South.

With a population of 3,916,632 (July 2005 estimate) and density of 1127 people per square mile (2004 estimate), Puerto Rico is one of the most densely populated islands in the world and is more densely populated than any of the states (Welcome to Puerto Rico: People, 2006). Some 71% of the population lives in urban areas. Approximately one third of the population is concentrated in the San Juan-Carolina-Bayamon metropolitan area; 80.5% are white, 8% are black, and the remainder are Asian, American Indian, or from other races. A total of 98.8% of the population considers themselves Hispanic (*World Almanac*, 2006). According to 2004 estimates, the birthrate is 14.1 per 1000, the average annual rate of growth is 0.49%, the infant mortality rate is 8.2 per 1000, and the life expectancy at birth is 78.4 years (74.46 years for males and 82.54 years for females) (Central Intelligence Agency, 2006; *Time Almanac with Information Please*, 2007; CultureGrams, 2002; Welcome to Puerto Rico: People, 2006).

Puerto Rico is a major hub of Caribbean commerce and tourism, boasting a diversity of attractions in an unvarying climate that ranges year round from 75° to 85°F (Porter & Prince, 2000). San Juan provides one of the world's busiest cruise ship ports and is among the most dynamic cities in the West Indies (Porter & Prince, 2000). Romantic resorts, private villas, and remote offshore islands offer attractive honeymoon destinations. The chief crops of Puerto Rico include coffee, plantains, pineapples, tomatoes, sugarcane, bananas, mangos, and ornamental plants. Chief industries are pharmaceuticals, manufacturing of electronics and apparel, and tourism. Some 19% of the labor force is employed by the government. In spite of marked success in Puerto Rico's developmental efforts, the per capita income (1999 estimate) of $9800 is low by U.S. standards, and the unemployment rate (2002) of 12% means some persons live off public assistance (Central Intelligence Agency, 2006).

MIGRATION TO THE UNITED STATES

The open borders allows migration of Puerto Ricans to the United States. As American citizens, they are neither immigrants nor aliens (Spector, 2004). Initial settlements of Puerto Ricans were in New York. In the 1950s, an average of 40,000 Puerto Ricans were migrating yearly, so that by 1970 more than 1.4 million Puerto Ricans lived in regions across the United States. When the economy in the United States declined in the 1970s, thousands returned to Puerto Rico. When the Puerto Rican economy declined, social programs from the U.S. government were provided.

In mainland United States, Puerto Ricans make up the second largest Hispanic subgroup in the United States and represent 9.7% of the country's Hispanic population (U.S. Department of Commerce, Bureau of the Census, 2004). Today, 3,406,178 Puerto Ricans reside in mainland United States, predominantly in the Northeast, with large numbers in New York and metropolitan New Jersey (*Time Almanac with Information Please*, 2007). As citizens, Puerto Ricans do not require a work visa to live or work in the United States, significantly simplifying travel back and forth. However, while travel can be done without difficulty, problems with the English language, lack of financial resources, and health problems can present significant acculturation problems that require assistance from culturally competent professionals (Cohen, 1972). Among the Puerto Rican population in the United States, 25.8% live in poverty, compared to 12.4% of the total population (U.S. Department of Commerce, Bureau of the Census, 2004). As an ethnic group and minority, Puerto Ricans in the mainland United States may encounter prejudice not experienced on an island where racial diversity is the norm.

COMMUNICATION

For many years Spanish and English were both designated as the official languages of Puerto Rico. Even though few Puerto Ricans spoke English, English was the official language of instruction and children were forced to learn it in school (Juarbe, 2005). In 1991, in response to pleas from the people, the Puerto Rican legislature passed a bill that made Spanish the island's official language. However, in 1993 the governor restored equal status to Spanish and English (Welcome to Puerto Rico: Description, 2006). Today, Spanish tends to be used at home and in schools, the mass media, and business, while English is used for all federal matters, is spoken in all major tourist areas, and is taught as the second language in most schools. Puerto Ricans from large cities are most likely to read, understand, and speak at least some English (Juarbe, 2005).

It is important for the nurse to appreciate that the Spanish spoken by Puerto Ricans may differ significantly from the Spanish spoken by individuals from other Hispanic cultures. An example of this is found in the use of *Escala de Inteligencia para Ninos*, which is a translation of the Wechsler Intelligence Scale for Children (WISC) developed in Puerto Rico but used widely for testing with many Spanish-speaking children. When Christine Miracle (1981) tried to use this test with Aymara children in Bolivia who were bilingual in Spanish and Aymara, a number of overt and covert problems were identified. The language presented overt problems, and differences in cultural heritage between the two groups taking the test presented covert problems. When a word was taken from American English to Puerto Rican Spanish to Bolivian Spanish and from White middle-class children in the United States to Puerto Rico to the poor rural American Indian children in Bolivia, both the word and the meaning changed.

Puerto Ricans are sensitive people and are quick to express feelings of love and affection, *carinosos*. They are known for their hospitality and desire warm and smooth interpersonal relationships, *simpaticos* (Juarbe, 2005). Gratitude and respect are often expressed to others, including health care providers, by gifts of homemade food. Since showing respect properly is highly valued in the culture, rejection of a gift can be interpreted as an insult.

Puerto Ricans are fond of fiestas (celebrations) and celebrate not only U.S. federal holidays but also many holidays unique to Puerto Rico, including Three Kings Day (January 6), the Discovery of Puerto Rico Day (November 19), and Constitution Day (July 25). Tourists can easily find festivals and carnivals to add to their holiday itinerary when visiting Puerto Rico (Porter & Prince, 2000). Many Puerto Ricans living in the United States continue to celebrate Puerto Rican holidays.

Tone of voice is important in communication for Puerto Ricans; their tone is typically melodic and peaceable (Juarbe, 2005). A Puerto Rican may misinterpret the nurse's use of high pitch and voice inflection as confrontation when this is not intended.

Puerto Ricans are generally accustomed to shaking hands when greeting people. Close friends may grasp shoulders and kiss each other on the cheek. While women may kiss women or men in this way, men do not greet other men with a kiss. However, a man may embrace a good friend or relative, *compadres*, after a long absence with a hug. It is common for females to touch each other with their hands during communication. In greeting, more traditional Puerto Ricans may avoid eye contact as a symbol of respect. Avoidance of eye contact may also be practiced when greeting the elderly as s symbol of respect.

For most Puerto Ricans, self-respect is communicated by pride in personal appearance, particularly by what is worn in public. In Puerto Rico, parties and social gatherings are occasions where formal dress is expected, with shirts and ties for men and dresses or skirts and blouses for women. Sloppy, overly casual, or revealing dress is not considered appropriate. The traditional clothing once associated with Puerto Rico is no longer worn, but *Espiritistas* or faith healers may wear white outfits, hats, and handkerchiefs on selected days.

When addressing others in formal situations, Puerto Ricans may use titles to show respect. A Puerto Rican may use a title recognizing the person's profession alone or in combination with a surname. It is most respectful to address an older person by combining the title with the person's first name.

Implications for Nursing Care

Lack of ability to speak English has been related to lack of adequate treatment for Puerto Ricans in the United States. While Spanish literature for teaching may be available, the literacy level of the patient may not permit the literature to be understood. When a Spanish-speaking translator is available, the dialect of the translator may be so different that the Puerto Rican patient does not clearly understand what is being explained. Rogler (1999) noted that translators can make many errors in translating a language they are familiar with. When a translator lacks the cultural and linguistic background to recognize words in a language that may change meaning from one culture to the next, the translation can lack accuracy (Bonder, Martin, & Miracle, 2002).

When interpreters are used, it is important to consider the topic to be discussed and the gender of the interpreter. If the topic carries a stigma such as AIDS, tuberculosis, or sexual behavior, a patient may be more likely to express concerns to an interpreter than to a family member and to express concerns to the interpreter that they do not want disclosed to the health care provider. Thus, it is necessary to convey to the patient that no information should be communicated to the interpreter that the patient does not want the health care provider to know. For some topics related to sexual matters, same-sex family members will be more effective translators than an interpreter of the opposite sex.

Ruiz (1983) noted that when dealing with Puerto Rican patients who have come from an agrarian society, even if the care provider or interpreter speaks Spanish, the patient may have difficulty with good control of the Spanish language. Additionally, in contrast with other Hispanic persons, it is essential to understand the nonverbal communication and symbolism that Puerto Ricans convey with hand gestures and facial expressions, which are critical to understanding the patient's communication.

It is important for the nurse to appreciate that a Puerto Rican patient may be very hesitant to use a bedside commode or bedpan and may refrain from having a bowel movement during hospitalization because of embarrassment. The nurse may be able to provide adequate privacy that enables a patient on bed rest to use a bedpan by being aware of the stress this causes the patient. Even when a Puerto Rican is sick, self-care for personal needs or care by a family member of the same sex may be preferred over having care provided by medical care providers. The nurse should be flexible and adapt care to be culturally appropriate.

The nurse must appreciate the value that Puerto Ricans place on saving face. For example, a patient who has limited grasp of the English language may be hesitant to ask a nurse to slow down or repeat what is said. The importance of respect in verbal and nonverbal communications should be recognized and accepted with cultural understanding, for example, accepting a patient's gift of homemade food to show appreciation and respect. Because Puerto Ricans are particularly sensitive to feeling slighted, the nurse should be attentive to actions that may be interpreted as rejection (CultureGrams, 2002).

SPACE

Puerto Ricans are accustomed to standing close together when talking. A Puerto Rican may feel insulted if the other individual in a social or professional interaction moves away even slightly during the conversation (CultureGrams, 2002). On the other hand, personal space can be a significant issue for some Puerto Rican women, who are conscious of maintaining a reasonable distance with persons of the opposite sex. Younger Puerto Ricans may relate distance to being stereotyped as nonassertive.

Implications for Nursing Care

Since special needs and interpretations vary, it is important to assess each individual in relation to special needs. Spatial needs will vary with sex, age, and position.

SOCIAL ORGANIZATION

The family, including both nuclear and extended members, is highly valued in the Puerto Rican culture. In fact, in most Puerto Rican families all activities, decisions, and social and cultural standards occur in the context of the family (Juarbe, 2005).

In Puerto Rico, the total fertility rate is 1.9 (2001 estimate), and 70% of Puerto Rican women report use of contraception to control family size. The average family size in Puerto Rico is 3.5 people. The marriage rate is 9.2 per 1000 persons, with a divorce rate of 4.47 per 1000 (Welcome to Puerto Rico: People, 2006). Older Puerto Ricans are often rejecting of nonheterosexual preferences, and subsequently gay and lesbian choices may not be revealed to older family members (Juarbe, 2005).

Puerto Ricans tend to rely on older adults and elder family when making decisions. In some families, the oldest son or daughter is the one with final decision-making authority over health matters (Juarbe, 2005). When a health-related decision is to be made, a wife will typically consult her husband. Even in an emergency situation, the nurse should be sure to ask a Puerto Rican woman if her husband needs to be consulted regarding consent for treatment of a Puerto Rican male when another family member should be included in the decision-making process. In some situations, an older woman in the family will have authority and a respected role in decision making. For younger families it will usually be the man who takes responsibility for decisions. Since generational differences may exist and also differences related to generation of migration to the United States, the nurse must be sensitive and assess each patient for decision-making responsibility within the family. Sick individuals are expected to assume a passive role in terms of care responsibilities and allow themselves to be taken care of by a family member. Family members generally prefer to provide support for individuals needing care in the home themselves rather than involving home care or homemaking services; for example, an elder daughter or son may assume care responsibilities for an elderly parent and a wife for the husband rather than involving an outside caregiver.

It is important to avoid stereotyping individuals who are Hispanic since many differences exist between Hispanic cultures. For example, Sokol-Katz and Ulbrich (1992) investigated family structure in relation to alcohol and drug use among Mexican, Puerto Rican, and Cuban American adolescents. Whereas Mexican American adolescents in female-headed households had higher rates of drinking, drug use, and overall risk-taking behavior, Puerto Rican adolescents in female-headed households had higher rates of overall risk-taking behaviors, and Cuban American adolescents' behavior did not show any relationship to family structure. Thus, relationships and influences within the family structure vary among different Hispanic groups.

Children are highly valued members of the Puerto Rican culture and represent a significant portion of the population: 22.4% of the population of Puerto Rico is 0 to 14 years of age, while 65.4% is 15 to 64 years of age, and 12.2% is 65 years and over (Welcome to Puerto Rico: People, 2006). Mothers assume the greater role in physical care of children, and a father's role is for financial needs. The socioeconomic environment of some Puerto Rican families places children at higher risk for health problems. Wasserman, Brunnelli, Rauh, and

Alvarado (1994) report that high rates of poverty, poor housing, violence, and high rates of mental illness in adults place children in Puerto Rican families at higher risk for both health problems and acquired disability, for example, head trauma, lead poisoning, and spinal injury. Research has provided data that suggest values of Puerto Rican parents may hamper optimal functioning of children with disabilities. Gannotti, Handwerker, Groce, and Cruz (2001) investigated sociocultural influences on disability status in Puerto Rican children. These investigators conclude that Puerto Rican values of interdependence, *anonar* (pampering or nurturing behaviors), and *sobre* protective (overprotectiveness) influence parental expectations for the capacity of children with disabilities and need to be taken into account when evaluating scores on the Pediatric Evaluation of Disability Inventory (PEDI) and in establishing plans of care.

When a family member is sick, it is expected that close and distant family members, as well as neighbors and friends, will visit to provide support. The nurse should attempt to accommodate the need of some Puerto Rican families to have someone with a hospitalized patient on an ongoing basis.

Attitude toward victims of child sexual abuse varies between cultures and has been found to be more positive in Puerto Rican families. Rodriguez-Strednicki and Twaite (1999) found that Puerto Rican adults evaluated victims more positively than did Cuban American adults and thus are less likely to stigmatize the child.

Pregnancy is a time for indulgence for many Puerto Rican women. Men are supportive and tolerant of pregnant women. While most Puerto Rican women follow a diet, exercise is viewed as inappropriate. Therefore, it is helpful for the nurse to encourage exercise and good nutrition in order to avoid excessive weight gain. During labor, fathers generally assume a passive supportive role, and many prefer not to be in attendance at the delivery. Vaginal delivery is preferred since there is some stigma that a cesarean section suggests a "weak woman" (Juarbe, 2005). Many women from rural areas prefer breastfeeding. Women who work may combine breastfeeding with formula. A tradition for the first meal after delivery for some Puerto Ricans is homemade fresh chicken soup. Some Puerto Rican women's birth recuperation includes avoiding housework and hair washing for 40 days. Male babies are traditionally circumcised at birth.

Researchers conducted a study to investigate the cultural differences in the relationship between maternal sensitivity, emotional expression, and control strategies during the first year of life, comparing middle-class island Puerto Rican and mainland Anglo mother–infant pairs. All mothers were interviewed in their homes by ethnically matched interviewers in their native language. According to the researchers, the Puerto Rican mothers used physical control in a meaningful and predictable manner in their interactions with their infants. The Puerto Rican mothers persistently and actively structured interactions with their infants in a manner consistent with their long-term socialization goal, teaching infants to be attentive, calm, and well-behaved, compared to teaching infants to be assertive and self-confident. The researchers concluded that their findings supported the need to explore the role of culture in early relationship formation and to define culturally specific definitions of sensitive caregiving (Carlson & Harwood, 2003).

In a small city in the northeastern United States, research was conducted to explore the experience of fatherhood among young Puerto Rican fathers whose sexual partners were teenagers when their first child was born. The setting was selected because of the persistently high adolescent birth rates in this urban environment. Of the 40% Hispanic population in the city, 90% are Puerto Rican. The 30 fathers participating in the study were Puerto Rican, ranging in age from 14 to 24 when their first child was born, and had an income below the federal poverty guidelines. Two findings were unanticipated by the researchers: (1) ten (33%) of the fathers interviewed reported that they had planned pregnancy with their partner for at least a year; and (2) children challenged the fathers to act more responsibly in the world on behalf of their children. The fathers acknowledged concern about how their children perceived them and that children made them aware of their mortality. The unexpected findings, although not generalizable, emphasize the importance for nurses to recognize that reproductive health behaviors occur beyond stereotypical assumptions. The positive and affirming component of identity helps to explain the persistence of adolescent pregnancy, in spite of health promotion messages to avoid it (Foster, 2004).

Since 85% of Puerto Ricans are members of the Roman Catholic church, beliefs related to Roman Catholicism are a significant influencing factor for many Puerto Ricans. For example, when a new store opens in San Juan, the owner often invites a priest to bless the business. When individuals plan a meeting, one may say, "*Si Dois quierre*," "If God wills" (Kent, 1992). The other 15% are Protestants (8%), nonreligious (2.3%), and others (3%) (Welcome to Puerto Rico: People, 2006). There is a separation of church and state; however, because of the high numbers of Catholics, Catholic traditions and customs prevail among the people. Puerto Ricans consider themselves a religious people and often attribute good fortune to the deity. However, while most Puerto Ricans and Puerto Rican Americans are Christians, many also practice *espiritismo*, or spiritualism, a blend of Indian, African, and Catholic beliefs. The belief that good and evil spirits are present and can be encouraged or warded off with the proper herbs and rituals is often still present among Puerto Ricans who live in the United States. Even if Puerto Ricans in the United States do not actively practice spiritualism, many respect the beliefs (Kent, 1992).

The literacy rate in Puerto Rico is 94.1% (2002) (Welcome to Puerto Rico: People, 2006). Puerto Ricans value education, and families encourage children to not only finish high school but also attend college. This importance is underscored by the fact that a teacher's salary in Puerto Rico in 1997 was $1500 a month, far above the mean income (McGovern, 2002). Puerto Rico has 50 institutions of higher education and rates sixth in the world for college education rates. Some 56% of college-age persons are attending institutions of higher learning (Welcome to Puerto Rico: People, 2006).

Implications for Nursing Care

The nurse should be aware that Puerto Ricans have a strong need for family support and that decision making usually occurs in a family context. The nurse should also be aware that Puerto Ricans in the United States are also likely to be strongly loyal to their country and to feel a strong sense of nationalism. Rather than calling themselves "*Americanos*," many Puerto Ricans prefer to call themselves "*Puertorriquenos*" or "*Boricuas*." When referring to "my country," the reference is usually to Puerto Rico rather than the United States. Some Puerto Rican descendants born in America refer to themselves as Puerto Ricans, saying, "I am Puerto Rican, but I wasn't born there." When the nurse is able to speak knowledgeably about Puerto Rican culture or has visited the country, even if only to get off a cruise ship at San Juan for a few hours to visit Fort San Cristobal or the El Yunque rain forest, this familiarity will facilitate a bond with the patient (Zbar, 2001). Puerto Ricans in the United States are generally eager to talk about their country and their plans for returning to visit when this is possible (Welcome to Puerto Rico: People, 2006). Thousands of Internet sites are available to keep Puerto Ricans in the United States in touch with what is happening in Puerto Rico and to provide opportunities to share thoughts and feelings. *The Puerto Rico Herald* is available in both English and Spanish online.

It is important for the nurse to consider that appropriateness of maternal responses and reproductive health behaviors is based in part on cultural factors. Assessment of mother–child interactions must be understood in terms of cultural beliefs about parenting and child development (Carlson & Harwood, 2003). The power of gender relations in adolescent health behavior must be considered an integral part of the solution to unintended pregnancy among teenagers. Male partners must be included in a comprehensive approach to contraceptive counseling and preparation for parenting (Foster, 2004). Health behaviors, as well as personal development, occur in a context of cultural values.

TIME

The Puerto Rican concept of time is generally relaxed and more social than clock oriented. In other words, the social interaction occurring at the moment is considered more important than scheduled appointments. If a friend, relative, or business associate drops by unexpectedly, a Puerto Rican will often stop what is being done in order to visit, regardless of other commitments.

Implications for Nursing Care

The social orientation to time sometimes serves as a barrier to punctuality with health care appointments at a predetermined time. It is important to emphasize to the patient that the office schedule is often not flexible and arriving late may mean that the appointment will have to be rescheduled.

ENVIRONMENTAL CONTROL

Puerto Ricans tend to have a serene rather than fatalistic view of life. Most Puerto Ricans feel that destiny, a Deity, spirits, or spiritual forces control events that occur, health, and death (Juarbe, 2005). Illness may be attributed to heredity, sin, lack of personal attention to health, an evil spirit, or a disharmony of environmental forces within the individual. A person under the control of an evil sprit or forces will seek a spiritualist to perform an intervention. A disharmony of environmental forces can be treated by foods, medicines, and herbs, which will restore a positive internal environment.

Some Puerto Ricans believe in *Santeria*, a belief that originated among the Yoruba people in Nigeria and was brought to Puerto Rico with the importation of the Yoruba slaves. In order to be compliant with the demand to practice the Catholic religion, the Yoruba identified their gods (*Orishas*) with names of Catholic saints (Gonzalez-Wippler, 1987). Certain saints were attributed with curative powers for various health conditions. The *Santeria* belief system is practiced by *santeros*, who are sought out by many Puerto Ricans for treatment of symptoms that are described by Western medicine as symptoms of mental illness. Mumford

(1973) reported that of Puerto Rican patients seen in an outpatient mental health clinic in New York, 73% had already sought out a *santero*. Ruiz (1983) reported that in the early 1970s, 85% of the Puerto Ricans seen with mental problems went to both Catholic church on Sunday and spiritualistic centers during the week. In fact, Puerto Ricans who seek Western medical treatment for mental illness may fear being rejected by their community for this action. Puerto Ricans have traditionally placed great faith in the power of the *santero* to listen and to perform an appropriate treatment that makes the person feel "special" and thus restores damaged self-esteem. *Santeria* can be practiced in any location, for example, the individual's home, a storefront, or a college dormitory (Spector, 2004). A *santero* may wear a white robe and beaded bracelet as a sign of identity and when ceremonies are performed.

Wearing amulets is a traditional healing practice that some Puerto Ricans still practice. A small black fist (*azabache*) or small black rabbit foot may be tied on a child to protect him or her from evil. Removal of the object may be thought to produce illness, misfortune, or even death, so it should not automatically be done by the nurse in the process of giving care. It is important to ask for permission before removing such objects and to be aware that in time of crisis amulets may provide hope and reassurance (Juarbe, 2005). For some families, a priest's benediction may be requested before removal of an amulet. The nurse should also ask permission before removing rosary beads from a patient's neck. The family or patient may agree to allow the rosary beads to be moved to the patient's hand if they interfere with care. The family or patient may also desire to have other items of religious significance near the patient, including candles, pictures or statues of saints, or holy water. The family may want to use aromatic oils and lotions to rub the body as a way to ward off evil spirits.

Whereas many Hispanics believe in hot and cold diseases, Puerto Ricans have further classified remedies (food and medications) as hot (*caliente*), cold (*frio*), and cool (*fresco*). Treatment of a hot disease is with a cold or cool remedy, while treatment of a cold disease is with a hot remedy (Spector, 2004). An example of a hot illness is constipation. An example of a cool medicine that can be used to treat this problem is milk of magnesia. Another hot illness is diarrhea, which may be treated with the corresponding cold treatment, bicarbonate of soda (Schilling & Brannon, 1986). Ear disorders or aches, which are considered cold illnesses, can be treated with olive oil, which is a hot treatment (Juarbe, 2005). Since penicillin is classified as a hot remedy, it should not be used to treat constipation or diarrhea, which are symptoms of a hot bodily condition (Harwood, 1971). If a baby is being given infant formula containing evaporated milk, which is classified as hot, use of whole milk should be avoided because it is classified as cool. In other words, hot and cold food and medications should not be combined (Harwood, 1971).

In a review of the literature on barriers to health care access for Latino children, the authors identify that children account for more that 39% of the major subpopulations of Latinos (Mexican American, Puerto Rican, and Cuban American) in the United States. Because children are a large, rapidly expanding population that are disproportionately likely to be poor, to be uninsured, and to have parents with limited educational attainment, they are at greater risk for poor health and underutilization of health services. The authors report that folk medicine practices may lead to delay or complication of conventional health care. The potential for folk practices to act as barriers to health care is described by an example reported from an inner-city Puerto Rican community in Connecticut: 64% of the children had experienced *empacho* (a gastrointestinal illness); 77% of the parents reported that they took their child to a *santiguadora* (a folk healer in the Puerto Rican community) for treatment, 58% used home remedies, and 37% visited a physician. While visiting a physician was the initial choice for only 9% of the parents, 85% sought another form of treatment afterward, primarily *santiguadora* (Flores & Vega, 1998).

Spector (2004) lists folk diseases described by Puerto Ricans, including (1) *susto*, a sudden fright causing shock; (2) fatigue, with asthma-like symptoms; (3) *empacho*, which is pain and stomach cramps caused by lack of food digestion; (4) *mal ojo*, a sudden, unexplained illness; and (5) *atoque*, falling to the ground with wild movements of arms and legs and screaming. Folk illnesses may be treated with folk medicine, by a relative or friend, or in some cases by Western-style medicine and health care providers.

Rituals Related to Death and Dying

Puerto Rican families can be expected to maintain cultural death rituals. Enabling Puerto Rican families to grieve and honor the dead in a culturally appropriate manner is essential to the delivery of culturally competent care (Munet-Vilaro, 1998). In some Hispanic families, there is a code of silence in which the dying individual is not informed of the impending death (Rivera-Andino & Lopez, 2000). If a family member is dying, the family may want to keep constant vigil in a waiting area. The spiritual leader is expected to be with the patient when death occurs. When death has occurred, the person who serves as a family spokesperson should be the one to receive this information. The family may want to kiss and touch the body to say goodbye. After a death, a private area should be available for discussion with and by the family and to allow for expressions of emotion, including crying, feeling faith, being nauseated, or vomiting (Juarbe, 2005). Puerto Ricans usually support organ donation since this is a way to help others. Nevertheless, the nurse should be sensitive to which family members in the family structure should provide authorization. Autopsies are generally viewed as a violation of the body. If an autopsy is necessary, it is essential that the requirement is explained and that the family spokesperson has given consent (Juarbe, 2005).

Since a large proportion of Puerto Ricans are Catholic, death rituals are described as heavily influenced by Catholic beliefs, wherein spirituality is important and there is a continuing relationship between the living and the deceased through prayer and visits to the gravesite (Lobar, Youngblut, & Brooten, 2006)

Implications for Nursing Care

The importance of family must be recognized by the nurse. Strong family ties and high levels of instrumental and affective support are characteristic in Hispanic subgroups (Talamantes, Gomez, & Braun, 2000). The potential for parental belief systems to act as an access barrier is an important consideration. It is important when responding to the concerns of a Puerto Rican patient and his or her family to explore what types of treatment interventions have already been attempted. Through respect and acceptance, alternative practices to treatment can be discussed and integrated into conventional management of childhood illness (Flores & Vega, 1998). In many cases, because of beliefs about the causes of illness, it is essential to combine both home remedies and other beliefs with use of Western medicine to obtain an optimal outcome.

When providing health teaching about health promotion activities, it is important to explain how the relationship works between health prevention activities and future health. When Puerto Rican patients believe they have control over future events, taking action will be more likely. The nurse should be aware that being underweight and thin tends to be associated with ill health, while being overweight is associated with health. It is important to realize that teaching about the need for regular exercise may contradict the value placed on being overweight, an indication of economic advantage.

On matters of end-of-life decision making, the nurse must be aware that collectivist rather that individualist decision making is supported by the values of *familismo* and *espiritismo*. When end-of-life care planning is considered, levels of acculturation, literacy, linguistic isolation, and values must be taken into account to promote open communication, mutual understanding, and cultural accommodation (Talamantes, Gomez, & Braun, 2000).

BIOLOGICAL VARIATIONS

Body Size and Structure

People in different racial groups vary according to body size and structure. Some examples of research involving Puerto Ricans will be noted. Cephalometric radiography is an important aspect of treatment for orthodontic deviations. Evanko, Freeman, and Cisneros (1997) noted that when norms for White European Americans and Black Americans of African descent were compared with those for Puerto Ricans, there were significant differences between ethnic groups in the dentoalveolar region. Similarities were noted in the upper face height and the anterior cranial base length. The purpose of this study was to facilitate the treatment of Puerto Ricans by means of the development of a standard mesh diagram.

Bermudez, Becker, and Tucker (1999) report the development of sex-specific equations for estimating stature of elderly Puerto Rican and other Hispanic persons by using knee height equations. Previously published equations significantly overestimated stature of Hispanic subjects. Estimated stature of frail elderly is influenced by socioeconomic status as well as ethnicity. Mott, Wang, Thornton, et al. (1999) investigated the relationship of age and body fat in four ethnic groups to test the hypothesis that body fat is lower in the elderly than in middle-aged persons. While Asians, Blacks, and Whites showed a highly significant curvilinear relationship between age and body fat, Puerto Rican men did not. Lauderdale, Jacobsen, Furner, et al. (1998) concluded that elderly Puerto Ricans are at less risk for hip fracture than Whites, Blacks, and other Hispanic populations studied.

Genetic Deviations

Santiago-Borrero and Valcarcel (1994) report that Puerto Rican infants are at higher risk for congenital malformation, particularly neural tube defects, and for genetic diseases such as hypothyroidism and abnormal hemoglobins than other Hispanic babies because of low birth weight.

Susceptibility to Disease

Major causes of death per 100,000 population in Puerto Rico (1993) included the following:
- 142.6 heart and cardiovascular disease
- 95.4 cancers
- 55.1 diabetes

- 38.0 cerebrovascular disease
- 29.2 pneumonia and influenza (Welcome to Puerto Rico: People, 2006)

Asthma. The 1982–1984 Hispanic Health and Nutrition Examination Survey (HHANES) reported high rates of asthma among Puerto Rican children in the Northeast when compared with Mexican and Cuban children (Carter-Pokras & Gergen, 1993). Crain, Weiss, Bijur, et al. (1994) reported high rates of asthma among Puerto Rican children in an inner city study. Ledogar, Penchaszadeh, Garden, and Acosta (2000) reported that in a study of Puerto Ricans and other Latinos in a New York metropolitan area, Puerto Ricans were more likely than other Latinos to have asthma. These researchers supported the suggestion of other researchers that gene–environment interactions may well play a part in asthma prevalence among Puerto Ricans (Colb, Pappas, Moran, & Lieberman, 1993). Other researchers have observed that the reasons for the significantly higher prevalence of active asthma for the Puerto Rican children may be key to improved understanding of asthma pathophysiology, prevention, treatment, and correlated social and environmental factors (Flores et al., 2002).

Asthma prevalence among U.S. adults was analyzed by specific variables, including age, gender, race, and ethnicity. Lifetime asthma was found to be significantly higher among Puerto Ricans (17%) than among any other racial/ethnic group. In an analysis where race/ethnicity were considered together with geographic region, Puerto Ricans in all regions of the U.S. had high rates of asthma. These researchers also concluded that further study of gene–environment interactions among Puerto Ricans is needed to explore the susceptibility to asthma-triggering responses (Rose, Mannino, & Lederer, 2006).

Visual Impairments. In a study by Lee, Gomez-Marin, Lam, Ma, & Vilar (2000), Puerto Rican children and adolescents in New York City were found to have a significantly higher prevalence of usual-corrected visual acuity impairment than Cuban Americans, Mexican Americans, and non-Hispanic Whites in samples drawn from Miami and five southwestern states. The findings suggest that compared with their counterparts, the Puerto

Rican children and adolescents may not be receiving similar corrective refractive care, may have more severe ocular diseases, or both. Awareness of visual impairment is important since it has been related to poor school performance, learning disabilities, and juvenile delinquency (Evans, 1968; Flax, 1970; Snow, 1983). In another study related to visual acuity, Lee, Gomez-Marin, and Lam (2000) investigated the relationship between lifetime history of depression and visual acuity in Hispanic adults. The data indicated that while there was a higher relationship between impaired acuity and Mexican Americans and Cuban Americans and incidence of depression, no significant relationship was found in Puerto Ricans.

Obesity. Childhood obesity has been described as a major health problem in the United States, affecting nearly 25% of American children. In a longitudinal health survey, it was found that among Hispanic adolescents aged 12 to 18 years, obesity patterns were greater among Puerto Ricans than among other Hispanic subpopulations. Childhood obesity has important health consequences for children, is a major precursor of adult obesity, and is an important risk factor for hypertension. Additionally, an acculturation and assimilation effect was identified by the researchers, indicating the significant effect that second- and third-generation Hispanics are more likely to be obese. The researchers remarked that during adolescence, constraints linked to the family may be overridden by peer and other effects in situations where shifts in diet and physical activity that promote obesity are influenced by acculturation and assimilation (Popkin & Udry, 1998).

Obesity is a risk factor for diabetes, cardiovascular disease, and some cancers. Obesity rates for Puerto Rican woman are high, at 28% to 39%. Dietary factors, including high intake of animal fat, may be associated with the increased risk (Glanz, Croyle, Chollette, & Pinn, 2003).

Diabetes. Type 2 diabetes mellitus, previously known as non–insulin-dependent diabetes, is a major health problem among Latinos. In a study involving Puerto Ricans in the United States and Mexican Americans with type 2 diabetes, Lipton, Losey, Giachello, et al. (1996) found while most patients spoke only or mostly Spanish, 14% had received instruction in English alone. Most have a basic understanding of the disease, and more than half reported positive health behaviors in the past year, but 54% of the Puerto Rican Americans and 26% of the Mexican Americans had been admitted to the hospital or had used the emergency room for diabetes-related conditions. Tucker, Bermudez, and Castaneda (2000) investigated prevalence of type 2 diabetes among Hispanic elders of Caribbean origin. The investigators found that prevalence was higher among Puerto Rican elders and noted that ethnicity was more strongly associated with diabetes status and control than were socioeconomic or measured health behavior variables.

The attitude of health professionals also affects treatment. For example, Lipton, Losey, Giachello, Mendez, and Girotti (1998) investigated attitudes and issues in treating Puerto Ricans in the United States with type 2 diabetes. The practitioners agreed that communication with patients was hindered by low reading levels, lack of proficiency in English, and an excessive respect for physicians. These emotional barriers to adequate treatment were often more important than financial concerns even among low-income patients. In this study, fear of insulin therapy was also a factor that contributed to use of folk remedies to treat diabetes. An additional cultural complication was that since many Puerto Rican individuals considered family needs to be more important than individual needs, adhering to a treatment regimen can be viewed as self-indulgence and thus not compatible with family values. This research illustrates the necessity of considering a variety of factors that may influence the delivery of culturally competent care, including communication, family values, and environmental control.

Overall, Latino subgroups (e.g., Puerto Ricans, Cubans, and Mexicans) have been described in recent studies as exhibiting differences in sociodemographic characteristics, health status, and use of health services that are often greater that differences between ethnic groups. The health disparities experienced by many Latino subgroups result from complex interrelated factors. In addition to being one of the most rapidly growing populations, the Latino population in the mainland is one of the youngest, with 36% under the age of 18 years. Barriers to health promotion and disease prevention can be reduced by addressing inadequate access to care related to a disproportionate poverty rate and level of uninsurance, as well as a shortage of Spanish-speaking health care workers. It is imperative to understand the issues related to access to health promotion and disease prevention for this vulnerable population in order to improve the quality of health care delivered and to help eliminate the racial and ethnic disparities (Betancourt, Carrillo, Green, & Maina, 2004).

Cancer. The burden of cancer is not distributed equally; many racial and ethnic minorities suffer disproportionately from cancer. Cancer-related health disparities are related to risk factors and early detection strategies. The most common cancers among Puerto Rican women from 1992 to 1998 were cancers of the breast and lung and non-Hodgkin's lymphoma. According to the National Cancer Institute, recent data suggest that rates of mammography have increased since the 1980s among Puerto Rican women—just under half of Puerto Rican women report having had a mammogram within 3 years—but Hispanic women in general are substantially less likely than their non-Hispanic counterparts to have had a recent Pap test. Higher smoking rates were found among Puerto Rican women (30.3%) on the mainland, more than most Hispanics and other ethnic groups, but studies suggest that women in Puerto Rico smoke less than on the mainland (National Cancer Institute, 2006; Glanz, Croyle, Chollette, & Pinn, 2003).

Implications for Nursing Care

It is important for the nurse to be aware that health and quality of life for Puerto Ricans are affected by a multifaceted combination of biological variations and demographic and socioeconomic factors. In a study conducted between 1996 and 2000 in Puerto Rico, lower income was positively correlated with self-reported decreased quality of life and increased mental and physical illness. Persons with higher income have fewer unhealthy days regardless of sex, while persons of low income have more unhealthy days. Older women, persons with less education, persons unable to work, and those who were overweight or who had diabetes or high blood pressure reported more days when they were physically or mentally unhealthy (Centers for Disease Control and Prevention, 2002). Nurses must respect the traditional beliefs and cultural contexts of illness and health-seeking behaviors. They must also understand the skepticism and distrust based on experience with discrimination and exclusion that minority groups may experience. Multidisciplinary and collaborative approaches with ethnic minority communities are important to develop relevant health improvement initiatives.

SUMMARY

The Puerto Rican population totals more than 7 million, with approximately 55% living in Puerto Rico and the remaining 45% living in the mainland United States. With an open border between Puerto Rico and the United States, Puerto Ricans are increasingly traveling back and forth. The nurse should be prepared for differences, which may challenge the nurse in the delivery of culturally competent care.

Case Study

Maria, a 24-year-old Puerto Rican, came to America with her husband 2 years ago. They both communicate in English and are employed at the local community college. Maria's mother recently has come to live with them so that she can "pamper" Maria and help when the baby is born.

Maria is 5 feet tall and weighs 110 pounds at her first visit to the clinic. The nurse determines that Maria is in the second trimester at about 20 weeks gestation. Maria states that she has not been eating very much lately because she is afraid she will get "too fat" like her older sisters did when they had babies. Her mother has told her about the cool and cold foods that she should eat during pregnancy and the hot foods that she should eat after the baby is born. Her mother has warned her not to mix hot and cold remedies. Maria wants to do what her mother tells her out of respect and feels guilty when she eats the wrong things.

Maria voices concern about her husband wanting to be with other women now that she is getting a bigger "belly." She states that she has seen other Puerto Rican men do this. She also wants her husband to be with her during labor and delivery.

CARE PLAN

Nursing Diagnosis: Altered nutrition, less than body requirements related to concern about weight gain and following traditional dietary requirement of culture of origin

Client Outcomes

1. Client will gain approximately 1 pound per week for the remainder of her pregnancy.
2. Client will maintain a hemoglobin level about 10.5 g/dL throughout her pregnancy.

Nursing Interventions

1. Take a diet history. Ask Maria to recall what she had to eat at meals and as snacks in the past 24 hours. Determine if this is a usual pattern. Give Maria a food intake record to list what she eats in the next 2 days. Have Maria complete a food frequency questionnaire and bring it to her next prenatal visit.
2. Use a U.S. Department of Agriculture (USDA) food pyramid to explain the recommended foods and serving sizes during the last weeks of her pregnancy and after the baby is born. Emphasize that it is possible to follow the traditions of her Puerto Rican heritage and still keep her figure after delivery. Encourage her to ask her mother to put in the names of foods to eat during pregnancy. Give her another food pyramid for

(Continued)

CARE PLAN — CONT'D

her mother to put in the foods to eat after the baby is born. Point out the serving sizes as well as the number of servings from each food group.

3. Explain the importance of keeping her appointments, having the lab work done, and eating foods rich in nutrients. These things are all important for the health of her developing baby, as well as for Maria's health during and following delivery.

4. Point out specific foods that she prefers to eat that are especially healthy for her and her baby. For example, corn tortillas and cheese are good sources of calcium, meat (beef, pork, chicken, fish) is rich in protein, and vegetables and fruits (chili peppers, tomatoes, beets, cabbage, chayotes, bell peppers, string beans, avocado, bananas, coconut, lima beans, white beans, barley water, raisins, watercress, onions, peas, kidney beans) are excellent sources of vitamins and minerals.

✳ *Nursing Diagnosis: Risk for altered health maintenance related to nonassertive communication patterns of family members, as evidenced by Maria's comments about her husband's sexual behavior in the last part of her pregnancy and her guilt when not eating what her mother says she should eat.*

Client Outcomes

1. During the first clinic visit, client will verbalize her plan for regular prenatal visits and explain the benefits of visiting the clinic regularly.

2. The client and family members will express concerns with the nurse and with each other.

Nursing Interventions

1. Encourage Maria and her husband to talk about their concerns about Maria's pregnancy by using broad opening statements, such as "Many couples have concerns about continuing sexual intercourse during pregnancy...."

2. Explain what will be done at the following prenatal visits and how these activities are important to the health of the baby and Maria.

3. Offer explanations for all aspects of the prenatal visit. Explain the size and development of the growing baby.

4. Explain how sexual activities between husband and wife can change during the pregnancy so that it is comfortable. Reassure them that it will not harm the baby.

5. Explain the dangers of unprotected sex with multiple partners for all members of the family. Sexually transmitted diseases can cause long-term illness and even death. The human immunodeficiency virus (HIV) is life-threatening for the father. It can be transmitted to Maria via sexual intercourse and then to the developing fetus through the placenta. Other diseases may be mild in adults but catastrophic for the developing fetus and the newborn, such as cytomegalovirus, rubella, herpes, and hepatitis B. Specific medications are used to treat sexually transmitted diseases, such as syphilis, gonorrhea, chlamydial infection, and trichomoniasis. If untreated, these diseases are also life-threatening for the developing baby.

6. Encourage Maria and her husband to write down their concerns, call the office any time, and talk about their feelings to each other.

7. Before leaving the room, ask Maria and her husband to state what their plan is in regard to future clinic visits.

8. Explain how they can be involved with childbirth classes and a tour of the hospital prior to delivery.

✸STUDY QUESTIONS

1. Describe the culturally based explanations of why some pregnant Puerto Rican women may be extremely concerned about their weight gain during pregnancy.
2. Explain possible correlations between cold and hot foods and diet during pregnancy discussed by Puerto Rican women.
3. List questions that may facilitate discussion between a Puerto Rican husband and wife and the nurse related to beliefs about sexual activities during pregnancy.
4. Relate the effect of beliefs related to environmental control and preventive health care for some Puerto Rican clients.
5. Explain the individuals, by family role assignments, who may be involved in decision making concerning child and infant care among some Puerto Rican families.
6. Describe the values and beliefs about pregnancy and children commonly held by Puerto Ricans.
7. Describe how stereotyping Puerto Ricans as similar to other Hispanic Americans can lead the nurse to errors in patient care.
8. Describe how a health care provider's approach to the patient by the health care provider can be individually and uniquely focused while still utilizing knowledge about common behaviors and beliefs held by some Puerto Ricans.

NCLEX-RN REVIEW QUESTIONS

1. A pregnant Puerto Rican client comes to the clinic. Because of the cultural implications, the nurse needs to consider which of the following for this client:
   A. Service lifestyle
   B. Including the extended family
   C. Diet and exercise
   D. Prayers and rituals

2. A Puerto Rican client is being scheduled for a follow-up visit to the clinic. For this client it is important for the nurse to:
   A. Emphasize to the client to be prompt as the office schedule often is inflexible.
   B. Emphasize the importance of coming for the appointment that day.
   C. Inform the client of the appointment in writing.
   D. Emphasize the importance of bringing the father to the next visit.

3. When using an interpreter for a Puerto Rican client, it is important for the nurse to:
   A. Convey to the client that no information should be communicated to the interpreter that the client does not want the nurse to know.
   B. Use a same-sex family member as the interpreter.
   C. Use a translator who is familiar with the language.
   D. Provide the interpreter with available Spanish literature for teaching.

References

Bermudez, O., Becker, E., & Tucker, K. (1999). Development of sex-specific equations for estimating stature of frail elderly Hispanics living in the northeastern United States. *American Journal of Clinical Nutrition*, 69(5), 992–998.

Betancourt, J. R., Carrillo, J. E., Green, A. R., & Maina, A. (2004). Barriers to health promotion and disease prevention in the Latino population. *Clinical Cornerstone*, 6(3), 16–29.

Bonder, B., Martin, L., & Miracle, A. (2002). *Culture in clinical care.* Thorofare, N.J.: Slack.

Carlson, V. J., & Harwood, R. L. (2003). Attachment, culture, and the caregiving system: the cultural patterning of everyday experiences among Anglo and Puerto

Rican mother-infant pairs. *Infant Mental Health Journal*, 24(1), 53–73.

Carter-Pokras, O., & Gergen, P. (1993). Reported asthma among Puerto Rican, Mexican-American, and Cuban children, 1982 through 1984. *American Journal of Public Health*, 83, 580–582.

Centers for Disease Control and Prevention. (2002, March 1). Health related quality of life—Puerto Rico, 1996–2000. *Morbidity and Mortality Weekly Report*, 51(8), 166.

Central Intelligence Agency. The World Factbook (2006). Retrieved May 9, 2006, from http://www.cia.gov/cia/publications/factbook/geos/rq.html.

Cohen, R. (1972, June). Principles of preventive mental health programs for ethnic minority populations: the acculturation of Puerto Ricans to the United States. *American Journal of Psychiatry*, 128(12), 79.

Colb, C., Pappas, J., Moran, E., & Lieberman, J. (1993). Variants of alpha 1-antitrypsin in Puerto Rican children with asthma. *Chest*, 103, 812–815.

Crain, E., Weiss, K., & Bijur, P., et al. (1994). An estimate of the prevalence of asthma and wheezing among inner-city children. *Pediatrics*, 94, 356–362.

CultureGrams. (2002). *Culture grams standard edition*, vol. 1. Salt Lake City, Utah: Brigham Young University.

Evanko, A., Freeman, K., & Cisneros, G. (1997). Mesh diagram analysis: developing a norm for Puerto Rican Americans. *Angle Orthodontist*, 67(5), 381–388.

Evans, J. (1968). Relationships between visual skills and behavioral disorders. *Journal of the American Optometry Association*, 39, 623–640.

Flax, N. (1970). The contribution of visual problems to learning disability. *Journal of the American Optometry Association*, 41, 841–845.

Flores, G., Fuentes-Afflick, E., Barbot, O., Cartrer-Pokras, O., Lara, M, et al. (2002). The health of Latino children: urgent priorities, unanswered questions, and a research agenda. *Journal of the American Medical Association*, 288(1), 82–90.

Flores, G., & Vega, L. R. (1998). Barriers to health care access for Latino children: a review. *Family Medicine*, 30(3), 196–205.

Foster, J. (2004). Fatherhood and the meaning of children: an ethnographic study among Puerto Rican partners of adolescent mothers. *Journal of Midwifery & Women's Health*, 49(2), 118–125.

Gannotti, M., Handwerker, W., Groce, N., & Cruz, C. (2001). Sociocultural influences on disability status in Puerto Rican children. *Physical Therapy*, 81, 1512–1523.

Gonzalez-Wippler, M. (1992). *Santeria-African magic in Latin America* (revised ed. 2). New York: Original Publications.

Glanz, K., Croyle, R. T., Chollette, V. Y., & Pinn, V. W. (2003). Cancer-related health disparities in women. *American Journal of Public Health*, 93(2), 292–298.

Harwood, A. (1971). The hot-cold theory of disease: implications for treatment of Puerto Rican patients. *Journal of the American Medical Association*, 216, 1154–1155.

Juarbe, T. (2005). Puerto Ricans. In Lipson, J., Dibble, S., & Minarik, P. (Eds.), *Culture and nursing care*. San Francisco: UCSF Nursing Press.

Kent, D. (1992). America the beautiful: *Puerto Rico*. Chicago: Children's Press.

Lauderdale, D., Jacobsen, S., Furner, S., et al. (1998). Hip fracture incidence among elderly Hispanics. *American Journal of Public Health*, 88(8), 1245–1247.

Ledogar, R., Penchaszadeh, C., Garden, C., & Acosta, L. (2000). Asthma and Latino cultures: different prevalence reported among groups sharing the same environment. *American Journal of Public Health*, 90(6), 929–935.

Lee, D., Gomez-Marin, Q., & Lam, B. (2000, February). Current depression, lifetime history of depression, and visual acuity in Hispanic adults. *Journal of Visual Impairment and Blindness*, 94(2), 85–96.

Lee, D., Gomez-Marin, Q., Lam, B., Ma, F., & Vilar, N. (2000, October). Prevalence of usual-corrected distance visual acuity impairment in Hispanic and non-Hispanic children and adolescents. *Pediatric and Perinatal Epidemiology*, 14(4), 357.

Lipton, R., Losey, L., Giachello, A., et al. (1996, October). Factors affecting diabetes treatment and patient education among Latinos: results of a preliminary study in Chicago. *Journal of Medical Systems*, 20(5), 267–276.

Lipton, R., Losey, L., Giachello, A., Mendez, J., & Girotti, M. (1998, January–February). Attitudes and issues in treating Latino patients with type 2 diabetes: views of healthcare providers. *Diabetes Educator*, 24(1), 67–71.

Lobar, S. L., Youngblut, J. M., & Brooten, D. (2006). Cross-cultural beliefs, ceremonies, and rituals surrounding death of a loved one. *Pediatric Nursing*, 32 (1), 44–49.

Miracle, C. (1981). Intelligence testing and the Aymara. In Hardman, M. J. (Ed.), *The Aymara language in its social and cultural context* (pp. 240–247). Gainesville: University Presses of Florida.

Mott, J., Wang, J., & Thornton, J., et al. (1999). Relation between body fat and age in 4 ethnic groups. *American Journal of Clinical Nutrition*, 69(5), 1007–1013.

Mumford, E. (1973, November–December). Puerto Rican perspectives on mental illness. *Mount Sinai Journal of Medicine*, 6(40), 771–773.

Munet-Vilaro, F. (1998, November–December). Grieving and death rituals of Latinos. *Oncology Nursing Forum*, 25(10), 1761–1763.

National Cancer Institute. (2006). *Cancer control and population sciences: Cancer in Puerto Rican woman.* Retrieved May 25, 2006, from http://dccps.nci.nih. gov/womenofcolor/puerto.html.

Popkin, B. M., & Udry, J. R. (1998). Adolescent obesity increases significantly in second and third generation U.S. immigrants: The national longitudinal study of adolescent health. *Journal of Nutrition*, 128, 701–706.

Porter, D., & Prince, D. (2000). *Frommer's Puerto Rico.* Chicago: IDG Books World Wide.

Rivera-Andino, J., & Lopez, L. (2000, July). When culture complicates care. *RN*, 63(7), 47–48.

Rodriguez-Strednicki, O., & Twaite, J. (1999). Attitudes toward victims of child sexual abuse among adults from four ethnic/cultural groups. *Journal of Child Sexual Abuse*, 8(3), 1–24.

Rogler, L. (1999). Methodological sources of cultural insensitivity in mental health research. *American Psychologist*, 54, 424–433.

Rose, D., Mannino, D. M., & Lederer, B. P. (2006). Asthma prevalence among US adults, 1998–2000: Role of Puerto Rican ethnicity and behavioral and geographic factors. *American Journal of Public Health*, 96(5), 1–9.

Ruiz, P. (1983). Cultural factors in diagnosis and treatment: transcript of the panel discussion. *ACP Psychiatric Update*, 3(2), 2–6.

Santiago-Borrero, P., & Valcarcel, M. (1994). Maternal and child health and health care in Puerto Rico. In Lamberty, G., & Coll Garcia, D. (Eds.), *Puerto Rican women and children: issues in health, growth, and development* (pp. 39–54). New York: Plenum Press.

Schilling, B., & Brannon, E. (1986). Health related dietary practices. In *Cross-cultural counseling: a guide for nutrition and health counselors.* Alexandria, Va.: U.S. Department of Agriculture and U.S. Department of Health and Human Services, Nutrition and Technical Services Division.

Snow, R. (1983). The relationship between visual and juvenile delinquency. *Journal of the American Optometry Association*, 54, 509–511.

Sokol-Katz, J., & Ulbrich, P. (1992, October). Family structure and adolescent risk-taking behavior: a comparison of Mexican, Cuban, and Puerto Rican Americans. *International Journal of the Addictions*, 27(10), 1197–1209.

Spector, R. (2004). *Cultural diversity in health and illness* (ed. 6). Upper Saddle River, N.J.: Pearson Prentice Hall Health.

Talamantes, M. A., Gomez, C., & Braun, K. L. (2000). Advance directives and end-of-life care: the Hispanic perspective. In Braun, K. L., Pietsch, J. H., & Blanchette, P. L. (Eds.) *Cultural issues in end-of-life decision making* (pp. 83–100). Thousand Oaks, Calif.: Sage.

Time almanac with information please. (2007). Boston: Information Please, Inc.

Tucker, K., Bermudez, O., & Castaneda, C. (2000, August). Type 2 diabetes is prevalent and poorly controlled among Hispanic elders of Caribbean origin. *American Journal of Public Health*, 90(7), 1288–1293.

U.S. Department of Commerce, Bureau of the Census. (2003). Hispanic population in the United States: March 2002. Retrieved May 9, 2006, from http://www. census.gov/prod/2003pubs/p20-545.pdf.

U.S. Department of Commerce, Bureau of the Census. (2004). We the People: Hispanics in the United States. December 2004. Retrieved May 9, 2006, from http:// www.census.gov/prod/2004pubs/censr-18.pdf.

U.S. Department of Commerce, Bureau of the Census (2006). Population estimates: 2000–2005 Puerto Rico municipios. Retrieved May 9, 2006, from http:// www.census.gov/popest/municipios/PRM-EST2005. html.

Wasserman, G., Brunnelli, S., Rauh, V., & Alvarado, L. (1994). The cultural context of adolescent childrearing in three groups of urban minority mothers. In Lamberty, G., & Coll Garcia, C. (Eds.), *Puerto Rican women and children: issues in health, growth, and development* (pp. 137–160). New York: Plenum Press.

Welcome to Puerto Rico. Description. (2006). Retrieved January 6, 2006, from http://welcome.topuertorico. org/descrip.shtml.

Welcome to Puerto Rico. Government. (2006). Retrieved January 6, 2006, from http://welcome.topuertorico. org/government.shtml.

Welcome to Puerto Rico. History. (2006). Retrieved January 6, 2006, from http://welcome.topuertorico.org/history. shtml.

Welcome to Puerto Rico. People. (2006). Retrieved January 6, 2006, from http://welcome.topuertorico.org/people. shtml.

Welcome to Puerto Rico. Puerto Rican Culture. (2006). Retrieved January 6, 2006, from http://welcome.topuertorico.org/culture.

World almanac. (2006). New York: World Almanac Books.

Zbar, J. (2001). *Explorer of the seas.* Miami, Fla.: Royal Caribbean International.

Appendix A: Answer Key

Chapter 2

1. Answer: A
Cognitive Level: Comprehension
NCLEX Category: Psychosocial Integrity
Nursing Process: Assessment

2. Answer: D
Cognitive Level: Application
NCLEX Category: Health Promotion
   and Maintenance
Nursing Process: Assessment

3. Answer: B
Cognitive Level: Knowledge
NCLEX Category: Psychosocial Integrity
Nursing Process: Implementation

Chapter 3

1. Answer: B
Cognitive Level: Application
NCLEX Category: Safe, Effective Care Environment
Nursing Process: Implementation

2. Answer: A
Cognitive Level: Application
NCLEX Category: Psychosocial Integrity
Nursing Process: Assessment

3. Answer: A
Cognitive Level: Knowledge
NCLEX Category: Psychosocial Integrity
Nursing Process: Analysis

Chapter 4

1. Answer: C
Cognitive Level: Knowledge

NCLEX Category: Psychosocial Integrity
Nursing Process: Planning

2. Answer: C
Cognitive Level: Knowledge
NCLEX Category: Physiological Integrity
Nursing Process: Analysis

3. Answer: D
Cognitive Level: Application
NCLEX Category: Health Promotion and Maintenance
Nursing Process: Planning

Chapter 5

1. Answer: C
Cognitive Level: Knowledge
NCLEX Category: Health Promotion
   and Maintenance
Nursing Process: Implementation

2. Answer: A
Cognitive Level: Knowledge
NCLEX Category: Health Promotion
   and Maintenance
Nursing Process: Planning

3. Answer: A
Cognitive Level: Knowledge
NCLEX Category: Health Promotion
   and Maintenance
Nursing Process: Implementation

Chapter 6

1. Answer: B
Cognitive Level: Application
NCLEX Category: Health Promotion
   and Maintenance
Nursing Process: Analysis

2. Answer: A
Cognitive Level: Application
NCLEX Category: Health Promotion
   and Maintenance
Nursing Process: Planning

3. Answer: A
Cognitive Level: Knowledge
NCLEX Category: Psychosocial Integrity
Nursing Process: Planning

Chapter 7

1. Answer: D
Cognitive Level: Knowledge
NCLEX Category: Health Promotion
   and Maintenance
Nursing Process: Assessment

2. Answer: A
Cognitive Level: Application
NCLEX Category: Health Promotion
   and Maintenance
Nursing Process: Assessment

3. Answer: A, C, & D
Cognitive Level: Knowledge
NCLEX Category: Health Promotion
   and Maintenance
Nursing Process: Assessment

Chapter 8

1. Answer: A
Cognitive Level: Knowledge
NCLEX Category: Health Promotion
   and Maintenance
Nursing Process: Analysis

2. Answer: D
Cognitive Level: Application
NCLEX Category: Health Promotion
   and Maintenance
Nursing Process: Implementation

3. Answer: A
Cognitive Level: Application
NCLEX Category: Physiological Integrity
Nursing Process: Assessment

Chapter 9

1. Answer: C
Cognitive Level: Knowledge
NCLEX Category: Health Promotion
   and Maintenance
Nursing Process: Implementation

2. Answer: B
Cognitive Level: Knowledge
NCLEX Category: Health Promotion
   and Maintenance
Nursing Process: Implementation

3. Answer: B
Cognitive Level: Knowledge
NCLEX Category: Psychosocial Integrity
Nursing Process: Planning

Chapter 10

1. Answer: C
Cognitive Level: Knowledge
NCLEX Category: Health Promotion
   and Maintenance
Nursing Process: Assessment

2. Answer: D
Cognitive Level: Knowledge
NCLEX Category: Health Promotion
   and Maintenance
Nursing Process: Analysis

3. Answer: B
Cognitive Level: Knowledge
NCLEX Category: Psychosocial Integrity
Nursing Process: Planning

Chapter 11

1. Answer: C
Cognitive Level: Knowledge
NCLEX Category: Physiological Integrity
Nursing Process: Analysis

2. Answer: B
Cognitive Level: Application
NCLEX Category: Health Promotion
   and Maintenance
Nursing Process: Implementation

3. Answer: D
Cognitive Level: Knowledge
NCLEX Category: Health Promotion
and Maintenance
Nursing Process: Assessment

Chapter 12

1. Answer: A
Cognitive Level: Application
NCLEX Category: Health Promotion
and Maintenance
Nursing Process: Implementation

2. Answer: B
Cognitive Level: Application
NCLEX Category: Health Promotion
and Maintenance
Nursing Process: Assessment

3. Answer: D
Cognitive Level: Knowledge
NCLEX Category: Psychosocial Integrity
Nursing Process: Analysis

Chapter 13

1. Answer: B
Cognitive Level: Knowledge
NCLEX Category: Physiological Integrity
Nursing Process: Planning

2. Answer: A
Cognitive Level: Knowledge
NCLEX Category: Psychosocial Integrity
Nursing Process: Assessment

3. Answer: D
Cognitive Level: Knowledge
NCLEX Category: Psychosocial Integrity
Nursing Process: Assessment

Chapter 14

1. Answer: A
Cognitive Level: Knowledge
NCLEX Category: Health Promotion
and Maintenance
Nursing Process: Assessment

2. Answer: A
Cognitive Level: Knowledge
NCLEX Category: Psychosocial Integrity
Nursing Process: Assessment

3. Answer: A
Cognitive Level: Knowledge
NCLEX Category: Psychosocial Integrity
Nursing Process: Assessment

Chapter 15

1. Answer: A
Cognitive Level: Knowledge
NCLEX Category: Psychosocial Integrity
Nursing Process: Implementation

2. Answer: B
Cognitive Level: Knowledge
NCLEX Category: Psychosocial Integrity
Nursing Process: Implementation

3. Answer: D
Cognitive Level: Application
NCLEX Category: Psychosocial Integrity
Nursing Process: Implementation

Chapter 16

1. Answer: A
Cognitive Level: Knowledge
NCLEX Category: Psychosocial Integrity
Nursing Process: Analysis

2. Answer: C
Cognitive Level: Knowledge
NCLEX Category: Physiological Integrity
Nursing Process: Assessment

3. Answer: B
Cognitive Level: Knowledge
NCLEX Category: Psychosocial Integrity
Nursing Process: Assessment

Chapter 17

1. Answer: A
Cognitive Level: Knowledge
NCLEX Category: Physiological Integrity
Nursing Process: Analysis

2. Answer: C
Cognitive Level: Knowledge
NCLEX Category: Psychosocial Integrity
Nursing Process: Assessment

3. Answer: C
Cognitive Level: Knowledge
NCLEX Category: Psychosocial Integrity
Nursing Process: Assessment

Chapter 18

1. Answer: A
Cognitive Level: Knowledge
NCLEX Category: Physiological Integrity
Nursing Process: Planning

2. Answer: B
Cognitive Level: Knowledge
NCLEX Category: Psychosocial Integrity
Nursing Process: Planning

3. Answer: D
Cognitive Level: Knowledge
NCLEX Category: Psychosocial Integrity
Nursing Process: Evaluation

Chapter 19

1. Answer: B
Cognitive Level: Application
NCLEX Category: Psychosocial Integrity
Nursing Process: Implementation

2. Answer: B
Cognitive Level: Knowledge
NCLEX Category: Psychosocial Integrity
Nursing Process: Assessment

3. Answer: A
Cognitive Level: Knowledge
NCLEX Category: Psychosocial Integrity
Nursing Process: Implementation

Chapter 20

1. Answer: D
Cognitive Level: Application
NCLEX Category: Psychosocial Integrity
Nursing Process: Planning

2. Answer: B
Cognitive Level: Application
NCLEX Category: Psychosocial Integrity
Nursing Process: Implementation

3. Answer: D
Cognitive Level: Knowledge
NCLEX Category: Psychosocial Integrity
Nursing Process: Assessment

Chapter 21

1. Answer: D
Cognitive Level: Application
NCLEX Category: Psychosocial Integrity
Nursing Process: Implementation

2. Answer: C
Cognitive Level: Application
NCLEX Category: Psychosocial Integrity
Nursing Process: Implementation

3. Answer: A
Cognitive Level: Application
NCLEX Category: Psychosocial Integrity
Nursing Process: Implementation

Chapter 22

1. Answer: A
Cognitive Level: Application
NCLEX Category: Psychosocial Integrity
Nursing Process: Implementation

2. Answer: D
Cognitive Level: Application
NCLEX Category: Physiological Integrity
Nursing Process: Planning

3. Answer: C
Cognitive Level: Knowledge
NCLEX Category: Psychosocial Integrity
Nursing Process: Assessment

Chapter 23

1. Answer: D
Cognitive Level: Application
NCLEX Category: Health Promotion and Maintenance
Nursing Process: Assessment

2. Answer: C
Cognitive Level: Application
NCLEX Category: Psychosocial Integrity
Nursing Process: Analysis

3. Answer: B
Cognitive Level: Knowledge
NCLEX Category: Physiological Integrity
Nursing Process: Implementation

Chapter 24

1. Answer: B
Cognitive Level: Knowledge
NCLEX Category: Psychosocial Integrity
Nursing Process: Assessment

2. Answer: A
Cognitive Level: Knowledge
NCLEX Category: Health Promotion and Maintenance
Nursing Process: Analysis

3. Answer: A
Cognitive Level: Application
NCLEX Category: Psychosocial Integrity
Nursing Process: Assessment

Chapter 25

1. Answer: A
Cognitive Level: Knowledge
NCLEX Category: Psychosocial Integrity
Nursing Process: Assessment

2. Answer: A
Cognitive Level: Application
NCLEX Category: Psychosocial Integrity
Nursing Process: Implementation

3. Answer: B
Cognitive Level: Knowledge
NCLEX Category: Health Promotion and Maintenance
Nursing Process: Assessment

Chapter 26

1. Answer: A
Cognitive Level: Knowledge
NCLEX Category: Physiological Integrity
Nursing Process: Analysis

2. Answer: A
Cognitive Level: Knowledge
NCLEX Category: Physiological Integrity
Nursing Process: Analysis

3. Answer: C
Cognitive Level: Knowledge
NCLEX Category: Psychosocial Integrity
Nursing Process: Assessment

Chapter 27

1. Answer: A
Cognitive Level: Knowledge
NCLEX Category: Psychosocial Integrity
Nursing Process: Planning

2. Answer: D
Cognitive Level: Knowledge
NCLEX Category: Psychosocial Integrity
Nursing Process: Planning

3. Answer: D
Cognitive Level: Knowledge
NCLEX Category: Psychosocial Integrity
Nursing Process: Assessment

Chapter 28

1. Answer: C
Cognitive Level: Knowledge
NCLEX Category: Psychosocial Integrity
Nursing Process: Assessment

2. Answer: A
Cognitive Level: Analysis
NCLEX Category: Psychosocial Integrity
Nursing Process: Assessment

3. Answer: C
Cognitive Level: Knowledge
NCLEX Category: Psychosocial Integrity
Nursing Process: Assessment

Chapter 29

1. Answer: C
Cognitive Level: Knowledge
NCLEX Category: Psychosocial Integrity
Nursing Process: Assessment

2. Answer: C
Cognitive Level: Comprehension
NCLEX Category: Health Promotion and Maintenance
Nursing Process: Assessment

3. Answer: B
Cognitive Level: Knowledge
NCLEX Category: Psychosocial Integrity
Nursing Process: Assessment

Chapter 30

1. Answer: B
Cognitive Level: Knowledge

NCLEX Category: Psychosocial Integrity
Nursing Process: Assessment

2. Answer: B, C, & D
Cognitive Level: Comprehension
NCLEX Category: Psychosocial Integrity
Nursing Process: Assessment

3. Answer: A
Cognitive Level: Knowledge
NCLEX Category: Psychosocial Integrity
Nursing Process: Assessment

Index

Note: Page numbers followed by "f" denote figure; "t" tables; "b" boxes.

A
Acetaldehyde dehydrogenase
   (ALDH), 156, 156–157
Acquired immune deficiency syndrome
   (AIDS), 167, 342, 485, 580
   African Americans, 221, 222t
   Filipino Americans, 485
   Haitian Americans, 580
   Irish Americans, 813
   Jews, 604
   Korean Americans, 635
   Mexican-Americans, 262
   Navajos, 292
   Nigerian Americans, 708b
   spatial behavior and, 56
   Ugandan Americans, 730
   Vietnamese Americans, 520
ADH. *See* Alcohol dehydrogenase
Afghanistan, 395
Afghans
   biological variations, 406
      nursing care implications, 406
   communication, 397
      nursing care implications, 399
   environmental control, 402
      death beliefs, 405
      death customs, 405
      health care access, 403
      illness/wellness behaviors, 403
      mental health issues, 404
      nursing care implications, 406
   social organization, 400
      acculturation, 400
      family roles, 400
      family system, 400
      immigration, 400
      nursing care implications, 401
      religion, 401
   space, 399
      nursing care implications, 399
   time, 402
      nursing care implications, 402
   in United States, 396

African Americans
   biological variations of, 209
      birth weight, 209
      body fat, 210
      body proportion, 210
      growth/development, 210
      skin color, 210
   communication and, 193
      Block English pronunciation, 194
      dialect, 193
      nursing care implications, 195
      origin of, 193
   disease susceptibility, 214
      AIDS (HIV) risk, 221, 222t
      cardiovascular disease, 214
         diabetes, 219
         hypertension, 216
         obesity/sedentary lifestyle, 219
         serum cholesterol levels, 217
         smoking, 218
         stroke, 220
         sudden cardiac death, 221
   environmental control, 201
      death/dying rituals, 207
      folk medicine, 203
      health care beliefs, 202
      health care benefits, 201
      nursing care implications, 207
      witchcraft, 204
   enzymatic variations, 214
   genetic differences in, 212
      apolipoprotein E, 213
      methylenetetrahydrofolate
         reductase, 212
      tumor necrosis factor alpha, 212
   health assessment of, 15t
   nutritional preferences of, 169, 170t
   overview of, 191
      education and, 191–192
      health problems of, 192–193
      infant mortality rate of, 193
      life expectancy, 193
      population, 191

African Americans (*Continued*)
   slavery and, 192
   psychological characteristics, 223
      chemical abuse, 224
      nursing care implications, 226
      posttraumatic stress disorder, 225
   social organizations, 197
      discrimination and, 197
      family characteristics, 199
      family role changing, 198
      nursing care implications, 200
      slavery and, 197
   space, 196
      nursing care implications, 197
   time and, 200
      nursing care implications, 201
AIDS. *See* Acquired immune deficiency
   syndrome
Air Force Health Study, 522
Alaska. *See also* American Eskimos
   overview of, 324
   land, 324
Alaska Native Claims Settlement Act
   (ANCSA), 327–328, 329
Alcohol, 156–157
   Filipino Americans and, 486
   French Canadians and, 658
   Irish Americans and, 813
   Irish Americans and 7, 813
   Japanese Americans and, 383
   Jews and, 611
   Navajos and, metabolism, 293
   Russian Americans and, 433
   Vietnamese Americans and, 525
Alcohol dehydrogenase (ADH),
   156–157
ALDH. *See* Acetaldehyde
   dehydrogenase
Alleles, 153
ALLHAT. *See* Antihypertensive and Lipid
   Lowering Treatment to Prevent Heart
   Attack Trial
Alzheimer's disease, 707, 791

Pages 689–821 (Chapters 25–30) can be found online at http://evolve.elsevier.com/Giger.

American Eskimos
  biological variations, 338
    blood variations, 345
    body size, 338
    body structure, 338
    disease susceptibility, 340
      anemia, 343
      arthritis, 345
      asthma, 345
      cancer, 344
      cardiovascular disease, 343
      communicable disease, 340
      diabetes mellitus, 342
      glaucoma, 342
      hepatitis B virus, 345
      STDs, 342
      tuberculosis, 341
    enzymatic variations, 340
    lifestyle preferences, 345
    Mongoloid heritage, 339–340
    nursing care implications, 347
    nutritional preferences, 345
    psychological characteristics, 345
    skin color, 339
  communication, 329
    kinesics, 331
    language, 329
    nursing care implications, 331
    silence, 330
    touch, 331
  culture of, 326
  environmental control, 337
    illness/wellness behaviors, 337
    nursing care implications, 338
  health assessment of, 15t
  heritage of, 326
  overview of, 325
  social organization, 333
    family, 333
      individual freedom, 334
      social status, 334
    nursing care implications, 335
    political structure, 335
  space, 332
    nursing care implications, 333
  time, 336
    nursing care implications, 337
American Indians 97. See also Navajos
  health assessment of, 15t
  nutritional preferences of, 172, 173t
Amish Americans
  biological variations, 790
    genetic variations, 792

Amish Americans (Continued)
    illness susceptibility, 790
      Alzheimer's disease, 791
      cancer, 791
      communicable diseases, 791
      diabetes, 791
      high blood pressure, 790
      obesity, 790
    nursing care implications, 792
  communication, 779
    nursing care implications, 780
  environmental control, 789
    death/dying rituals, 789
    nursing care implications, 790
  social organizations, 782
    Amish haystack dinners, 787b
    Amish youth, 785
    family roles, 782
    family systems, 782
    nursing care implications, 785
    religious principles, 783
    state and, 785
  space, 781
    nursing care implications, 781
  time, 788
    nursing care implications, 788
Amish, overview of, 777
Amok, 69
Amor propio, 473–474
Amyotrophic lateral sclerosis, 484
Anemia, 343
  pernicious, 261
  sickle cell, 165, 580, 730
Antihypertensive and Lipid Lowering
    Treatment to Prevent Heart Attack
    Trial (ALLHAT), 162
Antihypertensives, 157
Appalachia, overview of, 301
  core cultural patterns, 303
  economy, 302
  education, 303
  history, 302
  public services, 303
Appalachians
  biological variations, 314
    health disparities, 314
      cancer, 315
      coronary artery/heart disease, 314
      respiratory tract diseases, 314
      traumatic injuries, 314
    infant mortality, 315
    nutrition, 315
  communication, 304, 305t

Appalachians (Continued)
    nursing care implications, 305
  environmental control, 309
    care barriers, 310
    death rituals, 309
    death/dying, 309
    folk health system, 311
      beliefs, 311
      biomedical disease knowledge, 311
      lay practitioners, 312
      medicinal plants, 311
    health threats, 309
    illness/wellness behaviors, 312
      health screening, 313
      illness behaviors, 313
      nursing care implications, 314
      risk behaviors, 312
    locus of control, 310
  health assessment of, 15t
  social organization, 306
    family, 306
      nursing care implications, 307
    religion, 307
  space, 305
    nursing care implications, 306
  time, 308
    nursing care implications, 308
Arthritis, 292, 345
Ascariasis, 731
Asthma, 345, 681
Auditory perception, 48
Autosomes, 154–155

B
Baklava, 175
Bandhi, Mahatma, 546
Batista, Fulgencio, 758
Battering, 180
Behavioral Risk Reduction Strategies for
    Chronic Indicators and High Risk
    Factors for Premenopausal African-
    American Women (25-45) with
    Coronary Heart Disease, 16
Bergson, Henri, 110
Biocultural ecology, 145–146
Biological variations
  of Afghans, 406
    nursing care implications, 406
  of African Americans, 209
    birth weight, 209
    body fat, 210
    body proportion, 210
    growth/development, 210

Pages 689–821 (Chapters 25-30) can be found online at http://evolve.elsevier.com/Giger.

Biological variations (*Continued*)
skin color, 210
of American Eskimos, 338
blood variations, 345
body size, 338
body structure, 338
disease susceptibility, 340
anemia, 343
arthritis, 345
asthma, 345
cancer, 344
cardiovascular disease, 343
communicable disease, 340
diabetes mellitus, 342
glaucoma, 342
hepatitis B virus, 345
STDs, 342
tuberculosis, 341
enzymatic variations, 340
lifestyle preferences, 345
Mongoloid heritage, 339–340
nursing care implications, 347
nutritional preferences, 345
psychological characteristics, 345
skin color, 339
of Amish Americans, 790
genetic variations, 792
illness susceptibility, 790
Alzheimer's disease, 791
cancer, 791
communicable diseases, 791
diabetes, 791
high blood pressure, 790
obesity, 790
nursing care implications, 792
of Appalachians, 314
health disparities, 314
cancer, 315
coronary artery/heart disease, 314
respiratory tract diseases, 314
traumatic injuries, 314
infant mortality, 315
nutrition, 315
of Chinese Americans, 455
body size, 455
body structure, 455
death, leading causes of, 458
disease susceptibility, 456
cancer, 456
infectious diseases, 456
enzymatic variations, 456
genetic variations, 456
mortality, 458

Biological variations (*Continued*)
nursing care implications, 459
psychological characteristics, 458
skin color, 455
of Cuban Americans, 768
disease susceptibility, 769
diabetes, 769
low birth weight, 769
mental illness, 769
substance abuse, 769
vision impairment, 769
nursing care implications, 770
nutritional deficiencies, 769
nutritional preferences, 769
dimensions of, 147
body structure, 147
body weight, 149
disease susceptibility, 158
electrocardiographic patterns, 158
enzymatic variations, 152
genetic variations, 152
keloids, 152
metabolism of drugs, 156
Mongolian spots, 152
skin color, 151
of East Indian Hindu Americans, 555
disease susceptibility, 555
enzymatic variation, 555
genetic variation, 555
nursing care implications, 557
nutritional deficiencies, 556
nutritional preferences, 556
psychological characteristics, 556
racial strain and, 555
of Filipino Americans, 481
body size, 481
body structure, 481
cleft lip/palate, 482
disease susceptibility, 482
AIDS, 485
amyotrophic lateral sclerosis, 484
cancer, 484
cardiovascular disease, 482
diabetes mellitus, 484
gallbladder disease, 484
glaucoma, 485
hepatitis B, 485
hypertension, 483
palatal mucosal changes, 484
enzymatic variation, 482
genetic variation, 482
Mongoloid, 482
nursing care implications, 486

Biological variations (*Continued*)
nutritional preferences, 485
psychological characteristics, 486
alcohol use, 486
skin color, 482
of French Canadians, 656
disease susceptibility, 657
intravenously transmitted
diseases, 657
STDs, 657
genetic factors, 656
life expectancy, 656
nursing care implications, 659
psychological characteristics/
coping, 658
alcohol, 658
drug abuse, 658
mental health, 658
tobacco, 658
of Haitian Americans, 578
body size, 578
body structure, 578
childbearing dietary
habits, 582, 583*b*
disease susceptibility, 579
AIDS, 580
cancer, 580
high birth rate, 579
hypertension, 580
intestinal problems, 579
malaria, 580
malnutrition, 579
sickle cell anemia, 580
tuberculosis, 579
venereal disease, 579
ear wax, 578
nursing care implications, 583
nutritional deficiencies, 582
nutritional preferences, 582*b*
psychological characteristics, 582,
584*b*
skin color, 578
of Irish Americans, 811
genetic variations, 811
abdominal aortic aneurysm, 812
cystic fibrosis, 812
neural tube defects, 812
sarcoidosis, 812
Tay-Sachs disease, 812
teeth, 812
HIV risk, 813
nursing care implications, 815
psychological characteristics, 813

Pages 689–821 (Chapters 25–30) can be found online at http://evolve.elsevier.com/Giger.

Biological variations (*Continued*)
  adolescents, drinking behavior
    and, 814
    alcoholism, 813
    bipolar disorders, 814
    schizophrenia, 814
  of Japanese Americans, 376
    body size, 376
    disease susceptibility, 377
    drug interactions, 377
    enzymatic variations, 377
    eye shape, 376
    genetic variations, 377
    Mongolian spots, 376
    mouth/teeth, 376
    nutritional deficiencies, 380
    nutritional preferences, 380
    psychological change, 380
      alcohol use, 383
      folk traditions, 382
      internment trauma, 382
      mental health, 381
      nursing care implications, 383
      psychopharmacology, 383
      self cultural values, 380
      somatization, 382
      stress manifestations, 381
    skin color, 376
  of Jews, 606
    disease susceptibility, 607
      cancer, 607
      communicable disease, 611
      Crohn's disease, 609
      diabetes mellitus, 609
      heart disease, 608
      myopia, 609
      polycythemia vera, 609
      ulcerative colitis, 609
    enzymatic variations, 606
    genetic variations, 606
    nutritional deficiencies, 609
    nutritional preferences, 609
    psychological characteristics, 610, 611
      alcoholism, 611
      Holocaust survivors, 611
      mental health, 610, 612
      nursing care implications, 612
  of Jordanian Americans, 750
    genetic variations, 750
    nursing care implications, 751
    nutritional deficiencies, 750
    nutritional preferences, 750
  of Korean Americans, 632

Biological variations (*Continued*)
    body size, 632
    body structure, 632
    diet, 633
    disease susceptibility, 634
      body weight, 634
      cardiovascular disease, 634
      HIV/AIDS, 635
      smoking, 634
    enzymatic variations, 633
    genetic variations, 633
    metabolism of drugs, 634
    skin color, 632
  of Mexican-Americans, 260
    disease susceptibility, 260
      childhood obesity, 261
      communicable diseases, 261
      diabetes, 260
      hepatitis C, 261
      HIV/AIDS, 262
      hypertension, 261
      pernicious anemia, 261
    nursing care implications, 264
    psychological characteristics, 262
    skin color, 260
  of Navajos, 287
    alcohol metabolism, 293
    body size, 288
    body structure, 288
    disease susceptibility, 289
      arthritis, 292
      HIV/AIDS, 292
      hypertension, 291
      myocardial infarction, 292
      shigella, 291
      tuberculosis, 289
      type 2 diabetes, 289
    earlobe creasing, 289
    enzymatic variations, 289
    nursing care implications, 294
    nutritional preferences, 292
    psychological characteristics, 293
    skin color, 288
    uvula and, 289
  of Nigerian Americans, 705
    birth weight, 705
    disease susceptibility, 706
      AIDS/HIV risk, 708*b*
      Alzheimer disease, 707
      cancer, 706
      chemical abuse, 709
      epilepsy, 710
      hypertension, 706

Biological variations (*Continued*)
      lactose intolerance, 707
      malaria, 707
      nursing care implications, 711
      psychological characteristics, 710
      skin color, 706
  of Puerto Rican Americans, 680
    body size, 680
    body structure, 680
    disease susceptibility, 680
      asthma, 681
      cancer, 682
      diabetes, 681
      obesity, 681
      visual impairments, 681
    genetic deviation, 680
    nursing care implications, 682
  of Russian Americans, 430
    body size, 430
    dental needs, 431
    disease susceptibility, 430
      cancer, 431
      hypertension, 430
      tuberculosis, 430
    enzymatic variations, 430
    eye care needs, 431
    nursing care implications, 434
    nutritional deficiencies, 431
    nutritional preferences, 431
    psychological characteristics, 431
      alcoholism, 433
      illness/wellness behaviors, 431
      mental health, 432
    radiation accidents, 433
    toxic pollution, 433
  of Ugandan Americans, 729
    disease susceptibility, 730
      AIDS/HIV, 730
      ascariasis, 731
      brucellosis, 731
      cancer, 731
      chronic obstructive pulmonary
        disease, 730
      hypertension, 730
      leishmaniasis, 731
      malaria, 731
      mental diseases, 730
      nursing care implications, 732
      schistosomiasis, 731
      sickle cell anemia, 730
      tropical disease, 731
      typhoid fever, 731
    enzymatic variation, 729

Pages 689–821 (Chapters 25–30) can be found online at http://evolve.elsevier.com/Giger.

Biological variations (*Continued*)
  genetic variation, 729
  nutritional deficiencies, 729
  nutritional preferences, 729
  of Vietnamese Americans, 513
    blood type, 513
    body size, 513
    body structure, 513
    dioxin, 521
    enzymatic variations, 514
    genetic variations, 514
    noses, 514
    nutritional preference, 520
    psychological characteristics, 522
      adaptation, 524
      alcohol abuse, 525
      coping, 524
      mental health, 522
      metabolism of drugs, 527
      nursing care implications, 528
      posttraumatic stress disorder, 526
      refugees, emotional and behavioral
        manifestations of, 523
    refugees medical problems, 514
      cancer, 517
      hepatitis B, 515
      HIV/AIDS, 520
      hypertension, 514
      tuberculosis risk, 516
    skin color, 513
    teeth, 514
Black lung disease, 309
Blessingway, 285
Block English pronunciation, 194
Bock, Phillip, 110
Body posture, nonverbal communication
  and, 32
Body structure
  bone density, 147–148
  ears, 148
  face, 148
  mandibular/palatine torus, 148
  muscle size/mass, 148–149
  noses, 148
  stature, 149
  teeth, 148
Body weight
  childhood obesity, 149
  metabolic syndrome, 149
BRCA1, 154–155
BRCA2, 154–155
The Broken Heart: The Medical
  Consequences of Loneliness, 54

Brown lung disease, 309
Brucellosis, 731
Bulgogi, 633
Byssinosis, 309

C
Cafe con leche, 170–171
Caffeine, 157
Canadians. *See* French Canadians
Cancer, 344, 431, 456, 484, 580, 607, 682,
  706, 731
Cardiovascular disease, 634
  in African Americans, 214
    diabetes, 219
    hypertension, 216
    obesity/sedentary lifestyle, 219
    serum cholesterol levels, 217
    smoking, 218
    stroke, 220
    sudden cardiac death, 221
  in American Eskimos, 343
  of Filipino Americans, 482
CAS. *See* Cultural attitude Scale
Chemical abuse, 709
Childhood obesity, 149
  in Mexican-Americans, 261
China, 443
Chinese Americans
  biological variations, 455
    body size, 455
    body structure, 455
    death, leading causes of, 458
    disease susceptibility, 456
      cancer, 456
      infectious diseases, 456
    enzymatic variations, 456
    genetic variations, 456
    mortality, 458
    nursing care implications, 459
    psychological characteristics, 458
    skin color, 455
  communication, 445
    context, 446
    dialect, 445
    kinesics, 446
    nursing care implications, 447
    style, 445
    touch, 445
    volume, 445
  environmental control, 451
    death/dying issues, 454
    death/dying practices, 454
    illness behaviors, 452

Chinese Americans (*Continued*)
    wellness behaviors, 452
    folk practices, 454
      nursing care implications, 455
    folklore, 454
      nursing care implications, 455
    health assessment of, 15*t*
    overview of, 443
    social organization, 448
      family, 449
      immigration and, 448
      marital status, 450
      nursing care implications, 450
      religion, 450
    space, 447
      nursing care implications, 448
    time, 451
      nursing care implications, 451
Chlamydia, 342
Chloramphenicol-resistant Salmonella
  typhi, 264–265
Chronic obstructive pulmonary
  disease, 730
Circumcision, 137
Codeswitching, 244
Communicable disease(s), 261, 340, 611, 791
Communication
  Afghans and, 397
    nursing care implications, 399
  African Americans and, 193
    Block English pronunciation, 194
    dialect, 193
    nursing care implications, 195
    origin of, 193
  American Eskimos and, 329
    kinesics, 331
    language, 329
    nursing care implications, 331
    silence, 330
    touch, 331
  Amish Americans and, 779
    nursing care implications, 780
  Appalachians and, 304, 305*t*
    nursing care implications, 305
  barriers of, 21
  Chinese Americans and, 445
    context, 446
    dialect, 445
    kinesics, 446
    nursing care implications, 447
    style, 445
    touch, 445
    volume, 445

Pages 689–821 (Chapters 25–30) can be found online at http://evolve.elsevier.com/Giger.

Communication (*Continued*)
  Cuban Americans and, 761
    nursing care implications, 762
  culture and, 21
  definition of, 20
  East Indian Hindu Americans and, 542
    Hindustani dialect origin, 542
    kinetics, 543
    nursing care implications, 543
    style, 543
    touch, 543
    volume, 543
  factors influencing, 23*b*
  Filipino Americans and, 472
    context, 473
    dialect of, 472
    kinesics, 473
    language of, 472
    nursing care implications, 474
    style, 472
    tone, 472
  French Canadians and, 646
    behavior, 647
    culture, 646
    French, 646
    language, 646
    nursing care implications, 647
  functions of, 22
  Haitian Americans and, 569
    nursing care implications, 569
  Irish Americans and, 803
    nursing care implications, 804
  Japanese Americans and, 363
    culture and, 363
      context, 364
      linguistics, 364
      oral language, 364
      style, 363
      voice quality, 365
    nonverbal, 365
      kinesics, 365
      silence, 366
      touch, 366
    nursing care implications, 366
  Jews and, 595
    nursing care implications, 596
    style, 595
    touch, 596
  Jordanian Americans and, 743
    nursing care implications, 744
  Korean Americans and, 623
    culture, 623
    dialect, 624

Communication (*Continued*)
    eye contact, 624
    kinesics, 624
    language, 623, 625
    nursing care implications, 625
    social rank, 625
    style, 624
    verbal, 624
  language and, 21, 25
  linguistics and, 22
  Mexican-Americans and, 244
    context, 245
    dialect, 244
    English as a second language, 245
    kinesics, 245
    nursing care implications, 246
    touch, 244
  Navajos and, 279
    dialect, 279
    kinesics, 280
    language lateralization, 280
    names, 280
    nursing care implications, 281
    silence, 280
    style, 279
    touch, 280
  Nigerian Americans and, 693
    nursing care implications, 695
  nonverbal, 24*b*, 29
    body posture and, 32
    eye movement and, 32
    facial expression and, 31
    humor and, 33
    touch and, 29, 30*b*
    warmth and, 33
  nursing care communication, culture
    and, 34, 35*b*
    approach modification, 35, 36
    variables, 34, 35
  nursing care, culture and, 34, 35*b*
    case study example, 20
    communication approach
      modification, 35, 36
    communication variables, 34, 35
    interpreters, 39
    language differentiation, 35, 38
    nonthreatening communication
      manner, 35, 37
    personal beliefs, 34, 35
    plan of care, 35, 36
    respect, 35, 36
    sexual matters, 35, 38
    trust development, 35, 37

Communication (*Continued*)
  validating communication
    techniques, 35, 38
  people connection and, 20
  process of, 23
  Puerto Rican Americans and, 673
    nursing care implications, 674
  Russian Americans and, 418
    context, 419
    dialect, 418
    kinesics, 420
    nursing care implications, 420
    style, 418
    touch, 419
    volume, 418
  Ugandan Americans and, 721
    nursing care implications, 722
  verbal, 24*b*, 25
    grammatical structure and, 27
    humor and, 33
    intonation and, 28
    names and, 27
    pronunciation and, 28
    rhythm and, 28
    silence and, 29
    speed and, 28
    vocabulary and, 26
    voice qualities and, 28
    warmth and, 33
  Vietnamese Americans and, 497
    context, 498
    kinesics, 498
    language, 497
    nursing care implications, 499, 501*b*
    style, 497
    touch, 498
Community, Culture, and Care: A Cross-
  Cultural Guide for Health Workers, 4
Community Health: Education and
  Promotion Manual, 15–16
Compadrazgo, 250
Confianza, 243
Coronary Artery Risk Detection in
  Appalachian Communities
  (CARDIAC), 315
Coronary artery/heart disease, 314
Crohn's disease, 609
CSES. *See* Cultural Self-Efficacy Scale
Cuba, overview of, 758
Cuban Americans
  biological variation, 768
    disease susceptibility, 769
    diabetes, 769

Pages 689–821 (Chapters 25–30) can be found online at http://evolve.elsevier.com/Giger.

Cuban Americans (*Continued*)
  low birth weight, 769
  mental illness, 769
  substance abuse, 769
  vision impairment, 769
  nursing care implications, 770
  nutritional deficiencies, 769
  nutritional preferences, 769
communication, 761
  nursing care implications, 762
environmental care, 766
  death/dying rituals, 767
  nursing care implications, 768
immigration to United States, 760
social organization, 763
  education, 764
  family structure, 763
  nursing care implications, 765
  religion, 764
space, 763
  nursing care implications, 763
time, 766
  nursing care implications, 766
Cubans, nutritional preferences of, 171
Cultural assessment guide, 8, 13*t*
Cultural attitude Scale (CAS), 16–17
Cultural competence, 6–7
Cultural health practices
  dysfunctional, 131
  efficacious, 130
  medical health practices, 130
  neutral, 131
  uncertain, 131
Cultural Heritage Model, 8, 12*f*
Cultural Self-Efficacy Scale (CSES), 16–17
Culture
  nursing care communication and,
    34, 35*b*
  case study example, 20
  communication approach
    modification, 35, 36
  communication variables, 34, 35
  interpreters, 39
  language differentiation, 35, 38
  nonthreatening communication
    manner, 35, 37
  personal beliefs, 34, 35
  plan of care, 35, 36
  respect, 35, 36
  sexual matters, 35, 38
  trust development, 35, 37
  validating communication
    techniques, 35, 38

Culture (*Continued*)
  totality of, 68
    bicultural, 70
    biracial, 71
    culture-bound, 68
    culture-bound syndromes, 69
    disability and, 73
    ethnic minority, 72
    ethnicity, 70
    ethnocentrism, 69
    gender role, 72
    homogeneity, 70
    minority, 71
    race, 71
    stereotyping, 72
Culture and Disability Assessment
  Model, 73, 74*f*
Curanderismo, 256
Curandero/a, 140, 256, 260, 259, 265–266
Cystic fibrosis, 155
Cytogenetics, 152–153

D
Dawn Bible Students Association, 88–89
Death/dying, 138
  advanced directives, 138
  autonomy, 138
  truth-telling in, 138
Death/dying customs
  of Irish Americans, 811
  of Nigerian Americans, 703
Death/dying issues, 138
  advanced directives, 138
  of Appalachians, 309
  autonomy, 138
  of Chinese Americans, 454
  of Filipino Americans, 477
  of Japanese Americans, 374
  of Jewish client, 604
  of Korean Americans, 631
  of Mexican-Americans, 250
    nursing care implications, 251
  truth-telling in, 138
  of Ugandan Americans, 728
Death/dying rituals
  of African Americans, 207
  of Amish Americans, 789
  of Chinese Americans, 454
  of Cuban Americans, 767
  of French Canadians, 654
  of Haitian Americans, 577
  of Irish Americans, 811
  of Japanese Americans, 374

Death/dying rituals (*Continued*)
  of Navajos, 285
  of Nigerian Americans, 703
  of Puerto Rican Americans, 679
Dental hygienists, cultural assessment
  and, 15–16
Dharma, 540
Diabetes, 160, 219, 260, 681, 769
  type 2 diabetes, 289
Diabetes mellitus, 342, 484, 609
Directly observed therapy, 517
Disease(s), 130
  acquired immunodeficiency
    syndrome, 167
Disease susceptibility
  of African Americans, 214
    AIDS (HIV) risk, 221, 222*t*
    cardiovascular disease, 214
      diabetes, 219
      hypertension, 216
      obesity/sedentary lifestyle, 219
      serum cholesterol levels, 217
      smoking, 218
      stroke, 220
      sudden cardiac death, 221
  of American Eskimos, 340
    anemia, 343
    arthritis, 345
    asthma, 345
    cancer, 344
    cardiovascular disease, 343
    communicable disease, 340
    diabetes mellitus, 342
    glaucoma, 342
    hepatitis B virus, 345
    STDs, 342
    tuberculosis, 341
  blood groups, 159
  of Chinese Americans, 456
    cancer, 456
    infectious diseases, 456
  of Cuban Americans, 769
    diabetes, 769
    low birth weight, 769
    mental illness, 769
    substance abuse, 769
    vision impairment, 769
  diabetes, 160
  dimensions of, 158
  of East Indian Hindu Americans, 555
  of Filipino Americans, 482
    AIDS, 485
    amyotrophic lateral sclerosis, 484

Pages 689–821 (Chapters 25–30) can be found online at http://evolve.elsevier.com/Giger.

Disease susceptibility (*Continued*)
 cancer, 484
 cardiovascular disease, 482
 diabetes mellitus, 484
 gallbladder disease, 484
 glaucoma, 485
 hepatitis B, 485
 hypertension, 483
 palatal mucosal changes, 484
 of French Canadians, 657
  intravenously transmitted
   diseases, 657
  STDs, 657
 of Haitian Americans, 579
  AIDS, 580
  cancer, 580
  high birth rate, 579
  hypertension, 580
  intestinal problems, 579
  malaria, 580
  malnutrition, 579
  sickle cell anemia, 580
  tuberculosis, 579
  venereal disease, 579
 hypertension, 161
 of Japanese Americans, 377
 of Jews, 607
  cancer, 607
  communicable disease, 611
  Crohn's disease, 609
  diabetes mellitus, 609
  heart disease, 608
  myopia, 609
  polycythemia vera, 609
  ulcerative colitis, 609
 of Korean Americans, 634
  body weight, 634
  cardiovascular disease, 634
  HIV/AIDS, 635
  smoking, 634
 of Mexican-Americans, 260
  childhood obesity, 261
  communicable diseases, 261
  diabetes, 260
  hepatitis C, 261
  HIV/AIDS, 262
  hypertension, 261
  pernicious anemia, 261
 of Navajos, 289
  arthritis, 292
  HIV/AIDS, 292
  hypertension, 291
  myocardial infarction, 292

Disease susceptibility (*Continued*)
  shigella, 291
  tuberculosis, 289
  type 2 diabetes, 289
 of Nigerian Americans, 706
  AIDS/HIV risk, 708*b*
  Alzheimer disease, 707
  cancer, 706
  chemical abuse, 709
  epilepsy, 710
  hypertension, 706
  lactose intolerance, 707
  malaria, 707
 of Puerto Rican Americans, 680
  asthma, 681
  cancer, 682
  diabetes, 681
  obesity, 681
  visual impairments, 681
 Rh factor, 159
 of Russian Americans, 430
  cancer, 431
  hypertension, 430
  tuberculosis, 430
 sickle cell, 163*b*
  anemia, 165
 systemic lupus erythematosus, 166
 tuberculosis, 158
 of Ugandan Americans, 730
  AIDS/HIV, 730
  ascariasis, 731
  brucellosis, 731
  cancer, 731
  chronic obstructive pulmonary
   disease, 730
  hypertension, 730
  leishmaniasis, 731
  malaria, 731
  mental diseases, 730
  nursing care implications, 732
  schistosomiasis, 731
  sickle cell anemia, 730
  tropical disease, 731
  typhoid fever, 731
Distance receptors, 48, 48
 auditory perception, 48
 olfactory perception, 50
 visual perception, 48
Doble abrazo, 57
Dolma, 175
Domestic violence, 180
Dominant gene, 154
Double helix, 152–153

Double-step family, 77
Duchenne muscular dystrophy, 155
Duvalier, François, 565
Dysmetabolic syndrome, 216

E
Eakat, 93
East Indian Hindu Americans
 biological variations, 555
  disease susceptibility, 555
  enzymatic variation, 555
  genetic variation, 555
  nursing care implications, 557
  nutritional deficiencies, 556
  nutritional preferences, 556
  psychological characteristics, 556
  racial strain and, 555
 communication, 542
  Hindustani dialect origin, 542
  kinetics, 543
  nursing care implications, 543
  style, 543
  touch, 543
  volume, 543
 environmental control, 551
  death perception, 553
  folk medicine, 552
   belief sign, 552
   practitioner type, 553
  hygiene principles, 553
  illness perception, 551
  nursing care implications, 554
 health assessment of, 15*t*
 immigration to United States/
   Canada, 540
  first-wave, 540
  second-wave, 541
  third-wave, 541
 social organization, 544
  caste systems, 546, 547*b*
  family, 544
  immigration effect and, 548
  marriage, 545
  nursing care implications, 550
  religion, 547
  women's position, 546
 space, 543
  nursing care implications, 544
 time, 550
  nursing care implications, 551
EBV. *See* Epstein-Barr virus
Education
 African Americans and, 191–192

Pages 689–821 (Chapters 25–30) can be found online at http://evolve.elsevier.com/Giger.

Education (*Continued*)
    Appalachia and, 303
    Cuban Americans and, 764
    French Canadians and, 645
    Haitian Americans and, 571
    Japanese Americans and, 370
    Mexican-Americans and, 250–252
    Vietnamese Americans and, 505
Enculturation, 68
End-of-life decision. *See* Death/dying
Environmental control, 129–130
    Afghans and, 402
        death beliefs, 405
        death customs, 405
        health care access, 403
        illness/wellness behaviors, 403
        mental health issues, 404
        nursing care implications, 406
    African Americans and, 201
        death/dying rituals, 207
        folk medicine, 203
        health care beliefs, 202
        health care benefits, 201
        nursing care implications, 207
        witchcraft, 204
    American Eskimos and, 337
        illness/wellness behaviors, 337
        nursing care implications, 338
    Amish Americans and, 789
        death/dying rituals, 789
        nursing care implications, 790
    Appalachians and, 309
        care barriers, 310
        death rituals, 309
        death/dying, 309
        folk health system, 311
            beliefs, 311
            biomedical disease knowledge, 311
            lay practitioners, 312
            medicinal plants, 311
        health threats, 309
        illness/wellness behaviors, 312
            health screening, 313
            nursing care implications, 314
            risk behaviors, 312
        locus of control, 310
    case study, 129
    Chinese Americans and, 451
        death/dying issues, 454
        death/dying practices, 454
        illness behaviors, 452
        wellness behaviors, 452
    Cuban Americans and, 766

Environmental control (*Continued*)
        death/dying rituals, 767
        nursing care implications, 768
    East Indian Hindu Americans and, 551
        death perception, 553
        folk medicine, 552
            belief sign, 552
            practitioner type, 553
        hygiene principles, 553
        illness perception, 551
        nursing care implications, 554
    Filipino Americans and, 479
        folk medicine, 479
        illness/wellness behavior, 481
        nursing care implications, 481
    French Canadians and, 652
        death/dying rituals, 654
        health attitudes, 652
        health social environment, 652
        illness/wellness behaviors, 653
        nursing care implications, 655
        physical environment, 653
    Haitian Americans and, 574
        death/dying rituals, 577
        nursing care implications, 577
        Voodoo practices, 575
    Irish Americans and, 809
        death/dying customs, 811
        death/dying rituals, 811
        folk medicine, 810
        illness behavior, 810
        locus of control, 809
        nursing care implications, 811
        perception of illness, 810
        wellness behavior, 810
    Japanese Americans and, 372
        customs observed, 374
        death/dying, 374
        dying rituals, 374
        folk medicine, 373
        illness/wellness behaviors, 373
        locus of control, 372
        nursing care implications, 375
    Jews and, 600
        AIDS, 604
        circumcision, 605
        dying Jewish client, 604
        health care beliefs, 600
        illness, 602
        illness behaviors, 600
        Kosher diet, 602
        life-support measure, 603
        nursing care implications, 605

Environmental control (*Continued*)
        organ transplants, 603
        procreation, 603
        religious holidays, 602
        wellness behaviors, 602
    Jordanian Americans and, 747
        death customs, 749
        death rituals, 749
        folk beliefs, 748
        folk practices, 748
        illness behavior, 748
        nursing care implications, 749
        wellness behavior, 748
    Korean Americans and, 629
        death/dying issues, 631
        illness behaviors, 629
        nursing care implications, 631
        oriental herbal medicine, 629
        postpartum practices, 630
        pregnancy, 630
        preventive health practices, 630
        wellness behaviors, 629
    Mexican-Americans and, 253
        folk medicine, 256
        health care beliefs, 254
        locus of control, 253
        nursing care implications, 258
    Navajos and, 284
        death/dying rituals, 285
        illness and wellness behaviors, 284
        native healers, 285
        nursing care implications, 286
    Nigerian Americans and, 701
        death/dying customs, 703
        death/dying rituals, 703
        folk medicine, 702
        health care practices, 701
        nursing care implications, 705
    nursing care implications in, 139
    Puerto Rican Americans and, 678
        death/dying rituals, 679
    Russian Americans and, 427
        folk medicine, 428
        health treatment, 427
        locus of control, 427
        nursing care implications, 429
        time of death practice, 429
        wellness/illness behaviors, 427
    Ugandan Americans and, 727
        death/dying issues, 728
        nursing care implications, 728
    Vietnamese Americans and, 507
        death beliefs/practice, 510, 511*t*

Pages 689–821 (Chapters 25–30) can be found online at http://evolve.elsevier.com/Giger.

Environmental control (*Continued*)
illness concepts, 508
germs, 510
metaphysical causes, 508, 510*b*
natural causes, 508, 509*b*
supernatural causes, 508
nursing care implications, 511, 512*b*
Ephemeris time, 109
Epilepsy, 710
Epstein-Barr virus (EBV), 344
Eskimos. *See* American Eskimos
Espiritista, 140
Evil eye, 257
Exteroceptors, 51
Eye movement, nonverbal communication
and, 32

F
Facial expression, nonverbal
communication and, 31
Familismo, 249
Family function, 84
Family households, 75
Feldshers, 427
Feng shui, 452
Filipino Americans
biological variations, 481
body size, 481
body structure, 481
cleft lip/palate, 482
disease susceptibility, 482
AIDS, 485
amyotrophic lateral sclerosis, 484
cancer, 484
cardiovascular disease, 482
diabetes mellitus, 484
gallbladder disease, 484
glaucoma, 485
hepatitis B, 485
hypertension, 483
palatal mucosal changes, 484
enzymatic variation, 482
genetic variation, 482
Mongoloid, 482
nursing care implications, 486
nutritional preferences, 485
psychological characteristics, 486
alcohol use, 486
skin color, 482
communication of, 472
context, 473
dialect of, 472
kinesics, 473

Filipino Americans (*Continued*)
language of, 472
nursing care implications, 474
style, 472
tone, 472
environmental control, 479
folk medicine, 479
illness/wellness behavior, 481
nursing care implications, 481
health assessment of, 15*t*
immigration to United States, 469
first-wave, 470
second-wave, 470
third-wave, 470
social organizations, 475
birth rituals, 477
death/dying, 477
family, 475
family systems, 476
nursing care implications, 478
religion, 477
space, 475
nursing care implications, 475
time, 478
nursing care implications, 479
Folk beliefs, of Jordanian Americans, 748
Folk health system, Appalachians, 311
beliefs, 311
biomedical disease knowledge, 311
lay practitioners, 312
medicinal plants, 311
Folk medicine, 134
African Americans and, 203
definition of, 204
origins of, 205
perception concerning, 205
practice of, 203
practitioners of, 204
rationale for use of, 206
witchcraft and, 204
East Indian Hindu Americans, 552
belief sign, 552
practitioner type, 553
Filipino Americans, 479
Irish Americans, 810
Japanese Americans, 373
Mexican Americans and, 256
brujos/as, 257
caí da la mollera, 257
curandero/a, 256
empacho, 258
family folk healer, 256
illnesses, 257

Folk medicine (*Continued*)
mal ojo, 257
nervios, 258
religious views, 258
susto, 258
yerbero, 256
natural events, 134
natural illnesses, 135
Nigerian Americans, 702
Russian Americans, 428
as system, 134
alternative therapies and, 136
ecological model and, 136
religious systems, 137
Western Medical System and, 136
unnatural events, 134
unnatural illnesses, 135
Folk practices
Chinese Americans, 454
nursing care implications, 455
Jordanian Americans, 748
Folk traditions, Japanese Americans, 382
Folklore, Chinese Americans, 454
nursing care implications, 455
Food patterns. *See* Nutritional preferences
French Canadians
biological variations, 656
disease susceptibility, 657
intravenously transmitted
diseases, 657
STDs, 657
genetic factors, 656
life expectancy, 656
nursing care implications, 659
psychological characteristics/
coping, 658
alcohol, 658
drug abuse, 658
mental health, 658
tobacco, 658
communication, 646
behavior, 647
culture, 646
French, 646
language, 646
nursing care implications, 647
environmental control, 652
death/dying rituals, 654
health attitudes, 652
health social environment, 652
illness/wellness behaviors, 653
nursing care implications, 655
physical environment, 653

Pages 689–821 (Chapters 25–30) can be found online at http://evolve.elsevier.com/Giger.

French Canadians (*Continued*)
  political development, 644
    economy, 645
    education, 645
    health care, 645
    Quiet Revolution, 644
  social organization, 648
    church, 648
    family evolution, 649
    interdependence models, 649
    nursing care implications, 650
    population aging, 650
    religion, 650
    youth, 650
  space, 648
    conceptualization, 648
    interpersonal, 648
    nursing care implications, 648
    physical, 648
  time, 651
    nursing care implications, 652
    past and present, 651
Friendshaft, 138
Future shock, 114–115

G
G-6-PD, 176, 177
Gallbladder disease, 484
Genetic drift, 153–154
Genotypes, 152–153
Giger and Davidhizar's Transcultural
  Assessment Model, 5, 7*f*, 8*f*, 9*f*, 12*f*,
  73, 74*f*
  competent care defined, 6
  cultural behaviors, 11–12, 15*t*
  development of, 8
  diverse nursing care, 6
  refinement of, 8
  research and, 16
  sensitive environments, 7, 9*f*
  transcultural nursing defined, 5–6
  unique individuals, 7, 8*f*
Glaucoma, 342, 485
Grammatical structure, verbal
  communication and, 27
Greenwich, 108

H
Hae-Chan, Lee, 620–621
Haemophilus influenzae type B
  (Hib), 340–341
Haiti, overview of, 564
  life, 566

Haiti, overview of (*Continued*)
  social history, 564
Haitian Americans
  biological variations, 578
    body size, 578
    body structure, 578
    childbearing dietary habits, 582, 583*b*
    disease susceptibility, 579
      AIDS, 580
      cancer, 580
      high birth rate, 579
      hypertension, 580
      intestinal problems, 579
      malaria, 580
      malnutrition, 579
      sickle cell anemia, 580
      tuberculosis, 579
      venereal disease, 579
    ear wax, 578
    nursing care implications, 583
    nutritional deficiencies, 582
    nutritional preferences, 582*b*
    psychological characteristics, 582,
      584*b*
    skin color, 578
  communication, 569
    nursing care implications, 569
  environmental control, 574
    death/dying rituals, 577
    nursing care implications, 577
    Voodoo practices, 575
  health assessment of, 15*t*
  immigration to United States, 567
  social organization, 571
    education, 571
    family, 571
    nursing care implications, 573
    social class, 571
  space, 570
    nursing care implications, 570
  time, 573
    nursing care implications, 574
Hantavirus disease (HVD), 633
Haploid set, 153
Health care behavior, 130
Health care beliefs, of Mexican Americans,
  hot and cold theory, 254, 255*b*
Health care inequality, 147
Health care practices, values and, 131
  activity orientation, 132
  innate human nature, 133
  locus-of-control construct, 133
  people-to-nature, 132

Health care practices, values and
  (*Continued*)
  relational orientation, 132
  temporal orientation, 132
  value orientation, 132
Health Care Traveler, 15–16
Health disparity, 146, 147
Health status, 130
Health-Promoting Lifestyle Profile
  (HPLP), 253–254
Healthy People 2010, 20
Heart disease, 608
Hemoglobin electrophoresis, 166
Hepatitis B, 485
Hepatitis B virus, 345
Hepatitis C, 261
Heterozygous, 154
Hib. *See* Haemophilus influenzae type B
High birth rate, 579
Hinduism, overview of, 538
Hiragana, 363
HIV. *See* Acquired immune deficiency
  syndrome (AIDS)
Hmong, 97
Hogan, 246–247
Homozygous, 154
Honji, 363
Hôpital Albert Schweitzer, 566–567
Hospital Topics, 15–16
HPLP. *See* Health-Promoting Lifestyle
  Profile
Humor
  nonverbal communication and, 33
  verbal communication and, 33
HVD. *See* Hantavirus disease
Hwa-byung, 635
Hypertension, 161, 216, 261, 291, 430, 483,
  580, 706, 730
Hyun, Rih Moo, 620–621

I
Illness, 130
Immediate receptors, 48, 51
  skin membranes, 51
Immigration
  of Afghans, 400
  of Chinese Americans, 448
  of Cuban Americans, 760
  of East Indian Hindu Americans,
    540, 548
  first-wave, 540
  second-wave, 541
  third-wave, 541

Pages 689–821 (Chapters 25–30) can be found online at http://evolve.elsevier.com/Giger.

Immigration (*Continued*)
  of Filipino Americans, 469
    first-wave, 470
    second-wave, 470
    third-wave, 470
  of Haitian Americans, 567
  of Irish Americans, 802
  of Japanese Americans, 359, 367
  of Jordanian Americans, 742
  of Nigerian Americans, 693
  of Russian Americans, 415
    life in United States, 417
  of Vietnamese Americans, 496
    first-wave, 496
    second-wave, 496
    third-wave, 496
Incomplete dominance, 155
India, overview of, 538
Indians. *See* American Indians East Indian
    Hindu Americans
Infectious disease(s), 456
Inner personal space, 47
International Journal of Nursing
    Studies, 2
International Nursing Review, 2
Interpreters, nursing care communication,
    culture and, 39
Intestine, problems of, 579
Intonation, verbal communication
    and, 28
Intravenously transmitted diseases, 657
Inukitut, 330
Inupiat. *See* American Eskimos
Ireland, overview of, 800
Irish Americans
  biological variations, 811
    genetic variations, 811
      abdominal aortic aneurysm, 812
      cystic fibrosis, 812
      neural tube defects, 812
      sarcoidosis, 812
      Tay-Sachs disease, 812
      teeth, 812
    HIV risk, 813
    nursing care implications, 815
    psychological characteristics, 813
      adolescents, drinking behavior
        and, 814
      alcoholism, 813
      bipolar disorders, 814
      schizophrenia, 814
  communication, 803
    nursing care implications, 804

Irish Americans (*Continued*)
    environmental control, 809
      death/dying customs, 811
      death/dying rituals, 811
      folk medicine, 810
      illness behavior, 810
      locus of control, 809
      nursing care implications, 811
      perception of illness, 810
      wellness behavior, 810
    immigration to United States, 802
    social organization, 806
      adolescents, 807
      children, 807
      family, 806
      marriage, 806
        men's role, 807
        women's role, 806
      nursing care implications, 808
      political influences, 807
      religion, 807
    space, 805
      nursing care implications, 805
    time, nursing care implications, 809
Islamic social organizations, 92
    common phrases, 93, 94b
    cultural social differences, 94
    family emphasis, 94
    five pillars, 93
    infertility crisis, 95
    marriage, 96
    sex, 96
    social support, 95
    stereotypes, 96
    women's dress, 95
Isoniazid, 156

J
Japan, overview of, 358
Japanese Americans
  biological variations, 376
    body size, 376
    disease susceptibility, 377
    drug interactions, 377
    enzymatic variations, 377
    eye shape, 376
    genetic variations, 377
    Mongolian spots, 376
    mouth/teeth, 376
    nutritional deficiencies, 380
    nutritional preferences, 380
    psychological change, 380
      alcohol use, 383

Japanese Americans (*Continued*)
      folk traditions, 382
      internment trauma, 382
      mental health, 381
      nursing care implications, 383
      psychopharmacology, 383
      self cultural values, 380
      somatization, 382
      stress manifestations, 381
    skin color, 376
  communication, 363
    culture and, 363
      context, 364
      linguistics, 364
      oral language, 364
      style, 363
      voice quality, 365
    nonverbal, 365
      kinesics, 365
      silence, 366
      touch, 366
    nursing care implications, 366
  environmental control, 372
    customs observed, 374
    death/dying, 374
    dying rituals, 374
    folk medicine, 373
    illness/wellness behaviors, 373
    locus of control, 372
    nursing care implications, 375
  immigration, 359
  social organizations, 367
    education attainment, family role
      in, 370
    family systems, 367
    immigration effects on, 367
    nursing care implications, 371
    religion, 371
  space, 366
    nursing care implications, 367
  time, 372
    nursing care implications, 372
  in United States, 362
Japanese, nutritional preferences of,
    172, 173t
Jehovah's Witnesses, 88, 90b
    nursing care implication of, 89
Jewish Americans, health assessment
    of, 15t
Jews
  biological variations, 606
    disease susceptibility, 607
      cancer, 607

Pages 689–821 (Chapters 25–30) can be found online at http://evolve.elsevier.com/Giger.

Jews (*Continued*)
  communicable disease, 611
  Crohn's disease, 609
  diabetes mellitus, 609
  heart disease, 608
  myopia, 609
  polycythemia vera, 609
  ulcerative colitis, 609
  enzymatic variations, 606
  genetic variations, 606
  nutritional deficiencies, 609
  nutritional preferences, 609
  psychological characteristics, 610, 611
    alcoholism, 611
    Holocaust survivors, 611
    mental health, 610, 612
    nursing care implications, 612
  communication, 595
    nursing care implications, 596
    style, 595
    touch, 596
  environmental control, 600
    AIDS, 604
    circumcision, 605
    dying Jewish client, 604
    health care beliefs, 600
    illness, 602
    illness behaviors, 600
    Kosher diet, 602
    life-support measure, 603
    nursing care implications, 605
    organ transplants, 603
    procreation, 603
    religious holidays, 602
    wellness behaviors, 602
  overview of, 593
    in United States, 593
  social organizations, 597
    nursing care implications, 598
  space, 596
    nursing care implications, 596
  time, 598
    nursing care implications, 599
Jiabao, Wen, 443
Jinato, Hu, 443
Johnson, Anthony, 192
Johnson, Richard, 192
Jordan, overview of, 741
Jordanian Americans
  biological variations, 750
    genetic variations, 750
    nursing care implications, 751
    nutritional deficiencies, 750

Jordanian Americans (*Continued*)
    nutritional preferences, 750
  communication, 743
    nursing care implications, 744
  environmental control, 747
    death customs, 749
    death rituals, 749
    folk beliefs, 748
    folk practices, 748
    illness behavior, 748
    nursing care implications, 749
    wellness behavior, 748
  immigration to United States, 742
  overview of, 742
  social organization, 745
    nursing care implications, 746
    religion, 745
  space, 744
    nursing care implications, 744
  time, 747
    nursing care implications, 747
Jourard, Sidney, 21
The Journal of Transcultural Nursing, 2
Julius Caesar, 110

K
Kaffiyeh, 742
Kampo, 373
Kanji, 363
Karma, 373
Kata-kana, 363
Keloids, 152
KHF. *See* Korean hemorrhagic fever
Kimchi, 174, 633
Knowledge base questions, 16–17
Korea, overview of, 620
Korean Americans
  biological variations, 632
    body size, 632
    body structure, 632
    diet, 633
    disease susceptibility, 634
      body weight, 634
      cardiovascular disease, 634
      HIV/AIDS, 635
      smoking, 634
    enzymatic variations, 633
    genetic variations, 633
    metabolism of drugs, 634
    skin color, 632
  communication, 623
    culture, 623
    dialect, 624

Korean Americans (*Continued*)
    eye contact, 624
    kinesics, 624
    language, 623, 625
    nursing care implications, 625
    social rank, 625
    style, 624
    verbal, 624
  environmental control, 629
    death/dying issues, 631
    illness behaviors, 629
    nursing care implications, 631
    oriental herbal medicine, 629
    postpartum practices, 630
    pregnancy, 630
    preventive health practices, 630
    wellness behaviors, 629
  life in United States today, 621
  overview of, 621
  social organizations, 626
    family, 626
    nursing care implications, 627
    religion, 627
    social values, 627
  space, 625
    nursing care implications, 625
  time, 628
    nursing care implications, 629
Korean hemorrhagic fever (KHF), 633
Koreans, nutritional preferences of, 174

L
La Valley, William, 136–137
Lactose intolerance, 176–177, 707
Language
  communication and, 21, 25
  differentiation, nursing care
    communication, culture and,
    35, 38
Las Posadas, 250
Latinos, 241–242
Leininger, Madeleine, 2
Leininger's sunrise model, 4
Leishmaniasis, 731
Linguistics
  communication and, 22
  United States isolation of, 24
Low birth weight, 769

M
Machismo, 243
Malaria, 580, 707, 731
  combat of, 707

Pages 689–821 (Chapters 25–30) can be found online at http://evolve.elsevier.com/Giger.

Malaria (*Continued*)
  pathophysiology of, 707
  prophylaxis, 708
  travel hints, 708
Malnutrition, 579
Mano milagroso, 260
Marriage
  East Indian Hindu Americans and, 545
  Irish Americans and, 806
    men's role, 807
    women's role, 806
  Islamic and, 96
  Navajos and, 282
  Nigerian Americans and, 698
McPhee, Stephen, 516
Medical system, 135
Megatreds, 243
Mellon Foundation, 566–567
Mendel, Gregor, 153
Mendelian traits, 155
Mental diseases, 730
Mental illness, 769
Mestizos, 240
Metabolic syndrome (syndrome X),
  149, 216
Method of Advancing Dental Care, 15–16
Methylenetetrahydrofolate reductase
  (MTHFR), 212
Mexican American Prevalence and Services
  Survey (MAPSS), 263
Mexican-Americans, 240
  biological variations in, 260
    disease susceptibility, 260
      childhood obesity, 261
      communicable diseases, 261
      diabetes, 260
      hepatitis C, 261
      HIV/AIDS, 262
      hypertension, 261
      pernicious anemia, 261
    nursing care implications, 264
    psychological characteristics, 262
    skin color, 260
  communication and, 244
    context, 245
    dialect, 244
    English as a second language, 245
    kinesics, 245
    nursing care implications, 246
    touch, 244
  cultural uniqueness, 252
  death/dying, 250
    nursing care implications, 251

Mexican-Americans (*Continued*)
  education and, 250–252
  environmental control, 253
    folk medicine, 256
    health care beliefs, 254
    locus of control, 253
    nursing care implications, 258
  health assessment of, 15*t*
  health care system and, 248
  social organizations, 248
  space, 248
    nursing care implications, 248
  time, 252
    nursing care implications, 252
  workforce and, 253
Mexico, 240
Middle Easterners, nutritional preferences
  of, 175, 176*t*
Miller, William, 91
Minnesota Multiphasic Personality
  Inventory (MMPI), 225–226
Models
  Leininger's sunrise, 4
  of transcultural nursing
    analysis of, 4
    non-nursing, 3
    nursing-specific, 4
Molecular genetics, 152–153
Mongolian spots, 152
Monomorphic, 154
Mosby's Medical, Nursing, and Allied
  Health Dictionary, 12, 38–39
MTHFR. *See* Methylenetetrahydrofolate
  reductase
Mullen, Sharon S., 17
Muslim. *See* Islamic social organizations
Mutation, 153
Myocardial infarction, 292
Myopia, 609

N
Names, verbal communication and, 27
NANDA. *See* North American Nursing
  Diagnosis Association
National Heart, Lung, and Blood Institute
  (NHLBI), 161
National High Blood Pressure Education
  Program (NHBPEP), 161
Navajos
  biological variations, 287
    alcohol metabolism, 293
    body size, 288
    body structure, 288

Navajos (*Continued*)
    disease susceptibility, 289
      arthritis, 292
      HIV/AIDS, 292
      hypertension, 291
      myocardial infarction, 292
      shigella, 291
      tuberculosis, 289
      type 2 diabetes, 289
    earlobe creasing, 289
    enzymatic variations, 289
    nursing care implications, 294
    nutritional preferences, 292
    psychological characteristics, 293
    skin color, 288
    uvula and, 289
  communication of, 279
    dialect, 279
    kinesics, 280
    language lateralization, 280
    names, 280
    nursing care implications, 281
    silence, 280
    style, 279
    touch, 280
  environmental control, 284
    death/dying rituals, 285
    illness and wellness behaviors, 284
    native healers, 285
    nursing care implications, 286
  overview of, 277
  social organization, 282
    family, 282
    family roles/structures, 282
    marriage, 282
    nursing care implications, 283
    religion, 283
    traditional dress, 283
  space, 281
    nursing care implications, 281
  time, 283
    nursing care implications, 284
Neuroleptics, 157
NHBPEP. *See* National High Blood
  Pressure Education Program
NHLBI. *See* National Heart, Lung, and
  Blood Institute
Nigeria
  history of, 691
    British rule, 692
    early, 691
    Europeans, 691
    military rule, 692

Pages 689–821 (Chapters 25–30) can be found online at http://evolve.elsevier.com/Giger.

Nigeria (*Continued*)
  Nigeria Republic, 692
  overview of, 690
Nigerian Americans
  biological variations, 705
    birth weight, 705
    disease susceptibility, 706
      AIDS/HIV risk, 708*b*
      Alzheimer disease, 707
      cancer, 706
      chemical abuse, 709
      epilepsy, 710
      hypertension, 706
      lactose intolerance, 707
      malaria, 707
    nursing care implications, 711
    psychological characteristics, 710
    skin color, 706
  communication, 693
    nursing care implications, 695
  environmental control, 701
    death/dying customs, 703
    death/dying rituals, 703
    folk medicine, 702
    health care practices, 701
    nursing care implications, 705
  immigration to the United States, 693
  social organizations, 697
    family, 697
    marriage, 698
    nursing care implications, 699
    religion, 698
  space, 696
    childbearing and, 696
    nursing care implications, 697
  time, 700
    nursing care implications, 700
Non-sex chromosome, 154–155
Nonverbal communication, 24*b*, 29
  body posture and, 32
  eye movement and, 32
  facial expression and, 31
  humor and, 33
  touch and, 29, 30*b*
  warmth and, 33
North American Nursing Diagnosis
    Association (NANDA), 4–5
Nursing care communication, culture
    and, 34, 35*b*
  case study example, 20
  communication approach
      modification, 35, 36
  communication variables, 34, 35

Nursing care communication, culture and
    (*Continued*)
  interpreters, 39
  language differentiation, 35, 38
  nonthreatening communication
      manner, 35, 37
  personal beliefs, 34, 35
  plan of care, 35, 36
  respect, 35, 36
  sexual matters, 35, 38
  trust development, 35, 37
  validating communication
      techniques, 35, 38
Nursing care implications
  Afghans
    biological variations, 406
    communication, 399
    environmental control, 406
    social organization, 401
    space, 399
    time, 402
  African Americans
    communication and, 195
    environmental control, 207
    psychological characteristics, 226
    social organizations, 200
    space, 197
    time and, 201
  American Eskimos
    biological variations, 347
    communication, 331
    environmental control, 338
    social organization, 335
    space, 333
    time, 337
  Amish Americans
    biological variations, 792
    communication, 780
    environmental control, 790
    social organizations, 785
    space, 781
    time, 788
  Appalachians
    communication, 305
    environmental control, illness/
        wellness behaviors, 314
    social organization, 307
    space, 306
    time, 308
  Chinese Americans
    biological variations, 459
    communication, 447
    folk practices, 455

Nursing care implications (*Continued*)
    folklore, 455
    social organization, 450
    space, 448
    time, 451
  Cuban Americans
    biological variation, 770
    communication, 762
    environmental care, 768
    social organization, 765
    space, 763
    time, 766
  East Indian Hindu Americans
    biological variations, 557
    communication, 543
    environmental control, 554
    social organization, 550
    space, 544
    time, 551
  Filipino Americans
    biological variations, 486
    communication of, 474
    environmental control, 481
    social organizations, 478
    space, 475
    time, 479
  French Canadians
    biological variations, 659
    communication, 647
    environmental control, 655
    social organization, 650
    space, 648
    time, 652
  Haitian Americans
    biological variations, 583
    communication, 569
    environmental control, 577
    social organization, 573
    space, 570
    time, 574
  Irish Americans
    biological variations, 815
    communication, 804
    environmental control, 811
    social organization, 808
    space, 805
    time, 809
  Japanese Americans
    biological variations, psychological
        change, 383
    communication, 366
    environmental control, 375
    social organizations, 371

Pages 689–821 (Chapters 25–30) can be found online at http://evolve.elsevier.com/Giger.

Nursing care implications (*Continued*)
    space, 367
    time, 372
Jehovah's Witnesses, 89
Jews
    biological variations, psychological
        characteristics, 612
    communication, 596
    environmental control, 605
    social organizations, 598
    space, 596
    time, 599
Jordanian Americans
    biological variations, 751
    communication, 744
    environmental control, 749
    social organization, 746
    space, 744
    time, 747
Korean Americans
    communication, 625
    environmental control, 631
    social organizations, 627
    space, 625
    time, 629
Mexican-Americans
    biological variations in, 264
    communication and, 246
    death/dying, 251
    environmental control, 258
    space, 248
    time, 252
Navajos
    biological variations, 294
    communication of, 281
    environmental control, 286
    social organization, 283
    space, 281
    time, 284
Nigerian Americans
    biological variations, 711
    communication, 695
    environmental control, 705
    social organizations, 699
    space, 697
    time, 700
Puerto Rican Americans
    biological variations, 682
    communication of, 674
    space, 675
    time, 678
Russian Americans
    biological variations, 434

Nursing care implications (*Continued*)
    communication by, 420
    environmental control, 429
    social organizations, 425
    space, 422
    time, 426
    Seventh-Day Adventists, 91
    for social organizations, 98
    Ugandan Americans
        biological variations, disease
            susceptibility, 732
        communication, 722
        environmental control, 728
        social organizations, 725
        space, 723
        time, 726
    Vietnamese Americans
        biological variations, psychological
            characteristics, 528
        communication, 499, 501*b*
        environmental control, 511, 512*b*
        social organizations, 506
        space, 502
        time, 507
Nursing Management Skills: A Modular
    Self-Assessment Series, Module IV,
    Transcultural Nursing, 12
Nutritional deficiencies, 176
    of Cuban Americans, 769
    of East Indian Hindu Americans, 556
    of Haitian Americans, 582
    of Japanese Americans, 380
    of Jews, 609
    of Jordanian Americans, 750
    of Russian Americans, 431
    of Ugandan Americans, 729
Nutritional preferences, 168
    of African Americans, 169, 170*t*
    of American Eskimos, 345
    of American Indians, 172, 173*t*
    of Cuban Americans, 769
    of Cubans, 171
    of East Indian Hindu Americans, 556
    of Filipino Americans, 485
    of Haitian Americans, 582*b*
    of Japanese, 172, 173*t*
    of Japanese Americans, 380
    of Jews, 609
    of Jordanian Americans, 750
    of Koreans, 174
    of Middle Easterners, 175, 176*t*
    of Navajos, 292
    of Puerto Ricans, 170, 171*t*

Nutritional preferences (*Continued*)
    of Russian Americans, 431
    of Ugandan Americans, 729
    of Vietnamese Americans, 520

O
Obesity, 681
    childhood, 149
        in Mexican-Americans, 261
    Russian Americans, 430
Obesity/sedentary lifestyle, 219
Octoroon, 71
of Ugandan Americans
    AIDS/HIV, 730
    nursing care implications, 732
Old Farmer's Almanac, 140
Olfactory perception, 50
Operation Ranch Hand, 521–522
Orgullo, 243
Outline of Cultural Materials, 4

P
Palatal mucosa, changes of, 484
Pernicious anemia, 261
Personal beliefs, nursing care
    communication, culture and, 34, 35
Personal boundaries, 60
Personal space. *See* Space
Phenotype, 152–153
Philippines, overview of, 468
    economy, 468
    population, 468
Phillips, Carla G., 17
Piñata, 250
Plan of care, nursing care communication,
    culture and, 35, 36
Polycythemia vera, 609
Polymorphic, 154
Population genetics, 153
Posttraumatic stress disorder (PTSD), 179,
    241, 264, 404
Posture, nonverbal communication
    and, 32
Potlatch, 327
Potter and Perry's Fundamentals of
    Nursing, 8
Pronunciation, verbal communication
    and, 28
Proprioceptors, 51
Proxemics, 55
Psychological characteristics, 178
    of African Americans, 223
    chemical abuse, 224

Pages 689–821 (Chapters 25–30) can be found online at http://evolve.elsevier.com/Giger.

Psychological characteristics (*Continued*)
  nursing care implications, 226
  posttraumatic stress disorder, 225
  of American Eskimos, 345
  of Chinese Americans, 458
  of East Indian Hindu Americans, 556
  of Filipino Americans, 486
    alcohol use, 486
  of French Canadians, 658
    alcohol, 658
    drug abuse, 658
    mental health, 658
    tobacco, 658
  of Haitian Americans, 582, 584b
  of Irish Americans, 813
    adolescents, drinking behavior
      and, 814
    alcoholism, 813
    bipolar disorders, 814
    schizophrenia, 814
  of Japanese Americans, 380
    alcohol use, 383
    folk traditions, 382
    internment trauma, 382
    mental health, 381
    nursing care implications, 383
    psychopharmacology, 383
    self cultural values, 380
    somatization, 382
    stress manifestations, 381
  of Russian Americans, 431
    alcoholism, 433
    illness/wellness behaviors, 431
    mental health, 432
  of Vietnamese Americans, 522
    adaptation, 524
    alcohol abuse, 525
    coping, 524
    mental health, 522
    metabolism of drugs, 527
    nursing care implications, 528
    posttraumatic stress disorder, 526
    refugees, emotional and behavioral
      manifestations of, 523
Psychotropic drugs, 156
PTSD. *See* Posttraumatic stress disorder
Puerto Rican Americans
  biological variations, 680
    body size, 680
    body structure, 680
    disease susceptibility, 680
      asthma, 681
      cancer, 682

Puerto Rican Americans (*Continued*)
    diabetes, 681
    obesity, 681
    visual impairments, 681
  genetic deviation, 680
  nursing care implications, 682
  communication of, 673
    nursing care implications, 674
  environmental control, 678
    death/dying rituals, 679
  migration to United States, 672
  social organizations, 675
  space, 675
    nursing care implications, 675
  time, 678
    nursing care implications, 678
Puerto Ricans, nutritional preferences
  of, 170, 171t
Puerto Rico, overview of, 671

Q
Quèbec province 643. *See also* French
  Canadians
  culture of, 643
  people of, 643
Quebecers, overview of, 643
Quiet Revolution, 644

R
Recessive gene, 154
Relational orientation, 132
  collateral mode, 132
  individualistic mode, 132
  lineal mode, 132
Religion
  Afghans and, 401
  Appalachians and, 307
  Chinese Americans and, 450
  Cuban Americans and, 764
  East Indian Hindu Americans and, 547
  Filipino Americans and, 477
  French Canadians and, 650
  Irish Americans and, 807
  Japanese Americans and, 371
  Jordanian Americans and, 745
  Korean Americans and, 627
  Navajos and, 283
  Nigerian Americans and, 698
  Vietnamese Americans and, 505
Respect, nursing care communication,
  culture and, 35, 36
Respeto, 243
Respiratory syncytial virus (RSV), 340
Respiratory tract diseases, 314

Rh factor, 159
Rhythm, verbal communication and, 28
RSV. *See* Respiratory syncytial virus
Russia
  history of, 414
  immigration from, 415
    life in United States, 417
  life in, 412
  overview of, 411
Russian Americans
  biological variations, 430
    body size, 430
    dental needs, 431
    disease susceptibility, 430
      cancer, 431
      hypertension, 430
      tuberculosis, 430
    enzymatic variations, 430
    eye care needs, 431
    nursing care implications, 434
    nutritional deficiencies, 431
    nutritional preferences, 431
    psychological characteristics, 431
      alcoholism, 433
      illness/wellness behaviors, 431
      mental health, 432
    radiation accidents, 433
    toxic pollution, 433
  communication by, 418
    context, 419
    dialect, 418
    kinesics, 420
    nursing care implications, 420
    style, 418
    touch, 419
    volume, 418
  environmental control, 427
    folk medicine, 428
    health treatment, 427
    locus of control, 427
    nursing care implications, 429
    time of death practice, 429
    wellness/illness behaviors, 427
  social organizations, 422
    family, 422
    individualism, 423
    nursing care implications, 425
    religious beliefs, 425
    spirituality, 425
    women's position, 424
  space, 421
    nursing care implications, 422
  time, 426

Pages 689–821 (Chapters 25–30) can be found online at http://evolve.elsevier.com/Giger.

Russian Americans (*Continued*)
nursing care implications, 426
Rutherford, Dawn Bible, 88–89

S
Safrrito, 170–171
Santero, 140
Sawm, 93
Schistosomiasis, 731
Schizophrenia, 157–158, 179
Serum cholesterol levels, 217
Seventh-Day Adventists, 88, 91, 92*b*
nursing care implications of, 91
Sexual matters, nursing care
communication, culture and, 35, 38
Sexually transmitted diseases (STDs),
342, 657
Shigella, 291
Sickle cell anemia, 165, 580, 730
Silence, verbal communication and, 29
Skin color
of African Americans, 210
of American Eskimos, 339
of Chinese Americans, 455
dimensions of, 151
of Filipino Americans, 482
of Haitian Americans, 578
of Hatian Americans, 578
of Japanese Americans, 376
of Korean Americans, 632
of Mexican-Americans, 260
of Navajos, 288
of Nigerian Americans, 706
of Vietnamese Americans, 513
Skin membranes, 51
SLE. *See* Systemic lupus erythematosus
Smith, Linda, 16–17
Smoking, 218, 634
Social organization, 73
of Afghans, 400
acculturation, 400
family roles, 400
family system, 400
immigration, 400
nursing care implications, 401
religion, 401
of African Americans, 197
discrimination and, 197
family characteristics, 199
family role changing, 198
nursing care implications, 200
slavery and, 197
of American Eskimos, 333

Social organization (*Continued*)
family, 333
individual freedom, 334
social status, 334
nursing care implications, 335
political structure, 335
of American Indians, 97
of Amish Americans, 782
Amish haystack dinners, 787*b*
Amish youth, 785
family roles, 782
family systems, 782
nursing care implications, 785
religious principles, 783
state and, 785
of Appalachians, 306
family, 306
nursing care implications, 307
religion, 307
case study of, 68
of Chinese Americans, 448
family, 449
immigration and, 448
marital status, 450
nursing care implications, 450
religion, 450
of Cuban Americans, 763
education, 764
family structure, 763
nursing care implications, 765
religion, 764
of East Indian Hindu Americans, 544
caste systems, 546, 547*b*
family, 544
immigration effect and, 548
marriage, 545
nursing care implications, 550
religion, 547
women's position, 546
ethnic groups in United States, 97
family function, 84
family groups, 75
family location, 85
family organization, 81
functioning levels, 82
family roles, 80
family structure types, 75
alternative family, 77
communal families, 78
extended family, 76
gay families, 78
nuclear dyad family, 76
reconstituted/blended family, 77

Social organization (*Continued*)
single-parent family, 77
skip-generation family, 77
traditional nuclear family, 75
family system characteristics, 78
behavioral system, 79
boundaries, 80
environment, 80
independent units, 79
family system communication, 80
of Filipino Americans, 475
birth rituals, 477
death/dying, 477
family, 475
family systems, 476
nursing care implications, 478
religion, 477
of French Canadians, 648
church, 648
family evolution, 649
interdependence models, 649
nursing care implications, 650
population aging, 650
religion, 650
youth, 650
of Haitian Americans, 571
education, 571
family, 571
nursing care implications, 573
social class, 571
Hmong, 97
of Irish Americans, 806
adolescents, 807
children, 807
family, 806
marriage, 806
men's role, 807
women's role, 806
nursing care implications, 808
political influences, 807
religion, 807
Islamic, 92
common phrases, 93, 94*b*
cultural social differences, 94
family emphasis, 94
five pillars, 93
infertility crisis, 95
marriage, 96
sex, 96
social support, 95
stereotypes, 96
women's dress, 95
of Japanese Americans, 367

Pages 689–821 (Chapters 25–30) can be found online at http://evolve.elsevier.com/Giger.

Social organization (*Continued*)
    education attainment, family role
      in, 370
    family systems, 367
    immigration effects on, 367
    nursing care implications, 371
    religion, 371
  Jehovah's Witnesses, 88, 90*b*
  of Jews, 597
    nursing care implications, 598
  of Jordanian Americans, 745
    nursing care implications, 746
    religion, 745
  kinship, 84
  of Korean Americans, 626
    family, 626
    nursing care implications, 627
    religion, 627
    social values, 627
  of Mexican-Americans, 248
  of Navajos, 282
    family, 282
    family roles/structures, 282
    marriage, 282
    nursing care implications, 283
    religion, 283
    traditional dress, 283
  of Nigerian Americans, 697
    family, 697
    marriage, 698
    nursing care implications, 699
    religion, 698
  nursing care implications for, 98
  of Puerto Rican Americans, 675
  religious groups, 85, 87*t*, 88*t*
  of Russian Americans, 422
    family, 422
    individualism, 423
    nursing care implications, 425
    religious beliefs, 425
    spirituality, 425
    women's position, 424
  Seventh-Day Adventists, 88, 91, 92*b*
  special interest groups, 98
  of Ugandan Americans, 724
    nursing care implications, 725
  of Vietnamese Americans, 502
    Asian and Pacific Islanders, 506
    children, 504
    education, 505
    family, 502, 503*b*
    nursing care implications, 506
    religion, 505

Social organization (*Continued*)
  values, 506
Social time, structure of
  temporal orientation, 116
  temporal pattern, 113
    duration, 115
    periodicity, 113
    sequence, 116
    tempo, 114
    timing, 115
  temporal perspective, 117
Socialization. *See* Enculturation
Solar day, 109
Space
  Afghans and, 399
    nursing care implications, 399
  African Americans and, 196
    nursing care implications, 197
  American Eskimos and, 332
    nursing care implications, 333
  Amish Americans and, 781
    nursing care implications, 781
  Appalachians and, 305
    nursing care implications, 306
  body movement/position, 60
    adapters, 61
    affect displays, 61
    cultural implications of, 61
    emblems, 61
    illustrations, 61
    regulators, 61
  case study of, 47
  Chinese Americans and, 447
    nursing care implications, 448
  Cuban Americans and, 763
    nursing care implications, 763
  East Indian Hindu Americans and, 543
    nursing care implications, 544
  enclosed, 56
  environment objects, 58
    cleanliness and, 59
    color and, 60
    cultural implications of, 60
    disability and, 60
    restraints, 59
    structural boundaries, 59
  Filipino Americans and, 475
    nursing care implications, 475
  French Canadians and, 648
    conceptualization, 648
    interpersonal, 648
    nursing care implications, 648
    physical, 648

Space (*Continued*)
  Haitian Americans and, 570
    nursing care implications, 570
    interpersonal messages, 56
  Irish Americans and, 805
    nursing care implications, 805
  Japanese Americans and, 366
    nursing care implications, 367
  Jews and, 596
    nursing care implications, 596
  Jordanian Americans and, 744
    nursing care implications, 744
  Korean Americans and, 625
    nursing care implications, 625
  Mexican-Americans and, 248
    nursing care implications, 248
  Navajos and, 281
    nursing care implications, 281
  Nigerian Americans and, 696
    childbearing and, 696
    nursing care implications, 697
  nursing care implications, 61
    autonomy, 62
    privacy, 62
    security, 61–62
    self-identity, 62–63
  perception of, 48
    distance receptors, 48
    immediate receptors, 48, 51
  Puerto Rican Americans and, 675
    nursing care implications, 675
  Russian Americans and, 421
    nursing care implications, 422
  sensory stimulation, 56
  spatial behavior, 54
    abuse, 57–58
    cultural implications of, 49
    proximity to others, 55
    territoriality, 58
    violence, 57–58
  tactile, 53
  Ugandan Americans and, 723
    nursing care implications, 723
  Vietnamese Americans
    and, 501
    intimate zone, 501
    living, 502
    nursing care implications, 502
    personal zone, 502
    public zone, 502
    social zone, 502
  visual, 53
Spanish language, 254

Pages 689–821 (Chapters 25–30) can be found online at http://evolve.elsevier.com/Giger.

Spatial behavior, acquired immune
    deficiency syndrome and, 56
Special interest groups, 98
Speed, verbal communication and, 28
STDs. *See* Sexually transmitted diseases
Stroke, 220
Substance abuse, 769
Succinylcholine, 156
Sudden cardiac death, 221
Synchronization, 115
Syndrome X, 149
Systemic lupus erythematosus, 166
Systemic lupus erythematosus (SLE), 166

T
Taber's Cyclopedic Medical
    Dictionary, 38–39
Tactile space, 53
Tardive dyskinesia, 157–158
Tay-Sachs disease, 155, 812
Teenage pregnancy, Mexican-Americans
    and, 249–250
Thalassemia, 751
Theory of Reasoned Action, 253–254
Time
    Afghans and, 402
        nursing care implications, 402
    African Americans and, 200
        nursing care implications, 201
    American Eskimos and, 336
        nursing care implications, 337
    Amish Americans and, 788
        nursing care implications, 788
    Appalachians and, 308
        nursing care implications, 308
    calendar, 109
    case study on, 106
    children and, 107
    Chinese Americans and, 451
        nursing care implications, 451
    clocks, 108
        social vs, 110
    concept of, 106
    Cuban Americans and, 766
        nursing care implications, 766
    cultural perceptions of, 119
        future-oriented perceptions, 119
        present-oriented perceptions, 119
    East Indian Hindu Americans and, 550
        nursing care implications, 551
    Filipino Americans and, 478
        nursing care implications, 479
    French Canadians and, 651

Time (*Continued*)
        nursing care implications, 652
        past and present, 651
    Haitian Americans and, 573
        nursing care implications, 574
    human intervention and, 118
    infants and, 107
    Irish Americans and, nursing care
        implications, 809
    Japanese Americans and, 372
        nursing care implications, 372
    Jews and, 598
        nursing care implications, 599
    Jordanian Americans and, 747
        nursing care implications, 747
    Korean Americans and, 628
        nursing care implications, 629
    measurement of, 107
    Mexican-Americans and, 252
        nursing care implications, 252
    Navajos and, 283
        nursing care implications, 284
    Nigerian Americans and, 700
        nursing care implications, 700
    nursing care implications of, 122
    physiochemical influences and, 121
    Puerto Rican Americans and, 678
        nursing care implications, 678
    Russian Americans and, 426
        nursing care implications, 426
    social
        clock vs, 110
            worldview of, 111
        structure of, 113
    solar time, 109
    tropical years, 109
    Ugandan Americans and, 726
        nursing care implications, 726
    Vietnamese Americans and, 507
        nursing care implications, 507
Touch, nonverbal communication
    and, 30*b*, 29
Transcultural nursing
    culture and, 2
    culture values and, 2–3
    diagnoses, 4
    knowledge and, 3
    models
        analysis, 4
        non-nursing, 3
        nursing-specific, 4
    tools analysis, 4
Transcultural Nursing Society, 2

Transcultural Nursing Society
    Newsletter, 2
Tropical diseases, 731
Tuberculosis, 158, 289, 341, 430, 579
Tumor necrosis factor alpha (TNFα), 212
Tuskegee project, 225
Typhoid fever, 731

U
Uganda, overview of, 718
Ugandan Americans, 720
    biological variations, 729
        disease susceptibility, 730
            AIDS/HIV, 730
            ascariasis, 731
            brucellosis, 731
            cancer, 731
            chronic obstructive pulmonary
                disease, 730
            hypertension, 730
            leishmaniasis, 731
            malaria, 731
            mental diseases, 730
            nursing care implications, 732
            schistosomiasis, 731
            sickle cell anemia, 730
            tropical disease, 731
            typhoid fever, 731
        enzymatic variation, 729
        genetic variation, 729
        nutritional deficiencies, 729
        nutritional preferences, 729
    communication, 721
        nursing care implications, 722
    environmental control, 727
        death/dying issues, 728
        nursing care implications, 728
    social organizations, 724
        nursing care implications, 725
    space, 723
        nursing care implications, 723
    time, 726
        nursing care implications, 726
Ulcerative colitis, 609
Umiaks, 327
Unequal Treatment, 161

V
Venereal disease, 579
Verbal communication, 24*b*, 25
    grammatical structure and, 27
    humor and, 33
    intonation and, 28

Pages 689–821 (Chapters 25–30) can be found online at http://evolve.elsevier.com/Giger.

Verbal communication (*Continued*)
  names and, 27
  pronunciation and, 28
  rhythm and, 28
  silence and, 29
  speed and, 28
  vocabulary and, 26
  voice qualities and, 28
  warmth and, 33
Vergüenza, 243
Viandas, 170–171
Vietnam, overview of, 495
Vietnamese Americans
  biological variations, 513
    blood type, 513
    body size, 513
    body structure, 513
    dioxin, 521
    enzymatic variations, 514
    genetic variations, 514
    noses, 514
    nutritional preference, 520
    psychological characteristics, 522
      adaptation, 524
      alcohol abuse, 525
      coping, 524
      mental health, 522
      metabolism of drugs, 527
      nursing care implications, 528
      posttraumatic stress disorder, 526
      refugees, emotional and behavioral
        manifestations of, 523
    refugees medical problems, 514
      cancer, 517
      hepatitis B, 515
      HIV/AIDS, 520
      hypertension, 514

Vietnamese Americans (*Continued*)
    tuberculosis risk, 516
    skin color, 513
    teeth, 514
  communication, 497
    context, 498
    kinesics, 498
    language, 497
    nursing care implications, 499, 501*b*
    style, 497
    touch, 498
  environmental control, 507
    death beliefs/practice, 510, 511*t*
    illness concepts, 508
      germs, 510
      metaphysical causes, 508, 510*b*
      natural causes, 508, 509*b*
      supernatural causes, 508
    nursing care implications,
      511, 512*b*
  health assessment of, 15*t*
  immigration to United States, 496
    first-wave, 496
    second-wave, 496
    third-wave, 496
  social organizations, 502
    Asian and Pacific Islanders, 506
    children, 504
    education, 505
    family, 502, 503*b*
    nursing care implications, 506
    religion, 505
    values, 506
  space, 501
    intimate zone, 501
    living, 502
    nursing care implications, 502

Vietnamese Americans (*Continued*)
    personal zone, 502
    public zone, 502
    social zone, 502
  time, 507
    nursing care implications, 507
Vietnamese Community Health
  Promotion Project, 516
Virginia House of Burgesses, 192
Vision impairment, 769
Visual impairments, 681
Visual perception, 48
Visual space, 53
Vocabulary, verbal communication
  and, 26
Voice qualities, verbal communication
  and, 28

W
Warmth
  nonverbal communication and, 33
  verbal communication and, 33
Western Medical System, 136
White, Ellen G., 91
Wild type, 153

Y
Yang, 72–73
Yerbero, 140, 256
Yin, 72–73
Yom Kippur, 603
Yup'ik. *See* American Eskimos

Z
Zion's Watchtower Tract Society,
  88–89
Zygote, 153

Pages 689–821 (Chapters 25–30) can be found online at http://evolve.elsevier.com/Giger.